Pathophysiology

Concepts and Applications for Health Care Professionals

Third Edition

Thomas J. Nowak
British Columbia Institute of Technology

A. Gordon Handford
British Columbia Institute of Technology

In Consultation with
Geraldine M. Whitelegg, M.D.

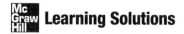 **Learning Solutions**

Boston   Burr Ridge, IL   Dubuque, IA   New York   San Francisco   St. Louis
Bangkok   Bogotá   Caracas   Lisbon   London   Madrid
Mexico City   Milan   New Delhi   Seoul   Singapore   Sydney   Taipei   Toronto

Pathophysiology: Concepts and Applications for Health Care Professionals, Third Edition

3 4 5 6 7 8 9 0 RJE RJE 12

ISBN-13: 978-0-07-804291-1
ISBN-10: 0-07-804291-7

Learning Solutions Manager: Heidi Freund
Production Editor: Carrie Braun
Printer/Binder: Von Hoffmann Press

*Dedicated to the thousands of students
with whom we have learned so much over
the years.
T. J. N.   A. G. H.*

Brief Contents

Contents

Preface

A Note from the Authors

Treating pathophysiology in a concise and focused manner that is suited to contemporary Nursing and Allied Health curricula continues to be the main goal and focus of this third edition of *Pathophysiology: Concepts and Applications for Health Care Professionals.* In preparing the text, we have included much new information while striving to retain the tightly focused presentation that was so well received by users of our first and second editions.

While emphasizing how the essential concepts of pathophysiology are immediately relevant to clinical practice, we have left specifics of clinical practice to the specialty courses and clinical experience that make up much of the preparation of health care professionals.

To promote clear understanding of the essentials of pathophysiology, the information in this text is presented in a logical progression of concept development. A core of foundation material is treated in the Introduction and the first six chapters, which constitute Part One. Part Two then goes on to explore the patterns of disease in the body's major organ systems. Most chapters provide a focused review of those aspects of normal anatomy and physiology required for an understanding of the pathophysiology that follows. If students are fresh from anatomy and physiology preparation, they may well forego reading these, but many students will find them useful.

We have taken care to sequence the text's content on the basis of a logically unfolding, conceptual framework. If your curriculum allows, we feel that following this sequence provides an optimal development of understanding that more effectively transfers to clinical situations.

Because the training of health care professionals involves a significant amount of clinical exposure, we include some references to diagnostic procedures and therapies. Our goal is not to provide clinical instruction in these areas, but to show how their clinical relevance logically emerges from the principles of pathophysiology. Also, linking clinical situations to their underlying pathophysiology provides for more meaningful learning and better retention of information.

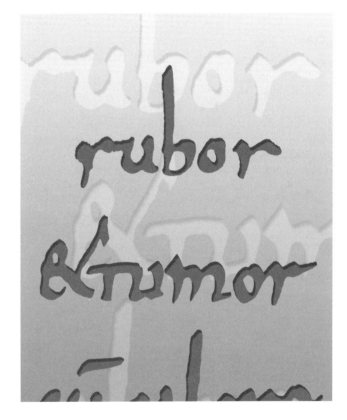

The calligraphy shown here and on the first page of every chapter is from a 15th-century Italian translation from the Latin of Celsus' *De Re Medicina,* written in A.D. 30. Celsus gathered together the best of Greek and Roman medicine at the beginning of the first millennium, including plastic surgery and surgical techniques for removing kidney stones from the bladder and urethra. This phrase (see chapter openers) translates as "redness and swelling with heat and pain" and describes the cardinal signs of inflammation (cú is an abbreviation of "cum," or "with"). His writing was eclipsed by the brilliant self-promotion and massive output of the great physician Galen (131–203 A.D.), whose ideas ruled medical thought for 1500 years. Rediscovered in 1440 and published in 1478, Celsus was highly revered throughout the Renaissance.

We adopted this calligraphy as a design element to draw attention to the fact that contemporary health care professionals deal with many of the same problems with which their predecessors had to grapple. We hope the quotations at the beginning of each chapter will serve a similar function. Embarking on a career in health care can be seen as joining a continuum of medical endeavor, with its roots in earliest times. Although the body of knowledge has greatly expanded, the motivating concern for those in need of care remains the same today.

Key Features of the Third Edition:

The Checkpoint—New! Each is a brief note that provides some additional context for the material just read, a look ahead to where the material is leading, or some additional insight, perhaps from a new perspective. We hope students will come to see these as a welcome "tap-on-the-shoulder" from the authors who briefly interrupt with a useful and interesting comment.

Patient Perspectives—Expanded! These short essays are written by actual patients who describe their experience of a particular disease with particular reference to the health care professionals providing their treatment. These essays are especially successful in enabling students to see beyond the details of pathogenesis, signs, and symptoms, to the more "human face" of the disease. The *Perspectives* are also useful as focal points for discussions in seminars or other settings, where aspects of practice beyond the purely medical are considered.

A Patient's Perspective

Focus Boxes—Updated! Special-interest content boxes are highlighted by icons to indicate the *focus* of the material. They are an ideal mechanism to allow students to pursue additional information on topics that interest them, to use as a stimulus to classroom discussion, or to assign for further exploration in term papers or class presentation.

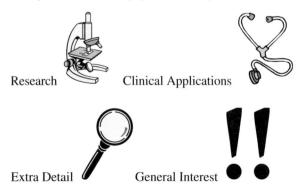

Research   Clinical Applications

Extra Detail   General Interest

*Concept Maps—*Every chapter contains several concept maps to help students understand the relationship of various events in a process or cycle. These not only crystallize the essence of pathogenesis for many students—they are excellent conceptual organizers that provide a convenient means of study and review.

*Case Studies—*Every chapter ends with a case study that provides some "real-world" reference to reinforce the information in the chapter and, at the same time, illustrate that the development and treatment of disease are often not as straightforward as one might hope. The case studies provide an insight into the way in which various imaging, diagnostic laboratory, and nursing fields combine to address a given patient's situation—a perspective easily lost among the details and restricted focus of day-to-day activity in one's particular field. They also serve as reminders that not all health care is provided in large metropolitan medical centers.

*Photo History—*Many specimen photos are accompanied by short histories that explain how the specimen came to be. In effect, these are "mini case studies" that heighten interest and augment understanding.

*Key Concepts—*Every chapter concludes with a set of key concepts. These highlight the central themes of the chapter and alert the student to the core ideas covered. Along with the concept maps, the key concepts provide an excellent study and review tool for students.

*End-of-Chapter Review Activities—*These critical-thinking activities require students to interact with the chapter content. Because an active approach is far more effective than memorization, or other similarly passive study practices, once students become familiar with this approach and experience its benefits, they should be able to generate similar review activities on their own.

Instructor Resources:

*Digital Content Manager—*A CD-ROM containing the text's line art and concept maps is available in jpeg format. We are confident that instructors will find this resource useful for lecture and other presentations.

*Test Bank—*A bank of examination questions is available to instructors who adopt our text.

Please contact your McGraw-Hill representative for details (*www.mhhe.com*).

SYNOPSIS OF REVISIONS FOR THE THIRD EDITION

Chapter	New Coverage	Revised/Expanded Coverage
1 Cell Injury	Cytoskeleton—normal function and injury effects.	Toxic injury, free radicals and their mechanism of injury, mechanisms of atrophy and apoptosis; updated illustrations and concept maps.
2 Inflammation	Cell-derived mediators of inflammation, table on inflammatory mediators, figures illustrating phagocytosis, specific COX-2 inhibitors.	Description of role of vasculature and loose connective tissue in the inflammatory response, chemotaxis, oxygen-dependent and -independent bactericidal action, acute phase proteins, prevention of reperfusion injury; updated illustrations.
3 Fever	Positive feedback, hyperthermia, hypothermia, acute phase reactions.	Regulation of body temperature, mechanisms of heat loss, fevers of undetermined origin, "exogenous agents," cooling effects on brain of cooling forehead; updated illustrations.
4 Healing	Traumatic neuroma, new concept map covering "Patterns of Regeneration."	The extracellular matrix—its composition and contributions to healing; updated illustrations and concept maps.
5 Diseases of Immunity	Origins of HIV, epidemiology of HIV/AIDS at North American and global scale, HAART therapy, role of co-receptor in disease progression, importance of HIV RNA levels, non-nucleoside reverse transcriptase inhibitors, ABO incompatibility as a complication of pregnancy, new illustrations and Focus essays.	T helper cells, T and B cell interactions, HIV incidence/prevalence, LAK role in cancer therapy; updated illustrations.
6 Neoplasia	Genes and cancer, new concept map covering "Apoptosis in Oncogenesis."	Oncogenesis and lymphadenopathy; updated illustrations and concept maps.
7 Blood Disorders	Role of R-binder protein in vitamin B_{12} absorption, anticoagulation therapy, nutritional deficiencies, new concept maps covering "Interaction between Extrinsic and Intrinsic Pathways," "Endothelial Mediation of Anticoagulation," and "Hemostasis Overview."	Interactions between the intrinsic and extrinsic coagulation pathways, endothelial mediation of anti-coagulation; updated illustrations and concept maps.
8 Hemodynamic Disorders		The pathogenesis of thrombosis, blood hypercoagulation, thrombus propagation, anti-coagulation therapy.
9 Vascular Disorders	Organization of arterial disease, role of homocysteine as a risk factor in atherosclerosis, nitrous oxide in hypertension.	Systemic hypertension, including therapy via diuretics, β-blockers, ACE-inhibitors and calcium-channel blockers, free-radical oxidation of LDL, contribution of diabetes mellitus to atherosclerosis; updated illustrations and concept maps.
10 Cardiac Pathophysiology	Cardiac vasculature and controls on perfusion (text and figures), role of endothelial injury in altered control of perfusion, table grading severity and progression of heart disease, 2 page box on ECG basics and selected arrythmias, section on stress and heart/vascular disease (text and figure), PCTA.	Relation of events of ECG to cardiomyocyte activity, precordial leads, cardiac artery disease, right sided vs left sided heart failure, autonomic effects on vascular and cardiac function, angina, variant and unstable angina, pain of acute MI, acute ischemia, antiplatelet and anticoagulant therapy, ACE inhibitors; updated illustrations.

Chapter	New Coverage	Revised/Expanded Coverage
11 Circulatory Shock	Shock in blood transfusion.	Role of endothelium in vascular shock, systemic effects of shock; updated concept maps.
12 Respiratory Pathophysiology	Retrolental fibroplasias and oxygen toxicity in NRDS.	Asthma, ARDS; updated illustrations and concept maps.
13 Gastrointestinal Pathophysiology		*H. pylori* in peptic ulceration, appendicitis, diverticular disease, intussusception, gluten-sensitive enteropathy; updated concept maps.
14 Hepatobiliary and Pancreatic Pathophysiology	HGV in viral hepatitis; new concept map covering "Sequelae of Bile Duct Obstruction."	Viral hepatitis, cholelithiasis, alcoholic cirrhosis, liver transplantation; updated illustrations.
15 Renal Pathophysiology	New concept map covering "Pathogenesis of Glomerulonephritis."	Acute and chronic glomerulonephritis, nephritic and nephritic syndrome, role of mesangial cells, nephrosclerosis, updated illustrations.
16 Fluid and Electrolyte Imbalances		Mechanism of ADH action; updated illustrations, concept maps, and tables.
17 Endocrine Pathophysiology	New concept map covering "Pathogenesis of NIDDM."	Mechanism of insulin action, etiology and pathogenesis of NIDDM, HHNK, microangiopathy; updated illustrations and concept maps.
18 Skeletal and Muscular Pathophysiology	HRT implications for osteoporosis, dual X-ray absorptiometry in diagnosis of osteoporosis, methotrexate therapy for rheumatoid arthritis.	Osteomyelitis, role of obesity in osteoarthritis, gout, muscle disorders; updated illustrations and concept maps.
19 Reproductive Pathophysiology	Breast feeding links to breast cancer, Patient Perspective: Breast cancer; new concept map covering "PCO Syndrome Pathogenesis."	Prostate cancer, PSA, endometrial carcinoma, PCO Syndrome, preeclampsia, breast fibrocystic change; updated illustrations and tables.
20 Disorders of Central Nervous System Development, Vascular Support, and Protection	New variant CJD, paretic neurosyphillis, Lyme disease, tumors of the pituitary, CMV, box on TIA, PRIN, and CVA, box on "brain attack."	Hemorrhagic CVA, lacunar syndrome, disc herniation treatment, NO in cerebral circulation, Kuru; updated illustrations.
21 Disorders of Movement, Sensation, and Mental Function	Brainstem and cord role in locomotion, essential/familial tremor, box on olfactory epithelial cells and repair in the CNS, box "The Dance with Madame Guillotine," table–Assessment of Movement Disorders, "Patient Perspective cartoons The Lighter Side of Living with Quadriplegia."	Brainstem anatomy and function, primary myopathies, Lambert-Eaton syndrome, dystonia, dying back, NOGO and oligodendrocytes, syringomyelia, Friedreich's ataxia, Alzheimer disease; updated illustrations.
22 Seizures and Epilepsy	Delirium-tremens.	Antiepileptic medications.
23 Pain and Pain Management	Descending pain processing (figure), specific COX-2 inhibitors, non-medical/alternative approaches to pain management.	Descending pain processing, migraine, COX inhibitors, scheme underlying perception of two types of pain (figure), central vs peripheral distinction in analgesics.
24 Trauma	"Patient Perspective: Severe Limb Trauma," links between ligament damage and fracture.	Updated illustrations.

Acknowledgments

The names on the title page of this book do not accurately reflect the many who have played a direct or indirect part in bringing this project to completion. We are pleased to acknowledge the contributions of the following:

The Department of Pathology in the University of British Columbia's Faculty of Medicine and, in particular, Dr. W. Chase for access to the specimens in the Boyd Museum used in the preparation of many of the photographs that augment the text.

The BCIT Department of Medical Radiography Technology, for use of its facilities and histological slide collection.

Ken Kajiwara, for his photographic skill and experience, delivered far beyond the degree indicated by the numbers on the invoice.

Dr. John H. Emes, Ph.D., who made an enormous contribution to the text's original graphics.

Our medical consultant, Dr. Geraldine Whitelegg, whose patience and guidance were invaluable assets in focusing our efforts.

Reviewers

We are also indebted to the reviewers whose knowledge and objective appraisal kept us to the straight and narrow:

Second Edition:

Elaine F. Betts
Central Michigan University

Paula A. Witt-Enderby
Duquesne University School of Pharmacy

Nora Howell
Mississippi University for Women

Lorrie Klosterman
Mount Saint Mary College

Marlene McCall
Community College of Allegheny

Donald Meyer
Eastern Virginia Medical School

Kathleen H. Murphy
Gateway Community Technical College

Claudia M. Williams
Campbell University

First Edition:

John Dziak
Community College of Allegheny County

Lois S. Ellis
Indiana Wesleyan University

Louis A. Giacinti
Milwaukee Area Technical College

Larry E. Hibbert
Ricks College

Larry S. Johns
Camosun College

Lori Kashuba
University of Alberta Hospitals School of Nursing

Holly J. Morris
Lehigh County Community College

William L. Teitjen
Georgia Southwestern College

James K. VanArsdel
Champman University

About the Authors

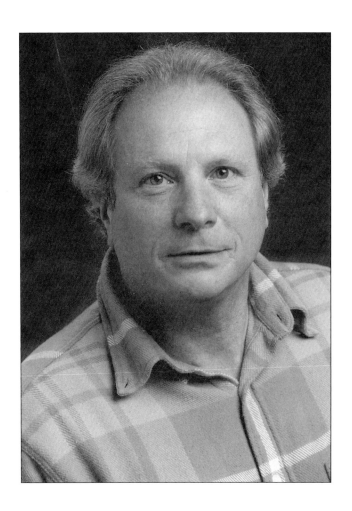

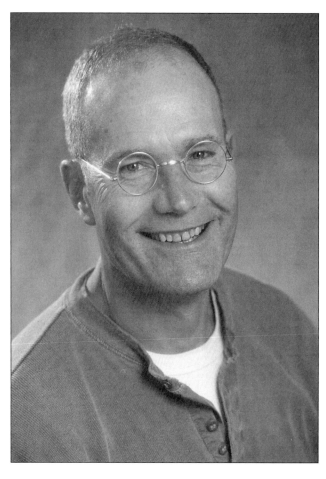

Thomas J. Nowak

After completing studies at the University of Minnesota, I joined the UM Department of Radiation Therapy. I was pleased when the opportunity to join the British Columbia Institute of Technology's faculty arose and I could explore the world of education (and escape Minnesota's winters). Since then, my "teaching gene" seems to have expressed itself fully and I've never been tempted to return to research. I've done additional studies in education and pathology and was drawn into the world of educational technology when serving on the BCIT team that developed an award-winning, computer-based interactive program that dealt with heart structure and function. Beyond teaching students for the last 36 years in virtually every School of Health Sciences program, I've also worked with our Faculty Association, been involved in institutional governance, and enjoyed collaborating with Gordon in bringing this text to its third edition.

A. Gordon Handford

In 1976, I began a temporary teaching job in the School of Health Sciences at the British Columbia Institute of Technology. I was quickly swept into the dialectic of teaching and learning and have never looked back. The School's focus is the widest assembly of two- and four-year health technology programs in Western Canada. I've taught both anatomy and physiology, neuroanatomy, and/or pathophysiology in most of them. Within days of my arrival at BCIT, Tom coaxed me out for a run, and I've been huffing to keep up with him ever since.

This book is a product of that pursuit. On the lifelong learning front, I'm currently assisting with research on a "brain-computer interface" that will allow people with profound paralysis to control a computer with their brain waves.

Introduction

Objection, evasion, distrust, and irony are signs of health. Everything absolute belongs to pathology.

FRIEDRICH WILHELM NIETZSCHE
BEYOND GOOD AND EVIL

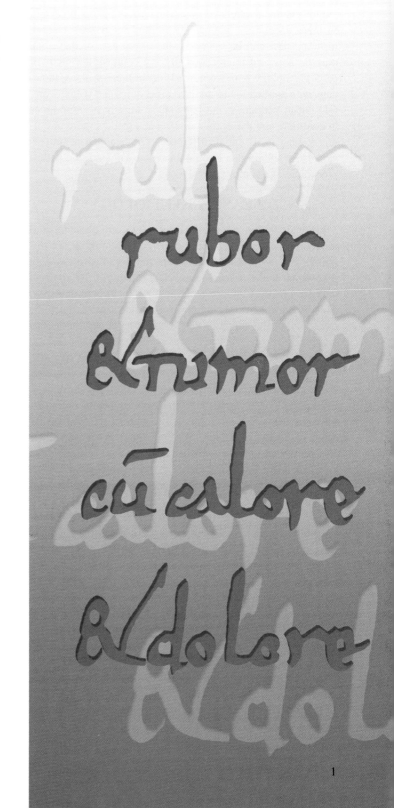

Before we proceed to study the specifics of patho-physiology, it will be useful to establish a core of fundamentals. These provide the context in which all subsequent text material is presented and introduce some essential terminology that is widely used by health care professionals.

First, we distinguish between the terms **pathology** and **pathophysiology.** While both terms refer to the study of disease, pathology is usually applied to the work of pathologists and physicians whose focus is on the physical changes present in diseased organs and tissues. These are often studied in specimens obtained **post-mortem,** or following death. In these specimens, abnormalities may be **grossly** visible, meaning they can be seen with the naked eye, or they may only be observed microscopically. By contrast, the focus of pathophysiology is the abnormal functioning of diseased organs with application to medical procedures and patient care. Of course, pathology and pathophysiology have large areas in common, and the distinction between them is more of emphasis than of essential difference. The health care professionals for whom this book is intended will find that pathophysiology is the more useful focus.

DISEASE AND ETIOLOGY

We consider that we are healthy when our physical and mental capacities can be fully utilized. When these are impaired, we say that disease is present. Broadly speaking, a disruption of the homeostatic balance required for optimal cellular function underlies the loss of functional capacity. This disruption at the cellular level will, sooner or later, be expressed at the somatic (whole body) level, and be recognized as disease.

The term **etiology** refers to the cause of a disease. Strictly speaking, etiology is the study of disease causation, but common usage equates the terms etiology and cause. For example, you might hear that some types of liver disease have a viral etiology, while others are caused by blockage of the bile ducts. When etiology is unknown, the disease is said to be **idiopathic.**

Considered broadly, there are three categories of etiology. Diseases are described as genetic, congenital, or acquired. In disease with a **genetic** etiology, an individual's genes are responsible for some structural or functional defect. The effects of that defect continue as the defect is passed by parents to their offspring, generation after generation. In **congenital** disease, the genetic information is intact, but other factors in the embryo's intrauterine environment interfere with normal development. Cystic fibrosis is a genetic disease, whereas fetal alcohol syndrome is the result of a mother's alcohol intake, which produces congenital abnormalities in a genetically normal infant. The third, and largest, category of etiology is **acquired** disease. In these conditions, genes and development are normal, but other factors, encountered later, produce the disease. Examples are tuberculosis, emphysema, or hepatitis.

SIGNS, SYMPTOMS, AND PATHOGENESIS

When indications of illness arise, the sufferer may seek medical assistance. Medical personnel respond by taking a medical history: the patient's description of the problem. The patient may describe sensations of abnormality such as pain or **malaise,** the generalized feeling of weakness or loss of well-being. These are known as **symptoms** because they reflect the patient's subjective experiences; no one else can feel the patient's pain or experience the malaise. By contrast, a **sign**—such as elevated body temperature or an irregular pulse—can be detected by an observer. Signs usually emerge during a **physical examination.** The results of laboratory tests, medical imaging, or exploratory surgery together make up the **findings** that clarify the clinical picture. Consider the situation of a patient's abdominal pain, which is a symptom, and abdominal tenderness, which is a sign. An observer can't feel the pain, but can easily see the patient's exaggerated response to abdominal pressure during a physical examination. Findings obtained later may provide insight into the reason for the pain.

The characteristic combination of signs and symptoms associated with a particular disease is called a **syndrome.** Some diseases present such typical patterns of signs and symptoms that the term **syndrome** is used in naming them. Examples are Down's syndrome (a genetic abnormality), adult respiratory distress syndrome (ARDS), fetal alcohol syndrome, and acquired immune deficiency syndrome (AIDS).

In assessing a patient's signs and symptoms, conclusions can often be drawn about the pattern of development of the disease: its **pathogenesis.** Typically, pathogenesis involves some initial damage that produces certain effects. These in turn produce other effects, and so on, as the disease progresses. Each stage in the development may produce characteristic signs and symptoms (fig. I.1). A condition resulting from a disease is a **sequela.** For example, thickening of arteriolar walls is a sequela of high blood pressure. Another aspect of pathogenesis is the time over which a disease develops. **Acute** conditions have a more rapid onset, develop quickly, and are usually of short duration. By contrast, a **chronic** disease is typically of longer duration, often lasting months or even years. Note, however, that in some chronic diseases the onset is abrupt, while in others the onset is more **insidious**—that is, with minor changes that don't arouse immediate concern.

The distribution of **lesions** (injury sites) in a particular disease may be described as local or systemic. If damage is defined as **local,** it is confined to one region of the body. In **systemic** disease, lesions are more widely distributed. For example, a cancer's early growth might be localized within the lung, but later in the course of the disease systemic effects result from its spread to other organs. Within a diseased organ, damage is said to be **focal** when limited to one or more distinct sites. If more uniformly distributed, damage is said to be **diffuse.**

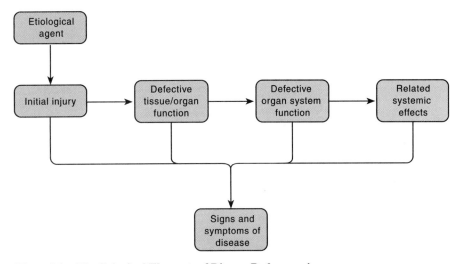

Figure I.1 **The Principal Elements of Disease Pathogenesis.**

DIAGNOSIS, THERAPY, AND PROGNOSIS

Analysis of the signs and symptoms, coupled with a consideration of pathogenesis, often leads to a **diagnosis,** the identification of the patient's specific disease. Once the diagnosis is established, **therapy** can proceed. Therapy is the treatment of disease with the aim of achieving a cure, or at least reducing the patient's signs and symptoms to a level where some near-normal function can be restored. For example, antibiotic therapy may completely destroy infecting organisms to effect a quick cure. By contrast, in certain heart diseases, one drug might be used to stabilize the heart's rhythm and another to promote loss of excessive body fluid. In this way they make the heart better able to pump efficiently, even though the underlying cause of the problem can't be corrected.

An assessment of the body's responses to therapy, knowledge of a disease's pathogenesis, and clinical experience can all combine to provide the basis for **prognosis.** This is the prediction of a particular disease's outcome (fig. I.2). Typically, early diagnosis and treatment of cancer are associated with a good prognosis. The prognosis is often poor if there is delay in its diagnosis and treatment.

With this background in basic concepts and terminology, we can turn to the study of cell injury. For those in need of a brief review of normal cytology, we start with a section on the normal cell.

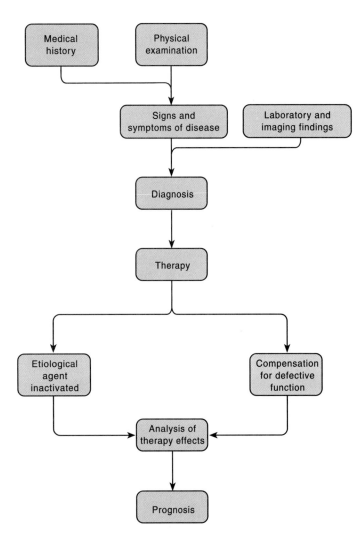

Figure I.2 **Medical Intervention in Disease.**

Chapter

1

Cell Injury

We do not die wholly at our deaths: we have moldered away long before.

WILLIAM HAZLITT
On the Feeling of Immortality in Youth

rubor
& tumor
cū calore
& dolore

In this chapter's analysis of the causes and mechanisms of cell injury, we often make reference to the "normal" cell, contrasting it with an injured or otherwise abnormal cell. For this reason, a brief review of normal cell structure and function follows. If your background is up to date, you may want to move directly to the discussion of cell injury. If you do, remember that the review material is here for reference if you need it.

THE NORMAL CELL

In the same way that body structure and function are based on the cell, cellular structure and function are based on subunits of the cell. At the subcellular level, specific cell structures called **organelles** perform the various tasks that contribute to the cell's overall functioning.

The general and specialized functions of the cell are the result of its organization at the chemical level. When left to themselves, atoms and molecules tend toward random patterns of organization. Cells counter this process, and their ability to do so is critical in the distinction between the living and the nonliving.

The Plasma Membrane

The **cell membrane,** or **plasma membrane,** is composed of phospholipid, cholesterol, glycolipid, protein, and glycoprotein. It is important to the cell in three ways. First, it defines the size and shape of the cell and acts as a container for all its components. Second, the membrane is able to influence the passage of various substances between the cell and its environment. The membrane is described as **selectively permeable** because some molecules, water for instance, pass freely through its pores, whereas others, sodium ion for example, are restricted in their transmembrane movement. This property of the plasma membrane is especially significant because the cell depends on transmembrane movement for the uptake of nutrients and the outward passage of cell products and wastes (fig. 1.1a). When the cell must expend energy to move molecules against a concentration gradient, the process is described as **active transport.** Because of the energy expenditure, the active transport systems that effect ion movement are known as **ion pumps.**

The properties of the cell membrane also provide for the larger-scale movement of material into or out of the cell. For inward movement **(endocytosis),** a region of the membrane first sags in and then pinches off, forming a vacuole within the cytoplasm. **Phagocytosis** is the type of endocytosis involved in the uptake of particulate matter, while fluids, and the molecules they contain, enter the cell by **pinocytosis.** The process is reversed in **exocytosis,** where cytoplasmic vacuoles merge with the membrane, passing their contents to the cell's exterior (fig. 1.1b).

The third function of the cell membrane derives from the fact that it provides the surface at which the cell interacts with its environment. Factors outside the cell can influ-

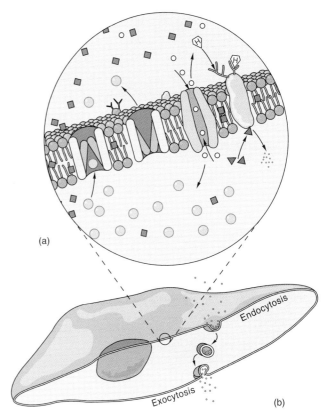

Figure 1.1   Movement Through the Cell Membrane.
(*a*) Magnified endothelial cell membrane, showing lipid-soluble molecules (small squares) passing through membrane by dissolving in membrane lipid. Larger circles represent transport via specific transport systems, while smaller circles move through pores. Binding of hormone (H) at receptor triggers degradation of intracellular molecule. (*b*) Endocytosis and exocytosis.

ence its activities by affecting membrane permeability or cellular metabolism. Such influence depends on the binding of specially structured control chemicals to correspondingly structured **receptors** in the plasma membrane (fig. 1.1a). These receptors are often formed by the carbohydrate component of membrane glycoprotein. This mechanism is the basis of most hormone-cell interactions, synaptic transmission between neurons, and much of the immune response. Binding at membrane receptors also provides for the uptake of specific molecules in some endocytosis.

The Mitochondrion

Many of the molecules entering the cell through its membrane serve as energy sources. Most cellular activity is driven by energy that the cell extracts from these energy-rich molecules. Glucose is the most common such molecule. Once glucose is inside the cell, enzymes break the six-carbon molecule into two three-carbon units. The organelle called the **mitochondrion** then extracts much of the energy in the chemical bonds in these units. The process involves a series of chemical changes that release the energy in small, easily handled amounts. The energy that is released is captured and

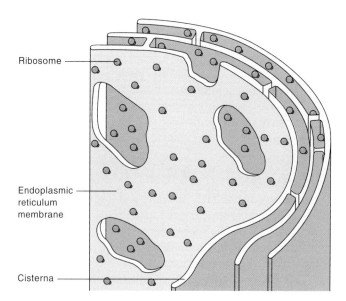

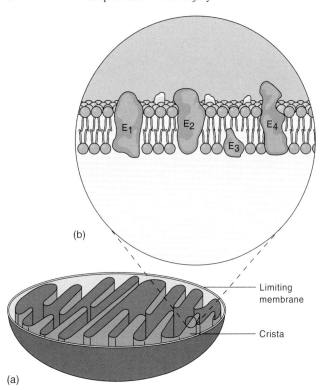

Figure 1.2   **The Mitochondrion.** (*a*) Section through a mitochondrion with (*b*) a portion of one of its cristae magnified to show the linear sequence of four representative enzymes. Held in this sequence, the enzymes function more effectively in the stepwise catalytic conversions that are involved in energy metabolism.

Figure 1.3   **Granular Endoplasmic Reticulum (GER).** Note the ribosomes at the surface and the interconnections among the cisternae.

stored in adenosine triphosphate (ATP). In ATP, the energy is present in the form of chemical bond energy, which is readily available for transfer to various other metabolic pathways as needed.

ATP is produced in the mitochondrion as a product of the **citric acid cycle,** which is also known as the **Krebs cycle.** It involves a sequence of energy-yielding chemical transformations that produce carbon dioxide (CO_2). Complete energy extraction requires that the Krebs cycle reactions be linked to other reaction systems that release energy, consume oxygen, and produce water. The inhalation of oxygen-rich air and the exhalation of CO_2-rich air reflect, at the somatic level, energy metabolism occurring at the cellular level. Because the mitochondrial reactions require oxygen, the energy metabolism of the mitochondrion is called **aerobic.**

The significance of the mitochondria as the sites of energy metabolism lies in their enzymes. Most enzymes specific to the energy-releasing reactions are found within the mitochondria. Depending on a cell's energy requirements, its cytoplasm may contain a few hundred or as many as thousands of mitochondria. Each of these is composed of two lipoprotein membranes (fig. 1.2*a*). The outer, limiting membrane provides the characteristic elongated shape of the mitochondrion. The inner membrane is less regular and is thrown into a series of folds, each called a **crista.** The

cristae provide a large membrane surface that can support enzymes in the order dictated by the reaction sequences. Thus, the mitochondrion not only houses the enzymes but organizes them as well (fig. 1.2*b*). Much of the ATP produced in mitochondria is used in joining chemical building blocks to form molecules needed by the cell. These are used in normal growth, reproduction, and for the replacement of damaged organelles.

Cells must also be able to synthesize the wide variety of enzymes needed for their membrane functions, energy metabolism, and the synthesis of cell parts and secretions. Because cell organelles are rich in protein, and because enzymes are made of protein, much cell activity is devoted to protein synthesis.

Granular Endoplasmic Reticulum

Protein synthesis occurs in the **cytoplasm,** or **cytosol.** This is the fluid of the cell, which consists of the cell water, its solutes, and the organelles. The physical characteristics of the cytoplasm shift between fluid and gel states as required. The cytoplasm contains an extensive membrane complex called the **endoplasmic reticulum** (ER). ER is normally present in the cytoplasm in two different configurations. One consists of long, parallel arrays of flattened membrane sacs called **cisternae.** The cisternae are interconnected and may have small, rounded masses called **ribosomes** associated with their cytoplasmic surfaces. The presence of ribosomes in this form of ER is indicated in the name **granular endoplasmic reticulum** (GER). The term **rough ER** is also used (fig. 1.3).

In supporting ribosomes, GER contributes to the synthesis of protein, because protein is formed on the surface of the ribosomes. After it is formed, newly synthesized protein may pass to the interior of the GER, for storage and

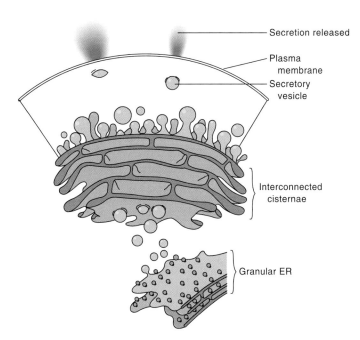

Figure 1.4 **Golgi Complex.** Cell product received from the GER is stored and/or modified prior to its transfer to the plasma membrane for release.

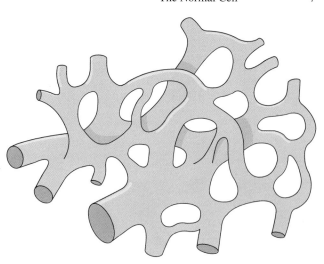

Figure 1.5 **Agranular Endoplasmic Reticulum (AER).** Note the lack of ribosomes and the tubular cisternae.

possible modification, until needed. This occurs not only for protein that is to be moved out of the cell for external use but also for protein that is to be incorporated into cell membranes. Soluble protein that is to be used directly within the cytoplasm is synthesized on the surfaces of free ribosomes that are not associated with ER membranes.

The Golgi Complex

Before secretion, the GER passes its newly synthesized product to another organelle in the cytoplasm called the **Golgi complex.** This organelle consists of a stacked cluster of membranous cisternae. Small pieces of GER membrane, containing newly synthesized protein, pinch off from the GER and merge with the membrane of the Golgi complex. On receiving this protein, the Golgi complex stores it until it is needed (fig. 1.4). Often carbohydrate or lipid is added to the stored protein to form a fully functional product for secretion. To pass the secretion to the cell's exterior, small sacs called **vesicles** separate from the Golgi complex and move to the plasma membrane. They merge with it, passing the secretion to the exterior where it may function locally or at some distant site to which a duct or the blood delivers it.

Agranular Endoplasmic Reticulum

The second ER configuration involves smaller, tubular cisternae, which are less uniformly arranged (fig. 1.5). They lack ribosomes at their membrane surfaces and are therefore described as **agranular,** or **smooth, endoplasmic reticulum** (AER/SER). AER contributes two important cell functions. One is **detoxification,** in which enzymes within the AER chemically degrade hormones, drugs, or toxins

that threaten the cell by their presence in the cytoplasm. AER cisternae also contain enzymes that function in the formation of the major lipid types: phospholipid, triglyceride, and steroid. A cell secreting steroid hormones would contain significant amounts of AER.

The Lysosome

Another of the cytoplasmic organelles is the **lysosome.** It is found freely distributed in the cytoplasm and consists of a membrane vesicle containing more than 30 different enzymes, which are capable of degrading most macromolecules. For this reason, lysosome membranes must have chemical properties that can resist the activities of the enzymes they contain. In the absence of this resistance, the enzymes would degrade the lysosome membrane and escape to destroy the cell of which they are a part. As foreign material enters the cell, some of the plasma membrane encloses it within a cytoplasmic bubble called a **digestive vacuole** or **phagosome.** Lysosomes move to the vacuole and, by merging with its membrane, empty their enzymes into it. Next, the pH is lowered, activating the enzymes. The enzymes then destroy the contents of the vacuole by digesting them (fig. 1.6). When cell organelles are damaged or are no longer required, they are eliminated by a similar process. The vacuole involved is then called an **autophagosome** because the cell is digesting part of itself.

The Cytoskeleton

The cells **cytoskeleton** consists of a complex of fine protein filaments and tubules distributed throughout the cytoplasm. The cytoskeleton makes several important contributions to the cell, including support and organization of the cell's organelles and movement of materials within the cell. Because the cytoskeleton is attached to the plasma membrane, it also plays a role in maintaining cell structure and in linking adjacent cells.

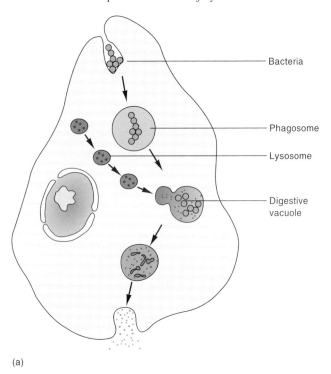

(a)

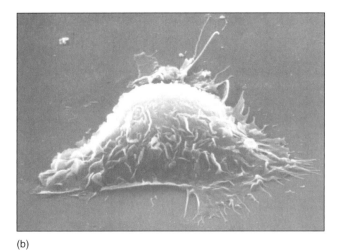

(b)

Figure 1.6   **Role of the Lysosome.** (*a*) Bacteria are destroyed by lysosomal enzymes after fusion of lysosome and phagosome. The resulting debris is expelled by exocytosis. (*b*) Phagocytic cell.

The Nucleus

The functioning of the various cell organelles is smoothly coordinated and highly efficient. Complex control mechanisms provide internal regulation of their function. The source of this control is found in the cell's **nucleus.** Separated from the cytoplasm by a two-layered membrane, the nucleoplasm contains long filaments of deoxyribonucleic acid (DNA) and protein that form the **chromosomes.** DNA structure incorporates a coding system that contains the information needed for producing the enzymes on which cellular metabolism depends. Thus, all cell function depends on the chromosomes.

Later in this chapter we will see how injury to cells affects the functioning of organelles. First, however, it will be useful to analyze the causes of cell injury.

 Checkpoint 1.1

Chapter 1 contains many references to the cell organelles just described. When you encounter them in the discussion of cell injury, you may want to return to this discussion for a quick review of their structure and function.

CAUSES OF CELL INJURY

In analyzing and classifying the causes of cell injury, it is common to identify a fairly large number of causes. For example, in one classification, hypoxia, chemicals, physical agents, infectious agents, immune injury, genetic defects, nutritional imbalances, and aging are cited as the causes of cell injury. Such a classification may be useful in providing the background needed for diagnosis, therapy, or day-to-day care in a particular disease. However, strictly speaking, there are only three essential ways that a cell can be injured. From the perspective of the cell, injury is the result of (1) the lack of a substance necessary to the cell—a **deficiency,** (2) the presence of a substance that interferes with cell function—poisoning, or **intoxication,** or (3) the loss of the cell's structural integrity—physical injury, also called **trauma.**

Deficiency

The life processes of the cell derive from its complex metabolism, presenting a great variety of specific chemical requirements as well as a general need for an energy supply. Any lack of these interferes with cell function and can therefore cause injury. The most common causes of death in Western societies—heart attack and stroke—are caused by oxygen and nutrient deficiencies in critical organs. Starvation involves a lack of dietary energy sources and of many molecules with specific roles in metabolism. In many cases, diets are ample and even excessive in providing energy sources, but for lack of a specific nutrient, cell injury may still occur. For example, a dietary deficiency of thiamin, one of the B vitamins, causes damage to nervous tissue because the vitamin is required for the normal carbohydrate metabolism of the tissue. A lack in the diet is called a **primary nutrient deficiency;** a **secondary nutrient deficiency** arises when substances are present in the diet but cannot be absorbed.

Genetic defects can also cause injurious deficiencies in cells. Many substances in the cell's metabolic pathways are synthesized on the basis of information encoded in the genes that are present in the chromosomes. As chromosomes are damaged, production of metabolic intermediates declines and cell function is compromised by the lack of

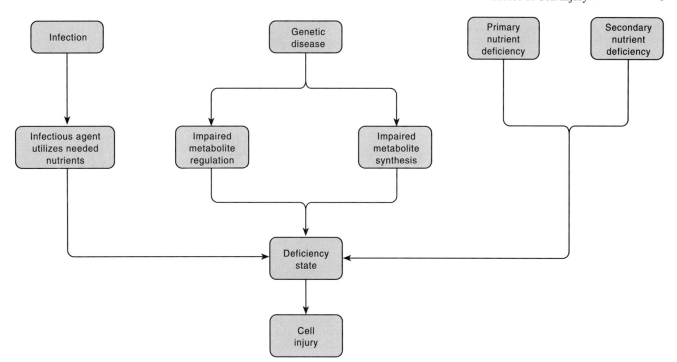

Figure 1.7 **Factors That May Produce a Deficiency of Essential Nutrients.**

these intermediates. Another problem can arise from inadequate genetic control of metabolism. We noted earlier the dependence of cellular metabolism on enzymes that control these complex reactions. It follows that even if adequate amounts of **precursors** (starting forms) and intermediates are available, improper regulation due to lack of controlling enzymes will disrupt cellular function (fig. 1.7).

Remember that our discussion is focused on injury to the cell that suffers the deficiency. In pernicious anemia, a secondary nutrient deficiency arises because gastric mucosal cells cannot synthesize the substance (intrinsic factor) that is needed for the absorption of Vitamin B_{12}. The stomach cells, which cannot produce the intrinsic factor, do not directly suffer for its lack. But without absorption of the vitamin, the marrow's rate of red cell production falls, and all body cells are threatened with a deficiency of oxygen. Note that the marrow itself is not injured; the damage occurs in the tissues deficient in oxygen that the blood is unable to deliver.

Viral action, too, can produce deficiency injury to a cell. Following infection of a cell by a virus, the virus causes the cell to produce new virus particles that are then released from the infected cell. Although the cell can survive for some time in this way, the heavy demand for key metabolites in the production of new viral particles disrupts the cell's metabolism, causing its injury.

Intoxication

The second mechanism of cell injury is poisoning. Many substances will interfere with normal function when present within cells. Such injurious substances are called **toxins,** and they are said to produce an **intoxication.** Toxins may originate outside the cell or they may arise internally. Toxins of external origin are called **exogenous** and can be characterized as being of biological or nonbiological origin.

Biological toxins are produced by living organisms, most commonly by microorganisms. As agents of **infection,** they gain access to body tissues and release injurious substances. The most common sources of biological toxins are bacteria, but other microorganisms, for example, fungi or protozoa, can also produce toxins.

Nonbiological exogenous toxins are injurious chemicals that originate outside the body. This large category contains a number of substances that are injurious if inhaled or swallowed. The degree of exposure is a critical factor in intoxication. Some toxins are injurious in small quantities while others are well tolerated except when exposure is high. In a medical context, many therapeutic drugs are highly effective at prescribed dose levels, but the same drugs can be fatal at higher doses. An example is toxic injury in suicidal barbiturate ingestion.

Injurious substances that arise inside the cell are called **endogenous** toxins. Essentially, they are formed in two ways. One way involves a genetic defect that directly causes a toxic substance to be produced. This is the underlying cause of Huntington's disease, in which a toxic substance causes neurological dysfunction. An indirect genetic intoxication can arise if the product of a genetic defect, while not itself toxic, activates an alternative metabolic pathway, the products of which are toxic. An example is phenylketonuria (PKU). In this condition, toxic phenylketones formed via such an alternative pathway interfere with normal neurological development.

Instead of producing toxic products, the principal effect of abnormal gene function might be the abnormal

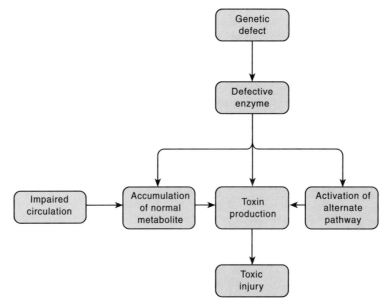

Figure 1.8   **Sources of Endogenous Toxins.**

accumulation of a metabolite. Normally, such accumulations do not occur because once formed, metabolites are promptly modified in a metabolic sequence. A genetically induced enzyme lack prevents the metabolite from moving along the metabolic pathway, while at the same time the metabolite continues to be formed. When it accumulates to toxic levels, cell injury is the result.

A second way in which endogenous toxins can arise involves impaired circulation that allows metabolic by-products to accumulate to toxic levels. Many substances produced by cells are not toxic at normal levels—CO_2 and bilirubin, for example. If they are not removed from the cell, however, their levels rise and damage can result. Note that cell injury from such a build-up of normally tolerated substances is secondary to the impaired circulation that has interfered with their normal removal (fig. 1.8).

In toxic injury, the toxin exerts its effects by binding to critical cell structures, disrupting their function. Cell membranes and various key molecules in the cell's energy production system are often affected. Note that a toxin may not be directly damaging. Instead, the damage can be done by the products formed by the cell's chemical breakdown of the toxin. Generally, cells most at risk of toxic damage are those with high exposure to the toxin. Example are cells of the intestinal mucosa that are exposed to ingested toxins and cells of the liver, where much detoxification occurs and toxic degradation products are first formed.

Note that there may be interplay between mechanisms of cell injury. For example, a genetic defect might cause a deficiency of a critical product. Now consider the case of a metabolic product that self-regulates its formation by feedback inhibition, i.e., when there is more of it, production slows, and when there is less, production increases. If a genetic defect results in a deficiency of such a product, inhibition is released and over-production can cause its precursors to accumulate to toxic levels.

Trauma

Trauma is physical injury. Many different agents are able to cause injury by physical disruption of cells. In some cases, the physical damage is so great that the cell's integrity is completely lost as its membranes rupture and its contents lose all organization. In other cases, the physical damage arises more gradually.

Trauma can be caused by physical agents. One is extreme cold, or **hypothermia,** which injures cells as a result of ice crystal formation in the water of the cytoplasm. This kind of damage is typical in frostbite.

On the other hand, extreme heat, or **hyperthermia,** damages cells by disrupting cell proteins. Initially, excessive heat causes proteins to **denature.** Most protein in cells is formed of a thin helix (a three-dimensional spiral) formed by a long chain of amino acids. The helix is held in a folded configuration by chemical bonds that join key sites along its length. When these bonds are disrupted by heat or other factors such as acid, the bonds break and the protein unfolds—it has been denatured. Of course, because the function of cell proteins is linked to their structure, denaturation is followed by significant functional disruption. At extremes of heat, protein is chemically transformed by combining with oxygen. This produces the blackening and charring characteristic of burned tissue. In burn injury, tissue destruction may involve charring at the site of highest temperature and damage due to protein denaturation in nearby areas where temperatures were lower.

Burns can result from direct or near contact with a hot object or from exposure to the sun's radiation. Electric currents also cause burning because, as electricity flows through tissue, substantial amounts of heat are released.

Ionizing radiation is another physical agent that causes traumatic injury. Ionizing radiation is the high-energy radiation associated with X-rays and nuclear radioactivity as opposed to the much lower-energy radiations that form the sun's rays: solar radiation. At very high exposures, ionizing radiation produces temperature increases in tissues that can produce burning. At lower levels, its damaging effects are less obvious but still quite significant at the molecular level, where they produce not a chemical alteration but physical break-up of large cell constituents. Ionizing radiation causes injury through the production of **free radicals.** These are highly energetic ions that form when ionizing radiation strips electrons from cell molecules. In this form, they interact vigorously with other cell constituents producing significant damage to them, and others, even to the point of breaking them into dysfunctional fragments. Cell membrane lipids, cell proteins (including enzymes), and DNA are especially vulnerable to free-radical damage. Various other aspects of free-radical formation are considered in the Focus box on p. 20. In the context of traumatic cell injury, you can appreciate the effect of free-radical damage to critical cell macromolecules, in particular the DNA that is responsible for all essential cell operations. Damage to DNA in the tissues that form ova or spermatozoa are especially significant in that offspring who inherit the defective DNA can develop a genetic disease and, in many cases, can transmit it to their children.

Mechanical pressure is another source of traumatic injury. In the face of increased pressure, cells are physically overwhelmed and can't maintain their structural integrity. Thus, pressure applied to a body surface, the pressure of a rapidly expanding tumor, or that of an abnormally bulging artery can subject adjacent cells to traumatic injury. Sound of high intensity can also cause injury because loud noises generate high pressures in the fluids of the delicate inner ear.

Physical injury may arise from the action of microorganisms. We noted earlier that some bacteria use toxins to damage cells, but bacteria can also cause physical damage in the infection process. Potent enzymes released by bacteria can break up the connective tissues that support the host's cells, as well as disrupt the cells themselves. Many viral infections commonly involve trauma. After infecting a cell, viruses take control of cell activity causing cells to produce many new viral particles. Also formed are viral proteins that bind to cell membranes forming gaps that prevent normal cell operation and, ultimately, causing cell rupture. This traumatic break-up destroys the cell, but for the viruses it is the means of achieving release, freeing them to infect other cells. Some larger microorganisms, such as the protozoa, can attack individual cells. For example, in malaria, a form of the infecting agent (genus *Plasmodium*) that is intermediate in the life cycle causes damage by entering and then rupturing red blood cells.

The immune system normally works to protect us, but sometimes its responses actually cause immune injury. In these cases, antigen-antibody interactions at cell surfaces lead to physical disruption of the cell membrane. An example involves viruses. After entering the cell, a virus can trigger production of many new viruses. The newly formed viruses are released from the cell without damaging it. But

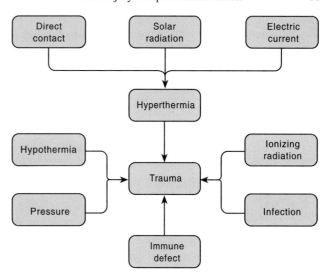

Figure 1.9   **Factors in the Etiology of Cell Trauma.**

in the process, some viral protein becomes incorporated into the plasma membrane. This allows specialized cells of the immune system to recognize the viral protein as foreign and to attack the cell by binding to the viral proteins. The result is membrane trauma and cell death.

Other viruses, the agent of hepatitis B, for example, activate another immune response that forms open channels in the cell membrane. These channels destroy the barrier and selective permeability functions of the membrane, and the cell's integrity is lost as movement through its membrane becomes unrestricted.

The factors that can produce traumatic damage are summarized in figure 1.9.

 Checkpoint 1.2

The essential point in the etiology of cell injury is that there are many diseases and many causes for them. From the perspective of the cell, however, it either lacks something, a toxin is present in it, or it is being physically damaged. Keep this in mind when your clinical experience brings you into contact with a variety of diseases. See if you can assess the situation from the cell's "point of view."

CELL INJURY: RESPONSES AND EFFECTS

Following injury, or even before injury when conditions start to deteriorate, cells can activate various adaptive responses that enable them to better cope with the situation. When injury occurs, its effects depend on a subtle interplay between structure and function. A structurally damaged organelle may function improperly, or altered function may arise first and then give rise to structural changes. Although changes in both structure and function are usually involved in cell injury, it is often quite difficult to pinpoint the initial change because the first identifiable disruption may be several steps removed from the original disturbance. It is also important to note that the effects of injury, and the cell's responses to it, are determined not only by the nature of the causative agent, but also by the intensity, the duration, and the number of exposures to it. The pulmonary effects of low-level exposure to an irritant inhaled over many months may produce the cough and chronic breathing difficulties seen in many coal miners, while a single exposure lasting only a few minutes may be life threatening, as in smoke inhalation in a burning building.

When normal conditions are restored, or when only moderate injury has occurred, the cell may return to normal levels of function. We will consider such reversible injury before going on to study the effects of more severe injury.

Reversible Changes: Functional

Adaptive Responses

Injury to the cell is often reversible, because the cell's adaptive responses enable it to cope with injury or adverse conditions. These can be used when needed and can be deactivated when the situation returns to normal. The following discussion describes the principal adaptive mechanisms that enable the cell to cope with injury. Note that not all cells have the full complement of adaptive mechanisms, described below. Lacking adaptive capability makes certain cells more vulnerable to specific forms of injury. Examples are presented later in the chapter.

Alternative Metabolism In confronting unfavorable conditions, a cell can employ alternative metabolic pathways that allow it to adjust to the conditions. For example, in conditions of hypoxia (oxygen deficiency), the major energy production pathway of the cell, **oxidative phosphorylation,** is threatened because it is oxygen dependent (aerobic). In the face of declining aerobic energy metabolism, some tissues can adapt by switching to **glycolysis.** This energy-yielding process is anaerobic, and since it can produce ATP without oxygen, a cell can rely on it until normal oxygen delivery is restored.

Similarly, should the supply of the body's principal energy source, glucose, be interrupted, many cells can turn to fat or protein as a fuel. The breakdown of these materials can produce enough energy to sustain cell activities until glucose levels return to normal.

Altered Size Size changes are another adaptive capability exhibited by cells. **Hypertrophy** is the process of cell and organ enlargement that occurs in response to increased demands. Enlargement of the remaining muscle fibers of a damaged muscle, endocrine cells chronically subjected to a secretion stimulus, and myocardial cells that increase in size and strength when required to pump through a narrowed heart valve are examples of adaptive hypertrophy.

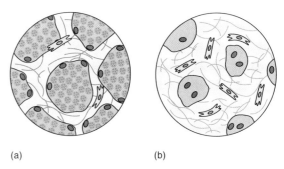

(a)   (b)

Figure 1.10 **Atrophy.** (*a*) Normal skeletal muscle fibers in cross section, showing the myofibrils so tightly packed in the sarcoplasm that the cell's multiple nuclei are forced to the periphery. (*b*) Polio blocks nerve stimulation to muscle, and atrophy results. Note the shrinkage and loss of myofibrillar organization.

In **hyperplasia,** new cells are formed by mitosis to respond to increased demand. This process is considered further in chapter 6 in the context of growth disorders.

The other size adaptation is **atrophy,** or shrinking. Various factors that reduce demand on a cell or decrease its normal input stimuli can produce shrinking. The most common cause is reduced workload, which produces the condition of **disuse atrophy.** Patients confined to bed for a prolonged period lose muscle and skeletal mass as a result of reduced weight bearing. The cell benefits because the reduction in size lowers its energy and other metabolic requirements and allows it to function more efficiently until demand increases. However, such patients can suffer fatigue and possible bone fractures if they resume normal activities before an adequate hypertrophy response can restore their strength.

Inadequate neurological or hormonal stimulus can also induce atrophy. The loss of strength and muscle mass seen in poliomyelitis is associated with significant muscle atrophy that is due to loss of nervous stimulus (fig. 1.10). Another example is the atrophy of the thyroid gland that follows a decline in the level of its regulating hormone TSH (thyroid-stimulating hormone).

The term **pressure atrophy** is applied to the shrinking of cells subjected to long-term pressure. Examples are cells that lie near an expanding tumor or an abnormally bulging artery (an aneurysm). Some deficiency-related damage may be a factor in pressure atrophy, as pressure can compress blood vessels, reducing blood flow and therefore nutrient delivery.

In undergoing atrophy, cells adapt to reduced demand by gradually shutting down their specialized functions and reverting to a low level of activity that sustains only their basic metabolic needs. This usually involves reducing organelle numbers by degrading them with lysosomal enzymes in autophagosomes. The response is reversible in that if demand is restored, cells can build up their normal organelle complement and reactivate normal specialized functions.

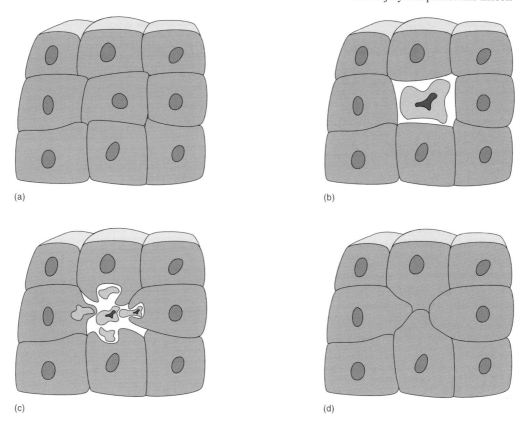

Figure 1.11   **Apoptosis.** (*a*) A representative normal tissue. (*b*) A damaged and weakened cell undergoing apoptosis. (*c*) Resulting cell fragments are engulfed by adjacent unaffected cells. (*d*) Reorganized tissue after loss of damaged cell.

Apoptosis (pronounced "ā-pop-tō′sis" or "āp-ō-tō′sis") is another adaptive response that involves a reduction in cell numbers by a process of self-destruction.

Because the process is genetically regulated, apoptosis is also known as **programmed cell death.** When cells are un-needed, weak, or damaged this orderly removal process is activated. The affected cell undergoes a systematic alteration of its cytoplasm and nucleoplasm, forming dense, dysfunctional masses. These are reorganize into membrane-bound fragments that are engulfed by adjacent cells. As the process continues, the engulfing cells slowly move in to fill the space formerly occupied by the fragmented cell (fig. 1.11).

Apoptosis operates in normal situations in which cell numbers are excessive. For example, in normal embryonic development, many cells are initially overproduced, then later reduced in number by apoptosis. It is also involved in the elimination of unneeded immune cells and to clear cells of the breast that are no longer needed when nursing stops. Certain cells of the immune system destroy other cells by inducing them to undergo apoptosis (cytotoxic T cells; see chapter 5). Since programmed cell death is also useful in dealing with damaged cells, we will encounter various ex-amples as we deal with specific disease processes in later chapters.

Cell Stress Proteins   When exposed to a wide variety of ad-verse conditions—for example, anoxia, toxins, elevated temperature, or trauma, cells respond with the production of **cell stress proteins.** Because they were initially discov-ered in experiments that used heat to stress cells, they were called **heat stress** or **heat shock** proteins. Although there is much to be learned about their adaptive role, they seem to help cells cope with injury. For example, heat or free-radical damage to cell proteins causes them to unfold (de-nature). This change is followed by their clumping together to form insoluble tangles of protein that accumulate in the cytoplasm, interfering with cell structure and function. The stress proteins that form in response to the adverse condition can help in at least three ways. One is by binding to the damaged proteins in a way that makes it easier for enzymes to destroy such proteins before they can form clumps. An-other is by stabilizing the proteins long enough to enable them to refold and become functional once again. Third, the denatured proteins, with stabilizing stress proteins bound to them, are more easily passed through the cell membrane, a change allowing them to be expelled before they can form clumps (see box).

Organelle Changes   By altering its complement of or-ganelles, a cell is better able to respond to unfavorable conditions. The liver, for example, employs enzyme sys-tems associated with its agranular endoplasmic reticu-lum to degrade toxic chemicals. When levels of such a substance rise, the liver responds by producing more AER, matching its detoxification capacity to the in-creased demand. Similarly, when a cell faces a sustained

Focus on Cell Stress Proteins in the Lab and Hospital

There are more than 30 recognized stress proteins. With increasing study, they are being implicated in the pathogenesis of some diseases. Atherosclerosis, the underlying cause of most heart attacks and strokes, and rheumatoid arthritis are examples. Continuing research also indicates that they have potential relevance to a wide variety of diagnostic or preventive procedures. For example, when produced following injury, stress proteins are picked up by the blood. Their presence in a blood sample therefore provides an early indication of cell injury that could enable some preventive response or more prompt therapeutic intervention.

Although the pattern is not yet clearly established, certain cell types may produce only certain stress proteins. This difference, if confirmed, would allow greater diagnostic accuracy at an earlier stage before more grossly detectable signs and symptoms develop. Another potential application is the possibility of preadapting cells to an anticipated stress, such as surgery. Experiments have shown that a mild stress triggers stress protein production. Perhaps if a patient's temperature were intentionally raised prior to surgery, the stress proteins produced in response to the heat stress would increase the patient's ability to cope with the stress of surgery.

Another possible application of stress proteins is in the field of environmental pollution. Because certain toxins, including heavy metals, induce stress protein production, their presence in the body could indicate exposure to pollutants that had yet to cause enough damage to produce more obvious signs and symptoms.

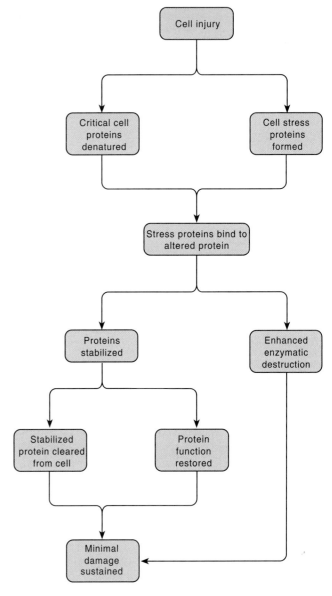

Box Figure 1.1   **Cell Stress Proteins.** The role of cell stress proteins in enabling cells to cope with damage.

---

increase in energy demand, it can form more mitochondria to boost ATP production. Note that these adaptations are seen only when altered conditions persist over an extended period. They do not come into play in the short-term.

Cell and Tissue Accumulations

Much injury directly or indirectly disrupts the cell's metabolism or its protein synthesis capability. As a result, various substances accumulate within the cell. Water is one such substance.

Hydropic Change   When damage reduces cellular energy production, membrane ion pumps, which are fueled by ATP, fail to eject sodium ions from the cell. Normally, leakage of sodium ions (Na^{++}) into the cytoplasm is countered by the membrane pumps, but without adequate ATP, they are slowed and sodium ions accumulate inside the cell. The rise in their concentration increases the osmotic pressure, and water inflow follows (fig. 1.12). The water that

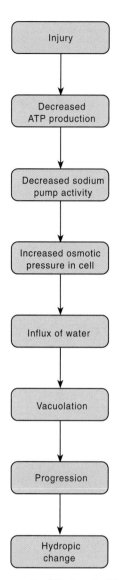

Figure 1.12   **Pathogenesis of Hydropic Change.**

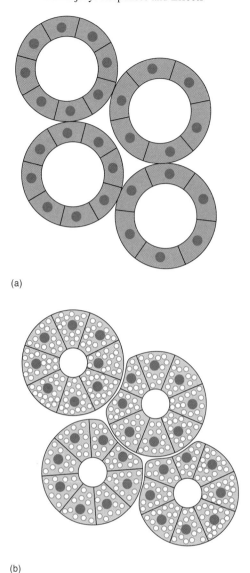

Figure 1.13   **Hydropic Change.** (*a*) Normal microscopic appearance of four representative renal tubules in cross section. (*b*) Appearance after exposure to an injurious toxin. The individual cells are swollen and pale because of the presence of water-filled cytoplasmic vacuoles. As its cells enlarge, the entire kidney appears swollen.

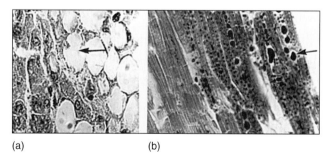

Figure 1.14   **Fatty Change.** (*a*) Liver damage from alcohol abuse. Compare normal cells at lower left with fat-filled, damaged cell indicated by arrow. (*b*) Cardiac muscle cells damaged by chronic oxygen deficiency. Darkly stained fat fills vacuoles in the cytoplasm of the injured cells (arrow). Compare these to the less damaged cells at left.

enters the cell by osmosis enters various membranous organelles, causing a generalized swelling. In response, endoplasmic reticulum cisternae pinch off to form water-filled vacuoles that accumulate in the cytoplasm. The vacuoles cause the cell's optical properties to change and the cytoplasm appears paler. When vacuolation is pronounced, the condition is called **hydropic change** or **hydropic degeneration** (fig. 1.13). In extreme cases, rupture of the cell may result, but this is unusual.

Fatty Change   Another intracellular accumulation is **fatty change,** in which cell injury causes fat to accumulate within the cell. First, small fat droplets and then larger masses form until the cell becomes swollen. Cytoplasm and nucleus are subjected to potentially damaging pressure as they are pushed to the periphery of the cell (fig. 1.14). As cells enlarge, so does the entire organ, which in extreme cases can triple in size (see fig. 14.16). With increasing severity of

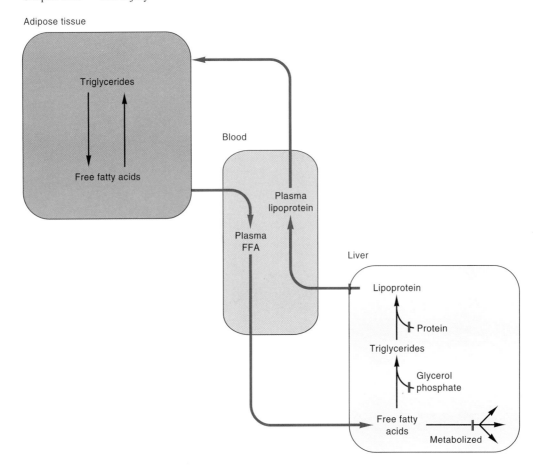

Adipose tissue

Triglycerides

Free fatty acids

Blood

Plasma
lipoprotein

Plasma
FFA

Liver

Lipoprotein

Protein

Triglycerides

Glycerol
phosphate

Free fatty
acids

Metabolized

Figure 1.15 **Pathogenesis of Fatty Change.** In liver, free fatty acids (FFAs) that are not metabolized are converted to triglycerides and combined with protein. The resulting lipoprotein is returned to adipose tissue stores. Only lipoprotein can be cleared from the cell. The bars indicate the points at which injury can interfere with the process to cause fat accumulation.

injury, the accumulated fat may cause rupture of cells, which is followed by the coalescence of fat from adjacent cells to form fatty deposits within the damaged organ. Kidney, heart, and liver commonly demonstrate fatty change in response to injury. Hypoxia (abnormally low oxygen in the tissue) and intoxications—especially in the case of alcoholic liver damage—are typical causes of fatty change.

Tissues susceptible to fatty degeneration are those that utilize fat as an energy source or those involved in the synthesis of lipids. For example, the liver receives free fatty acids (FFAs) from fat stores throughout the body. Within the liver the FFAs may be metabolized to various products, for example, cholesterol or phospholipid, or they may be used in energy metabolism. However, most FFAs are combined with glycerol phosphate to form triglycerides. These, in turn, are used to form lipoprotein by combination with protein that the hepatocyte (liver cell) has produced. The lipoprotein is then passed to the exterior of the cell, where it is taken up by the blood, which returns it to adipose tissue. It is significant that hepatocyte membrane transport systems can export lipid only in the form of lipoprotein. When injured, the hepatocyte may have difficulty coping with the continually arriving FFAs. It may be unable to

metabolize them adequately, or it may be unable to form triglyceride or to produce lipoprotein. Finally, it may not be able to clear lipoprotein from its cytoplasm by passing it to the exterior. Whatever the specific derangement, the result is a build-up of fat within the cytoplasm as FFAs continue to be delivered to a cell that can't handle them (fig. 1.15).

Residual Bodies The intracellular accumulation of **residual bodies** is related to the cell's capacity to cope with potentially threatening bacteria or to deal with damaged organelles. Residual bodies are derived from phagosomes whose contents are not expelled, but instead are retained when lysosome numbers are inadequate to complete digestion or when damaged cell structures are resistant to lysosomal enzyme attack. The term **lipofuscin granule** is applied to residual bodies that contain undigested cell membrane lipids (fig. 1.16). These dark-staining bodies are most often found in neurons, liver, and myocardium. As more and more of these bodies accumulate with increasing age, they can be interpreted as an indication of the cell's history of injury, but note that their presence causes no harm to the cell (fig. 1.17).

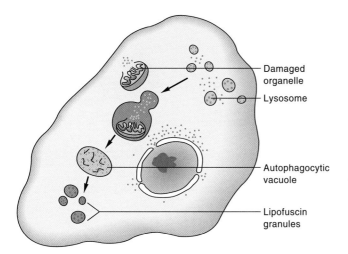

Figure 1.16   **Formation of Lipofuscin Granules.**

- Damaged organelle
- Lysosome
- Autophagocytic vacuole
- Lipofuscin granules

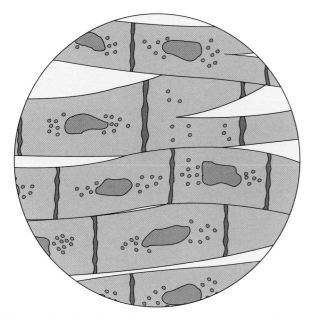

Figure 1.17   **Lipofuscin.** Diagrammatic representation of lipofuscin granules in cardiac muscle tissue of an elderly person.

Hyaline Change   In typical light microscope sections of damaged tissue, a pink-staining, glasslike substance may be seen in or between cells. This material is called **hyaline,** and the condition in which it is present is referred to as **hyaline change** or **hyalinization.** The material deposited is usually protein and may be found in damaged arterioles, renal tubules, damaged liver cells, and neurons. Pathogenesis of protein accumulation is specific to each tissue in which hyaline is present. In some cells infected with viruses, newly formed viral particles appear as hyaline. In other cases, the accumulated protein may derive from plasma proteins, the cytoskeleton, or the basement membrane.

 Checkpoint 1.3

The idea, then, is that cells aren't to be seen as passive sufferers of stress and injury. They have a variety of coping mechanisms that give them a chance to deal with unfavorable conditions. They can often "weather the storm" to carry on when more favorable conditions are restored.

Reversible Changes: Structural

Depending on the nature and duration of injury, cells suffering damage exhibit various structural alterations. The plasma membrane is quick to show effects. For example, it may become stretched and distorted, producing cytoplasmic bulges called **blebs,** which project from the surface of the cell. In some cases, the membrane may exhibit focal coiling, producing forms that resemble the whorled pattern seen in the myelin that wraps neuron processes. Such membrane abnormalities are called **myelin figures.** In other cases, damage may cause specialized membrane structures, such as microvilli or desmosomes, to become distorted and functionally deficient.

In the earlier discussion of hydropic change, we noted that an injured cell may enlarge as the result of osmotic water inflow. Injury-related changes in organelle membranes also allow water to leak into the organelles, causing them to become enlarged and distorted. This change is seen in the Golgi complex, ER, and mitochondria. Swollen mitochondria may also develop densely stained regions within their internal matrix, and as GER cisternae swell, ribosomes are lost from their surfaces. Ribosomes can be seen dispersed in the cytoplasm of an injured cell, but when conditions are restored, they can reaggregate at ER membrane surfaces.

In reversible injury, the nuclear structure appears unchanged in light microscope views, although the nucleolus may show some loss of organization (fig. 1.18).

Irreversible Injury and Necrosis

Structural Changes

The severely injured cell, which cannot recover its normal functions, shows structural changes that are more extreme than those seen in the reversibly injured cell. The plasma membrane exhibits more extreme distortions, accompanied by varying degrees of increased permeability. The latter change allows a more rapid inflow of sodium, calcium, and water. Gaps in the membrane also allow escape of vital cell constituents. In extreme cases, the cell membrane ruptures and its contents spill into the exterior. Mitochondrial and ER membranes undergo similar breakdown. The mitochondria may greatly enlarge and exhibit bizarre structural

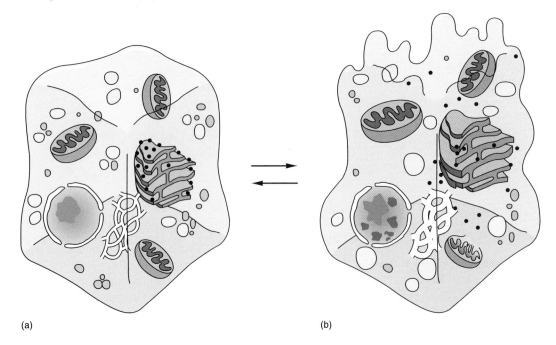

(a)   (b)

Figure 1.18   **Reversible Structural Change Following Cell Injury.** (*a*) A normal cell and (*b*) an injured cell. In the injured cell, note the blebs in the plasma membrane, swollen and distorted mitochondria and ER, ribosomes lost from ER surfaces, vacuolated cytoplasm, and nuclear clumping.

distortions, often developing focal deposits of calcium in their interior. The ER often develops myelin figures. In severe irreversible injury, ER cisternae may also rupture and disperse in the cytoplasm.

The irreversibly injured cell also has fewer lysosomes because lysosomal membranes lose their stability when severely injured. Normally, these membranes isolate their potent lysosomal enzymes from the cytoplasm, but in irreversibly injured cells, the less-stable membranes break open, releasing their destructive contents.

The single, most significant indicator of irreversible cell injury is an altered nucleus. Housing the vital chromosomes, the nucleus must remain intact and functional if the cell is to have any chance of recovery. Following cell death, in some cases nuclear DNA is degraded, and with less material to stain, the nucleus seems to fade and melt into the cytoplasm. This condition is called **karyolysis** (fig. 1.19). In other cases, the nucleus may shrink and condense **(pyknosis),** or it may break up into densely staining fragments that disperse in the cytoplasm **(karyorrhexis).**

Mechanisms of Irreversible Injury

In irreversible injury, a small number of derangements have widespread and devastating effects. One of these is damage to cell membranes—both the plasma membrane and those forming the cellular organelles. When membranes are damaged, their permeability and cytoplasm-organizing functions are compromised. The result is severe swelling from sodium influx, loss of cytoplasmic constituents to the cell's exterior, and a large flow of calcium into the cell with devastating effects. In high concentration, calcium causes

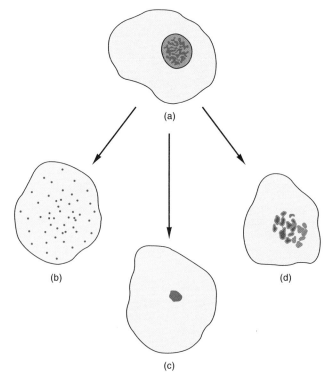

Figure 1.19   **Nuclear Changes in Irreversible Injury.** (*a*) A representative normal cell, with translucent cytoplasm and a nucleus showing typical chromatin staining. The nature and intensity of injury produce different nuclear effects in necrosis: (*b*) karyolysis, (*c*) pyknosis, and (*d*) karyorrhexis.

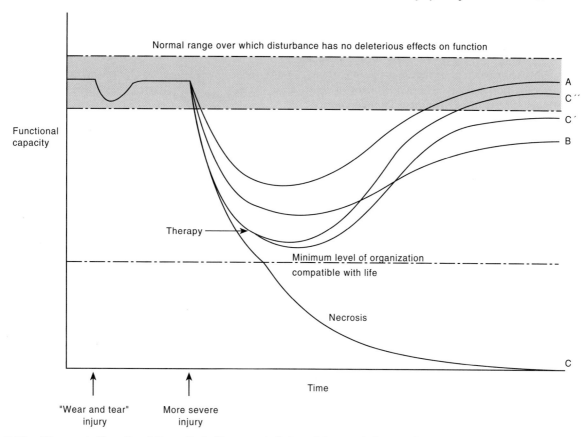

Figure 1.20 Changes in Functional Capacity in Response to Injury. Therapeutic intervention may fully or partially restore function, but if it is ineffective, cell death may be unavoidable. See text.

protein denaturation, resulting in critical loss of enzyme function. The excessive calcium also forms insoluble masses in mitochondria and causes activation of enzymes that further damage cell membrane systems, generally. The result is disruption of permeability, declines in mitochondrial ATP production, and flawed protein synthesis on deranged endoplasmic reticulum surfaces. Note the positive feedback cycling that operates here: Increased calcium causes damage that affects membrane permeability. This allows further calcium inflow resulting in further damage. As noted earlier, when energy levels fall, cells can respond by switching to glycolysis for ATP production. However, this anaerobic energy metabolism produces high levels of acid products. These lower the pH, a change that triggers the activation and release of lysosomal enzymes that can degrade important cytoplasmic and nuclear structures.

Severely damaged cells also suffer disruption of their **cytoskeleton.** Recall that this is the system of protein filaments that maintains overall cell shape and provides much of the cell's internal structural organization. In damaged cells, its components may form extensive tangles that interfere with normal functioning. When dysfunctional, the cytoskeleton's links to the internal surface of the plasma membrane may be affected, allowing the membrane to form the blebs often seen in damaged cells. In more serious injury, the disrupted cyoskeleton allows membrane stretching to the point of complete rupture.

✔ *Checkpoint 1.4*

Injury occurs when a cell is pushed beyond its ability to adapt. This may be a reversible condition, but when the situation is severe or prolonged, the cell reaches levels of disruption from which it can't recover. Cell death follows at some point thereafter.

Cell Death

Depending on the nature and intensity of injury, its timing, and the innate resistance of the cell, different cells may respond in different ways when exposed to the same injurious agent. They may adapt within a normal range of wear and tear. They may be reversibly injured and recover, or they may be permanently affected and forced to function at a less than normal level. In the extreme case, injury can result in cell death.

These concepts are presented in figure 1.20. The vertical axis represents the cell's level of functional capacity, with the normal range indicated by shading. Time is represented by the horizontal axis. During the life of the cell, various injuries occur. Minor, well-tolerated injuries represent a normal wear-and-tear level of demand to which the

Focus On Free Radicals

Current research is uncovering the important role of free radicals as a major factor in cell membrane damage. The phospholipid core of the membrane is highly sensitive to damage by free radicals; the process is known as **lipid peroxidation.** Free radicals can be produced by ionizing radiation, as the products of the metabolism of exogenous chemicals, or when iron and copper levels in the cell are elevated. They can also be produced by normal metabolic reactions that release hydroxyl radicals (—OH) or the molecular-oxygen free radical called **superoxide.** The superoxide and hydroxyl radicals are known as **activated oxygen species.**

An important aspect of free-radical formation is **self-propagation,** or **autocatalysis.** This means that the formation of one free radical leads to its interaction with other molecules, not only causing damage but producing a new free radical, which can then repeat the cycle to produce a self-catalyzing chain reaction. In this way, a single event forming only one free radical can produce far-reaching effects (box fig. 1.2*a*). On the other hand, the cell is not completely at the mercy of free radicals. Some reaction chains may be interrupted when free radicals interact to produce stable forms. Various specific enzymes (catalase, superoxide dismutase) promote such reactions and serve to limit free-radical formation. Other substances may take up (scavenge) free radicals to interrupt the chain sequences. Vitamins A, C, and E are examples of such scavengers as are the systems that bind iron and copper to limit free-radical formation. Substances that oppose the effects of oxygen-free radicals are called **antioxidants.** They convert activated oxygen species to harmless water (box fig. 1.2*b*).

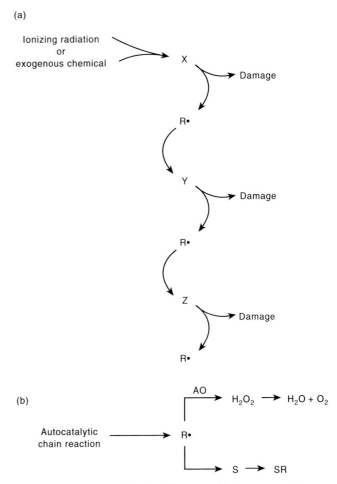

Box Figure 1.2   **Free Radical Damage.** *(a)* An autocatalytic chain reaction produces damage to critical cell constituents X, Y and Z, while generating a new free radical, R•, at each step. *(b)* The cell's antioxidants, AO, or scavenger molecules, S, interact with free radicals to produce stable forms, terminating the chain reaction.

---

cell can adapt and still maintain normal function. Cell activities are not significantly affected by these physiological stressors. For example, the hepatocyte can adapt to a chronic, low-level intoxication by producing more AER.

Figure 1.20 also shows a later, more severe injury that significantly affects cellular function, and indicates three possible outcomes of exposure to such an injurious stressor. In one (curve A), the cell overcomes the effect of the injury and returns to a normal functional level. Another possibility (curve B) is that the cell recovers, but not at its normal functional level; the injury effects are nonreversible. Curve C shows the third possible outcome. The functional capacity

of the cell has fallen to a level below which no recovery is possible (dashed line in the figure) and cell death results. But notice that cell death may not be immediate. Even though the cell has dropped below the critical point of no return, some time may pass before the loss of functional capacity is complete. Also note that the "point of no return" is a theoretical point not clinically definable or detectable by laboratory or other tests. Therapeutic intervention seeks to interrupt the decline in functional capacity. The timing and effectiveness of the intervention determines whether partial or complete function is restored. These possibilities are represented by curves C′ and C″. Note that following injury,

Tissue Vulnerability to Injury   21

cells that survive but are unable to return to normal (curves B and C′) may be eliminated by apoptosis.

The condition of cell death is called **necrosis.** It is accompanied by substantial changes in the cell and in the tissue of which it is a part. The contents of the cell are broken down by its endogenous enzymes and by the enzymes of phagocytic cells that arrive at the scene to assist the process. The resulting debris is removed and healing of the tissue usually follows.

The cell enzymes involved are primarily those of the lysosomes. When, and only when, a cell suffers a lethal injury, lysosomes release their enzymes into the cytoplasm, and these initiate the chemical breakdown of cell constituents. Note that this event is nothing like the cell's using its lysosomes in some suicidal impulse. Lysosomal enzymes are released only after the point of lethal injury. The cell is, in effect, already dying, and the lysosomes are simply speeding the breakdown and removal of nonfunctional tissue from the scene.

Following their death, most tissues become somewhat firm for a period of a few days. This is referred to as **coagulation necrosis** (fig. 1.21). In coagulation necrosis, cell proteins are quickly denatured by the high levels of acid and calcium and the otherwise abnormal conditions that exist in the dead or dying cell. Lysosomal enzymes are also affected and are unable to digest the cell. This delays complete breakdown of a damaged tissue until the arrival of phagocytic blood cells whose enzymes accomplish the final tissue breakdown. Until the arrival of the phagocytes, the tissue retains its overall organization; its denatured proteins are responsible for the tissue's coagulation.

In certain cases, coagulation necrosis may produce unusual characteristic features. **Caseous necrosis** is an example that is often seen in tuberculosis. In this infection, the necrotic tissue has a pale, granular, cheeselike appearance. (The word "caseous" comes from the Latin for cheese.) In this case, the coagulated cells remain although the overall tissue organization is lost.

Gangrene, or **gangrenous necrosis,** is another subtype of coagulation necrosis. It is characterized by the presence of noxious products of anaerobic bacterial metabolism. If these organisms, which can thrive without oxygen, gain access to an area of damage caused by reduced blood flow **(ischemia),** they can proliferate in the oxygen-deprived necrotic tissue. This process is often referred to as **putrefaction.** In some cases, foul-smelling gases are produced. If the enzymes of invading phagocytic cells break down the necrotic debris and produce some liquefaction, the descriptive term **wet gangrene** is applied. More typically, coagulation is sustained and the condition is called **dry gangrene.**

In some cases, coagulation does not occur. Instead, the necrotic tissue breaks down quite promptly. This is known as **liquefaction necrosis.** For reasons that are unclear, it typically follows brain necrosis due to ischemic injury. In

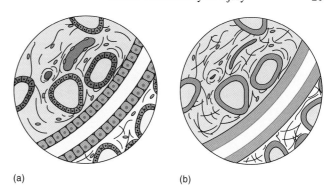

Figure 1.21   Coagulation Necrosis. (*a*) A section of kidney, showing the normal arrangement of tubules, ducts, vessels, and supporting connective tissue. (*b*) Oxygen deprivation has caused cell death, but the tissue's essential organization is retained. Note the loss of nuclei in the necrotic cells.

this case, it is possible that lysosomal enzymes are able to resist denaturation long enough to produce a quick breakdown of the tissues. The other occurrence of liquefaction involves certain bacterial infections wherein the microorganisms possess potent enzymes that quickly liquefy the necrotic cells at the infection site.

Calcification   At sites of necrosis, regardless of type, calcium deposition often occurs. This is especially the case in persistent injury or where damage effects are slow to develop. Indeed, early injury that affects membrane function allows calcium into the cell. There it condenses in mitochondria to contribute to the cell's ultimate death.

Initially, the calcium crystals that form are tiny, but progressive deposition produces larger masses that can lead to significant rigidity and brittleness in the affected tissue. The process, called **dystrophic calcification,** often serves to indicate necrosis and little else. In some cases, however, calcification can produce its own complications—for example, in heart valves whose calcified leaflets cannot fully open or close, or in calcified arteries that lose their elasticity.

Metastatic calcification also involves calcium salt deposition but differs from dystrophic calcification in two ways: (1) it occurs in otherwise normal, as opposed to necrotic, tissue, and (2) the deposition is a consequence of an excessive systemic calcium level, or **hypercalcemia.** Although generally widespread, calcium deposits are most often found in lung, kidney, blood vessels, and the mucous membrane of the stomach. If severe, metastatic calcification may interfere with lung or kidney function, but generally its consequences are minimal.

TISSUE VULNERABILITY TO INJURY

Because the various cells of the body have different characteristics, they differ in their vulnerability to injury. Consider the following examples.

Ischemia

Central nervous system (CNS) neurons are highly sensitive to ischemia because they have a high metabolic rate and are dependent on glucose as their only energy source. Thus, the brain can tolerate loss of blood supply for only a few minutes before a lack of ATP permanently injures its neurons. This type of cell injury is the underlying cause of **stroke,** which kills millions of people every year. In contrast, kidney or liver cells are less sensitive to ischemia. At body temperature, these tissues can tolerate up to 60 minutes of interrupted blood flow without permanent damage. By cooling the kidney to lower its metabolic rate and thereby reduce its energy demand, this time can be extended considerably. This tolerance is a significant factor in being able to transplant a kidney from a healthy donor to a patient whose kidneys are damaged beyond saving. Even more tolerant of ischemia are fibroblasts. These connective tissue cells can tolerate ischemia for prolonged periods, far longer than neurons or kidney and liver cells. This proves valuable when fibroblasts must form scar tissue at injury sites, where oxygen levels remain low until new blood vessels can form.

Intoxication

Carbon tetrachloride (CCl_4), an exogenous toxin that causes liver damage after it is inhaled, provides another example of differential cell vulnerability to injury. From the respiratory passages, CCl_4 enters the blood and ultimately reaches the liver. Although the lining of the respiratory passages, the lung tissue, and blood cells are all exposed, the CCl_4 causes greatest damage in the much more susceptible hepatocytes. The breakdown of CCl_4 by liver cells produces a toxic free radical. Because the other tissues can't break down CCl_4, they are little affected by their exposure to it.

Ionizing Radiation

When the body is exposed to ionizing radiation, many different tissues are damaged. As we noted earlier, DNA is especially sensitive to high-energy radiation damage. In particular, actively dividing cells that are undergoing DNA replication are susceptible to injury from this source. For this reason, areas of rapid mitosis—skin, red bone marrow, and gastrointestinal mucous membranes—show the greatest disruption of function after exposure to radiation. Such disruption underlies the problems of nausea, diarrhea, gastrointestinal hemorrhage, hair loss, and bone marrow effects typically associated with radiation exposure.

Viral Infection

A last example of differential vulnerability is viral infection. Viruses enter and then disrupt cells from within. However, most viruses can't simply enter any cell they happen to contact. A specific interaction between the virus and the host cell is involved, so that each virus can infect only a specific type of cell. A particular case of such specificity is seen in the polio virus, which infects neurons in the gray matter of the spinal cord. The virus attacks only the cells of the anterior horns, which supply stimulation to skeletal muscle. Several other types of neurons are immediately adjacent but they are not affected. The specificity of viral attack seems to be based on the fact that the susceptible cell has membrane surface receptors to which the viral particle can bind. This binding is the critical step that allows the virus to enter the cell. Tissues lacking specific receptors provide no easy access to the cell's interior and so are much less vulnerable to attack.

DETERMINATION AND MONITORING OF CELL INJURY

We have seen that cells are subject to injury and that in response they undergo certain changes in their function and structure. As we noted in the Introduction, successful outcome of a particular medical problem requires that the problem be correctly identified so that appropriate therapy can be undertaken. In other words, one needs to know not just that something is wrong, but the precise nature of the defect. The problem is to determine which of the many body cells have been injured, and to what degree. There are four common approaches to this problem: assessments of functional loss, detection of cell constituents released from injured cells, monitoring of electrical activity, and direct tissue examination.

Functional Loss

The loss of mobility suffered from a leg fracture is obvious. Functional deterioration of internal organs may not be so easily apparent, but it can be assessed in various ways. These usually reveal subtle changes in the body fluids, which reflect the functional deterioration. For example, the liver normally removes the pigment bilirubin from the blood and excretes it into the bile. Thus, the finding of elevated plasma levels of bilirubin may indicate functional deterioration of liver cells. Similarly, hydrogen ion (H^+) is normally excreted by the kidney. When the kidney suffers damage, its excretion of H^+ is likely to be reduced. A clue to this functional loss appears in a decrease in the concentration of H^+ in the urine. In another case, alterations from the normal values of oxygen and carbon dioxide in the blood can be a sign of functional decline in the respiratory system.

Release of Cell Constituents

A second means of determining cell injury is based on the release of cell constituents by injured cells. Normally, substances confined to the cell's interior, such as potassium ions (K^+) and cell enzymes, leak to the exterior at a slow,

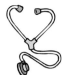

Focus on Serum Enzymes in Diagnosis

Diagnosis is often complicated by the fact that a given pattern of signs and symptoms may be associated with more than one disease. In such cases, serum enzyme levels can sometimes be used to differentiate among several possibilities. The following example illustrates the principle. Several different liver diseases produce an accumulation of bile pigments that discolors the skin and whites of the eyes—the condition called jaundice. The diagnostic challenge is to identify which disease is responsible for a given patient's jaundice. The problem can be solved because different types of liver cell damage lead to different levels of release into the blood of the enzyme alkaline phosphatase (ALP). Box figure 1.3 shows that in liver damage caused by bile duct obstruction (obstructive jaundice), the enzyme is present at almost five times its normal level. But it is present at only twice the normal level in cirrhosis or viral hepatitis. Now consider the case of viral hepatitis, in which the damage releases over 15 times the normal level of aspartate amino transferase (AST). If such high levels of AST occur, it is easy to exclude obstruction or cirrhosis as contributing to the patient's jaundice, because in these conditions, AST doesn't usually exceed four times normal.

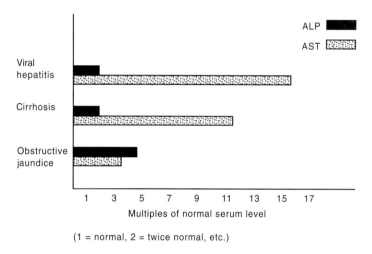

Box Figure 1.3 **Serum Enzymes in Diagnosis.** Different liver diseases produce varying patterns of enzyme loss to the blood. Assessing serum levels of appropriate enzymes is a valuable diagnostic aid.

---

steady rate, establishing a normal plasma level. Injury-related permeability changes or complete cell rupture release constituents in larger quantities. High plasma levels of these substances can therefore be taken as indications of cell injury.

Because potassium ions are much more concentrated in the cell than in its exterior, a rising level of plasma potassium indicates widespread tissue damage. For example, elevated plasma potassium is a typical result of hemolysis, which involves the often large-scale rupture of red blood cells.

In muscle tissue that is damaged, a component of its contractile system, troponin, escapes and can be detected in the blood. It is an important indicator of myocardial injury in cases of heart attack.

The other substances that may also escape through ruptured or damaged membranes are intracellular enzymes; for example, creatine phosphokinase (CPK). This enzyme is abundant in skeletal and cardiac muscle and in the brain. In the necrosis that follows a heart attack or stroke, the tissues release CPK. Thus, a high plasma level of CPK can initially indicate, or later confirm, that skeletal, cardiac, or brain tissue damage has occurred. Similarly, an increased plasma level of the enzyme gamma-glutamyl transferase (GGT) is an indication of liver damage, because large quantities of this enzyme are normally present in hepatocytes.

High liver enzyme levels in the plasma do not necessarily indicate liver damage; instead they may signal a high rate of production of detoxification enzymes in response to the threat of some poison. On the other hand, a decline in plasma enzymes is not a good sign either. It may be that so much tissue damage has already occurred that in the remaining cells, normal enzyme leakage is insufficient to maintain even the normally low plasma level.

Tumor cells tend to overproduce their intracellular enzymes. For example, the cells of prostate gland cancer, upon spreading to other body sites, produce large amounts of the enzyme acid phosphatase. Without this indication of

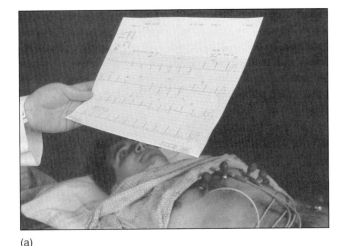

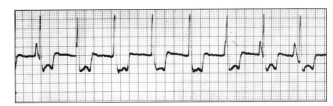

(a)

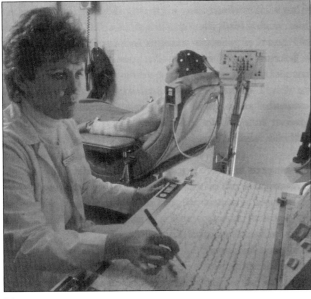

(b)

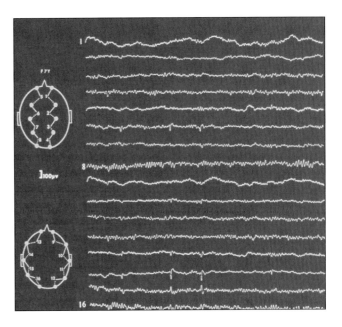

Figure 1.22   **Monitoring Cell Injury.** (*a*) Electrical monitoring of the heart, shown beside an electrocardiogram (ECG) that indicates an unusually rapid heart rate. (*b*) The placement of scalp electrodes used for monitoring brain activity. The accompanying electroencephalogram (EEG) is one that indicates seizure activity.

its activity, the presence of the tumor might go undetected for a dangerously long time.

In a few cases, an enzyme is present in significant quantities in only one tissue. When the plasma level of that enzyme is increased, the finding points directly to the site of the damage. An example is the enzyme alcohol dehydrogenase, produced only in the liver.

Electrical Activity

A third approach to assessing cell injury involves the monitoring of electrical activity to detect changes from the normal. The effects of much of the electrical activity in the in-

terior of the body are detected at its surface by specialized electronic equipment, which then visually displays the results. Any change from the normal electrical pattern can be interpreted in terms of altered functioning. This approach is used most commonly in studying the heart, for which the **electrocardiogram** (ECG or EKG) is used (fig. 1.22*a*). Similarly, the electrical activity of the brain can be displayed in an **electroencephalogram** (EEG) to assess seizure activity (fig. 1.22*b*) or to monitor a patient in a coma. Electrical activity associated with muscular contraction is displayed in the **electromyogram** (EMG), which can yield useful information regarding muscle weakness or paralysis. The conduction times of the action potentials that elicit muscle contraction responses can also indicate abnormality. If conduction times increase, the reason may be neuron injury or defective synaptic transmission.

Biopsy

A fourth means of determining cell injury is direct microscopic examination of the tissue in which damage is suspected. A small portion of tissue is removed from the body in a minor surgical procedure called a **biopsy.** The tissue is then prepared for microscope study. Biopsies are also often done to study tissue organization and cell characteristics. The goal is to determine whether a tumor is present and, if present, whether it is a benign or more threatening malignant tumor.

Checkpoint 1.5

If you're wondering why imaging techniques such as X-ray, nuclear isotope, computerized tomography (CT), magnetic resonance image (MRI), or positron emission tomography (PET) scans were not mentioned in this section, it is because the emphasis has been on cell injury. The imaging techniques noted are primarily directed at detecting gross structural changes that are usually several steps removed from the initial cell injury.

Case Study

A 54-year-old man came to his general practitioner for a physical examination. He was found to be in good health overall, but the physician thought he detected alcohol on the man's breath. This particularly concerned him because the patient had a history of alcoholism, although he had abstained from drinking for the past three years. In response the physician's general question on his continuing to avoid alcohol, the man denied any alcohol use.

As part of the patient's general blood analysis, the physician requested that the serum level of gamma-glutamyl transferase (GGT) be measured. The blood tests confirmed the general good health of the patient, but GGT was clearly elevated above normal. With this evidence, and no other indication of liver damage, the doctor called the patient in for a consultation, during which the patient admitted his recent return to drinking in response to work-related stresses. He agreed to enter and follow through with a medically supervised alcohol rehabilitation program.

Commentary

In this all-too-common situation, the outcome may well be a positive one. Too often the alcoholic denies excessive drinking and strongly resists efforts to interrupt it.

Because the elevation of serum GGT is a sensitive indicator of alcohol abuse, it is often used in establishing the presence of covert drinking. In the case of this enzyme, a high serum level is due, not to its release from damaged liver cells, but rather to the high cellular levels formed in response to high alcohol intake. The physician's evidence of drinking, which could not be refuted, effectively undercut any inclination to denial and may have been a factor in the agreement to enter the rehabilitation program. There is also a good chance that the serum GGT would be used in the patient's rehabilitation program to monitor alcohol abstinence.

Key Concepts

1. Although many different agents or mechanisms may be involved in causing cell injury, from the cellular perspective injury is essentially the result of (1) a deficiency of a necessary metabolite, (2) the presence of a toxic substance, or (3) disruption of the physical integrity of the cell (pp. 8–11).

2. The intensity, duration, and number of exposures to an etiological agent determine the degree of cell injury, but the resulting signs and symptoms may reflect effects that are several steps removed from the initial biochemical disturbance (p. 12).

3. Cells may adapt to injury by temporarily altering their size, their mix of cytoplasmic organelles, or their metabolism in order to cope better with unfavorable conditions. They may also activate systems that cope with free radicals or denatured proteins or may self-destruct. (pp. 12–14).

4. A common, reversible effect of cell injury is the abnormal intracellular accumulation of certain substances, most often water, fat, or proteins of various types (pp. 14–17).

5. Injured cells may demonstrate reversible structural changes, most often involving membrane malformations, swelling and distortion of cellular organelles, and the disaggregation of ribosomes from endoplasmic reticulum surfaces (p. 17).

6. Severe injury can irreversibly damage cells, producing more extreme intracellular changes such as pronounced disruption or rupture of cytoplasmic structures, loss of cell constituents through damaged membranes, the release of lysosomal contents, protein denaturation, and nuclear degeneration (pp. 17–19).

7. Many variables combine to determine the outcome of cell injury, which may be (1) relatively mild and reversible damage, (2) more severe damage, with some lingering functional deficit, or (3) cell death. Therapeutic intervention can often improve the outcome (pp. 19–21).

8. The features that are characteristic of coagulation necrosis, liquefaction necrosis, caseous necrosis, or gangrene reflect differences in combined effects of lysosomal enzymes on extracellular proteins, peculiarities of the necrotic debris, and the action of bacterial products (if infection is involved) (p. 21).

9. Variations in tissue characteristics determine the observed differences in their susceptibility to injury (pp. 21–22).

10. Cell injury can be assessed by direct and indirect analysis of altered function, by detection of cell constituents or abnormal enzyme levels in the plasma or urine, by monitoring of electrical activity, or by examination of a tissue sample (pp. 22–25).

REVIEW ACTIVITIES

1. Look back to figure 1.7. Be certain that you know the difference between primary and secondary nutrient deficiency and that you could give an example of how an infectious agent might contribute to the deficiency problem.

2. Lay out a flow chart that indicates clearly the pathogenesis of fatty change. Start with: "FFAs enter cell" and end with "lipid accumulation." Check back in the text to verify that you've got the whole story.

3. In figure 1.18, without consulting the legend, for each organelle in (a), identify how it has changed in the postinjury state (b). Check pages 17–18 for verification.

4. Complete the table on the right by providing information on the body fluid or region analyzed in diagnosis and on a possible cause of an abnormal value of the variable. Pages 22 to 24 may be worth consulting if blanks remain after your initial attempt.

5. Look back to the case study at the end of the chapter. In the commentary, note that the GGT level was elevated not because of damage, but in response to a potentially injurious agent. Is this a useful adaptive response? Is it

Abnormal Variable	Fluid/Region Assessed	Possible Problem
Bilirubin		
CO_2		
K^+		
CPK		
H^+		
O_2		
EEG		

a specific example of the general case described on pages 17–18? Would you expect a liver biopsy (if one were done) to reveal increased AER in the patient's hepatocytes? Would the liver cells be different sometime after a successful rehabilitation program? Is the GGT increase a reversible or irreversible adaptation?

Inflammation

. . . people in good health were all of a sudden attacked by violent heats in the head, and redness and inflammation in the eyes, the inward parts, such as the throat or the tongue, becoming bloody . . .

THUCYDIDES
THE PELOPONNESIAN WARS

rubor

&tumor

cū calore

&dolore

Injury to the body or a breach of its defensive barriers triggers a versatile, localized response called **acute inflammation.** The response involves a dramatic increase in blood flow to the injury site, which causes it to become red and warm. Local swelling also occurs, as a result of the movement of fluid and cells to the intercellular spaces, and the site becomes painful. These signs and symptoms were recorded as early as 2,000 years ago by the Roman physician Celsus. For this reason, they are often referred to by the original Latin terms **rubor** (redness), **calor** (heat), **tumor** (swelling), and **dolor** (pain). You see these terms to the side of the title page, in Italian, in the hand of a Renaissance translator. Later, Virchow added a fifth classic sign: loss of function (**functio laesa**). You will still come across these terms in modern medical literature and practice. Because acute inflammation arises in response to many types of injury, it is very common. All those conditions whose names end in the suffix "itis"—for example, dermatitis, meningitis, pericarditis—are inflammatory conditions. Inflammation is a complexly orchestrated response to injury that serves to destroy the source of injury, remove the accumulated debris, and trigger the repair process.

Before moving to the study of inflammation, you may find it useful to review the following information on normal vascularized connective tissue and the formation of tissue fluid.

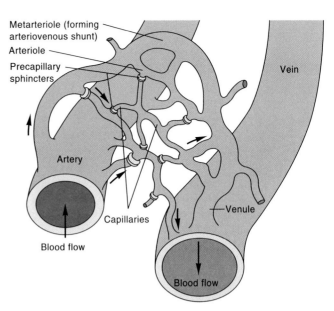

Figure 2.1   **The Relationship of Artery, Arteriole, Capillaries, Venules, and Veins in the Microcirculation.** Relaxation of precapillary sphincters permits blood flow through portions of the capillary bed. Metarterioles can shunt blood past the tissue when the precapillary sphincters, which regulate blood flow through the tissue, are closed.

NORMAL VASCULARIZED CONNECTIVE TISSUE

The inflammatory response is focused in the vascularized connective tissue present throughout the body. This tissue is called **loose** or **areolar connective tissue** in anatomy and physiology texts. One important location is in the dermis of the skin. Loose connective tissue is also the principal component of the lamina propria that underlies the mucosa lining the gastrointestinal and urinary tracts; it supports the epithelium of the respiratory tree; it provides the supportive and mechanical context of muscle fibers; and it forms the lining of joint capsules. You can see that this tissue is well placed to encounter any breach of the surface covering of the body or its communicating internal spaces and to respond to mechanical injuries of muscle and joints as well. The vessels that participate in the inflammatory response are the postcapillary venules (fig. 2.1). **Capillaries,** which convey blood into the venules and are in intimate relation to the injured tissue to which inflammation is a response, are short tubes (perhaps 1–2 mm) formed of flattened endothelial cells supported by a basement membrane on their tissue surfaces. The basement membrane is composed of collagen fiber bundles embedded in a gel of **proteoglycans,** compounds that contain protein and sugar.

Functionally, the **capillaries** are significant because they provide for the exchange of oxygen, nutrients, and wastes between the blood and tissue spaces. This exchange occurs via some combination of diffusion and active transport *through* the endothelial cells with selective fluid movement *between* them. Flow through a network of capillaries is controlled by groups of smooth muscle cells located in the walls of the smallest arterioles, the vessels that supply the capillaries. These smooth muscle sphincters can alter their degree of constriction, allowing more or less blood to perfuse the capillaries as demand changes. For this reason, they are known as **precapillary sphincters.** Beyond a bed of interconnected capillaries lie the vessels that drain them, the **postcapillary venules.** These venules have somewhat thicker walls than capillaries because smooth muscle and some protective connective tissue are also present. These venules are the normal site at which cells bound for the tissue space leave the bloodstream. They are also the region where most fluid leaves the vascular compartment during an inflammatory response.

Normal vascular permeability is determined by the cells of the endothelium. These flattened cells fit together tightly like tiles as they line the vessel lumen. Where two adjacent endothelial cells meet, forming an **endothelial junction,** their edges overlap and a thin layer of intercellular substance (glycoprotein) fills the gap. Most substances entering the tissue must pass through the endothelial cells either by diffusion or in transfer vesicles. Open channels formed by temporary merging of vesicles may contribute to the process (fig. 2.2). The endothelial junctions found in loose CT tend to be "intermediate" in the range of junctions found in different tissues. Inflammation

A simple point needs to be made. The vessel relations we are discussing here, among precapillary arterioles, capillaries, and postcapillary venules, are microscopic in nature. And while we talk about and diagram them in linear sequence, remember that all cells within the loose connective tissue (CT) or the tissue to which it is adjacent and that may be the primary site of the injury, are very close to a precapillary arteriole or a capillary. Any chemicals that could initiate some aspect of an inflammatory response in the tissue space will tend to diffuse. This will allow them to interact with the smooth muscle of the precapillary sphincter, promoting relaxation and increased perfusion of the capillary bed. In like manner, these chemicals can diffuse into a capillary and then be carried downstream with the blood. Chemicals released from the capillary endothelium itself will follow the same course. The first larger vessel these chemicals encounter will be the postcapillary venule, whose endothelium is richly supplied with receptors to a variety of these inflammation- and injury-related chemicals. Wherever the injury occurs, there will be a downstream venule waiting to get involved. Tissues that contain either little loose CT (like bone) or dramatically different CT (like the liver) can produce inflammatory responses that are more muted or require the participation of some of the inflammatory cells we will describe shortly.

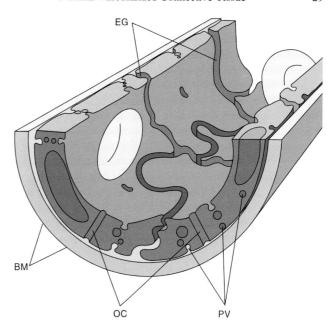

Figure 2.2   **The Endothelium in Vascular Permeability.**
EG: The endothelial gap between adjacent cells; PV: pinocytotic vesicles carrying fluid between the blood and tissue spaces; OC: open channels formed by the merging of pinocytic vesicles; BM: basement membrane.

Macrophages (a kind of phagocytic cell) may be present to engulf any debris formed by normal tissue wear and tear. **Mast cells,** which have various roles in mediating inflammation, are also typically scattered through the extracellular matrix of a connective tissue, particularly in association with small blood vessels.

The formation of tissue fluid and its return to the blood depend on the balance of pressure across the capillary wall. Because **blood hydrostatic pressure** (BHP), the fluid pressure of blood confined within vessels, is high near the arterial end of the capillary, fluid is forced out of the vessel to form **tissue fluid.** A slight **tissue osmotic pressure** (TOP), which derives from the solute molecules in the interstitial spaces, assists this outward flow. Near the venous end of the capillary, blood hydrostatic pressure is lower, but the osmotic attraction of the blood for water, called **blood osmotic pressure** (BOP), is higher because the loss of fluid to the tissue spaces concentrates the plasma proteins. As well, fluids driven into the interstitium are confined within its spaces, producing a **tissue hydrostatic pressure** (THP) that adds to blood osmotic pressure. Together, blood osmotic pressure and tissue hydrostatic pressure force the fluid back into the capillary to complete the exchange (fig. 2.3*a.*) Because the pressures that produce tissue fluid are slightly greater than those that return it to the blood, some excess extracellular fluid results. This is normally drained off by the lymph capillaries and returned to the venous circulation. We will return to this model in the next section, Acute Inflammation.

will loosen these junctions within the postcapillary venules. Vascular endothelial junctions in adjacent tissues—for example, the normally "tight" junctions found within the capillaries and venules of the brain—will also loosen in response to the signals produced in inflammation. This moves the inflammatory response from the loose CT into the parenchymal tissue of the organ with which the CT is associated. In this way, inflammation can deal with tissues that, although injured, don't possess the mechanisms to orchestrate an inflammatory response. As we will see much later in this book, this can create additional problems for the brain.

Surrounding the vessels in vascular connective tissue is a complex consisting of the **extracellular matrix** (ECM) and the various cells and fibers contained within it. The extracellular matrix consists largely of proteoglycans. These provide anchorage for the collagen and elastic fibers present in connective tissues, as well as for capillaries, whose basement membranes bind to proteoglycans. **Fibroblasts** in connective tissues are the cells that produce the proteins of the extracellular matrix and many of its fibers.

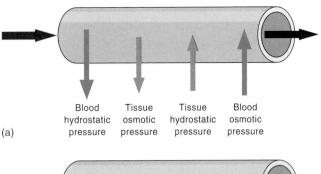

(a)

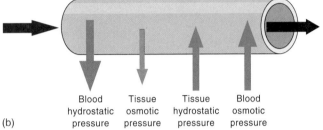

(b)

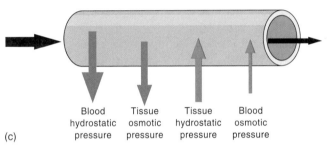

(c)

Figure 2.3 **Tissue Fluid Formation.** (*a*) The diagram shows the pressures across the capillary wall that normally contribute to the formation of tissue fluid and its return to the plasma. Gray indicates the pressures whose contribution is minor. (*b*) Under conditions of arteriolar dilation, blood hydrostatic pressure predominates, forcing more fluid through the capillary or venule endothelium. (*c*) Increased permeability at the venule allows the escape of plasma proteins, which reduces blood osmotic pressure while increasing tissue osmotic pressure. While (*b*) produces largely a transudate and tissue edema, (*c*) produces the protein-rich exudate characteristic of inflammation. Note that inflammation combines the vasodilation of (*b*) with increased venule permeability.

ACUTE INFLAMMATION

The acute inflammatory response has two distinct components. One is its vascular component, which consists of an increased blood flow to the damaged tissue and an increase in venule permeability. This component leads to the redness and warmth that are so often observed at the site of injury, and to the swelling that follows as fluid increasingly moves to the tissue spaces.

The second component is cellular. Large numbers of specialized leukocytes (white blood cells) move to the tissue spaces, where they inactivate certain disease agents (e.g., bacteria) and remove debris. This movement of fluid, suspended substances, and cells is generally called **exudate** formation (as it is the small proteins that characterize it)

Focus on Exudate versus Transudate

Increased flow without increased permeability, such as occurs in an active muscle, moves more fluid to the tissues, but this fluid simply represents an increase in volume and not a change in the nature of the fluid. Such a fluid is called a transudate. It has relatively little protein, and has a specific gravity of 1.012 or less. The exudate that forms with increased permeability is rich in proteins and cells, and has a specific gravity of 1.020 or greater.

and depends on both the increased blood flow through the capillary bed and the increased permeability of the vasculature as just described.

The Formation of Exudate: Vascular Factors

Hyperemia and Stasis

In response to injury, blood flow changes at the scene occur almost immediately. After an initial fleeting constriction, arterioles and precapillary sphincters supplying the damaged tissue dilate. This change has the effect of reducing vascular resistance, and blood flow to the area increases greatly. The increased blood flow is called **hyperemia.** Shortly after hyperemia develops, capillaries and venules dilate as well. This response is largely a passive yielding to the increased blood pressure caused by the large volume of blood entering these vessels from their dilated supply arterioles (fig. 2.4).

Inflammation brings about an alteration in the pattern of movement of fluid from the vascular compartment to the tissue space and a change in the nature of that fluid. Two factors come into play: The first is indistinguishable from the hyperemia in a vascular bed that normally follows a natural period of hypoperfusion or a period of intense activity. Chemicals cause the precapillary sphincters to relax, leading to increased flow and increased blood hydrostatic pressure—more blood at greater pressure. This increases the forces driving fluid out of the vessel, particularly the capillary, as it is the usual site of fluid and dissolved nutrient, metabolite, and gas exchange. This fluid, called **transudate,** is the same in composition as the fluid that was passing out at a much slower rate before arteriolar dilation (see fig. 2.3*b*) This is one source of the swelling noted in inflammation. The second factor, which is unique to inflammation, involves changes in the permeability of the endothelium, particularly of the postcapillary venules. Following injury, chemicals cause the endothelial cells to contract slightly so that junctions loosen. Fluid, called exudate, containing an assortment of small plasma proteins that are usually confined to the vessel, passes at a much

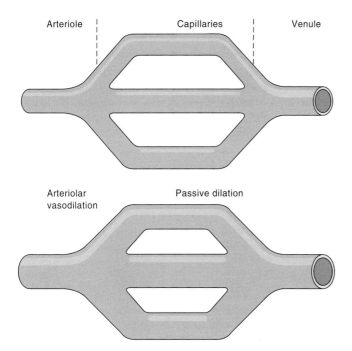

Arteriole | Capillaries | Venule

Arteriolar vasodilation | Passive dilation

Figure 2.4 **Passive Dilation.** In inflammation, arteriolar dilation allows increased blood flow, which causes passive dilation of the capillaries and venules.

greater rate than normal into the tissue spaces (fig. 2.5). This increases tissue volume and contributes to swelling in two ways: It increases the osmotic pressure within the tissue space, which retains water. It also subtracts from the osmotic pressure within the vessels, thereby impeding fluid return from the tissue compartment into the vascular compartment (see fig. 2.3c). The net effect of these altered fluid movements is that the blood volume drops and what remains becomes more viscous. RBCs respond by aggregating, increasing viscosity even more. Stasis (temporary cessation of blood flow) may be observed. Stasis can exaggerate the blood hydrostatic pressure by temporally blocking the venules. Figure 2.6 gives an overview of these processes. These hemodynamic forces affect not only the flow of blood in the postcapillary venule, but alter the usual laminar flow of blood cells in the center of the column of blood. Large cells tend to move out of the mass of RBCs and travel close to the endothelial wall. This makes them available for attachment and movement out of the vessel into the tissue spaces, which will be described later.

What has just been described occurs when the tissue injury is mild, such as might occur in a mosquito bite. Mild to moderate injury elicits a two-phase permeability change: first, a rapid and brief (peaks at 5–10 minutes, over by 30 minutes) increase in permeability of venules, then a second increase that develops more slowly (hours) and is sustained longer (several hours up to days). If the injury that triggers the inflammation is more intense, as might occur in burns or infection with a bacterium that is directly toxic to vessels, like beta-hemolytic strep A, the endothelia of all the microcirculation may be injured. This will lead to an

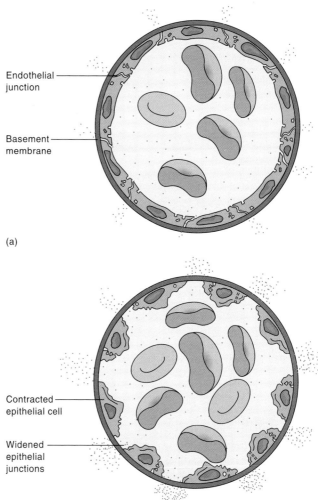

Endothelial junction

Basement membrane

(a)

Contracted epithelial cell

Widened epithelial junctions

(b)

Figure 2.5 **Permeability Changes in the Postcapillary Venule in Acute Inflammation.** Compare the normal movement of fluid through the vessel in (*a*) with the flow typical of acute inflammation in (*b*), where the widened endothelial junctions allow more fluid to escape to the tissue spaces.

immediate and prolonged (lasting one to several days) process of exudate formation. In this case, the exudate may contain RBCs as well as leukocytes.

Inflammatory exudate may contribute to the pain of inflammation by increasing the pressure and tension applied to nerve endings in the inflamed tissue (as well as introducing chemicals that trigger pain receptors). The throbbing nature of some inflammatory pain results from arterial pressure pulses that are transmitted to the swollen tissues, alternately increasing and decreasing the pain-causing pressure.

Having considered the formation of a fluid exudate in acute inflammation, you may well ask, What good comes from the accumulation of fluid and plasma proteins at an injury site? We can identify four benefits. One is dilution of toxins. The accumulating fluid dilutes any harmful substances at the scene, reducing the further damage they might do. A second benefit is the increased pain caused by the swelling. The pain forces limits on use of the affected part and, thus, may prevent additional injury. The third

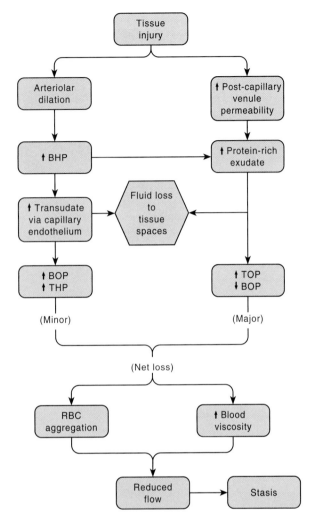

Figure 2.6 **Blood Flow in the Microcirculation Following Injury and the Commencement of an Inflammatory Response.** Loss of both transudate and exudate from the vessels can greatly reduce the rate of flow, even to the point of complete stoppage, or "stasis."

benefit is the presence, at the injury site, of antibodies that would be retained in the blood without a change in vascular permeability. In the tissue spaces they can act against disease-causing microorganisms. A fourth beneficial effect of the fluid exudate is its content of proteins, which contribute to amplifying the response, killing organisms, and fostering the phagocytosis of microorganisms, cellular debris, and various other particles associated with tissue damage. The mechanics of phagocytosis are described in some detail in a later section, Phagocytosis.

Descriptive Classification

Acute inflammations can be classified on the basis of differences in the nature of their fluid exudates. These differences are linked to the severity of injury. This means that a single descriptive term provides information about both the intensity of injury and the nature of the tissue's response.

Serous inflammation is the response to a mild injury in which only fluid is allowed to escape to the interstices (another term for intercellular spaces). In such cases, the endothelial cells contract only slightly, so that more fluid escapes but protein is retained. The watery fluid seen in the blistering of mildly burned skin is an example of a serous inflammation. At inflamed mucous membrane surfaces; for example, in mild upper respiratory infections, fluid exudate also contains mucus.

Increased levels of tissue damage cause increased permeability, allowing protein molecules, notably fibrinogen, to leave the blood. In the tissues, the fibrinogen is converted to strands of fibrin, which cause the fluid to coagulate. The affected tissue will have masses of gelled exudate covering its surface. Such a fibrinous exudate may be seen in various forms of pericarditis or in the pleurae in pneumonia.

More severe injury, causing greater necrosis or involving a more potent toxin or irritant, causes a **purulent** or **suppurative inflammation.** Here, the exudate contains large numbers of leukocytes called neutrophils, which accumulate at the scene of damage. These cells, both living and dead, along with the necrotic debris and fluid exudate, form the thick, white or greenish fluid called **pus** that is common to many acute inflammations. Diffuse suppurative inflammation is called **cellulitis.** An **abscess,** on the other hand, is a localized accumulation of pus that develops at a focus when an agent of injury cannot be neutralized quickly. When the inflammatory response finally removes the threat, a fluid-filled sac called a **cyst** may remain. Ultimately, the cyst may diminish as the fluid is resorbed or replaced by connective tissue. In extreme cases, a subsurface abscess can enlarge and spread. As tissue becomes necrotic, many cell constituents are released into the abscess. This change increases the osmotic attraction for water from surrounding tissues into the pus-filled area. The result is physical pressure that tends to expand the abscess along lines of least resistance into the surrounding tissues.

Where injury is of great intensity, capillary damage allows the escape of blood to the tissue. This **hemorrhagic inflammation** is characterized by the presence of large numbers of erythrocytes (red blood cells) in the interstices. Thus, there is an increase in the amount of debris that must ultimately be removed to allow healing to restore the tissue.

The descriptions we have just given indicate general characteristics. Because injury will vary in the nature and intensity of damage it may cause, more than one of the various types of acute inflammation will often be represented in any particular case.

The Formation of Exudate: Cellular Factors

The outpouring of large numbers of white blood cells from the blood is called **leukocyte emigration.** Normally, about half of the leukocytes in the blood move with the flowing plasma. Others move more slowly, rolling along the surface of the endothelium that lines the lumen of the vessels. Occasionally these rolling cells will pass from the blood to the

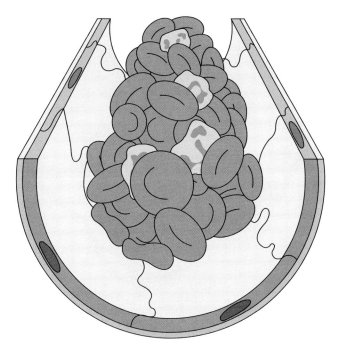

Figure 2.7   **Axial Flow of Blood.** The formed elements cluster around the long axis of the vessel to form a central column that is surrounded by the plasma. This is the pattern of small vessel blood flow in normal, noninflamed tissues.

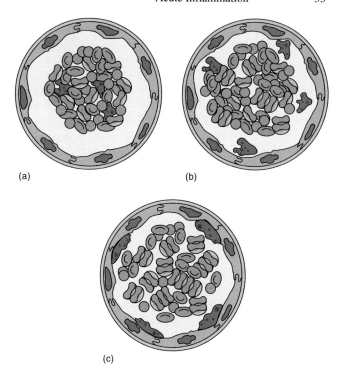

(c)

Figure 2.8   **Margination and Pavementing of Leukocytes as Blood Passes through the Capillaries to the Venule.**
(*a*) Slowing blood flow allows margination as leukocytes move to the margins of the central column. (*b*) Margination is well advanced, allowing contact with endothelium. (*c*) The transition to the reaction in the postcapillary venule during inflammation: first rolling and then adhesion preparatory to leukocyte emigration.

tissue spaces, where most survive for only a day or so. The majority of the circulating leukocytes are neutrophils, and it is the neutrophils that have this short tissue life span. Monocytes, by contrast, may live in the tissue for years. Leukocytes lost from the blood in this way are replaced from bone marrow and lymphoid tissue. During an inflammatory response, the emigration of leukocytes is greatly increased, an effect due in part to changes in the normal pattern of blood flow.

Margination

Blood flowing at normal rates demonstrates the phenomenon of **axial flow.** This means that the moving blood distributes itself in the vessel so that its formed elements (erythrocytes, leukocytes, platelets) move in a central column parallel to the long axis of the vessel. The largest of the formed elements, the leukocytes, are nearest to the center, with the smaller red cells and platelets forming the outer layers. Plasma surrounds this column of formed elements and flows smoothly along the endothelial lining of the vessel (fig. 2.7).

As fluid is lost and flow rate decreases in an inflamed tissue, the central column of formed elements enlarges so that its borders move nearer to the endothelium. In addition, the loss of plasma fluid to the tissues causes erythrocytes to aggregate. These clumps of cells now constitute the largest units in the column of formed elements and, as such, they assume a more central location within it. In consequence, the leukocytes are forced to assume peripheral po-

sitions at the margins of the column, near the vascular endothelium (fig. 2.8*a,b*). The phenomenon is called **margination.**

Rolling, Pavementing, and Adhesion

As a result of margination, leukocytes are much more likely to contact endothelium. For a brief distance, they tumble over the endothelium ("rolling"). In the vasculature of injured tissue, they are able to adhere to the endothelial surface and resist being moved by the flowing plasma. As they adhere along the surface, they flatten to suggest the appearance of paving stones; hence, this phenomenon is called **pavementing** of leukocytes (fig. 2.8*c*).

The importance of leukocyte pavementing is that it provides for the transition of leukocytes from a state of motion to a state of attachment to the venule endothelium at an injury site. This is the essential step that precedes leukocytes leaving the blood for the tissue spaces (fig. 2.9).

Transmigration

The transmigration or emigration of leukocytes from the blood to the tissue spaces occurs in stages. After initially adhering to the endothelial surface, they start to slide along the surface in an amoebalike fashion. This movement continues

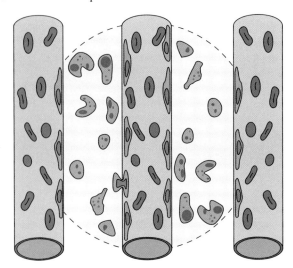

Figure 2.9 **Pavementing of Leukocytes at an Injury Site (Circled Area).** Only in the injured area are endothelial leukocyte receptors exposed to allow adherence to the surface of the postcapillary venules. No cells can stick to the endothelial surfaces outside the injured area. (Note: This is entirely diagrammatic.)

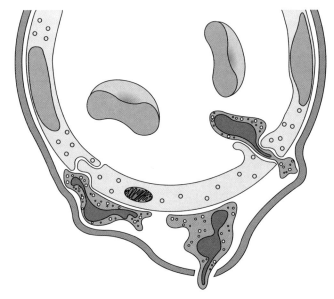

Figure 2.10 **Leukocyte Transmigration.** One polymorphonuclear cell (neutrophil) is shown emigrating via an endothelial gap. A second cell, at lower left, pauses after leaving the lumen. At lower right, a third cell passes through the basement membrane to reach the tissue spaces.

until an endothelial junction is reached. There, the leukocyte forms a slender extension of its cytoplasm, which it insinuates into the gap between the cells. Probably by physical pressure, but perhaps by enzymatic or other chemical means, the gap is widened just enough for the leukocyte to squeeze past the endothelium. After a pause, the cell continues by traversing the basement membrane and the rest of the wall, finally reaching the tissue space (fig. 2.10). The process takes about ten minutes. Other leukocytes will often follow at the point where a given junction has been "eased" by the passage of the first leukocyte. During the inflammatory response, emigration occurs at the endothelial gaps of postcapillary venules. Emigration is not seen in capillaries or in the arterial system.

While hemodynamic forces set the stage for rolling, pavementing, adhesion, and transmigration, molecular changes take over to achieve close association of the leukocytes and the endothelial walls. A variety of adhesion molecules on the leukocyte's surface bind to corresponding molecules on the endothelial surface causing it to roll over the endothelium, adhere, and finally move through a cell junction. This is a subtle dance, with signals generated at the site of injury ensuring the display of appropriate endothelial anchoring molecules in the appropriate locations along the venule wall. As leukocytes pass through the capillaries and into the venules of the injured site, they are gently bound which slows their rolling. This exposes them to signals that activate the leukocytes, causing them to increase the avidity of their binding molecules, leading to adhesion and pavementing. Some of these molecules are preformed and take only minutes to redistribute to the cell's surface. Others are "induced" and require one to two hours to be displayed. The details are outside our scope, but a few names are

selectins, intercellular adhesion molecule **ICAM-1,** and vascular cell adhesion molecules **VCAM-1,** all on the endothelium. Leukocytes bear receptors, a few being sialyl-Lewis X and integrins. Individuals with mutations in the genes producing one of these adhesion or receptor molecules suffer recurrent bacterial infections.

Sometimes the active process of emigration is called **diapedesis,** but the use of this term should be limited to describing the passive movement of red cells that may occur at the same site. In such cases, blood hydrostatic pressure forces red blood cells into the tissue spaces, particularly where there has been extensive endothelial damage. These cells then die, releasing hemoglobin, which is converted to hemosiderin. Macrophages stained with hemosiderin at the site of inflammation bear witness to red blood cell extravasation (i.e., movement out of the vessel into tissue interstices).

Two types of leukocytes are dominant in the acute inflammatory response. The earliest cells arriving at the scene of injury are the neutrophils. On reaching the tissue spaces, they are often described as **polymorphonuclear cells** (PMNs) because of their multilobed nuclei. (Strictly, the term PMN also includes leukocytes called eosinophils and basophils.) A later phase of emigration delivers larger numbers of leukocytes to the tissue spaces. These cells, lacking segmentation in their nuclei, are called **mononuclear** cells or monocytes. In the tissue spaces, they are called **macrophages,** because of their large size and phagocytic capability.

Over the period of an acute inflammatory response (6–24 hours), PMNs are initially the most numerous leukocytes on the scene. Their numbers then decline and macrophage numbers increase until, later in the response, the mononuclear cell dominates in the area of injury. There are four principal reasons for this observed pattern. One is the much greater number of neutrophils in circulation, as compared with monocytes; there are more of them available to emigrate. Second, outside the bloodstream the polymorphonuclear leukocytes survive for only a short time, often only a matter of hours (up to 48), and then undergo apoptosis. This pattern may be related to the lower pH and higher temperature of damaged tissue. In contrast, the macrophage can survive for much longer periods and, hence, will outlive polymorphonuclear leukocytes at the scene. A third factor is the difference in agents that attract macrophages into the tissue (chemotactic agents) and further agents that keep them resident at the site. Chemotactic agents that attract both neutrophils and monocytes predominate early, while those selective to monocytes persist. Fourth, there is evidence that macrophages can replicate within the tissue. This may be an unusual event, but it has been documented. Experimental evidence indicates that peak polymorphonuclear leukocyte levels are reached at about 12–24 hours after injury. These levels decline 24–48 hours postinjury as mononuclear cell numbers simultaneously increase to reach a maximum after about two to three days. In viral and rickettsial infections and in acute dermatitis, lymphocytes are the predominant cell type in the site of inflammation. With allergy and some parasitic infections, eosinophils are the major cell throughout the response. Typhoid fever generates mainly a macrophage infiltration.

Phagocytosis

As we have seen, one aspect of exudate formation is the delivery of great numbers of phagocytes to the site of inflammation. In the tissue spaces, particles such as dysfunctional cells, infectious agents (fungi or bacteria), immune complexes, or the debris that results from tissue damage are phagocytized. Removal of the injurious agent is an obvious advantage. Less obviously, the phagocytosis of debris is beneficial in removing material that might be subject to bacterial action, causing putrefaction.

Effective phagocytic activity involves several steps. Once in the tissue, a phagocyte must become activated and move to the immediate vicinity of its target; then it must recognize and attach to it. Finally, it must engulf and destroy the target by releasing enzymes and other toxic substances that it has produced and stored in its lysosomes. These are required to kill the pathogen and/or break down the target molecules. The following discussion describes the events of phagocytosis in more detail.

Chemotaxis

When a phagocyte enters an inflamed tissue and encounters an increased concentration of some chemical attractant, a **chemotactic agent,** it exhibits **chemotaxis.** This is a directed migration of the leukocyte toward regions of increas-

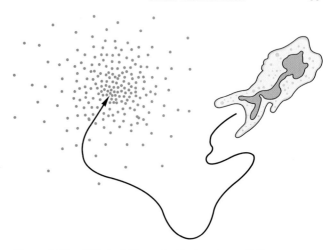

Figure 2.11 **Effect of Chemotactic Agents on Cell Movement.** The initial random movements of a phagocytic cell are altered when it encounters chemotactic agents. Its movement becomes focused, moving up the concentration gradient to the source of the agent.

ingly high concentrations of the agent (see fig. 2.11). Exogenous chemoattractants include certain bacterial products, both peptides and lipids. Endogenous chemicals include components of the complement system particularly C5a, leukotriene B4, and interleukin 8 (these will be described shortly). The process of chemotaxis is based on the presence of specific receptors for the chemotactic agent on the surface of the leukocyte. The binding of the agent to the receptors triggers a complex chain of biochemical events whose net effects change the cell into a larger, more active phagocyte with high levels of destructive agents stored in its intracellular granules. In this state the cell is said to be activated. Binding also mobilizes and directs the phagocyte's movement. This is achieved through the rapid assembly of actin molecules (remember the actin and myosin of muscle contraction) into linear polymers at the leading edge of the advancing pseudopod. Leukocytes tend to "hone in on" one attractant at a time, flexibly utilizing signals generated by the invading organism or the body's own cells. Confusing competition between signal sources is avoided by exogenous chemotactic agents taking precedence.

Recognition and Attachment

Although phagocytosis of "naked" particles may occur (e.g., latex beads are engulfed by neutrophils in a test tube), it tends to be a slow and inefficient process. **Opsonization** greatly enhances phagocytosis. Opsonins are substances from the plasma that have particular affinity for the surface features of foreign particles. Leukocytes are able to respond to opsonins because they display opsonin binding sites. Once an opsonin-coated particle is bound to the surface receptors of the phagocyte, the particle is readily engulfed. Examples of opsonins include pathogen-specific antibodies, C-reactive protein, a complement fragment called C3b, and plasma proteins called "collectins" that bind to microbial

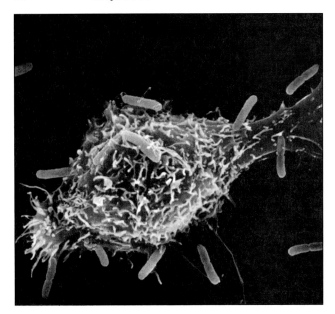

Figure 2.12   **Macrophage in Action.** Scanning electron micrograph of a macrophage engulfing several bacteria (in this case E. coli).

cell walls. Other opsonizing proteins will be mentioned later in the focus box Acute Phase Proteins (p. 43).

Engulfment and Destruction

Binding of a particle to the phagocyte membrane elicits the next step, engulfment (fig. 2.12). In this step, the phagocyte membrane flows around the particle to enclose it in a cytoplasmic phagosome. Granular-appearing lysosomes that contain destructive agents then merge with the phagosome membrane, thereby bringing their contents into contact with the particle. As lysosomes merge with the phagosomes, their numbers within the phagocyte are reduced and the phagocyte is said to have *degranulated.*

If a particle is too large to be easily engulfed, for example, a multicellular parasite or a long asbestos fiber, there may be regurgitation of the granule contents into the tissue spaces. The same thing may happen when immune complexes are deposited on an exposed basement membrane, as occurs in certain immune-mediated diseases of the kidney and lung. The leukocyte attempting to engulf this flat surface experiences "frustrated phagocytosis" and releases toxic and degradative substances that damage the basement membrane and the surrounding cells and matrix. Persistent infection with resistant microorganisms—for example, the tuberculin bacillus, which frustrates eradication by dwelling intra-cellularly—can result in extensive tissue damage as is seen in tuberculosis-related damage to the lung or bone. The agent in this case, is the host inflammatory response.

The killing of microorganisms, the destruction or inactivation of toxic agents, and the degradation of macromolecules are the specialized tasks of phagocytes. Although some of the specifics differ, many basic mechanisms are shared between neutrophils and macrophages, and this discussion will not differentiate between them. Killing is accomplished by two broad classes of mechanisms: oxygen-independent and oxygen-dependent. **Oxygen-independent** mechanisms involve the release of preformed substances that damage bacterial cell walls, disrupt bacterial replication, and produce a low pH, which may be directly toxic and may indirectly aid the function of other enzymes. Bacterial cell walls are attacked by bactericidal permeability-increasing protein (**BPI**), **lysozyme** (the same bacterial coat-digesting enzyme as found in tears and nasal secretions), and **major basic protein,** which is more toxic to parasites. Bacterial replication is impaired by the release of **lactoferrin,** which reduces the free iron necessary for mitosis in many bacteria. "**Defensins**" are toxic to many bacteria. As well as killing, phagocyte enzymes can digest bacteria and tissue debris, an action that promotes healing. Elastase, a proteolytic enzyme that breaks down elastin, and collagenase, an enzyme that degrades collagen, are examples of lysosomal enzymes active in removing intercellular debris. (In sterile inflammation such as occurs in a burn, the removal of damaged tissue is the principal role of phagocytes.) **Oxygen-dependent** killing, which is more important than the oxygen-independent agents just described, is accomplished by the creation and release of oxygen free radicals: hydrogen peroxide, superoxide, hydroxyl radicals, and so-called "singlet-oxygen." The action of these toxic radicals was described in chapter 1. Neutrophils also produce and contain an enzyme that facilitates the combination of hydrogen peroxide with any of the halides that are available (Cl^-, I^-, Br^-) to produce, for example, HOCl (hypochlorous acid—the substance used to disinfect swimming pools). This "halogenation" is the most potent bactericidal agent produced by neutrophils. By being contained within lysosomes, its destructive potential is focused on the engulfed organism. The enzyme is myeloperoxide (MPO), which imparts the greenish color to pus and neutrophil-rich mucus.

In the case of regurgitation or frustrated phagocytosis, the destructive capacity of oxygen free radicals can be turned on the host tissues (so-called "bystander injury"). When these effects are combined with those of oxygen-independent processes, the enzymes, toxins, and inflammatory mediators, the potential for damage is clear (fig. 2.13).

Bacterial Defenses

Bacteria have evolved a variety of defenses against phagocytosis. Some bacteria produce exotoxins that kill leukocytes or inhibit chemotaxis. Some produce a slimy coat to which opsonins have difficulty binding. Some forestall phagocyte binding by shedding substances that bind opsonins so that they cannot attach to the bacterium. And some have tough capsules or can produce cytotoxins to protect them against destruction if they are engulfed.

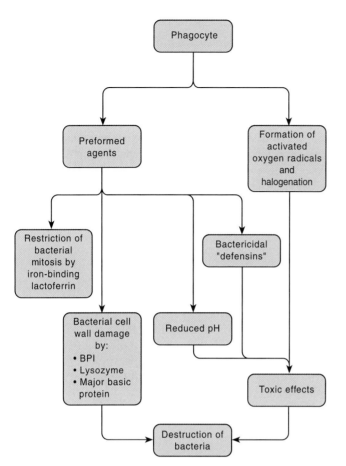

Figure 2.13   **Mechanisms Underlying the Destruction of Bacteria by Phagocytes at an Injury Site.** Note: Oxygen-free radicals and halogenation are by far the most potent agents.

Defects in Leukocyte Function

Effective phagocyte function depends on a chain of events that begins with margination and pavementing and culminates in removal of the injurious agent, healing, and return to the preinjury state. Defects at any point in the chain will impair host defenses. A number of conditions can produce such defects.

Certain leukocyte defects are associated with chronic or recurrent infections, often involving bacteria with low infection potential. An example is **chronic granulomatous disease of childhood,** a rare genetic defect in phagocyte killing that is due to impaired production of oxygen free radicals. Affected children develop persistent and widespread suppurating infections and often die at an early age. In another rare autosomal recessive genetic disease, **Chédiak-Higashi syndrome,** there are defects in both phagocyte motility and degranulation, often leading to early death. In a more common example, diabetics suffer defects in phagocytosis that are derived from circulatory problems secondary to changes in their blood vessels. These problems prevent inflammatory cells from being effectively delivered to the site of inflammation. Active motility in neutrophils may also be impaired. Leukemias may prevent mobilization of leukocytes from the bone marrow, and other diseases may affect opsonization or formation of chemotactic factors. In some diseases (e.g., arteriosclerosis, malnutrition), the formation of an adequate exudate is compromised. Finally, many drugs (e.g., steroids, morphine, tetracycline, chloramphenicol) also interfere with phagocyte function.

Focus on Reperfusion Injury

There are some endogenous sources of free radicals. The electron transport chain that is linked to ATP synthesis in mitochondria constantly leaks electrons that generate toxic free radicals. Some enzymes are directly oxidative, for example, xanthine oxidase, which is formed in hypoxic conditions. It is apparently one of the agents responsible for the damage that occurs in an ischemic tissue when its blood supply is restored. In such **reperfusion injury,** the tissue survives the initial anoxia but is damaged by the production of radicals, when oxygen becomes available again. Use of the antioxidants allopurinol and bucillamine have been effective experimentally in treating reperfusion injury. However, the injury that may be triggered by ischemia and/or referusion is much broader than the production of oxidants. Programmed cell death by apoptosis is a factor, as are leukocyte accumulation, macrophage activation, and the selective/upregulation of COX-2 enzyme (discussed later). Protection of organs in transplant or ischemic heart or brain tissue in IHD and stroke, require a comprehensive approach.

✓ *Checkpoint 2.2*

The vascular component of the inflammatory response involves dilation of the precapillary sphincters and hyperemia combined with increased permeability, normally at the postcapillary venules. Together, these convey masses of protein-rich exudate to the site of injury. Changes in hemodynamics and the display of adhesion molecules on the venule endothelium and corresponding receptors on the leukocytes arrest the passage of leukocytes through the tissue and ensure their transmigration into the tissue spaces. Chemotactic agents produced by both the foreign pathogen and the body's own defenses guide leukocytes to pathogens that have already been labeled with a variety of opsonins that facilitate phagocytosis. Ingestion into a phagosome elicits a variety of oxygen-independent and -dependent mechanisms that limit pathogen replication, destroy bacterial walls and membranes, and usually achieve killing and removal. Defects in any of these stages result in impaired capacity to deal with infections.

Table 2.1	Factors that Can Act as Initiators in the Chemical Mediation of the Inflammatory Response

Substances released from injured cells
Direct stimulus to mast cells (trauma, heat, cold)
Microbial products
Exposure of basement membrane or connective
    tissue components
Complement activation
Deposition of antigen/antibody complexes
Disruption of vascular integrity
Products of the breakdown of thrombi

Chemical Mediation of Inflammation

To this point in our consideration of acute inflammation, we have been content to examine the particulars of its vascular and cellular components. We can now address the question: What causes these events to occur? More specifically, what triggers the dilation and permeability changes that occur, what activates phagocytic cells and, further, how are these responses linked to the injury that induces them? The answer, in essence, is the process of chemical mediation. That is, injury initially causes certain chemical substances to be produced or released at the site of injury, and these substances then bring about, directly or indirectly, the assortment of specific changes we group under the term *acute inflammation.*

A variety of different triggering events, often called **initiators,** produce essentially the same vascular and cellular responses; for this reason, acute inflammation is said to be **nonspecific.** Traumatic injury, substances released from infective agents, immune complex deposition, and other factors (table 2.1) all induce essentially the same response. What they hold in common is that they all signal a risk of cellular injury.

Initiators achieve their results indirectly, through a larger number (and the list is growing) of **chemical mediators** that work directly to elicit the vascular and cellular events that make up the inflammatory response. A given initiator often activates several mediators, whose effects may overlap and intertwine, but ultimately achieve a response that focuses inflammation on the injurious or potentially injurious agents. Many of the component mediators of the inflammatory response are presented in physiology texts as classic examples to illustrate healthy "positive feedback" regulatory processes (feedback systems are discussed briefly in chapter 3). In positive feedback, a small deviation in some factor is rapidly amplified into a large deviation. For example, in blood coagulation, the formation of the first tiny thrombus in the wall of a torn vessel sets into motion a rapid escalation of clotting that quickly seals the opening. To work this efficiently, positive feedback has

certain requirements, all of which apply to the collective response called *inflammation.* The ingredients for the response are largely made in advance and held in an inactive form, waiting to be deployed. There is redundancy of signaling, so that a variety of stimuli can elicit a common reaction. One dramatic positive feedback avalanche tends to trigger a contradictory avalanche that carries the system in the opposite direction, thereby limiting and quenching the initial response. The signals that mediate the positive feedback system tend to be very short-lived. And, finally, the reactions tend to take place in a "favored environment" that permits and supports the response, surrounded by a generally hostile or inhibiting environment. If this limiting of the response breaks down, it threatens the entire system. A painful bump in response to a bee sting is appropriate inflammation. But if an inflammatory response gets established in too much of the body, as might happen in a systemic allergic reaction to that same bee sting, the result is anaphylactic shock: Life is at risk. Likewise, if the inflammatory response is steadily triggered at a low level, as happens in tuberculosis, severe damage to the system can occur. So, with this perspective, let's look at the chemical mediators of inflammation. Although many and complex, mediator systems can be classed as cell derived or plasma derived.

Cell-Derived Mediators

While many of the mediators we present in this section are produced by a variety of cells, we will only mention what are thought to be the most important sources. We will also only report on the predominant effect of a mediator and only for mediators that have a significant role in inflammation. Even with these provisos, this is an impressive list (fig. 2.14).

Histamine, which is familiar to allergy sufferers who take *anti*histamines, rapidly but briefly increases vascular permeability by inducing venule endothelial cell contraction. This, of course, allows exudate to form. Histamine is released from **mast cells** and also from **platelets.** Mast cells are leukocytes with very specialized location and function. They are, you may recall, richly distributed in the loose CT that supports epithelial membranes: the skin, GI tract mucosa, and respiratory tree. Here, they are in an excellent position to encounter pathogens that have breached the body's barrier defenses. They are also first in line for exposure to traumatic injury and excesses in temperature. So what might trigger their **degranulation** (their release of mediators from preformed granules)? Cold, heat, trauma, and encounters with foreign antigen (features of an introduced substance or pathogen that bind to antibodies adhering to the outer membrane of the mast cell, antibodies that the body's immune system produced after a previous exposure) all trigger degranulation. In this role, they probably play an important part in dealing with parasites and worms in the skin and GI tract mucosa. The downside is in their being triggered by allergens and producing the immediate symp-

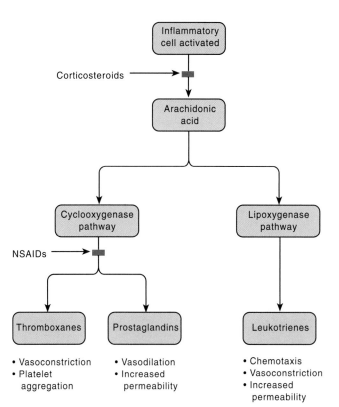

Figure 2.14   **Membrane-Derived Mediators.** The formation of arachidonic acid and some of the inflammatory roles of its principal derivatives. Also indicated are the sites of blocking action by corticosteroids and nonsteroidal anti-inflammatory drugs (NSAIDs).

toms associated with allergies: swelling and mucous secretion. Histamine binds to H_1 receptors on vascular endothelia. Therefore, to be effective, an antihistamine, which binds to and blocks the same receptors, has to be taken before exposure to allergen.

Serotonin is released, along with histamine, from platelets when they aggregate after encountering collagen in the basement membrane or extravascular space, ADP, thrombin (one of the triggers of clotting), or antibody-antigen complexes (which would be produced in an immune response to an infection). Serotonin has the same effect as histamine.

Eicosanoids are products of the metabolic transformation of the membrane phospholipid-derivative **arachidonic acid** (AA). This large eicosanoid family of mediators, some of which are involved directly in inflammation, plays a wide set of roles, some of which superficially seem contradictory. Biosynthesis of many of these compounds is initiated by injury, so their production is slower that of histamine and serotonin. All leukocytes and, especially, **mast cells,** produce these eicosanoids. Metabolism of AA passes through either of two enzyme-mediated pathways—the **lipoxygenase** route producing leukotrienes (looko-try-eens) and the **cyclooxygenase** route producing prostaglandins and thromboxanes. **Leukotrienes** take up the role of increasing vascular permeability that was left off

by fast-acting histamine and serotonin. But some also produce vasoconstriction (you were warned!) and bronchospasm. They also trigger leukocyte adhesion and chemotaxis. **Prostaglandins,** in general, contribute to inflammation in two ways: specifically, by producing vasodilation and, generally, by potentiating (enhancing) the effect of other mediators. An example of the latter is the role of **prostaglandin E_2** (PGE_2). Its presence makes the permeability-increasing effects of leukotrienes or serotonin much more intense. In chapter 3, we will see that both fever and pain are mediated indirectly by PGE_2. Therefore, controlling PGE_2 production is a way of controlling inflammation, fever, and pain. Figure 2.15 illustrates two ways that chemicals can interrupt the production of eicosanoids. **Corticosteroids,** like cortisone or prednisone, shut off the supply of AA by blocking the action of phospholipase A_2, the enzyme that releases AA from membrane phospholipid. Blocking phospholipase A_2 interrupts the production of all the eicosanoids, a very broad effect. Corticosteroids can usually be counted on to shut down an inflammation in the event that it is out of control, as it might be in asthma, or doing focused damage, as it might in a severe case of bursitis. On the other hand, **nonselective cyclooxygenase (COX) inhibitors** inactivate only the pathway that leads to the production of prostaglandins and thromboxanes. **Acetylsalicylic acid** (ASA), **acetaminophen,** and **NSAIDs** are all nonselective COX inhibitors (fig. 2.15). If prostaglandins were only involved in inflammation, fever, and pain, then blocking COX might be an entirely desirable thing. However, these products participate in a variety of other roles, two being the production of a hydroxyl-rich mucus covering for the GI tract and the responsive perfusion of the kidneys. So, all nonselective COX inhibitors interfere to varying degrees with GI tract lining protection and maintenance and kidney perfusion.

Nitric oxide (NO) is recognized as an important signal in the nervous system, the vasculature, and in the inflammatory response. In the vasculature, NO is a potent vasodilator. In the nervous system, it plays both a neurotransmitter-like role and participates in the targeted management of local perfusion, in much the same way it does in the rest of the body. In the inflammatory response, its main source is activated macrophages and it performs many functions. As a vasodilator it is important, in fact, in modulating the intensity of the inflammatory response by generating the familiar vasodilation we expect, making it harder for leukocytes to roll and attach. In like fashion, it interferes with platelet aggregation (reducing the release of both histamine and serotonin). When secreted by macrophages during inflammation, NO has a generally favorable antibacterial effect. However, when multitudes of macrophages are activated in response to circulating toxins, the release of NO can produce such vasodilation that the affected person can go into shock **(toxic shock syndrome).**

Platelet-activating factor (PAF), which is released by basophils and mast cells, macrophages, neutrophils, platelets, and endothelial cells, causes platelets to aggregate and degranulate, as its name implies, but is also modulates

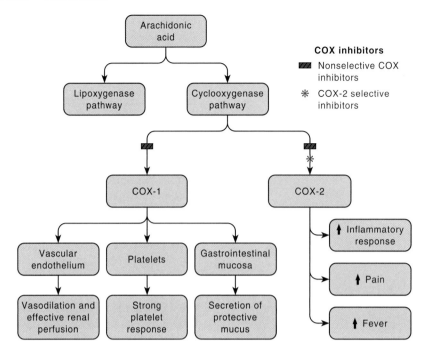

Figure 2.15   Mechanisms of COX Inhibitors. Sites of action of nonselective COX inhibitors and COX-2 selective inhibitors. "Inhibition" means the normal downstream effect is blocked.

Focus on the Targeted Use of COX-2 Inhibitors

Cyclooxygenase comes in two isoforms. These isoforms are distributed differentially in tissues. COX-1 is found in the gastric muscosa, where it is responsible for healthy maintenance including the secretion of protective mucus, in the kidneys where it regulates perfusion, and in platelets where it is involved in platelet aggregation, a key event in coagulation. COX-2 is richly available at sites of inflammation where it mediates, among other things, prostaglandin production. Aspirin, acetaminophen, and NSAIDs are nonselective blockers of COX activity. Hence, they tend to damage the gastric mucosa—in the case of acetaminophen, toxicity to the kidneys at doses over 4 g per day, and, in the case of aspirin, to irreversibly impair platelet function (the mechanism that allows aspirin to be used effectively to reduce the formation of platelet aggregates to impede atherosclerosis but predisposes the susceptible person to bleeding). COX-2 selective inhibitors leave COX-1 uninhibited and, therefore, don't have these specific downsides. Despite their immediate popularity, these COX-2 inhibitors do not have greater anti-inflammatory effects than do NSAIDs, and may not be entirely safe for the renal and cardiovascular systems. They are probably best used for control of inflammation in patients who have a high risk of gastric bleeding.

vascular tone and facilitates a variety of other inflammatory processes.

Macrophages, in interaction with other cells involved in defense, release **interleukin 1** (IL-1) and **tumor necrosis factor** (TNF). These produce the acute phase reactions detailed in the section Focus on Acute Phase Proteins in chapter 3. **Chemokines** are produced by all the leukocytes and have, among other functions, an activating and chemotactic function.

Plasma-Derived Mediators

Most plasma-derived mediators of inflammation are formed at the end of a sequence of activation steps called a **cascade,** an excellent example of a positive feedback system in oper-

ation. In essence, a number of inactive proteins circulate in the plasma. Following an initial activation event, one of these proteins is activated. It is then able to activate a second protein, which in turn activates a third, and so on. There are four interrelated cascades: the blood coagulation cascade, the kinin cascade, the fibrinolytic cascade, and the complement cascade (fig. 2.16). All four can be directly or indirectly triggered by the presence of the active form of a circulating protein known as **Hageman factor** (also called clotting factor XII).

The **coagulation** and **fibrinolytic** cascades function in inflammation and blood loss prevention, and the **complement** cascade is linked both to inflammation and to the immune system. In other words, only the **kinin** cascade seems to restrict its role to mediating inflammation. Split products

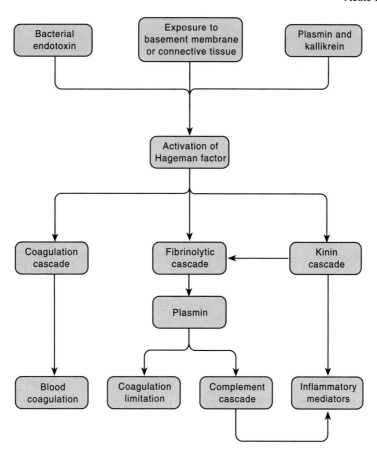

Figure 2.16   **Hageman Factor.** Four cascades with a role in coping with injury are related through their dependence on Hageman factor.

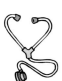

Focus on New NSAIDs—They Are Easier on the GI Tract, but . . .

A very serious side effect common to all NSAIDs is injury to the gastric and intestinal mucosa. A healthy adult will show bleeding of the gastric mucosa an hour after taking two ASA. The strategy of "enteric coating," which postpones breakdown of the capsule until it readies the duodenum, only postpones the site of inflammation or ulceration. As noted in this text, two independent cyclooxygenase enzymes operate: COX-1 produces prostaglandins involved in mucosal maintenance and other roles; COX-2 produces the prostaglandins involved in the inflammatory response. Agents are now widely prescribed (celecoxib and rofecoxib) that selectively block COX-2 blocking inflammation but leaving mucosal maintenance intact. These are an important alternative for people who cannot toler-

ate ASA, acetaminophen, or NSAIDs because of gastric or intestinal tract bleeding. NSAIDs with specific advantages in the management of pain or inflammation may be better tolerated if taken with misoprostol, a synthetic PGE_2. This diffuses into the mucosa and replaces endogenous PGE_2, which has been depleted by the nonselective COX inhibitor. A variety of other strategies are being explored. Adding lecithin (a waxy phospholipid) to aspirin appears to augment a phospholipid component of stomach mucosal mucus normally reduced by aspirin. Its presence repels water and thereby acid. Alternatively adding a nitric oxide producing chemical group to aspirin may facilitate local perfusion offsetting the usual effect of aspirin: reduced prostaglandins, reduced local perfusion, adherence and activation of white blood cells, release of ulcer producing chemicals. Look for safer NSAIDs in the near future.

from the breakdown of a clot by plasmin (fibrinolysis) are powerfully chemotactic. More detail on the coagulation and fibrinolytic cascades is presented in chapter 7.

The kinin cascade is significant in that one of its components, **bradykinin,** is a contributing factor to the pain of inflammation. (Incidentally, bee stings contain mostly

bradykinin.) Other factors, noted earlier, are the tension and pressure produced by the accumulation of inflammatory exudate at the damage site. Lowered pH and potassium released from damaged cells also play a role.

The **complement system** consists of 20 circulating proteins. Their sequential activation produces a complex of

Table 2.2   Important Mediators of the Inflammatory Response, the Cells That Produce Them, and Their Main Effect

Chemical Mediators	Produced by	Main Contribution to Inflammation
Cell-Derived Mediators		
Histamine	Mast cells, platelets	Increased permeability (rapid)
Serotonin	Platelets	Increased permeability (rapid)
Leukotrienes	Mast cells and all leukocytes	Increased permeability (sustained; some vasoconstriction and bronchospasm)
Prostaglandins	Mast cells and all other leukocytes	Vasodilation and potentiation of effects of other mediators PGE_2—above plus pain and fever
Nitric oxide (NO)	Activated macrophages, vascular endothelium	"Tempers" inflammatory response, bactericidal, can produce "toxic shock"
Platelet-activating factor (PAF)	Platelets, leukocytes, vascular endothelium	Platelet degranulation, leukocyte activation, and adhesion
IL-1 and TNF	Macrophages	Acute phase reactions
Chemokines	Leukocytes	Leukocyte activation and Chemotaxis
Plasma-Derived Mediators		
Fibrin-split products	Original source is the liver	Chemotaxis leukocyte activation
Bradykinin	Original source is the liver	Pain
Complement	Original source is the liver	Chemotaxis, opsonization

five proteins called the **membrane attack complex** (MAC), which can destroy invading microorganisms by punching holes in their membranes. Beyond this, various of the activated intermediate complement proteins (C3a and C5a, particularly, are called *anaphylatoxins* because of their important role in inflammation and, potentially, "anaphylaxis" or shock) act as mediators of inflammation, with specific roles in promoting dilation, permeability, chemotaxis, phagocytosis, and histamine release from mast cells, as well as enhancing the kinin cascade. Activation of the complement cascade may be triggered by microorganism surfaces and by antibody in conjunction with its defensive role of the immune system (see chapter 5).

The chemical mediators that produce acute inflammation tend to be formed or released in a rapid, dramatic fashion and thereby orchestrate an appropriately aggressive response to injury. In the same manner, the concentration of these mediators drops suddenly after a time, ending the acute inflammation. This drop results from a combination of the following: mediator release is exhausted or terminated, cascades are triggered that reverse the mediating cascades, anti-inflammatory, antioxidant, and antiproteolytic agents are delivered to the site of former injury. The result is a quenching of the acute inflammation that is analogous to the processes that limit coagulation of blood. It also sets the stage for the healing process.

Antibody is the plasma-derived mediator that is not formed by a cascade. This key element of the immune system may be the initiator that activates the complement cas-

 Checkpoint 2.3

Einstein said that we should strive to make things as simple as possible, but not *too* simple! Table 2.2 presents the essential list of inflammatory mediators, their main sources, and effects. This is as simple as possible.

cade. Its role in triggering the release of cell-derived mediators in allergy disorders is described in chapter 5.

Systemic Effects of Acute Inflammation

Most of us are only too familiar with some of the systemic effects of inflammation: fever, loss of appetite, increase in very deep sleep, perhaps a rapid weight loss, and residual weakness. We may have experienced the reaction of our lymphatic system to infection. Perhaps our axillary or neck lymph nodes were swollen and sore to the touch (the condition called **lymphadenitis**). If the inflammation was related to a localized bacterial infection, we may have noted reddened streaks moving slowly proximally as lymph vessels in an inflamed state (**lymphangitis**) attempted to cope with a spreading infection. The thin, loose-walled capillaries of the lymph system aid in draining off the exudate (edema fluid) formed in an inflammation, but can pass bacteria

Focus on Acute Phase Proteins

Another set of systemic effects of inflammation is the rapid increase in **acute phase proteins** (also called acute phase reactants), some to levels 500 to 1,000-fold higher than normal. Produced largely by the liver, these proteins prime the plasma for contributing to the inflammatory response. **C reactive protein** (CRP), **serum amyloid associated protein** (SAA), and **serum amyloid P** protein (SAP) bind directly to the surface of pathogens, particularly bacteria, to enhance phagocytosis **(opsonization)**. A further contribution to opsonization (and bactericidal action) is made by facilitating the binding of complement. The DNA that is exposed during the destruction of microorganisms or leukocytes is bound by these three agents, making it easier to clear with the other debris of inflammation. As is the case in other aspects of inflammation, the story is not without problems. In a chronic inflammation, the prolonged presence of SAA leads to the deposition, in certain individuals, of amyloid A fibrils. This **secondary amyloidosis** interferes with the function of the organ within which it is deposited. Constituent proteins of both the coagulation and complement cascades are increased to facilitate coagulation and the bactericidal, inflammatory mediator, opsonization, and chemotactic effects of activated complement.

---

into the blood, producing **bacteremia,** and thereby spread the infection.

Some systemic effects are less readily observable. **Leukocytosis** is a two- to threefold increase of circulating leukocytes (up to 30,000/mm³ in contrast to normal levels of about 7,000/mm³). This change is rapid and involves both the release of stored neutrophils, largely from the lung capillaries and bone marrow, and an increase in leukocyte production by red bone marrow. The latter is in response to "colony stimulating factors" released from activated macrophages and T lymphocytes. (For more about T lymphocytes, see chapter 5.) Laboratory blood tests not only indicate the presence of leukocytosis but can differentiate among the various white cell types. These **differential white cell counts** are useful in diagnosis. For example, bacterial infection and ischemic damage produce elevated neutrophil counts **(neutrophilia)**. On the other hand, viral infections stimulate **lymphocytosis** (an increase in the number of lymphocytes), while allergic reactions or parasitic infections produce a relatively greater rise in eosinophils **(eosinophilia)**.

Therapeutic Modification of Acute Inflammation

This section describes the rationale for limiting inflammation and the essential concepts of anti-inflammatory therapy. It may seem strange to consider limiting the inflammatory response when we've just identified its beneficial role in dealing with the agents that produce tissue damage. However, even though acute inflammation accomplishes this task, there are some problems associated with excessive or inappropriate inflammation.

The first of these is pain, a benefit to some degree in signaling the fact of tissue damage and in limiting use of an injured tissue. But when pain is intense and prolonged, it can present significant problems to the patient. Second, sometimes swelling is so great that it impairs function, perhaps by limiting joint mobility or obstructing some anatomical passage. An example of the latter case would be acute pancreatitis, where the swollen pancreas can compress the common bile duct. Remember also that swelling can produce pain as tissue pressures impinge upon nerve endings and pain-producing mediators accumulate. So when swelling is excessive, excessive pain may also be present. A third problem arising out of the acute inflammatory response is tissue damage. A good example is a type of glomerulonephritis in which immune complexes are present in renal basement membranes. These complexes are chemotactic for neutrophils, which move to the scene and attempt to engulf them, but this event promotes frustrated phagocytosis and the release of substances that damage the basement membrane, leading in many cases to the threat of renal failure. The overall situation is summarized in figure 2.17.

You can see, then, that the inflammatory response has the potential to further complicate the patient's problems rather than reducing them. For this reason, therapy to limit the inflammatory response may be necessary. The challenge, of course, is to apply therapy in such a way as to limit inflammation, thus preventing excessive pain and tissue damage, while allowing a sufficient response to deal effectively with the problem. We will now consider some specific ways of modifying the inflammatory response. Broadly, there are both physical approaches and those that use therapeutic drugs.

Temperature

It has long been recognized that temperature manipulation is effective in coping with excessive inflammation. Application of cold to the damaged area causes a reduction of swelling. This effect is probably due to a vasoconstriction reflex in arterioles to prevent heat loss. Of course, at the scene of damage, the reduced blood flow has the effect of reducing formation of fluid exudate and swelling is relieved. Application of cold must be done with attention to one of the important cells involved in mediating inflammation—the mast cell. Application of cold for more than ten minutes will trigger mast cell degranulation and worsen the inflammation—hence, the general rule "10 on and 10 off" for cold. Alternating cold and heat (ten minutes each) is also done. The opposite situation, heat application, is also helpful in that an elevated temperature favors phagocytosis. In

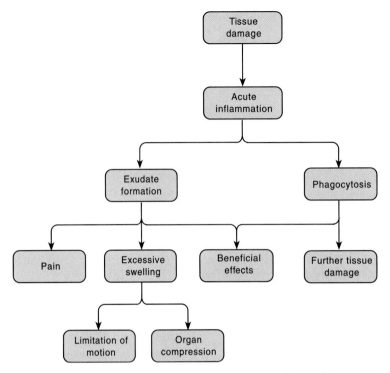

Figure 2.17 **Inflammation Management.** The rationale for therapeutically limiting inflammation is based on its excessive or inappropriate effects. Therapy seeks to minimize these without limiting the beneficial aspects of inflammation.

this context, you can understand the logic of temperature therapy in typical muscle and connective tissue injury. Cold is applied early, to limit swelling; then later, when phagocytes have accumulated at the scene, heat is applied to stimulate phagocytosis. One of the beneficial effects of fever, which is often associated with inflammation, may be the enhancement of phagocytosis that occurs as body temperature rises. Note that heat application is one of the few methods of enhancing a beneficial aspect of inflammation. Most often, suppression of an excessive response is the basis for therapy.

Elevation and Pressure

Another physical approach to dealing with an excessive inflammatory response is aimed at limiting swelling. In the case of damage involving the limbs, elevation is often successful in promoting drainage to reduce swelling. More importantly, blood flow is slowed, because the blood must oppose gravity in flowing to an elevated point, so fluid exudate formation, and therefore swelling, can be conveniently reduced. In some cases, constrictive wrappings may be applied to the inflamed area. These will prevent exudate formation by increasing the pressure in the tissues so that fluid is prevented from leaving the blood vessels. The higher tissue fluid pressures also promote lymphatic drainage.

Drug Therapy

In addition to altering the physical conditions just described, a major approach to anti-inflammatory therapy is directed at the chemical mediation system that underlies it. A variety of chemicals called **antihistamines** block the action of histamine at its blood vessel receptors. We have already mentioned the roles of nonsteroidal anti-inflammatory agents and corticosteroids, but a few further comments are appropriate. By blocking cyclooxygenase activity, agents like ibuprofen and acetylsalicylic acid (ASA, more commonly known as aspirin) block prostaglandin synthesis and thereby remove an important inflammatory mediator. To the extent that they successfully suppress the inflammation, they also bring pain relief by blocking the formation of pain mediators like bradykinin and prostaglandins, and suppressing K^+ and acid stimuli.

Steroid therapy has broad anti-inflammation effects because it interferes with the release of arachidonic acid from inflammatory cells. As a result, prostaglandin synthesis is reduced, and vasodilation and swelling are suppressed. And because arachidonic acid is the precursor of the leukotrienes, their vascular and cellular stimuli are also limited. The net effect is to reduce swelling and minimize damage from phagocytic cells. Another beneficial steroid effect involves lysosomes. By stabilizing lysosomal membranes, steroids can limit the release of enzymes and thereby reduce damage at the scene of inflammation. The anti-inflammatory effects of corticosteroids can be quite potent. For example, after injection into an inflamed joint, vessel permeability is so reduced that normal joint fluid production declines. This decline can result in exquisite pain, but it is relatively short-lived, lasting perhaps a few days, until fluid levels rise enough to allow normal joint movement.

Before leaving this section, let us note two potential complications of anti-inflammation therapy. One involves healing. Because some anti-inflammatory drugs, steroids for example, interfere with healing, incautious use can extend and complicate tissue restoration. A second problem has to do with infection. In damping the acute inflammatory response, we limit a major defense against infection. This means that therapy can induce a greater susceptibility to infection at the same time it seeks to reduce inflammatory damage or other problems arising from an excessive inflammatory response.

CHRONIC INFLAMMATION

Description

In some cases, when the acute inflammatory response is unable to remove or neutralize an injurious agent, the response is modified to forms called *subacute* or *chronic*. The distinctions between these are not well defined, but general guidelines indicate that the term **subacute** applies in inflammations lasting beyond one week. After six weeks' duration, the term **chronic** is applied. It is not unusual for a chronic response to last many months, even years. However, more than duration differentiates these responses. The nature of the response also changes. As the inflammatory process continues, fluid exudate diminishes in significance and the cellular response assumes dominance; whatever the nature of the inciting agent, the chronic response is dominated by a massive build-up of cells in the affected tissue. These cells are primarily macrophages and lymphocytes (cells normally involved in mediating immune system responses). The transition between the subacute and the chronic patterns is variable and, hence, not easily identified, so our consideration will emphasize the chronic inflammatory response.

In chronic inflammation there is, in essence, a standoff between the attack of the injurious agent and the counterattack mounted by the defenses of the host. The agent and the host are just capable of resisting each other's attacks, but neither is strong enough to overwhelm the other. The agents involved are typically of low invasive ability. They are unable to penetrate deeply into or spread rapidly throughout the body of the host. Such agents might be certain bacteria, fungi, or larger parasites. Some are organisms that can shelter from the immune system by living, at least part of the time, within macrophages. Some of the microorganisms involved in chronic inflammation are listed in table 2.3. Foreign bodies that are insoluble in the body's

Table 2.3   Selected Agents Typically Involved in Chronic Inflammation

Inflammatory Agent	Disease
Microorganisms	
Mycobacterium tuberculosis	Tuberculosis
Mycobacterium leprae	Leprosy
Listeria species	Listeriosis
Treponema pallidum	Syphilis
Brucella species	Brucellosis
Foreign Bodies	
Asbestos	Asbestosis
Silica	Silicosis
Beryllium	Berylliosis
Various organic dusts	Specific to the agent

fluids, although nonliving, can also elicit a chronic inflammatory response (table 2.3). Because talc powder, composed of magnesium silicate, used to be used to dust surgical gloves, it sometimes made its way into surgical wounds, stimulating a chronic foreign-body response. Intravenous drug abusers may use talc to carry or dilute a drug and thereby introduce it into the body. The talc tends to be trapped in the capillaries of the lung and can initiate a chronic inflammation there.

Regardless of the specific nature of the inciting agent, its presence in the tissues promotes a long-term conflict with the phagocytic cells of the host. This conflict typically proceeds at the expense of normal tissues. Their heavy infiltration by inflammatory cells progressively interferes with normal function. When the process continues over months and years, function deteriorates as tissue is destroyed, accumulating inflammatory cells replace functional tissues, and scarring develops. This deterioration can ultimately lead to somatic death—ironically, an ultimate victory for the biological agent at the expense of the host on which it depends.

Pathogenesis

Chronic inflammation is initiated by a typical acute response. However, the response is unable to eliminate the injurious agent or resolve the effects of injury. As we have seen, by the later stages of acute inflammation, macrophages are the dominant leukocytes at the scene, with some lymphocytes now present as well. In chronic inflammation, the highly active macrophages are also unable to remove the agent, and it persists in spite of their efforts at phagocytosis.

The long-term presence of the irritant may allow its antigenic properties to stimulate the host immune response. In the case of inert, nonbiological irritants (e.g., asbestos

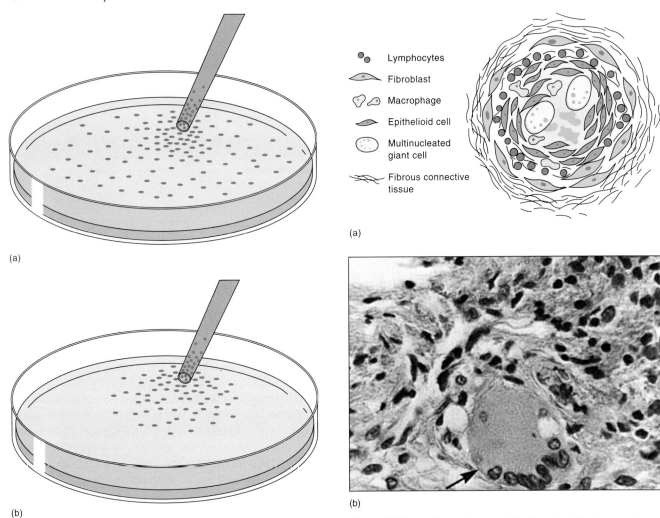

(a)

(b)

Figure 2.18   **Action of Migration Inhibition Factor (MIF).**
(*a*) Phagocytes introduced to the surface of a growth medium move out from the point of introduction. (*b*) When the medium contains MIF, their migration is greatly suppressed.

Lymphocytes
Fibroblast
Macrophage
Epithelioid cell
Multinucleated giant cell
Fibrous connective tissue

(a)

(b)

Figure 2.19   **A Granuloma and Its Principal Components.**
(*a*) Components diagrammed and labeled. (*b*) Close-up of a multinucleated giant cell (arrow) at the center of a long-standing granuloma.

particles), products of damaged tissue may provide the stimulus. In any case, stimulation of the immune system leads to activation of its lymphocytes, which respond by releasing substances called **lymphokines.** These have various specific effects on macrophages that contribute to the chronic inflammatory response. This situation is in contrast to acute inflammation, wherein chemical inflammatory mediators are responsible for neutrophil activation. The predominant cells of chronic inflammation, the macrophages, are under the more direct control of a subpopulation of lymphocytes called T_H cells (helper T cells). T_H cells and macrophages establish an interaction whereby the macrophages inform the lymphocytes as to the immune nature of the inflammatory initiator. The T_H lymphocytes then release substances that activate macrophages (MAF—macrophage-activating factor) and keep them at the site of inflammation (MIF—migration inhibitory factor), where their efforts can be best focused (fig. 2.18). Another con-

trast with acute inflammation concerns the sequencing of healing. In acute inflammation, the initial response is usually effective and healing follows. In chronic inflammation, inflammatory and repair processes occur at the same time so that neither is effective.

Classification

Two patterns of chronic inflammation can be distinguished. In one, called **nonspecific chronic inflammation,** a diffuse accumulation of macrophages and lymphocytes develops at the site of injury. Most chronic inflammations are of this type. A less common but distinctive form of the process is seen in the second pattern of chronic inflammation, **granulomatous inflammation.** This condition is characterized by a focal response that leads to the formation of a specific lesion, the **granuloma** (fig. 2.19). This roughly spherical mass is formed by hundreds of trans-

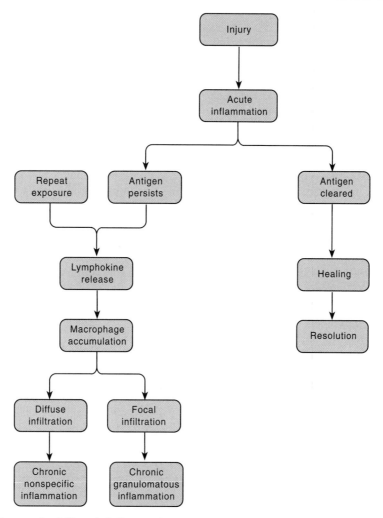

Figure 2.20   **Essential Pathogenesis of Chronic Inflammation.**

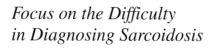

Focus on the Difficulty in Diagnosing Sarcoidosis

Sarcoidosis is a granulomatous disease that is relatively uncommon, but can have devastating consequences for about 20% of its victims. Its small, scattered, noncaseating granulomas can affect the eye, liver, skin, lymph node, lungs, spleen, or bone marrow. Sarcoidosis typically affects young people (age 20 to 35) and is ten times more common in blacks than whites, while it is very rare in Asians. Its cause is unknown.

formed macrophages called **epithelioid cells.** These have more cytoplasm than typical macrophages and are heavily granulated. They are surrounded by lymphocytes and fibroblasts. There may also be a central mass of necrotic tissue that has been "walled off," often containing the injuri-

ous agent. Also present in many instances are very large, multinucleated cells. These are formed by the merging of macrophages or the coalescence of several (a dozen would not be unusual) to form very large cells with phagocytic capabilities. They are descriptively termed **multinucleated giant cells.**

Typically, foreign-body granulomas are centered on the particle involved. Granulomas that arise in an allergic reaction to persistent bacterial, viral, or fungal agents tend to develop a necrotic center as they get larger. Those that develop with an intracellular bacterium (e.g., tuberculosis, syphilis, leprosy) show the characteristic pattern of necrosis referred to earlier as caseous necrosis. In this case, the center of the granuloma produces a crumbly, cheeselike breakdown product (casein is the phosphoprotein constituent of cheese).

Figure 2.20 provides an overview of the mechanisms underlying chronic inflammation. Here, immune-mediated processes are emphasized, although, as we have already noted, nonimmunogenic stimuli are often involved. The emphasis here is on the central role of the lymphocyte in mediating the response.

Case Study

A 25-year-old construction worker came to a general practitioner because of a painful, red swelling over his patella, which had been bothering him in his work for the past three days. Nothing in his medical history seemed likely to be a contributing factor, other than that he had recently been camping and had been badly bitten by mosquitos.

The examination revealed an area of 5 cm diameter that was swollen, red, and hot, with a central accumulation of pus. The lesion was strongly suggestive of a mosquito bite that had become infected, forming a large boil.

The boil was incised and drained, and a sample of pus was sent for laboratory culture and sensitivity studies to determine the organism involved and its antibiotic sensitivities. Pending results of these studies, Cloxicillin was prescribed on the assumption that *Staphylococcus aureus* was likely to be found. A dressing was applied to the patient's knee. Two days later, lab results confirmed that cloxicillin-sensitive *Staph. aureus* was involved.

Over the following months, the patient suffered recurring boils, which were presenting problems in his work. Blood sugar tests were done and found to be normal. A nasal culture revealed *Staph. aureus* to be resident in the nasal passages. An appropriate course of antibiotic therapy was instituted to eradicate the staph organisms and the patient has had no further problems with recurring boils.

Commentary

This is a situation in which resident nasal organisms provide a source of reinfection, which in this case was dealt with relatively easily.

Because draining a boil is usually adequate, prescribing an antibiotic is normally not necessary. However, in this case, several factors indicated that antibiotic therapy was prudent: the size of the lesion and its location, where it was subject to bending of the knee and friction from clothing, the risk of further irritation on the job site, and the physician's assessment of the patient's inadequate hygiene.

The blood sugar test was done in the face of recurring boils to determine whether an early diabetes mellitus condition might be contributing to the ease with which organisms were becoming established. In diabetics, elevated glucose levels provide a nutrient medium for infecting organisms at the same time as a compromised circulation limits the ability to cope with infection. Fortunately, no diabetes was present and the situation was resolved with relative ease.

Key Concepts

1. The cardinal signs of inflammation are redness, heat, swelling, pain, and loss of function (p. 28).

2. Increases in blood pressure and capillary permeability associated with the inflammatory response lead to accumulation of fluid exudate and phagocytic cells at the site of injury (pp. 28–29).

3. Changes in vascular flow and the stickiness of postcapillary venules ensure the delivery of appropriate numbers of leukocytes to the site of injury (pp. 30–31).

4. The type of exudate formed is related to the nature of the injury and affects the pattern of healing (p. 32).

5. An initial wave of neutrophils is followed by a later wave of monocytes capable of being focused by the lymphocytes, thereby staging the cellular response to injury (pp. 32–35).

6. The destruction of pathogens and the removal of debris are accomplished by phagocytic cells, which enter the tissue, become activated, move toward the target, recognize and attach to it, and then engulf and destroy it (pp. 35–36).

7. A variety of cell-derived and plasma-derived chemical mediators orchestrate, maintain, and then quench the acute inflammatory response (pp. 38–42).

8. Cold or heat, elevation and pressure, antihistamines, corticosteroids, and nonsteroidal anti-inflammatory agents can be used to control excessive or inappropriate acute inflammation (pp. 43–45).

9. Chronic inflammation develops when some persistent infection or foreign substance stimulates a lymphocyte-mediated accumulation of activated macrophages (pp. 45–47).

REVIEW ACTIVITIES

1. Diagram the sequence of events that starts with cell injury and leads to increased vascular permeability.

2. Explain how phagocytosis, chemotaxis, emigration, pavementing, and margination are related.

3. Describe the role of four types of chemical mediators thought to contribute to acute inflammation.

4. Construct a table relating a type of acute inflammation with its corresponding exudate characteristics.

5. Sketch a flow chart that traces the development of a granuloma.

6. List four methods of suppressing the inflammatory response and indicate the mechanism that operates in each case.

7. Corticosteroids and NSAIDs act to quench the production of certain delayed mediators. Get as fanciful as you like and invent a new way of controlling the acute inflammatory response (remember, this is purely theoretical). Is there anything else you could do to knock out a chronic inflammatory response, other than treating the tissue with corticosteroids or NSAIDs?

Chapter

3

Fever

So when a raging fever burns
We shift from side to side by turns;
An 'tis poor relief we gain,
To change the place to keep the pain.

Isaac Watts
Some Thoughts of God and Death

rubor
&tumor
cū calore
&dolore

Inflammation is often accompanied by elevation of the body temperature above its normal range. This condition is known as **fever** or **pyrexia.** The association of fever with disease, especially infection, has been recognized for hundreds of years. Indeed, many infectious diseases are named fevers (e.g., typhoid fever, rheumatic fever, cat-scratch fever) because fever dominates the clinical pattern of the disease. Rather than a defect in the system that regulates body temperature, fever represents an upward adjustment of the temperature level that the system seeks to establish and maintain. This point is better appreciated in the context of normal thermal regulation.

NORMAL THERMOREGULATION

At rest, normal oral temperature varies within a surprisingly narrow range of values whose average is about 36.7° C. Temperatures normally do not vary more than 0.5° C (1° F) above or below this value. A similar range is observed for rectal temperature, with its average values elevated about 0.5° C above oral, while the average axilla's (armpit) temperature is about 0.5° C lower than oral temperature. Rectal temperature is the most accurate, normally accessible estimate of "core temperature," which really means the temperature of the essential major organs: the heart and lungs, the liver, kidneys, and brain. Oral temperature is affected by ingestion of cold or hot substances or by breathing pattern (oral versus nasal). Tympanic temperature may be muted by accumulated cerumen (wax). Taking the temperature in the axilla, while the least accurate measure, is sometimes the most acceptable method in a very sick or restless patient. Body temperature varies throughout the day, with lowest temperatures in the early morning and highest around 4 P.M. (table 3.1). The normal body temperature value most often used is 37° C (98.6° F). The regular diurnal (24-hour) fluctuations, the range in "normal" temperature found in different individuals, and the common observation that fevers tend to peak in the evening, require that temperature be taken several times over at least 24 hours to definitively establish or rule out fever.

Body temperature is closely regulated because temperature changes can significantly affect cellular functions. Most cell enzymes function optimally within the normal body temperature range. Warm-blooded animals dedicate extensive metabolic, sensory, and regulatory resources to create, distribute, and dispel or conserve heat to maintain a stable temperature throughout the body. Significant deviation affects function. For example, a cranial temperature of 40.5° C (105° F) will disturb brain function, producing bewilderment and confusion. However, changes in function don't necessarily reflect structural alteration. People appear to be able to tolerate quite high body temperatures without significant tissue damage. In the days before antibiotics, "fever therapy" was sometimes used, with temperatures as high as 41.7° C (107.1° F) being induced with no problems resulting. People have died with much lower fevers, but the likelihood is that the tissue and organ damage resulted from

Table 3.1	Daily Temperature Fluctuation: Average Rectal Temperatures of a Group of Adults Taken at Intervals over 24 Hours

Time	Temperature (° C)
Midnight	36.7
0200	36.5
0400	36.4
0800	36.6
Noon	37.0
1600	37.4
2000	37.2
2200	37.1

underlying pathology; for example, local coagulation or hypoxia or cardiac arrest, rather than from the fever itself. However, with an increase to 43° C (109° F) for only a few hours, death usually follows. In the other direction, if temperature falls below normal, it can also affect enzyme function and slow metabolism, resulting in what we will later describe as hypothermia.

Maintenance of a given body temperature is achieved by balancing heat production against heat loss. All cells produce heat in the course of normal metabolism because energy conversions are considerably less than 100% efficient. This means that energy in the form of heat is constantly produced and released from living tissues. The amount of heat varies with normal fluctuations of metabolic activity related to each tissue's characteristic functions. For example, at rest, the liver and heart have higher metabolic rates than does skeletal muscle. Thus, at rest, the liver and heart are the source of most of the body's heat. During exercise, however, muscle heat production rises dramatically, consequently warming the muscle and the blood perfusing it and thereby warming the body core. When activity diminishes, heat production, and therefore muscle temperature, fall to resting levels.

Heat loss is achieved primarily by the delivery of heat energy to the surface of the body, where any excess can be lost to the environment. The delivery is accomplished by the blood, which picks up heat as it passes throughout the body and then carries it to the skin.

Mechanisms of Heat Production

As we noted earlier, heat is constantly being produced by cellular metabolism and must continually be lost to prevent overheating. On the other hand, if body temperature should fall, additional heat production is required. Heat production comes about by a variety of physiological reflexes and various appropriate behavioral responses.

An important heat-production mechanism reflex involves shivering. Both peripheral and central temperature receptors signal net heat loss to the hypothalamus in the center of the base of the brain. The hypothalamus triggers the autonomic nervous system, which interacts with motor neurons in the cord that generate shivering. Shivering entails a pattern of rapidly alternating skeletal muscle contractions that produce no skeletal motion. While inefficient for movement, shivering dramatically increases the amount of heat liberated by the contracting muscle. The muscle converts chemical energy in its fuel molecules, principally glucose, to the mechanical energy needed for the contraction. As this occurs, heat energy is released because of the inefficiency of the conversion process. Heat production behaviors also include conscious movements that also utilize muscle contractions to produce heat, such as arm waving or jumping in place.

 Checkpoint 3.1

In muscle, approximately 25% of the energy available in glucose is expressed in force generation, while the remaining 75% is given off as heat. This becomes a major issue in temperature regulation because basal/resting ATP production in skeletal muscle can increase over 20-fold in vigorously active muscle. Physical activity is therefore a major factor in temperature regulation as a source of heat, as just noted in the example of increasing movements as a way of keeping warm. Can you anticipate a way this heat production potential might produce *excessive* temperature? What factors might impair heat production in muscle to the detriment of returning a *lowered* core temperature to normal?

Mechanisms of Heat Loss

The skin, which accounts for about 90% of heat loss, is well suited to temperature regulation because it has a large surface area from which heat can be lost. Heat loss through the skin is accomplished by four mechanisms: radiation, evaporation, conduction, and convection. In loss by **radiation,** heat energy moves directly away from the warm skin surface. When you place a hand near a red-hot cooking element, you feel heat without actually touching the element, because of energy radiating from it.

In **evaporation,** which accounts for perhaps 30% of heat loss at rest, water at the skin surface is converted from a liquid to a gaseous state. The process consumes heat energy from the surrounding skin, causing body temperature to fall. The water that evaporates is secreted by the skin's sweat glands. It is moved to the surface by contraction of smooth muscle in the ducts that drain the glands. The openings of these ducts at the surface are called **pores.** Heat loss by evaporation from pulmonary surfaces occurs, but is not nearly as significant in humans as it is in some animals, whose panting is an important means of increasing heat loss.

Conduction is a third means of losing heat. About 70% of heat loss from the skin is by conduction. It involves direct transfer of heat by physical contact between the body and a cooler surrounding medium. When heat is carried away by movement of the air or water surrounding the body, the mechanism is called **convection.** In humans, this situation arises most dramatically when the body is immersed in water. Immersion can be used therapeutically to reduce fever.

The main mechanism of heat loss will depend upon the circumstances. In a hot environment or during intense exercise, sweating and evaporation will predominate. Convection, which is usually a minor mechanism, takes precedence in exposure to a cold wind. Heat loss by evaporation through the lungs, usually accounting for about 10%, becomes a dangerous mechanism of continued heat loss in a person who has become hypothermic, a topic that will be discussed shortly.

The mechanisms just described depend upon the physical circumstances the person encounters. But active behavioral responses can increase heat loss. For example, moving to a cooler location promotes heat loss, as does increasing skin surface exposure by rolling up shirt sleeves or wearing shorts rather than full-length slacks. Similarly, loosening the clothing promotes air flow to increase evaporation and convection losses.

Regulation of Heat Loss

At rest, metabolic heat production is relatively constant. Variations in the metabolic rate are only used as a means of regulating temperature in dire circumstances. In mild hypothermia or when a fever is being generated, increased thyroid hormone is released, turning up the rate of metabolism and, thereby, heat production. In "normal" temperature regulation, heat loss mechanisms are modified to achieve the required body temperature. Body temperature increases trigger accelerated heat loss, whereas temperature decreases below the normal range cause heat loss mechanisms to be inhibited. In other words, the system functions by allowing either more or less heat loss to the environment as required. At extremes of temperature, reflex shivering, thyroid activation, or behavioral responses are brought into play. Behavioral heat conservation measures include adding insulating layers of clothing or blankets and reducing the body surface area by curling into the fetal position or clenching the hands.

Heat loss occurs at the skin's surface and depends primarily on two easily altered mechanisms. One involves heat loss at the skin's surface, based on the transfer of heat from the blood. Dermal blood vessels are so arranged that, depending on the pattern of arteriolar constriction, blood can be distributed to vessels that are either nearer the surface or farther from it below the insulating layer of subcutaneous fat. When blood is moved near the surface, more heat is lost. When blood is moved farther from the surface, less heat is lost (fig. 3.1). At least as important as dermal redirection, there is a generalized increase in arterial resistance

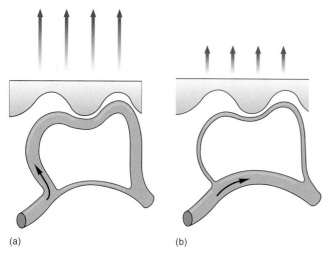

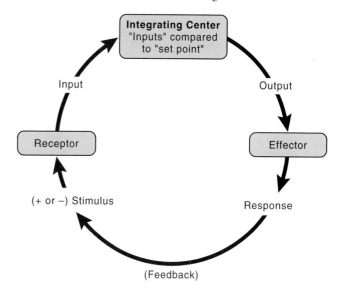

Figure 3.1 **Heat Loss and Dermal Blood Flow.** (*a*) Blood moving near the skin's surface loses body heat. (*b*) Heat loss is reduced when more blood is diverted from the surface.

Figure 3.2 **Essential Elements and Interrelationships of a Negative Feedback Control System.**

in the extremities, conserving blood for the core. No new heat is produced, but temperature is maintained by cutting losses.

The second mechanism used to regulate heat loss involves sweat production at the skin's surface. Changes in sweat production cause greater or less heat loss. The skin usually feels dry because perspiration fluid is quickly evaporated from it after reaching the surface. Loss of heat by evaporation from the skin and lungs is called "**insensible loss.**" When temperature rises, production rates exceed evaporation rates, and fluid accumulates.

Having considered the sources of heat and the mechanisms of heat loss, let us now take a closer look at the responses of the tissues involved. What are the factors that determine the appropriate response in the tissues that affect heat loss and heat production? In other words, what controls and coordinates the blood vessels, sweat glands, shivering, and the various behavioral responses, so that temperature is maintained at the desired level?

Negative Feedback Control of Body Temperature

A control system is a collection of components that function to maintain some variable at a particular value. Control systems are used extensively in engineering applications, and they function in biological control as well. To maintain control of a variable such as temperature, the control system must have one or more components that can respond to bring about changes in the variable (fig. 3.2). These responding tissues are called **effectors.** In a physiological control system, there is often more than one effector, and each of them must receive controlling input information. This information will stimulate them to increase or decrease their particular response. Control of the effectors is achieved by a second control system component called an **integrator,** or **integrating center** (IC). It is here that con-

trol "decisions" are reached on the basis of information regarding body temperature. This information is sent to the integrating center by specialized receptors called **sensors,** which are sensitive to changes in temperature. The system maintains the particular variable close to a certain value called the system's **set point.**

As body temperature changes, sensors alter their output to the integrating center, which then compares the information with its set point. If the difference between the two values falls outside an acceptable range, the integrating center institutes a corrective response by the system's effectors. The response tends to restore the set point value and therefore decrease the stimulus to the sensors. Because the system's response is monitored and acted upon in further corrective action, this type of control system is said to operate according to the principle of feedback. Because the corrective response is always in a direction opposite to the direction of change from the set point, such control is said to be **negative feedback control.** Thus, if temperature is too high, the negative feedback system will cause it to be lowered; if too low, the system will raise it. In this way correction for changes from the set point is always achieved.

Positive feedback takes place when a stimulus condition elicits a response that exaggerates the original condition. This system operates healthfully in the inflammation discussed in chapter 2 and in healing, which is the topic of chapter 4. In temperature regulation, positive feedback only occurs when there has been a failure of homeostatic responses. In hypothermia, lowered temperature leads to a drop in basal metabolism, which lowers heat production. The reverse occurs in hyperthermia. In these cases, positive feedback worsens the deviation from normal temperature.

In humans, the major temperature regulation effectors are dermal arterioles, sweat glands, and the skeletal muscles involved in both shivering and the various temperature-related behavioral responses. All of these receive controlling input from the **thermoregulation center** in the

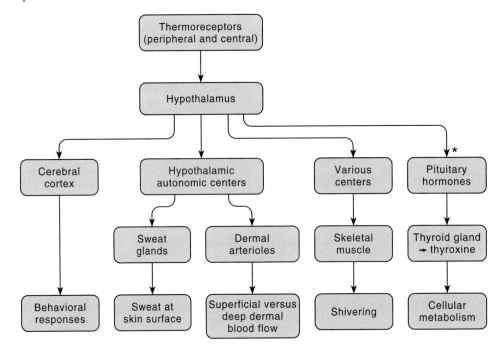

Figure 3.3   Principles of Normal Thermoregulation. A cold stimulus would produce increased activity, decreased sweating, diversion of dermal blood flow to deep vessels, shivering, and increased rate of cellular metabolism. (*Only occurs in mild hypothermia.)

preoptic nucleus of the anterior hypothalamus, which functions as integrating center. Temperature information is detected in all parts of the body by sensors called **thermoreceptors.** From these, the temperature information is relayed to the hypothalamus for analysis. Some neurons in the hypothalamus are also directly sensitive to temperature. These provide an important contribution to the process because they directly monitor levels of heat in the blood that flows through the brain. This process reflects the core temperature of the trunk from which this blood was immediately delivered. Normal human thermoregulation is summarized in figure 3.3.

 Checkpoint 3.2

The general regulatory framework just described is basic to all homeostatic controls systems. Pathophysiology is the study of its disorder. If the location and function of the hypothalamus is not clear to you, you might want to turn forward to that section in chapter 20.

FAILURE OF NORMAL THERMOREGULATION

The homeostatic mechanisms just described are supported by a host of sociocultural (clothing, housing, diet, geographic distribution, etc.) and behavioral (adjusting activity

level, exposure, wearing appropriate clothing, etc.) adaptations. This combination normally maintains critical core temperature so effectively that death through failure of normal thermoregulation is the tragic exception, rather than the rule. Humans have successfully colonized climatic extremes from the Namib desert to the Arctic tundra. And, unprotected, we easily tolerate, even enjoy, the roasting heat of the sauna or the cold of a dip in a glacial pool. The circumstances that push people outside this adaptive window are usually extreme: prolonged exposure to extreme heat or immersion in cold water. But more subtle factors can lead to loss of homeostatic control in less than hostile conditions: wet clothing, intoxication leading to impaired judgment or neural function, competitive exertion, abnormally low body fat, dehydration, illness or poor nutrition, for example. While the focus of this chapter is on fever, a brief examination of the two major ways temperature regulation can fail will serve to reinforce the core concepts and, at the same time, treat two conditions of major clinical importance.

Hyperthermia

A healthy person sitting in a sauna at anywhere between 60–100° C (140–212° F) maintains an essentially normal core temperature. Even the person's extremities, because of effective sweating and blood flow, are only gently warmed. If he stayed there long enough, however, this would change. A loss of homeostatic control that results in rising body core temperature is called **hyperthermia.** Heat accumulation, whether due to excessive heat production, factors that impair heat dissipation, heat from the environment, or primary hypothalamic dysfunction, increases the metabolic rate of tissues, producing more heat. This is a pathological example of positive feedback.

Perhaps 700 people die every year in North America due to **heatstroke.** Most succumb to **classic heatstroke.** The very young or old, the debilitated, or people who venture out into severely hot climates without sufficient water, shade, and food are the typical victims. Combine a humid heat wave (humidity counteracts much of the effect of sweating), a poorly ventilated room, insufficient fluid intake, and a pre-existing heart condition, perhaps with the use of diuretics, and you have heatstroke waiting to happen. The major predisposing condition in classic heatstroke is **dehydration,** which leads to **anhydrosis,** the absence of sweating. **Exertional heatstroke,** by contrast, is usually seen in the young, notably competitive male athletes, whose intense activity in a hot environment generates heat faster than it can be cleared. Health care resources in Saudi Arabia have developed expertise in dealing with both forms of heatstroke, which are common in that country during the annual pilgrimage to Mecca—the hajj. **Heat exhaustion** is a milder form of hyperthermia.

Characteristically, the classic heatstroke victim's skin feels hot and dry, rather than the cool, moist skin of the person who is sweating healthfully, while the skin in exertional heatstroke is hot and clammy. Most importantly, victims have experienced a rapid elevation in temperature (most above 40.5° C [105° F]). Most are confused or delirious and may be in coma or seizures. Tachycardia is common. As well as the accumulating heat, the depleted fluid volume puts strain on the heart and can lead to hypoperfusion of critical organs, perhaps renal failure, and heart failure. Heatstroke is a medical emergency. Physical cooling by spraying with lukewarm water, or even immersion in an ice water bath, and careful rehydration are generally effective treatments. The antipyretic medications that are so useful in treating fever are irrelevant here, as will become clear when we discuss fever.

We should mention **malignant hyperthermia of anesthesia.** This results when a genetically predisposed individual is given certain anesthetic agents or surgical muscle relaxants. Usually immediately after administration, but sometimes after a delay of several hours, the person develops muscle rigidity and severe hyperthermia. Immediately after the reaction is noted, anesthetic is discontinued and dantrolene sodium and physical cooling are administered. A number of other conditions produce hyperthermia, including aspirin intoxication, an interesting effect from a drug that is used to treat the overheating of fever.

Hypothermia

Prolonged or extreme exposure to cold can overwhelm the mechanisms normally effective in maintaining core temperature. **Hypothermia** is the term applied to a core temperature below 35° C (95° F). **Mild hypothermia,** a core temperature between 35–32° C (95–90° F), produces intense shivering and muscle cramping that may impair efforts at self-rescue. Rescue to a warm environment, nourishment, warm fluids, and physical activity will usually restore normal body temperature. However, at temperatures below 32° C (90° F), shivering is less effective or stops, the pulse and respiratory rate slow, blood pressure drops, judgment is impaired, consciousness may be altered, and many experience a sense of euphoria. Hypothermic individuals may act in highly maladaptive ways—tearing off clothing and diving into icy water. This is **severe hypothermia.**

The mechanism for the heat loss will depend upon the circumstances. In the water, heat loss through convection is 30 times faster than heat loss to the same temperature of air. On "dry" land, conduction accounts for much heat loss. Victims who avoid sitting or lying on the ground can extend survival. Wet, noninsulating clothes add a huge evaporative factor. Blue jeans are common apparel on hypothermic victims. And, of course, the wind can turn convection against someone stranded in the outdoors. The 10–35% heat loss through evaporation in the lungs can be a critical factor in the survival of someone with hypothermia (the person should be placed in a very warm environment).

The mechanism leading to a spiraling down of core temperature may be either the hypothermia itself (remember positive feedback and energy production) or the exhaustion of energy reserves that leave the person unable to deal effectively with the cold stress. But when the thermoregulatory center, cortex, and brain stem cool sufficiently, the body can no longer react adaptively. Shivering stops. Blood that was conserved for the core and deep dermal vessels now flows unrestricted, radiating further heat. Below 30° C (86° F), cerebral blood flow and oxygen requirements drop, cardiac output and arterial pressure decrease, and the person may appear dead. The instances of people, mostly small children, surviving drowning in icy waters can be explained by some of these changes. If the temperature-mediated metabolic demands of the brain and heart fall faster than the oxygen delivery to these tissues, the victim may survive unharmed for long periods. Resuscitation may require prolonged heavy sedation to keep the metabolic requirements of the brain, in particular, below the heart's ability to deliver. While ventricular fibrillation is a common mechanism of death in hypothermia victims, below 30° C (86° F), they may not respond to defibrillation as a means of resuscitation.

Emergency treatment in the first half hour is life-essential in extreme hypothermia. Moving the victim to a warm environment will not be sufficient. Active rewarming is required. In this context, the recent use of inhalation re-warming, in which the person is ventilated with warm (43–45° C [107–122° F]), water-saturated air, is interesting. This approach directly warms the head, neck, and critical thoracic core, including the heart. The effect on the brain is such that the temperature-regulating center in the hypothalamus, the cardiovascular centers in the medulla, and the centers involved in shivering return to functional temperatures. Active heat production resumes, as does the adaptive direction of blood flow to conserve the heat produced. And a word of caution: many persons experience **"after drop"**—that is, continued cooling of core temperature after rescue. Some of that may be due to premature activity by the victim: muscular activity returns cold peripheral blood to the body core and results in decreased core temperature.

FEVER

Fever is most commonly a prominent manifestation of inflammation. While itself a consequence, fever is part of a broad, integrated **acute phase reaction.** Chapter 2 dealt in some detail with the role of acute-phase proteins secreted by the liver (e.g., C-reactive protein). In fever, the hypothalamus orchestrates endocrine responses that include the release of glucocorticoids (stress response) and the decrease in vasopressin (ADH), which reduces body fluid volume and, therefore, the volume that requires warming in fever. The autonomic responses are cardiovascular (blood directed to deep dermal and body core vessels, increased heart rate and blood pressure) and decreased sweat production. Purely reflexive (shivering or "rigors") and higher-order behavioral responses are also triggered (the "chills" that prompt warmth seeking, loss of appetite, general malaise which in turn leads to lowered activity and involvement).

In a **febrile** (feverish) patient, elevated temperature would seem to suggest some defect in the temperature-regulating control system. In fact, the system is functioning normally, but on the basis of a new set point. In fever, the IC's set point is adjusted upward, causing the effectors to raise body temperature in response. Signs and symptoms prior to the onset of fever are consistent with the responses expected when body temperature is below the set point. Pallor (paleness) and chills are the result of dermal vasoconstriction, which is a means of reducing heat loss in support of the new, higher temperature setting. Shivering and huddling under bed covers are additional means of raising temperature to the level of the new set point. When the normal set point is restored, either by resolution of the infection or the administration of antipyretic drugs, heat-loss mechanisms come into play and fever subsides. Profuse sweating, dermal flushing, and throwing off of bed covers are all means of reducing temperature to the now lower set point value.

Mechanisms Underlying Fever

Pyrexia is associated with many different disease conditions. From this, you might assume that various external factors can directly influence the thermal regulation center in the hypothalamus to elevate the set point. However, this is not the case. It appears instead that the several external factors all stimulate a single, common pattern of response, which results in set point elevation. The body's response is a complex sequence of interrelated events involving several

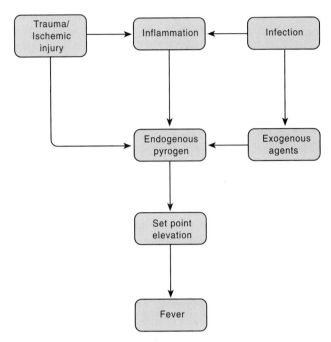

Figure 3.4   **The Role of Endogenous Pyrogen (EP) in the Pathogenesis of Fever.**

chemical mediators that affect the hypothalamus, altering its temperature set point. Although there is much that is unclear about the intermediate steps in the process, it is known that various fever-producing factors all cause the production and release of internally produced **pyrogen** (fever-causing substance). Once released, this **endogenous pyrogen** (EP) triggers the remaining events, which lead to upward readjustment of the temperature set point of the hypothalamus (fig. 3.4).

A host of exogenous substances are capable of inducing fever by stimulating EPs if introduced to the body. These used to be collectively termed **exogenous pyrogens.** We now understand that these agents provoke fever indirectly, via the endogenous system that will be described next. Therefore they are not "pyrogens" in the true sense. The prototype exogenous agent is **endotoxin,** a lipopolysaccharide (LPS) component of the cell walls of Gram-negative bacteria. In these bacteria, LPS forms an outer lipid membrane that is released only if the bacterium is injured or killed. Because LPS is heat stable, even heat sterilization of substances containing Gram-negative bacteria does not eliminate its pyrogenic effects. If injected into human subjects, the functional LPS can cause "injection fevers." These were a common complication of the administration of intravenous fluids, particularly in the early days when less was known of the mechanisms underlying fever. They can be prevented if fluids are prepared in sterile conditions and then specifically treated to remove LPS. While humans are exquisitely sensitive to LPS, a wide range of other organisms and substances can trigger fever, including viruses, bacteria, fungi, antigen-antibody immune complexes (see chapter 5), and various forms of tissue injury.

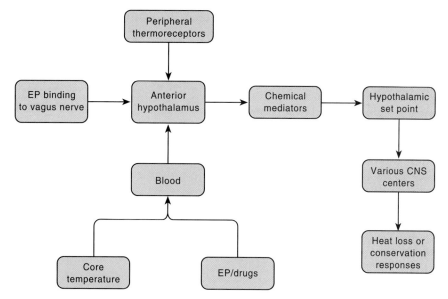

Figure 3.5   **Hypothalamic Processing in Thermoregulation.**

Many therapeutic agents, either because of excess dosage (e.g., aspirin, atropine, chlorpromazine) or a particular patient sensitivity (e.g., cimetidine, ibuprofen, bleomycin, penicillins) may be pyrogenic. Aspirin is interesting in this context since it is commonly used as an antipyretic agent.

Endogenous Pyrogens

As we have seen, a variety of exogenous agents generate fever through their capacity to stimulate the production and release of endogenous pyrogens (EPs). These are substances produced particularly in an inflammatory response that act on receptors in the hypothalamus to cause an upward alteration of its temperature set point. The clinically relevant sources of EPs that have been identified include principally the **mononuclear phagocytes.** This family of cells includes the monocytes/macrophages, which constitute the second wave of cells in acute inflammation and which are important in chronic inflammation. Mononuclear phagocytes capture and "process" pathogens (much more of this is discussed in chapter 5), and release EP.

The EPs include IL-1 (interleukin-1), TNFα (tumor necrosis factor), IFNα (interferon alpha), and TL6 (interleukin-6). The best-characterized are IL-1 and TNFα. IL-1 is produced by a wide number of cells in response to injury or inflammatory activation, and especially by activated macrophages, which appear to be the principal source of IL-1 in its role as an endogenous pyrogen. Certainly, the fever spikes noted in bacteremia are best explained by EP production related to the activation of free monocytes and macrophages resident in the liver, spleen, lymph nodes, lungs, and brain.

Essentially, then, endogenous pyrogens are produced and released by the body's phagocytic cells. In response to pyrogenic stimuli, these cells produce and release EPs. A notable exception exists in certain malignant tumors. The nonphagocytic cells of these tumors (e.g., leukemia and Hodgkin's disease) are able to release EPs. This mechanism may explain the fever commonly seen in some tumor patients, but other mechanisms may well be involved.

EPs are released only after a delay that follows the initial stimulation of phagocytic cells. This lag period lasts about one hour, after which body temperature starts to increase. Release of EPs after stimulation can continue for up to 15 hours. EPs are potent—only minute amounts are required to initiate pyrexia.

There is still work to do in clarifying hypothalamic temperature-regulation mechanisms. A thermosensitive nucleus (the preoptic nucleus) in the anterior hypothalamus receives stimulatory inputs from warm and cold receptors in the skin, the body core, and the preoptic nucleus itself, as well as being the site of action of at least some EPs. This combined sensor/thermostat puts out a signal to the system's set point (fig. 3.5). The hypothalamus gets constant feedback about surface and core temperatures, detects deviations from set point, and then adjusts output to cortical, hypothalamic, and brain stem centers that can generate an appropriate corrective response. It appears that there are a number of ways that EP can signal the preoptic nucleus. Low-level EP production (related to mild or "smoldering" infection) can bind to receptors on terminals of the vagus nerve in the thoracic and abdominopelvic cavities and, through the vagus, signal the hypothalamus. Higher levels of EP, produced anywhere in the body, travel in the vasculature to the hypothalamus where EP is either transported by specific transport molecules or enters through "leaky" areas in the vasculature of the preoptic nucleus, lacking the usual blood-brain barrier. Finally, so-called exogenous pyrogenic agents can travel to the preoptic nucleus where it is admitted and interacts with local mononuclear phagocytes (microglia and tissue macrophages), which produce the EP in situ.

Temperature-related intrahypothalamic signaling depends on several intermediary steps involving prostaglandin E (PGE), monoamines (particularly serotonin), cAMP (cyclic adenosine monophosphate), and perhaps cGMP (cyclic guanosine monophosphate). IL-1, IL-6, TNFα, and IFNα all act through a pathway mediated by prostaglandin synthesis. In fact, increased prostaglandin levels in the blood (which might be associated with inflammation) trigger a set point rise in the same way that serotonin or cAMP injected into the hypothalamus does. (Previously, this observation led to the erroneous idea that PGE was an endogenous pyrogen.) Substances that interfere with prostaglandin synthesis (e.g., nonsteroidal anti-inflammatory agents) act as antipyretics. That is why ASA and acetaminophen are commonly used to reduce set point and, thereby, control fever.

The Role of Fever

Fever is a common response to infectious, toxic, immunologic disease or injury among warm-blooded animals. Even cold-blooded creatures like lizards and snakes "treat" infection by lying in the sun and raising their body temperatures. If this response or mammalian fever is experimentally interfered with, the result is increased disease and death rates. Recent *in vitro* studies that allow control of other factors have shown that temperatures typical of fever enhance many aspects of immune function and phagocytosis. Conversely, some bacteria and viruses have been shown to reproduce more slowly when temperature is elevated. In experiments with AIDS patients, when the temperature of the blood was raised by circulating and heating it outside the body (albeit at temperatures exceeding those routinely observed in fever), there were decreases in indicators of infection. It also appears that, in certain bacteria, temperature elevation interferes with the uptake of iron that the bacteria require for proliferation.

Taken together, these seemingly small individual gains from a rise in temperature seem to provide a significant overall benefit. Thus, the idea that fever is "bad" and that it should always be reduced is oversimplified. In many cases, a moderate degree of fever may enhance the patient's defensive responses, providing more real benefit than would be gained by limiting the fever to provide a bit of comfort. On the other hand, modern interventions like antibiotics tend to offset the argument. Antibiotics are available to counteract the potential negative effects of fever suppression. However, the growing problem of antibiotic-resistant bacterial strains has again raised the debate around sacrificing the comfort that antipyretic agents offer.

Harmful Effects of Fever

There are very few situations in which fever is actually dangerous. One of these arises in patients with compromised cardiac function. Fever results from increases in both heat retention and production. As well, warmer tissues increase their metabolic rate during a fever. This change is reflected

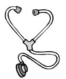

Focus on Febrile Seizures

Certain young children can respond to fever with convulsions, much to the horror of their parents. For the vast majority, these **febrile seizures** are quite benign. Of children who have experienced a fever-associated convulsion, about 35% will have a second (or more), and most of these will occur within a year. Of those children experiencing febrile seizures who are neurologically normal, perhaps 1% will go on to develop epilepsy. On the other hand, children with neurological abnormalities stand an increased chance of both febrile seizures and subsequent epilepsy. Those children who develop convulsions at lower temperature thresholds (38° C/100.5° F) tend to be more at risk. At one time, chronic anticonvulsant therapy (usually with phenobarbital) was recommended for any child who had two febrile seizures. Now such intervention is restricted to those children with neurological abnormalities, those with prolonged seizures, or those with a family history of seizure disorders. The simple administration of acetaminophen is usually very effective in controlling fevers and associated seizures.

in a 13% increase in oxygen consumption (and cardiac output) per a 1° C (1.8° F) rise in temperature. In high fevers, this can amount to a large increase in cardiac workload, a situation poorly tolerated by a person with heart disease. Patients who have suffered a stroke, particularly recently, are put at risk of more brain damage by a fever.

Normally, fever peaks at a maximum of about 40.5° C (105° F) following resetting of the hypothalamic set point as the infection has been dealt with and release of EP by mononuclear phagocytes has declined. This maximum assumes a healthy, functioning hypothalamus. In cases of head injury that compromises hypothalamic functioning, fever can climb to dangerous levels, perhaps requiring emergency application of cooling blankets, ice baths, or even iced gastric washing and cold intravenous fluids. Such dramatic intervention is necessary, in part, because of the harmful accelerating effect that fever has on the formation of extracellular fluids in the brain, which can raise cranial pressure.

Fever can also pose a threat during pregnancy. There is evidence that an excessive body core temperature, **hyperthermia,** either from fever or other causes like saunas or heat, may be harmful to the fetus.

Generally, any patient with hyperpyrexia—fever over 41° C (106° F)—requires emergency medical care.

Fever of Undetermined Origin

The decision to treat a fever is made after determining its cause. Failure to identify and treat the underlying pathology will, at best, result in only temporary relief and, at worst, mask a progressive disease. Sometimes health care professionals must deal with **fevers of undetermined origin**

(FUO). In these cases, the fever of at least 38.3° C (101.0° F) continues for at least three weeks while a week's routine diagnostics fails to determine a cause. Careful follow-up eventually identifies the agent in perhaps 88% of cases. Infections (31%) malignant tumors (21%), and collagen-vascular diseases, often autoimmune (14%), are the most common causes of FUO. Another 22% is ultimately attributed to other specific identified causes.

Infections may be either local (e.g., hepatic abscess or abscess beneath the diaphragm or surrounding the gall bladder) or systemic (e.g., widespread "miliary" tuberculosis or infective endocarditis). Viral infections usually produce mild and short-lived fevers. However, Epstein-Barr virus (EBV) and cytomegalovirus (CMV) can produce intense and persistent infections that frustrate easy diagnosis. Fever is extremely common in HIV/AIDS. In this circumstance, the difficulty is in deciding which of the possible organisms is the principal cause of the fever.

FUO is, by definition, a diagnostic challenge. Identification of the cause and possible therapeutic course involves the activities of medical and nursing staff, and a range of medical laboratory and other diagnostic modalities including radiography, nuclear medicine, and ultrasonography, and sometimes frustrating trials with antibiotic and other therapeutic agents. In the 10–15% of patients with FUO that is never successfully diagnosed, most live with their fever, taking NSAIDs for symptomatic relief.

Antipyretic Therapy

Assuming the underlying cause has been identified and appropriate treatment is underway, the question arises, "What about the fever itself?" When the decision to treat the fever is made, the common antipyretic agent is either aspirin (**acetylsalicylic acid** [ASA]) or acetaminophen, which has the same antipyretic potency as aspirin. ASA should not be used with children because of its association with Reyes syndrome, especially in children with flu or measles. These antipyretics create their effects by inhibiting prostaglandin production in the hypothalamus (fig. 3.6), which has the effect of blocking set point elevation and maintaining the set point at nearer normal levels. Note that ASA and most antipyretics reduce the set point only in febrile conditions, probably because it is only in those cases that prostaglandins are the intervening signal. When the same agents are used for their pain suppression effects in nonfebrile patients, no prostaglandins are involved, so no temperature reduction occurs. When fever is the result of damage to the hypothalamus, antipyretic agents are less effective, or ineffective, because the focus of their action is unresponsive to them.

Earlier, we referred to more aggressive physical antipyretic approaches; for example, ice baths. With these therapies there is often a parallel administration of antipyretic drugs to offset the body's attempts to maintain temperature at the altered set point. This might include administering other agents to reduce shivering.

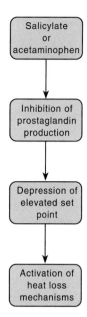

Figure 3.6   Pharmaceutical Intervention in Fever.

Elevated brain temperature is poorly tolerated and produces intense discomfort and irritability for many. A cool hand or cloth on the forehead; a welcome, cooling breeze—all of us know how comforting these can be during a fever. There is good evidence that these are something more than simply local comforts. Cooling applied to the forehead can reduce brain temperatures and ease discomfort seven times more effectively than cooling applied to other body surfaces.

The key to this cooling efficiency lies in the arrangement of some of the cerebral blood vessels. Most of the blood drained from the forehead, and from the triangle around the nose, passes to a complex of veins at the base of the brain called the *cavernous sinus.* Cooling the blood from these areas, either by breathing cooled air or cooling the forehead, significantly reduces the temperature of the blood perfusing the brain. This is because the internal carotid arteries, which provide 70% of the brain's blood, pass through the cavernous sinus on their way to the circle of Willis. This means that blood that has been cooled at forehead and face, and is traveling away from the brain via the cavernous sinus, surrounds warm arterial blood in the internal carotids. This arrangement allows heat to pass to the cooler venous blood, efficiently reducing brain temperature.

 Checkpoint 3.3

To ensure that you have a sound understanding of the difference between hyperthermia and fever, describe and explain the treatment of both. In what ways is the treatment of hypothermia like the treatment for hyperthermia?

Focus on the Mechanism behind the "Cooling Touch"

Blood and brain temperature reductions of 1–2° C have been experimentally achieved by cooling the forehead. This is sufficient to cool the brain below the core body temperature and provide a significant sense of relief. Cooling the body in a febrile person (in the absence of the administration of antipyretics) will induce intense shivering and discomfort. Why doesn't this brain cooling lower the temperature in the hypothalamic thermoregulatory center and thereby trigger the temperature sensors located there to induce the same effect? It may depend upon the nature of the perfusion (and therefore heating) of the hypothalamus. There is evidence that the preoptic nucleus, which *is* cooled in this circumstance through its perfusion by the anterior cerebral artery, is the center that produces responses consistent with overheating: sweating and di-

lation of peripheral and superficial-dermal arterioles. Neither of these occurs, in this case, because the preoptic nucleus is not being signaled of overheating. The posterior hypothalamus, on the other hand, is responsible for responses to cooling (shivering and cutaneous vasoconstriction). But it is perfused by blood from the feverish body via the posterior cerebral arteries. Therefore there is no signal from the posterior hypothalamus for shivering, blanching, and discomfort such as would normally occur in the presence of cooling of the body surfaces of a feverish person in a cold bath. Or it may simply reflect the fact that the hypothalamus receives temperature inputs from sensors in a variety of locations, and discounts or ignores information from one (preoptic nucleus) that is out of synch with the general picture (coming from the peripheral, body trunk, posterior hypothalamus) and the set point elevated by fever.

Case Study

A 10-year-old girl complained of vague periumbilical pain, intermittent nausea, and appetite loss. Her parents had measured her temperature and found it fluctuating between normal and 38.5° C (101.3° F) over a period of five days. The family physician then saw her, and found her temperature to be 37.5° C (99.5° F). Her pharyngeal tonsils were slightly enlarged, with no evidence of pus. No neck or other lymph node enlargement was detected, nor were there any signs or symptoms that suggested an abdominal abnormality. The physician ordered blood counts and a urinalysis, and suggested to the parents that the problem was probably a mild viral infection that would soon pass. The laboratory results were normal, supporting the doctor's assessment.

A week later the parents and child returned. They reported that little had changed: Temperatures remained intermittently elevated, the child ate poorly, and she had added generalized joint pains to her list of complaints. Examination revealed that nothing had changed and that all joints appeared normal, providing little basis for diagnostic insights. Further laboratory tests were ordered: another blood count, as well as a throat culture and determination of the erythrocyte sedimentation rate (ESR). These were again normal, except for a markedly elevated ESR, supporting the tentative diagnosis of infection. The parents were advised to monitor the situation and administer acetaminophen to reduce the fever and joint pain.

After five more days without improvement, the child's abdominal pain intensified and a skin rash developed over her buttocks and legs. Alarmed and frustrated with the inability of their family doctor to solve the problem, they took the child to the hospital emergency room. Examination there revealed a temperature of 38.0° C (100.4° F), normal joints, and diffuse abdominal tenderness. The character of the rash suggested that it was linked to the seepage of blood from small vessels into the skin. A series of lab tests, including cell and platelet counts, an ESR, and a uri-

nalysis were ordered and the parents were advised to continue acetaminophen, pending the results of the tests.

Test results indicated all blood counts to be normal with an elevated ESR. From the pattern and duration of the child's signs and symptoms, a diagnosis of Henoch-Schönlein purpura was finally made. This was suggested by the persistently elevated ESR amid an array of otherwise normal results.

Commentary

In this case, fever of unknown origin and various other signs and symptoms persisted for three weeks before the nature of the disease fully emerged. The natural anticipation that some typical childhood infection was at fault was the reason for the initial examination of the child's tonsils. The absence of any localizing signs in the abdomen indicated that acute appendicitis or other specific abdominal problems were probably not involved.

The ESR is the time it takes for red cells to settle out of a blood sample. Increased times are taken to be caused by a higher plasma fibrinogen content, which makes the plasma more viscous. This is apparently part of a generalized response to stress, such as an infection.

Henoch-Schönlein purpura is relatively rare and seems to involve a defect of the immune system that produces a generalized vasculitis. This irritation and inflammation of the blood vessel linings gives rise to patchy blood loss into the skin (purpura), as well as into the abdomen and joints. The laboratory findings don't point specifically to the disease, but are primarily used to exclude other possible diagnoses. For example, platelet counts were needed to eliminate the possibility of a bone marrow defect, which would reduce platelet numbers and impair blood clotting.

The mild form of this relatively rare disease is usually self-limiting and typically resolves in a few weeks.

Key Concepts

1. Long recognized as linked to disease, fever is not an abnormality of thermoregulation but rather is an upward adjustment of its set point (p. 51).

2. The skin's blood flow and sweat gland activity can be altered to cause loss of heat by way of radiation, convection, conduction, and evaporation or to foster heat retention (pp. 51–53).

3. Negative feedback control serves as the integrating principle in the operation of the thermoregulatory system's sensors, integrator, and effectors (pp. 53–54).

4. Hyperthermia results when essentially normal regulatory mechanisms are overwhelmed by excessive environmental or activity-generated heat or abnormal reactions to chemicals. (pp. 54–55).

5. "Hypothermia" indicates a core temperature below 35° C (95° F). Severe hypothermia will result in death in the absence of appropriate emergency care (pp. 55–56).

6. Endogenous pyrogens induce fever by elevating the temperature set point of the thermoregulation center in the hypothalamus (p. 56).

7. Various injuries or substances (including components of infectious agents) trigger phagocytic cells to release a variety of endogenous pyrogens (pp. 56–58).

8. Fever may enhance host capacities to resist infection or better cope with other forms of injury (p. 58).

9. Extreme or prolonged fever may result from long-standing injury or from a damaged hypothalamus, posing particular risk to individuals with heart disease or stroke (p. 58).

10. Commonly used antipyretic agents work by suppressing the production or action of the chemical mediator that upwardly adjusts the temperature set point in the hypothalamus (p. 59).

REVIEW ACTIVITIES

1. Analyze the data in table 3.1 to verify that they correspond to the statement on page 50 regarding oral temperature variation. Do they agree?

2. On figure 3.3, using a light pencil, add "Increased Body Temperature" at the top, draw an arrow to "Thermoreceptors" and then add up or down arrows to indicate more or less sweat at the skin surface, more or less dermal surface blood, or more or less shivering. Do the directions your arrows point reflect the information on pages 51 to 53? If not, think it over and make appropriate modifications.

3. Lay out a flow chart that relates an EP and its source, prostaglandins, set point change, and the effects of ASA. Have your chart start with an infection and build up a fever. Then indicate how therapeutic intervention might restore normal temperature.

4. Convince yourself that you know how an antipyretic agent like acetaminophen can lower body temperature, and why it works only in fever but not when temperature is normal. A small collection of brief, written phrases will be more convincing than a few vague thoughts.

Chapter

4

Healing

What wound did ever heal but by degrees?

WILLIAM SHAKESPEARE
OTHELLO

Table 4.1 Some Essential Features of the Three Regeneration Categories

Tissue Class	% Cells in Mitosis	Representative Examples
Labile	>1.5	Epithelium, red bone marrow
Stable	<1.5	Gland, fibroblasts
Permanent	0	Neurons, skeletal and cardiac muscle

In response to tissue destruction, the body has a remarkable ability to replace lost tissue—restoring structure, strength, and sometimes function. This restoration process is called **healing,** and it allows us to confront with greater confidence the rather hazardous world in which we live. In coping with injury and its immediate effects, the acute inflammatory response provides a transition between injury and healing. Inflammatory exudate provides an appropriate medium in which healing can occur, and phagocytosis clears the area of injurious agents and debris that would prevent or delay healing. Thus, inflammation and healing are closely related, and there is considerable overlap between the two responses following injury.

COMPONENTS OF THE HEALING PROCESS

The healing process provides for the replacement of lost tissue through the proliferation of adjacent undamaged tissue. Most organs of the body are formed of characteristic functional cells, the **parenchyma,** which are bound together and supported by connective tissue and blood vessels that combine to form the **stroma.** Healing takes one of two forms. When tissue is replaced from parenchyma, the process is called **regeneration.** When fibrous scar tissue fills the gap left by the loss of damaged tissue, it is called **repair.** Because the replacement tissue must have a blood supply, the formation of new vascular channels is an important aspect of healing. Much injury occurs at body surfaces, either internal or external, so it is also important that the protective epithelium be reestablished at damaged surfaces. Now let us consider these four major components of healing— regeneration, repair, revascularization, and surface restoration— in more detail.

Regeneration

Cells lost through injury may be replaced by cell division (**mitosis**) of the adjacent uninjured parenchymal cells. The process continues until the volume of newly formed tissue approximates the volume of tissue that was lost to injury. The new tissue assumes normal functions, and for this reason, regeneration offers the ideal response to tissue loss. However, not all tissues of the body possess the same degree of regenerative capacity. In terms of their regeneration

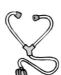

Focus on Tissue Regeneration and Medical Therapy

The differing regeneration capacities of the body tissues have significant implications for medical therapy. For example, much surgical intervention is possible because an incision in the skin or gastrointestinal mucosa is quickly followed by regeneration of the surface. Bone marrow or blood can be donated to someone in need because the tissue surrendered by the donor will soon be replaced. On the other hand, therapy aimed at central nervous system damage can't overcome the essential inability of neurons to regenerate, and will therefore be much less effective, if not impossible.

pattern, there are three types of tissue: labile, stable, and permanent (table 4.1).

The cells of **labile** tissues must divide continually to replace cells that are constantly being depleted by normal processes. Examples of such continuously dividing tissues are the epithelia of the skin, mucous membranes, the linings of various ducts (oviducts, urethra), red bone marrow, and lymphoid tissues. In these tissues, regeneration involves accelerating the normal mitotic rate to replace tissue lost through injury.

Stable tissues are those whose cells divide, but only slowly, beyond adolescence, when normal development is complete. These cells are able to function throughout life, so that high mitosis rates are not normally required. However, stable tissues can increase their mitosis rate when damaged tissue must be replaced. Glands are formed of stable tissue, with the liver demonstrating an especially well-developed regenerative capacity. Other stable cells are osteoblasts, smooth muscle fibers, and vascular endothelium. Regeneration in stable tissues usually proceeds in an orderly fashion, as newly formed cells organize according to a pattern dictated by the remaining undamaged stroma. This pattern of regeneration occurs, for example, in toxic or anoxic injury, to which the parenchymal cells are more sensitive than those of the stroma. When the stroma is also disrupted, the lack of an organizing framework leads to a

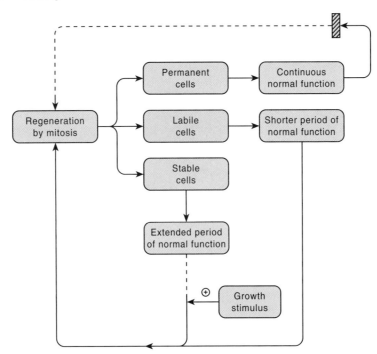

Figure 4.1   **Patterns of Regeneration.** Labile cells engage in a continuing cycle of divisions. Permanent cells are blocked from further mitosis. Stable cells exhibit only low levels of replacement by mitosis but more rapid divisions can be triggered by an appropriate growth stimulus.

disorderly regeneration process. The resulting abnormal tissue configuration typically involves functional deficiency. Regeneration, therefore, can produce a tissue with nearly normal functions or one with some degree of functional loss. In either case, the ability to provide some degree of function restoration is the significant factor in healing by regeneration.

For a sense of perspective on the distinction between labile and stable tissues, consider their relative rates of mitosis in adults. In a labile tissue, the number of actively dividing cells exceeds 1.5% of the total number of its cells. By contrast, in a stable tissue, fewer than 1.5% of the cells are undergoing a division at any given time.

The third pattern of regeneration is demonstrated in tissues that are termed **permanent.** Soon after birth, such tissues lose all mitotic ability, never to regain it. This means that loss of permanent tissue usually results in functional loss. The most common permanent tissues are nervous tissue and cardiac and skeletal muscle. In these tissues, cells lost to injury are replaced by scar tissue.

Figure 4.1 illustrates the cell division patterns in the three categories of regeneration. Labile cells divide continually because they can function for only relatively short periods before they need to be replaced. Once formed, stable cells divide at very low rates. After formation, they carry out their normal specialized activities; for example, gland cells secrete some useful product. Note that stable cells can reenter the division cycle, but only in response to an appropriate growth stimulus. Permanent cells continue to perform their specialized functions for a very long

✓ *Checkpoint 4.1*

From your study of mitosis in previous courses, you may be wondering how the mitotic stage of interphase fits into this business of regeneration. Essentially, interphase is the time between divisions when a cell goes about the everyday business of doing whatever it is specialized to do: protecting surfaces, contracting, secreting, etc. The idea of interphase is used in studying mitosis because the emphasis is on the particulars of the division process and all other cell considerations are less immediately relevant. For our purposes, we need to focus less on the details of division and more on what happens when everyday functions are interrupted by injury: Can a cell be replaced by mitosis of the remaining cells or not?

time. They are unable to divide again and, if lost, they cannot be replaced.

Repair

Healing by repair is the process of laying down fibrous connective tissue to restore the strength and structural integrity of damaged tissues that cannot regenerate. Strong, collagen-rich replacement tissue forms a **scar** by the process of **fibrosis.**

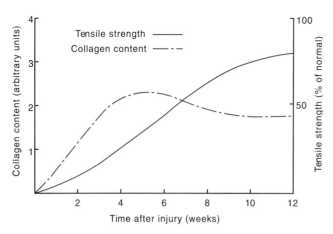

Figure 4.2 **Development of Tensile Strength in a Healing Skin Wound.** After collagen synthesis stops, strength continues to increase because of cross-linking between collagen fibers.

The principal event of fibrosis is the formation of collagen fibers. The **fibroblast** is the cell specialized for this task. It is normally present in the connective tissues of the organ's stroma. Fibroblasts are quite resistant to damage and, hence, are likely to survive at the scene of injury to initiate repair. In addition, migration of fibroblasts from adjacent areas and their mitotic division (remember, they're stable) both contribute to the steady increase in the number of fibroblasts available for collagen formation at the damage site.

The formation of collagen starts with the secretion of its fundamental subunit, **procollagen.** Outside the cell, procollagen molecules are enzymatically altered so that they can link together, end to end, forming long filaments of collagen. These join together to form thicker collagen fibers, which in turn group together to form a collagen fiber bundle. The process can be compared to the production of a thick, strong rope from tiny and individually weak strands of plant fibers or nylon.

Newly formed collagen is quite weak until about five days postinjury. Strength rapidly increases after this, as the fibers cross-link within collagen fiber bundles. Cross-linking occurs by means of chemical bonds that form between adjacent fibers. The resulting bundles have great **tensile strength**—the ability to resist being pulled apart. The tensile strength of collagen is greater than that of most plastics and approaches that of cast iron. After initial formation, collagen steadily increases in strength as cross-links between fibers continue to develop. As strength in individual collagen fiber bundles increases, the scar's strength also develops as a result of a change in the orientation of the bundles within the repair tissue. In response to the tensions and pressures existing at the injury site, the bundles realign along lines of stress to provide greater strength even though no additional collagen has been formed. For these reasons the repair site tensile strength continues to develop even after new collagen production stops (fig. 4.2).

The process of scarring occurs in the **extracellular matrix** (ECM), much of which is secreted by fibroblasts. In

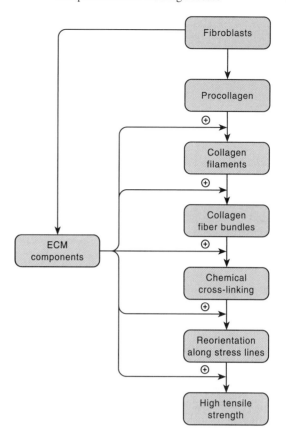

Figure 4.3 **Scarring and the ECM.** Collagen and the development of tensile strength in scar tissue. Note that the fibroblast secretes procollagen and much of the extracellular matrix enhances the process at various stages.

addition to collagen, the ECM contains elastic fibers in a medium formed of complex molecules structured of protein and sugar. The **glycoproteins** consist of protein with a small number of sugar units (up to a dozen or so) joined to it. The **proteoglycans** are the reverse, with a dominant carbohydrate component linked to a smaller protein or protein fragment. (Note that proteoglycans were previously known as *mucopolysaccharides,* a term that you may still encounter in your studies.) Rather than a passive medium into which collagen is secreted, the ECM directly contributes to the formation of a strong and well-anchored scar. The essential points of interaction are indicated in figure 4.3. We will return to other important aspects of the ECM's function later in this chapter and in the context of tumor growth in chapter 6.

When tissue damage occurs, blood usually escapes from disrupted vessels to flood the area. Plasma fibrinogen is converted to fibrin, forming a mesh that entraps blood cells and tissue debris. This gelled mass is called a **clot.** It must be removed before healing can be completed. The elimination of the clot by phagocytosis and its replacement by scar tissue are described as **organization.** The same term is applied to the removal of necrotic debris and its replacement by fibrous connective tissue. For example, because cardiac muscle tissue is permanent, a necrotic region

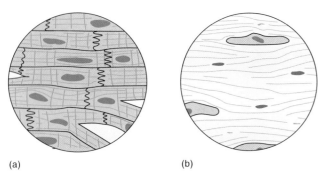

Figure 4.4 **Organization in the Myocardium.** (*a*) A microscopic view of normal myocardial tissue. (*b*) Following prolonged reduction of blood flow, the damaged myocardium has been organized. A few surviving muscle fibers remain scattered in the fibrous scar tissue.

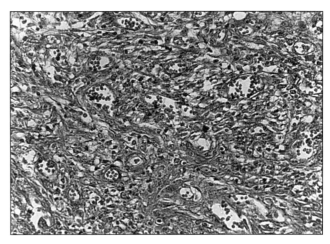

Figure 4.5 **Granulation Tissue.** Shown here are newly formed vessels in recently gelled exudate. Clear spaces are the lumina of these vessels, in which red blood cells can be seen.

of myocardium will be organized by macrophages and fibroblasts to form a scar tissue (fig. 4.4).

Revascularization

Whether regeneration or repair provides the replacement tissue, blood supply to the area must be restored. Initially, blood is required to supply the specialized activities related to healing (e.g., phagocytosis, mitosis, and collagen and ECM synthesis). After formation, the replacement tissue must be provided with a blood supply to meet its normal maintenance requirements. The production of new blood vessels to supply and drain the site of damage is called **revascularization,** or **angiogenesis.** It occurs in the loosely gelled, protein-rich exudate that forms at the damage site. As new blood vessels develop, the exudate takes on a characteristic pink and granular appearance under magnification. For this reason, it is called **granulation tissue** (fig. 4.5). The process of scarring that we described in the previous section, Repair, is actually dependent on the organization of granulation tissue.

Granulation tissue does not in itself provide strength to a healing wound. Rather, it is a transition material in which fibrosis and the completion of revascularization are favored, and in which macrophages complete the clearing of debris and fibrin from the wound site.

In revascularization, new capillaries are formed from intact vessels adjacent to the wound site. Dividing endothelial cells from these vessels project into the damaged area to form endothelial buds, or cords, extending from the parent vessel. Figure 4.6 illustrates the development of new vessels from these early buds. An elongating bud may loop back to reestablish contact with its parent vessel. When this happens, a lumen forms within the bud and merges with the parent vessel to form a continuous, new blood channel. Similarly, buds from different parent vessels may meet, fusing to form a new blood channel joining the previously isolated parent vessels. In some cases, an elongating cord may advance some distance without contacting another vessel or bud. If it extends beyond the point of obtaining

adequate nutrient supply from its parent vessel, the cord degenerates. The resulting cellular debris will be cleared by macrophages still at work in the granulation tissue matrix.

Lumen formation in an advancing vascular bud involves enlargement, mitosis, and vacuolation of its endothelial cells. As they migrate into an injury site, the cells enlarge and then divide. The resulting daughter cells develop cytoplasmic vacuoles that progressively enlarge and then merge with the vacuoles of adjacent cells. With continued fusion of adjacent vacuoles in the advancing cord, the new lumen is formed (fig. 4.7).

Once formed, the new blood vessels are slowly modified. They differentiate and rearrange to form a vascular pattern that more nearly approximates that of normal tissues. Some of the newly formed capillaries acquire the wall structure and flow patterns of arterioles, whereas others are modified to become venules. This means, in effect, that from a common starting structure, an endothelial tube, the different vessel walls are built up from inside out. Of course, some of the initially formed vessels become mature capillaries, but note that at the outset they are leaky and highly permeable, so that much fluid and even intact red blood cells can escape from them. The continued swelling seen at an injury site, even after the inflammatory response has faded, is explained by the higher permeability of the newly formed vessels of the healing wound.

As the process of revascularization continues, lymphatic drainage is reestablished along with blood supply, although this process starts later and is slower than the formation of new blood vessels. New lymphatic capillaries also arise from endothelial buds and ultimately differentiate to form larger lymphatics as necessary. Although the underlying mechanism is unclear, it is interesting that the new endothelial buds of blood capillaries never link up with those originating from a lymphatic vessel.

Final changes in blood vessel distribution involve an overall reduction in vessel numbers and, hence, flow, to the

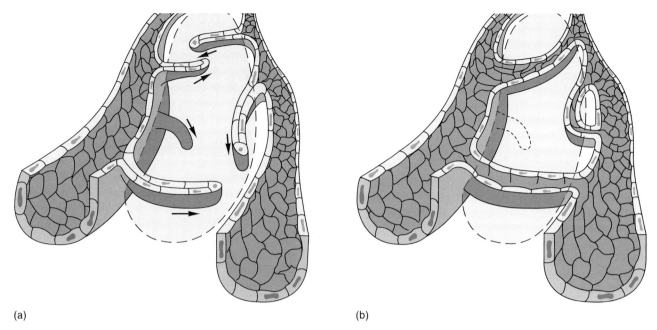

(a)

(b)

Figure 4.6   **Revascularization.** Blood vessels have been destroyed in the region between two undamaged vessels. (*a*) Endothelial buds form from undamaged endothelia. (*b*) Three new channels have formed while an isolated bud degenerates.

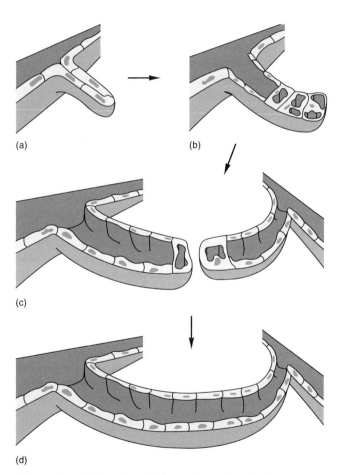

(a)

(b)

(c)

(d)

Figure 4.7   **Mechanism of Revascularization.** (*a*) Bud arises from normal endothelium adjacent to damage site. (*b*) Cells divide, enlarge, and develop vacuoles in their cytoplasm. (*c*) Vacuoles merge to form the lumen of the new vessel. The new channel extends by merging with another advancing bud. (*d*) The new vessel.

healing tissue. The healing region has an initially higher metabolic demand, which is due to the intense activity of cells involved in phagocytosis, fibrosis, and cell division. With healing completed, these activities decline and vascular supply is correspondingly reduced. For this reason, scar tissue initially has a pink appearance whereas an older scar, with its reduced vascular supply, is more pale. As revascularization proceeds over the following months, links to vasomotor neurons develop. This restores nervous control of the new vessels.

Surface Restoration

In healing, it is important to restore the protective epithelium that covers body and organ surfaces. This surface restoration is possible because epithelial tissues are labile and, hence, readily able to supply replacement cells by mitosis.

In surface restoration (fig. 4.8), a zone of active mitosis develops near the wound edge. Newly produced cells, and those originally at the edge of the damaged area, move away from the edge onto the denuded surface. This motion is not the ameboid motion normally used by phagocytes. Instead, it involves a characteristic ruffling of the membrane on the advancing side of the cell, which seems to draw the cell over the surface. In most cases, cell migration occurs on the surface of organizing granulation tissue. In the case of a superficial **abrasion** (scraping injury) of the skin, where only the epidermis is lost, sliding of epithelial cells occurs at the surface of the underlying dermis, which has remained intact.

Epithelial migration continues, with the cells secreting a new basement membrane as they proceed. When the sheets of cells advancing from opposite wound edges meet, they become anchored to the basement membrane and alter

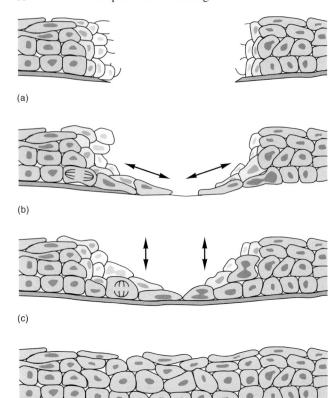

(a)

(b)

(c)

(d)

Figure 4.8 **Surface Restoration.** (*a*) Damaged epithelium. (*b*) Newly formed cells migrate across wound surface. (*c*) On contact, migrating cells alter their plane of division. Basement membrane is restored. (*d*) The restored epithelium.

their plane of division. Newly formed daughter cells now move up, away from the wound surface, rather than along it (fig. 4.8*b,c*). Differentiation accompanies these divisions to replace the specialized cell types that were lost. In skin injuries where parts of hair follicles and sweat glands remain intact, they serve as points from which new epithelial growth can spread. Mitosis in these structures provides new cells that migrate away from the follicle or gland to contribute to restoration of the epithelial surface. Note, however, that damaged follicles and skin glands cannot regenerate to form functional replacements.

 Checkpoint 4.2

In surface restoration and revascularization, new functional replacement tissue is produced by mitosis of undamaged cells. Thus, these two processes are, strictly speaking, special cases of regeneration. We have considered them separately in the context of their special relevance to the healing process.

WOUND HEALING: THE SKIN

Wounds of the skin are the most common type seen by medical personnel. For this reason, and because the skin is easily accessible, the healing of skin wounds has been intensively studied. The studies provide insights into how the various elements of healing contribute to the restoration of structure and function after an injury. Depending on the nature of the wound, healing is said to be either primary or secondary.

Primary Healing

Primary healing, and **healing by first intention** are the terms used to describe healing of an **incision,** or severing wound of the skin. In such a wound, the damage is minimal and the wound edges lie close to each other. This is the type of wound resulting from a surgical incision, where surgical closures—sutures—secure the wound edges, or from a cut where skin tension is low and the wound edges remain close together.

After an incision, bleeding into the narrow gap between the tissue surfaces is quickly followed by clot formation (fig. 4.9*a*). The clot serves not only to limit further blood loss but also to seal the wound from dehydration and invasion by infective microorganisms. It also provides early stabilization of the wound as its fibers bind to elements of the intercellular matrix adjacent to the wound. Once the clot has formed, its surface dries and, together with some tissue debris, produces a **scab.** As in any injury, the acute inflammatory response forms a fluid exudate and delivers numerous inflammatory cells to the scene of the incision. The phagocytes quickly go to work removing tissue debris. They also loosen and digest the clot by releasing enzymes into it. In this process, hemoglobin released from entrapped red cells is broken down to yield pigments that contribute to the early discoloration sometimes seen at the wound site.

By two to three days after injury, granulation tissue is present and both fibroblast activity and revascularization are well under way (fig. 4.9*b,c*). New blood channels form as previously described, and blood supply to the wound is restored. The blood provides nutrients to the fibroblasts, which are secreting new matrix and procollagen. Initially formed collagen fibers assume a vertical orientation at the margins of the wound, but by the sixth postinjury day, responding to normal skin stresses, the fibers align horizontally to bridge the gap and join to the adjacent undamaged dermis, thus binding the opposite sides of the wound together. After six to eight days, the wound is usually strong enough to allow removal of surgical stitches. Collagen continues to form and increases in strength as a dermal scar is formed.

As these events proceed in the dermis, new epithelium forms at the surface of the wound to restore the epidermis. As the migrating cells slide across the wound gap, they liberate enzymes that aid in loosening the clot, which pre-

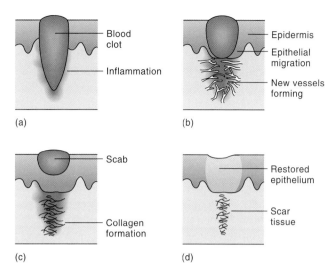

Figure 4.9 **Primary Healing.** (*a*) Incised wound filled by blood clot. (*b*) Surface restoration and revascularization are under way. (*c*) Collagen formation builds strength. (*d*) Healing is complete. Note lack of pigment above scar.

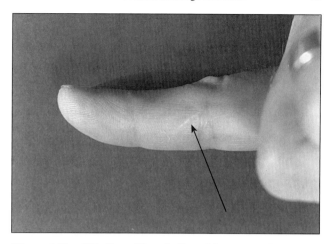

Figure 4.10   **Skin Scar.** The pale line of the scar can be seen at the site of an old skin wound.

The index finger of the senior author showing a more than 20-year-old scar. Note the paleness due to the underlying scar tissue and lack of pigment in the replacement epithelium. The scar's shape matches that of a serrated knife edge that was clumsily driven through the skin while cutting a banana. The senior author is more than 20 years older, but probably not much wiser.

sents an obstacle to their passage. When the opposing sheets of cells meet, after about two days, they differentiate to restore the epidermis that was lost. The newly formed epidermis now completely separates the healing dermis from the overlying scab. Resumption of keratin formation causes loosening of the scab, allowing it to easily separate from the newly restored surface (fig. 4.9*d*). Although disruptive to healing, premature scar removal provides an opportunity to see granulation tissue. It's the pink, probably bleeding bed exposed when its covering of new epidermis is torn away.

As surface restoration proceeds, pigment-producing cells (melanocytes) cannot regenerate and so they are not replaced. Their lack contributes to the lighter color of the epidermis overlying the scar. As we indicated earlier, reduced blood supply in the underlying mature scar tissue also contributes to its paler than normal appearance (fig. 4.10).

By the second postinjury week, inflammatory swelling and phagocytic cell numbers are reduced. Organization of granulation tissue is complete and vascularity is greatly reduced. Fibroblasts continue to proliferate and collagen bundle formation proceeds, producing an increasingly dense and pale scar mass spanning the original incision site.

The strength of fully healed skin, although adequate, never reaches its preinjury level. When the supporting sutures are removed, usually after five to seven days, skin strength is only about 10% of normal. A rapid increase in strength follows over the next two to four weeks as new collagen fibers continue to be laid down. By two months, strength is about one-third of normal, and continued collagen cross-linking yields further increases, to about 70–80% of normal, after three months. This is the maximum strength that the scar will achieve.

Secondary Healing

Secondary healing, or **healing by second intention** (fig. 4.11), is seen in wounds whose edges are not closely apposed. Such wounds are common in skin and in the mucous membranes of the gastrointestinal tract; a duodenal ulcer is an example. These wounds are larger than incised wounds and produce more debris. They also require formation of more granulation tissue as well as a more extensive restoration of the surface. For these reasons, secondary healing takes longer than primary healing. The same mechanisms that operate in primary healing are involved, with two additional distinguishing characteristics. One of these characteristics is the much larger quantity of granulation tissue that is needed to fill the larger wound gap. The second is **wound contraction.**

In secondary healing, soon after granulation tissue forms, the wound edges draw in toward the center. This contraction reduces both the size of the gap that the granulation tissue must fill and the area that new epithelium must restore (fig. 4.12). The mechanism underlying wound contraction depends on a specialized cell found only at secondary healing sites. It is called a **myofibroblast** because it exhibits contractile capability while resembling a fibroblast. The origin of myofibroblasts is unclear. They may be modified fibroblasts that have acquired contractile capacity or they may be derived from **pericytes.** Pericytes normally associate with capillaries and venules and may have the ability to contract.

Myofibroblasts function by first anchoring themselves to other cells or fibrous structures at the margins of the

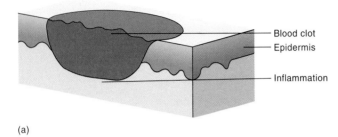

(a)

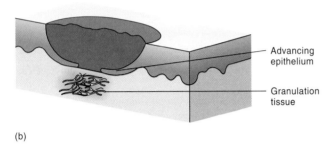

(b)

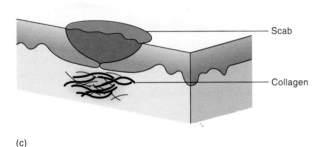

(c)

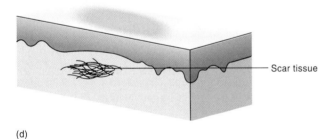

(d)

Figure 4.11   Secondary Healing. (*a*) Blood clot fills wound.
(*b*) Granulation tissue fills gap and surface restoration starts.
(*c*) Granulation tissue is organized. (*d*) Healing is complete.

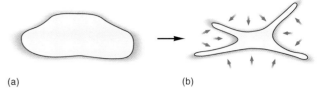

(a)   (b)

Figure 4.12   Wound Contraction. (*a*) Initial wound.
(*b*) Smaller wound after contraction.

wound. They then slowly contract, drawing in the edges to reduce the size of the wound. The process is initiated two or three days postinjury and can continue for weeks, ultimately reducing the size of the wound by 80% or more.

The original shape of a wound is often quite different from its final scar because of a peculiarity of the wound contraction process. The myofibroblasts align themselves so that they contract in a direction at right angles to the wound's margin—that is, toward the geometric center of the wound. As the contraction process draws in the edges, a point is reached where the myofibroblasts can no longer overcome the resistance offered by the crowding of wound edge structures. As contraction proceeds, near edges meet first, then those farther apart come together, with the farthest points on the edges joining last. Because of this, a scar's final configuration can be predicted on the basis of the wound's original shape (fig. 4.13*a*). Note that because edge contact occurs earlier, a circular wound leaves more surface to restore. A model that reflects the wound contraction mechanism that produces differently shaped scars is illustrated in figure 4.13*b,c*. The small insects shown in figure 4.13 represent tissue elements at the wound's edge. Like the wound edges, the insects move in toward the wound's center. As the insects approach each other, their rigid bodies impede progress and movement stops. Depending on their starting position, some are able to move farther in than others. The result is a scar with a shape that differs from the original wound shape. In round wounds, the advancing insects are impeded more quickly than in wounds with straight edges. The result is a larger surface that requires more time to restore.

HEALING: THE MAJOR TISSUES

Connective Tissues

Because of their comparatively limited blood supply, healing in the connective tissues tends to be a prolonged process. Faced with such delayed healing, an injured individual often becomes impatient and prematurely stresses the healing tissue. Re-injury, often more severe than the first injury, often results.

Bone

Osseous tissue has well-developed powers of regeneration. When bone is fractured, new bone tissue is formed and eventually restores the original structure and strength at the point of damage. After the edges of the fractured bone are properly positioned (**reduced**) and movement is restricted by a splint or cast, the healing of the bone proceeds in three stages.

Immediately after a bone fracture, there is bleeding into the gap between the bone ends and, when the periosteum is torn, into the surrounding muscle mass. The first stage of healing involves the early removal of clotted blood, bone fragments, and other tissue debris. As phagocytic cells clear the area, granulation tissue forms and be-

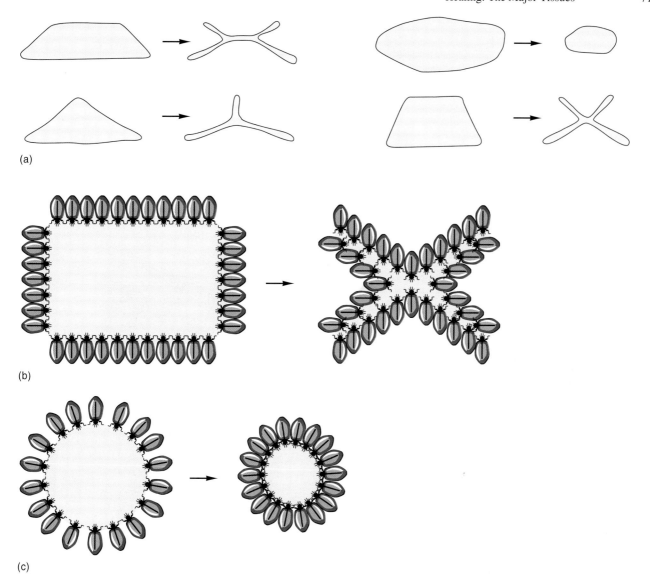

Figure 4.13   **Wound Contraction.** (*a*) The shape of the scar is determined by the movement of the wound's edges toward its center. (*b*) In comparison with (*c*), this rectangular wound will have a smaller scar because the edges are able to draw in more closely. (*c*) A circular wound doesn't fully close because of earlier crowding as the edge nears the center.

comes organized. Its capillaries develop from undamaged vessels in adjacent tissues. Also in this initial stage of healing, **osteoblasts** (bone-forming cells) held in reserve in the periosteum and endosteum are activated. They migrate to the fracture site to initiate the second stage of the process.

Early in the second stage of bone healing, osteoblasts lay down heavy deposits of dense collagen and form some cartilage as well. The resulting fibrocartilaginous mass spans the break and provides early stabilization of the fracture. This tissue is called **osteoid,** or **soft callus.** It is soon ossified by osteoblasts to form a loosely organized mass of woven bone that resembles cancellous bone (spongy bone). This **hard callus** is structurally weak and, because its production is excessive, there is local enlargement at the fracture site.

The third stage involves the remodeling of the hard callus to restore the characteristic architecture of normal bone. The remodeling is accomplished jointly by osteoblasts and **osteoclasts** (bone-dissolving cells). These cells build up and break down the hard callus, modeling the bone to finally restore its normal structure. Restoration of the overlying periosteum accompanies that of the bone (fig. 4.14).

The first stage of healing occurs in the four to five days following fracture. The second stage follows over the next three weeks, with final remodeling sometimes continuing over many months or even years. During this extended period of remodeling, the bone is strong enough to accommodate normal loading stresses and continued remodeling of the bone goes unnoticed.

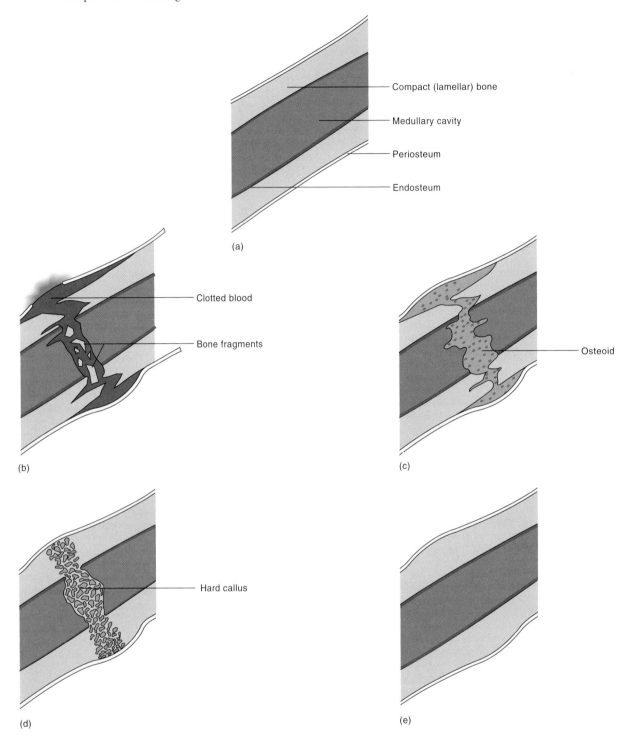

Figure 4.14   **Bone Healing.** (*a*) Section through the intact bone. (*b*) Following the fracture, clotted blood and bone fragments are cleared by phagocytes. (*c*) and (*d*) Formation of callus from osteoid. (*e*) Modeling of hard callus restores bone to near normal.

Tendon/Ligament

Regeneration of tendon and ligament is usually successful in injuries where relatively regular edges can be closely approximated and tightly sutured. Fibroblasts can then produce densely packed collagen bundles that span the damage site to restore tensile strength. If the edges of the damaged tissue are not held tightly together, or if a crushing injury produces irregular, roughened surfaces, scar tissue forms in the intervening spaces. The result is a weaker union with less tensile strength and reduced functional capacity.

Cartilage

When damaged, cartilage heals by fibrous repair. Scar tissue is supplied by fibroblasts from the protective sheet of perichondrium that covers cartilage surfaces. The scarring that follows cartilage damage can produce some loss of function, a persistent complication for those who suffer athletic and fitness-related injuries.

Adipose Tissue

Although the cells of adipose tissue cannot themselves undergo mitosis, their precursor cells are widely distributed and these cells are able to differentiate to produce new replacement tissue.

Epithelial Tissues

As we have seen, some epithelia are labile and, hence, readily able to regenerate. This characteristic is of great value in restoring protection at body surfaces, which are frequently subjected to injury. As previously described, epithelial cells reestablish the covering over a damaged surface by regenerating new cells that move across the gap in the tissue. This process occurs not only in the skin, but in mucous membranes and many other epithelial surfaces. An exception is the epithelium of respiratory surfaces in the adult. In these tissues, regeneration can take place if the damage to the epithelium is superficial, but not if the basement membrane and underlying intercellular matrix are disrupted. In the latter case, proliferating fibroblasts repair the damage by forming scar tissue.

Glandular Tissues

Most glands are formed of stable tissue. When they are damaged, the lost cells are readily replaced by new growth of functional tissue. The liver is notable in having prodigious powers of regeneration. Animal experiments indicate complete restoration of lost tissue when as much as 90% of the liver is surgically removed. Similar levels of regeneration are likely in humans. When tissue damage is extensive, however, the arrangement of the newly regenerated tissue may vary somewhat from the normal, causing some functional loss. In the kidney, cells of the nephron tubule are able to regenerate if damaged. However, no replacement of glomerular or Bowman's capsule cells is possible. When nephrons are lost, the remaining tubules compensate by hypertrophy.

In liver and kidney, severe injury sustained over an extended period can destroy both parenchymal cells, their supporting stroma, and ECM. In such cases, the lost tissue is replaced by a smaller volume of dense scar tissue. The contracted scar masses draw inward, producing a pattern of irregular surface depressions. The characteristic appearance of the kidney in chronic glomerulonephritis and that of the liver in hepatic cirrhosis are good examples (fig. 4.15).

There are some exceptions to the usual pattern of regeneration in glandular tissue. The parathyroid glands possess only minimal regenerative capacity. Similarly, tissues of the adrenal medulla and the posterior pituitary gland are unable to produce new functional cells when damaged. This inability seems related to their derivation from nervous tissue, which is permanent.

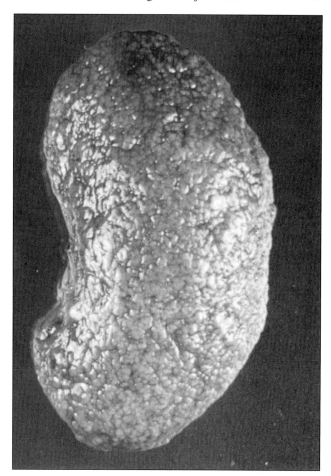

Figure 4.15   **Chronic Glomerulonephritis.** Long-term damage followed by scarring has produced the roughened surface of this kidney.

 Checkpoint 4.3

A great deal of current medical activity is based on the underlying issue of the healing capacity of our tissues. Much medical intervention is simply a matter of assessing and then stabilizing the situation until healing can occur—easing pain, preventing blood loss, reducing fractures, etc. Think of the enormous array of surgical interventions in which tissues are intentionally cut through for purposes of repair or removal. The entire approach depends utterly on the severed tissues being able to heal. Note as well how medical practice continues to grapple with the problems presented by damage to permanent tissues: the inability of myocardium to regenerate following heart attack and the lack of neuronal regeneration following stroke or CNS traumatic injury.

Nervous Tissues

Since neurons are permanent cells, no mitosis is possible after birth. In nervous tissue, damaged neurons are replaced by **gliosis**—the proliferation of **neuroglia.** These cells are abundant in nervous tissue and provide support, phagocytosis, and repair functions that white blood cells and fibroblasts perform in other tissues. In the central nervous system, if neuron cell bodies remain intact, some initial regeneration of axons may occur. But after 10 to 14 days, the proliferating glial cells form a scarlike mass that blocks any further growth of the damaged axons. Thus, no function can be restored by this partial and inadequate axon regeneration.

In the peripheral nervous system, when only part of a myelinated neuron process is lost through damage, the lost portion can regenerate if the supporting connective tissue and **Schwann cells** (a type of glial cell) remain intact along the original path of the neuron process. This is often the case because the Schwann cell is more resistant to injury than is the neuron process. After injury, the process distal to the point of injury degenerates, and the resulting debris is removed by macrophages (fig. 4.16a). Regeneration replaces any Schwann cells lost at the injury site (fig. 4.16b). Next, a tuft of newly formed sprouts grows out from the proximal end of the neuron process (fig. 4.16c). One of these finds its way into the tube of connective tissue and continues to grow along the tube until it reaches the point served by the original process (fig. 4.16d). The remaining sprouts are lost, and myelination of the newly formed process follows. This pattern of regeneration is relatively slow and may take weeks to complete. It cannot replace any specialized sensory receptors at the ends of sensory neuron dendrites. The result is some loss of sensation even though motor function is restored. When a nerve's connective tissue is lost through injury, the necessary guidance for the growth of new sprouts is lacking and the regeneration of the axon or dendrite does not occur. When an entire nerve is severed, regeneration of its neuron processes may occur if the opposite ends of the nerve are carefully aligned and promptly sutured. If the nerve ends remain separated, the distal processes degenerate. At the proximal end, numerous regenerating processes emerge from the severed nerve stump. These penetrate into the new scar tissue formed by fibroblasts from the nerve's fibrous stroma. The result is a disorganized tangle of axons and scar tissue called a **traumatic neuroma,** which is typically quite painful.

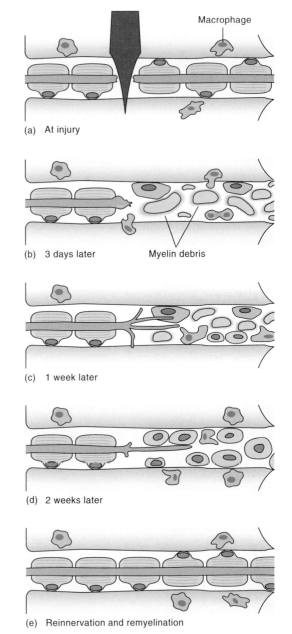

Figure 4.16   **Regeneration of a Neuron Process.** (*a*) Severing injury. (*b*) Debris is cleared by phagocytosis and undamaged Schwann cells proliferate. (*c*) Buds emerge from stump of axon. (*d*) A single bud extends along the cylinder of Schwann cells. Other buds have degenerated. (*e*) Myelin sheath restored and regeneration complete.

Muscle Tissues

Skeletal muscle and cardiac muscle are permanent tissues. When they are lost, healing is accomplished through fibrous repair. As we have seen, this process implies loss of function, in this case a decline in the contractile strength of the injured muscle. However, muscle tissue possesses a highly developed compensation capability. Its cells can increase in size and strength. This hypertrophy results in an increased muscle mass in response to demand. Weightlifters produce no new cells as their training proceeds; rather, existing cells hypertrophy. Not only can skeletal muscle and the muscle of the heart restore their strength to preinjury levels, but they can increase their strength to levels higher than any previously achieved. Therefore, a patient whose heart has been damaged need not become an invalid. Full recovery is possible if hypertrophy is cautiously induced by presenting the myocardium with a gradually increasing workload.

Like neurons, muscle fibers can regenerate a portion of their structure under certain circumstances. In the case of damage from a crushing injury, the muscle's stroma remains largely intact. The sheaths of connective tissue remain to act as guides for the growth of the ends of the damaged muscle fibers. On the other hand, when a severing injury cuts through the supporting stroma, the muscle fibers draw back from the point of injury. With loss of stromal guidance the potential for regeneration is lost.

In the case of smooth muscle tissue, there are indications that some regeneration does occur. Mitotic capability is quite limited, however, and fibrous repair is common. A notable exception is the wall of the uterus, which has the capacity for significant cell division. During pregnancy, some cells enlarge while others undergo mitosis to produce new tissue. Of course, this is not a response to injury. It is a normal response that anticipates the extra strength required for delivery of an infant. After delivery of the child, the uterine tissue that is no longer required is reduced by means of apoptosis (chapter 1).

COMPLICATIONS OF HEALING

The healing process occasionally goes astray, so that healing is inadequate, is delayed, or has other undesirable consequences. The following are the most common complications of healing.

Contracture

When damage is extensive, newly formed collagen demonstrates an exaggerated wound contraction response as it matures. This process is called **contracture.** It can be so pronounced that significant tissue distortion results. For example, in widespread skin burns, contracture can cause substantial disfiguration (fig. 4.17). The change from normal appearance can have significant psychological impact, especially when the face is involved. Contracture may also limit mobility. For example, contracture following burns of the skin of the neck may limit motion of the head. When the skin of the hand is involved, the motion of wrist and finger joints can be restricted. Inceased incidence of contracture occurs in the skin of the palms, soles, and anterior thorax.

In repair of damage to the walls of tubular organs, contracture presents another type of problem. As the excessive contraction proceeds, it produces a narrowing or **stricture** in the lumen of the organ. The consequences can be serious because normal motion of the organ contents is slowed or even stopped (stasis). In the intestine, a stoppage can lead to infection, which can in turn lead to perforation of the wall and the rapid spread of infection throughout the abdomen. Stricture of the ureter will also predispose to infection, which can affect the kidney, and stricture of the Fallopian tube can lead to sterility. Much infertility in females is the result of the stricture that follows venereal disease damage to the oviducts.

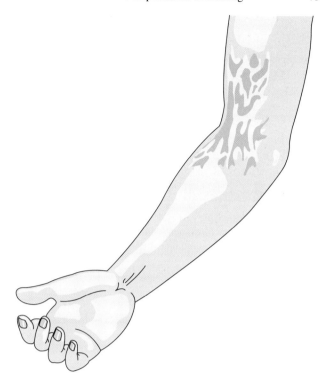

Figure 4.17 **Contracture.** Following a skin burn, contracture may produce distortion of body contours and may restrict motion of joints.

Adhesions

Another complication of healing can arise as a result of the organization of inflammatory exudate between serous membranes. The resulting repair produces a firm union of the two membranes, which normally move freely against each other. Such joining of serous membranes is called an **adhesion.** The major effect of adhesions is the restriction of movement in structures that must move freely. In injury or surgical intervention involving the heart, lungs, or most abdominal organs, the possibility of developing adhesions is always present. After abdominal or thoracic surgery, it is relatively common for a patient to be readmitted to the hospital because of problems related to adhesions (fig 4.18).

Dehiscence

Dehiscence is the breaking open of a healing wound. The essential cause is pressure applied to the healing tissues, which interferes with the development of normal strength. The abdominal wall is the most common site of dehiscent wounds because of the relatively high pressure in the abdomen. Following abdominal surgery, both skin and abdominal musculature are sutured and healing is uncomplicated, but if sutures are faulty or are removed prematurely, abdominal pressure is fully applied to the healing site, interfering with the formation of fully mature collagen. The result is a weekend abdominal wall that may rupture. Paroxysms (acute, violent episodes) of coughing, vomiting,

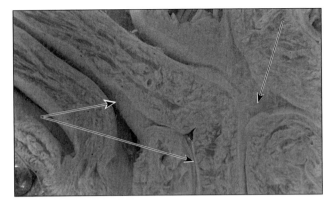

Figure 4.18   Adhesions. Arrows at left show free intestinal surfaces, which allow movement without restriction. Arrow at right shows adhesion binding intestinal surfaces and restricting normal movements.

These adhesions developed in the bowel of an elderly woman following rupture of her diseased colon. She had been convalescing in the hospital for a fractured hip, when a weak point in her colon ruptured, causing the peritonitis that led to her death. The adhesions had formed as the irritated peritoneal sheets were undergoing repair, but extensive damage to various abdominal structures overwhelmed her weakened defenses and she died.

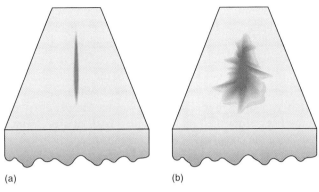

Figure 4.19   Keloid Formation. (*a*) A section of skin in which an incision is healing normally. (*b*) The irregular piling up of excessive scar tissue forms the keloid.

or diarrhea can greatly raise abdominal pressure and increase the chances that the wound will burst. Another factor that may contribute to dehiscence is any compromise of collagen formation such as a deficiency of vitamin C would cause, (see the Requirements for Healing section).

Dehiscence presents two principal risks. One is the exposure of the abdominal contents to infection as the wound breaks open. The second is that a loop of intestine will be squeezed into the open wound, so that its blood supply is threatened as its blood vessels are compressed at the point of the healing wound's rupture. Loss of blood supply may be followed by gangrenous necrosis. The displacement of an organ from its normal body cavity position is called **herniation.** Dehiscence following abdominal surgery may produce an incisional hernia.

Keloids

Keloids are irregular masses of scar tissue that protrude from the surface of the skin. They result from the overproduction of dermal collagen during healing. Keloids usually arise on the upper body and are seen more frequently in blacks in Africa and the Caribbean, especially among young women. If disfiguring, they may be surgically removed, but they have a tendency to recur after removal (fig. 4.19).

Keloid formation may be due to excessive release of a particular growth factor known to promote fibroblast proliferation. This factor, TGF-β (transforming growth factor beta), is secreted by macrophages and platelets at the scene of damage. Even the secretion of normal amounts of TGF-β may produce keloids in individuals who are highly sensitive to its effects.

Proud Flesh

The overproduction of granulation tissue is called **proud flesh.** It presents a problem in that the excess granulation tissue can protrude from the wound to interfere with surface restoration. This condition, is sometimes referred to as exuberant granulations.

Suture Complications

Minor punctures of the skin heal quickly and with minimal scar tissue formation. Thus, puncture scars from therapeutic injections or from tissue biopsies tend to be of little consequence. However, in healing of a surgical incision, a minor complication can arise because of the stitching used to secure the wound edges. At the surface, where the suture material enters the skin, the epithelium is interrupted. This condition stimulates epithelial mitosis and migration, but the cells cannot spread across the intervening suture material. Instead, they migrate into the dermis along the suture channel. Later, when the stitches are removed, most of the new epithelium is carried off with the suture material and the surface regenerates normally. In some cases, however, keratin from the epithelium, which is normally restricted to the surface of the skin, is sealed within the suture tract deep in the dermis. Its presence causes a pronounced fibrosis response in the dermis. This explains the somewhat more prominent scarring seen at the points where sutures have passed through the skin.

Therapy

Some therapy can have an inhibitory effect on healing. For example, anticancer therapy using radiation or chemicals, or both, suppresses tumor cell division, but can also suppress the mitosis needed for normal healing. Various anti-inflammatory drugs or immune system suppressants interfere with processes important to healing, such as protein synthesis, wound contraction, and regeneration of new epithelium. Corticosteroid preparations used to limit inflammation can also interfere with healing, perhaps by interfering with the migration of fibroblasts to injury sites. Another problem is the immune system suppression that corticosteroids can produce. This can increase the risk of infection at the wound site.

REQUIREMENTS FOR HEALING

Clearance of Debris

For optimal healing to occur, the scene of damage must be cleared of debris, tissue remnants, pus, and any extraneous matter—for example, sand, small pieces of glass, or bullet fragments. Inability to remove such material will increase the likelihood of infection and delay and complicate the healing process.

Immobility

Movement near wound edges delays or prevents healing because it interferes with the joining of tissues across the damaged area. For example, consider what happens with bone fractures that have not been immobilized. In this case, constant motion prevents normal calcification, so that a fibrocartilaginous mass resembling osteoid is formed and maintained without becoming ossified. This condition is called **non-union** or **fibrous union.** Obviously, the replacement tissue in this case is much weaker than the original tissue. Immobility is also especially important in tendon and nerve regeneration, where accurate alignment of newly forming structures is critical.

Blood Supply

Adequate blood flow is required for the delivery of oxygen and nutrients to the area that must be healed. Many of the healing problems so commonly seen in the elderly are the result of age-related circulation deficiencies. For example, even with adequate immobilization, fibrous union often occurs in the healing of hip fractures of older persons. In diabetics, even trivial peripheral skin injuries may heal poorly because of the faulty circulation associated with the disease.

Nutrients

Specific nutrient requirements for healing are relatively few. Although much new protein is synthesized during healing, dietary protein deficiency will depress the healing response only if prolonged. The amino acid methionine is required for normal healing. This might seem surprising in that this amino acid does not occur in collagen. It is, however, required for the production of proteoglycans in forming new extracellular matrix. Zinc is also required for normal healing. Although its function is not clearly understood, it is known to be required for the normal function of several enzymes.

In forming collagen, vitamin C (**ascorbic acid**) is required for the conversion of an amino acid in the production of procollagen. Without this conversion step, fibro-

Table 4.2	Factors that Stimulate or Inhibit Various Components of the Healing Process

Name	Standard Designation
Epidermal growth factor	EGF
Transforming growth factor	TGF-β*
Platelet-derived growth factor	PDGF
Fibroblast growth factors	FGFs
Interferon alpha	INF-α*
Interleukin-1	IL-1
Tumor necrosis factor	TNF
Vascular endothelial growth factor	VEGF

*Inhibition is the dominant effect.

blasts cannot secrete procollagen. Another essential nutrient is copper. It is a component of the enzyme that facilitates the cross-linking upon which collagen fiber bundles depend for added strength. Deficiencies of either vitamin C or copper will result in the formation of weakened scars.

CONTROL AND REGULATION OF HEALING

The processes that contribute to normal healing are closely regulated. When injury occurs, cells begin to divide to form replacement tissue. When sufficient tissue is formed, cell division stops. New growth is orderly and is limited to the replacement of lost tissue only.

There is much about the control of the healing process that is not well understood, but an array of chemical control factors is being carefully studied. These can be identified in the plasma and at healing sites. They have the ability to promote and inhibit many of the processes known to be involved in healing. Generally, two broad categories are recognized: **growth factors,** which promote growth, and **growth inhibitors,** with the opposite effect. These widely distributed substances regulate the processes vital to normal healing: migration of fibroblasts and epithelial cells, formation of new blood vessels, mitosis, and collagen formation. The principal growth factors are listed in table 4.2.

Many critical aspects of healing depend on specific cell interactions with the extracellular matrix. Surface receptors on fibroblasts, and on other cells involved in healing, enable them to bind to elements of the complex intercellular material. Interactions with the matrix affect cell proliferation and migration, as well as differentiation. Thus, rather than being an inert filler, the extracellular matrix has a specific role in regulating regeneration and repair. This is the likely explanation for the scarring that follows the destruction of the extracellular matrix in stable tissues. Although remaining cells are able to undergo mitosis, they

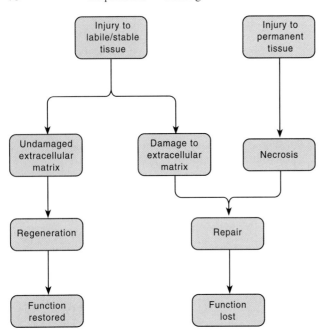

Figure 4.20   Role of the Extracellular Matrix in Determining Functional Loss.

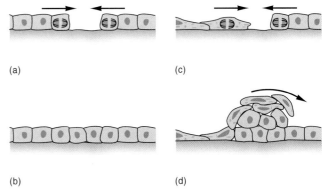

Figure 4.21   Contact Inhibition. (*a*) Similar cells reproduce and move over surface. (*b*) When they come into contact, mitosis stops. (*c*) Different cell types approach each other. (*d*) When these come into contact, no inhibition results.

fail to do so for lack of regulatory input from extracellular matrix interactions. Healing then proceeds by repair. When the extracellular matrix is undamaged, regeneration proceeds normally (fig. 4.20). An example is the liver, which can readily regenerate after an hepatitis A infection. The virus affects hepatocytes only, leaving the stroma and ECM intact to support regeneration. However, in the case of liver damage caused by parasites, cells and stroma are both damaged so that healing can only proceed by fibrous repair. In another case, lung airway epithelium readily regenerates after an acute viral infection because damage is confined to the airway's surface. When long-term lung accumulation of silica crystals produces silicosis, lung tissue stroma, ECM, and epithelial basement membranes are all destroyed. As a result, no regeneration occurs and fibrosis and loss of function follow.

Physical contact between cells is a factor that seems to regulate the mitosis of epithelium. When dividing cells

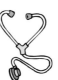

Focus on Growth Factor Therapy

Study of the factors that control healing has the potential for great therapeutic benefit. For example, knowledge of the factors that stimulate the healing process would speed the recovery of burn victims and could reduce the length of postsurgical hospitalization. Several preparations containing various tissue growth factors are currently being studied to assess their therapeutic potential. Unfortunately, the wide array of side effects found in these early trials is likely to delay the use of growth factors as therapeutic agents.

contact each other, mitosis stops. This phenomenon, called **contact inhibition** (fig. 4.21), can be demonstrated by cells grown in laboratory cultures. On surfaces, cells starting from two points will divide and migrate until the two sheets of cells meet. Following contact, their mitosis rate drops markedly. Note, however, that this response occurs only when the advancing sheets of cells are of the same tissue. Contact with other tissues or nonliving barriers does not affect the mitosis rate.

Case Study

A 27-year-old woman came to her general practitioner because of mild but persistent pain in her lower abdomen. A pelvic examination revealed a mildly purulent cervical discharge. Samples for culture were obtained. She was otherwise healthy, and no indications of other problems were evident. The woman was sexually active, not using birth control pills, and was not pregnant. When the culture results were returned, they indicated the presence of *Chlamydia trachomatis,* and the physician recalled the patient to begin therapy.

She could not at first be reached, but returned ten days later, explaining she had been forced to leave town on short notice to attend a business meeting for another manager who had been in an auto accident. She was concerned because while away she had developed a fever and her lower abdominal discomfort had worsened. These problems had no sooner subsided than another emerged. For the previous three days she had been experiencing more pronounced pain in her right upper abdominal quadrant. She explained that it was especially severe when taking a deep breath. On examination, her right upper quadrant was quite tender but she seemed otherwise normal. She had no other complaints, and verified that her upper quadrant pain wasn't aggravated by fatty meals. She was admitted for an exploratory laparoscopy, and tetracycline antibiotic therapy was started.

The exploration of the abdomen revealed some postinflammatory adhesions at the openings of the right Fallopian tube. Also present were elongated strands of fibrous adhesions joining the abdominal wall and the surface of the liver. These were surgically cleared, as were the adhesions at the Fallopian tubes.

Recovery from the procedure was uneventful. The patient was released with instructions to return for monitoring over the next three weeks. She was advised that the adhesions at the opening of the Fallopian tube might reduce the chances of her becoming pregnant. She was also advised to discuss the situation with her sexual partner and to encourage him to get treatment since he was the likely source of her infection. Males are typically asymptomatic when carrying *C. trachomatis* and are unlikely to be aware of their infectious state.

Commentary

Many cases of salpingitis (inflammation of the Fallopian tubes) arise as the result of infection that is sexually transmitted, often producing only mild symptoms. *Chlamydia trachomatis* is increasingly involved, but tetracycline therapy is quite effective in dealing with this organism. The less common complication seen in this case is the spread of the organisms, by blood, lymph, or over connecting peritoneal surfaces, to reach the peritoneal capsule of the liver. The resulting inflammation produces a condition known as **perihepatitis,** or the **Fitz Hugh-Curtis syndrome.** The irritated liver capsule initially develops a fibrinous surface exudate, which later forms characteristic "violin string" adhesions to the anterior abdominal wall, producing pain as respiratory or other motion applies tension to the liver surface.

The low probability that a gall bladder problem was causing abdominal pain in a woman of this young age was supported by the lack of any increased discomfort after a fatty meal that would trigger gall bladder contraction. The possibility that other potentially more serious problems could involve similar signs and symptoms made the laparoscopy decision a sound one. The fact that this patient was not using birth control pills was a factor to consider given the increased incidence of gall bladder problems in users of the "pill."

The antibiotic therapy was successful and the fact that only one Fallopian tube had been involved decreased the chance that fertility had been impaired.

Key Concepts

1. Following injury and the inflammatory response, the healing process replaces lost tissue (p. 63).

2. Healing involves four components that combine to restore lost parenchyma, replace stroma, and reestablish blood supply and surface integrity (p. 63).

3. The ability of the healing process to restore function in the face of tissue loss is determined by the differing regenerative capacities of the body tissues (pp. 63–64).

4. Scarring is the result of the repair process, which employs fibroblasts to lay down high-tensile-strength collagen as a strong replacement tissue (pp. 64–65).

5. The healing process, and the replacement tissue it forms, are both dependent on the prompt restoration of blood supply via revascularization, which forms new flow channels that are derived from undamaged vessels adjacent to the injury site (pp. 66–67).

6. Damage at internal and external surfaces is restored by mitosis of undamaged cells at the wound edges (pp. 67–68).

7. Primary and secondary healing are different patterns of wound healing that are elicited as a function of wound size and the distance between the wound's opposite edges (pp. 68–69).

8. Patterns of healing among the various tissues and organs differ on the basis of several factors, such as tissue regenerative capacity, basement membrane restoration, and the status of the intercellular matrix (pp. 70–75).

9. Healing may be complicated by various derangements that limit normal motion of joints or internal organs, interfere with the healing process itself, allow a wound to reopen, or produce significant skin irregularities (pp. 75–77).

10. For healing to proceed optimally, various physical, vascular, and nutrient requirements must be met (p. 77).

11. The precise control required for the initiation, orderly development, and appropriate cessation of the healing response is provided by a complex of closely interrelated chemical mediators and interactions with the intercellular matrix (pp. 77–78).

REVIEW ACTIVITIES

1. Link the following scrambled elements in a flow chart that reflects the sequence of events in revascularization. Pages 66–67 should be your guide.

   Bud degenerates

   Arteriole formation

   Lumen formation

   Advancing buds contact

   Differentiation of new capillaries

   New capillaries formed

   Buds emerge from intact vessels

   Lymphatic vessel formation

   Venule formation

   No bud contact

2. Study figure 24.2. Make a rough sketch or tracing to show what the damaged skin in the diagram would look like after completion of healing. Which skin structures will you leave out of your sketch? Pages 69–70 have the answer if you need it.

3. Locate a few of your own skin scars. Study the shape of each and relate it to the original wound shape. (Don't forget your scalp. Hair can hide some fascinating scars.) Analyze how wound contraction produced the transition from the original to the final shape. A water-soluble marker pen might be useful in marking the original wound edges and tracing their movements. Check with a friend so that you can verify each other's assessments. Figures 4.12 and 4.13 may be helpful in this exercise.

4. Be certain that you understand the use of the term *organization* in the context of healing. To help, jot down its essential definition and then list how it applies to scarring, primary healing, and adhesion formation. If unsure, check pages 65, 68–69, and 75.

5. In the section on how therapy can interfere with healing (p. 76), note the references to the effects of corticosteroids and NSAIDs. Now locate the flow chart in chapter 2 that indicates specific points at which those therapeutic agents produce their effect.

6. Two of the key concepts in this chapter refer to the role of the intercellular matrix in healing. Find three flow charts in this chapter that specifically refer to this role (you may need to consult the legend to identify one of them). Reflect on the content of the flow charts.

Diseases of Immunity

Chapter

5

Half the secret of resistance is cleanliness, the other half is dirtiness.

ANONYMOUS

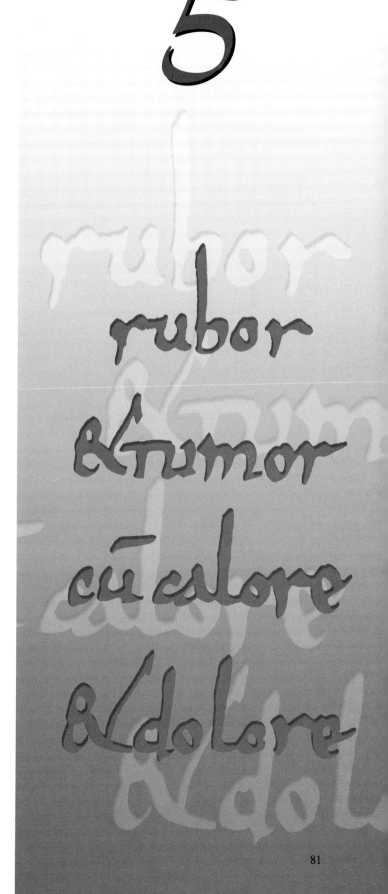

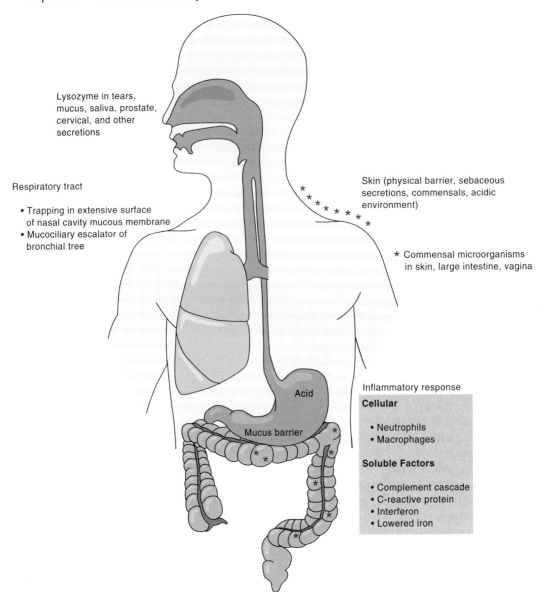

Lysozyme in tears,
mucus, saliva, prostate,
cervical, and other
secretions

Respiratory tract

- Trapping in extensive surface
  of nasal cavity mucous membrane
- Mucociliary escalator of
  bronchial tree

Skin (physical barrier, sebaceous
secretions, commensals, acidic
environment)

* Commensal microorganisms
  in skin, large intestine, vagina

Acid

Mucus barrier

Inflammatory response

Cellular

- Neutrophils
- Macrophages

Soluble Factors

- Complement cascade
- C-reactive protein
- Interferon
- Lowered iron

Figure 5.1   **Summary of Mechanisms of Nonspecific Defense.**

IMMUNITY

A casual glance at a magazine or a few hours of TV would convince a visitor from another planet that North Americans are obsessed with sterilizing, deodorizing, sanitizing—in a word, cleanliness. Indeed, basic modern sanitation preserves us from many of the plagues that carried away one-third of the population of medieval Europe. The defensive mechanisms described in chapters 2 and 3 (and outlined in figure 5.1 and table 5.1) are assailed by many of the microorganisms to which we are exposed. It makes sense that the more times these defenses are breached, the more likely we are to be colonized by one of these invading microorganisms. Figure 5.1 and table 5.1 concentrate on antimicrobial defense mechanisms that are always in place or that can be rapidly mobilized, and that require no previous contact with a specific microorganism to be effective in neutralizing it. They are often collectively termed natural

nonspecific defenses or **innate** or **nonspecific immunity.** (The Latin term *immunitas* means "freedom from public service." It was a special honor bestowed upon highly regarded individuals, exempting them from the usual burdens of citizenship in Rome such as taxes and military service.) In this scheme we have included so-called barrier defenses that are designed to block, inactivate, or destroy pathogens (disease producers) before they can enter the body. So, in terms of "cleanliness," barriers prevent entry of organisms, and the complement cascade, neutrophils, macrophages, and so on clean up any organisms that breach the barriers.

Fundamentals of Specific Immunity

In contrast to our innate defenses against infection, there is another kind of resistance that is acquired after birth. It is here that dirtiness has its place. A population's lack of exposure to a microorganism might make first contact devas-

Table 5.1	Essential Elements of Nonspecific Defenses

Physical Barriers

Skin
Mucous membranes: GI, respiratory, genitourinary tracts
Mucociliary blanket of respiratory passages
Surface flushing: tears, urine, GI contents

Antibacterial Agents

Acidity of stomach, skin, urinary tract, vagina
Various secretions; e.g., lysozyme in tears
Rapidity of pH change in GI tract

Commensal Microorganisms

Growth provides an environment that is inhospitable to competing, potentially pathogenic, organisms

Ongoing Phagocytosis

Phagocytic cells routinely destroy threatening organisms

Inflammatory Response

Destruction and phagocytosis by neutrophils, macrophages, and natural killer cells
Direct and indirect pathogen destruction by the complement cascade
Promotion of phagocytosis by C-reactive protein
Resistance to viral infection mediated by interferon

Fever

Temperature elevation enhances phagocytosis
Inhibition of mitosis by iron depletion

tating. A clear example is the experience of native North Americans, whose first contact with measles and smallpox came with the European explorers, traders, and settlers. This example tells us several things about acquired immunity. First, it is specific: Native Americans coped quite effectively with the spectrum of diseases they had experienced before contact with Europeans. They were probably, by and large, healthier than the tattered sailors who gladly left their ships to come ashore and mingle, but they were devastated by the diseases that the sailors carried because they'd had no previous exposure to them. The specific nature of their vulnerability implies the second feature of acquired immunity: the immune system's capacity to recognize a microorganism. A third feature is the system's more effective response to second and subsequent exposures to the same pathogen. This demonstrates learning, and the long-term retention of the improved response demonstrates memory. Finally, our immune system is able to discriminate between foreign substances and those that make up our own body, and to direct its attack only against intruders. It can even detect and attack abnormal cells of the body such

as tumor cells or those harboring viruses. These four processes (recognition, learning, memory, and self-discrimination) are characteristic of **acquired immunity,** also called **adaptive** or **specific immunity.** The components of this system normally work effectively in direct attack on invading pathogens or in collaboration with the components of nonspecific immunity to ensure the ultimate survival of the individual. In practice, there is no neat boundary between nonspecific defenses and specific immunity. Survival would be impossible without nonspecific defenses but, as is demonstrated in AIDS, paralysis of acquired immunity is also incompatible with life. The basic function of specific immunity is to focus and reinforce nonspecific defenses. Its capacity to discriminate "self" from "nonself" adds some potent weapons to our defensive arsenal.

T Lymphocytes, B Lymphocytes, Antibodies, and Third Population Cells

Lymphocytes, the cells that mediate specific immunity, fall into three distinct populations: T lymphocytes, B lymphocytes, and the so-called third population cells.

T Lymphocytes T lymphocytes are cells produced in the bone marrow or thymus. Wherever they originate, they migrate to the thymus, where they mature (the T is for thymus). T-cell surfaces are studded with molecules called **T-cell receptors,** which are the key to their function in the immune system. T lymphocytes are able to "recognize" the molecular aspects of a wide variety of foreign substances, particularly the surface features of microorganisms, because their receptor shapes match, allowing them to bind together. Three regions within the T-cell DNA (V for "variable," D for "diversity," and J for "joining") contain a few hundred genes that can undergo DNA rearrangement. This allows the production of as many as a billion distinct populations of T cells, each of which bears a unique T-cell receptor. It is this receptor that interacts with ("recognizes") the foreign substance (fig. 5.2). The general shape of all T-cell receptors is the same, but fine details of structure make them different for each clone. These fine structural differences determine the shape and the distribution of electrical charges on the recognition site and thereby the shape and characteristics of the substance with which it will bind.

Anything the specific immune system is able to recognize and to which it responds is called an immunogen or antigen (for antibody generator—antibodies will be discussed shortly). Only parts of a microbe are antigenic (immunogenic), and within the antigen there may be different regions with which a T-cell receptor can bind. These specific regions are called **antigenic determinants,** or **epitopes.** Our immune system has the capacity to recognize a billion epitopes. This enormous variety of recognition codes means that sometimes we will produce a response to something harmless (the basis of allergies). At other times we may confuse nonself-antigens with self-antigens (part of the basis of autoimmune diseases).

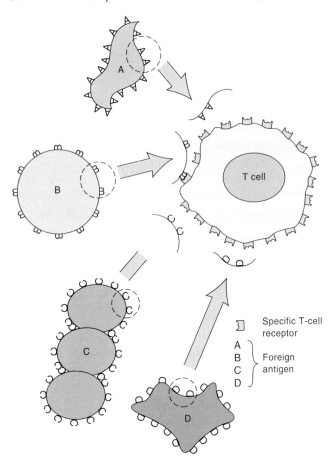

Figure 5.2 **Interaction Between T-Cell Surface Receptors and the Molecular Features of a Foreign Substance.** (In this case, parts of the surface proteins of an invading microorganism.) Note that this particular T cell binds only to B-surface antigen. Lack of a match to A, C, and D means no binding can occur. Binding is critical because this "recognition" triggers an immune response to the microbe.

As we noted, T cells are capable of generating a wide variety of receptor molecules (many more than the million-plus we normally produce). The genetic processes that lead to this diversity are thought to be fairly random. Presumably, there are occasions when receptors to self-antigens are produced along with receptors to foreign antigens. After all, we have a lot in common at the molecular level with the pathogens that invade us. To cope with this situation, T cells mature and display their clonal receptors in the thymus. A process called **positive selection** goes on as recently produced T cells pass through the thymus. To understand this process, we need to introduce a characteristic of T-cell interaction that will be explained in more detail later. T cells can only react to antigens that are in association with self-antigens called **MHC** (major histocompatibility complex). In the thymus, all of those T cells that bind moderately to MHC on thymic cells are therefore "positively" selected. They are, at that time, also differentiated into one of two classes of T cells (T_4 and T_8), which we will discuss later. T cells that have weak or no affinity to MHC self-

antigens undergo apoptosis and cell death. On the other hand, T cells with a high affinity for MHC, whether on thymic cells or cells in the peripheral lymph nodes, undergo **negative selection.** The interaction triggers apoptosis in them as well. In this way, we develop an immune system that attacks only foreign antigens while accepting (tolerating) those recognized as self-antigens. This feature, known as **self-tolerance,** works well enough to make autoimmune disease the exception rather than the rule.

B Lymphocytes The T-cell receptor is very closely related to the antibody. Antibodies are produced by a class of cells called **B lymphocytes.** These cells arise in the red bone marrow. In birds, the animal in which B-cell maturation was first described, B lymphocytes migrate to a region of the cloaca (a common intestinal and urogenital duct) called the bursa of Fabricius; the B comes from bursa. In humans, maturation proceeds in the bone marrow. Much of what we have said about T-cell receptors holds here as well, including the deletion or suppression of any emerging B cells that are specific to self-antigens. The surface of a particular B lymphocyte is dotted with copies of the antibody it produces. Through these, a mature B lymphocyte can react to a specific epitope. Its response is to produce antibodies that have affinity with that epitope. To understand why this might be helpful, we should look at the structure and function of antibodies.

Antibodies **Antibodies** are Y-shaped protein molecules that provide a flexible means of linking our relatively limited repertoire of defenses to the host of invaders that threaten us (fig. 5.3). They are a remarkably simple solution to the problem of defending against a large variety of specific pathogens without developing undue complexity. Part of the secret is in the Fab portion of the antibody. Fab stands for **antigen-binding fragment,** and the end part of the structure is analogous to the T-cell receptor binding site (and is produced by DNA rearrangement in the V, D, and J regions we noted with T cells). Through the Fab, the immune system can attach to and mark any of a billion foreign epitopes. It can also attach to and neutralize toxic substances produced by microorganisms. Through the Fc (for **crystallizable fragment**) component, which forms the stalk of the Y, the immune system gets a single, common handle on all this diversity. The antibody response to an antigenic stimulus will be the production of masses of antigen-specific antibody that can bind to the antigen.

Macrophages, PMNs, and eosinophils have Fc receptors on their membranes. These allow them to carry surface antibody to tissues where invading organisms are present. When the antigens of the infecting agent bind the membrane antibody, phagocytosis and cytotoxicity of antibody-labeled pathogens follow (fig. 5.3). Binding of the Fc region by platelets, mast cells, and complement is an initiating factor in the release of various of the mediators of inflammation described in chapter 2.

There is more to the subject of antibodies than appears in the simple diagram of figure 5.3, but for our purposes

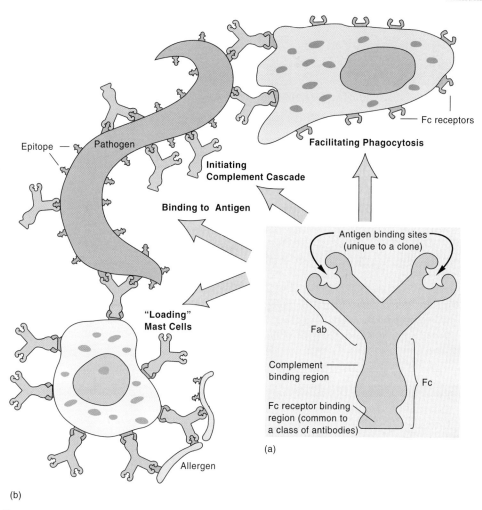

(a)

(b)

Figure 5.3   **The Structure and Various Roles of the Antibody Molecule.** (*a*) The structure of an antibody molecule. The variable antigen-binding regions (Fab) and the common stalk (Fc), which mediates the interaction of the antibody with components of the nonspecific defenses. (*b*) Antibody binding has a wide range of effects. Complement deposition damages microorganisms directly and produces products that enhance inflammation. Along with antibody, complement enhances phagocytosis. Binding of antibody to mast cells "loads" (sensitizes) them.

only a brief review of this topic is needed. There are five classes of antibodies. Two have relevance to antibody labeling of bacteria. In a normal immune response, an activated clone of B cells first produces **IgM** class (for immunoglobulin M) antibodies and then shifts its production to **IgG** class antibodies (this is called class switching). IgM antibodies have a different shape (actually five Y's in a wheel), but the Fab binding site is exactly the same (fig. 5.4). IgG is the principal immunoglobulin circulating in the blood. A third class of antibody, **IgE,** is mainly involved in antigen triggering of mast cells and is of clinical significance in allergies and in parasitic worm (helminth) infestations. **IgA** is the secreted antibody and is found in saliva, breast milk, and respiratory and genitourinary tract secretions. **IgD** seems to serve as an antigen receptor on lymphocyte membranes. These five types of antibody form a first line of protection along with the nonspecific defenses. Collectively, antibodies used to be called gammaglobulins. Figure 5.5 pictures a routine, normal pattern of serum electrophoresis

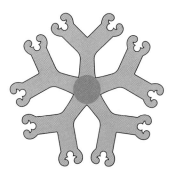

Figure 5.4   **The Structure of an IgM Antibody.** Essentially, it consists of five IgG-type units joined at the Fc regions.

that indicates the location of the antibody classes relative to the other major plasma proteins.

Natural Killer Cells Natural Killer cells also called **non-T, non-B,** or **null cells** are large, granular lymphocytes. They are capable of three distinct patterns of cell-killing activity.

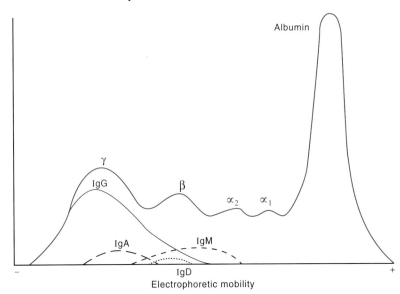

Figure 5.5   **Graph of Plasma Electrophoresis, Showing the Relative Location of Four Immunoglobulins.** IgE is in too low a concentration to be evident. Plasma proteins migrate in a charged field in a way that depends on their size and charge. The peaks have been arbitrarily named α_1, α_2, β, and γ. IgG contributes the bulk of protein in the γ peak. For this reason, in the past the immunoglobulins have been called "gammaglobulins."

Focus on Monoclonal Antibodies: A Breakthrough in Research and Therapy

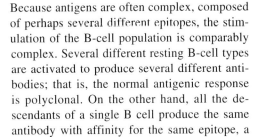

Because antigens are often complex, composed of perhaps several different epitopes, the stimulation of the B-cell population is comparably complex. Several different resting B-cell types are activated to produce several different antibodies; that is, the normal antigenic response is polyclonal. On the other hand, all the descendants of a single B cell produce the same antibody with affinity for the same epitope, a so-called monoclonal antibody. Say we are interested in labeling a particular epitope because that epitope is unique to a line of cells we are studying and we wish to identify those cells among a complex culture. We could produce a monoclonal antibody (Mab) to that epitope, label it in some way we could detect, expose the culture to the labeled antibody, and simply pick out our target cells. Alternatively, we could use a Mab to identify the cellular distribution of a particular protein.

Monoclonal antibodies can be used therapeutically in a wide variety of ways: to carry bound toxins exclusively to a tumor cell that displays a unique antigen, to block a receptor-mediated process, or to neutralize some substance released by cells in the body that is causing disease. Today the production of Mab has become routine technology.

The first, **antibody-dependent cellular cytotoxicity** (ADCC), is important in some forms of autoimmune disease. Lymphocytes that employ this pattern have numerous Fc receptors; they attach to a cell that has been covered with an antibody and kill it. This is now seen to be a specialized function of natural killer cells, but ADCC is shared by neutrophils, macrophages, and eosinophils. **Natural killer** (NK) cells are also capable of a second form of cytotoxic activity that is quite different. It seems to be important in the control of tumor development, since NK cells can recognize a cell that is becoming abnormal, then engage and kill it (see fig. 5.6). This capacity is called **tumor surveillance.** NK cells are also capable of lysing virally infected cells, a third distinct pattern of cellular cytotoxicity. In ADCC, antitumor, and antiviral cytotoxicity, the target cell membrane forms blebs and ruptures, while the DNA

fractures. NK cells are innately endowed (hence, the term "natural") with an ability to recognize ill-defined molecules on a cell's surface. The appearance of these abnormal molecules is a product of tumor transformation or viral infection. Although NK Cells lack T-cell receptors; they do display receptors for MHC class I molecule. Binding firmly to MHC I inhibits their cytotoxic activity. Viral infection or neoplastic transformation reduces MHC I production, removing this inhibitory signal and releasing NK cytotoxic activity.

Lymphoid Tissue

The primary lymphoid tissues (red bone marrow and thymus) house the lymphoid stem cells, which produce immature T and B cells. After the selective deletion of any

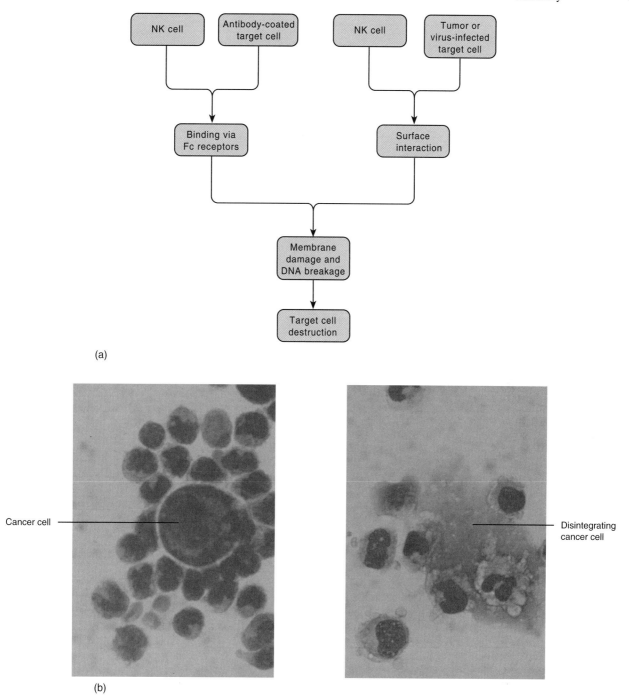

Figure 5.6   Monoclonal Antibodies. (*a*) The Fc receptors of NK cells enable them to bind and destroy antibody-coated target cells. This feature is called antibody-dependent cellular cytotoxicity (ADCC). Natural killer (NK) cells can also interact with target cells whose surfaces are altered. The target cell is destroyed as a result. (*b*) Two steps in the cytoxic T cell-mediated destruction of a cancer cell: *the left image* shows the cell surrounded by NK, T$_{HI}$, and cytotoxic T cells; *the right image* shows the cancer cell undergoing the bleb formation and nuclear dissintegration associated with NK, T$_{HI}$, and cytotoxic T cells-mediated destruction.

self-antigen-reactive lymphocytes that may arise, these T and B cells move out to the secondary lymphoid tissues, which include the lymph nodes, spleen, tonsils, and Peyer's patches in the intestines. Lymphocytes from the primary lymphoid tissues leave the bloodstream from the postcapillary venules in the secondary lymphoid tissues and take up temporary residence. They can then leave the secondary lymphoid tissues in the draining lymph to reen-

ter the blood circulation and begin another circuit of lymphocyte traffic (fig. 5.7*a*).

This constant migration serves two purposes. First, the lymphoid tissues are strategically located to encounter antigen shortly after it violates the body's outer defenses. In figure 5.7*c*, note the concentrations of nodes where the limbs join the trunk, as well as the masses of lymphoid tissue that are associated with the mouth and gut. Lymphocytes are

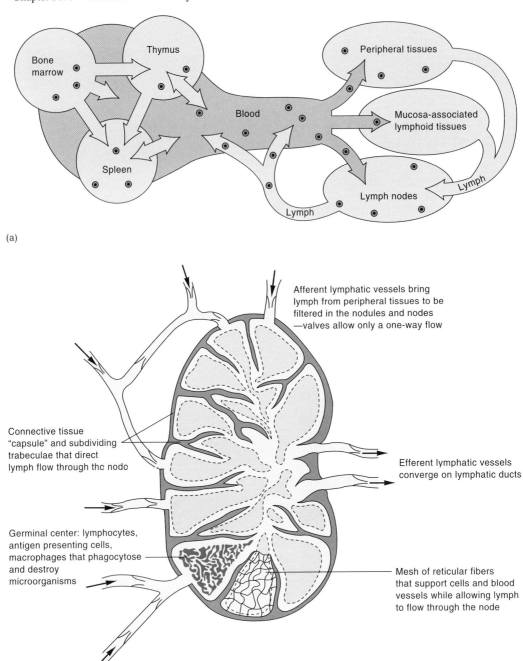

(a)

(b)

Figure 5.7   **The Origin and Movement of Lymphocytes, the Structure of a Lymph Node, and the Lymphatic System.** (*a*) Course of "lymphocyte traffic." Arrows indicate the direction of movement of lymphocytes. Stem cells reside in bone marrow and produce immature lymphocytes that migrate to the thymus and spleen to mature and replicate. Migration into lymphoid tissues is facilitated by the presence of specialized regions of postcapillary venules. Inflammation greatly enhances immigration into peripheral tissues. (*b*) Lymph node. Afferent lymphatic vessels bring lymph from peripheral tissues to be filtered in the nodules and nodes. Valves in the lymph vessels impose a one-way flow. (*c*) Major concentrations of lymphoid tissue, principal drainage routes, and major lymphatic vessels.

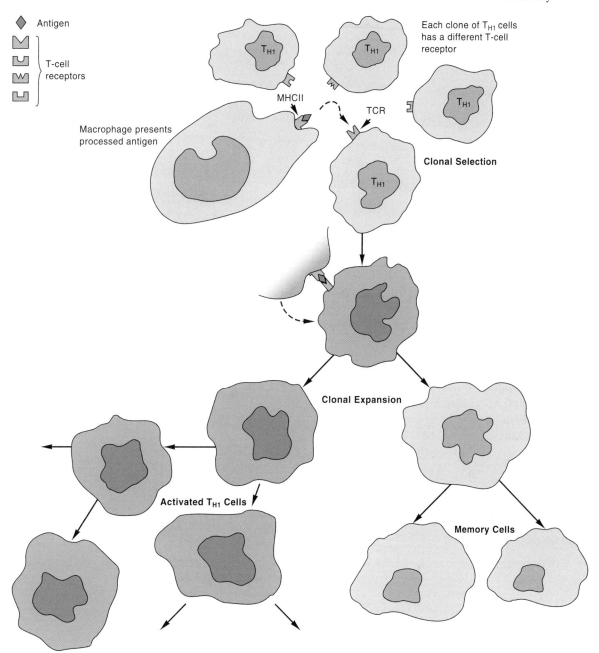

Figure 5.8   **T$_{H1}$ Cell Function.** In clonal selection, an antigen-presenting cell interacts with an antigen-responsive helper T cell, (T$_{H1}$). Activation and proliferation of the responsive clone results in clonal expansion, producing many activated T$_{H1}$ cells and a reserve of memory T cells. (For simplicity's sake, we have not drawn in the CD4 and other co-receptors on the T cells.)

In actual circumstances, usually one or the other response is dominant (because of the T$_H$–T$_{H2}$ interaction noted above).

The first antibody response to an antigen takes about a week to mobilize. IgM production is followed by class switching to IgG, which peaks at about 12 days and then tapers off. Compared with this primary antigen "challenge," the second and subsequent challenges produce a faster rise in antibody production, which is retained at higher levels for a longer time. As well, the secondary response is predominantly IgG and the individual antibodies have a higher

affinity for antigen (fig. 5.10). The effect is that both the specific immune response and the nonspecific defenses it supports are stronger and more effective.

Communication between the cells involved in the immune response is mediated by factors called **cytokines** (literally, "cell movers"). Most cytokines act on cells in the immediate vicinity of the secreting cell or even on themselves, but some—for example, interleukin-1, which we encountered as a mediator of fever in chapter 3—act on distant target organs. Research on the

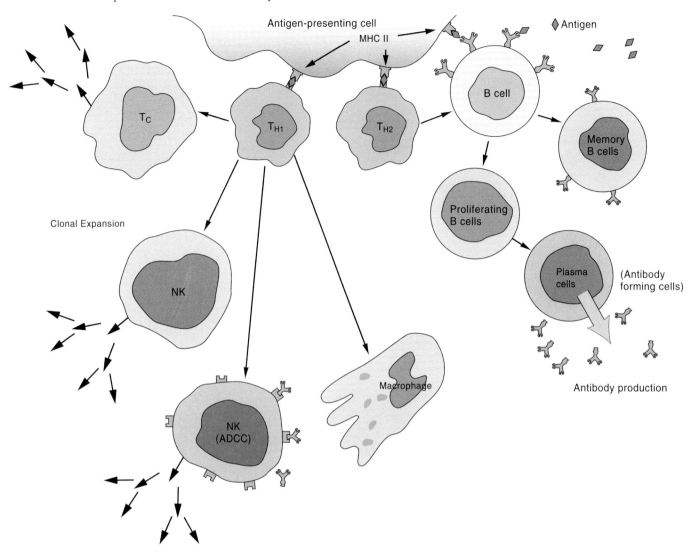

Figure 5.9   D$_4$ and other co-receptors on the T and B sensitized T$_{H1}$ cells orchestrate cellular immunity (T$_c$ cells, NK cells, NK$_{ADCC}$ cells).

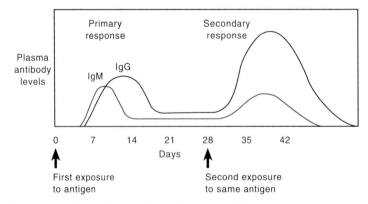

Figure 5.10   **Comparison of Primary and Secondary Antibody Responses.** The second exposure to a specific antigen produces a more rapid, extensive, and prolonged antibody production. IgG can permeate tissues more readily and binds to antigen with greater affinity.

Focus on Economy of Size and Delayed Response

Reflect for a moment on the significance of memory cells and the secondary response. The alternative approach to the problem of coping quickly with a threatening antigenic challenge would be to produce and hold the responsive T- and B-cell clones in reserve. An analogy might be the musculoskeletal system, in which our peak strength greatly exceeds the ordinary demands of activities like walking and breathing, in order to cope with the extraordinary challenge of running for a bus.

To match our equivalent muscle mass, the lymphoid tissues, which collectively account for about 2% of our body weight, would have to weigh perhaps 100 times as much, with an attendant increase in food requirements. So the trade-off for this incredible economy of size is the five- to seven-day lagtime for clonal expansion of antigen-specific memory T- and B-cell lines. Of course, while we suffer for a week with our cold or flu, it may be difficult to derive comfort from the fact that, by and large, our immune system can take credit for our survival!

Table 5.2   The Principal Cytokines

Cytokine	Source	Principal Effects
Interleukin-1 (IL-1)	Antigen-presenting cells	Immune response activation, enhancement of inflammation
Interleukin-2 (IL-2)	Helper T cells	Immune response activation, some tumor therapy applications
Interleukins 3–11	Various cells	Of this group, IL-4 is perhaps the most important in mediating a broad array of immune and chronic inflammatory responses
Interferon (IFN)	Various cells: leukocytes, fibroblasts, epithelia	Direct inhibition of viral replication, promotion of the destruction of virally infected cells
Tumor necrosis factor (TNF)	Macrophages, T cells	Antiviral/antiparasite action, tumor cytotoxicity, enhanced phagocytosis, some cancer side effects
Colony-stimulating factor (CSF)	Various cells	Division and differentiation of hemopoietic stem cells

These are water-soluble molecules that typically exert their effects on adjacent cells in mediating their various contributions to body defenses.

---

cytokines has progressed like the investigations by the proverbial blind men who touch and describe an elephant, each perceiving an entirely different phenomenon. The result was a welter of names that were based on what the discoverer initially thought the function of a factor to be. Recently, at least for those factors originally thought to be produced by active leukocytes (the interleukins), such names have been replaced by numbers based on order of discovery.

Table 5.2 presents a selected list of cytokines for reference. For our purposes, IL-1 is important. Besides being an endogenous pyrogen, it is released by the antigen-presenting cell at the same time as it presents processed antigen to the T_H cell. These two stimuli (IL-1 and appropriate antigen) are necessary to activate the T_H cell, which responds by producing IL-2. This interleukin then acts on adjacent T and B cells of the same clone, stimulates the T_H cell itself, and is responsible for clonal expansion. (We have already described how IL-2 is used to stimulate the proliferation of NK cells into LAK cells.) IL-4 (B-cell growth factor) and IL-6 (B-cell differentiation factor) are also released by T_H cells to foster clonal expansion of B and

 Checkpoint 5.1

Take some time to familiarize yourself with the cast of characters diagrammed in simplified form in figure 5.12 (p. 95). What you see are cellular and humoral "agents" with a range of response potentials. These are programmed into their cellular structure and primed DNA, in the case of cellular agents, or into their elaborately interacting biochemistry, in the case of plasma agents. It is tempting to characterize individual agents in anthropomorphic terms, as "soldiers" or "spies," but everything simply behaves as its biology dictates. That is the strength of this system. But as we shall see, it is also its weakness.

T cells. Figure 5.11 diagrams these interactions and figure 5.12 presents an overview of this section. We will now look at some of the ways an understanding of normal immune function can be used to avoid disease.

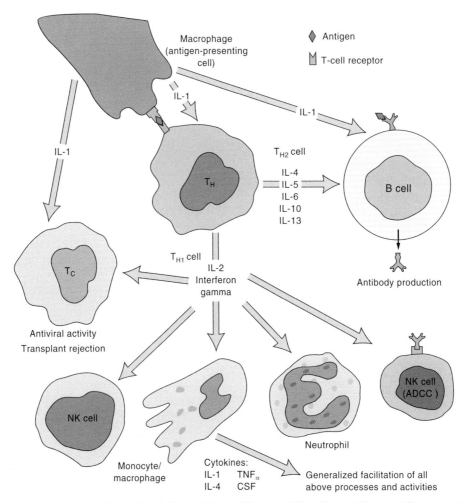

Figure 5.11   **Interactions Between Activated T$_H$ Cells and Other Effectors of Specific and Nonspecific Immunity.** The role of specific cytokines is noted. (Only the MHC class II molecule on the antigen-presenting cell and the T-cell receptor have been drawn in.)

THERAPEUTIC APPLICATIONS OF IMMUNITY

Immunization

Immunization is the prophylactic (preventive) technique of artificially inducing an immune response. The technique seeks to stimulate the immune system without exposing the body to an infection. The means is most commonly a preparation of the antigenic components of a microorganism, or of its toxins. This preparation is called a **vaccine.**

It is interesting to note that the technique of vaccination was developed well before the essentials of immune function were understood. In 1796, the British physician Edward Jenner took advantage of the antigenic similarity between the relatively harmless cowpox virus and the deadly smallpox virus to invent vaccination. Smallpox was declared eradicated worldwide in 1979. Vaccines have been developed for a wide range of both viral and bacterial infections (table 5.3).

Vaccines may include killed microorganisms, attenuated (weakened) microorganisms, or inactivated microbial

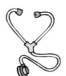

Focus on Failure to Immunize

Recently there has been concern because a routine immunization has been too effective! Following the introduction of the Salk vaccine against the crippling and potentially fatal disease poliomyelitis in the 1950s, a generation of children grew up for whom polio was just a scary memory. But memory fades and so did full compliance with public health expectations of routine immunization. In the late 1980s, sporadic cases of polio were showing up in unimmunized children.

toxins. The basic principle of a vaccine is that it is harmless, while still containing antigenic material that can induce a primary antibody response with the long-term retention provided by memory T and B cells. Subsequent encounters with the same antigenic determinants will elicit a brisk and usually effective secondary immune response.

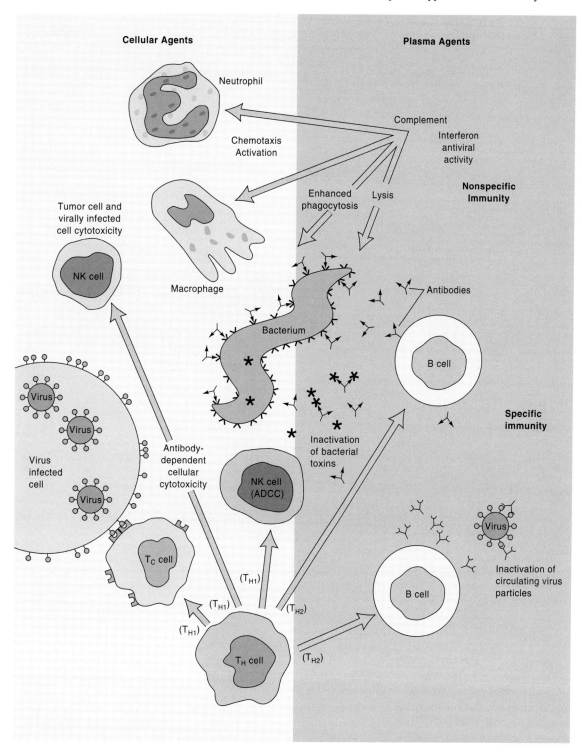

Figure 5.12   **Overview of Nonspecific and Specific Immunity.** (For simplicity's sake, T_{H1} and T_{H2} presented together.)

An interesting variant of vaccination occurs with the treatment of suspected rabies infection, where the immunization vaccine is given *after* the primary infection. Rabies has a long (at least two weeks) and variable incubation period, and once symptoms are displayed the disease is almost invariably fatal. Between infection and disease there is a window during which repeated inoculation of attenuated rabies virus triggers an immune response that copes with the incipient infection. Previously, a course of 14 to 21 injections was required, but recent improvements in techniques have reduced the number to 4 to 6.

Table 5.3	A Selection of Vaccines Commonly Used against Viral and Bacterial Diseases in Humans		
Disease	**Vaccine**	**Recommendation**	**Booster**
Viral Diseases			
Hepatitis B	Viral antigen	High-risk medical personnel	None
Influenza	Inactivated virus	Chronically ill individuals and those over age 65	Yearly
Measles Mumps Rubella	Attenuated viruses (combined MMR vaccine)	Children 15–19 months old	None
Poliomyelitis	Attenuated or inactivated virus (oral poliomyelitis vaccine [OPV])	Children 2–3 years old	Adults as needed
Rabies	Inactivated virus	Individuals in contact with wildlife, animal control personnel, veterinarians	None
Yellow fever	Attenuated virus	Military personnel and individuals traveling to endemic areas	10 years
Bacterial Disease			
Cholera	Fraction of *Vibrio cholerae*	Individuals in endemic areas	6 months
Diphtheria Pertussis Tetanus	Diphtheria toxoid, killed *Bordetella pertusis,* tetanus toxoid (DPT vaccine)	Children 2–3 months old	10 years
Haemophilus influenza	Polysaccharide-protein conjugate	Children under 5 years of age	None
Plague	Fraction of *Yersinia pestis*	Individuals in contact with rodents in endemic areas	Yearly
Pneumococcal pneumonia	Purified *S. pneumoniae* polysaccharide	Adults over age 50 with chronic disease	None
Tuberculosis	*Mycobacterium bovis* BCG (attenuated)	Individuals exposed to TB for prolonged periods of time	3–4 years
Typhoid fever	Killed *Salmonella typhi*	Individuals in endemic area	3–4 years

From Lansing M. Prescott, John P. Harley, and Donald A. Klein, *Microbiology.* Copyright © 1990 The McGraw-Hill Companies, Dubuque, Iowa. All Rights Reserved. Reprinted by permission of The McGraw-Hill Companies.

The Use of Antisera

The immunity induced by vaccination is called **active** because it is indistinguishable from a normal primary immune response; it requires the full participation of the immune system. **Passive** immunity, by contrast, is protection that is imported in the form of ready-made antibodies from outside the system. Characteristically, this immunity lasts only a short while (weeks or months). Natural passive immunity is transferred to a fetus with the already formed maternal antibodies that are transported across the placental barrier to the infant. In breast milk, antibody transfer continues this passive support of the very young infant's relatively incompetent immune system. Artificial passive immunity is conferred by the transfer of antibodies from a sensitized host (in the past often a horse, but increasingly monoclonal antibodies are used) to a nonimmune recipient so that those an-

tibodies can interfere with or interrupt a pathological process already underway. The serum injected for this purpose is rich in the antibody of interest and is called an **antiserum.** The term continues to be used with artificially produced antibodies that are not carried in serum.

Antisera can be used in different circumstances. In suspected rabies infection, for example, rabies antiserum is used to infiltrate the wound and neutralize the virus before it can enter tissues and replicate. In another approach, antiserum is introduced into the bloodstream of infected individuals before they have developed an immune response to neutralize virulent pathogens. In effect, the antiserum buys time for activation of the immune system. A third application of antisera is in the neutralization of bacterial toxins. For example, improperly preserved food may host a bacterium (*Clostridium botulinum*) that produces a dangerous

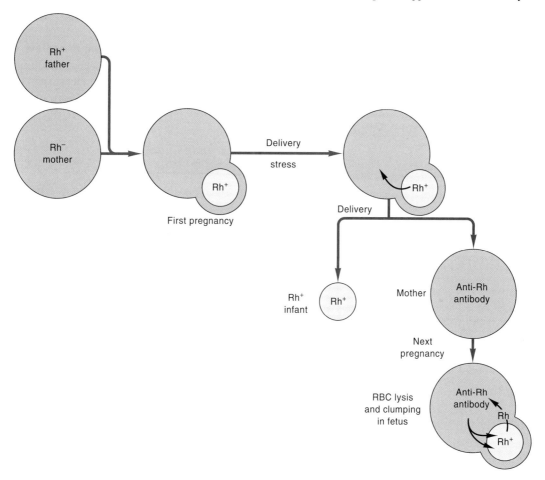

Figure 5.13   **The Immunology of Erythroblastosis Fetalis.** Delivery stresses allow the Rh antigens of a Rh⁺ fetus to cross to its Rh⁻ mother. Anti-Rh antibody production follows the delivery. In the second and subsequent pregnancies with an Rh⁺ fetus, the antibody can cross to the fetus, causing potentially serious damage.

poison called botulinum toxin. Antibotulinum toxin antiserum will effectively neutralize the toxin before it can have a devastating effect on neuromuscular and nervous system function.

The fourth application is interesting in that it is intended to prevent a normal immune response rather than to support a weak or absent one. If a pregnant woman who is negative for the Rh factor on her red blood cells (about 15% of women) carries a fetus who inherited Rh factor from an Rh-positive father, she is at risk of becoming exposed to her fetus's Rh-positive blood and developing an immune response to it. This is of little consequence to her directly, since she encounters only tiny amounts of Rh-positive RBCs. The situation for the fetus is different. The most usual circumstance is that the original antigen exposure occurs during labor with the first child, when its Rh antigens are more likely to gain access to the maternal circulation. Even a minute transfer of fetal RBCs mobilizes maternal antibody production. During a following pregnancy these antibodies cross the placenta, attach to fetal red blood cells, and induce lysis of RBCs or their clumping followed by destruction in the liver. The resultant anemia and jaundice in the in-

fant, called **erythroblastosis fetalis** or **hemolytic disease of newborns** (fig. 5.13), is potentially fatal.

In current medical management, routine maternal blood tests detect pregnancies that pose such risks. Within 48 hours of delivery (or at any other point that fetal blood transfer is suspected), anti-Rh antibodies are administered to the mother in the form of **Rho(D) immune globulin.** These bind to fetal RBCs in the mother and tag them for phagocytosis in the liver or spleen. By preventing immune sensitization in the mother, this approach, where used, has virtually eliminated the risk of erythroblastosis fetalis.

Partly because care in cases of potential Rh incompatability is so good, a different blood group incompatibility is now clinically recognized. This derives from incompatibilities within the ABO blood group system. Problems may occur when the mother is type A and the fetus is type B (by inheritance from a type B father) or when the mother is type B while the fetus (and father) are type A. A person with type A carries type A antigen on her RBCs and circulating anti-B antibodies in her plasma. Conversely, type B individuals have B-antigen positive RBCs and circulating anti-A antibodies. The problem occurs if there is a placental breakdown, which sensitizes the mother to the antigen of her fetus. In the first case (mother–A; fetus–B), the masses if anti-B antibody can cross the placenta, and attach to the fetuses RBCs, causing RBC aggregation and lysis or occlusion of vascular beds. This disorder is milder than Rh incompatibility but more common. In an Italian study, 2.7% of pregnancies were associated with "alloimmunization" and, of those, 82% were ABO. Only 1.3% of the 2.7% (i.e., 0.04%) needed transfusion therapy at birth. In another study of 135 newborns with ABC (A or B incompatible) incompatibilities, 21% had significant hyperbilirubinemia. Why don't O or AB mothers have a problem? O-types produce mild amounts of both anti-A and anti-B antibodies while AB-types produce neither.

IMMUNE-MEDIATED TISSUE INJURY

We now turn to diseases of immunity, beginning with conditions that have as their basis "too much immunity." We will deal with four broad patterns of immune-mediated injury called hypersensitivity reactions (including allergies) and then discuss a therapeutic intervention that is made problematic by the normal functioning of the immune system: transplantation.

Hypersensitivity Reactions

Our skin and intestine and our respiratory and other mucosal barriers are richly supplied with mast cells that are studded with IgE antibodies. In these locations, mast cells are ideally situated to detect the entry of parasitic worms (helminthic infections), which shed antigen as part of their attempt to confuse the host immune system. If all goes according to *our* schedule, these parasitic antigens bind to IgE on mast cells, causing the cells to degranulate and triggering a localized inflammatory response. Some of the mediators released by activated mast cells attract eosinophils, which are specially adapted to engage and kill the threatening parasitic worms.

Western sanitation and personal hygiene are such that most of you reading this book have never been made ill by parasitic worms. However, about 15% of you will be familiar with the misery of "pollen season." The same system that improves the chances of survival against parasitic infection sets up certain individuals for allergies; that is, an inherently harmless antigen (allergen) activates a bothersome and potentially fatal **anaphylaxis.** The Greek roots here are *ana* ("without") and *phylaxis* ("watching" or "guarding"), and the term implies a dramatic reaction that occurs without warning. **Immediate hypersensitivity** and **anaphylactic (type I) hypersensitivity** are terms applied to this pattern of immune system response, in which the cure (immune response) is worse than the disease. There are three other broad patterns of hypersensitivity in which immune system overactivity causes tissue damage: antibody-dependent cytotoxicity (type II), immune-complex-mediated hypersensitivity (type III), and cell-

mediated, delayed-type hypersensitivity (type IV). Figure 5.14 presents the key features. Because these reactions are central to many diseases of immunity and are significant in other disorders, we will discuss each in a little more detail. Note, however, that we describe them separately for convenience only. Seldom does one pattern occur in complete isolation from others.

Type I: Immediate Hypersensitivity (Anaphylaxis)

In this pattern of hypersensitivity, the first exposure to antigen, which may be through the skin or at a mucosal surface, produces no noticeable reaction. Nevertheless, antigen-presenting cells have captured and processed the allergen and presented it to B and T cells, and cell production of the corresponding IgE antibodies has been launched. The IgE antibodies bind to the Fc receptors on local mast cells and spill over into the circulation to bind on mast cells throughout the body. They are now primed for the next contact with the allergen (this sensitization can last for months). When the next exposure occurs, allergen binds to the Fab, cross-linking adjacent antibodies and causing mast cell degranulation and mediator release (fig. 5.14*a*). The immediate (5–30 minutes) response is largely due to the release of preformed histamine. It consists of an increase in vascular permeability as well as the constriction of bronchial muscles and a narrowing of airways. Histamine also stimulates increased secretion from nasal, bronchial, and gastric glands. Other specific reactions are associated with the degranulation of mast cells in the skin (**hives**), the eye (**conjunctivitis**), and the mucous membranes of the nasal cavity (**rhinitis**). This early reaction can be over in an hour. Other mediators—those responsible for the cellular infiltration and tissue damage that accompany more extensive allergic reactions—take longer to be released or to act. They include chemotactic factors for eosinophils and neutrophils, leukotrienes, prostaglandins, platelet-activating factor, and protein-digesting enzymes. These mediators account for the second wave or late phase reaction of immediate hypersensitivity, which occurs in two to eight hours and may last for two or three days (fig. 5.15). The symptoms of the first wave may be subdued if the person has been taking antihistamines. On the other hand, epinephrine (a beta-adrenergic compound) can block mast cell degranulation by interfering with ability of the mast cell to respond. Another approach is the use of corticosteroids and nonsteroidal anti-inflammatory agents that block the synthesis of leukotrienes and prostaglandins, and thereby the late phase reaction, while leaving the early phase unaffected.

Localized anaphylaxis can take many forms: allergic asthma, hay fever, eczema, and urticaria (hives). The name **atopy** is sometimes applied to this constellation of symptoms in individuals with a family history of allergies. Although these people tend to have elevated plasma IgE levels, only with atopic eczema is there any good correlation between allergic symptoms and measured IgE. Allergy sufferers also tend to have both an inherited general hyper-

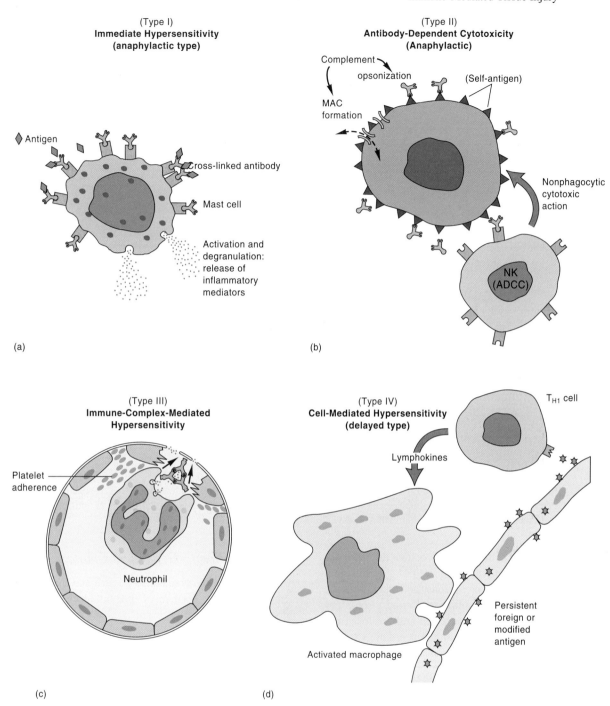

(Type I)
**Immediate Hypersensitivity
(anaphylactic type)**

◆ Antigen

Cross-linked antibody

Mast cell

Activation and
degranulation:
release of
inflammatory
mediators

(a)

(Type II)
**Antibody-Dependent Cytotoxicity
(Anaphylactic)**

Complement

opsonization

(Self-antigen)

MAC
formation

Nonphagocytic
cytotoxic
action

NK
(ADCC)

(b)

(Type III)
**Immune-Complex-Mediated
Hypersensitivity**

Platelet
adherence

Neutrophil

(c)

(Type IV)
**Cell-Mediated Hypersensitivity
(delayed type)**

T$_{H1}$ cell

Lymphokines

Persistent
foreign or
modified
antigen

Activated macrophage

(d)

Figure 5.14   **Overview of Hypersensitivity Reactions.**

responsiveness and an inherited antigen-specific response. Lowered numbers and depressed activity of suppressor T cells play an important role. Even with a genetic predisposition, however, the allergy tends to develop only after repeated exposure to low doses of allergen presented (usually) at a mucosal barrier.

One way to control an allergy is to avoid the allergen, whether in foods, the droppings of dust mites in house dust, animal dander, and so on. It will also be helpful

(though difficult) to avoid exposure to environmental pollutants. Sulfur dioxide, nitrogen oxides, fly ash, and diesel fumes can make the mucosa more permeable and thereby worsen ordinary allergic reactions. Instead of avoidance, the physician may try injections of the same allergen, in low and increasing doses, to reduce sensitivity. Injection tends to increase IgG, which acts as a blocking antibody, removing antigen from tissue fluids before it can interact with mast cells.

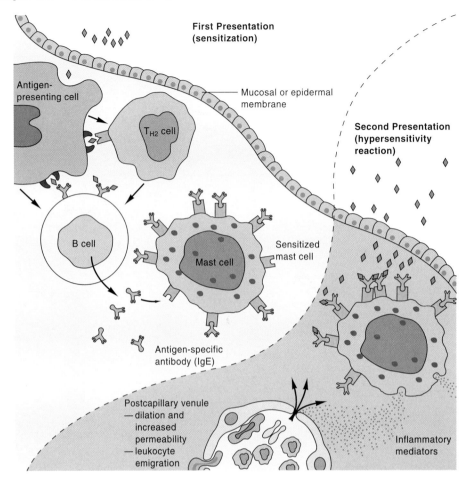

Figure 5.15   **Immediate Hypersensitivity.** First contact with antigen results in plasma cell production of antigen-specific (IgE) antibody. This binds to the Fc receptors on mucosal, dermal, or perivascular mast cells, thus arming them (sensitizing them to antigen). The second and subsequent contacts result in mast cell degranulation and synthesis of secondary mediators.

Unfortunately, desensitization procedures are not risk-free. Sometimes they trigger a generalized or systemic anaphylaxis. In this case, widespread mast cell degranulation with histamine release can result in profound circulatory shock as fluids pool in the capillary bed and are lost from the vascular compartment; other symptoms are also present (fig. 5.16). Systemic anaphylaxis can also be brought on by drugs (e.g., penicillin or sulfonamides), insect venoms (e.g., bees, wasps), or foods (e.g., peanuts, seafoods). Whatever the triggering allergen, the pattern is the same. Within minutes the person experiences pruritus (intense itching), urticaria, erythema (red rash), wheezing, and dyspnea (labored breathing). The larynx swells, and there may be vomiting, cramps, and diarrhea. In the worst case, laryngospasm may lead to suffocation and death. To counter the reaction, histamine competitors (e.g., epinephrine or isoproterenol) and antihistamines are administered parenterally (by injection). Systemic anaphylaxis is mediated by IgG as well as IgE antibodies. The term *anaphylactoid* is applied to conditions that are clinically identical to anaphylaxis but are due to the direct action of chemicals or drugs on mast cells, causing degranulation without the mediation of IgE. In these cases, usually large amounts of drugs are involved and the reaction is dose-related.

Type II: Antibody-Dependent Cytotoxicity

This pattern of hypersensitivity is triggered when antibodies attach to the surface of individual cells, such as red blood cells, or to cells or surfaces associated with a solid tissue, like the glomerular basement membrane of the kidney (fig. 5.14*b*). The antibody acts as an anchor and activator for K cells that then engage in antibody-dependent cellular cytotoxicity (ADCC). As well, antibody Fc components assist in the phagocytic activity of other cells whose surfaces bear Fc receptors (neutrophils and macrophages). Antibody attachment to a cell surface forms a favored site for the precipitation of complement—an event leading to activation of the complement cascade. As we noted in chapter 2, this cascade is associated with assembly of a membrane attack complex (MAC) and lysis of cell membranes; with chemotaxis of neutrophils, eosinophils, and macrophages; with activation of phagocytic cells and their release of mediators; and with facilitation of phagocytosis through opsonization.

From this brief summary of the usually beneficial effects of antibody binding, you can see how potent a weapon antibodies might be when turned against our own cells. There are several different diseases in which this takes

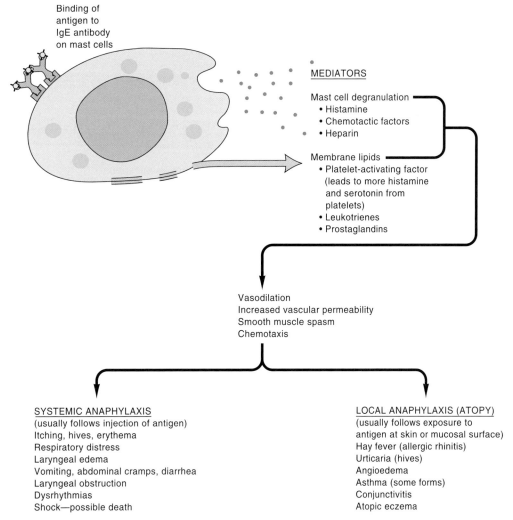

Figure 5.16   Symptoms Associated with Immediate Hypersensitivity. Systemic anaphylaxis and local anaphylaxis both result from antigen activation of sensitized mast cells.

place (table 5.4). Some of these are genuine autoimmune disorders in which errant or uncontrolled plasma cells produce antibodies against self-antigens (e.g., myasthenia gravis or Goodpasture's syndrome). Some involve drugs combining with antibody. The complexes thus formed then attach to adjacent tissues, instigating the cytotoxic mechanisms just described. Since the tissues themselves are not involved in initiating the reaction, this has been called the "innocent bystander" mechanism.

Type III: Immune-Complex-Mediated Hypersensitivity

Immune complexes are simply aggregations of antigen and their corresponding antibodies. When there is a good match between the concentration of antigen and the antibody produced to deal with it, such as occurs in a healthy immune response to infection, large complexes are formed and carried in the bloodstream (many attached to red blood cells). These are quickly removed in the liver and spleen, and the infective organism is thereby neutralized. When antigen is in excess, as it might be in lungs subjected to continuous inhalation of antigenic dust, or when antibody is in excess, as in autoimmune disease, smaller complexes are formed. It is these that produce the damage in immune-complex-mediated hypersensitivity. When they deposit in blood vessel walls, the small complexes mediate the formation of microthrombi and cause endothelial damage (fig. 5.14c). The deposition in vessel walls also triggers a variety of inflammatory processes involving complement activation, vasodilation, increased permeability, phagocyte chemotaxis, and frustrated phagocytosis followed by basement membrane damage.

Where the antibody is specific to a tissue, as it is in arthritis, deposition tends to occur in that tissue. In the case of a large burden of exogenous antigen, as occurs in various inhalation diseases called pneumonoconioses, the area of exposure (the lung) tends to be the area of deposition.

Table 5.4	Diseases in Which Type II Hypersensitivity (Antibody-Dependent Cytotoxicity) Plays a Major Role

Antiglomerular Basement Membrane Nephritis

Antibodies to glomerular basement membrane can severely damage the kidney and threaten renal failure.

Goodpasture's Syndrome

Characterized by pulmonary hemorrhages combined with glomerular damage caused by cross-reacting antibodies.

Transfusion Reactions

Cells of an incompatible donor are destroyed by complement-dependent lysis and opsonization.

Erythroblastosis Fetalis

Maternal antibodies cross the placenta to destroy the cells of her Rh^+ fetus via complement-mediated processes.

Autoimmune Hemolytic Anemia; Agranulocytosis; Thrombocytopenia

Self-reactive antibodies attack a population of cells via complement-dependent mechanisms.

Drug-Related Anemias

Complexing of a therapeutic drug and red cell antigens induces immune-mediated hemolysis and indirect organ damage.

Graft Rejection

Foreign tissue destruction by immune-mediated cellular attack on antibody-coated cells: antibody-dependent cellular toxicity (ADCC).

Myasthenia Gravis

Autoimmune destruction of acetylcholine receptors in muscle produces greatly weakened muscular responses.

Grave's Disease

Antibodies that bind to thyroid gland receptors induce excessive thyroxine secretion and hyperthyroid effects.

Table 5.5 presents some of the disorders that principally involve the type III mechanism; figure 5.17 summarizes the relevant pathophysiology.

Type IV: Cell-Mediated, Delayed-Type Hypersensitivity

This is the principal mechanism of damage in tuberculosis, contact dermatitis, many fungal, viral, and parasitic infections, and acute and chronic transplant rejection. The mediating cells are cytotoxic T cells, activated macrophages, K cells (ADCC), and also NK cells. Helper T cells orchestrate the attack against a resistant, largely intracellular bacterium (in tuberculosis and leprosy), against a persistent immune complex (in contact dermatitis), or against foreign tissue (in transplantation) (fig. 5.14*d*). Antigen presentation and T_H sensitization are prerequisites. In the tuberculin test for TB and in contact dermatitis, subsequent exposure to the antigen activates responsive T_H cells, which produce a variety of cytokines. These attract and mobilize "angry" macrophages, which attempt relatively indiscriminate phagocytosis and, along with lymphocytes and fluid, form an exudate that peaks at about 48–72 hours (hence, delayed). In contact dermatitis,

Table 5.5	Disorders That Result from Immune-Complex-Mediated (Type III) Hypersensitivity

Serum Sickness

Damage from frustrated phagocytosis of immune complexes deposited in capillaries following large transfusions of foreign serum (e.g., horse antidiphtheria serum).

Immune Complex Glomerulonephritis

Damage to the glomerulus following deposition of immune complexes that may form as a result of certain viral or bacterial infections.

Neurological Disorders; Skin Rashes

Immune complex deposition in various brain or nerve sites or the skin.

Rheumatoid Arthritis

Local production and deposition of antibodies against the synovial membrane elicit type III hypersensitivity responses leading to joint inflammation and damage.

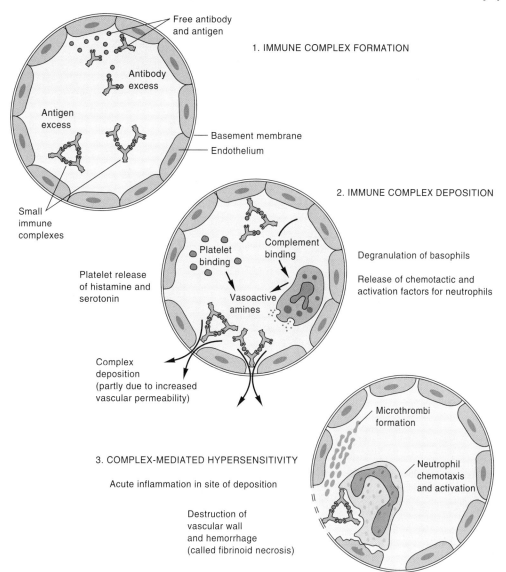

Figure 5.17 **Steps Involved in Immune-Complex-Mediated Hypersensitivity (Type III).** The vessels involved may be specialized, as are those in the glomerulus or the choroid plexus, or deposition may reflect hemodynamic factors, as in the accumulation of complexes on the heart valves.

 Checkpoint 5.2

As was pointed out at the beginning of this section on hypersensitivity, many specific diseases of immunity are mediated by more than one of these mechanisms. Before you leave this section, return to figure 5.14 and make sure you are comfortable explaining each of the four types of hypersensitivity responses. Although two of three may occur in concert, you will still be expected to describe the triggers and mechanisms of each component.

the antigen, perhaps nickel, rubber, or poison oak or ivy, is usually deposited superficially in the epidermis, whereas in the tuberculin test, the inoculant, derived from the tubercle bacillus, is introduced into the dermis and the infiltrate is largely dermal. Figure 5.18 provides an overview of type IV hypersensitivity.

The Major Histocompatibility Complex

Surveillance for intruding microorganisms that have evaded nonspecific defenses may be based on either of two strategies. The first involves the production of molecules that recognize or have an affinity for parts of other molecules that are not normally encountered in the body. The antibodies

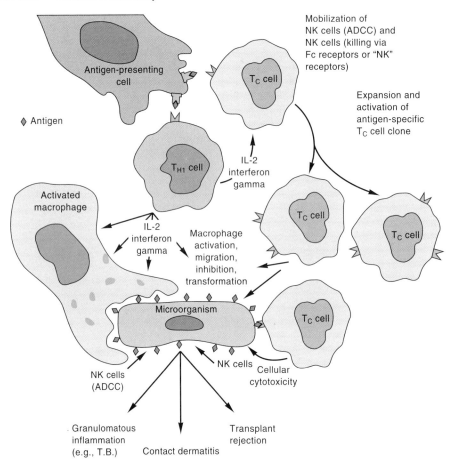

Figure 5.18   **Cell-Mediated, Delayed-Type Hypersensitivity (Type IV).**

and T-cell receptors that we have discussed are examples of this approach. In essence, it involves the recognition of "foreignness": this substance is nonhuman, it is potentially dangerous and must be destroyed. This is an excellent strategy—none of us would have survived to adulthood without it—but it has a significant flaw, similar to one that human spies exploit. A microorganism skilled in the art of disguise, which displayed surface features that closely resembled the surface features of human cells, could escape detection. Such a perfect pathogen could sweep through the human population in a devastating plague.

Fortunately, there is no such thing as a typical human cell. As we all know from hearing about the problems of transplant rejection or about campaigns to find suitable bone marrow donors, human cells (in fact, those of most animals) have features that are virtually unique to each individual. This opens the possibility of a second strategy for immune defenses: the recognition of "nonself." This strategy is utilized when our immune system identifies and attacks a virally infected cell. In becoming a factory for viral production, the cell has been altered, allowing it to be discriminated from normal "self" and killed. The immune system has the capacity to recognize the individual's unique cell surface features. This cell surface protein "fingerprint" is determined by a region on chromosome 6 called the

major histocompatibility complex (MHC). The membrane protein products of the MHC genes are involved in the rejection (or acceptance) of transplanted tissues, hence the term histocompatibility. In the transplantation of cells producing elements of the immune system—for example, bone marrow—a very close match is crucial, so the antigens on the surface of leukocytes are carefully characterized or "typed" in the process of selecting a donor. This practice has given rise to the term **HLA (human leukocyte antigen),** which is essentially interchangeable with the term MHC. Typing the leukocyte antigens will indirectly identify the antigens found on other tissues, so this approach is also used for kidney and other transplants. Note in passing that while the MHC is a major determinant of transplant success, many other factors play important roles—for example, ABO and other blood group compatibility, age, previous transfusions, further disease, and the response to and tolerance of immunosuppressive drugs.

MHC Class I and Class II: Antiviral Activity Disease Susceptibility, APC, Tissue Typing

Two MHC subtypes have been identified. The MHC class I surface proteins function as the essential self-marker. The MHC class II antigens are less widespread, playing recogni-

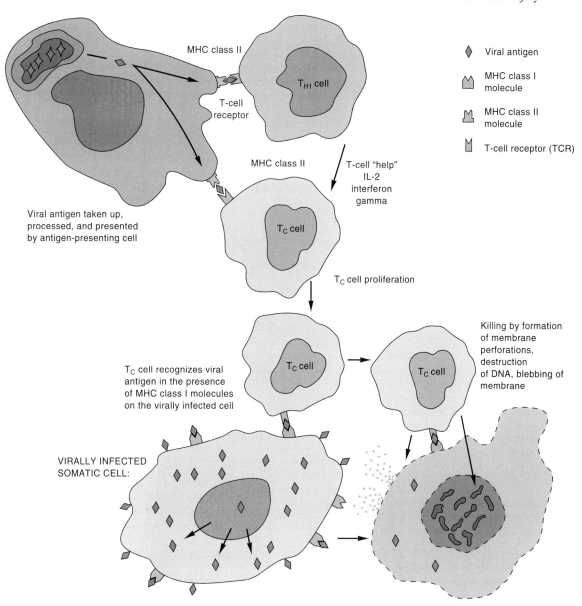

Figure 5.19   **Antiviral Activity of Cytotoxic T Lymphocytes (T_C Cells).** (Co-receptors have not been drawn to maintain clarity.)

tion and communication roles among cells of the immune system. We will present just the highlights of these functions.

Antiviral Activity You will recall our description of the antiviral activity of NK cells. Cytotoxic T cells (T_C) also play a crucial role in our resistance against viruses. Viruses are intracellular parasites unable to reproduce without the assistance of a cell. They enter a cell by first attaching to surface molecules that the cell developed for quite other purposes. Once inside, the virus is hidden from immune detection and can, using the metabolic machinery of the cell, assemble new virus particles that can exit the cell to infect other cells. The shedding of virus particles may kill the host cell. Fortunately, antigenic elements of the virus are usually displayed on the surface of an infected cell. T_C cells can detect these viral antigens but require that the antigen be associated with an MHC class I molecule. This association is

interpreted by the T_C cell to mean that although this cell is "self," it is infected and must be destroyed. The T_C cell then attacks and kills the cell and its viral contents (fig. 5.19). Requiring both MHC class I recognition and viral antigen recognition ensures that the receptors on T_C cells do not become blocked with free virus particles.

Disease Susceptibility Certain diseases are more common in individuals bearing certain HLAs or patterns of antigens. The increase in relative risk of developing the disease varies (see table 5.6). These findings argue for a direct or indirect role of immune system function in many very significant diseases, a topic that we will discuss later. As well, the intensity of immune responses appears to be based on MHC. This is good news for the person who "never gets a cold" but a great burden for the hay fever victim, both of whom display strong immune responses.

Table 5.6   Selected HLA Antigens and Their
Associated Diseases

Disease	HLA Allele	Risk Increase
Rheumatoid arthritis	DR4	5.8x
Dermatitis herpetiformis	DR3	56.4x
Chronic active hepatitis (autoimmune)	DR3	13.9x
Celiac disease	DR3	10.8x
Sjögren's disease	DR3	9.7x
Addison's disease (adrenal)	DR3	6.3x
Type I diabetes mellitus	DR3/4	14.3x
Goodpasture's syndrome	DR2	13.1x
Ankylosing spondylitis	B27	84.4x
Myasthenia gravis	B8	4.4x

x represents risk in the normal population. The risk of contracting the
disease is greater when the antigen is present, but note that in no case is
the disease certain to develop. These data hold for those of European
Caucasian extraction.

Data derived from Roitt, I., *Essential Immunology,* Seventh Ed.,
Blackwell Scientific Publications, London, 1991.

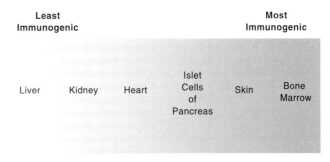

Figure 5.20   **Tissues Vary in Their Tendency to Generate
Immune-Mediated Rejection.**

✓ *Checkpoint 5.3*

The distinction between MHC class I and class II
molecules, like the four types of hypersensitivity reactions, is difficult to learn initially. Take the time
now to consolidate the information presented here.
Otherwise, when you encounter the terms later, you'll
be back!

Antigen-Presenting Cells As we described earlier, before the immune system can mount a response, antigen
must be presented to T$_H$ (helper T) cells. You may also recall that only T cells from a specific clone will recognize
a particular antigen. The cells that process and display
antigens for T$_H$ cells are known as **antigen-presenting
cells** (APCs). These express high levels of MHC class II
antigens, which allow them to interact with the T-cell receptor molecule in antigen presentation. The dominant
APCs are probably cells of the monocyte/macrophage cell
line: macrophages in tissues, monocytes in the blood,
Kupffer cells in the liver, resident macrophages in the
spleen and lymph nodes, and microglia in the brain.
The term also applies to various nonphagocytic cells
(e.g., dendritic cells) in the skin, lymphoid tissue, and
other tissues; and both B and T cells can function as
APCs. In the central area of lymph nodes and in the
spleen, APCs called **interdigitating dendritic cells**
(IDCs) are found. They are considered the most important
APC in inducing a primary immune response. APCs can
interact with microorganisms shortly after they enter the
body and process their antigenic components so they are
capable of stimulating T$_H$ cells. They then enter the lymph
drainage, move to the appropriate part of the lymph node,
and select and interact with the T$_H$ cells. This last step is
effected through the association of the antigen with an
MHC class II molecule. These are expressed only on
APCs and are the essential recognition factor between
APC and T$_H$ cells. Therefore, T$_H$ recognition of antigen is
said to be class II restricted.

Tissue Transplantation

Tissue matching and the development of selective immune
suppression have led to dramatic improvements in the success of transplant therapy. The following sections deal with
some general issues in transplant rejection and some approaches that seek to improve graft survival.

Transplant Rejection

Tissues vary in their tendency to generate an immune-
mediated rejection, whatever their particular HLA match
(fig. 5.20). One factor involved is the density of the dendritic cells present: both skin and bone marrow are rich in
these APCs and are better able to mount a vigorous reaction. A second factor is the variation in the expression of
the class II MHC. Some tissues (e.g., liver and kidney) produce relatively little antigen and thereby generate milder reactions. In the case of the liver, its large volume of tissue
can act like a sponge for the antibody, causing its distribution in low concentrations throughout.

Very rapid (hyperacute) rejection can occur if an individual has had previous contact with specific foreign tissue
antigens, usually by transfusion or previous transplantation.
In such a sensitized individual, it may be only minutes before preformed antibodies initiate complement-mediated
destruction of the transplanted tissue. As a result, a transplanted kidney, for example, rather than being firm, pink,
and producing ample urine, would be soft and pale and
would produce only drops of bloody urine. The antibodies
appear to attach to the vascular endothelium, triggering

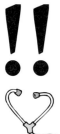

Focus on MHC: Tissue Typing

The MHC occupies a significant part (1/3,000th) of our entire genetic endowment (the human genome). The varied combination of alternate alleles gives rise to a great deal of variability from individual to individual in HLA type, in excess of perhaps one million! On average, you would have to test over 50,000 people from the general population before encountering a workable HLA match (in the range of 1/450 for a common match, 1/750,000 for a rare match). Of course, the odds are greatly improved in related individuals and identical twins, who have identical or very similar HLA.

In practice, MHC antigens are not randomly distributed and selected in the population. Certain genes are more commonly found associated with each other, and certain constellations of HLA antigens are more common in specific racial groups. This pattern sometimes helps focus the search.

---

complement deposition, neutrophil infiltration, platelet and fibrin adhesion, and the formation of thrombi in the arterioles and glomerular and peritubular capillaries. In the more usual transplant rejection problem, where there is some degree of MHC incompatibility, the reaction takes longer to develop.

Although the mechanism of rejection probably varies with the nature of the tissue and the degree of incompatibility, all the mechanisms require that the host T_H cells (helper T cells) come into contact with the graft tissue's MHC antigens. This contact is probably mediated by the dendritic cells of the graft tissue itself. These cells can interact directly with host T_H cells via their class II molecules or can process graft antigen and then present it to T_H cells in association with class II molecules. Either method will strongly activate T_H cells.

At this point, three different possibilities exist. In the first, antigen-specific T_H cells stimulate the activation and proliferation of appropriate T_C cells, which then mount a focused attack on the transplant tissue. In the second, responsive antigen-specific T_H cells move to the graft site, where they release lymphokines. These recruit monocytes/macrophages and T_C cells to the graft site and maintain them at the scene while they destroy the tissue. (You may recognize this as a delayed-type hypersensitivity reaction.) As well as these direct cell-mediated mechanisms of graft rejection, there is a third mechanism in which antibodies play a role. The responsive T_H cell interacts with the appropriate B cell clone, producing a shower of antibodies to the implanted tissue's MHC antigens. These can trigger either complement-mediated graft damage or antibody-mediated cellular cytotoxicity. The latter is accomplished by K or killer cells.

Antibodies generated by MHC incompatibility can produce an acute rejection, either hours or days after transplantation or much later, when immunosuppressant therapy is terminated. Fortunately, HLA cross-matching has largely eliminated this pattern of rejection. There still remains the risk of chronic rejection, which is typically cell-mediated. It can be prevented only by very close cross-matching or continued immunosuppression. Sometimes purging the graft tissue of potential APCs; for example, by infusing the donor kidney with cytotoxic drugs or by subjecting skin grafts to ultraviolet light, enhances transplant acceptance.

Bone marrow transplantation presents a special rejection problem. In this case the graft is being done because there is a serious defect in the person's own bone marrow—for example, leukemia or perhaps radiation damage that has reduced the numbers of blood-producing cells. Preliminary to the injection of donor bone marrow, the patient's bone marrow is destroyed in order to remove the offending tumor cell lines in the case of leukemia. If the donor marrow contains mature competent T_H cells, these can set up an assault on the patient's cells because the donor T_H cells recognize the host tissue as foreign. This potentially fatal rejection of the host cells by the donor tissue is called **graft-versus-host disease.** It typically affects the host liver, skin, and GI mucosa. Close MHC matching and selective T-cell depletion of donor marrow are often effective in preventing this major problem. Figure 5.21 presents an overview of the mechanisms of graft rejection.

Improving Graft Survival

The goals for improving graft acceptance and survival are to avoid T_H cell sensitization and to suppress the response of any sensitized T_H cells that already exist. As we have just seen, the first goal is approached by careful tissue matching and by using cytotoxic agents to clean the donor organ of resident APCs. The pool of previously sensitized T_H cells can be reduced by administering cytotoxic or specific anti-T-cell agents—for example, antithymocyte globulin (ATG) or antilymphocyte globulin (ALG)—to the recipient.

Drugs are also routinely used to suppress the immune response to transplanted tissue. Corticosteroids (e.g., prednisone) have potent anti-inflammatory and immunosuppressant effects. By blocking the metabolic pathways that produce long-acting inflammatory mediators, they dramatically mute or reverse the rejection reaction.

Other drugs have a more focused effect. The commonly used immunosuppressant drug cyclosporin A (CSA) blocks the production of interleukin 2 (IL-2) in a T_H cell. As a result, the T_H cell can't communicate with itself; that is, the IL-2 can't feed signals back to the T_H cell and so the cell does not proliferate. Thus, there is blockage of the stimulation of related B cells (suppression of antibody production) and cytotoxic T cells (suppression of T_C-mediated graft rejection). Cyclophosphamide, another immunosuppressant drug, has its effect through a quite different route.

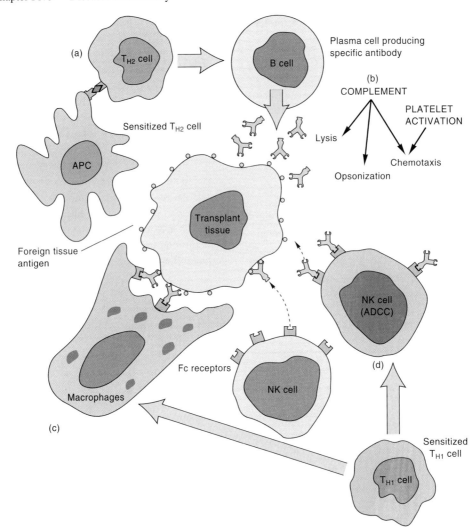

Figure 5.21 **Overview of Mechanisms of Graft Rejection.** (*a*) Antigen-presenting cells facilitate T-cell sensitization, which enhances complement deposition and platelet aggregation (*b*) and, in turn, phagocytosis. Antibody binding makes possible antibody-dependent cellular cytotoxicity by NK cells (*c*). NK cells attack the transplant tissue (*d*), while sensitized and activated T cells mobilize a chronic attack on the graft tissue.

It interferes with the normal cycling of surface receptors, limiting T_H and B-cell responses to activation and proliferation signals. Figure 5.22 summarizes the approaches to improving graft survival.

Although corticosteroids, cyclosporin A, and cyclophosphamide greatly improve graft survival rates by suppressing a major protective response, they share the unfortunate side effect of making a person more vulnerable to infection. If the recipient develops an infection that is unresponsive to antibiotics, the immunosuppressant drugs must be discontinued, which means that the graft may be rejected.

IMMUNE DEFICIENCY SYNDROMES

Just as an immune system that functions too intensely can create problems, one that functions poorly can impair our capacity to deal effectively with infection. Much of our understanding of basic immune system function has been de-

rived from observing the disease states that occur when one or more components of the immune system are congenitally absent or malfunctioning, usually through a genetic abnormality. These primary immunodeficiencies—B-cell deficiencies, T-cell deficiencies, combined B- and T-cell deficiencies, defects in phagocytosis or cytotoxicity, deficiencies in complement components—have provided "experiments in nature" from which scientists have drawn conclusions about the contribution of specific immune system components. The following discussion is organized in terms of such components. However, as you can now appreciate, normal function depends on an interaction among them. As we will see, immune deficiency diseases often produce widespread and complex effects.

Primary Immune Deficiencies

Primary immune deficiencies are often genetically determined. They usually become apparent from recurrent or

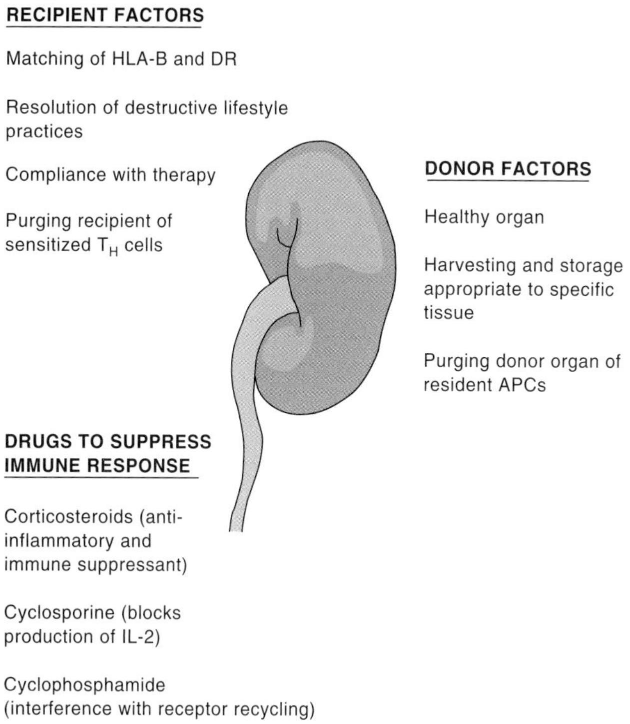

RECIPIENT FACTORS

Matching of HLA-B and DR

Resolution of destructive lifestyle practices

Compliance with therapy

Purging recipient of sensitized T_H cells

DONOR FACTORS

Healthy organ

Harvesting and storage appropriate to specific tissue

Purging donor organ of resident APCs

DRUGS TO SUPPRESS IMMUNE RESPONSE

Corticosteroids (anti-inflammatory and immune suppressant)

Cyclosporine (blocks production of IL-2)

Cyclophosphamide (interference with receptor recycling)

Figure 5.22   **Strategies Used to Improve Graft Survival.**

persistent infections suffered by infants beyond six months of age. This pattern suggests that the passive immunity conferred on an infant by the mother has not been replaced by normal active immune responses. Treatment of these individuals must take into account their extreme vulnerability to infection; for example, a child may have to live in a completely isolated environment. Vaccines may present an infection risk despite the fact that the virus has been attenuated. Even blood transfusions may be the cause of graft-versus-host disease, because the donor T cells are not resisted in their attack on what is, to them, foreign tissue.

B-Cell Deficiencies

In very general terms, B-cell deficiencies result in recurrent or overwhelming infections by viruses that are normally neutralized by antibody (e.g., the virus that causes rubella) or by bacteria that can resist phagocytosis unless they are well opsonized by antibody (e.g., *Staphylococcus* or the *Haemophilus influenzae* responsible for meningitis in very young children). The B-cell deficit produces lowered or absent gammaglobulin levels (**hypogammaglobulinemia**). In **Bruton's agammaglobulinemia,** the antibody levels are variable and may be profoundly depressed. This is an X-linked disease and therefore affects primarily males. The lymphoid tissues, with the exception of the thymus, are poorly developed. These are presumably the bursa-equivalent tissues, and their absence interferes with the maturation of the pre-B cells produced in bone marrow in normal numbers. T-cell numbers and function are normal, as is their coping with most viral and fungal infections. For unknown

reasons, many individuals with Bruton's agammaglobulinemia develop autoimmune connective tissue diseases like rheumatoid arthritis and systemic lupus erythematosus.

T-Cell Deficiencies

In general, T-cell deficiencies result in chronic or recurrent infections with viruses (recall that T_C cells destroy virally infected cells) and yeasts/fungi (such as *Candida* and *Histoplasma*) or intracellular bacteria (such as the mycobacterium responsible for tuberculosis). Such deficiencies are one characteristic of the **DiGeorge syndrome.** This disorder is accompanied by various nonimmune abnormalities, in varying degrees. They include small jaw and cheeks, turned-down mouth, partial or complete absence of parathyroids, and heart defects. Because these structures all derive from associated embryonic structures, they point, together with the absent or incomplete thymus, to a common developmental problem occurring about the seventh week of gestation. Depending on the particular developmental deficits, the newborn may face immediate, life-threatening disorders that derive from an interrupted aortic arch or hypocalcemia from impaired parathyroid hormone secretion. The failure of normal thymus development, which, like the other defects, may be due to viral infection, trauma, or perhaps a blood clot, leads to a profound T-cell deficit. The thymic hypoplasia is sometimes treated by transplantation of fetal thymic tissue. If blood products are given, they need to be irradiated to prevent donor T cells from engrafting and producing graft-versus-host disease.

In some cases of T-cell deficiency, people lack a specific clone of T cells, and therefore they cannot recognize and respond to the antigen specific to that T-cell receptor. Such is the case in **chronic mucocutaneous candidiasis.** People with this disorder suffer mild to severe *Candida* infections of the mucous membranes and skin without mounting an effective immune response because their T cells don't recognize this antigen. The candidiasis may appear as thrush, an infection of the tongue or oral cavity involving ulcers and white spots. The vagina is also commonly colonized, and the esophagus is a less common but very serious target. The consequences of T_H-cell deficiency are shown in figure 5.23.

Severe Combined Immunodeficiency (SCID)

As the name implies, SCID is a very serious disorder of both T-cell and immunoglobulin production and function. It is inherited, either through autosomal recessive or X-linked transmission, and is typically a common (T and B) stem cell disorder. Without a successful bone marrow transplant, children with SCID succumb to opportunistic infections during their first year of life. The microorganisms involved include those that affect the AIDS patient: *Pneumocystis carinii, Candida, Pseudomonas,* cytomegalovirus, and the virus that causes herpes simplex. Marrow transplantation may fail, either because of NK-cell-mediated rejection or

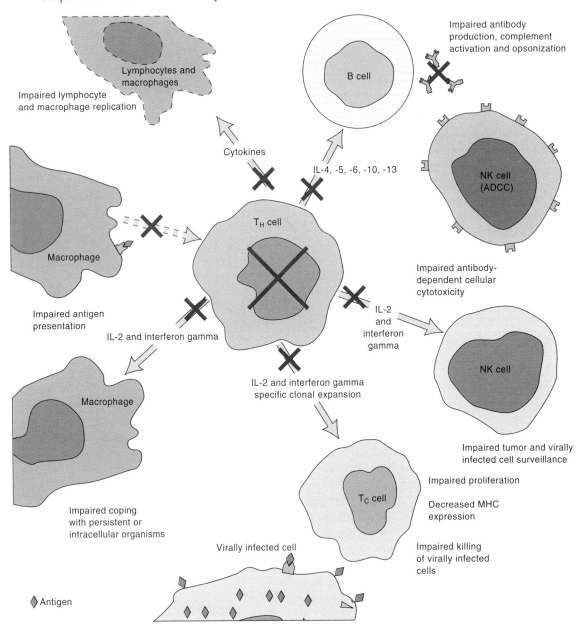

Figure 5.23 **Summary of the Impact of Drastically Reduced T$_H$ Cell Numbers.** Note that, for simplicity's sake, T$_{H1}$ and T$_{H2}$ have been collapsed into a T$_H$ cell.

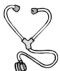

Focus on Gene Therapy for SCID

In the spring of 1991, the first results were announced for new and exciting therapy. A little girl with the ADA deficiency form of SCID had responded well and was maintaining adequate lymphocyte counts and producing functional immune responses. In the treatment, doctors separated circulating lymphocytes from her blood and had introduced a functional ADA gene into them by infecting them with an ADA-bearing virus. Then they expanded the isolated lymphocyte pool by treating it with interleukin-2 to promote proliferation; and finally they reintroduced these cells to her body. If it were possible to isolate lymphocyte stem cells and treat them in this way, a permanent cure could be achieved. Very active research proceeds in this and other directions. This is the first example of effective human gene therapy and holds great promise.

Table 5.7   Key Features of Selected Immunodeficiency States

Deficiency/Disease	Comments
B Cells	
Bruton's agammaglobulinemia (or Bruton's panhypogammaglobulinemia)	Recurrent pyogenic (pus-forming) infections at 5 to 6 mo of age
	No B cells in peripheral blood
	X-linked genetics; more boys affected
	IgG levels variable, others absent
	Lack of "bursa-equivalent tissue"
Isolated IgA deficiency	Most common immunodeficiency condition (other than AIDS)
	Absence of secretory IgA
	Some may have more GI, pulmonary, and urogenital infections
	Transfusion may induce severe anaphylaxis
Acquired hypogammaglobulinemia (common variable immunodeficiency)	Depressed antibody levels
	Recurrent pyogenic infections from 15–35 yr
	Higher incidence of autoimmune disease
T Cells	
DiGeorge syndrome	Extreme T-cell deficit
	Associated with facial abnormalities, parathyroid and cardiac defects
	Chronic/recurrent viral, yeast, fungal, bacterial infections
Chronic mucocutaneous candidiasis	Chronic mild/severe *Candida* infections: thrush, vaginal, and esophageal infections
B and T Cells	
Severe combined immunodeficiency (SCID)	Genetic defect causing inadequate B/T-cell production
	Early onset (6 mo)
	Chronic/recurrent viral fungal infections
	Susceptible to graft-versus-host disease
Wiskott-Aldrich syndrome	X-linked; mostly boys affected
	Severe eczema, thrombocytopenia, allergies, recurrent infections
Ataxia-telangiectasia	Autosomal recessive inheritance
	Cerebellar degeneration (ataxia) and telangiectasia (small vessel dilation)
	Decreased antibody production and T-helper activity

because of fatal graft-versus-host disease. About half the children with the autosomal recessive pattern of transmission lack an enzyme in their red and white blood cells called ADA (adenosine deaminase). Its absence leads to the accumulation of substances toxic to lymphocytes.

Table 5.7 summarizes the features of the disorders we have been discussing. It also gives information about several other primary immune deficiency diseases. These are quite rare, often genetic disorders whose signs and symptoms are related to the lack of a particular component of the immune system.

Secondary Immune Deficiencies

The thymus achieves its peak size during adolescence, the time during which we contact and establish immunity against a wide variety of pathogens. After that it gradually atrophies, and by middle age it is only a fraction of its for-

mer size. Although the number of circulating T cells doesn't drop significantly, the capacity to mount a T-cell-mediated immune response does decrease with increasing age. (For example, there is a reduction in delayed-type hypersensitivity reactions in the tuberculin test.) At the same time, there is an increase in the levels of circulating autoantibodies. These are self-reactive antibodies and are involved in a variety of autoimmune diseases, to be described in some detail at the end of this chapter. Thus, there are age-related trends in immune system function that may be associated with impaired immunity and the development of autoimmune disorders.

Diet can also affect immune function. Those subjected to severe caloric or protein malnutrition, particularly children, suffer impaired T-cell, complement, and neutrophil function. They are therefore particularly vulnerable to bacteria that require opsonization and phagocytosis or T-cell-mediated cellular immunity. Selective deficiencies can also lead to impaired immunity. For example, a zinc deficiency, which might be caused by a failure to absorb zinc, by zinc loss through diarrhea, by severe burns, or by renal disease, can severely impair both T- and B-cell function.

Besides opening the barrier to infection that the skin usually provides, extensive burns can lead to both a generalized suppression of immune function and focal, antigen-specific immune suppression. Complement levels are depressed and neutrophil chemotaxis and cytotoxicity are reduced, so that the burn victim is more vulnerable to infection by bacteria that are difficult to engulf without opsonization (e.g., *Haemophylus influenzae* or *Staphylococcus*).

Impaired immunity can be secondary to a number of other disorders. For example, diabetes mellitus produces vascular changes and impaired leukocyte function, which together reduce both inflammatory and specific immune responses and contribute to the recurrent and prolonged infections characteristic of that disease. Malignancies of bone marrow (leukemia and myeloproliferative disorders) and lymphoid tissues (lymphoma) can suppress immune function, as can certain infections (e.g., congenital rubella, cytomegalovirus, tuberculosis, coccidiomycosis).

Deficiencies may also be associated with medical treatments (iatrogenic deficiencies). The most obvious example has been mentioned: infections associated with the use of immunosuppressant drugs in transplantation. Chemotherapeutic agents and radiation used for treating cancer differentially affect rapidly replicating cells such as blood-forming cells in bone marrow and lymphoid tissues. Besides producing a generally lowered white blood cell count, tumor suppression therapy can paralyze both T- and B-cell responses to a specific pathogen by blocking clonal expansion. Other drugs (e.g., some anticonvulsants, antimicrobials, tranquilizers, or analgesics) are directly toxic or produce immune-mediated effects on mature lymphocytes. Depression of immune function is a potential side effect that must be monitored routinely with many medications. In the same vein, surgery and anaesthesia can depress T- and B-cell function and induce severe lymphocyte deficiency for up to a month.

The correlation between presumably stressful life events (divorce, death of family member, promotion, job loss, etc.) and the incidence of disease (including infection) was noted 20 years ago. Stress appears to reactivate latent viral infections and may have a role in making individuals more vulnerable to new infection. There is evidence for interaction between the neuroendocrine and immune systems: Many lymphoid tissues are innervated, and immune system cells can both produce and respond to agents with neuroendocrine activity (e.g., endorphins, ACTH, TSH, interleukin-1). Corticosteroids produced during stress reactions depress macrophage production of interleukin-1, and this change could interfere with antigen presentation and initiation of the immune response. As well, corticosteroids can have the effect of depressing IL-2 production by helper T cells, thereby affecting the primary immune response and subsequent sensitization. The interactions in stress are complex and only partially understood. From what is known, stress could be the basis of either immune system hyperactivity or hypofunction. For vulnerable individuals, stress may play an important role in immune-mediated illness (e.g., autoimmune disease) or immune deficiency.

Acquired Immune Deficiency Syndrome (AIDS)

Over two decades have elapsed since the United States Centers for Disease Control (CDC) identified a cluster of five cases of *Pneumocystis carinii* pneumonia (PCP) among young homosexual males in the Los Angeles area, two of whom soon died. To monitor this flare-up of a usually rare disease, the CDC quickly established a category for people who acquired diseases that were rare except in those with profoundly depressed cellular immune function. This included people with Kaposi's sarcoma (a rare skin cancer) or any of a limited number of opportunistic infections, particularly PCP. Opportunistic implies that the infection flourishes because of defects or impaired function in an individual's immune system. With this surveillance definition, the era of AIDS was born. By 1984, the **human immunodeficiency virus** (HIV) had been isolated and described, and mechanisms of transmission were being identified: intimate sexual contact; direct contamination of blood as occurs between intravenous drug abusers using contaminated equipment, or hemophiliac or transfusion recipients of contaminated blood or blood products; passage of virus from mother to a fetus, at birth or through breast milk.

The Epidemiology of HIV/AIDS

The population distribution of HIV/AIDS varies from country to country, reflecting complex interactions between how and through which group the infection entered the population, the social/cultural/economic forces that supported its dissemination, and the nature and vigor of the medical, governmental, and societal responses to the epidemic. Within a society, this distribution also changes dynamically over time. The reporting on HIV/AIDS assumes an understanding of HIV and AIDS definitions and of some basic epidemiology. The "HIV+" designation is given to an individual who has tested positive for HIV infection. An "AIDS" diagnosis implies a positive HIV test and the progression of the disease to the point at which the person has developed the opportunistic infections and/or other symptoms that fit the diagnosis "AIDS." The criteria for this diagnosis are set by the agency to which health personnel file any "reportable diseases." In the United States, this is the CDC (Centers for Disease Control) and in Canada it is the Centre for Infectious Disease Prevention & Control. (Named reporting of HIV and AIDS in adults is mandatory in 36 states and territories in the United States, eight of which have begun this program since 1997. The rest have their own regulations regarding anonymity, and simply remove patients names from the files they report to the

CDC). The evolving CDC surveillance definition was expanded in 1993 to include AIDS-related neurological conditions. This created an immediate rise in the number of identified cases, which took about three years to settle down. "HIV/AIDS" includes all those with confirmed HIV infection. "Cumulative cases" includes all identified cases, alive and dead, since the original disease definition in 1982. "Incidence" is the number of new cases identified in a year, while "prevalence" is the total number of people affected with a disorder. So, the incidence of HIV is the number of people reported to have been newly diagnosed HIV positive in a particular year. The prevalence of HIV is the total number of people living with HIV infection, but does not include those who have gone on to develop AIDS. Incidence or prevalence "rate" is the number of cases per 100,000 of the general population. These terms may be further focused by restricting the population compared against—for example, the prevalence of HIV-positive status among men who have sex with men (which one might expect to be higher than the prevalence in the general population). As an indicator of disease trends, the incidence of HIV, presuming widespread and representative testing, is a more sensitive statistic than AIDS incidence or prevalence because of the variable lag time between HIV seroconversion and development of "full-blown AIDS" (there is on average about a ten-year lag between HIV and AIDS). The math can be puzzling. In the United States, there was a 42% drop in the 1996–1997 deaths from AIDS due to the beginning of **highly active antiretroviral treatment** (HAART). This led to a sharp rise in the prevalence of AIDS, something we might not, at first blush, think of as very positive. With this background in mind, let's look at HIV/AIDS in the West.

The first 100,000 AIDS cases recorded in the United States take us back to the first eight years of the epidemic: The risk group breakdown was 61% men who have sex with men (MSM), 20% intravenous drug users (IDUs), and 5% through heterosexual transmission. For the same group, 62% were white, 27% African American, and 15% Hispanic. Males composed 91% of all cases. As of December 2000, 775,000 AIDS cases were diagnosed and about 450,000 deaths had occurred. The historic complexion of the epidemic is somewhat modified in the breakdown of these cumulative deaths: 46% were white, 35% African American, and 17% Hispanic, while 85% were males and 15% females.

To bring this into the present, in the United States in 2002, about 930,000 people are living with HIV, and of those, about 350,000 are living with AIDS. The incidence of new infections is around 40,000 per year (this includes those who although newly diagnosed have already progressed to AIDS), with 70% male and 30% female. Although 4,000 children under the age of 13 are living with AIDS (just over 1% of all cases), the incidence of new cases has dropped dramatically, mostly attributable to the prenatal use of antiretrovirals by the mother and the administration of antiretroviral drugs to the baby for up to 6 months. (Currently, about 90% of HIV in children was transmitted parentally—i.e., during gestation, during labor, or perhaps with breastfeeding. The risk of transmission to the baby is about 20–30%. Caesarian section reduces transmission by about 50% while perinatal use of antiretroviral drugs reduces incidence in the newborn from 25% to perhaps 8–10%.) The incidence of HIV infection attributable to transfusions or contaminated blood products has virtually been eliminated (the risk is about 1 per 525,000 for blood transfusion). HIV-1 has been tested for in blood since 1985 and HIV-2 since 1992 (we will describe these later). The 2001 statistics for HIV incidence (males and females together) were 42% of cases in men who have sex with men (MSM), 33% of cases associated with heterosexual transmission, followed by intravenous drug use at 25%. African Americans (constituting only 13% of the American population) form 54% of the 40,000 newly diagnosed HIV cases, while 26% are white, and 19% Hispanic. It is revealing to contrast the HIV incidence in men and women. Speaking only of men who have been newly infected, 50% are black, 30% white, and 20% Hispanic. Considered by risk group, the breakdown is 60% men who have sex with men, 15% contracted through heterosexual contact, and 25% intravenous drug users. Of women, 64% are black, with the remainder split evenly (18%) between Hispanic and white. By risk group, 75% contracted HIV through heterosexual activity and the rest (25%) were IDUs.

Although no pattern of incidence should be taken as grounds for either complacence or paranoia, the dramatic drop in death rate that coincided with the advent of HAART was part of a general trend of dropping incidence of both HIV and AIDS since the peak in AIDS incidence in 1993. (The peak in deaths due to AIDS was in 1995). The incidence of both HIV and AIDS has dropped for the general population and across risk groups (MSM, IDU, heterosexual transmission) and ethnic grouping (white, African American, and Hispanic) significantly between 1993 and 1997, and slowly since. And to put AIDS into some crude perspective, about 55 times as many people die of heart disease and stroke combined, and six and one-half times as many die in accidents. (To balance this, AIDS is typically a disease of the young and, among young males, constitutes a major killer, thereby generating disproportionate "years of life lost"). This good news of decreased general incidence and death rate is balanced by the trends just noted. At the level of proportions, HIV/AIDS has shifted into the minority populations. Proportionally more people living with HIV/AIDS are African American or Hispanic, female, residents of the South, and are infected by heterosexual contact. So the wedge of heterosexual transmission is entering to an unbalanced extent in the African American and Hispanic communities. And studies have shown a frightening prevalence of 7% in young (ages 15–22), black, MSM men and double this for African American MSMs (14%) as a group (compared to 3% for white MSMs). A wild card added to this is the estimated one-quarter of persons living with HIV/AIDS who are unaware of their infection and the

Focus on 2002 International AIDS Conference Opens with Bleak News

The keynote address painted a discouraging picture of the international progression of HIV/AIDS. With 40 million people currently infected, AIDS is growing faster than ever in its history. In the previous year, over 3 million people died of AIDS and an estimated 16,000 contract the disease every day. Globally, of those infected, 44% are women and 4% are children (only 1% of total infections in the West are children). The risk of transmission to the fetus/baby varies from 7–49%, depending to a large extent on the health of the mother and the coexistence of veneral disease. There has been a dramatic rise in infections in the Middle East and Eastern Europe, particularly among the young, with the fastest growth rate in the world in the Russian Federation. In Russia, the number of new cases reported in the year 2000 exceeded the total number of cases reported previously. Here, the first wave of the epidemic is being driven by young, male intravenous drug users, a sign of a society in crisis. In sub-Saharan Africa, 25 million people are living with HIV and perhaps 2.5 million will die in 2002. Some countries in this region have an infection rate of 50%. The strain on the local economies is extreme, with a drop in GDP estimated to be in the vicinity of 20% for 2002. The Caribbean, while having low absolute number of HIV-positive individuals, has a prevalence rate second only to Africa. The beneficial impact of the aggressive use of antiretroviral drugs has been confined to the wealthy nations, while 90% of the infections are taking place in the developing world. In the West, the good news of HAART (highly active antiretroviral therapy) has been balanced by an upswing in high-risk sexual practices among young, gay men. And an effective vaccine looks to be at least ten years in the future. Twenty years after the CDC identification of the disease, prevention still holds the greatest promise for control of this epidemic. The tailored campaigns that might make the difference hinge upon AIDS groups and governments receiving the annual $10 billion (US) pledged to the Global AIDS Fund—pledges that are not being fully honored.

---

further one-third who, while aware, are not receiving care. These findings collectively mean that this illness is increasingly afflicting segments of the population that are poorer and have traditionally had less access to medical and preventive services. HAART has demonstrated the impact that more appropriate care can have on delaying both AIDS and death. But its most effective application is treatment as early after HIV infection as possible. The intense need for continued, effectively targeted public health campaigns and appropriate funding for drug therapies is clear.

In Canada, approximately 50,000 persons are living with HIV/AIDS; approximately 59% are MSM, 4% MSM-IDUs, 20% IDUs, and 16% through heterosexual contact. With about 10% of the U.S. population, this means that both the Canadian incidence and prevalence of HIV/AIDS are about half those of the United States. Like the U.S. statistics, there has been a downswing in Canadian HIV/AIDS incidence since 1993 and a steady increase in prevalence due to HAART. In Canada, the introduction of HIV was more concentrated in the MSM population, which is reflected in MSM accounting for 78% of the cumulative number of AIDS cases reported through the end of 2000 (prior to 1995 this was 81%) and 72% of the cumulative reports of HIV (reflecting the historic decline in incidence within this population). Newly diagnosed HIV runs at about 4,400 cases per year in Canada, and, as in the United States, the risk group characterization is changing. The breakdown by risk group (1999 stats) is MSM 38%, MSM-IDU 7%, IDU 34% (this peaked at 47% in 1996), and heterosexual transmission 21%. The drop in incidence since 1992 to 1994 was driven principally by changes within the MSM population, which until 1988 formed about 80% of AIDS incidence. This drop within MSM initially represented a combination of returns for the intense, community-based efforts toward education and intervention and perhaps the "maturation" of the disease among this population (the most at-risk individuals become affected and the "plague" runs its course). Then, in 1996, there was the same dramatic drop in progression to AIDS noted in the United States due to HAART, but this encouraging trend within MSM has recently reversed. While the percentage contribution to incident AIDS cases by MSM dropped fairly steadily from 1988 until 1999, it took a sudden upswing in 2000. MSM-IDU attributed 6.5% of AIDS cases (up from 5% before 1995). And HIV incidence, which is sensitive to emerging trends, increased in 1999 and again in 2000. These increases were particularly evident in the major metropolitan centers of Toronto and Vancouver. As an indication of an alarming trend among MSM, a Vancouver study reported that while 32% of respondents engaged in unprotected anal intercourse (a very high-risk behavior) with regular partners and 15% with casual partners, this had changed to 72% and 47%, respectively, one year later! In another study in Vancouver, of those who claimed to practice safe sex, 26–30% had relapsed to unprotected anal sex in 6–12-month follow-up. Of the 21% of HIV infections in women, 54% were attributed to IDUs and 46% to heterosexual transmission. The relatively small aboriginal population of Canada is at particular risk—there was a 91% increase in HIV prevalence within the aboriginal peoples. The 9% of all new HIV infections that are accounted for by this group were attributable to IDUs (64%), heterosexual transmission (17%), MSM (11%), and MSM-IDUs (8%). Isolation of aboriginal communities, limited access to health resources, and problems of stigmatization not limited to this community, raise grave concern over these trends.

The Focus box (2002 AIDS Conference) presents a very brief account of HIV/AIDS in the rest of the world. Bear in mind, as you read, that some of the details have been blunted in the service of the larger message—that AIDS is a very threatening international crisis that is not getting sufficient resources fast enough. There are "bright spots" in the center of the crisis. Changes in incidence in sub-Saharan Africa indicate very tentatively that the epidemic there may be taking the turn it appears to be taking in North America. But the aching need created by the current crisis and the long-term repercussions far outweigh any impulse to complacency.

Theoretical Sources of HIV Infection

Retrospective studies of banked blood indicate that HIV was present in North America by 1967. There are two strains of the HIV virus, which is an enveloped RNA virus and a member of the lentivirus family. The virus particles contain reverse transcriptase that after entry into cell produces a "provirus" that can integrate into host DNA, thereby establishing a "viral factory." HIV-1 is responsible for most of the international epidemic while HIV-2, which remains uncommon in North America, arose in West Africa and passed, with immigration, into Europe. HIV-2 appears to produce immunodeficiency and AIDS with lower frequency than does HIV-1. Analyses of HIV RNA link this virus to strains of simian immunodeficiency virus (SIV). Apparently, HIV-1 arose in chimpanzees while HIV-2 passed to humans from the sooty mangabey monkey. Evidence exists, again based on tiny differences in RNA, for several independent passages from primates to humans. It is thought that HIV-1 first showed up in humans in Africa in 1931 or earlier. There are three different groups of HIV-1 virus, with the M (main) group responsible for most of the worldwide epidemic. Within the M group, there are ten distinct subtypes or "clades" (designated A to J). This genetic diversity creates severe challenges to groups attempting to develop effective vaccines.

HIV-1: The Major AIDS Virus

Almost all researchers accept the central importance of the human immunodeficiency virus in the development of acquired immune deficiency syndrome. Several features that are essential to our understanding of the transmission and replication of HIV are depicted in figure 5.24. To reproduce themselves, viruses must gain access to the genetic and metabolic machinery of a host cell. The knobs on the surface of the virus particle, called gp120 (for glycoprotein of 120,000 gram molecular weight), have affinity for a molecule called CD4, which is produced and displayed on the surface of selected cells of the body. Helper T cells (recall that they are also called T_4 because of the presence of CD4) are richly covered, as are monocyte/macrophage cells

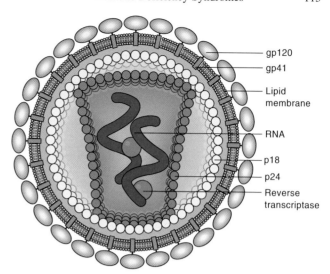

Figure 5.24   **Structure of the HIV Virus Particle.**

and their lineage, including Langerhans cells (in the loose connective tissue supporting the gastrointestinal and genital mucosa) and dendritic cells (residing within lymph nodes and nodules), and some B cells. There is evidence that other cells in the body have gp120 receptors—for example, glial (support) cells in the brain and chromaffin (unicellular glandular) cells in the duodenum, colon, and rectum. The binding of the gp120 "knobs" to T-cell receptors, whether on T helper cells or the various cells of the monocyte line (macrophages, Langerhans cells, dendritic cells), is not sufficient to allow integration with the membrane of the host cell. The second requisite binding proteins are part of the family of chemokine receptors. Chemokines are relatively small chemicals released by lymphocytes to influence the function of related cells. This influence can be either paracrine (acting on different cells in the immediate vicinity) or autocrine (acting on themselves or immediately adjacent cells of the same type). In this case, the chemokine receptor plays an essential role as a co-receptor by increasing the intimacy of the contact between the HIV-1 particle and the surface of the cell with which it is about to merge. There are two chemokine co-receptors of relevance. One sort, the CCR5 or "R5," is displayed on the surface of all the cells with which HIV can merge. The second, CXCR4 or "R4," is restricted to the CD4 + T-cell lineage. Briefly, after binding to the T-cell receptor, the gp120 engages R5 or R4, is pulled closer to the phospholipid membrane of the host cell, merges with it, and empties its contents of RNA—reverse transcriptase, viral core protein gp24 (which is the target of the usual ELISA antibody test for HIV infection), and "integrase" (which helps integrate the provirus into host DNA) into the interior of the host cell (fig. 5.25). This understanding of chemokine co-receptors has provided an explanation for the observation that some persons appear to have a very slow progression to AIDS with HIV-1 infection and some show an apparent resistance to HIV infection. There is natural genetic variability in the R5 co-receptor. If

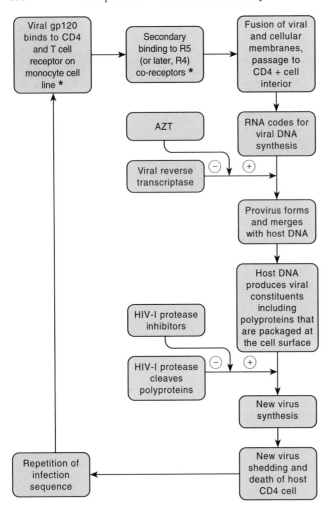

Figure 5.25 **Sequence of Events in HIV Infection.** The key function of viral reverse transcriptase is blocked by AZT to prevent synthesis of new viral particles.

*Later in the progression of HIV infection, binding is increasingly to R4 co-receptor, positive T-helper cells, rather than the monocyte cell line.

a person is homozygous for the variant, he or she produces abnormal R5 co-receptors that do not function in the role of bringing the virus particle into close association with the CD4 cell and thereby create resistance to infection. It has been estimated that 1% of the population has this protective homozygous condition. Heterozygous individuals, with a slightly modified CCR5 receptor, experience normal infection but much delayed progression.

The differential distribution of R5 and R4 is responsible, to some extent, for the progressive stages of the disease. HIV-1 produces two major variants: an R5 strain and an R4 strain. Early in the infection, it is the R5 variant that is produced preferentially. It binds very effectively to cells of the monocyte cell line, facilitating its dissemination around the body, particularly seeding the lymphoid tissues that are rich in these R5 receptor-exclusive cells. Later in the infection, R4 variant is produced in greater proportions, which moves the infection into the CD4 T-cell line. This accounts, to some extent, for the delay in the profound

paralysis of the immune system that results when CD4 T cells are massively attacked and depleted.

You will note in figure 5.24 that the core contains two strands of RNA (rather than the DNA we usually associate with genetic information storage) and two molecules of **reverse transcriptase.** It is these features that give HIV its designation as a **retrovirus:** Replication of HIV requires that RNA first be transcribed back into a DNA form (hence, the reverse transcriptase enzyme). The viral DNA formed in this way is then incorporated into the host cell chromosomes and, in this form, is known as a **provirus.** It stays here until cycling of the host cell is triggered, at which point the provirus elements are replicated, producing hundreds or thousands of copies of HIV RNA plus all the requisite components to form the HIV **virion** (virus particle). **Zidovudine** (also called AZT, azidothymidine, or retrovir) is an antiviral drug that delays the development of AIDS and slows its progression. It acts by interfering with the normal action of reverse transcriptase (see fig. 5.25).

One of the elements produced by the normal transcription of HIV, gp120, is exported to the surface of the host cell. The virion is shed from a cell through the budding of an assembled viral core in a sheath of host cell plasma membrane studded with gp120 molecules. The virion can then go on to infect other CD4-bearing cells. Again, the distribution of R4 co-receptors plays a role in HIV progression. Early in the infection, when principally R5 cells are involved, the infected cells remain distinct one from another. R4 cells, by contrast, tend to stick to one another when infected, forming what is called a "syncitium." (The same term is used to describe the cells of the myocardium that are branching and linked to one another by ion channels.) Through this mechanism, infected R4 host cells readily stick to and fuse with other host cells that display CD4 and R4 to form **giant cells.** These are particularly noted in brain biopsies of advanced AIDS-associated neurological disease. Their role in the pathophysiology of AIDS is not clear, but the process of giant cell formation also provides a means whereby uninfected cells can incorporate HIV. It also produces complexes of infected cells that can in turn deposit in tissues that individuals cells would pass through.

Why does full-blown AIDS occur one year after infection in one person, but not for 12 or 15 years in another? When an infected CD4 cell proliferates, it duplicates its DNA, including the perhaps multiple provirus inclusions, thereby replicating the virus. The provirus also contains a segment with affinity for IL-2 that triggers viral transcription. As you will recall, activated T_H cells produce IL-2, providing another stimulus to viral replication. These mechanisms might be important for individuals with a larger exposure to pathogens, who have more T_H activation and therefore more IL-2 stimulus. This would be the case, for example, in intravenous drug users or people with weakened primary nonspecific resistance.

Before leaving the description of the AIDS virus, let us comment on the role of the monocyte/macrophage in the development of HIV infection. Recall that the monocyte is a freely traveling cell found in the bloodstream. After about three days, monocytes pass into the tissues and take on the morphology and phagocytic function of macrophages (see chapter 2). Studies have shown these cells to have a higher rate of HIV infection than T_4 cells early in the progression of HIV infection, as mentioned. However, they appear not to be involved in a major way in the immune defects of HIV infection. They serve as an early reservoir of HIV infective particles and play a role in the spread of HIV into tissues, particularly the central nervous system.

The Pathogenesis of AIDS

The current understanding is that there is really no **latent period,** a theoretical period during which the HIV virus is present but inactive. With more precise ways of monitoring the progression of HIV infection, it is apparent that there is no period when viral replication does not occur. The clinical picture, on the other hand, supports and is the original source of the idea of a latent, inactive infection. Infection is followed in seven days (range of 4–11 days) by an early **acute phase** in 40–70% of people. This lasts perhaps a few weeks and resembles influenza or infectious mononucleosis. Acute HIV infection produces nonspecific symptoms and is often missed by a diagnosing physician. The symptoms include sore throat, muscle aches, fever, swollen glands, and perhaps, rash. Nervous system symptoms ranging from headache to meningitis may be present. At some point, for most people between 3 and 17 weeks after infection, **seroconversion** occurs—that is, HIV proteins reach the blood. Blood is tested for the presence of these antigenic elements of the HIV virus with the **enzyme-linked immunosorbent assay** (ELISA). While the ELISA, if correctly done, detects 99% of individuals in whom the virus is replicating and is 99% specific to HIV, a positive ELISA is followed by a more complex and costly procedure called a **Western blot assay** to confirm the presence of specific HIV proteins; for example, p24 or gp120.

Studies that identify the plasma HIV RNA levels provide a strong predictor of the course of HIV infection in an individual. After an initial surge of plasma HIV RNA, levels of circulating HIV drop to significantly lower levels that are then maintained fairly consistently until the disease progress into AIDS. This reduced level is termed the **HIV set point.** It reflects the vigor of the HIV-specific cytotoxic T-cell response in the given individual. The stronger the cytotoxic T-cell response, the more intense the attack on HIV-infected CD4 cells, and the lower the levels of circulating HIV.

Cytotoxic T cells are part of the CD8 T-cell lineage. As such, their numbers depend upon complex interactions between CD4 T cells and related CD8 clones. When CD4 T cells are depleted sufficiently due to HIV infection (to levels below 200), this facilitation of cytotoxic T cells is paralyzed and the relatively effective attack on HIV-infected CD4 cells, particularly T cells, breaks down. This allows the infected person to slip across the line into AIDS.

The middle or **chronic phase** of the disease can last for years. Some people are asymptomatic for much of this time, but for many others it is characterized by chronic lymphadenopathy (swollen lymph nodes). This may be the only symptom in an otherwise apparently healthy person. The swelling reflects chronic immune stimulation, particularly of B cells. These produce antibodies, but they are ineffective in neutralizing HIV. During this period, HIV continues to replicate, possibly being held in check by HIV-specific cytotoxic T lymphocytes. HIV-infected T cells are possibly sequestered in the lymph nodes. Throughout this phase there is a gradual drop in T_4 cell concentration in the blood (from the normal $800/mm^3$). As well, there is a progressive increase in the proportion of circulating T_4 cells that are infected with HIV, from perhaps 1/100,000 to 1/100 in full-blown AIDS. The rate of infection of T_4 cells in the lymph nodes is considerably higher. These changes are often clinically silent until the T_4 levels drop below $200/mm^3$.

At about this point ($T_4 < 200/mm^3$), HIV infection enters the final or **crisis phase.** The already established chronic lymphadenopathy is complicated by long-lasting fever (three months or longer), persistent night sweats, weight loss, and diarrhea. Skin tests that measure delayed hypersensitivity—that is, the individual's ability to generate a cellular immune response against specific immunogenic proteins injected under the skin—will be negative or weak. This result indicates a profound breakdown in T_H-cell-mediated immunity. T_4 counts are reduced significantly, and the normal 2:1 ratio of CD4 to CD8 is reversed. This stage of the disease has been called **ARC (AIDS-related complex)** and is designated **CDC class IVa** (for the U.S. Centers for Disease Control). In this stage, the person probably has persistent viral or fungal infection of the skin and mucous membranes, including thrush, herpes simplex (a viral infection producing painful and persistent sores in the anal, genital, and mouth areas), and infection of the vagina by *Candida albicans* (the same fungus that causes thrush). Oral hairy leukoplakia (fuzzy, adherent, white patches, usually on the tongue) may also be observed.

AIDS is diagnosed when a person positive for HIV develops any of a variety of infections or neoplasms that are highly unusual in people with normal immune function (see table 5.7). **PCP,** pneumonia caused by the protozoan *Pneumocystis carinii,* is the most common life-threatening opportunistic infection contributing to the definition of AIDS. It appears in up to 50% of AIDS victims. Even with prophylactic use of inhaled pentamidine, an antiprotozoal agent, many patients develop pneumocystis pneumonia, and of those, 5–30% will experience often fatal respiratory failure. The pathogenesis of AIDS is presented in figure 5.26.

Kaposi's sarcoma (KS), a skin cancer causing dark, splotchy lesions, develops in 15–25% of HIV-positive individuals, in whom it often follows an aggressive course. It is far more common among HIV-positive homosexual men than among intravenous drug users or other risk groups and may develop while the person is otherwise relatively

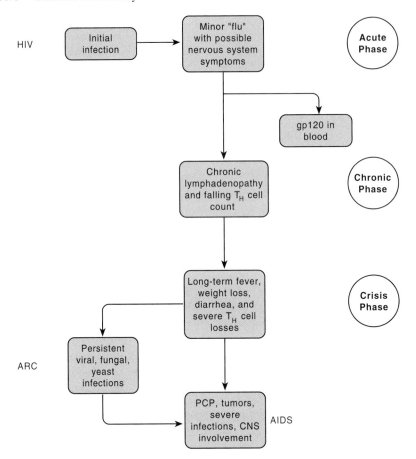

Figure 5.26   **The Pathogenesis of AIDS.** The chronic phase follows several weeks after the initial infection and may last from months to years.

healthy. Kaposi's sarcoma may be more likely to develop in HIV infection because the function of antitumor natural killer (NK) cells is impaired. There is also growing evidence that factors released by a variety of cells, including activated T_H cells and the tumor cells themselves, are responsible for fostering dramatic tumor growth. The fact that KS can arise in the absence of HIV infection, among other evidence, raises the possibility that KS develops from a cancer-causing virus that infects people independently, but that its action is promoted by the development of HIV infection.

Some otherwise rare opportunistic infections associated with AIDS bear noting. The parasitic protozoan *Toxoplasmosis gondii* often infects the brain and can lead to seizures and coma. The fungus *Cryptococcus* not only can cause meningitis but may damage the liver, bone, skin, and other tissues. **Cytomegalovirus,** a viral agent to which 70% of us have been exposed, can cause pneumonia, encephalitis, blindness, and inflammation of the gastrointestinal tract in AIDS.

While various factors probably play a role in the development and progression of HIV infection, the current, widely accepted view is that there is an unavoidable continuum progressing from HIV infection to ARC and then to AIDS.

Antiviral and Protease Inhibitor Therapy

All therapeutic agents identified to date, including AZT (zidovudine), have potential toxic side effects and these must be balanced against anticipated benefits. Trials with zidovudine published in 1990 indicate a delay in the onset of AIDS with patients started on the drug when they experienced mild symptomatic illness and T_4 cell counts of 200–499/mm³ A second study began therapy in asymptomatic patients with counts below 500/mm³ Progression to symptomatic illness was delayed, the decline in T_4 counts slowed, and the drug was better tolerated than it was by patients with full-blown AIDS. An added benefit of early treatment may be in reducing the infectivity of the HIV positive person. Extensive use of a medication on an actively mutating microbial strain increases the likelihood of developing resistant strains, and this has been observed in *in vitro* testing of zidovudine. Antiviral agents act in one of three ways:

1. Nucleoside reverse transcriptase inhibitors (NRTIs—which include zidovudine, abacavir, didanosine, lamivudine, stavudine, and zalcitabine) interfere by becoming incorporated into viral DNA in the place of a normal DNA building block (thymidine in the case of AZT). Other DNA constituents cannot attach to the nu-

cleoside analogue (building block) molecule, so transcription effectively terminates at that point. Zidovudine has a similar (and thereby potentially harmful) effect on host DNA replication, but only at concentrations much greater than normal therapeutic doses. In some patients, even the lower therapeutic doses produce progressive bone marrow toxicity. This usually leads to anemia, depressed neutrophil counts, and some bleeding abnormalities.

2. Non-nucleoside reverse transcriptase inhibitors (NNRTI's—which include delavirdine, efavirenz, and nevirapine) do not act as chain terminators. Instead, they directly inhibit the functioning of the reverse transcriptase enzyme.

3. The recent development of HIV-specific protease inhibitors has given new hope to people infected with HIV-1. In the production of viral particles, host DNA produces chains of nonfunctional viral polypeptide (called polyprotein) that are packaged at the cell membrane. At the same time, "immature" (nonfunctional) viral particles, missing key protein components, are released. At this point, HIV-1 protease cleaves the polyproteins into smaller, functional units, which are incorporated into the viral particles making them infective. Protease inhibitors (PIs) bind to the active site of HIV-1 protease, preventing it from doing its job of cutting the polyproteins. Noninfective, "ghosted" viral particles are the result. Currently available protease inhibitors include amprenavir, indinavir, lopinavir, nelfinavir, ritonavir, and saquinavir. PIs are combined with both nucleoside and nonnucleoside reverse transcriptase inhibitors to greatly improve the suppression of HIV particle production and increase the T_4 counts. These results have been dramatic when patients have received a three-drug cocktail of AZT, 3TC (lamivudine), and indivar (an HIV-1 protease inhibitor). In one study, over 80% of participants had undetectable levels of HIV in the blood for one year. There isn't sufficient experience with these drugs (saquinavir mesylate, ritionavir, indinavir sulfate, and nelfinavir mesylate) to understand their long-term impact on disease progression or their ultimate toxicity. By late 1997, some patients who had responded well to the "cocktail" were showing lowered T_4 counts and increasing HIV loads. Individuals who establish a higher set point of circulating HIV after the initial phase of viremia that characterizes acute HIV progress more quickly to AIDS. It is now clear that early and aggressive antiretroviral therapy helps people maintain a more effective cytotoxic T-cell response, thereby restraining the progression to AIDS. So, as soon as HIV infection is confirmed, antiretroviral therapy should be commenced. It is now common to engage in **structured treatment interruption.** In this approach, the person is cycled off antiretroviral medications and HIV (monitored through plasma HIV RNA levels) is allowed to rebound. Presuming the person was treated appropriately in acute HIV and still has a pretty intact cytotoxic T-cell capacity, this escalation of HIV triggers a robust cytotoxic T-cell response. When HIV RNA peaks, antiretroviral therapy is recommenced until HIV RNA is brought down again and held at low plasma levels for a period of time, after which it is again allowed to escalate. This is far more effective than simply maintaining antiretroviral dosing constant because it takes advantage of the body's relatively effective innate defenses.

Why doesn't this work forever? The evolution of R4-specific HIV-1 strain is part of the explanation. In addition, HIV-1 strains can develop resistance to antiretroviral drugs in a way analogous to the development of antibiotic resistance in bacterial strains. This issue may be a more significant problem with the advent of structured treatment interruptions. Opportunistic infections take a heavy toll on body tissues and systems as well. Much of the rest of the failure of therapy lies in the wily way the HIV-1 virus mutates elements of its viral core. This rapid evolution of different antigens outstrips the beleaguered capacity of the decimated CD4 T-cell clones and finally overwhelms the immune defenses (more on this later).

To reiterate the importance of early diagnosis in the treatment of HIV infection, there are three impacts to the early use of antiretroviral agents. The first is an immediate decrease in the viral load. This leads to fewer infectious CD4 cells within the infected person's body, but it also means that the person is less infectious to unprotected sex partners or to those with whom the person might share a contaminated needle. Early diagnosis also catches the person before he or she slips into the long "chronic phase" when the person has fewer symptoms and is less likely to be diagnosed. Diagnosis also increases the likelihood that the person engages in safe sex practices and thereby reduces the passage of HIV. Perhaps the most beneficial effect for the infected person whose condition has been diagnosed is the opportunity to engage in HAART, with its clear impact on preserving intact cytotoxic T-cell responses.

HIV and the Nervous System

Earlier, we referred to the CNS manifestations sometimes accompanying or following the period of seroconversion and acute HIV infection: headache and a condition called *aseptic meningitis*—"aseptic" because no microbial agent can be recovered from the cerebrospinal fluid (CSF). At the other end of the spectrum is the finding that 70–90% of those dying with AIDS or ARC show brain and spinal cord pathology at autopsy. CNS or neuromuscular abnormalities can be found in up to 80% of infected adults, so the CDC in 1993 recognized dementia in HIV-positive adults as an indicator of AIDS, even without the presence of other secondary infections or tumors. Other CNS disorders include primary CNS syndromes associated with HIV, opportunistic viral and nonviral CNS infections and neoplasms, and HIV-related neuromuscular diseases. Many of these conditions are described in more detail in Chapters 20 and 21. Here, we will consider only the major problems.

The most common primary CNS syndrome associated with HIV in adults is chronic HIV encephalopathy, widely called AIDS dementia complex. While uncommon (2–3%) in asymptomatic HIV-positive people, as many as 50% of those with lymphadenopathy experience symptoms such as difficulty concentrating and slowing of verbal and motor responses. As HIV infection progresses, there is an increasing incidence of withdrawal, personality changes, clumsiness, mutism, seizures, partial paralysis, psychosis, incontinence, eventual confinement to bed, and relative unresponsiveness. The direct role of HIV is implicated by the presence of HIV in monocytes, macrophages, microglia, and multinucleated giant cells in the brains of people with AIDS dementia complex and other CNS changes. Although astrocytes, oligodendrocytes, and neurons possess CD4 and co-receptor molecules, there is no evidence of them being infected by HIV particles. Among other explanations being explored, a number bear noting. First, the dysfunction may be due to cytokines and other agents released from macrophages or astrocytes, perhaps in response to direct infection of astrocytes. Second, it is possible that gp120 alters neuronal regulation of neural function. The presence of HIV may instigate immune-mediated "bystander" injury. Alternatively, cross-reacting antibodies to an HIV protein may bind to receptors and produce neurotransmitter blockade. Some other CNS complications of AIDS are presented in table 5.8.

Impact of HIV Infection on Helper T Cells

In a strict sense, people do not die of HIV infection. They die of the opportunistic infections and neoplasms that thrive when normal helper T-cell function is paralyzed. What we know about HIV-associated alterations in immune function is, to a large extent, conjecture based on our understanding of normal function. As noted earlier, the initial infection and early replication of HIV probably are focused in the monocyte-macrophage cell line (including Langerhans and dendritic cells). The impact on immune function is minimal at this phase. In time, particularly, as cytotoxic T-cell, responses decline, the infection shifts to include T_4 cells (CD4 T cells). In many people, T_4 counts are at less than 100/mm^3 when AIDS is diagnosed, and they subsequently fall lower. This reduction in T_4 counts is central to the pathophysiology of HIV infection. Recall that a specific antigen is presented to the members of the responsive clone of T_H by APCs, which at the same time release IL-1. The T_H cell then becomes activated, produces IL-2, and subsequently proliferates. Equally important are the other cytokines released by T_H cells, those that cause activation and proliferation of B cells, stimulate lymphocyte and macrophage production, induce MHC class I and II, recruit

Table 5.8   Nervous System Disorders Associated with HIV Infection and AIDS

Central Nervous System

Disorders probably attributable to HIV infection
  Meningitis—in acute stage of HIV infection
  Spinal cord disease—principally motor disorders
  Progressive brain damage in children (2 mo–5 yr)—impaired growth, motor dysfunction, death
  Progressive brain damage in adults—behavioral, cognitive, and motor impairment (AIDS dementia complex)
Opportunistic infections
  Viral—fatal demyelinating diseases and other infections
  Nonviral—fungal and/or bacterial infections causing meningitis and/or abscesses
Neoplasia
  Lymphomas infiltrating CNS

Peripheral Nervous System

Diseases Affecting Peripheral Nerves
  Various demyelinating diseases
  Various motor and sensory disorders

and focus the activities of macrophages, and so on. In turn, cells that respond to T_H cytokines produce cytokines of their own.

The chronic reduction of T_H cell cytokines leads to a depletion of monocytes/macrophages (reduced production of IL-1 and TNF) and neutrophils (decreased inflammatory response). With the reduction of antigen-specific antibodies, a host of secondary defects appear: decreased function of antibody-dependent cellular cytotoxicity (ADCC), decreased complement fixation to pathogens, with consequent impaired inflammatory response and decreased opsonization, and less effective phagocytosis. Also involved is a decreased expression of MHC antigens, causing impaired antigen presentation and natural killer cell (NK) function; decreased chemotaxis, activation, and phagocytic activity by macrophages and neutrophils; and failure of NK cells to proliferate and activate, causing less effective killing of tumor cells. In the face of this hypofunction, how do we reconcile the lymphadenopathy and hypergammaglobulinemia (excess antibodies in circulation)? Two explanations are probable. First, opportunistic infection with certain agents such as Epstein-Barr virus (EBV) and cytomegalovirus (CMV) causes generalized direct stimulation of B cells to produce antibodies and, as a consequence, lymph nodes swell. Second, certain proteins or glycoproteins produced when HIV replicates may stimulate B cells. The overview in figure 5.27 provides a helpful summary.

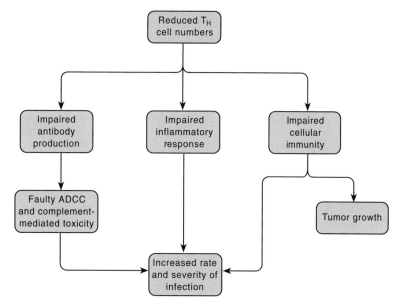

Figure 5.27   **Consequences of T$_H$ Cell Depletion in AIDS.**

Transmission of HIV Infection

HIV has been demonstrated in the saliva, tears, urine, CSF, serum, T$_H$ cells, and macrophages of infected people. Semen and vaginal secretions are particularly rich in HIV and infected lymphocytes. At this point, it seems likely that these T$_4$ cells are the principal vehicle for transmitting HIV from one person to another. The HIV virus itself is relatively fragile, so casual contact (shaking hands, eating together, living in close association) is not likely to cause infection.

What activities do carry a high risk of transmission? Any activity that can pass large numbers of infected CD4 cells directly into the bloodstream or to areas that bear receptors for HIV and HIV particles are high risk. Sexual activity, especially if mucous membrane damage from trauma or an infection is present, is the most common mode of transmission. Direct injection of infected lymphocytes or HIV is also a very effective means of infection, which occurs among intravenous drug users who share contaminated needles, syringes, or other drug paraphernalia. It is also the mechanism affecting recipients of transfusions of blood or blood products derived from pooled blood components from many donors. AIDS cases have been traced to a single unit of transfused blood, and, even with screening, a slight risk remains. The screening tests used have a very slight false-negative rate and, more significantly, there can be a window of infectivity (perhaps longer than four months) before an individual shows seroconversion and gives a positive test. This means that blood can test negative prior to a transfusion and still carry the virus to a transfusion recipient.

To put the problem into perspective, anyone who is infected is producing HIV particles. Infectivity probably increases with the number of HIV particles and number of infected CD4 cells produced and passed, and therefore in-

fectivity is initially very high in acute HIV when virions are being produced at high rates. Infectivity declines somewhat during chornic HIV infection and then increases as the HIV infection progresses into AIDS. The wild card in this game is that apparently some individuals are inherently more infectious, perhaps because they carry a variant HIV strain that is more resilient and virulent. As we have noted, some evidence suggests that treatment with zidovudine may decrease infectivity. Worldwide, sexual contact is the principal route for infection (75%). Anything that weakens the mucosal barrier facilitates transmission. This includes rough sexual activity that causes mucosal bruising or tears, and inflammation resulting from genital ulcers, urethritis, or cervicitis. In this context, STDs, especially herpes simplex, potentiate the transmission of HIV (and vice versa). Oral sex, while less risky than genital sex, still poses a significant risk of HIV transmission.

The chief targets of efforts to contain the spread of HIV continue to be the established North American risk groups—homosexual and bisexual men, intravenous drug users, and their sexual partners. However, spread of the virus in the heterosexual population has now become a major concern as well. AIDS is growing fastest among young, sexually active adults, and teens are at a growing risk. While condom use should be routine, this precaution merely reduces the risk of infection; some risk still remains. Of course, it makes sense to avoid sexual contact with individuals who belong to, or are in intimate contact with the members of, one of the high-risk groups. But it isn't always easy to get an accurate idea of the background of a potential sex partner. A study published in the *New England Journal of Medicine* (March 15, 1990) points out the difficulty of establishing risk if the people you ask tell lies (see the focus box "Sex, Lies, and HIV").

Focus on Sex, Lies, and HIV

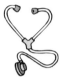

A group of 665 18- to 25-year-old college students in southern California completed anonymous questionnaires assessing sexual behavior, HIV-related risk reduction, and their experiences with deception when dating. Of the 422 who were sexually active (196 men, 226 women), the following percentages reported dishonesty.

	Men	Women
Has told a lie in order to have sex	34%	10%*
Has been sexually involved with more than one person	32%	23%*
Has had sex with a partner who did not know HIV status	68%	59%
Has been lied to for purposes of sex	47%	60%*
Would lie about having negative HIV-antibody test	20%	4%*
Would understate number of previous partners	47%	42%
Would never disclose a single episode of sexual infidelity	43%	34%*

"The implications of our findings are clear. . . . Patients should be cautioned that safe-sex strategies are always advisable, despite arguments to the contrary from partners."

* Responses of men significantly different from responses of women.

Source: from *New England Journal of Medicine*, Vol. 322, No. 11, March 15, 1990, pp. 774–775.

Focus on Call by Nelson Mandela and Scientists for Broader Approaches in Africa

In July 2002, the anti-apartheid leader and former President of South Africa made an impassioned plea to the people of Africa to end the stigmatization that smothers the victims of HIV/AIDS. Shortly after the announcement of a multi-billion dollar fund from the G8 to support African development, he identified this prejudices as the essential impediment to progress in dealing with the devastating impact of HIV/AIDS on Africa. The shame around HIV/AIDS is such that women may breastfeed a baby, knowing of the risk of transmitting their infection to the infant, rather than be discovered to be HIV positive. Taboos around the open discussion of sexuality and sexual matters compound the problems. The social ostracism of gays infected with HIV that has been tackled in films and television in the West is being played out with women as the victim in other countries. In the same vein, Corbett et al., in *The Lancet,* June 2002, pointed out that "the high prevalence of untreated STD infections has been a major factor facilitating the spread of HIV-1 in Africa, with the synergistic interaction between HIV transmission and genital herpes being of special concern for control of both diseases." They also point out "increased susceptibility to tuberculosis after infection with HIV-1 has led to a rising incidence and threat of increased transmission of tuberculosis. Clinical malaria occurs with an increased frequency and severity in HIV-1-infected individuals, especially during pregnancy." Benatar (*J.Med.Philos,* April 2002) painted the AIDS "pandemic as a reflection of a complex trajectory of social and economic forces that create widening global disparities in wealth and health and concomitant ecological niches for the emergence of new infectious diseases. While the biomedical approach to HIV/AIDS is necessary . . . it cannot, in isolation, improve the health of populations (without) addressing the deeper social causes of pandemics." The common thread might be that the legacy of a colonial history needs to be recognized through support from the former colonial powers but addressed by the people themselves.

Health Care Workers and the Risk of HIV Infection

HIV infection rates and individual HIV burdens will vary among populations with which a health care worker may come in working contact. At the extreme of exposure are those nurses and doctors whose professional work is exclusively with AIDS patients. The chief source of risk for them is direct, accidental inoculation of contaminated blood or tissues by needle, wire, bone, or scalpel punctures, or exposure of blood to the delicate membranes of the eye. Bites by infected persons have not been shown to transmit HIV, and contact with body fluids other than blood also carries relatively low risk. Pricking with a needle is estimated to lead to HIV infection in about 0.3% of these cases (about 1/100 the risk of hepatitis B infection after a single exposure!). This may be considered low, and, in fact, relatively few health care workers have contracted AIDS. However, compared with the estimated risk of a woman being infected through a single incident involving vaginal sex with an infected man (0.2%), it is significant. As of July 1, 2000, 56 documented cases of occupational transmission were reported to the CDC, with another 138 cases of possible transmission. The majority (80%) were due to needle stick, cut, or other skin exposure. Recommendations in case of an incident are to cleanse the site of exposure and begin antiretroviral prophylactic therapy as soon as possible with two or three agents administered simultaneously.

Cardiac surgeons, assistants, and scrub nurses can experience a risk of HIV infection in the range of 0.5% per year or greater, depending on the nature of the surgery and the patient group. Saws and drills can produce tiny airborne fluid droplets containing infective HIV particles or lymphocytes, another source of risk for surgical or dental personnel.

As the number of AIDS cases increases, it becomes clear that health care workers must take routine precautions with all patients. And this, of course, is a two-way street: 1991 marked the first case in which a patient sued a health care worker (in this case an infected dentist) for liability in transmitting HIV. To date this is the only documented incident of caregiver to patient transmission.

 Checkpoint 5.4

We have dedicated more space to HIV/AIDS than to any of the primary immunodeficiencies. This reflects its prevalence; its impact on the health care system, the economy, and society at large; and both its infectivity and, at present, bleak outcome. Before we leave this section, you might wish to return to table 5.7 to review the primary immunities. Which would you have to put together, and in what order, to arrive at end-stage AIDS?

AUTOIMMUNE DISEASES

Autoimmune diseases are distinguished by several criteria, which are listed in table 5.9. Applying these criteria strictly, we would arrive at a very short list; but as you may be aware, many disorders are said to be probably or possibly autoimmune. The two best candidates are strangely at opposite poles of a continuum, ranging from organ-specific to systemic. They are also at the extremes of autoantibody specificity. **Hashimoto's thyroiditis,** one of the first diseases to be associated with autoantibodies, affects mostly middle-aged women, causing goiter and hypothyroidism. In affected patients, the serum usually has high titers of anti-

Table 5.9	The Criteria Applied in Determining That a Given Disease Is an Autoimmune Disorder

1. Antibody or T cells against self-antigens have been demonstrated.
2. Specific interaction between antibody or T cells and tissues involved in the disease process has been demonstrated.
3. Immune dysfunction is the primary factor in the disease.
4. Other possible nonimmune causes do not induce the immune defect.
5. Disease is transferable to others via antibody or T cells only.*
6. Autoimmune characteristics of the disease can be duplicated in experimental systems.*

*Asterisks indicate more stringent criteria applied by some, but not all, investigators.

bodies to thyroglobulin, the protein in the thyroid follicles that binds and stores thyroid hormones, and the immune-mediated disease is restricted to the thyroid gland. Systemic lupus erythematosus (SLE), on the other hand, is a systemic disease with a bewildering assortment of autoantibodies. Arthritis, skin lesions, fever, and kidney disease are some of the disorders that recur in individuals affected by SLE.

The best-defined autoimmune diseases are also clearly influenced by genetics, as shown by familial trends toward increased autoantibodies and increased incidence of autoimmune disease. Genetics also appears to strongly influence the specific nature of the autoimmune disease; that is, there seems to be a general familial tendency toward elevations of particular autoantibodies. On the other hand, various environmental factors, including diet, drugs, chemicals, and viruses, are also implicated in the etiology of autoimmune disorders. Genetics sets a predisposition, perhaps expressed in elevated specific autoantibodies, but (in most cases) the environmental factors must also intervene to produce the immune system derangement that results in autoimmune disease. The tendency for women to be more affected than men (e.g., SLE afflicts ten times as many women of childbearing age as men) presents an ongoing puzzle. Estrogen is implicated, but a satisfactory explanation is lacking.

Table 5.10 lists the more commonly encountered diseases that probably have a basis in autoimmunity. We will deal with many of these in some detail in later chapters, in connection with the pathology of the system in which they primarily occur. The remainder of this chapter deals with some largely multisystem autoimmune disorders: SLE, progressive systemic sclerosis, dermatomyositis, and Sjögren's syndrome.

Table 5.10 Selected Disorders with an Autoimmune Etiology or Pathogenesis. Also Indicated Are the Tissues Affected by Self-Antibodies or Immune Complexes.

Disorders	Target Tissues
Widely Accepted as Autoimmune	
Hashimoto's thyroiditis	Thyroid gland
Grave's disease	Thyroid, eyes, skin
Systemic lupus erythematosus	Systemic
Goodpasture's syndrome	Lung, kidney
Autoimmune thrombocytopenia	Platelets
Autoimmune atrophic gastritis of pernicious anemia	Gastric mucosa
Myasthenia gravis	Acetylcholine receptor
Insulin-dependent diabetes mellitus	Pancreatic islet cells
Rheumatoid arthritis	Systemic
Systemic sclerosis	Systemic connective tissues, especially skin
Sjögren's syndrome	Systemic
Probably Autoimmune	
Polymyositis-dermatomyositis	Muscle, skin
Chronic active hepatitis	Liver
Ulcerative colitis	Colon, small intestine
Primary biliary cirrhosis	Liver

Table 5.11 Criteria for the Diagnosis of SLE. The Disease Is Deemed to Be Present When Four of These Eleven Criteria Are Met.

Criterion	Comment
Malar rash	Erythema over the cheekbones
Discoid rash	Raised scaly patches on skin
Photosensitivity	Skin rash on exposure to sunlight
Oral ulcers	Ulcers in oropharynx and/or nasopharynx (usually painless)
Arthritis	Acute inflammation in two or more peripheral joints
Serositis	Acute inflammation in pleurae or pericardium
Renal disorder	Loss of protein in urine; blood cells or hemoglobin in tubule
Neurologic disorder	Seizures or psychoses without other identifiable cause
Blood disorder	Deficiency of platelets or white cells, anemia from red blood cell lysis
Immune disorder	Various antibodies identifiable
Antinuclear antibody	Antibodies to DNA in 50% of non-drug-induced SLE

Systemic Lupus Erythematosus

Systemic lupus erythematosus (SLE) is an autoimmune disorder characterized by acute or insidious onset with widely variable systemic effects. Also typical are periods of remission and intense exacerbation, especially in the initial stages of the disease. However, there are so many different signs and symptoms that diagnosis is difficult. The name lupus, which means wolflike, comes from a rash over the cheeks and the bridge of the nose, which appears in some patients. SLE affects 1 in 700 women aged 20 to 64 and 1 in 245 American black women, but it can strike anyone at virtually any age.

Diagnosis has been made easier by the fact that virtually every SLE patient is positive for antinuclear antibodies (ANAs)—antibodies directed against a variety of nuclear components including DNA. With immunofluorescence tests, it is possible to identify such antibodies adhering to nuclear features. While high proportions of patients with other systemic autoimmune disorders also are positive for ANAs, this test is one of the 11 criteria proposed for the identification of SLE patients (table 5.11). A person is said

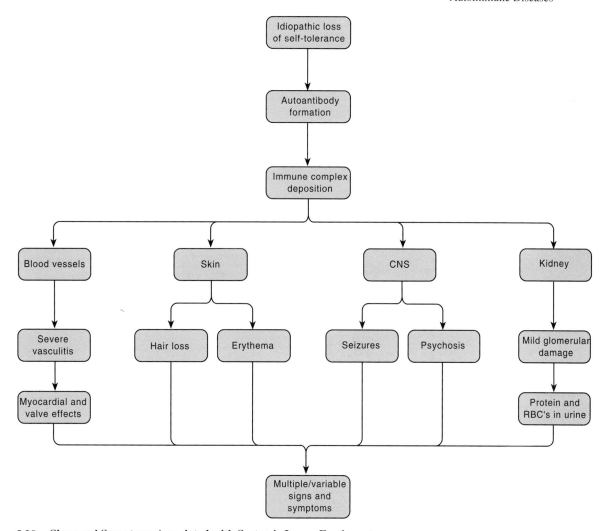

Figure 5.28   **Signs and Symptoms Associated with Systemic Lupus Erythematosus.**

to have SLE if any four or more criteria are met together or in sequence at any time.

SLE occurs when, for unknown reasons, there is a breakdown of the mechanisms that maintain self-tolerance (fig. 5.28). Genetics and environmental factors probably combine as etiological factors. Estrogens may also be involved; that would explain the greater incidence of SLE in women. Whatever the cause, the resultant production of autoantibodies to a wide variety of targets, including nuclear antigens and cytoplasmic and membrane components, leads to the formation of immune complexes that can deposit in vessel walls and vulnerable organs (glomeruli of kidneys, choroid plexus of the brain, the skin, perhaps joint connective tissue). There, they activate complement, whose breakdown products mediate neutrophil attack on endothelia and basement membranes (type III hypersensitivity). Although the ANAs do not appear to have a direct role in pathology in this case by binding to nuclear proteins, other antibodies do. Those against erythrocytes, leukocytes, or platelets can produce serious blood disorders (type II hypersensitivity). IgG and IgM

autoantibodies bind to the cell surface and result in cell death by any of three routes: enhanced phagocytosis through opsonization, lysis through the membrane attack complex, or antibody-dependent cellular cytotoxicity.

Pathogenesis

The criteria for diagnosing SLE are listed in table 5.11. Chronic fever and fatigue and weight loss are experienced by the vast majority of patients. Widespread vasculitis, secondary to the immune complex deposition, affects small arteries and arterioles. Vasculitis is particularly evident in the skin and muscles and may be responsible for the muscle aching noted by one-third of patients. Immune complex disposition is probably responsible for the butterfly rash (erythema) over the cheeks and bridge of the nose, as well as for the raised, scaly, discoid rash found on the scalp and other parts of the body. Hair loss (alopecia), sometimes permanent, may accompany the disfiguring discoid lesions.

The kidney is involved, at least minimally, in almost all cases of SLE. Mild glomerular damage can give rise to

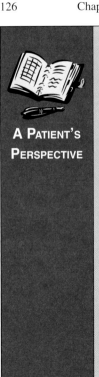

Systemic Lupus Erythematosus

"My Body Has Turned against Me"
—Anonymous

They tell me that my immune system has turned against me. They don't actually use those words; they say my SLE problems are "rooted in an autoimmune attack on my tissues." But I get the picture: a part of me has somehow turned against me. And not just one or two parts of me, but lots of me. So far it's mostly been joint, muscle, and skin problems, but I know the more serious threat that my heart, kidneys or brain might be affected is always there. At least I'm OK in those area(s) so far, but it's hard not to look over my shoulder and wonder. Apart from specific pains and skin rashes, my immune system must be on the prowl in a lot of tough to pinpoint areas because a lot of times I feel generally weak, feverish, and ill. It's hard to describe, but that's basically it. I just don't feel healthy.

Another bothersome thing about this lupus disease is the flare-ups when everything gets a lot worse at times that I can never predict. More pain in my muscles and joints and outbreaks of discoloration and scaly patches in my skin. These times can be tough, but I know they will pass and I'll have a remission period when everything quiets down. Problem is, it's sure hard to plan anything too far in advance because I never really know what shape I'll be in at any time down the road. At least there's a chance I won't be flaring up when the date arrives.

I've had it for about eleven years now. Anyone can get it, but I'm in the most likely category: a black woman of childbearing age. It's easier today, but back then, when I first started having problems, it took almost a year before they could tell me what I had. They say lupus is like that. It looks like it could be a lot of things, so it's hard to figure, but finding out is quicker these days.

It was hard at first because I know some people thought I was just making it up. They couldn't feel how weak and achy I felt and the rashes hadn't come along then. My husband was pretty good, but I know some people just thought I was some kind of hypochondriac. It was really hard at work where you had to keep up. As I got worse, I had to move to easier work, part-time, and that's worked out pretty well, though I do miss the extra money, especially with the cost of some of these new drugs.

Over the years I've learned to cope pretty well with the ups and downs of my condition. I've adjusted and know my limitations. But there's a lot I can still do and I hate being pitied or fussed over. And I know when I look terrible, so don't tell me I "look fine" when I know I don't.

I guess the most precious thing to me was learning to rest; not sleep but getting out of the habit of always having to be doing something. It's made a big difference. Part of it is learning to listen to my body when it says "take it easy . . . moderation in all things."

---

the passage of large molecules (proteinuria) and cells (hematuria) into the urine, where they can be identified by routine urinalysis. One cause of death in SLE can be renal failure. Heart problems can include pericarditis, myocarditis secondary to acute vasculitis, and the development of small (1–3 mm), warty, sterile vegetation anywhere on the valve leaflets. The basis for the disturbance of central nervous system function is not well established. Although some patients experience seizures or psychosis, many more have subtle mental and psychological disorders. Autoantibodies to neurons and to endothelial phospholipids have been demonstrated. Those to endothelia appear to initiate a thickening of the vessel intima that can limit blood flow to brain tissues and may explain some of the CNS symptoms. The arthritis, while causing pain and discomfort, doesn't damage the joint as it does in rheumatoid arthritis, and joint swelling is variable.

Treatment As our understanding of autoimmune disorders improves, a variety of treatments, now being experimentally explored, will be used with SLE. In the meantime, two principal approaches are employed. Corticosteroids, including topical creams, are used as sparingly as possible to alleviate acute symptoms but limit the harmful side effects. In patients with serious life-threatening symptoms, cytotoxic immunosuppressants like cyclophosphamide and azathioprine can be used. These drugs can have serious side effects (e.g., increased risk of cancer for both drugs, and bladder damage for cyclophosphamide).

Drug-Induced Systemic Lupus Erythematosus

Certain drugs can induce a lupuslike syndrome in susceptible individuals. In this case, the reason is probably a genetically determined metabolic deficiency that results in the accumulation of products that adhere to nuclear and cellular molecules. The accumulation produces antigenic alterations that set off an immune-mediated, SLE-like production of autoantibodies. From that point, the two conditions are essentially indistinguishable except for one dramatic difference—drug-induced SLE completely remits when the offending drug is stopped. Some of the many drugs implicated are procainamide (an anti-hypertensive), isoniazid (an antitubercular agent with liver and CNS toxicity), and D-penicillamine (a chelating agent used to treat copper, lead, or mercury poisoning and Wilson's disease, a disorder involving copper metabolism).

Progressive Systemic Sclerosis (Scleroderma)

This chronic, progressive disease of connective tissue involves the excessive deposition of collagen and affects about three females to one male. It usually emerges in early middle age and is most apparent in the skin. When well advanced, the disease results in clawlike, inflexible fingers and a face like a drawn mask. It is a systemic disorder primarily affecting the gastrointestinal tract, the heart and its vasculature, and the kidneys, lungs, and musculoskeletal system. The pathology arises both from the increased activity of fibroblasts laying down collagen and from impaired local circulation. Together these lead to intense fibrosis that interferes with organ function. Formerly called **scleroderma** because of the widespread involvement of the skin, the disease is increasingly known as **progressive systemic sclerosis** (PSS).

Pathogenesis

The pathogenesis of PSS is poorly understood. There appears to be dysfunction at the level of both the fibroblasts and the microvasculature. The triggering antigen or immune defect is unknown, but apparently collagen-reactive T cells and B cells mediate the pathology. The response of autoreactive helper T cells to their encounter with collagen sets up a cycle of progression. The delayed hypersensitivity reaction (type IV) generates mediators that attract and stimulate the division of fibroblasts. These produce more collagen that is antigenic for more T cells, stimulating them to additional mediator release, and so on.

Collagen-reactive B cells could produce antibodies that form complexes and mediate vascular damage, or other autoantibodies may be involved. The vascular derangements affect small arteries and arterioles, which are subject to intimal thickening and narrowing of the lumen, both by deposition of mucinous or collagenous material and by proliferation of intimal cells. These processes set the stage for scar formation because the tissue is robbed of adequate blood supply. Platelet adherence in the injured vessels contributes to the stimulation of fibroblasts because of the factors released. As in other diseases identified as autoimmune, there are abnormalities of immune function, such as circulating antinuclear antibodies.

Polymyositis-Dermatomyositis

This usually chronic weakness of proximal musculature affects twice as many women as men and usually appears in middle age, although a variant affects children. Half the patients experience rashes, classically in the eyelids and the extensor surfaces of joints including the fingers, elbows, and knees. While abnormalities are found in many systems (e.g., vasculitis, lung fibrosis, transitory arthritis), it is the muscle weakness that produces most difficulty. Initially, patients have difficulty raising their arms or climbing stairs. This weakness can progress to weakness of neck muscles, impaired swallowing, and difficulty breathing as intercostals and diaphragm are involved. Occasionally, a fulminant case will rapidly lead to death, perhaps due to vasculitis-induced heart failure. The presence of muscle enzymes in the plasma (e.g., creatine kinase and lactic dehydrogenase) is evidence of the muscle cell destruction that takes place.

The association of this disease with others of presumably autoimmune origin (e.g., SLE, Sjögren's syndrome, and PSS) and the presence of ANAs in many of the patients argue for this being an autoimmune disease. What elicits the autoreactive response is unknown, although, as with many other of its autoimmune relatives, a virus (in this case, perhaps Coxsackie virus) is suspected. There is evidence that muscle-antigen-reactive T cells may be the immune agent.

Sjögren's Syndrome

A presumed autoimmune disease with almost as wide an assortment of autoantibodies as occurs in SLE, **Sjögren's syndrome** involves destruction of the salivary and lacrimal glands and their ducts. The resultant dry eyes cause blurred vision, burning and itching, and inflammation of the conjunctiva and corneal epithelium, followed by erosion of the cornea. The dry mouth becomes cracked and fissured and ulcers develop. Food can't be tasted and swallowing of solids is difficult. In about 40% of patients this is the extent of their lesions. They are said to have primary Sjögren's syndrome or **sicca (dry) syndrome.** The other 60% have this disorder along with some other autoimmune disease, often rheumatoid arthritis. Most (90%) of the patients are middle-aged women. People with Sjögren's also have an increased risk of developing lymphoid malignancies.

Case Study

A 28-year-old black woman came to her general practitioner because she was alarmed by recent signs of blood in her urine. She explained that she had been feeling increasingly tired at her work as a nurse, and for the past five months had been troubled by periods of stiffness and swelling in her hands, mild fevers, appetite and weight loss, and a rash over her cheeks, which worsened when she was out in the sun. On examination she was otherwise normal, but reported that

she was taking isoniazid, a widely used antibacterial agent that is effective against tuberculosis. Her most recent routine tuberculin test at the hospital where she was employed had been positive, and the house physician had prescribed the drug. She was also using birth control pills.

The patient was taken off isoniazid and switched to another antibacterial agent. Laboratory studies were ordered and revealed some small loss of protein and blood to the urine. They also revealed the presence of antinuclear antibodies. On the basis of these factors, a diagnosis of systemic lupus erythematosus was made.

The patient was advised to avoid stress and exertion at work and to get as much rest as possible. Prednisone, a corticosteroid anti-inflammatory agent, was prescribed for her joint pain and kidney problems. Avoidance of sun exposure was also advised, and when exposure was inevitable, the use of an effective sun-blocking agent was counselled. It was also recommended that she stop using birth control pills.

Her symptoms improved and she continued to be monitored for any side effects of her therapy.

Commentary

The signs and symptoms in this patient pointed fairly clearly to SLE and were confirmed when the tests for antinuclear antibodies were returned as positive. It was necessary to stop the use of isoniazid because in some sensitive individuals it induces anti-DNA antibodies. When the possible role of the drug was removed and the antinuclear antibodies remained, the SLE diagnosis was relatively straightforward. The suggestion to abandon the use of birth control pills was based on indications that, in many cases, estrogen use can worsen SLE symptoms.

Prednisone is likely to suppress the glomerular inflammatory damage that is disrupting renal function, but other agents with similar effects are available should side effects become a problem. If episodes of more severe signs and symptoms develop, more aggressive immunosuppressive therapy may be indicated, but the side effects of such agents would be carefully weighed against expected benefits.

Generally, prognosis in such relatively mild cases of SLE is optimistic when the diagnosis is promptly made. Unfortunately, the variation and complexity of SLE signs and symptoms often offer a confusing picture, which delays diagnosis and prompt therapeutic intervention.

Key Concepts

1. Vaccines build up immunity to a pathogen by exposing the immune system to some dependably recognizable but harmless feature(s) specific to that pathogen; subsequent exposure to the pathogen results in a rapid and intense immune response (pp. 94–96).

2. Antisera can be used to neutralize pathogens at the infection site or, once the pathogens are in the bloodstream, to neutralize bacterial toxins or to avoid immune sensitization (pp. 96–98).

3. In hypersensitivity reactions, damage to tissue function and/or structure arises out of immune responses to harmless antigenic stimuli, to self-antigens, to deposited immune complexes, or to persistent foreign or modified self-antigens (p. 98).

4. Allergies are an example of type I immediate hypersensitivity: the exposure of sensitized mast cells in the skin and mucosal barriers to a specific allergen elicits immediate inflammation, bronchoconstriction, and increased secretion, as well as delayed reactions (pp. 98–100).

5. Aberrant antibody production or chemical alteration of self-antigens can elicit antibody-dependent cytotoxicity (type II hypersensitivity), in which K cells, phagocytes, and complement can injure tissues (pp. 100–101).

6. Exposure to masses of foreign antigen (e.g., pneumonoconiosis) or excessive production of antibody (autoimmune disease) can lead to the formation and deposition of small immune complexes that trigger a range of inflammatory and immune processes destructive to tissue (type III immune-complex-mediated hypersensitivity) (pp. 101–102).

7. Cell-mediated, delayed-type hypersensitivity (type IV) results when helper T cells mobilize a macrophage response to a persistent foreign antigen (e.g., tubercular bacillus or fungi) or an altered self-antigen (e.g., contact dermatitis) (pp. 102–103).

8. Each individual has a combination of cell surface proteins that is more or less unique, called human leukocyte antigens (HLA) or self-antigens. These make possible the identification and destruction of virally infected cells but also make tissue transplantation problematic (pp. 103–104).

9. The genes that produce HLA proteins (the MHC complex) are also responsible for other surface antigens and aspects of immune system function that may be the basis of autoimmune diseases. Certain specific HLAs are more commonly identified in individuals with particular autoimmune diseases (pp. 104–106).

10. Strategies for improving transplant graft survival include careful tissue matching, use of cytotoxic drugs to reduce the pool of sensitized T_H cells, and use of immunosuppressant drugs such as prednisone, cyclosporin A, or cyclophosphamide (pp. 106–108).

11. Primary immune deficiencies result when one or more components of immune system function are deficient or lacking, often because of a genetic defect, with a resulting characteristic pattern of infection (pp. 108–111).

12. Secondary immune deficiencies can arise from a wide variety of infections or as a toxic effect of drugs or other medical treatments (pp. 111–112).

13. Molecular characteristics of the HIV virus particle explain its absorption, replication, and spread (pp. 115–117).

14. HIV infection classically passes through three phases. Infection is followed in weeks to months by a brief acute phase resembling mononucleosis or flu; a prolonged chronic phase, accompanied by swollen glands and gradually dropping T_4 cell counts; and a crisis phase that includes ARC and AIDS (pp. 117–118).

15. The AIDS phase of the disease is diagnosed when the HIV-positive person develops any of a variety of opportunistic infections (particularly PCP), otherwise rare neoplasms (e.g., Kaposi's sarcoma), or dementia. Women with advanced HIV infection may show only highly resistant candidiasis and other infections (pp. 117–118).

16. HIV infection can result if HIV particles or infected lymphocytes, which are present in large numbers in semen, vaginal secretions, and blood, and in lower numbers in other body fluids, are passed into the bloodstream or to areas that bear receptors for HIV (pp. 121–123).

17. In autoimmune disease, a primary immune defect allows the development of self-reactive antibodies or T cells (loss of tolerance) that mediate tissue destruction (pp. 123–127).

REVIEW ACTIVITIES

1. Describe the steps involved in effective immunization, from the first step, vaccination, when antigenic features are engulfed and processed by an antigen-presenting cell, to the last step, when pathogen-specific antibodies and cytotoxic T cells mediate destruction of the naturally encountered pathogen.

2. Explain the feature that the four hypersensitivity reactions have in common. Construct a table briefly describing the principal mechanisms of injury in each case, and name a disorder in which that reaction plays a key role.

Hypersensitivity	Mechanism	Example
Type I		
Type II		
Type III		
Type IV		

3. Using figure 5.27 as a guide, explain the various ways in which depressed T_4 numbers can result in impaired immunity (both specific and nonspecific) and tumor growth. Although the distinction is not made in the figure, you should be able to distinguish between the primary role of T_{H1} and T_{H2} cells.

4. What signs and symptoms would you expect to note in the case history of each of the following? (a) a child with severe combined immunodeficiency disease, (b) an adult with Sjögren's syndrome, (c) isolated IgA deficiency, (d) dermatomyositis, (e) DiGeorge syndrome.

5. You are probably familiar with the use of universal precautions when handling body fluids of someone who is HIV positive. These decrease the likelihood that the health care worker will contract the disorder. What do they do for the person with AIDS?

6. Based on the information presented on the populations affected, the means of transmission, and the treatments available, design a prevention and treatment strategy for a particular region.

7. You have read that genetics may play a role in individual cases of diseases like rheumatoid arthritis or diabetes mellitus. What group of genetically programmed characteristics is thought to account for these differences? The mechanisms are not well understood. Can you suggest how these genetic patterns are expressed in intensified or inappropriately focused immune system function?

8. "Systemic lupus erythematosus is a model for the loss of self-tolerance." What is meant by this statement?

Chapter

6

Neoplasia

On some a relentless cancer has fastened its envenomed teeth.

JAMES HERVEY, *MEDITATIONS AND CONTEMPLATIONS*

rubor

rubor

&tumor

cū calore

&/dolore

Neoplasia is a potentially grave growth abnormality whose more serious form is known as cancer. Neoplasia is the second-ranking cause of death in North America, with over 30% of the population suffering some form of the disease. Approximately 25% of North American adults die of cancer, and it kills more people under the age of 15 than any other disease. The high incidence of neoplasia is indicated by autopsy studies that find many people who do not die *of* the disease have a good chance of dying *with* it. For this reason, and because of pain and serious functional complications that accompany the disease, as well as the many severe side effects associated with therapy, neoplasia is widely recognized as a major threat to our health and well-being.

TISSUE GROWTH DISORDERS

"Neoplasia" means new tissue formation and involves the overgrowth of a tissue to form a neoplastic mass, or **neoplasm,** which is called a **tumor.** (Although "tumor" was originally used to denote any abnormal swelling, the term is now restricted to use in the context of neoplasia.) To put this excessive growth into perspective, let us first review some nonneoplastic growth disorders.

Adaptive Growth Responses

When demand increases, but cells cannot divide, hypertrophy produces enlarged cells with increased functional capacity; skeletal muscle is one example. If demand is low, atrophy reduces cell size in response, while cell numbers are retained to provide for future demand increases. In healing, regeneration of labile and stable tissues produces new cells to replace those lost to injury.

In **hyperplasia,** mitosis produces new cells, but only in response to a particular growth stimulus and only in limited numbers. For example, focal hyperplasia of the epidermis is a response to increased pressure and friction at the skin's surface. The newly formed epidermal tissue provides a thicker, more protective callus, which regresses when demand is reduced. Similarly, endometrial hyperplasia plays a role in the normal menstrual cycle. These adaptive responses are the result of closely balanced control factors that produce a growth response carefully matched to demand. The swollen lymph nodes seen in patients suffering chronic infections are the result of hyperplasia. Substances drained by the lymph flow from infected tissues presumably trigger hyperplasia in both the lymphoid tissue and the phagocytic reticuloendothelial cells of the lymph nodes.

When disease requires surgical removal of a kidney, some cells of the remaining kidney undergo hypertrophy and others become hyperplastic. Both responses compensate for the loss of one kidney by increasing the functional capacity of the remaining organ.

Metaplasia and Dysplasia

When demand is more intense or prolonged, altered tissue growth can produce structural and functional abnormalities. These are seen most often in the epithelia, which are exposed to injurious agents at body surfaces.

Metaplasia is the conversion of one cell type to another. Chronic exposure to some unfavorable condition usually brings on the change. Connective tissues occasionally undergo metaplasia, but usually an epithelium is involved. For example, respiratory epithelium undergoes metaplasia in response to inhaled irritants, usually inhaled cigarette smoke or industrial pollutants. The process involves replacement of the normal ciliated, pseudostratified epithelium with a thicker, tougher lining that is better able to stand up to the irritants. The new stratified epithelium is well organized and its cells have a normal appearance (fig. 6.1). Metaplasia in epithelia is usually reversible. Note that in adapting to chronic irritation, the tissue loses its cilia and goblet cells. This means the tissue suffers a much reduced ability to clear inhaled particles and microorganisms and to maintain normal mucus secretion.

Dysplasia is seen in an epithelium when irritation is more severe and prolonged. As with metaplasia, the replacement tissue is a tougher, stratified tissue. However, its architecture is disordered and its cells demonstrate **pleomorphism.** Pleomorphic cells are variable in their size and shape, in contrast to the regular cell structure seen in normal tissues. They also have larger, more darkly stained nuclei and increased mitosis rates (see fig. 6.1). Dysplasia is also a reversible condition but is less so than metaplasia. It is associated with the chronic bronchitis commonly seen in cigarette smokers, and also in prolonged inflammations of the uterine cervix. Severely dysplastic tissues often resemble tumors (fig. 6.2), and it is generally accepted that dysplasia often precedes a tissue becoming neoplastic. Some forms of dysplasia are known as **precancerous** lesions.

In the case of neoplasia, the formation of the tumor mass represents an irreversible alteration in a cell's growth pattern. Normal formation of new tissue represents a fine balance between growth stimulation and growth inhibition; the body produces only the tissue necessary to meet demand, and no more. In a tumor, tissue production continues beyond the body's needs and, in many cases, continues until the resulting disruption of function causes the victim's death (fig. 6.3). Clearly, the growth of a tumor represents a dramatic departure from the normal pattern of tissue formation.

This concept of the balance of stimulus and inhibition is presented in figure 6.4. Genetic or developmental abnormalities produce the problems of **aplasia**—lack of organ development—and **hypoplasia**—development that is inadequate, so that the resulting tissue is immature and functionally deficient. Adaptive responses to changing

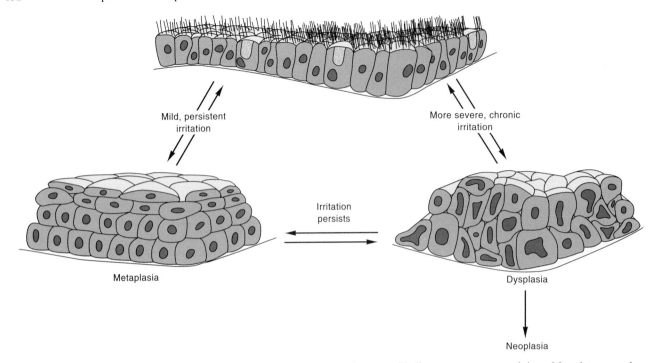

Figure 6.1   **Metaplasia and Dysplasia.** These reversible changes to respiratory epithelium are responses to injury. More intense and prolonged exposure to the injurious agent can produce the irreversible transformation to neoplasia.

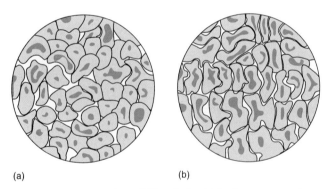

(a)   (b)

Figure 6.2   **Dysplasia and Neoplasia.** (*a*) In the representative microscope field, the dysplastic cells show varying degrees of pleomorphism, with some cells appearing to be near normal. (*b*) The neoplastic (tumor) cells are all abnormal, with enlarged nuclei and more pronounced pleomorphism.

demand—atrophy, hypertrophy, hyperplasia, and regeneration—are reversible. In neoplasia, the transformation is irreversible and the newly formed tissue continues to grow without control. It is the imbalance between growth stimulus and growth inhibition that produces the inappropriate tissue overgrowth.

The tumor's ability to avoid growth inhibition factors means that it has escaped the controls that limit growth to the degree necessary for normal function. Having escaped these controls, we say that the tumor's growth is

autonomous—that is, it is growing independently. Without the usual restraints, the resulting tissue is excessive in quantity and also inappropriate in that it makes no contribution to any functional need.

The regulation of tissue growth was introduced in chapter 4. There, we considered contact inhibition, cell interactions with components of the extracellular matrix, and various growth factor (GFs) (table 4.2) in the context of tissue regeneration following injury. These regulatory inputs are shown in figure 6.5*a*. Generally, derangements of tissue growth may result from flawed regulatory input due to inadequate levels of growth factors, from damage or loss of cell surface receptors, or from defective links to key elements of the extracellular matrix (ECM) (fig 6.5*b*).

TUMOR TERMINOLOGY

The study of tumors is called **oncology,** from the Greek word *oncos,* meaning tumor. In describing a tumor, two distinguishing characteristics are relevant: its pattern of growth and its tissue of origin.

In terms of its growth pattern, a tumor falls into one of two broad categories. It is said to be **benign** if its growth is relatively slow and orderly and if the tumor remains localized. A **malignant** tumor, by contrast, is characterized by more rapid, disorderly growth and by aggressive invasion into adjacent normal tissues. The term **cancer,** from the Latin word for crab, refers to malignant tumors, generally. (It is unclear whether the term arose because of the clawlike

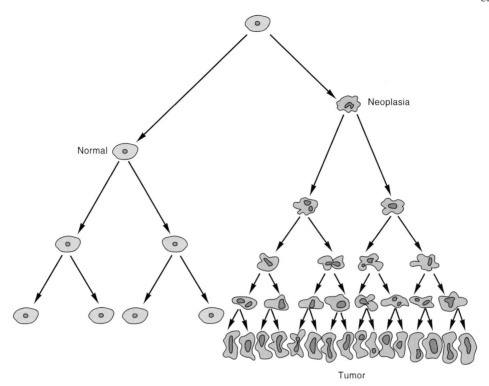

Figure 6.3   **Growth of a Neoplasm.** Tumor growth outstrips that of normal tissue, forming a neoplastic mass.

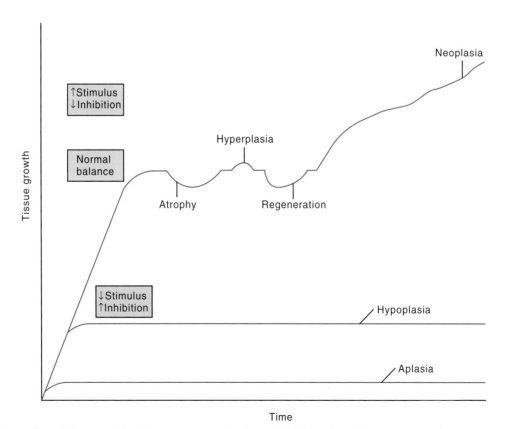

Figure 6.4   **Tissue Growth Patterns.** The balance between stimulus and inhibition determines the pattern of tissue growth. See text.

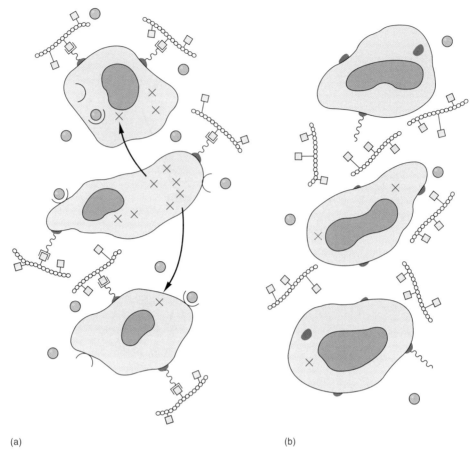

(a)   (b)

Figure 6.5   **Cell Growth Regulation.** (*a*) Extracellular matrix components bound by surface receptors and plasma-borne and cellular growth factors provide appropriate growth control. (*b*) Damaged receptors reduce normal interaction with ECM components. Lack of adequate growth factors alters growth regulation. ⊔: ECM receptor; ●: GF from plasma; ×: from cells.

growth extensions of malignancies, the crab-claw appearance of some tumor blood vessels, or the crablike tenacity with which the disease belabors its victims.) The invasiveness of a malignant tumor is usually accompanied by spread to other, distant points in the body. These differences in tumor behavior underlie the more favorable prognosis associated with benign tumors. Malignant tumors, if untreated, inevitably lead to the death of the host.

The suffix "-oma" may be used to designate any tumor. In naming benign tumors, a root word indicating the type of tissue that has become neoplastic is used. For example, where glandular tissue is involved, the benign tumor is called an adenoma. In the case of bone, the benign tumor is called an osteoma. Other examples are given in table 6.1.

Malignant tumors are classified according to the embryonic origin of the tissue in which the tumor arises. During development of an embryo, three primary tissue layers form. **Ectoderm** lines the outer surface of the body, whereas **endoderm** provides the protective lining for its internal surfaces. Malignant tumors arising in tissues derived from these primitive layers are known as **carcinomas.** Generally, carcinomas are malignant tumors of the skin and the epithelial linings of the alimentary canal and the respiratory passages. Because glandular tissue is derived from ecto-

derm or endoderm, malignant glandular tumors are included with the carcinomas and are called **adenocarcinomas.** If a benign **adenoma** contains pockets of tumor secretions (cysts), it is called a **cystadenoma.**

The third embryonic tissue layer is **mesoderm.** Malignancies developing in tissues that derive from mesoderm are called **sarcomas.** Specific sarcoma terminology makes reference to the particular tissue of origin; for example, tumors of cartilage and fibrous connective tissue are called chondrosarcoma and fibrosarcoma, respectively.

There are a few cases in which traditional but less precise usage persists. For example, you might think that a melanoma, lymphoma, or hepatoma is benign because of its name, but all three are actually quite malignant. The more accurate terms are malignant melanoma, lymphosarcoma, and hepatocellular carcinoma, respectively.

Table 6.1 lists only the most frequently encountered terms describing tumors. Many other terms are used to provide more specific insight into the origin and other characteristics of a given tumor. For example, in malignant tumors of stratified epithelium, usually in the skin, a tumor might involve different cells. When the cells in the deepest layer become neoplastic, the tumor is called a **basal cell carcinoma.** If cells nearer the surface of the skin or other epithelia are in-

Table 6.1   Tumor Terminology and Classification

Tissue of Origin	Benign	Malignant
Ectoderm/Endoderm		
Epithelium	Epithelioma (papilloma if projecting from surface)	Carcinoma
Gland	Adenoma (if cysts present; cystadenoma)	Adenocarcinoma
Melanocytes		Malignant melanoma
Neuroglia	Glioma	Glioma
Embryonic nervous tissue*		Neuroblastoma
Embryonic retinal cells*		Retinoblastoma
Mesoderm		
Adipose tissue	Lipoma	Liposarcoma
Cartilage	Chondroma	Chondrosarcoma
Bone	Osteoma	Osteosarcoma
Fibrous tissue	Fibroma	Fibrosarcoma
Lymphoid tissue		Lymphosarcoma
Smooth muscle	Leiomyoma	Leiomyosarcoma
Embryonic skeletal muscle*		Myoblastoma
Multiple tissues (usually gonadal)*	Teratoma	
Leukocyte-Producing Tissues		
Red bone marrow		Myeloid leukemia
Lymphoid tissue		Lymphocytic leukemia

* Less well-differentiated cells not normally present in adults

volved, the term **squamous cell carcinoma** is used. Further complexity in terminology arises when other factors are used to expand the basis of tumor classification. Most of these have clinical relevance that lies beyond the scope of this text.

 Checkpoint 6.1

In the rest of this chapter and throughout the remaining chapters, there is frequent use of the tumor terminology just described. When you encounter a term whose meaning you've forgotten, do a quick check back to table 6.1. It will aid your understanding and help you to remember.

TUMOR STRUCTURE

Neoplastic Tissue

A principal constituent of a typical tumor is neoplastic tissue with varying degrees of resemblance to its tissue of origin. The degree of resemblance is greater in benign tumors than in malignancies. A benign tumor contains cells of near-normal size and shape, arranged in a manner that closely resembles normal tissue architecture. Occasionally, a cell in the process of dividing can be seen in microscopic studies. A malignant tumor is usually quite different (fig. 6.6). Its

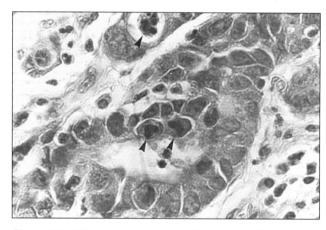

Figure 6.6   **Tumor Pleomorphism.** Shown are malignant cells from a gastric carcinoma. Arrows indicate large pleomorphic cells with irregular and deeply staining nuclei. Normal tissue architecture is lost and the cells bear little resemblance to their tissue of origin.

cells are highly pleomorphic, with enlarged, unusually shaped nuclei and abnormalities of chromosome structure and number. Some cells are very large due to a failure of separation following mitosis. The tissue configuration is disordered, and mitotic cells are seen more frequently than in benign tumors. The irregular and often bizarre configurations seen in tumor cells provide the basis for tumor diagnosis in cases where tissue samples are available. An application of

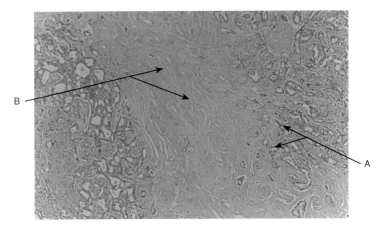

Figure 6.7   **Scirrhous Tumor.** Although tumor cells (A) are evident in this view, the dominant feature is fibrous tissue (B), which tightly binds the neoplastic cells. The fibrous tissue produces the characteristic firmness of the scirrhous tumor.
A 50-year-old assembly line worker discovered a lump in her breast during a regular breast self-examination. On the follow-up, her physician found a very firm lump of 2 cm diameter. It was joined to the skin and underlying pectoral muscle, indicating that it had invaded locally. The mass and adjacent tissue was surgically removed. Later, microscopic study revealed a significant fibrous tissue component, which accounted for the tumor's firmness. The woman suffered no further complications.

this is seen in the **Papanicolaou,** or **Pap, test.** In this test, named for its originator, George Papanicolaou, a microscopic study is made of epithelial cells that have been gently removed with a swab from the lining of the cervix. Cell size and shape as well as nuclear size, shape, and number are studied for indications of neoplasia.

Biochemical changes can also be detected in cancers because the enzyme complement of a malignant cell resembles that of more primitive, undifferentiated cells. The malignant cells demonstrate a greater use of anaerobic glycolysis as an energy source, regardless of oxygen availability. Also, malignant cells typically lose some of the specialized functional capabilities characteristic of their tissue of origin. The pattern of change that reflects an earlier cell form is called **anaplasia.** As tissues develop normally, differentiation yields a highly specialized cell whose reproductive capability is usually reduced in comparison with its earlier, less-specialized forms. The anaplastic cell, however, seems to have regained reproductive capacity at the expense of functional specialization.

Anaplasia is not an all-or-nothing phenomenon. Rather, it is a characteristic present to different degrees in different tumors. Generally, the degree of anaplasia and the degree of malignancy are directly linked. At the extreme, highly malignant tumors may be so undifferentiated that they lack resemblance to any particular tissue and, hence, cannot be classified except in their general resemblance to embryonic tissue. In such cases, broadly descriptive terminology, emphasizing some obvious characteristic, is often used—for example, **giant cell carcinoma.**

Fibrous Stroma

Another major component of a tumor is the fibrous stroma (connective tissue framework) that supports the tumor cells. It is important to note that this tissue is in itself not neoplas-

tic. It is formed in response to the increased amount of new tumor tissue. Malignant tumors have been shown to secrete factors that stimulate fibroblasts to produce collagen and other stromal components. Tumors vary in their ability to induce this response. The result is a broad range in a tumor's physical properties. When there is little stroma, the tumor has a softer, fleshy consistency, which is typical of sarcomas. At the other extreme is a **scirrhous** (ski′rus) tumor. In this case, the stromal response is exaggerated and a densely collagenous tumor, hard to the touch, results. The fibrous tissue that is newly formed may undergo contracture to add to the density of the tumor mass. Scirrhous tumors are typical of adenocarcinoma of the breast and may have as much as 90% of their volume formed of stromal elements (fig. 6.7).

Vascular Stroma

A tumor also contains vascular stroma. Its blood vessels, like a tumor's fibrous stroma, are nonneoplastic and are formed in response to the increased demand for blood flow to the developing tumor. Initially, a tumor can derive its nutrients from adjacent normal tissues by diffusion, but after the tumor reaches a diameter of about 1 mm, it requires additional vascular supply. Note that although this seems a minute size, over such distances diffusion is too slow to sustain tissue growth. Consider also the high metabolic demand of the one million growing cells that might be present in the tumor this size, and you can better appreciate the need for new blood vessels.

The process of new vessel formation (**angiogenesis**) in tumors seems essentially the same as in the revascularization of a healing tissue. That is, it is closely regulated by a group of tissue growth and inhibition factors. One of these is called **vascular endothelial growth factor** (VEGF; see table 4.2). Although widely distributed in normal tissues, it is also present in many tumors. It is thought that the large quantities of

Focus on Growth Factors in Antitumor Therapy

Growth factors are the focus of much research in the field of antitumor therapy. Under particular study is the role of vascular endothelial growth factor in promoting vessel growth in tumors. After its secretion by the tumor, VEGF binds to specific receptors on the surfaces of adjacent blood vessel endothelia. This binding triggers increased mitosis and the formation of new vessels needed by the growing tumor. (This process is described in the context of healing on pages 66–67.)

One research approach involves use of a therapeutic agent that can bind to endothelial VEGF receptors without triggering the cells to divide. While bound to the receptor, such an agent also blocks VEGF access to the receptors and mitosis rates remain low. The resulting lack of blood vessel development significantly retards tumor growth.

Other research takes a different tack based on laboratory production of an antibody that selectively binds to VEGF that is already bound to the antibody's endothelial receptors in a growing tumor. The key to this technique is that the antibody is prepared with a toxin molecule joined to it. The toxin damages the endothelial surface, which, in turn, triggers the formation of a mass of blood platelets and coagulated blood. This mass, a thrombus, blocks blood flow to the tumor, slowing its growth or destroying it completely.

The ultimate usefulness of these approaches depends on resolving a number of technical difficulties and side effects. But they indicate the direction much research is taking.

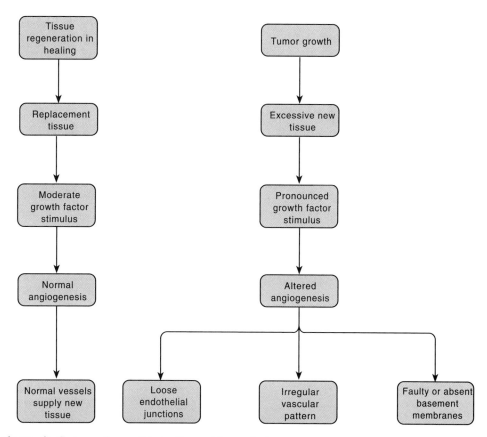

Figure 6.8   **Angiogenesis.** Compare the result in healing and in neoplasia.

VEGF secreted by growing tumors overcome the effects of inhibitory factors. The result is a strong stimulus to the formation of new vascular channels (see focus box).

Tumors vary in their ability to induce new vessel formation. Generally, the newly formed vessels have a less-regular pattern compared with those at healing sites. Newly formed tumor capillaries also have looser endothelial junc-tions and may lack basement membranes. They are more highly permeable as a result (fig. 6.8).

Tumor Products

Many cells produce some product in the course of their normal activities. Hormones and mucus are examples, as is the

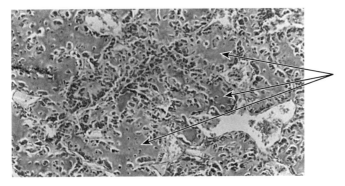

Figure 6.9   Tumor Product Formation. The arrows indicate the bone matrix substance being produced by the cells of this bone tumor (osteogenic sarcoma). Note the lack of similarity to normally structured bone.

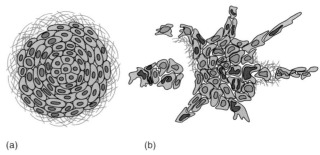

(a)   (b)

Figure 6.10   **Typical Tumor Structure.** (*a*) A benign tumor, in which near-normal cells slowly undergo expansile growth, enclosed by a connective tissue capsule. (*b*) A malignant tumor, characterized by abnormal cytology and irregular, invasive growth.

keratin formed by dry-surfaced stratified epithelium. Other examples of cell products are the intercellular materials of connective tissues and the basement membranes produced by epithelia.

On becoming neoplastic, the cells typically continue such production. The tumor that emerges contains a large tumor product component. The product's properties depend on the degree of the tumor's anaplasia. Products of a benign tumor tend to closely resemble the normal product. Those of malignant tumors may sufficiently resemble the normal to allow some degree of normal function or physiological potency (fig. 6.9). In other cases, the products of malignant tumors may be completely nonfunctional. A squamous cell carcinoma produces excessive keratin, much of it lying below the surface of the skin. Tumor diagnosis may be aided by a tumor's overproduction of enzymes. As they are picked up by the blood, their high levels may betray the presence of a tumor that would otherwise be unnoticed.

Tumor products may also contribute to differences in the physical characteristics of a tumor. For example, tumors secreting large quantities of serous fluid (**serous tumors)** may form cysts, while overproduction of mucus leads to the loose, gelatinous texture of a **mucoid tumor** such as colon carcinoma.

TUMOR BEHAVIOR: BENIGN VERSUS MALIGNANT

Benign

Benign tumors grow more rapidly than normal tissues, but more slowly than malignant tumors. In a benign tumor, the production of new tissue proceeds in an orderly pattern of expansion to form a generally regular tumor mass. Another characteristic of benign tumors is the presence of a fibrous connective tissue capsule that surrounds the tumor mass and provides a distinct line of separation between the tumor and the adjacent normal tissue in which it is growing. The capsular tissue is derived in part from newly formed connective tissues and in part from the stroma of the normal

tissue that has been replaced by the tumor. Both the slower, measured, expansile growth and the surrounding capsule contribute to the more favorable prognosis typical of benign tumors. Slower growth means there is less damage to the surrounding normal cells, and the presence of the capsule makes surgical removal easier (fig. 6.10*a*).

Malignant

The behavior of a malignant tumor is a different matter. Its more rapid rate of growth can produce a larger tumor mass, but more significant is its pattern of growth, which is aggressively invasive. The tumor sends columns of cells into adjacent normal tissues, causing disruption of their structure and function (fig. 6.10*b*). The occurrence of a capsule is rare. When present, it is usually incomplete and irregular. The blurred lines of demarcation between malignant tumor and adjacent normal tissue complicate surgical removal (see fig. 6.11).

An even greater factor in the poor prognosis of a malignancy is its ability to spread to distant points in the body. This type of spread is called **metastasis.** In metastasis, the original tumor mass, growing at its **primary site,** is able to shed cells that become established as tumors at one or more distant **secondary sites.** There is no physical continuity between tumors at primary and secondary sites. However, the secondary tumor is the same tissue as that growing at the primary site. That is, the normal tissue of the secondary site has not become neoplastic; rather, tumor cells have been transported to the secondary site and have resumed growth there (fig. 6.12).

Metastasis is a major problem in dealing with tumors. There is often doubt over whether metastasis has already occurred. On the other hand, a secondary tumor may be the first to produce signs or symptoms, in which case the problem lies in determining the location of the primary tumor from which it arose. For example, a bone that fractures after relatively slight strain may have been weakened by tumor growth within it. (This is known as a pathologic fracture rather than one caused by trauma.) When a biopsy re-

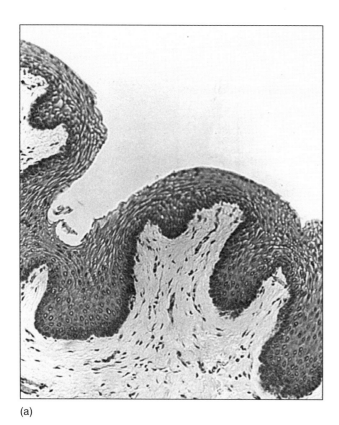

(a)

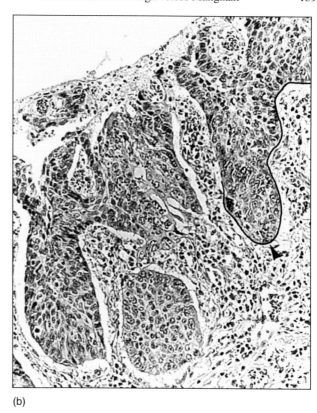

(b)

Figure 6.11   **Malignant Tumor Growth.** (*a*) Normal esophageal epithelium. (*b*) A squamous cell carcinoma of the esophagus. The solid line at upper right (arrow) indicates an area where the tumor is still confined within the tissue's basement membrane. In the central portion of the photo, the tumor is present in cords and islands of cells that have broken through to the underlying submucosa.

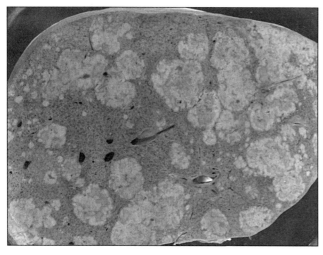

Figure 6.12   **Liver Metastasis.** This section through the liver reveals numerous secondary tumor masses. They originated as multiple tumor emboli that were shed by a colon carcinoma. The site at which they lodged in the liver was determined by the flow pattern of the hepatic portal blood arriving from the colon.

The extensive secondary tumors visible in this liver section originated in the colon of an elderly man. His tumor had been assessed as inoperable when he developed signs and symptoms of liver malfunction. His damaged liver was unable to excrete bile pigments and his serum alkaline phosphatase level was elevated. He died soon after these problems developed.

Table 6.2	Characteristics of Benign and Malignant Tumors	
Characteristic	**Benign**	**Malignant**
Cell structure	Near normal	Abnormal shapes, larger cell and nucleus
Tissue structure	Orderly	Disordered, irregular
Growth rate	Above normal	Rapid
Invasive growth	Uncommon	Typical
Metastasis	Never	Typical
Capsule	Typical	Rare, incomplete if present
Anaplasia	Minimal	Typical
Prognosis	Good	Poor

veals the tumor to be an adenocarcinoma, the problem is to locate the unknown gland bearing the primary tumor in the hope of intervening before further metastasis can occur.

The ability to metastasize is the single characteristic that clearly differentiates the malignant from the benign tumor (table 6.2). Also, even though malignant growths both invade and metastasize, the two characteristics are not

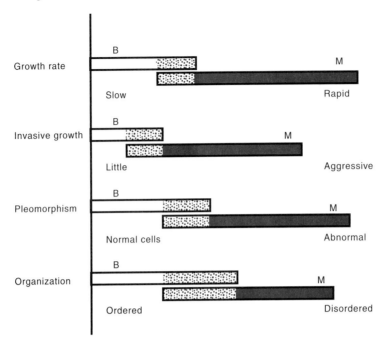

Figure 6.13 **Characteristics of Benign and Malignant Tumors.** B: benign; M: malignant. Note the stippled areas where the upper end of the B scale overlaps the M scale. These overlaps can complicate diagnosis.

necessarily present to the same degree. That is, highly invasive tumors may metastasize to only a limited degree, and tumors that are minimally invasive may metastasize extensively.

Any tumor that metastasizes is, by definition, malignant. This is the only tumor characteristic that clearly distinguishes benign from malignant tumors. All other tumor characteristics are expressed over a range, usually with an area of overlap between the extremes of benign and malignant tumor behavior. For example, some tumors that do not metastasize, and are therefore benign, might demonstrate an invasive pattern of growth. In comparison, a metastasizing—and therefore malignant—tumor might grow in a manner that is only mildly invasive. A similar overlap exists in tumor tissue architecture. The most precisely ordered malignant tumors may be more regularly arranged than the least orderly benign tumors (fig. 6.13). This overlap has important implications for diagnosis because therapy and prognosis depend on the early determination of whether a tumor is benign or malignant. Unless metastasis has clearly occurred, any tumor whose observed invasiveness or tissue architecture or other characteristics fall into the area of overlap between benign and malignant presents a problem. On the one hand, it would be regrettable to subject a person with a benign tumor to the rigorous and often unpleasant therapies intended for a malignant tumor. On the other hand, treating a malignant tumor as though it were benign could tragically shorten the patient's life.

Increasingly, cancer diagnosticians are using specialized staining, electron microscopy and sophisticated techniques based on the use of monoclonal antibodies (Mab, see p. 86). The Mabs reveal the tumor's identity by binding to antigens that are unique to a given tumor. Still many histopathologists would agree that the process of establishing a tumor's identity is far from precise and, in some ways, is more of an art than a science.

Tumor Growth Rate

Tumor growth rates also overlap: the most rapidly growing benign tumors have growth rates that surpass those of the slowest-growing malignancies. Although higher than normal, tumor growth rates are not strikingly rapid. Normal fetal growth and regeneration in healing tissues have growth rates that are significantly higher than those found in most tumors. However, a clear understanding of tumor growth rates requires a precise distinction between two growth-related concepts. The first is **generation time**—the time between successive cell divisions. Generation time includes the time taken for mitosis itself, as well as the time when the cell rests, undergoes preparatory metabolic changes, and then synthesizes the molecules needed for its next mitotic division. The second concept is **doubling time**—the time required to double the number of tumor cells or the size of the tumor.

You might assume that generation time and doubling time would be the same, but clinical experience indicates that doubling times for tumors are much longer than generation times. In fact, doubling times actually increase as a tumor ages. How can this be? The reason has to do with the fate of newly produced cells—not all go on to reproduce, forming new cells that reproduce in turn, and so on. Some of the newly formed cells lose their mitotic ability, some enter a nondividing resting phase, while still others die. It is

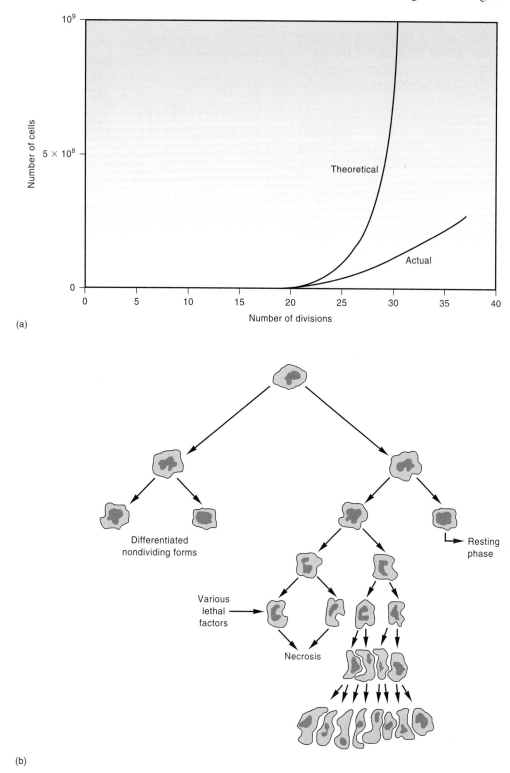

Figure 6.14   **Tumor Growth.** (*a*) Theoretical versus actual tumor growth. (*b*) After six divisions of a single tumor cell, the number of surviving cells is significantly lower than the 64 that are theoretically possible.

estimated that in tumors, as many as 90% of the newly formed cells do not immediately go on to divide. This means that many cycles may be required to double the amount of tumor tissue. Also, as a tumor ages, reduced blood supply, nutrient depletion, and host responses can re-

duce the number of actively dividing cells so that doubling times increase and the rate at which new, viable tumor tissue is produced decreases (fig. 6.14).

The number of a tissue's cells that are dividing is the tissue's **growth fraction** (GF). It is usually presented as a percentage. In slowly growing tumors, studies indicate growth fractions under 10%, while the most rapidly growing malignancies have growth fractions that approach 20%. Note also that normal intestinal epithelium has a growth fraction of about 15%, a more rapid growth than is seen in many tumors.

Another factor may extend a tumor's doubling time. In certain tumors, the generation time increases due to an extended period in the mitotic stage of the cell's reproductive cycle. For human tumors, laboratory studies produced generation times ranging from one to five days. Rapid doubling times were as low as 30 days, while the longest extended to over a year. On this basis, you can appreciate that a tumor may be growing for many months, or even several years, before its presence is detected.

In normally dividing tissues, precise growth controls match cell loss to new cell production. In tumors, although all daughter cells don't survive, there is still a net increase in cell production over cell losses. The problem of neoplasia emerges from this fundamental imbalance.

Tumor Invasion

There are several essential factors involved in a tumor's invasion of the normal tissue that surrounds it. One is pressure atrophy. As a tumor expands, it puts pressure on adjacent normal cells and their blood vessels. Tissues vary in their ability to tolerate such pressure, but ultimately they undergo apoptosis and are eliminated. The tumor can then more easily fill the newly available space (see fig. 1.11). However, pressure atrophy is a relatively minor factor in tumor invasion, and growth rate and invasion are not linked directly. For example, a type of benign breast tumor grows relatively rapidly, yet invades only minimally. In contrast, a malignant form of breast cancer invades extensively even though it grows more slowly than the benign tumor.

More important to a tumor's invasive capability is tumor cell motility. Especially in malignant tumors, some cells develop the ability to separate from the primary tumor mass and move into surrounding tissues. Several factors contribute to this pivotal invasive capability. One is reduced intercellular adhesion. Unlike normal cells, which are tightly bound together, malignant cells can separate from neighboring cells and actively move into adjacent normal tissues. The extracellular matrix (ECM) and, in the case of epithelial tumors, the basement membrane (BM), may restrict this motility. But this restriction is met by a second adaptive capability that now comes into play.

In becoming malignant, cells acquire surface receptors that enable them to bind to particular elements of the extracellular matrix or basement membrane. Once bound to these, the tumor cells release an array of enzymes. These degrade and loosen the ECM, or BM, to provide low-resistance invasion paths through the disrupted tissues. The result is easier penetration and infiltration by the aggressive tumor cells.

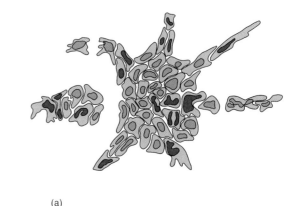

(a)

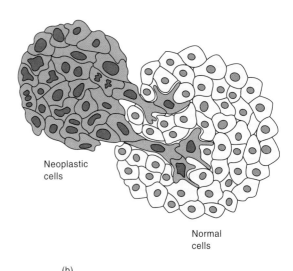

Neoplastic cells

Normal cells

(b)

Figure 6.15 **Tumor Invasion.** Malignant tumor cells grown in tissue culture. In (*a*), tumor in isolation produces randomly directed cords of cells. In (*b*), an adjacent sheet of normal cells draws the tumor to it.

Another key aspect of tumor invasiveness is the process of chemotaxis, which draws cells from the tumor into the adjacent tissues. That is, the tumor cells respond to chemical stimuli from the nearby normal tissues. These chemical signals speed up and direct the tumor's invasion. This property can be demonstrated in the laboratory. When tumor cells are grown adjacent to normal cells in tissue culture, they don't spread uniformly in all directions and encounter the normal cells by chance. Instead, they grow toward the normal cells to a greater extent than they do in other directions, appearing to preferentially invade the normal tissue (fig. 6.15). Chemotaxis explains this phenomenon. Chemotactic factors for tumor cells are formed in the normal tissue, and these focus and accelerate tumor cell motility and invasion.

There are three sources of such chemotactic factors. Some products of normal cell metabolism are chemotactic for tumor cells. Some of the products of ECM and BM

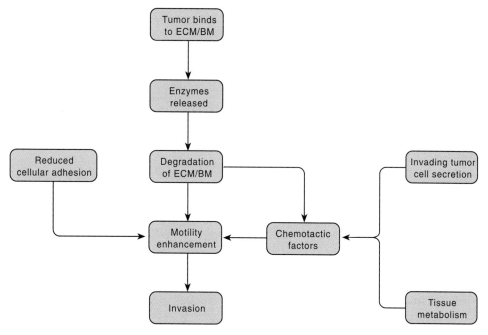

Figure 6.16   The Mechanisms of Tumor Invasion. Factors underlying a tumor's invasive growth capacity.

degradation are tumor attractants. The third source is the tumor cell itself. In becoming neoplastic, many tumors acquire the ability to secrete substances called **autocrine motility factors** that are chemotactic to other tumor cells. The earliest invading cells secrete these, actively drawing other cells from the primary tumor mass. Figure 6.16 summarizes the mechanisms that underlie tumor invasion.

Patterns of Invasion

At the microscopic level, we have seen that the breakdown of the BM and ECM provides paths along which invading tumor cells can more easily penetrate. Similarly, at the gross level, tumors will invade along planes of low resistance. Fascia, bone, thick-walled arterioles, and the pericardial sac are examples of tissues resistant to invasion. Rather than penetrating, advancing tumors will grow around or along the low-resistance planes between an organ and its neighbors (fig. 6.17). This pattern is seen in the abdominal cavity, for example, where sheets of tumors grow along peritoneal surfaces. On the other hand, a tumor originating within an organ and unable to break through its connective tissue capsule, might extend its growth along a low-resistance plane within the organ, just deep to the capsule.

After invading through the wall of a vein or lymphatic vessel and gaining access to the lumen, the tumor cells lie within a channel that offers a low-resistance path favoring growth along the lumen. However, this pattern does not seem to occur with any significant frequency. Exceptions are renal carcinoma and the relatively rare primary hepatic tumors. These may grow along the veins that drain the organ to form elongated, cordlike tumor masses that can

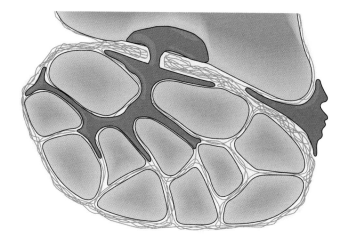

Figure 6.17   Invasion Planes. Initially impeded by the capsules of the organs, the growing tumor (at right) extends along low-resistance paths between them. Even when penetration of the capsule is achieved (at left), growth proceeds along the internal subdivisions of the organ.

reach the heart via the inferior vena cava. As with their other characteristics, tumors vary greatly in their invasive capability. In the case of highly invasive malignant tumors, organ capsules may only temporarily slow invasive spread before the tumor penetrates into adjacent structures.

Tumor Metastasis

Malignant tumors typically couple localized invasion with metastasis to secondary sites. This spread increases the damaging effects of the tumor because after metastasis, destructive invasive growth can proceed at other, often widely separated locations. Although this is the usual pattern, invasion and metastasis are not necessarily linked. Some malignant tumors invade extensively but metastasize only rarely—for example, basal cell carcinoma of the skin and brain glioma.

Metastasis via Embolism

Most often, metastasizing tumor cells are carried to secondary sites by the blood or lymph. The initial event in a typical metastasis is the invasion of a vein or lymphatic vessel by a growing tumor. Once within the vessel, some further tumor growth is followed by small clumps of cells separating to form emboli. (Recall the low intercellular adhesiveness among tumor cells that favors this separation.) The emboli formed in this way are carried along with the moving blood or lymph until they reach some part of the vascular system that prevents their passage. At such points, they become trapped and resume growth. As growth proceeds, the tumor invades the vessel wall, gaining access to the tissue at the secondary site, where further invasive growth continues (fig. 6.18). After developing at secondary sites, the tumor can repeat the sequence to produce further metastatic dispersion.

Blood Vessel Metastasis The thin walls of capillaries and veins seem to allow easy penetration by aggressively invasive tumor cells. Once within a vein, a tumor embolus passes through successively larger veins, which ultimately deliver it to the right heart. The embolus then enters the pulmonary arterial system, whose branches at some point become sufficiently small to block its passage. Lodged in a small blood vessel within the lung, the tumor cells become actively invasive, secreting the enzymes and motility factors that promote passage through the vessel wall into the surrounding lung tissue. By this mechanism, the lungs trap emboli arising from many widely dispersed, primary tumor sites. The lung is therefore a very common site of secondary tumor growth. The major exception to this general pattern is the venous drainage of the abdominal organs. This blood passes directly to the liver in the vessels of the hepatic portal system. In the liver, vessels branch to form small-diameter sinusoids that can trap tumor emboli; for this reason, the liver is a common secondary site for primary tumors of the intestines and stomach (fig. 6.19).

Arterial metastasis is much less common, probably because the thick arterial walls are harder to penetrate. Primary lung tumors provide a special case, however, in that tumor emboli that form in the pulmonary veins are carried back to the left heart, which ejects them into the systemic arterial flow. The emboli are then widely disseminated, and extensively dispersed metastases can result. Of course, the organs that receive a larger arterial flow—the brain and kidney, for example—are particularly vulnerable.

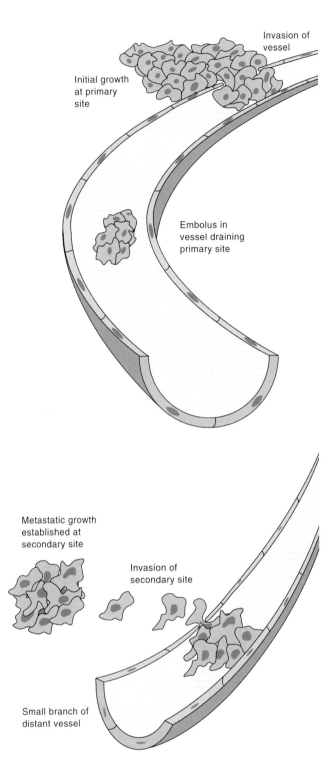

Figure 6.18 **Metastasis by Embolism.** Penetration of a blood or lymphatic vessel is followed by the formation of an embolus and its trapping at some distant site. Invasion of the secondary site is followed by growth of the secondary tumor.

Lymphatic Vessel Metastasis Like veins, lymphatic vessels are easily invaded by malignant tumors, particularly carcinomas. Because lymph must pass through a succession of lymph nodes before reaching the blood, you might think that tumor emboli would be trapped, preventing metastasis.

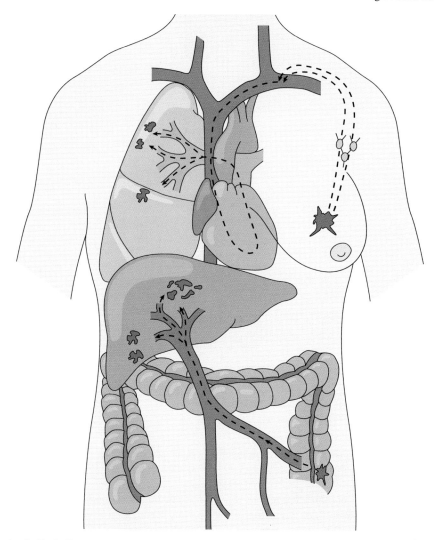

Figure 6.19 **Metastasis via Embolism.** Lymph drainage carries emboli from primary breast tumor to blood, which then carries them to lungs, where they form secondary tumors. Emboli from various abdominal organs are typically delivered to the liver via the hepatic portal system.

Unfortunately, this is not the case. Instead, lymph node involvement seems to actually promote metastasis. Three principal mechanisms are at work.

The first involves growth of a tumor within the lymph node. Trapped in the lymph node's reticular tissues, the tumor cells grow invasively, often completely replacing normal node tissues. In effect, each lymph node becomes a small secondary site. Tumor tissue in each node becomes a source of new emboli, which are then carried by the efferent lymph to the next lymph nodes in the chain, where the process repeats.

Second, tumor growth in the lymph nodes blocks normal lymph flow, causing lymph to be redirected through alternative channels. The result is that tumor emboli can be dispersed over a wider field of secondary sites. Lymphatic vessels blocked by tumor tissue can cause retrograde flow leading to unusual and unexpected embolus

dissemination that can complicate diagnosis, therapy, and prognosis.

The third factor that favors metastasis via the lymph nodes is their vascular arrangement, which provides close intercommunication between lymph and blood vessels. This means that tumor cells arriving at the node via the lymph can gain easy access to the blood after growth is established. Once a tumor has reached a lymph node, you can assume that if blood metastasis has not yet occurred, it is soon likely (fig. 6.20).

The enlargement of regional lymph nodes is often an indication of metastatic tumor growth within the node. In some cases, however, the enlargement (**lymphadenopathy**) is due to a hyperplasia response. This proliferation of lymph node cells may be a response to substances, some antigenic, that are produced by the tumor cells and then carried to the nodes by lymph flow. Nodal hyperplasia of

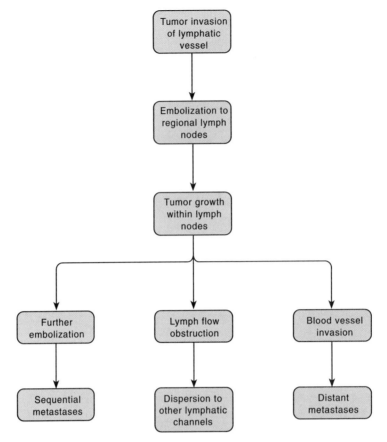

Figure 6.20   **Lymphatic Metastasis.** Consequences of lymphatic invasion and embolization.

this sort is completely reversible and nonthreatening, but it can suggest a more extensive metastasis than has actually occurred. Recall from chapter 2's consideration of the inflammatory response that lymphadenopathy may also be the result of an infection. Lymph nodes may undergo hyperplasia in response to infectious agents or their products. For example, various sexually transmitted diseases produce swelling in the inguinal lymph nodes. One can't assume, therefore, that all lymphadenopathy is linked to the presence of a metastasizing tumor.

Generally, once metastasis has occurred, it is much more difficult to effect a cure. In some cases, the initial diagnosis is complicated by the difficulty of distinguishing between primary and secondary growth. Even when a primary tumor is diagnosed, there is always the concern that metastasis has already occurred and that small groups of tumor cells, at one or more distant sites, will develop to cause additional problems after months or even years.

Factors Affecting Secondary Tumor Growth

It is significant that not all tumor cells that gain access to the blood or lymph survive to grow at secondary sites. Only a small fraction, some evidence suggests one in 1000, of the emboli formed from a primary tumor survive transport to secondary sites. The poor survival rate of circulating tumor cells is probably due to physical disruptions arising from turbulent blood flow and to host defense mechanisms. In the blood, tumor emboli may also pick up circulating lymphocytes, platelets, and coatings of fibrin that mask their surfaces. Their presence on the embolus may be related to the observation that single cells and large emboli are less likely to establish metastases than small clumps of five to ten cells. It may be that the intermediate-size embolus is protected by the fibrin, lymphocytes, and platelets at its surface. Perhaps the single cells are destroyed by blood turbulence, while larger clumps can't be completely masked by platelets and fibrin, allowing host defenses to be more effective.

While the distribution of secondary growth sites reflects blood and lymph flow patterns, a significant number of secondary tumors, as many as 40%, cannot be explained on this basis alone. Certain tumors seem to establish preferentially at secondary sites other than those that would be predicted by blood or lymph drainage. For example, the venous drainage of prostate, thyroid, and kidney tumors should predispose to secondary growth in the lung, but these tumors all preferentially metastasize to bone. And note, as well, that tumor emboli that are widely dispersed by arterial blood rarely establish secondary growth in skin or in skeletal or cardiac muscle.

Four factors combine to determine a tumor's success in becoming established at a secondary site. The first involves specific binding of the tumor cells to the endothelium of the

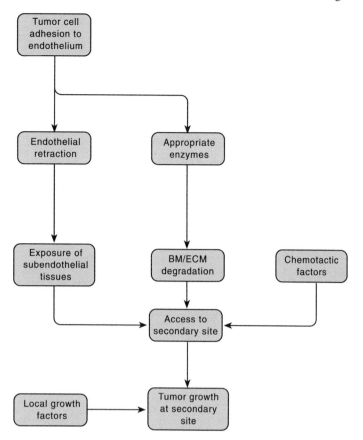

Figure 6.21   **The Process of Tumor Metastasis.** Requirements for successful metastasis of a tumor cell embolus.

vessel in which they are lodged. Those tumors with surface receptors that match particular endothelial adhesion molecules can bind at the surface. Those lacking the receptors cannot adhere. The significance of surface binding is that it triggers a critical response in the underlying epithelial cells. Binding of their surface adhesion molecules cause them to retract their edges, exposing the underlying basement membrane. This exposure allows easier movement of tumor cells out of the vessel **(extravasation).**

The second factor is the differing complements of enzymes that tumors can produce to degrade vessel basement membranes and the extracellular matrix of the secondary site. A given tumor's enzymes will permit the tumor access to certain tissue quite easily while allowing the tumor to invade other secondary sites only with great difficulty.

Third, normal metabolic activity at a secondary site produces substances that act as attractants for certain tumor cells, while other tumor types are unresponsive to them. Thus, various tissues will differ in the chemotactic coaxing they offer to cells lodged in their small vessels.

The fourth factor is variation in the growth factors present in the body tissues. If a given tissue has the growth factors needed to support the particular type of tumor that has been delivered to it, then metastatic growth is more easily established. If the necessary factors are absent, growth at the secondary site will be less likely to occur.

In summary, for secondary tumor growth to succeed, tumor emboli must be able to adhere selectively to vascular endothelium. Once they achieve adhesion, the cells must be able to release the enzymes that will allow them to escape from the vessel and infiltrate the adjacent tissue. Then, sufficient tissue chemotactic and growth factors must be present to promote invasion and support secondary growth. Where any of these factors is lacking or deficient, secondary tumor growth is much less likely (fig. 6.21).

Metastasis via Body Cavities

The second major mechanism of metastasis involves tumor spread by way of the body's cavities. In such cases, tumors can invade out through the surface of the primary site organ and spread to other sites. For example, adenocarcinoma cells may be shed from the pancreas and move to the inferior extremes of the pelvic cavity, where they grow to form a shelflike mass of tumor that surrounds the rectum. In the case of a neuroblastoma whose primary site is the medulla oblongata, cells shed from the primary tumor may "seed" down the subarachnoid space to resume growth at inferior regions of the spinal canal.

Another example is the extensive dispersal of ovarian carcinoma over peritoneal surfaces. In these cases of metastasis through body cavities, gravity is a factor in the movement of tumor cells that detach from their parent tumor.

Table 6.3   Typical Sites of Metastasis for Selected Primary Tumors

Primary Tumor	Typical Sites of Metastasis
Carcinoma and breast adenocarcinoma	Bone (especially vertebral column), brain, liver, adrenals, regional lymph nodes
Bronchogenic carcinoma	Brain, spinal cord, bone, regional lymph nodes
Osteosarcoma	Lung, brain
Renal carcinoma	Lung, liver, bone, brain
Prostatic carcinoma	Bone (especially vertebral column)
Colon carcinoma	Liver, brain, ovary, lung, regional lymph nodes
Neuroblastoma	Bone, regional lymph nodes
Malignant melanoma	Lung, liver, spleen, regional lymph nodes

The spread of abdominal tumors may be aided by peristaltic motions or by movements of the abdominal organs caused by movements of the diaphragm in normal breathing. Respiratory pressure changes also affect the cerebrospinal fluid and may be a factor in the movement of tumor cells through the subarachnoid space.

Metastasis via Natural Passages

The term *natural passages* is used here to refer to the lumina of the numerous hollow organs of the body, excluding blood and lymphatic vessels. The gastrointestinal tract and various ducts (i.e., ureters and bile ducts) are examples. Because tumors are known to arise in the epithelia lining these passages, it is natural to assume that tumor cells would be carried along to distant points of the passage where they establish secondary sites of tumor growth. However plausible this might seem, there is little evidence that it occurs. The principal reason probably has to do with the generally unfavorable conditions that exist in these lumina. As noted earlier, tumor cells have difficulty surviving in fluids as benign as the blood and lymph. Most of the lumina we are considering here present quite harsh conditions to any cells they might contain. Consider the extreme acidity of the stomach, the high concentrations of bicarbonate ion in pancreatic secretions, enzymes in the small intestine, bile salts and toxic bilirubin in bile, and the microorganisms and their metabolic products that populate the colon. All of these present a hostile challenge to the survival of any tumor cells that might detach from a primary tumor in an organ's wall. Again, however likely it may appear, metastasis via natural passages doesn't seem to occur.

Iatrogenic Metastasis

Another mechanism of metastasis is **iatrogenic** (due to medical intervention) and is probably very rare. In obtaining a biopsy for diagnostic purposes, or during surgical excision of a tumor, it is possible that a surgical instrument could introduce tumor tissue to a site where it might develop into a secondary tumor. The incidence of iatrogenic metastasis is difficult to determine. However, the surgical team's awareness of this danger is probably sufficient to keep the incidence extremely low. Table 6.3 indicates some typical tumors and the tissues to which they characteristically metastasize.

TUMOR EFFECTS

Tissue Destruction

The presence of a tumor growing at a primary and perhaps one or more secondary sites can be expected to affect normal functions. The tumor's autonomous growth produces a wide range of local and systemic effects. In the case of benign tumors, these effects may be relatively minor and slow to develop. For the malignant tumor, invasion and metastasis tend to produce an increasing burden of damage, whose effects may ultimately overwhelm the host in spite of vigorous therapeutic intervention.

The expanding tumor mass applies pressure to adjacent normal cells, distorting them and interfering with their normal activities. Blood vessels supplying the area may also be compressed by the tumor. This reduces the tissue's nutrient supply and waste removal. (This is the pressure atrophy described in chapter 1.) Loss of normal parenchyma may also be related to the tumor's release of destructive enzymes that disrupt the extracellular matrix that is necessary for normal function. These mechanisms combine to destroy normal tissue, which is then replaced by the expanding tumor mass. Steady deterioration of normal function is the result.

A further local complication can arise when a highly malignant tumor in one organ penetrates its capsule to invade an adjacent structure. For example, a common cause of death in cervical carcinoma is renal failure. The kidney damage is the result of tumor invasion from the cervix to the adjacent ureter and then to the kidney. Not only does such invasion from one organ to another broaden the functional deficit, but normal motion—for example, respiratory or

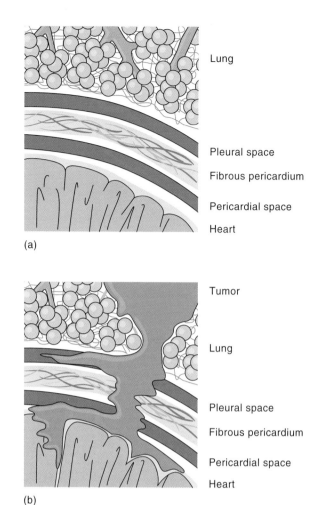

(a)

Lung

Pleural space

Fibrous pericardium

Pericardial space

Heart

(b)

Tumor

Lung

Pleural space

Fibrous pericardium

Pericardial space

Heart

Figure 6.22   **Tumor Joining Adjacent Organs.** (*a*) Normal heart and lung motion is unrestricted because these organs are isolated by the pericardial sac in the pleural membranes, (*b*) An invading lung tumor has penetrated to the heart, joining the two organs and restricting their normal freedom of movement.

peristaltic—may be restricted by tumor tissue that joins the two structures. Another example is shown in figure 6.22.

Organ Compression

Even if no invasion occurs, an expanding tumor may compress adjacent structures with harmful effect. The central nervous system is especially vulnerable in being soft and easily distorted and in being housed within the rigid skull and vertebral column. Intracranial tumors can cause damage as their expansion compresses brain tissue. The spinal cord may be compressed by primary or secondary tumors within the vertebral canal, and the intervertebral foramen may provide an opening through which an adjacent tumor can reach the spinal cord and compress it.

Obstruction

Depending on its location, a tumor may cause less damage through tissue destruction or compression than it does by obstructing a duct or other passage so as to interfere with normal movement or flow. Such obstruction may arise from a tumor's growth within a duct lumen, as typically occurs in carcinomas arising in mucosal epithelia. On the other hand, a growing tumor may apply external pressure to a duct or blood vessel, narrowing its lumen and restricting flow (fig. 6.23). Examples of internal obstructions are tumors of the bronchi, which can block air flow (fig. 6.24), intestinal tumors that obstruct motion, and **pharyngeal** or **esophageal carcinomas,** which interfere with swallowing. The ureters are especially vulnerable to obstruction from the external pressures produced by ovarian, prostatic, rectal, and cervical tumors.

A small but critically situated benign tumor can be particularly dangerous in spite of its relatively low invasive capability and its inability to metastasize. For example, a benign glioma growing adjacent to the cerebral aqueduct,

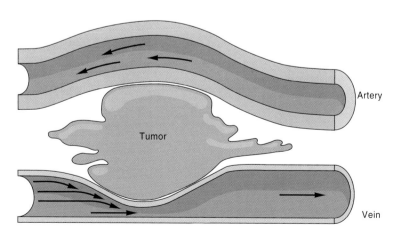

Artery

Tumor

Vein

Figure 6.23   **Flow Obstruction.** Tumor growth can compress adjacent vessels, obstructing flow. Because of their thinner walls, veins are more vulnerable than arteries.

Focus on Melanoma Metastasis

The deeply pigmented masses in these various organs are the result of the widespread metastasis of a malignant melanoma. The victim was a 52-year-old man who first noticed numerous small lumps in the skin over various parts of his body. They were not painful, and in some their dark coloration was visible through the skin. He also had noticed that his urine was quite dark.

One of the lesions was biopsied and was identified as metastatic melanoma. The primary site could not be identified, but the search for it revealed numerous secondary sites of tumor growth. For some reason, the spleen and liver were not involved, although they normally support secondary tumor growth quite well. Large amounts of melanin were being excreted in the urine, which explained its coloration.

The patient died six months later. At autopsy, the extensive metastases shown here, as well as numerous others in the skin, lymph nodes, and lung mucosae, were found.

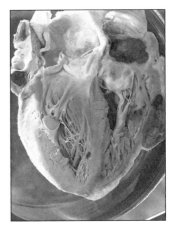

Heart

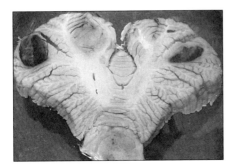

Brain

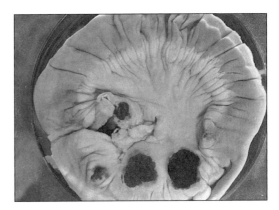

Intestine

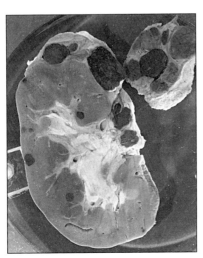

Kidney and adrenal gland

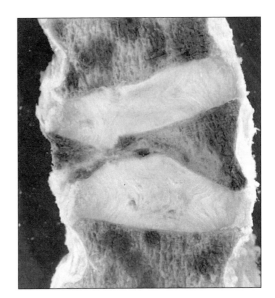

Vertebral column

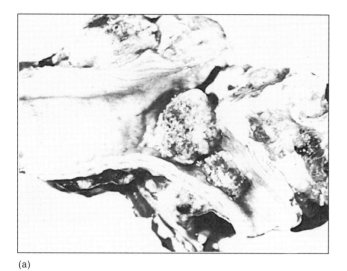

(a)

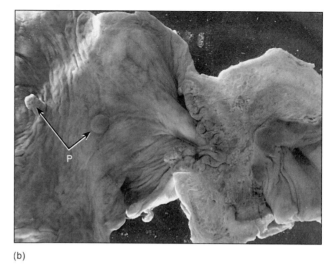

(b)

Figure 6.24   **Tumor Obstruction.** (*a*) Growth of a carcinoma in the trachea and primary bronchi can greatly obstruct the flow of air. (*b*) A colon carcinoma. Note the dilated proximal segment of the colon, where its contents accumulated behind the obstructing tumor. Note also the two polyps (P). The malignant and fatal tumor shown may well have arisen from such growths.

Acute, intense abdominal cramping and paroxysms of diarrhea were the result of the tumor shown here. It has severely restricted the lumen of this patient's colon. Scans of the lower GI tract revealed air and fluid accumulating proximal to the point of obstruction. These distressing events were superimposed on this patient's numerous other problems, stemming from a lung tumor and a damaged heart, which finally caused his death.

which connects the third and fourth ventricles of the brain, need only expand a small amount before completely stopping the flow of cerebrospinal fluid. The resulting pressure increase within the third and lateral ventricles poses a serious threat to the brain, especially since it is confined within the unyielding bone of the skull. Similarly, a rather small papilloma within the bile duct system can produce significant effects by interfering with bile flow to the duodenum.

Flow in the superior vena cava may be obstructed by growth of an adjoining lung tumor, or by a tumor in the lymph nodes that surround the vessel. Such tumors can press the vena cava against the adjacent sternum and right primary bronchus. The low pressure and thin wall of the vena cava make it especially vulnerable to compression, and interference with its large blood flow can have acute and serious consequences.

Infection

Infection is often associated with the presence of a tumor and several mechanisms are involved. One is the general suppression of the immune system that is seen in some malignancies. Another involves marrow suppression that reduces production of our principal phagocytic cells: neutrophils and monocytes. Also, where a tumor grows near a body surface, whether internal or external, the surface may be penetrated by invading tumor tissue. This disruption of the surface interferes with one of its essential functions: providing a barrier to infective organisms. When the barrier is damaged, microorganisms have easier access to the tissues and a greater chance of becoming established.

Infection may result from a tumor's blockage of the ureters, the gastrointestinal tract, or respiratory passages.

The tumor's presence disrupts normal patterns of motion that inhibit bacterial proliferation and infection. For example, normal movement of mucus produced by ciliary action in the respiratory mucosa restricts access of microorganisms to the lungs, and continuous flow of urine in the ureter prevents urethral organisms from reaching the kidney. When a tumor interferes with these normal preventive mechanisms, the risk of infection—pyelonephritis in the case of the urinary passages, bronchopneumonia in the case of the lungs—rises greatly. Infections in the small intestine or colon can erode the bowel wall to the point of perforation, posing the threat of peritoneal irritation. Peritonitis is a common complication of such tumor-related abdominal infections.

Anemia

Several tumor effects work directly or indirectly to produce **anemia:** a lack of oxygen delivery caused by a deficiency of hemoglobin or by too few circulating red blood cells. The reduced oxygen delivery in anemia can further weaken a person already suffering from various tumor-related problems.

A direct cause of anemia is the chronic bleeding associated with many malignant tumors. This bleeding is the result of the tumor's invasive growth that disrupts vessels and body surfaces. Blood loss linked to gastrointestinal carcinomas can be particularly threatening because bleeding into the lumen can go unnoticed.

While compensation for some blood loss is available through increased red marrow activity, tumor growth often interferes with marrow function to add to the anemia problem. Most tumor-related anemia is caused by such marrow

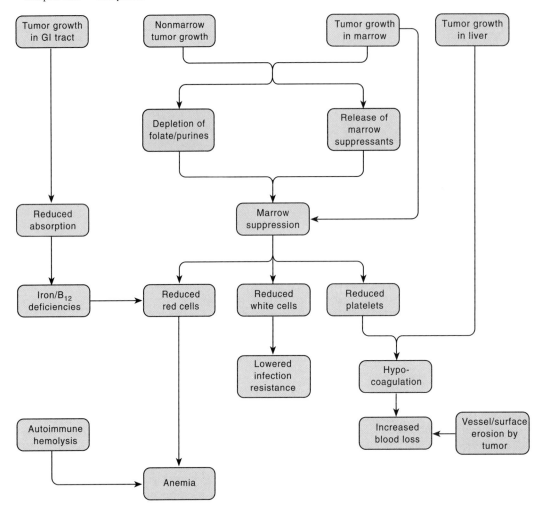

Figure 6.25   **Tumors and the Blood.** Principal effects of tumor growth on the blood.

suppression effects. When primary and, more commonly, secondary tumors grow in marrow, they replace functional tissue and red cell production falls. Loss of normal marrow also means a decline in platelet production. This reduces the coagulation capacity of the blood at that very time that tumor-related bleeding requires a vigorous coagulation response. Note that coagulation may also be compromised by liver tumors that interfere with the production of the clotting factors that cause the blood to coagulate.

Although primary or metastatic tumor growth within the marrow can produce the suppression, other tumor-related factors also contribute. One is the production of marrow-suppressant substances by tumors growing in other tissues. These enter the blood at their site of production and are then delivered to the marrow. Other factors are the infections that often accompany tumor growth and the marrow-suppression effects of radiation and chemotherapies used in treating patients with malignant tumors.

Two other tumor-related mechanisms can produce anemia. In the case of renal tumors, the kidney's normal production of **erythropoietin** may decline. Erythropoietin is the principal stimulus to red cell production, and any decline in its delivery to the marrow will significantly affect such

production. The second mechanism involves tumor activity that limits the supply of substances the marrow needs to maintain normal red cell output. Gastrointestinal tumors that interfere with normal absorption can significantly reduce the availability of iron and vitamin B_{12}. These are essential to maintain red cell production. Note also, that any tumor-related bleeding that is also present exaggerates the loss of iron in the blood's hemoglobin. The marrow's high mitosis rates also demand a steady supply of **purines** and **folate.** Growing tumors, which also require these substances, are able to accumulate and store large quantities of them, thus depriving the marrow of an adequate supply.

Apart from causing blood loss and affecting the marrow, tumor growth can produce anemia by the destruction of circulating red cells. Particularly in the elderly, some tumors—for example, leukemia and some lymphomas—can induce an autoimmune response directed against normal erythrocytes. This disrupts red cell membranes; they rupture **(hemolysis)** and are quickly cleared from the circulation. Anemia is the result. Figure 6.25 summarizes the links between tumor growth and anemia.

Polycythemia, in which excessive production of erythrocytes occurs, may be caused by a benign renal tumor.

Checkpoint 6.2

The two situations involving erythropoietin that were noted in the previous section reflect a renal tumor's degree of anaplasia. In the first case, a more anaplastic tumor has lost the ability to secrete functional erythropoietin, and anemia results. In the second case, a much less anaplastic benign tumor retains the ability to secrete functional hormone, and polycythemia results. The degree of anaplasia is the key to the difference.

Here, a tumor secretion is produced to excess, with harmful effect. The secretion is the hormone erythropoietin, which stimulates the marrow. As a result, the rate of erythropoiesis is increased, and excessively large numbers of red cells pour into the blood.

Pain

It is well known that pain, intermittent or constant, and often severe, is associated with tumor growth. Much of this pain is caused by the aggressive, invasive growth of malignant tumors, particularly in bone, where invasion can produce fractures, and in hollow organs, where obstruction stretches and distorts their walls. In some cases, direct invasion of nerves is the cause of pain. In the case of tumors of the spinal cord (glioma, meningioma), the rigid vertebral column or skull restricts the tumor mass, causing pain as the cord or brain is compressed. This topic is treated in more detail in chapter 23.

✓ **Checkpoint 6.3**

Before proceeding, it might be a good idea to review some of the basics of hormone action and terminology in the Endocrine Specificity section in chapter 17. The basic ideas will be useful in the next section, Hormonal Effects, and also in the consideration of cancer genetics in a later section of this chapter, Genes and Cancer.

Hormonal Effects

Tumors of endocrine tissues produce their effects through abnormal and uncontrolled hormone secretion. Improper regulation of various body tissues follows, with potentially serious systemic consequences. In the case of benign tumors or malignancies that are less anaplastic, functional hormone may be produced, with hypersecretion and overstimulation of target tissues the result. In the case of more anaplastic malignancies, hormones may function only partially or not at all. Target tissue hypofunction results. In either case, the result can present a serious threat to the host.

In pancreatic islet cell adenoma, hyperinsulinism results and can cause hypokalemia followed by coma and death. Adenoma in the adrenal cortex can lead to systemic hypertension, the result of excessive sodium and water retention, and to hypokalemia from excessive potassium losses. Both conditions are the result of hypersecretion of aldosterone.

A phenomenon seen in the case of some tumors is **ectopic secretion.** This means that tumors of nonendocrine origin develop the ability to secrete functional hormones. For example, lung carcinomas may secrete insulin, parathormone, antidiuretic hormone, and others. (Some recent evidence indicates that the lung normally secretes certain hormones in minute amounts.) Parathormone may also be secreted by breast, ovarian, or kidney tumors. Adrenocorticotropic hormone, a normal secretion of the pituitary gland, may be secreted by tumors of the lung, parathyroids, or kidneys. Such abnormalities of secretion may be indications that the tumor cell has access to genetic information that is normally masked. On the other hand, they may be related to abnormal differentiation—the anaplasia associated with malignancy. Whether deriving from endocrine or nonendocrine tissues, a relatively small hormone-secreting tumor can cause large systemic effects.

The principal tumor effects are summarized in figure 6.26.

Paraneoplastic Syndromes

The term **paraneoplastic syndromes** refers to the wide variety of tumor-related effects whose pathogenesis is poorly understood. The presence of the tumor and the paraneoplastic effects are easily established, but the links between them remain obscure. An example is the occurrence of leg vein thrombosis in cases of pancreatic or lung tumors. Tumor or necrotic tissue products might be implicated in damaging the endothelia of the veins that drain the region of tumor growth, but the relationship to the leg vein thrombosis is unexplained. Some lung and breast carcinomas are associated with muscle and peripheral nervous abnormalities, whereas other tumors, although not situated in the head, produce symptoms of increased intracranial pressure. Ectopic secretion of unidentified hormones, circulating toxic tumor products, and the deposition of tumor-derived antigen-antibody complexes are possible mechanisms underlying paraneoplastic syndromes. Further research is expected to clarify the pathogenesis of these puzzling situations.

Cachexia

The condition known as **cachexia** is seen most often in advanced malignancies. Cachexia is a syndrome involving generalized weakness, fever, wasting (weight loss), **anorexia** (loss of appetite), and pallor (paleness). This pattern of signs and symptoms is probably not the result of any single cause but rather the cumulative impact of the multiple tumor effects over the course of the disease. Thus, infection might contribute to weakness and fever, and hemorrhage and anemia add to the weakness and pallor. Loss of

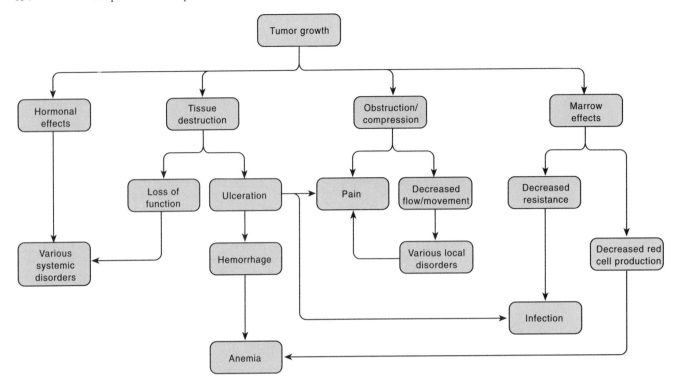

Figure 6.26   **Tumor Effects.** A summary of the local and systemic effects of tumor growth.

body mass in cachexia is due to the loss of both fat and muscle. Other factors in wasting are endocrine dysfunctions and tumor-induced nutritional imbalance or intestinal malabsorption, in the case of small bowel tumors. Also, pain, depression, and anxiety may well produce appetite loss and a reduced food intake. A specific growth factor, **tumor necrosis factor**-alpha (TNF), may play a role in cachectic wasting. It may be produced by tumor cells or by the host's phagocytes. The speculation is that it contributes in some way to the increased consumption of nutrients that is characteristic of cachexia. In combination with the loss of muscle tissue and reduced nutrient intake, loss of body mass can be quite dramatic.

Other factors contributing to cachexia might be toxins and the necrotic debris released from damaged tissues. These substances would ordinarily be detoxified by the liver, but hepatic metastases might depress such functions. As the various aspects of cachexia worsen, death may follow, with its specific cause remaining obscure. The tumor's growth, its spread, and then the multiple effects that produce cachexia increase to the point where the victim is overwhelmed.

✓ *Checkpoint 6.4*

Many patients with advanced malignancies typically suffer from the effects of several of the problems described in the previous sections. Keep this in mind when you read this chapter's case study.

ONCOGENESIS

As indicated earlier, tumor formation (**oncogenesis**) involves a fundamental alteration of cell reproduction and differentiation. Tumor cells seem unable to maintain a state in which they can carry out normal functions without dividing. Consider the fact that most tumors arise in tissues that have high normal rates of reproduction, namely, epithelia and marrow. Consider also that permanent tissues that have lost their reproductive capacity almost never become neoplastic. For example, tumors of skeletal muscle and neurons are extremely rare, and may not exist at all. It is difficult, however, to be absolutely certain because tumors that are highly anaplastic may closely resemble each other, even though originating in different tissues. Also, unusual differentiation patterns, seen in some tumors, might produce characteristics similar to those of muscle or neurons. The rare primary tumors thought to derive from skeletal muscle or neurons probably originate in embryonic cells that haven't fully differentiated.

Genes and Cancer

A detailed treatment of the genetics of cancer is beyond the scope of this text. However, a consideration of some of the basic principles involved can provide useful insights into the process.

The formation of new tissue is based on the balance of new cell formation versus cell losses. New cell production is the result of cell divisions that occur at rates that offset cell losses caused by typical "wear-and-tear" or more se-

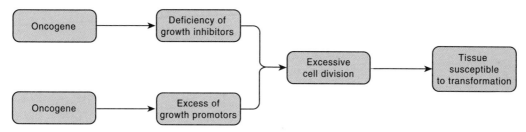

Figure 6.27 **Oncogenes and Growth Factors.** Oncogenes can cause excessive tissue formation by failure to produce inhibitory GFs or by overproducing GFs that stimulate mitosis.

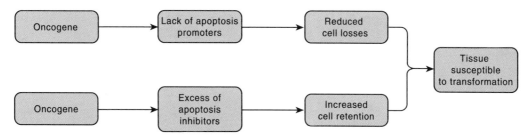

Figure 6.28 **Apoptosis in Oncogenesis.** Inadequate stimulation of apoptosis or excessive inhibition of apoptosis means more survival of cells susceptible to transformation.

vere injury. Cell division is regulated by exogenous **growth factors** (GFs) that may stimulate or inhibit mitosis. GFs and hormones accomplish this control by means of binding to cell surface receptors. Following binding, complex sequences of intracellular activation steps ultimately produce the appropriate alterations in mitosis. When a cell's DNA is damaged, it may be repaired. If repair is impossible, apoptosis eliminates the affected cells.

The genes that regulate these processes are known as **protooncogenes.** They code for the proteins that indirectly regulate mitosis, DNA repair, and apoptosis. When defective, they are known as **oncogenes** because their abnormal proteins cannot maintain the elegantly balanced regulation needed for normal tissue formation. If this balance is disrupted, tumor development follows. Oncogenes are known to be implicated in many human tumors. For example, the p53 gene is thought to contribute to over half of all human tumors.

As research continues, new insights into the mechanisms of oncogene operation are uncovered. An example is an oncogene that is unable to code for the production of cell growth inhibitors. Their lack means growth is unrestrained, forming an excess of tissue with the potential for tumor transformation. Alternatively, if an oncogene produces excessive quantities of growth promoters, high rates of mitosis generate the inappropriate tissue excess (fig. 6.27).

Another system of oncogenes is involved in the misregulation of the critical process of apoptosis. When an oncogene causes overproduction of apoptosis promoters, cell elimination is slowed and cells that would have been eliminated are retained. If an oncogene instead codes for insufficient apoptosis inhibitors, cell losses are reduced and cell retention is again the result. In both cases, cells with

damaged DNA that should be eliminated are retained. They can go on to divide and so form an increasing pool of genetically unstable cells likely to undergo transformation into a tumor (fig. 6.28).

Other oncogenes operate in the production of the cell membrane receptors that bind the growth factors that determine normal tissue formation. In cases where an oncogene codes for defective receptors, they might induce high mitosis rates even when GFs bind infrequently. In other cases, an oncogene might drive the production of excessive receptor numbers so that even small amounts of GF would produce exaggerated cell divisions. Excess tissue formed by these mechanisms is more likely to become neoplastic.

Most oncogenes form as the result of DNA damage caused by chemical agents or ionizing radiation. In the relatively few tumors with known viral etiology, the underlying mechanism seems to be based on viral DNA being inserted into the host cell's DNA, converting the affected protooncogene into a tumor-causing oncogene.

Mechanisms of Oncogenesis

Although oncogenesis is complex and difficult to study, some insights into its mechanisms are emerging. It appears that two distinct processes are involved. The process in which oncogenes are produced is known as **initiation.** Oncogenes give rise to an accumulation of excessive tissue. This tissue is typically unstable and susceptible to the action of various chemical agents that stimulate cell division. Such agents are called **promoters.** They act on initiated cells that are particularly sensitive to their action. Note that promoters have much less effect on normal cells; they are

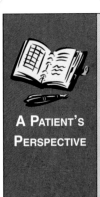

Liposarcoma

"You can't take my leg. You can't!"
—Russell Kelly

"**Y**ou have a liposarcoma," said my doctor, "a malignancy of tissue that resembles fat."

Oh my god, I thought. *Cancer. How long do I have to live?*

"We will have to take out some calf muscle, so there will be some loss of function. If the tumor were to recur, we would have to amputate. However, the success rate with removing these kinds of tumors is 90 percent."

Loss of function. Amputate. My brain reeled. I slowly replaced the handset on the receiver and looked out the window. I went down to the living room, lay on the couch, hugged my knee to my chest and cried. "No. You can't take my leg. You *can't!*"

That was the beginning of this cancer odyssey, over three years ago. I investigated and tried 12(?) distinct complementary cancer therapies. I received all three conventional therapies, including: 59 doses of high-voltage x-radiation and gamma radiation; four full anesthetic surgeries; and 18 weeks of chemotherapy. For a brief time I entertained the idea that there is a "cancer personality," that cancer reveals something singular about the person inflicted. I never went so far as to believe God punished me with cancer. I did, however, entertain for a short time the notion that I had led an "inauthentic" life. In the course of many counseling and therapy sessions, I went over and over my life history, my story. With their help I surveyed my emotional landscape. I concluded that my life had been adequately authentic, thank you. At this stage a very useful notion was: when I felt swamped in self-loathing for some past deed or some past negligence, I countered the feeling with the thought "With the knowledge and experi-ence I possessed at the time, I did my best. I forgive myself for any mistakes." Forgiveness is the begin-ning of self-love.

The denial phase, the why me? carved time out to sort through raging emotions. Not long after came a form of acceptance. "I don't know why me, but I've *got* cancer." From there it is a small step to: "Now that I've got it, I've got to *do* something about it." Moreover, to live successfully with cancer is to learn to live each day fully; to live, as Buddhists put it, "mindfully," in the present.

One of the most consistently helpful activities has been the relaxation sessions offered by the Cancer Agency. Sitting in a circle, the patients, support people, and facilitators took turns saying who they were, whatever seemed appropriate. The degree of honesty was remarkable. The opening circle lasted half an hour, at which time everyone except facilitators and volunteer "foot strokers" moved to the mats. Lights were dimmed. Soft guitar music was played while Lis and her helpers began a series of soft, slow medi-tations designed to induce a state of relaxation. She wove into her monologue every image and theme raised in the opening circle. As she spoke, foot stro-kers moved silently in pairs from mat to mat. One gently stroked me from knee to foot, cradling the foot. The other stroked my shoulders and brow. (This therapeutic touch was optional. Virtually everyone reported that they plunged even deeper into relaxation following the touch.)

For my tumors to shrink and disappear, for me to survive this cancer, would require a spontaneous "miracle cure." But by letting loved ones and fellow patients know that I needed help, and by asking di-rectly for it, I tapped an enormous wellspring of goodwill, support, and love among strangers, friends, and family.

---

not, by themselves, oncogenic. When cells are exposed to both initiator and promoter, transformation to neoplasia is greatly favored. Usually, prolonged application of the pro-moter is required. Tumors result even when exposure to the promoter is delayed after initiation. Promotion before initi-ation results in no tumor formation because uninitiated cells are not susceptible to the promoters action (fig. 6.29).

The action of initiators and promoters may provide the explanation for certain long-observed characteristics of tumors in humans. For example, most tumors occur in old age. This may be the result of a long period of pro-motion required for tumor formation or of low rates of exposure to promoters after initiation. Many tumors are hormone-dependent. That is, their growth is greatly in-creased when certain hormones (usually the sex hor-mones) are present. These hormones may be acting as promoters in such cases. The concept of promotion may also explain why tumor incidence varies in a given fam-ily or the general population, because individuals experi-ence differing patterns of exposure to promoters. Numer-ous studies have shown that increased tumor incidence is linked to various dietary factors—for example, increased protein, fat, and caloric intake—as well as to occupa-tional exposure, sex, smoking, and age. Some aspect of these conditions may act as a promoting agent that en-hances the development of neoplasia. Currently, only a few specific substances can be positively identified as being initiators or promoters. Until further insights are gained, we identify those agents as oncogenic without knowing their exact role in the process. With this back-ground we can proceed to an analysis of the principal factors in oncogenesis.

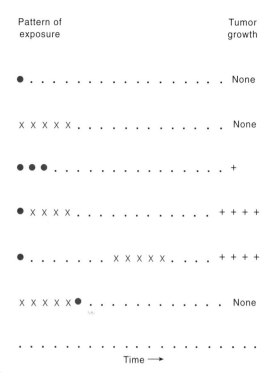

Pattern of exposure — Tumor growth

● . . . . None

X X X X X . . . . None

●●● . . . . +

● X X X X . . . . + + + +

● . . . . X X X X X . . . . + + +

X X X X X ● . . . . None

. . . .

Time →

● Initiator

X Promoter

Figure 6.29   **Chemical Oncogenesis.** The sequence and timing of exposure to initiators and promoters determines tumor development.

Heredity

Because cell growth and differentiation are governed by information contained in the chromosomes, it is here that the fundamental neoplastic transformation must arise. Such changes in genetic makeup raise the question of transmitting tumors to future generations: the role of heredity in oncogenesis.

Little is known of the role of heredity in oncogenesis because of the great difficulties associated with human genetic studies. Only a small number of tumors can be ascribed to directly transmitted genetic defects. In these cases, a family pattern of tumor incidence provides the basis for fairly accurate prediction of tumor occurrence in future generations. The relatively rare **polyposis coli, xeroderma pigmentosum,** and **retinoblastoma** are examples of such directly transmitted tumors. In some tumors, such as breast cancer (when it occurs before menopause) and ovarian and colon carcinoma, heredity appears to be a factor, but its role is not well understood. Familial patterns of incidence seem to occur but prediction is much less precise. In such cases, it can only be said that close relatives of a cancer patient are more likely to develop the same tumor than more distant relatives, or those unrelated. Similarly, differences in tumor incidence seem related to racial background. However, because racial and ethnic differences are often accompanied by environmental or cultural differences, the hereditary effects are difficult to isolate. As with

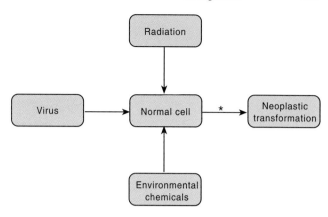

Figure 6.30   **Etiological Factors in Oncogenesis.** Asterisk represents mediation of the process by hereditary or hormonal factors.

any cellular or somatic characteristic, there is an interplay between hereditary and environmental factors in oncogenesis (fig. 6.30).

Environmental Factors

A great deal is known of the role of environmental agents in tumor formation. Experimental evidence derived from oncogenesis studies strongly supports the concept that tumor formation can result from exposure to agents in the cell's environment. These interact with and alter the DNA of the cell's chromosomes to bring about transformation from normal to neoplastic. The following are the principal environmental agents known to be capable of inducing tumor formation.

Physical Agents

Energy in the form of solar or ionizing radiation can induce tumor formation. Evidence clearly shows that increased exposure to radiation yields increased rates of **carcinogenesis,** or cancer production (the terms *carcinogenesis* and *oncogenesis* are often used interchangeably). Both solar radiation and ionizing radiation are known to damage cells and especially DNA (see chapter 1). On the other hand, in addition to causing DNA damage, radiation may activate other oncogenetic factors or suppress antitumor defenses (discussed in a later section, Antitumor Therapy). The result in either case would be increased tumor incidence. A lag period of many years is usually involved before radiation-induced tumors are discovered.

There are two major sources of exposure to radiation. One is the ultraviolet radiation of the sun. Those who work in the sun for long hours over many years show increased rates of skin cancer. The disease is often preceded by a dry, flaky, thickened condition of the skin called **actinic keratosis.** The second source of exposure is ionizing radiation from industrial or medical sources. Those working with industrial or medical X-ray equipment or radioactive materials in mining, manufacturing, or medicine are at risk

Table 6.4   Viruses Associated with Human
                       Tumors

Virus	Associated Tumor
Hepatitis B (HBV) and hepatitis C virus (HCV)	Hepatocellular carcinoma
Human papilloma virus (HPV)	Skin and cervical carcinomas
Epstein-Barr virus	Burkitt's lymphoma* and nasopharyngeal carcinoma
Human T-cell leukemia virus	Some leukemias
Cytomegalovirus	Kaposi's sarcoma*

* AIDS-related tumors

The role of these viruses in tumor etiology, if any, and their links to tumor pathogenesis are not well understood.

of increased tumor incidence. Any unnecessary exposure to medical or dental X-rays adds to the total burden of carcinogen exposure and should be avoided.

Viruses

Viruses are the only biological agents implicated in carcinogenesis. Viruses are known to interact with the chromosomal DNA of the cells they infect, converting protooncogenes into oncogenes. Although a few human tumors strongly suggest viral involvement, specific mechanisms of initiation and promotion are unclear. The principal human tumors and their suspected viral agents are presented in table 6.4.

Environmental Chemicals

For over 100 years it has been recognized that tumors can be induced by chemicals that originate in our environment. During this time, many specifically carcinogenic substances have been recognized and studied. As new chemical structures are produced and marketed, many inevitably reach body tissues by direct or indirect routes. Those substances are either industrial by-products or consumer products specifically intended to provide some benefit. Pollutants that are inhaled or ingested (e.g., in water supplies) or substances in foods, cosmetics, clothing, or medicines may be carcinogenic. The list of chemical carcinogens has increased dramatically and will probably continue to do so. Note that exposure to a chemical carcinogen is usually prolonged before actual tumor formation occurs. In other words, a few brief encounters with a carcinogen are unlikely to produce a tumor. This may explain, in part, why most tumors arise in a person's later years. Over 80% of all tumors are diagnosed in those past 55 years of age.

Chemical carcinogens alter DNA, typically by binding to it. The result is a change in the cell's information pool that may give rise to the formation of the tumor. It is difficult to determine, but it may be that in some cases a particular chemical is only indirectly carcinogenic. For example, the chemical might activate a virus already present in the cell, or by interacting with DNA or other cell constituents, it might make the cell more susceptible to initiation or promotion by other agents.

Because certain enzymes and other adaptive systems have variable occurrence within the population, some individuals have a higher risk of developing a tumor than do others. This important factor may well explain the variations in tumor incidence in groups whose individual members have similar exposure to carcinogenic chemicals.

Certain classes of chemicals are known to have many carcinogenic members, although it should be noted that oncogenic potency varies within each class of carcinogenic compounds. The following are some of the major classes of chemical carcinogens.

Polycyclic Hydrocarbons

Polycyclic hydrocarbons are a class of substances primarily derived from the combustion of organic compounds. Their name is descriptive in that they consist only of hydrogen and carbon. The carbon atoms are joined to form closed rings, with three or more such rings forming the molecule. Typical exposures are the result of inhaling smoke or ingesting smoked foods (e.g., smoked fish). The potent carcinogen **benzopyrene,** for example, is a common constituent of cigarette smoke. It is thought to act as an initiator in carcinogenesis. At the same time, tobacco combustion also produces tumor promoters, so the delivery of cigarette smoke to the respiratory passages is a highly efficient carcinogenic process. Historically, it was the polycyclic hydrocarbons that were first linked to chemical carcinogenesis in chimney sweeps, who developed higher rates of scrotal tumors than those not exposed to the polycyclic hydrocarbons of chimney soot.

Aromatic Amines

Aromatic amines are carbon ring structures to which an amino group is linked. Many are carcinogenic. These are substances used as dyes for fabrics or as coloring agents in foodstuffs. One of this group, **methylaminobenzene,** is metabolized in the liver to produce a carcinogenic agent that causes primary hepatic tumors. Another, **II-naphthylamine,** has its carcinogenic metabolites altered in the liver to a form that can be cleared by the kidney and excreted in the urine. Unfortunately, the urinary bladder's mucosa contains an enzyme that converts the excreted form back to the carcinogenic form. The result is a high incidence of bladder carcinoma in those exposed to II-naphthylamine.

Focus on Chemical Oncogenesis and DNA Damage

Box figure 6.1 provides some additional detail on the process of chemical oncogenesis. Note that exposure to an initiator need not produce permanent changes. The cell's enzymes, its stress protein response (see chapter 1), or other adaptive mechanisms may allow it to cope with the reactive intermediates formed by the initiator's interaction with cell components.

A cell may be exposed to the initiator but recover from its effects. If the cell is unable to clear the reactive intermediates, their binding to DNA poses a serious threat. If the cell lacks the needed DNA repair systems, the damage may destroy the cell or cause it to be permanently susceptible to neoplastic transformation by the later action of a promoter.

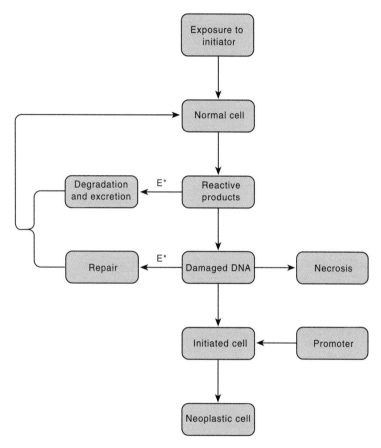

Box Figure 6.1   **Initiation and Promotion in Oncogenesis.** E* represents the role of adaptive enzyme responses in coping with the initiator's effects.

Nitrosamines

This is another class of compounds that can induce tumors. In cells, **nitrosamines** form products that interfere with DNA replication. The result is errors of DNA replication that, in some way, bring about the neoplastic transformation. Nitrosamines can form when nitrite ion reacts with amino acids. The process is favored by heat and acidity. Because nitrite ion is commonly used as a meat preservative, and because Western diets are rich in amino-acid-containing protein, people whose diets contain large

amounts of bacon, ham, sausage, or canned meats may be at risk, especially since the high acidity of the gastric secretions would favor nitrosamine formation even if the nitrite-containing meats were not cooked. The actual risk is not known, and since nitrite is a normal constituent of saliva as well as other substances that are commonly ingested, there may be protective mechanisms operating to reduce nitrosamine formation or to minimize the effects when nitrosamines do form. It is known that ascorbic acid (vitamin C) inhibits nitrosamine formation. Perhaps the traditional vitamin C-containing orange juice before a breakfast of bacon has for many years provided unsuspected anticancer benefits.

Aflatoxin

A carcinogen of biological origin called **aflatoxin** is produced by fungi of the genus *Aspergillus.* These fungi are widely distributed and grow on the surfaces of numerous vegetable products. While these products are growing or being stored before distribution for consumption, conditions of dampness and warmth favor production of the toxin. Animal experiments indicate that aflatoxin acts as a hepatocarcinogen, since liver tumors develop when it is converted to a form that binds to DNA. Improperly stored peanuts, cotton seeds, and corn are examples of farm products subject to aflatoxin contamination.

Inorganic Carcinogens

To this point, the carcinogens described have all been organic chemicals, but inorganic substances are also capable of inducing tumor formation. Cadmium, cobalt, and lead are known to be carcinogenic. Workers involved with nickel are at increased risk of lung cancer, as are those exposed to asbestos, a complex inorganic molecule used in fireproofing insulation and various other applications.

Note that chronic exposure to cobalt can lead to tumor formation. Inhaled or ingested cobalt can be carcinogenic as it interacts with body tissues. This effect should not be confused with the beneficial therapeutic effects of ionizing radiation derived from a radioactive form of cobalt. The radioactive cobalt is typically housed in a system that can focus and deliver its ionizing radiation to a tumor to destroy it. (See the Antitumor Therapy section later in this chapter.)

The conclusion to be drawn from the preceding information on carcinogenesis is that many cancers are preventable. Although viruses are impossible to avoid because of their extremely wide distribution and ability to remain within cells without destroying them, their carcinogenic role seems limited to only a few tumors. However, in the case of radiation and carcinogenic chemicals, it seems clear that minimizing their introduction to the environment will reduce tumor incidence. The reduction of exposure to those carcinogens that cannot be eliminated is, of course, also indicated. For example, lung cancer, the most common North American tumor, would become a rare disease if cigarette smoking were discontinued. After only 20 years, this change would result in a major reduction of all cancer-related deaths.

TUMOR IMMUNOLOGY

The fact that individual cells each carry a particular array of membrane surface antigens is well established. It is now recognized that some normal cells have surface antigens that are also present on tumor cells. These are **tumor-associated antigens** (TAAs). Other antigens occur only on tumor cells and are thus described as **tumor-specific antigens** (TSAs). The implication to be drawn is that the immune system should be able to recognize these antigenically altered cells and destroy them. This concept is referred to as **immune surveillance** in the sense that the immune system is constantly on guard and ready to act against newly arising tumor cells. There is evidence that immune destruction of tumor cells does occur, but the effects seem to be limited to small and isolated masses of tumor cells. The limited survival of tumor emboli, although they form in great numbers, is thought to be the result, at least in part, of immune destruction. Immune attack on larger tumor masses may occur but known instances are few and the evidence is weak. For example, some cases of certain tumors (breast, prostate, melanoma) demonstrate a heavy infiltration of lymphocytes. These are thought to be an immune response to TSAs, and so an improved prognosis might be expected. Unfortunately, prognosis is only slightly improved in such cases. Early studies of tumor incidence seemed to indicate a higher tumor incidence in those with an immune deficiency. This would seem to support the immune surveillance theory. Patients studied were those with immune deficiencies caused by genetic defects, with immune suppression to limit transplant rejection, or with impaired immune responses caused by a virus, as in AIDS. However, more recent studies indicate that the tumors that develop in immune-deficient people are not the most common types such as lung, prostate, breast, and colon cancers. This suggests that factors other than failure of immune surveillance are involved.

The inability of the immune system to easily suppress tumor growth likely has several components. It may be that a reduced immune capability allows the tumor to survive. An infection, some nutritional deficiency, or other factors might cause a disturbance in the normal immune response, allowing tumors to evade recognition and destruction. Furthermore, some tumors have specific immune suppression abilities that may help to increase their chance of survival. They may secrete immune suppressors or induce apoptosis of attacking immune system lymphocytes. Another possibility is suggested by the fact that some highly anaplastic tumors lose their TSAs. This would enable them to escape the immune component of the host's antitumor defenses. Also, because most TSAs are only weakly antigenic, the immune system may have difficulty in mounting an adequate response. Figure 6.31 summarizes these factors.

ANTITUMOR THERAPY

The essential approach in antitumor therapy is the removal or destruction of the tumor. Several quite different techniques are commonly employed, but all face an essential difficulty—that of confining their effects to the tumor while sparing normal tissue. Antitumor therapy may also involve significant and unpleasant side effects. The following sections describe the major antitumor therapies currently in use.

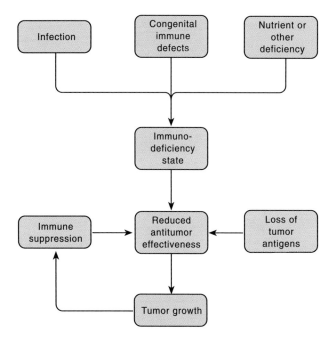

Figure 6.31 **Factors That Limit the Ability of the Immune System to Suppress Tumor Growth.**

Table 6.5   Selected Tumors Grouped According to Their Relative Radiosensitivity

Radiosensitive

Neuroblastoma
Chronic leukemia
Lymphomas
Wilm's tumor (renal tumor of childhood)

Moderately Radiosensitive

Squamous cell carcinoma
Genital carcinomas
Esophageal carcinoma
Bronchogenic carcinoma

Nonradiosensitive

Fibrosarcoma
Osteogenic carcinoma
Various adenocarcinomas

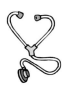

Focus on Fetal Antigens

Another aspect of tumor immunology has been useful in the diagnosis of tumors. Some tumors carry antigens that are not normally present beyond the time of birth. These are **fetal antigens** that are normally suppressed following birth. Some highly anaplastic tumors express and shed fetal antigens. Fetal antigens elicit only weak immune responses, but they can be detected in the plasma of tumor-bearing individuals. When found, they indicate the presence of a tumor. The two fetal antigens most widely used for diagnosis are carcinoembryonic antigen (CEA) for tumors of the lung, pancreas, and gastrointestinal tract and alpha-fetoprotein (AFP) for primary hepatomas.

Surgery

The surgical approach to therapy is simple and direct. It seeks to physically remove the tumor mass and thus eliminate the problem. However, the nature of tumor growth and metastasis presents certain, often major, difficulties. These are minimal in the case of a well-defined, encapsulated, benign tumor growing in a noncritical tissue. In such cases, the tumor can usually be removed easily, with only minor disturbance to adjacent normal tissue. By contrast, the irregular, invasive growth of malignant tumors can present great difficulty. Because the edge of the malignant tumor is not well defined, it is not possible to excise all of it without also removing some of the adjacent normal tissue that might contain invading tumor cells. Thus, depending on the size and growth pattern of the tumor, varying amounts of normal tissue will inevitably be lost. This loss can present significant difficulties where the nervous system or a small gland is involved.

If the tumor has spread from the primary site along lymphatic channels, these channels must be removed along with any involved lymph nodes that contain tumor tissue. Lymph node removal continues along the channels that drain the region until no further tumor is found. The lack of tumor is not necessarily a positive sign, however, since metastasis via blood embolization may have already occurred by tumor cells that have invaded blood vessels in the lymph nodes. Surgery is also complicated by the possibility that surgical manipulation of the tumor may produce large numbers of tumor emboli, which can metastasize to produce secondary growths. In cases in which the tumor is large, invasion to adjacent organs is extensive, or tumor growth involves a critical organ, the tumor may be judged to be inoperable. Other therapies must be used in such cases.

Radiation Therapy

Radiation therapy seeks to deliver a destructive dose of ionizing radiation to the tumor mass. Of course, normal tissue is also susceptible to damage from ionizing radiation (see chapter 1), and this presents the major difficulty in radiation therapy. Many complex and sophisticated techniques are used to maximize the dose reaching the tumor, while minimizing destructive effects on normal tissues. Some tumors are **radiosensitive;** that is, they are much more susceptible to radiation damage than are other tumors. These are best suited to radiation therapies because dose levels can be restricted and side effects held to a minimum (table 6.5).

Table 6.6	Tumor Susceptibility to Chemotherapeutic Agents

Highly Susceptible

Retinoblastoma
Hodgkin's disease
Wilm's tumor (renal tumor of childhood)
Testicular tumors
Acute lymphoblastic leukemia
Choriocarcinoma

Moderately Susceptible

Small cell carcinoma of lung
Lymphocytic lymphoma
Leukemia: acute and chronic myeloid
Carcinoma of breast and ovary

Resistant

Malignant melanoma
Carcinomas generally
Lung cancer
Soft tissue sarcomas

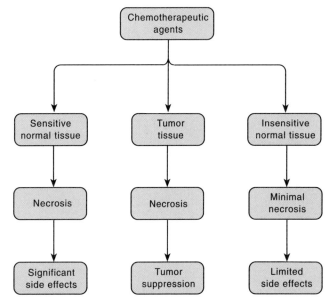

Figure 6.32 **Chemotherapy Outcomes.** Effects of chemotherapeutic agents on the tumor-bearing host.

Because rapidly dividing cells are most sensitive to radiation damage, most radiation side effects involve the rapidly dividing epithelia of the skin, hair, and gastrointestinal tract. Another problem in radiation therapy is the heat that develops in the skin as radiation passes through it to reach an underlying tumor. Such heat may cause skin burns. Sources of ionizing radiation are radioactive isotopes such as cobalt-60 and devices that produce X-rays.

Chemotherapy

In **chemotherapy,** toxic chemical substances are used to destroy the tumor. Their principal mode of action is via DNA, directly damaging it or inducing faulty division. See table 6.6 for some examples of tumor susceptibility to chemotherapeutic agents. The essential difficulty in chemotherapy is that the therapeutic agent is not able to selectively damage only tumor cells. Normal tissues are also damaged to varying degrees, causing many and often severe side effects (fig. 6.32). These can not only injure, but tend to demoralize the patient undergoing therapy. Although effective in treating a few primary tumors, such as acute leukemia, most chemotherapy aims at the smaller tumor mass found at metastatic sites.

Unfortunately, chemotherapeutic agents induce a tolerance on the part of the tumor victim. That is, a slowing of tumor growth may occur initially in response to chemotherapy, but after this early period of approximately several months, the antitumor effects seem to fade and tumor growth resumes at its previous higher rate. Such drug toler-

ance may be related to the presence in the tumor of a population of cells that are resistant to the drug's effects. On first exposure, the more numerous, drug-sensitive cells are destroyed and tumor growth is restricted. During this time, however, the resistant cells continue to divide until the tumor is large enough to again cause noticeable signs and symptoms.

Tumor resistance to both radiation and chemotherapy appears to be related to the oncogenes that contribute to the initial development of the tumor. Recall from the section on Genes and Cancer that the p53 protooncogene triggers the elimination of cells by apoptosis when their DNA is damaged. Because both radiation and chemotherapy exert their effects on DNA, a tumor with a defect in p53 can't clear damaged cells. Even though damaged, the tumor cells remain alive and are able to divide and resist the action of the therapeutic agent. By contrast, when other oncogenes are involved in tumor formation, but p53 is intact, damaged cells are promptly eliminated and the tumor shows much more susceptibility to radiation or chemotherapy.

Immunotherapy

Immunotherapy seeks to utilize the immune system to combat a growing tumor. Although early attempts to utilize this therapeutic approach seemed promising, its effectiveness has been disappointing. Initial attempts involved administering a substance with potent antigenic properties. The result was a strong, general stimulus to the immune system. The hope was that such a stimulus would increase the antitumor activity of host defenses along with the other parts of the immune response and thus increase tumor destruction. A common immune stimulant used in immuno-

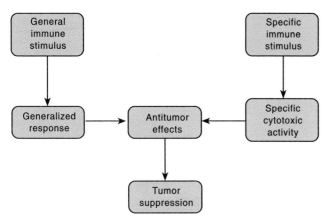

Figure 6.33 **Immune Therapy.** Specific and nonspecific stimuli may be used in the hope that the immune response will act against the tumor.

therapy was the **BCG** (bacillus Calmette-Guérin) antigen, which is derived from mycobacteria. More recently, attempts to activate specific cytotoxic cells of the immune system using interleukin-2 (IL-2) have been pursued with some success. Figure 6.33 illustrates the immunotherapy rationale.

As in the other antitumor therapies, there are some side effects and potential problems associated with immunotherapy. They include nausea, fever, liver damage, and inflammation and abscess formation at the sites of antigen injection. Also, potent stimulation of the immune system creates the risk of inducing such a strong response that autoimmune destruction of normal tissue results.

Combination Therapy

The most widely used therapeutic approach in neoplasia is **combination therapy.** This technique involves the use of two or more therapeutic modes in combination. The hope is that tumor destruction can be maximized by attacking the tumor on more than one front. At the same time, side effects are kept to a minimum because doses of each agent, for example, drugs or radiation, can be reduced while maintaining the same or even increased lethal effect on the tumor.

Particular therapy combinations are determined by each tumor's pattern of sensitivities to the different agents available. Typically, surgery, and in some cases radiation, is first used to reduce the tumor mass, followed by chemotherapy or radiation therapy in an attempt to destroy those cells that could not be surgically removed. For example, surgical removal of a primary tumor might be followed by radiation therapy aimed at the smaller masses of tumor cells that might have spread to adjacent lymph nodes or vessels, or surgery might be followed by both radiation and chemotherapy. The term *combination therapy* is also used when two or more chemotherapeutic agents are used. For example, one agent might have the most effect on dividing cells while a second might disrupt the metabolism of nondi-

viding cells. The result is more tumor cell destruction than if only one drug had been used. Whether combining different therapies or using multiple chemotherapeutic agents, the goal is the same: maximum therapeutic benefit with minimum side effects for the patient.

TUMOR STAGING AND GRADING

Tumor staging and grading are means of classifying malignant tumors for the purpose of simplifying description and aiding communication between health professionals.

Tumor Staging

Tumor staging is a system of categorizing malignant tumors in terms of their potential for invasion and metastasis. Because it facilitates description and discussion, it has proved useful in assessing prognosis, selecting appropriate therapy, and carrying out **epidemiological studies**—that is, studies that consider the relationships between tumors, their host populations, and relevant environmental factors.

Tumor staging is generally applied only to a solid tumor. In the simplest system, a tumor is said to be in stage I if its growth is restricted to its primary site, and in stage IV if it has grown and invaded extensively and shows wide metastatic spread. Stages II and III describe tumors that fall between these extremes.

Various other staging systems have been developed, but because of differing clinical perspectives, degree of complexity, and areas of overlap, they have sometimes introduced confusion instead of clarifying. Here we will deal only with one internationally recognized and widely used malignancy staging system, the TNM system. Again, its use is confined to discrete, solid tumors; it is less applicable to diffuse malignancies—for example, leukemia (described in chapter 7).

In the TNM system, three tumor criteria are assigned a modifying subscript number related to size, or degree, with lower numbers indicating low degree and higher numbers referring to increasing degrees. The T component refers to the size of the primary tumor. T_0 indicates that no tumor can be found at the primary site, while T_1, T_2, and T_3 indicate tumors of increasing size. The degree to which regional lymph nodes are involved is indicated by the N element. N_0 means there is no evidence of regional lymph node enlargement, while N_1, N_2, and N_3 reflect increasing degrees of node involvement. M refers to tumor metastasis, with M_0 meaning that no indications of metastasis are present, while M_1, M_2, and M_3 denote progressively more extensive spread. Figure 6.34 illustrates the TNM system as applied to three different lung cancer patients.

Tumor Grading

Following a biopsy, various histological characteristics of a tumor are assessed and the tumor is then assigned a

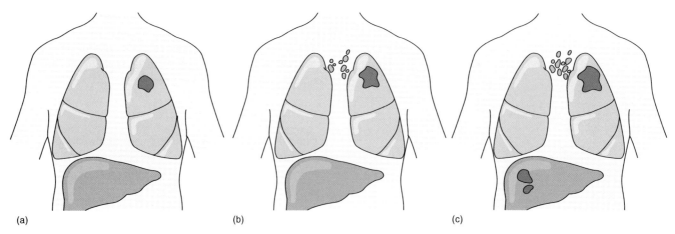

(a)   (b)   (c)

Figure 6.34   **The TNM Staging System** (*a*) $T_1N_0M_0$: This patient has a single primary tumor in the lung. It is less than 3 cm in diameter and there is no lymph node involvement or metastasis. (*b*) $T_2N_1M_0$: In this patient, the primary tumor is enlarged and adjacent lymph nodes are involved. (*c*) $T_3N_2M_1$: In the third patient, the primary tumor is large, mediastinal lymph nodes are involved, and there is metastasis to the liver.

descriptive designation, or grade. The degree of differentiation, the extent of pleomorphism, and the frequency of mitosis are typically studied as a means of judging the degree of malignancy that a particular tumor has achieved. A grade I tumor exhibits highly differentiated cells, is well ordered, and has few, if any, mitoses visible. At grade IV, the cells are poorly differentiated, pleomorphic, and mitoses are increased. Grades II and III represent intermediate degrees of malignancy between these extremes. In general, a low grade indicates a slow-growing tumor with limited tendencies to invade and metastasize. A low-grade tumor, therefore, usually has a good prognosis. For tumors of grades III or IV, the prognosis is less optimistic (table 6.7).

Grading of tumors is of limited use in dealing with any individual patient's tumor. Not only is it time-consuming, but it can be misleading since different regions of a given tumor can exhibit different histologic characteristics. It is, however, a useful tool for studying groups of cases with regard to the effectiveness of therapy or other clinical criteria.

Table 6.7   The Relationship between Tumor Grade and Prognosis in Selected Tumors

Tumor Site	Grade	% Survival 5 Yrs after Diagnosis
Thyroid gland	I	85
	II	55
	III	11
Salivary gland	I	85
	II	80
	III	38
	IV	18
Testis	I	85
	II	55
	IV	7

Case Study

The family of an 80-year-old woman noticed that, in contrast to her usual mental acuity, she had recently showed signs of being confused. The woman agreed with this assessment and stated further that she had been having difficulty in selecting appropriate words when speaking. Even more disturbing to her were the problems she had experienced in doing her favorite crossword puzzles. She had been reluctant to see a doctor because her own physician had recently retired and she was uncertain about going to a new one. On her family's urging she did consent to be examined.

Her new general practitioner found her to have the dry, hacking cough predicted by her 60 years of moderate to heavy smoking. She also had a history of long-standing social alcohol use, but was not an alcoholic. When young she had suffered two bouts of occupational radiation exposure as a radiographic technician during World War I. On both occasions reduced platelet counts had been noted, but she had recovered fully.

Her G.P. also noted that she was taking a variety of medications (a diuretic, an anti-inflammatory, a barbiturate, and a tranquilizer) that did not seem indicated by her otherwise apparently good health. She said her previous physician had prescribed them "because she was getting on," but that she used them only sporadically when she "was having a bad day" or when she felt guilty about not following her doctor's orders.

The doctor ordered a complete blood count and plasma assessments of the BUN (blood urea nitrogen), electrolytes, and vitamin B_{12}, as well as an ECG, all of which were normal. Her liver function tests were also normal and her urine was negative.

On the basis of these findings, the doctor explained that he felt she had had a mild stroke, and because routine tasks could be performed but processing new information was difficult, it might be located in the frontal lobes. Because of her previous training as an X-ray technician, she asked if a chest X-ray might be a good idea. The physician agreed and it revealed the presence of a mass in the middle lobe of her right lung. A bronchoscopy, airway washings, and a transbronchial biopsy were done, but failed to confirm the nature of the mass. A follow-up CT scan of the brain indicated the presence of multiple sites of secondary tumor growth in both frontal lobes.

In the following weeks, her condition worsened, with her speech and general condition deteriorating rapidly. She died ten weeks after her initial presentation. No postmortem examination was performed, but the presumed cause of death was the effects of bronchogenic carcinoma and its brain metastases.

Commentary
Diagnosis based on an elderly patient's confusion and disrupted cognitive functioning is always difficult because of the potential overlapping effects of senility, depression, social isolation, and the multiple side effects of the numerous medications prescribed to alleviate these and other problems associated with old age. If the diet is inadequate, a deficiency of vitamin B_{12} may produce dementia to further complicate diagnosis.

This case is unusual in that a single disease process seemed solely responsible for an elderly patient's demise. More typically in the elderly, death is due to the combined effects of at least two and often several conditions such as infection, heart disease, lung disease, or arteriosclerosis, to cite a few.

The initial suspicion of a frontal lobe cerebrovascular accident (CVA, or stroke) was based on the patient's altered mental functions, which are common to such conditions. The patient had no chest-related symptoms beyond the cough, which had been present for 40 years, and it is quite unusual for a bronchogenic carcinoma not to reveal its presence in the chest in some way before age 80. The lowered platelet counts noted in the patient's history were presumably related to marrow suppression caused by the early radiation exposure.

Once the tumor's presence was established, the doctor attempted to obtain a sample of the tumor tissue by biopsy or airway washings in the hope that it was an oat cell carcinoma, because they are highly sensitive to chemotherapy.

The final rate of decline was also unusual. The patient was spared the 6 to 12 months of slow deterioration that is typical in such cases.

Key Concepts

1. Because of its high incidence, the serious functional disruptions it causes, and the potentially severe side effects of therapy, neoplasia is a major threat to our health and well-being (p. 131).

2. Changing functional demands or exposure to injurious agents can induce adaptive changes in tissues, some of which involve structural and functional changes from normal (pp. 131–132).

3. The name given to a tumor usually makes reference to its benign or malignant character and to its embryonic tissue of origin (pp. 132–135).

4. A tumor consists of (1) neoplastic cells, usually exhibiting some degree of anaplasia and pleomorphism, (2) stroma induced by the increased tissue mass, and (3) some quantity of an often dysfunctional tumor product (pp. 135–138).

5. A benign tumor usually has a better prognosis because of its slower, more regular growth, which is confined to its site of origin (p. 138).

6. In comparison to benign tumors, malignant tumors grow more rapidly, invade aggressively at the primary site, and spread to distant sites to establish secondary growth (pp. 138–140).

7. Diagnosis and therapy in neoplasia are complicated by the fact that, apart from the capacity for metastasis, the characteristics of the many different tumors are expressed over a range, with overlapping at the extremes of benign and malignant behavior (pp. 139–140).

8. Although tumor growth rates are higher than normal cell growth rates, most tumor cells do not actively divide, so that doubling times may be as long as one year, and many years may pass before signs and symptoms appear (pp. 140–142).

9. The capacity of tumors to invade is based on their ability to detach from adjacent cells and move into normal tissues, using enzymes to disrupt basement membranes and intercellular matrix (pp. 142–143).

10. At the gross level, typical tumor invasion patterns are based on extension along paths of low resistance—that is, along and between structures, rather than penetrating resistant surfaces such as fascia, bone, or the pericardium (pp. 142–143).

11. Tumor metastasis arises primarily by invasion of blood or lymphatic vessels, followed by embolism and outward invasion to establish growth at the secondary site (pp. 143–146).

12. The pattern of growth in vascular metastasis is determined by the type of vessel and the tissues to which it delivers blood or lymph (p. 146).

13. Various factors contribute to the successful establishment of a tumor embolus at a secondary site. Among these are plasma survival, binding to vascular endothelia, and tissue conditions at the secondary site (pp. 146–147).

14. Metastasis via body cavities occurs with some frequency, but iatrogenic metastasis is assumed to be rare (pp. 147–148).

15. Tumor growth produces a broad range of physical and functional disruptions, both locally and systematically (pp. 148–154).

16. The autonomous growth of neoplastic tissue is based in large part on defects in the genes that regulate the fine balance of cell production versus cell loss by apoptosis. The defective genes, known as oncogenes, are derived from normal regulatory genes called protooncogenes (pp. 154–155).

17. In oncogenesis, an initiating agent predisposes DNA to the effects of promoters, which then greatly favor tumor formation (pp. 155–156).

18. Direct genetic transmission of neoplasia is limited to a few rare tumors, but less precisely defined familial factors may play a part in the emergence of some other, more common tumors (p. 157).

19. Given the effects of physical, chemical, and viral agents on cellular DNA, it appears that environmental agents are the most important factor in oncogenesis (pp. 157–160).

20. The immune system response to a tumor's characteristic surface antigens has implications for tumor diagnosis and therapy (p. 160).

21. In tumor therapy, the difficulty of removing or destroying only neoplastic tissue, while preserving normal cells, reduces success rates and introduces often unpleasant side effects (p. 160).

22. Antitumor therapy is based on surgical removal of neoplastic tissue or its destruction by chemicals, radiation, or the immune response, alone or in combination (pp. 161–163).

23. For purposes of description and ease of communication, systems of tumor staging, to assess prognosis, and tumor grading, to express the degree of malignancy, are in common use (pp. 163–164).

REVIEW ACTIVITIES

1. Examine each of the diagrams in this chapter (not flow charts or photos) and note those that clearly contain pleomorphic cells. The authors count eight; what count do you get? List the figure numbers.

2. Provide a name for each tumor characterized:

Malignant/lymphoid	Malignant/fibrous tissue
Benign/bone	Benign/gland
Benign/projects from surface	Benign/adipose
Malignant/red marrow	Malignant/gland

3. Using a sheet of graph paper, continue figure 6.13 by adding the characteristics prognosis, anaplasia, and metastasis. Indicate overlaps as in figure 6.13. If there is overlap in your graph for all three, see page 140.

4. On 18 small pieces of paper, copy the elements of the flow chart in figure 6.25 and sketch the connecting arrows on a blank sheet of paper. Now drop your 18 bits of paper into a container, pick them out at random, and position them to build up the flow chart. Do it, as much as possible, without referring to the figure.

5. Convince yourself that Key Concept number 8 is reflected in figure 6.14. If you're not convinced, read pages 140–141.

Blood Disorders

She was very anemic. Her thin lips were pale, and her skin was delicate of a faint green color, without a touch of red even in the cheeks.

W. Somerset Maugham
Of Human Bondage

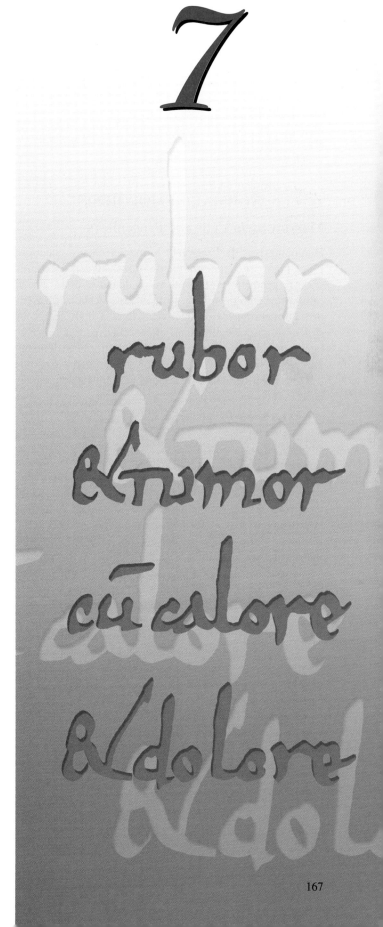

The blood is a complex fluid consisting of plasma and the formed elements: erythrocytes, leukocytes, and platelets. Chapter 7 deals with derangements of the formed elements only. Disorders of plasma volume and concentration are better considered in chapter 16, which deals with fluid and electrolyte imbalance.

We also consider here the blood coagulation system and its abnormalities, as well as the bleeding disorders that follow from such coagulation defects. The first two sections, Normal Hemopoiesis and Blood Coagulation, provide the basis for the later discussion of coagulation disorders. A knowledge of coagulation and anticoagulation is also the foundation for much of the material on thrombosis, which we discuss in chapter 8.

NORMAL HEMOPOIESIS

Marrow Stem Cells and Progenitors

Hemopoiesis is the process of formed element production. It combines sequential mitotic divisions and cell differentiation to produce large numbers of daughter cells. These cells differ significantly from their less-specialized parent cells. Generally, the product cells show a high degree of structural specialization that reflects their particular functional capabilities. As well, most of the formed elements have very limited, or completely lack, reproductive capability. This means that as they age and accumulate damage related to their various roles, or simply because of the "wear and tear" associated with rapid movement through narrow, branching blood vessels, they become dysfunctional or die and must be replaced.

For the most part, hemopoiesis occurs in red bone marrow. The average adult's approximately 2 liters of red marrow is distributed within the bones of the axial skeleton and the proximal heads of the humerus and femur. It includes a supporting stroma of fibroblasts, macrophages, fat cells, and blood vessels, in particular the thin-walled and loosely joined **marrow sinusoids,** which allow mature formed elements to enter the blood by squeezing through their large endothelial gaps. On this supporting stromal network are found the parent cells and various intermediate forms (known generally as **precursors**) involved in hemopoiesis. The earlier forms of these cells are of two types. **Stem cells** are those that can differentiate into all of the mature hemopoietic cells. They can also form new stem cells; that is, they have the capacity for self-renewal. **Progenitor cells** derive from stem cells but lack their self-renewal capability. They have become committed to a given cell line. That is, a mature cell of a given type can be traced back to only one parental cell type: its progenitor. (Note that many stem cells, progenitors, and early cell forms can't be easily distinguished on the basis of their structure; they can only be identified in complex tissue culture studies.) So, with minor exceptions, each mature formed element has a single progenitor from which it is descended. It is for this reason that abnormalities of hemopoiesis can often be identified as

arising at a certain point in the hemopoietic sequence. Figure 7.1 illustrates the general scheme of hemopoiesis. The control and regulation of this process depend on a variety of circulating and locally produced growth factors (GFs), which will be noted in the sections that follow.

Erythropoiesis

The formation of red blood cells, **erythropoiesis,** involves several linked mitotic divisions. Beyond a certain point in the sequence, the cells become smaller and smaller, and the nucleus shrinks and condenses until it is finally extruded from the cell. Hemoglobin synthesis commences relatively early in the developmental sequence. During the later stages, the cell loses its organelles and retains only the metabolic capacity to maintain its membrane, hemoglobin structure, and anaerobic energy metabolism. Before it completely matures, a red cell contains a residual network of cytoplasmic RNA, and is called a **reticulocyte.** The network is lost after three days and the fully mature erythrocyte is the result. Because final reticulocyte maturation occurs in the bloodstream, normal blood contains about one reticulocyte for every 100 erythrocytes. The entire red cell production sequence takes about eight days to complete.

As the erythrocyte circulates, it is subject to mechanical deformation as it is squeezed through small capillaries. It is also subject to various metabolic stresses. Together these present a challenge that the red cell, lacking a nucleus and possessing only a limited adaptive capacity, can tolerate for only four months. After about 120 days, it is dysfunctional and is removed from the circulation by macrophages in the spleen, liver, and marrow. Aging RBCs are cleared from the blood at the rate of about 1% per day. As a percentage, the loss is small, but since there are approximately 5 million RBCs per milliliter in the adult's 5 liters of blood, the daily loss is 25 billion erythrocytes—about 174 million per minute.

The red marrow must produce a corresponding number of replacement RBCs. This enormous task requires not only a high rate of mitosis but an adequate supply of iron for hemoglobin synthesis, as well as the vitamin B_{12} and folic acid needed for DNA synthesis in the rapidly dividing erythrocyte precursors.

The process of red cell production is controlled by the hormone **erythropoietin** (EPO) and two or more growth factors. Erythropoietin is required at several points in the red cell's maturation sequence (fig. 7.1). It is secreted by the kidney in response to changing oxygen levels detected by its oxygen-sensitive juxtaglomerular cells. Lower oxygen delivery to the kidney causes increased EPO secretion that stimulates RBC production in the marrow (fig. 7.2). This mechanism provides a useful corrective response to conditions in which the blood's oxygen delivery capacity is reduced. In extreme cases, erythropoietin can generate as much as an eightfold increase in red cell production.

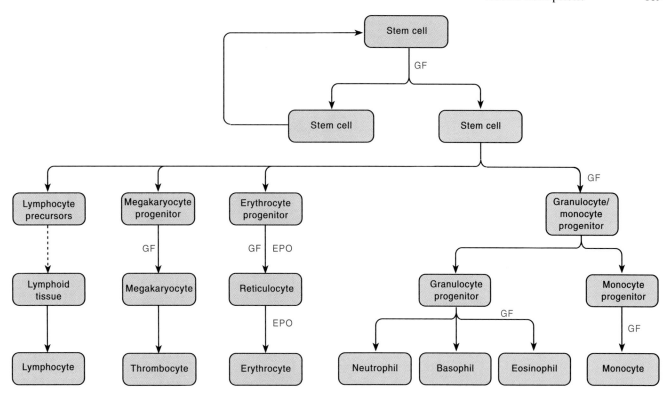

Figure 7.1   **Generalized Scheme of Hemopoiesis.** Mature formed elements derive from a single marrow stem cell in red bone marrow, which is self-renewing. Known points at which erythropoietin (EPO) and other growth factors (GFs) have effects are also indicated. Broken line denotes lymphocyte precursors' migration to lymphoid tissue for final maturation.

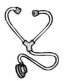

Focus on Red Cell Units

Formed element counts have traditionally been recorded as the number of cells per cubic millimeter (mm³) of blood. The increasingly favored SI (Système International) units use the number of cells $\times 10^9$ per liter for white cells and platelets, and the number of cells $\times 10^{12}$ per liter for red cells. A normal red cell count, therefore, might be expressed as 5,000,000/mm³ or 5×10^{12}/liter. 250×10^9 platelets/liter would indicate a normal thrombocyte count. Note further that because 1 mm³ equals 1 μl, or 1 millionth of a liter, a typical neutrophil count might be represented as 5,000/mm³ or 5,000/μl, and in SI units as 5×10^9/liter.

Apart from the hormonal control supplied by erythropoietin, various growth factors are required for erythropoiesis. They are locally derived from the marrow's stroma. Their exact roles and significance have yet to be precisely determined.

Leukopoiesis

This discussion of leukocyte formation will be confined to granulocytes and monocytes. The migration of lymphocyte progenitors to widespread lymphoid tissue sites in the body and the later maturation of lymphocytes is described in chapter 5.

The approximately 7 million leukocytes present in each milliliter of blood are in transit from their production sites to the various tissues in which they perform their essentially defensive functions. In the case of granulocytes and monocytes, an approximately equal number of cells are at work in the tissues. This means that the actual total of these cells is roughly twice their circulating number. Their life span is considerably shorter than that of the erythrocytes, with granulocytes living from just hours to as long as a few days and monocytes perhaps as long as two to three months. Note also that the circulating granulocytes are mature and able to commence their defensive tasks upon entering the tissue spaces. By contrast, the monocyte is an immature cell and must complete its development into a macrophage in the tissues before it can proceed with phagocytosis or immune system functions (see chapter 5).

The regulation of granulocyte and monocyte production depends on various growth factors, which interact in subtle and complex ways. As in erythropoiesis, interactions with the marrow's stroma also play an important role in the process (fig. 7.1).

Thrombopoiesis

The **thrombocyte,** or platelet, is derived from its marrow precursor, the **megakaryocyte** (fig. 7.1). **Thrombopoiesis,** the formation of platelets, occurs not by mitosis but,

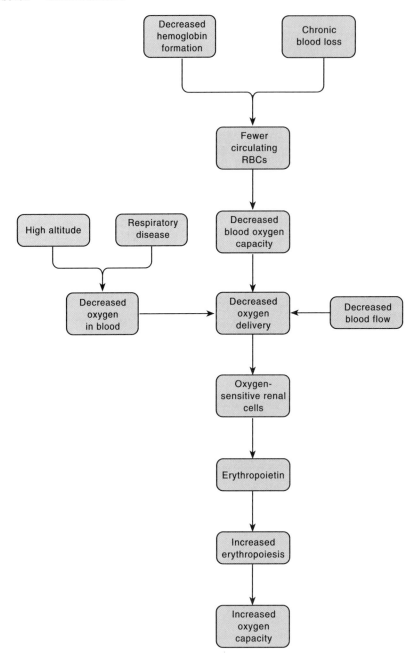

Figure 7.2 **Erythropoiesis.** The role of erythropoietin in erythropoiesis.

instead, by fragmentation. As the megakaryocyte matures, its cytoplasm develops numerous vesicles that give it a granular appearance. Its membranes also become discontinuous, forming gaps similar to the perforations in a sheet of stamps. The large megakaryocyte extends elongated extensions of its perforated membrane into the lumen of the marrow sinusoids, through their loose endothelial junctions. It then sheds cytoplasmic fragments into the blood. These assume the platelet's characteristic flattened, disklike shape. Some initially larger fragments may split off smaller portions while circulating through the lungs. After losing most of its cytoplasm in this way, the megakaryocyte's nuclear remnant is cleared by marrow macrophages.

The circulating blood contains about 250 million platelets in each milliliter. Their average life span is about four days, with about one-third of the total held as a reserve in the spleen, whose specialized **red pulp** takes up and stores platelets. They form a reservoir that can be released when demand is high.

Control of thrombopoiesis depends on several growth factors. The most important, **thrombopoietin,** is formed in the liver and is structurally related to erythropoietin. Thrombopoietin's principal effects are in the critical stages of platelet progenitor formation, with several other growth factors contributing to the final formation of mature platelets.

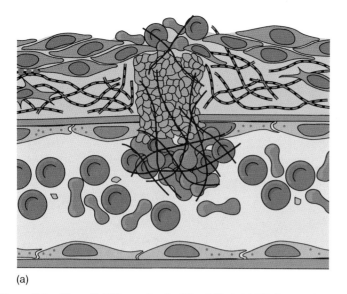
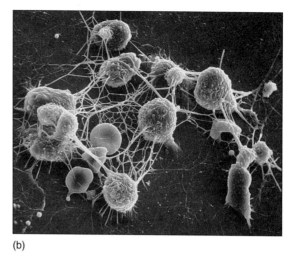

(a)   (b)

Figure 7.3   **Essential Elements of a Blood Clot.** (*a*) Fibrin strands entrap red cells where a platelet plug has formed at the site of vessel wall injury. (*b*) Scanning electron micrograph of a clot fragment containing fibrin strands, red cells, and platelets.

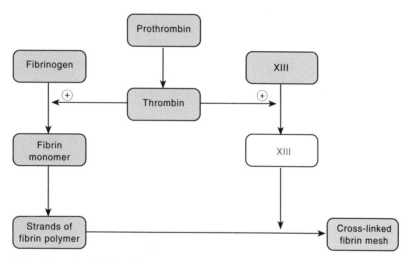

Figure 7.4   **Blood Coagulation.** A mesh of fibrin polymer strands is formed. Thrombin and activated clotting factor XIII act as catalysts in the process. White box indicates the activated form of factor XIII.

BLOOD COAGULATION

The importance of the blood is indicated by the elaborate mechanisms that are brought to bear when blood loss is threatened. The process of stopping blood loss is called **hemostasis,** and the principal hemostatic mechanism is blood coagulation. Essentially, this process involves converting the fluid blood into a nonflowing gel to prevent its escape from damaged blood vessels.

When blood coagulates, many long protein filaments form a tangled mesh within the blood. This mesh of filaments traps the blood's formed elements to form a red, gelatinous mass called a **blood clot.** The blood clot usually forms in the tissue spaces immediately adjacent to a damaged blood vessel and blocks further loss of blood from it (fig. 7.3). Note, however, that this mechanism is effective only in veins, capillaries, and small arterioles. The high blood pressure of the larger arteries interferes with clot for-

mation. This is why it is usually necessary to apply external pressure to stop bleeding in all but the smallest arterioles.

The blood clot's filaments are composed of the protein fibrin. Fibrin is derived from a plasma protein called **fibrinogen.** When two small fragments of the fibrinogen molecule are split off, the remaining portion is called fibrin. It is able to link with other fibrin units to form long strands. (This process is called polymerization; the single fibrin unit is known as a monomer, and the long fibrin strand, formed of hundreds of linked monomers, is called a polymer.)

The enzyme **thrombin,** derived from its inactive precursor, **prothrombin,** is the enzyme that splits fibrinogen to trigger the formation of fibrin and its polymerization. Thrombin also catalyzes the activation of factor XIII, which stabilizes fibrin by promoting chemical cross-linking between the newly formed fibrin filaments. This process converts a loose tangle of strands into a more tightly organized and stabilized mass (fig. 7.4). Thrombin can't normally

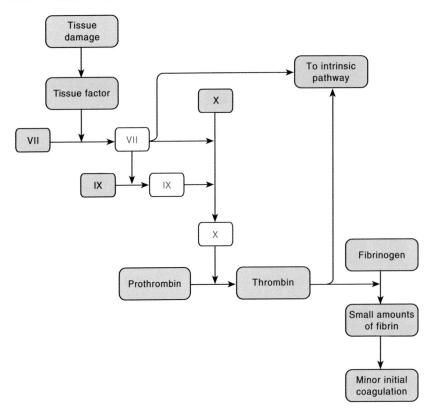

Figure 7.5   **The Extrinsic Pathway.** This is the initiating sequence in blood coagulation. White boxes indicate activated clotting factors.

Table 7.1	Clotting Factor Terminology. The Roman Numeral Designations Are More Commonly Used

Factor Name	**Roman Numeral**
Fibrinogen	I
Prothrombin	II
Tissue factor	III
Preaccelerin	V
Proconvertin	VII
Antihemophilic factor	VIII
Christmas factor	IX
Stuart-Prower factor	X
Plasma thromboplastin antecedent	XI
Hageman factor	XII
Fibrin-stabilizing factor	XIII

be present in the blood, but must be activated only when there is need for blood coagulation. The activation of prothrombin is accomplished by another enzyme, which is itself activated by another enzyme, which in turn depends on yet another activation step. Thus, fibrin formation depends on several linked enzyme activations. Such a sequence of reactions is called a **cascade.** The components of the coagulation cascade are called **clotting factors.**

Each of the components of the coagulation cascade has a name, but many of these are cumbersome, so a system of Roman numerals is more widely used in designating them (table 7.1). The exceptions are fibrinogen, thrombin, and prothrombin, whose names are used more frequently than their assigned numbers. Unfortunately, the various clotting factors were discovered and numbered before their positions in the cascade were fully understood. For this reason, they appear in the clotting sequence in an order different from their numerical sequence.

The plasma, then, contains clotting factors normally circulating in an inactive form. When the first in the sequence is activated, it activates the next member of the cascade and so on, until the fibrin strands form a tangled mass that coagulates the blood. We need now to consider the obvious question: What initiates the activation of the coagulation cascade?

At an injury site, endothelial cells, fibroblasts, and other affected cells, undergo a membrane change that exposes a protein known as **tissue factor** (TF, also called **tissue thromboplastin**). This substance activates the first component of the coagulation cascade called the **extrinsic pathway** (the name refers to the origin of TF outside the blood.) The extrinsic pathway's activation results in the initial formation of small amounts of fibrin that starts the coagulation response (fig. 7.5). More significantly, the thrombin generated by the extrinsic pathway has a powerful stimulating effect on a second cascade known as the **intrinsic pathway** (its activator is in the blood; hence, the

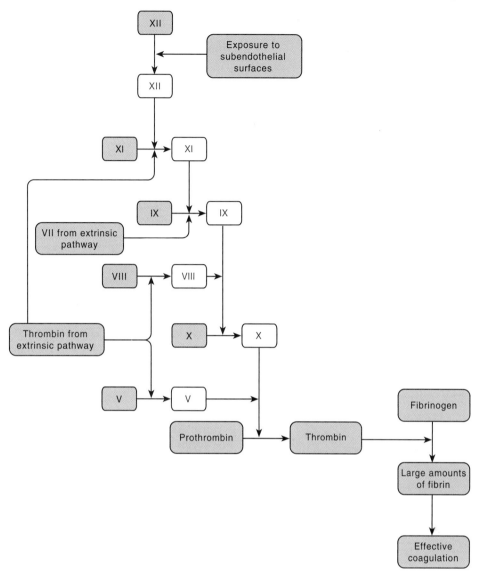

Figure 7.6   **The Intrinsic Pathway.** White boxes indicate activated clotting factors. The key to effective coagulation lies in the strong stimulus provided by thrombin and factor VII from the extrinsic pathway.

name "intrinsic"). Activated by thrombin at several key points, the intrinsic pathway yields larger amounts of fibrin that effectively counter the threat of blood loss (fig. 7.6). Of course, the thrombin produced by the intrinsic pathway promotes further intrinsic pathway activity with more thrombin formed in a continuing positive feedback cycle. Factor VII, also activated in the extrinsic pathway, provides further stimulus to the intrinsic pathway (fig. 7.5 and 7.6). The number of clotting factors and the complexity of their interactions may seem daunting at first. Figure 7.7 shows the essence of the two pathways' interaction and should help to clarify the matter.

As shown in figure 7.6, there is an alternate trigger to the intrinsic pathway: factor XII, also known as **Hageman factor.** Factor XII becomes activated when it is exposed to subendothelial surfaces. This activation mechanism is only a minor factor in clot formation when injury threatens

blood loss. It is very important, however, in the context of thrombosis, which is described in chapter 8.

Several steps of the coagulation cascade require the presence of calcium ion. Only minute amounts are required, and patients with calcium deficiencies do not suffer for lack of an adequate coagulation response. **Chelating agents** are often used to prevent the clotting of blood withdrawn for laboratory examination. They avidly take up calcium, preventing it from contributing to the coagulation cascade. Examples are oxalate and citrate ion preparations and EDTA (ethylenediaminetetraacetic acid).

The liver makes an important contribution to blood coagulation. Fibrinogen, prothrombin, and other clotting factors are synthesized in the liver by a process requiring vitamin K. This is a fat-soluble vitamin and, thus, its availability for absorption depends on the fat-emulsifying action of bile.

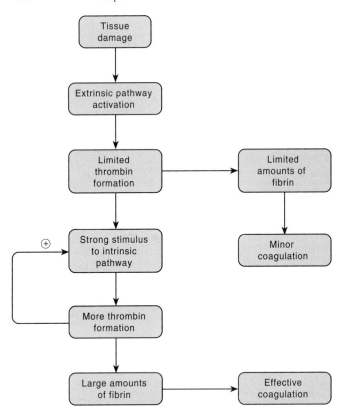

Figure 7.7   **Interaction between Extrinsic and Intrinsic Pathways.** Note the positive feedback cycling that generates rapid, large-scale fibrin production by the intrinsic pathway.

The Role of the Platelet

Platelets make an important contribution to hemostasis. At the site of vessel damage, subendothelial collagen is exposed to the blood. Circulating in it is a complex of factor VIII and another substance called **von Willebrand factor** (vWF). vWF can bind to exposed collagen and also to receptors on the surface of platelets. As flowing blood delivers platelets to the damage site, they bind to the vWF that is anchored there (fig. 7.8). Platelet binding is a key step in that it triggers a complex of platelet responses known collectively as **platelet activation.** These responses contribute to the massing of platelets at the site of vessel damage, to the promotion of blood coagulation, and to the control of these processes so that an excessive or inadequate response is prevented. Let us now consider in some detail the principal elements of the platelet activation response.

Platelet Plug Formation

The first platelets to arrive at a site of vessel damage bind to the vWF that has anchored to exposed endothelial collagen. This binding triggers a platelet membrane change that exposes receptors that can bind other platelets. As newly arriving platelets are bound to the first platelets, their membranes expose platelet receptors, and the process is repeated

again and again until an aggregation of platelets bound to the damage site is formed. This mass, called a **platelet plug,** contributes directly to hemostasis by acting as an obstruction to the flow of blood through the gap in the vessel wall (fig. 7.3).

The Platelet Release Reaction

Platelets store several regulatory substances in cytoplasmic vesicles. When activated, platelets release these substances. As the release reaction continues, platelets lose their granular appearance. For this reason the process is known as **platelet degranulation.** The substances released directly and indirectly promote hemostasis.

One of the substances released is ADP, **adenosine diphosphate.** It has the effect of promoting platelet activation and therefore more aggregation and further degranulation with the release of additional ADP to further increase the response, and so on. Another substance released by platelets is **thromboxane A_2** (TxA$_2$). Like ADP, it is a derivative of arachidonic acid, which is also the precursor of the leukotrienes. These play an important role in the mediation of the acute inflammatory response (see chapter 2). Like ADP, TxA$_2$ functions to promote further platelet activation, aggregation, and release. It also causes the injured vessel to constrict, reducing the size of the gap through which blood might be lost. As ADP and TxA$_2$ are released, they also interact with thrombin, which is simultaneously formed by the coagulation cascade. The three substances combine their effects in triggering clot retraction.

Activated platelets also release growth factors that play a role in the later stages of the process. When blood loss has been stopped, the gap in the wall must be repaired. The growth factors act to attract fibroblasts and promote healing by fibrosis. The effects of platelet activation are summarized in figure 7.9.

Exposure of Surface Receptors

Activated platelets bound to a damaged vessel also expose a membrane receptor called **platelet factor 3** (PF-3). It binds clotting factor V, which in turn binds factor X. In this way, PF-3 acts to localize factor X at the injury site where coagulation is needed.

Activated platelets also expose receptors specific to the binding of fibrinogen and fibrin. In this way, fibrinogen is positioned at the point where factor X will produce thrombin. As thrombin catalyzes fibrin formation, the resulting polymer filaments are anchored to the platelet surfaces, forming a localized mass of coagulated blood (fig. 7.8).

Clot Retraction

As coagulation proceeds, fibrin forms a tangle of filaments that are anchored at the surfaces of the platelet plug. The filaments trap red cells to form a loose, gelatinous mass at

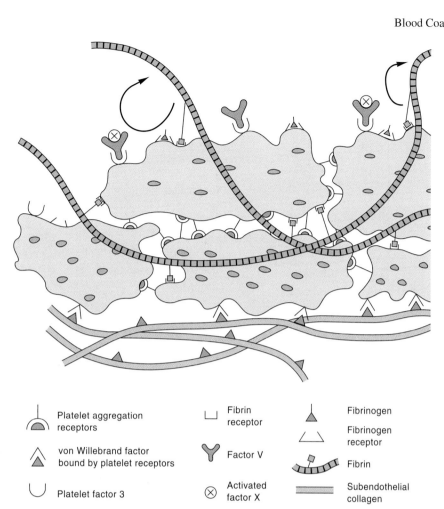

Figure 7.8 **Platelets and Coagulation.** Platelets bind to von Willebrand factor (vWF) on exposed subendothelial collagen. Platelet activation follows, exposing platelet factor 3, which binds factor V, which in turn binds activated factor X. Arrows represent the sequence of steps that convert fibrinogen to fibrin. Note the receptors localizing fibrinogen and fibrin at the surface of aggregated platelets.

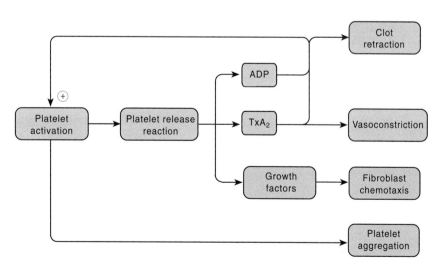

Figure 7.9 **Platelet Activation.** Principal effects of platelet activation and the platelet release reaction.

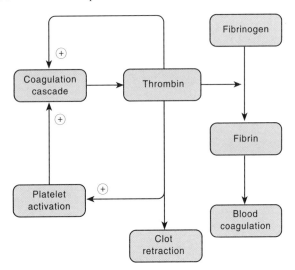

Figure 7.10   **The Role of Thrombin.** Positive feedback amplification of blood coagulation is mediated by thrombin. Recall the potent effects in the intrinsic pathway of the coagulation cascade.

the site of the vessel wound. At this stage, platelets make another contribution. Their internal system of contractile proteins, similar to those in muscle fibers, is activated by thromboxane, ADP, and thrombin. The platelets contract, pulling the fibrin strands into a more tightly packed mass. Plasma trapped in the mix of platelets, red cells, and fibrin is squeezed out and a denser, more firmly seated hemostatic gel results.

The Role of Thrombin

By now you may have been struck by the number of times thrombin has been cited as having a critical role in blood coagulation. Recall its central action in the conversion of fibrinogen to fibrin. Beyond this, we noted its important catalytic role in the intrinsic system that ultimately produces amounts of fibrin that can cope adequately with blood loss and its positive feedback effects in the intrinsic system. Thrombin also acts in another self-stimulating positive feedback system. Following platelet activation, the thrombin that initially forms stimulates further platelet activation, which results in further cascade activation and thrombin production, then more platelet activation, and so on. Finally, thrombin also contributes to effective blood clotting by contributing to clot retraction. These multiple thrombin functions are summarized in figure 7.10.

The Anticoagulation System

The positive feedback amplification of blood coagulation must be controlled or it could trigger widespread clotting, far beyond the amount needed to prevent blood loss. Such extensive coagulation would greatly impede blood flow with serious consequences, especially in critical organs like the brain. The fact that there is enough prothrombin in a few milliliters of blood to coagulate all the blood in the body emphasizes the need for fine control of the coagulation response. There are three major factors that limit clotting: hemodynamics, endothelial mediation, and the fibrinolytic system.

Hemodynamics

One factor limiting coagulation is the movement of the blood itself (**hemodynamics**). As clotting factors are activated, many are carried off by the flowing blood before they can activate others or be bound to surfaces at the injury site. At the same time, newly arriving blood dilutes the region's activated factors, slowing the coagulation cascade's reactions. Activated factors removed from the area are inactivated in the liver. This prevents their returning to the scene to continue to speed coagulation on later circulatory passes.

Endothelial Mediation

The endothelium adjacent to the site of vascular damage plays an important role in limiting clotting. It accomplishes this by secreting agents that oppose platelet aggregation and by blocking the action of key components of the coagulation cascade. Platelet aggregation is opposed by the action of **nitric oxide** (NO), a normal secretion of endothelium. After injury, as thrombin is formed, it triggers endothelial release of **prostacyclin** (also known as **prostaglandin I$_2$; PGI$_2$**), which also inhibits platelet aggregation at uninjured endothelial surfaces adjacent to an injury site. This confines adherence to the areas where platelets are needed to prevent blood loss, but prevents their massing at normal surfaces. The other anticoagulation agents are **tissue factor pathway inhibitor** (TFPI), which blocks the extrinsic pathway by interfering with TF activity; **thrombomodulin,** which works to indirectly block the action of factors V and VII; and **antithrombin III** (AT-III), whose action is directed against thrombin and several other clotting factors. Endothelial mediation in the case of AT-III is indirect. Although it is a circulating protein, AT-III is activated only when bound to the **heparin** that is present at endothelial surfaces.

Endothelial cells possess enzymes that degrade thrombin and the ADP released from platelets. ADP loss means less aggregation and activation of platelets, but beyond that, its breakdown products are known to specifically interfere with coagulation. Obviously, degradation of thrombin directly interferes with fibrin formation.

Another way that vascular endothelia limit the coagulation process is by activating enzyme systems that degrade clotting factors. These systems are dependent on endothelial membrane receptors, which bind key elements to activate them, confining them to the site where coagulation promoters are also confined.

Endothelia have receptors that bind **antithrombin III** (AT-III), which has a potent proteolytic effect on thrombin and various other clotting factors. It is intriguing to note that AT-III is effective only in degrading factors that are not

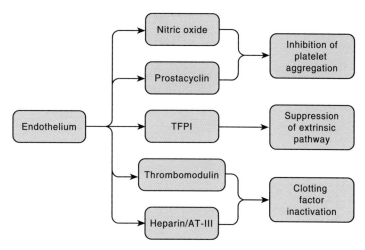

Figure 7.11   **Endothelial Mediation of Anticoagulation.** Heparin at the endothelial surface binds AT-III. Inactivation of clotting factors results.

bound to platelet surfaces. Those that are bound and participating in the coagulation cascade are in some way protected from AT-III's attack. A second type of endothelial receptor binds thrombin, which in turn activates another proteolytic enzyme. This one, called **protein C,** inactivates factors V and VIII to inhibit the coagulation cascade (fig. 7.11).

☑ *Checkpoint 7.1*

Squamous cells that line blood vessels are typically presented as the protective inner lining of the vessel wall. We can now appreciate how oversimplified this description is. Many endothelial surface components make subtle, but crucial, contributions to both coagulation and anticoagulation.

The Fibrinolytic System

As hemodynamics and endothelium-dependent enzyme systems counter the factors promoting coagulation, a fine balance is struck. This allows sufficient coagulation for hemostasis but prevents a potentially troublesome overresponse. The **fibrinolytic system** is an important factor in providing a transition between the hemostatic response and repair of the vessel wall. It provides a means of clot breakdown, allowing phagocytosis of its remnants and clearing the area for fibroblast activity and regeneration of various vessel wall elements.

The key to the system is its end product, **plasmin.** This proteolytic enzyme degrades fibrinogen, fibrin, and several clotting factors. By so doing, it not only attacks already coagulated blood but also opposes further clotting. The fibrinolytic system is quite complex and many of its details remain unclear. It is a cascade system, apparently with fewer components than the coagulation cascades and with many control-

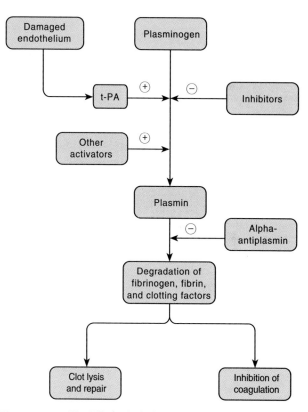

Figure 7.12   **The Fibrinolytic System.** t-PA: tissue plasminogen activator.

ling factors that balance its activation and inhibition. The best known of these activators is called **tissue plasminogen activator** (t-PA). You probably won't be surprised to learn that t-PA is yet another control molecule produced by endothelial cells. Its name describes its function. In the last step of the fibrinolytic cascade, t-PA acts on the circulating protein **plasminogen** to produce its active form, plasmin (fig. 7.12).

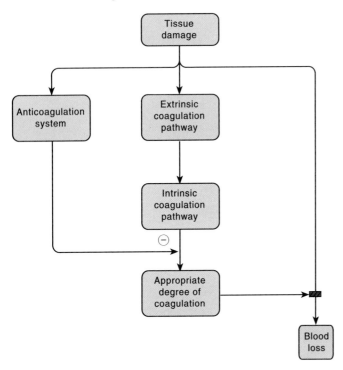

Figure 7.13 **Hemostasis Overview.** The system's finely balanced controls generate only the degree of coagulation needed to prevent blood loss.

As fibrin is formed and localized at the injury site, circulating plasminogen binds to it. In this way, as the clot forms, the plasminogen is directly incorporated into its structure. When t-PA is released, it also binds to fibrin. This means that the t-PA and plasminogen are held at the scene to facilitate the formation of plasmin, which is then in a position to directly attack the immediately adjacent fibrin. In this way the clot is lysed from within, and repair of the damaged vessel can proceed.

Of course, if the fibrinolytic process is not closely controlled, an excessive response could overwhelm the coagulation system's hemostatic effects to produce massive bleeding. Such overreaction is prevented by a circulating factor called **alpha$_2$-antiplasmin.** It has an antiplasmin action that moderates the fibrinolytic response (fig. 7.12).

Striking a Balance

The previous sections have explored the complexities of the coagulation system. We've considered the crucial role of the platelet and the two coagulation cascades. As well, the anticoagulation system's various elements were noted to be diverse and closely interrelated. Overall, the central idea is that although complex, the system's opposing interactions are finely balanced to yield only the degree of coagulation needed to prevent blood loss. At the same time, excessive coagulation is avoided and required blood flow to dependent tissues is not reduced (fig. 7.13).

The complexities of the mechanisms that produce effective coagulation and fine-tune the response are still being

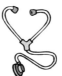

Focus on Anticoagulation Therapy

When coagulation occurs within blood vessels it can interfere with blood flow. This can be particularly threatening to vital structures like the brain or heart, and is often the underlying cause of heart attacks and strokes. Knowledge of the mechanisms of coagulation and anticoagulation provides the basis for intervention when the risk of coagulation in vessels is increased. **Oral anticoagulants** are agents that indirectly oppose coagulation by blocking the absorption of vitamin K. Reduction of clotting factor formation results and coagulation is inhibited. A more direct approach is taken by the common analgesic and anti-inflammatory drug aspirin (ASA). The basis for its action is blockage of the production of Tx-A$_2$, the agent that promotes platelet aggregation and therefore the coagulation that typically follows. Note that aspirin doesn't interfere with the production of PG-I$_2$, the normal aggregation inhibitor. Heparin therapy is based on increasing heparin levels so that more is present at endothelial surfaces to maximize binding of AT-III to increase its anticoagulation effects.

A recent treatment approach has proven very useful in cases in which a heart attack or stroke has already occurred. Prompt intervention with t-PA can generate sufficient fibrinolytic activity to break down coagulated masses that have narrowed heart or brain vessels. t-PA preparations are produced using advanced DNA-engineering techniques. Another proteolytic agent, streptokinase, has also been successful in heart attack intervention.

studied. The goal is to identify those points in the various systems where, by therapeutic intervention, it may be possible to restore fine control that has been lost and to correct responses that have become inadequate or excessive.

Blood Coagulation Tests

Information on the effectiveness of a patient's coagulation response can be gained from a variety of tests. These are usually aimed at measuring the time required to produce fibrin or a specific amount of an activated factor in the coagulation cascade. If the time is abnormally long, the assumption is that the inactive factor is deficient in the plasma or that the anticoagulation system is dominant. Currently used tests can pinpoint specific parts of the cascade to aid diagnosis. Some common coagulation tests are described in table 7.2.

BLEEDING DISORDERS

Loss of blood results if hemostatic mechanisms are defective. This section describes bleeding problems linked to defects in both the platelet and clotting factor components of the hemostatic response. In addition, we consider bleeding that results from abnormal fragility of fine blood vessels.

Table 7.2   Selected Laboratory Tests of Blood Coagulation

Test Name	Comments
Partial thromboplastin time (PTT)	Normal: 25–40 sec. Longer times usually indicate fault at some point in the coagulation system.
Prothrombin time (PT)	Normal: 9–12 sec. Tests extrinsic system. Can indicate low levels of factors I, II, V, VII, and X.
Thrombin time (TT)	Normal: 16 sec. Indicates time to convert fibrinogen to fibrin.
Fibrin-fibrinogen degradation products (FDPs)	Also called FSP (fibrin split products). Uses immune methods to test fibrinolytic system.
Fibrinogen	Chemical analysis to indicate amount in plasma. Normal range: 200–400 mg/dl.
Bleeding time	Longer times indicate low platelet numbers, delaying coagulation. Aspirin increases bleeding time.
Platelet aggregation	Platelet aggregometer uses optical means to measure aggregation. Indicates faulty platelet function.

Terminology

As blood escapes from the blood vessels, it is often trapped in the surrounding tissues. These accumulations may be visible at skin and mucous membrane surfaces. Pinpoints of hemorrhage seen in the skin, or in a post-mortem organ section, such as the brain, are called **petechiae** (fig. 7.14). They typically follow rupture of a capillary or small arteriole. Larger and sometimes less-regular areas of bleeding in the skin are called **purpura.** Still larger (over 2 cm) areas of bleeding are known as **ecchymoses.** These are commonly called bruises. Their characteristic coloration, involving the progression from purple, through blue/black, to green, and finally yellow, reflects changes in the hemoglobin released from ruptured RBCs. A large volume of blood trapped in a soft tissue is a **hematoma.** Hematomas present the risk of compressing an adjacent organ or duct, and can pose a serious threat by directly compressing brain tissue.

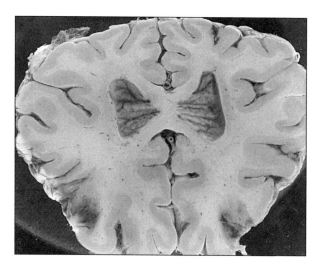

Figure 7.14   **Petechiae.** The tiny, dark spots in this brain section are the sites of petechial hemorrhages.

Platelet Disorders

Thrombocytopenia

Inability to mount an adequate hemostatic response may be the result of **thrombocytopenia,** the condition of insufficient circulating platelets. The problem can arise because platelet production has decreased or because platelets are being cleared from the blood at higher than normal rates. In either case, hemostasis is compromised and bleeding from minor vascular pressure or trauma produces petechiae and purpura. Platelet counts under $100,000/mm^3$ indicate thrombocytopenia but bleeding problems only arise with counts below $50,000/mm^3$.

Impaired platelet production may result from marrow suppression, in which case reduced red and white cell numbers would also result. Microscopic study of marrow biopsy verifies a hypoactive marrow in revealing a lack of megakaryocytes, the platelet's precursor cell. Some thera-peutic agents are specific in selectively inhibiting platelet formation; thiazide diuretics, gold and phenylbutazone (commonly used by arthritics), and certain antibiotics are examples. Chronic alcohol abusers may exhibit thrombocytopenia because of ethanol's marrow-suppression effects. Thrombocytopenia may also result if the marrow is unable to sustain normal mitosis rates because of rare congenital defects or because of more common dietary deficiencies of folic acid and vitamin B_{12}. Suppression may also be due to marrow replacement by tumor metastases, whose growth is well supported by marrow.

Excessive clearance of platelets may result from immune-related destruction or from nonimmune mechanisms. In these conditions, even though platelet counts are low, a marrow biopsy shows that normal numbers of megakaryocytes are present. A major nonimmune cause is **disseminated intravascular coagulation** (DIC), which is described in chapter 11. Essentially, widespread systemic

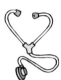

Focus on Thrombocytopenia and Blood Transfusion

A relative thrombocytopenia can result from large-scale blood transfusions. When blood is stored for prolonged periods, platelet numbers rapidly decline. Transfusion with such blood can dilute the recipient's platelets so that a relative thrombocytopenia results. Normally this is avoided by transfusing only blood and platelets that have been stored in a way that maintains their viability.

---

coagulation removes large numbers of platelets from the blood, producing thrombocytopenia. A related phenomenon is seen in certain hemangiomas, benign tumors originating in the cells of blood vessels. The numerous vessels have a large combined endothelial surface area that is defective and readily binds platelets so they are unavailable to participate in coagulation when needed. Some protozoan infections damage platelets, causing them to be removed from the plasma at an accelerated rate.

An interesting nonimmune mechanism causing thrombocytopenia involves the spleen. Normally, its vascular channels hold about 25% of circulating platelets. These provide a reserve that can rapidly enter the circulation, along with an erythrocyte reserve, in times of demand. When the spleen enlarges (splenomegaly), as it often does in cirrhosis and congestive heart failure, it can take up and hold additional platelets (hypersplenism). In extreme cases of splenomegaly, up to 80% of platelets may be held in the enlarged organ.

Most thrombocytopenia is caused by immune mechanisms that involve the binding of antibodies or antigen-antibody complexes to platelet surfaces. This hastens the removal of platelets from circulation and their phagocytosis by macrophages in the spleen. The causes of such an abnormal immune response are unknown. For this reason, the most common disorder involving this mechanism is called **idiopathic thrombocytopenic purpura** (ITP). Its two forms are characterized by petechial and purpuric bleeding in the skin and mucous membranes. In acute ITP, children under the age of 6 years are affected, but most of these cases are benign and spontaneously resolve in a period of a few weeks to six months. ITP often arises following a viral infection, a fact suggesting that the virus might interfere with immune recognition. In chronic ITP, adults, and women in particular, are affected.

Certain drugs are able to induce thrombocytopenia by an immune mechanism. Thiazide diuretics, quinidine, quinine, and heparin in some way disrupt the immune response, causing antibodies to the drug to complex with it and then bind to platelet surfaces. The result is a condition that presents in much the same way as ITP.

Another platelet deficiency disease is called **thrombotic thrombocytopenic purpura** (TTP). It is thought to involve an antibody that damages endothelium. Widespread platelet adherence to the damaged surfaces not only produces thrombocytopenia but also induces widespread coagulation in small blood vessels. The factors that predispose to thrombocytopenia are summarized in figure 7.15.

Impaired Platelet Function

Platelet function disorders are less common than low circulating platelet numbers, and involve abnormal platelet membranes. The platelets are unable to bind at damage sites to participate in the hemostatic response. As you can appreciate, these conditions are characterized by bleeding even though platelet counts are normal. Impaired platelet function may arise through genetic or acquired mechanisms.

The genetic impairment of platelet function is quite rare, with acquired conditions occurring more frequently. In marrow tumors, abnormal megakaryocytes may produce platelets with defective membrane receptors. Also, certain drugs, such as penicillin in large doses, can bind to platelets and reduce their functional capacity, as can the antibodies that are present in the plasma in multiple myeloma.

Patients with uremia may also suffer from platelet function loss. The plasma in such patients is a harsh environment, as it contains toxins normally excreted by the kidneys. When renal dysfunction prevents toxin clearance, platelets can be damaged.

Clotting Factor Disorders

As established earlier, the interplay between platelets and circulating clotting factors produces an integrated hemostatic response. With adequate numbers of normally functional platelets, bleeding disorders may arise if clotting factors are deficient. For all the seeming complexity of the coagulation cascades, you might expect many opportunities for the system to malfunction. In fact, the cascades are quite reliable and malfunctions are relatively rare. Clotting factor deficiencies may be of genetic origin or they may be acquired.

Genetic Clotting Factor Disorders

These disorders will arise early in life and are characterized by larger amounts of blood loss. Ecchymoses and hematomas are typical, as opposed to the smaller petechiae and purpura seen in platelet disorders. Bleeding may arise without warning, or excessive bleeding may follow minor trauma and dental or surgical procedures.

Von Willebrand's Disease Genetic deficiency of von Willebrand factor (vWF) interferes with platelet binding to subendothelial surfaces at the site of blood vessel damage. This is particularly significant in vessels where blood flow rates are high. Because the defect is transmitted by autosomal dominant inheritance, an affected individual will always have an affected parent. Factor VIII is normally carried in plasma complexed with vWF, so this disease may also produce defects in the coagulation cascade.

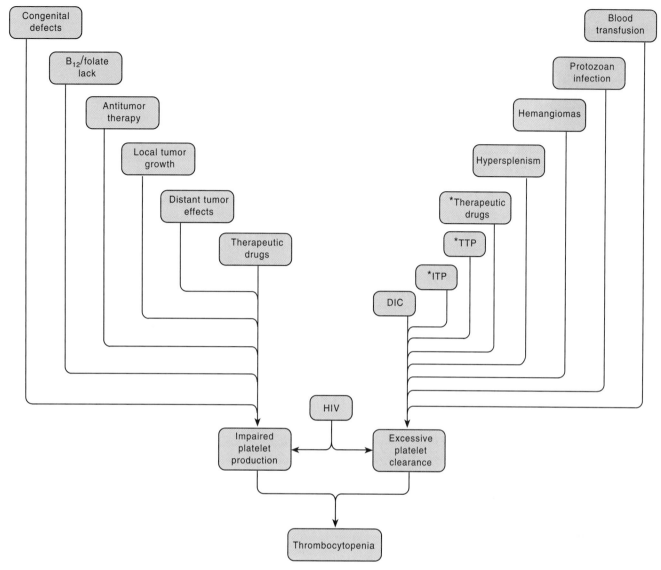

Figure 7.15   **Factors Predisposing to Thrombocytopenia.** Factors at left affect the marrow. Asterisks denote that an immune mechanism is involved.

Sufferers of von Willebrand's disease experience recurring bouts of gastric and intestinal bleeding, and women are subject to excessive menstrual hemorrhage (**menorrhagia**). Treatment of the disease is by transfusion with vWF derived from normal blood donors.

Hemophilias Although genetic deficiencies of all of the clotting factors exist, the most common involve inherited defects of factor VIII, called **hemophilia A,** or factor IX, in which the disease is called **hemophilia B.**

Because the genes coding for factors VIII and IX are located on the X chromosome, hemophilias A and B exclusively affect males, whose parents are unaffected by a bleeding disorder. Both conditions present similar patterns of abnormal bleeding. They can be distinguished only by analyzing the plasma to identify the deficient, or absent, clotting factor. Sufferers are subject to pronounced hemorrhage after trauma. Even relatively minor surgery presents a serious bleeding threat. As opposed to victims of von Willebrand's disease, hemophiliacs suffer less GI mucosal

Focus on Christmas Disease

Hemophilia B is also known as Christmas disease, since factor IX is also known as Christmas factor (table 7.1). You may, perhaps, be imagining that the name of this factor is related to a dedicated researcher's toiling late on Christmas eve to finally achieve its discovery. If so, you'll be disappointed to learn that it was named after the patient in whom its lack was first identified.

bleeding. They do, however, suffer from bleeding into the larger weight-bearing joints. Trauma in these structures is normally well tolerated, but hemophiliacs suffer repeated episodes of joint hemorrhage. Over time, joint deformities and fusion of the bones (**ankylosis**) are the result. Therapy

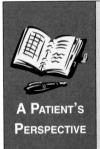

A PATIENT'S PERSPECTIVE

Idiopathic Thrombocytopenia

"I went from perfect health to death's door."
—Sylvia McFadyen Jones

The onset was absolutely sudden. One day, when getting home from a long walk, I noticed a rash on my legs. I thought "This looks serious!" and went to the doctor. He took a blood test and I went into town for the day. When I came home there was a note stuck on my door saying I was to contact the police urgently. I thought they were finally catching up to me for my speeding record. "It's absolutely urgent that you contact your doctor immediately." The doctor said "Get yourself to the hospital. Your platelet count is almost zero." I went from perfect health to death's door.

In the Emergency Room they said "It's all set up. We were expecting you. We are checking for possible donors." So I thought I must have leukemia and they were looking for marrow donors. (In retrospect, it was *platelet* donors they were talking about.) The hematologist had gone home (it was now 10:30 at night) so I had to stew all night wondering what was going on. I'm saying to myself "This is it! I'm dying!" When he arrived in the morning and took the bone marrow sample, I felt some satisfaction when the blood spurted on his beautiful grey suit. I was admitted to wait for the results. It felt like forever, waiting until 4 o'clock that afternoon. There was no malignancy in the bone marrow. So it wasn't leukemia, but what was it? This began two months of hospitalization and test after test. They tried chemotherapy and Prednisone in case it was an immune-mediated process. I had a violent reaction to the first IV administration so they switched to oral medications which I tolerated a little better. I lost my hair and I even lost nails! And through this experience in the hospital, of the transfusions, the people coming for chemo, I've come to realize that there's a community of people with serious illness, there's this unspoken knowing.

I had lots of visitors. People just couldn't believe what was happening. So I felt I had to deal with people's emotions, their confusion, trying to explain something I didn't understand myself. They were very supportive, but it's interesting, when you're fighting for your life you become very selective in your relationships. I was exhausted. My intimate friends became very important to me. One is a human rights lawyer. That was very validating. I felt that I wasn't alone, I had someone looking out for my rights.

I wasn't responding to treatment and I was spending time in the hospital medical library, desperately trying to get some idea what might be going on. My hematologist's response was "I'm the doctor, you don't have to know all this stuff! You are your own worst enemy because you build up this tension for which there is no answer. Just keep your spirits up!" It was like it was my own fault, that I was eating up my own platelets! On top of that, I felt we were locked in a struggle. When discussing the possibility of surgery, he blurted "I'll pick the surgeon!" That was the last straw for me. It was like they were just waiting for me to die! So I decided to take a chance and headed for the Faber Institute in Boston. Someone had told me they were experts and I was desperate for a diagnosis, some hope!

I had experienced bruising before, but when I was getting ready for the plane I had these dramatic bumps from subcutaneous bleeding. I remember just standing in the kitchen and my friend was saying "We really have to hurry, get your things, we have to catch a plane" and I'm looking at my hand and a purple bump is forming before my eyes. And then I'm bleeding from the cuticles in the Boston airport and I'm thinking "This is where I'm going to die!" I couldn't afford to redo the tests (my doctor wouldn't forward my records) so there was no clear diagnosis from the Faber, but they did give me the name of someone back home who was a research associate.

So I repacked and came home to a new GP and a new hematologist, a whole new team. And this time my experience was very different. The hematologist did new tests and tried gamma globulin. This doctor took very, very careful records and established some sort of a pattern. I went in twice a week for platelet transfusions and everything was done very precisely. I began to trust. This is also where I experienced an emotional rapport with an unknown donor. The platelets were the product of somebody else's, the donor's, body. A nuclear medicine scan established that the spleen was active, a hot spot, so they decided to operate. In the hospital I experienced a team approach. Everybody was working together. The meetings were held at my bedside. I could say "I don't feel up to doing that" and they would handle it. That was a tremendous relief to give up some of the control. But I felt ultimately no one was going to take over. The surgery was performed, my spleen removed, and my condition suddenly, and, touch wood, permanently returned to normal. I'm now focussed on rebuilding the strength and muscle mass I lost in the hospitalization and chemotherapy.

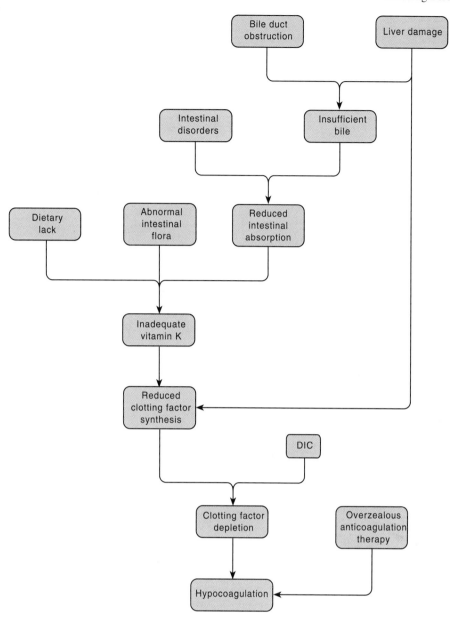

Figure 7.16   **Hypocoagulation Etiology.** Acquired clotting factor depletion or excessive anticoagulation therapy can produce an inadequate coagulation response.

typically involves transfusion with concentrates of the deficient factor from the blood of normal donors.

Acquired Clotting Factor Disorders

Given a normal genetic capacity to produce clotting factors, various acquired conditions can compromise clotting factor synthesis or function. These acquired disorders are much more likely to arise at later ages than are the genetic diseases. The most common etiologies of the acquired clotting factor disorders involve impaired hepatic synthesis, disseminated intravascular coagulation, and anticoagulant therapy.

Impaired Hepatic Synthesis Most clotting factors are produced in the liver, so clotting abnormalities may accompany liver disease. In practice, this problem is typically

seen only when liver damage is severe, as in advanced hepatic cirrhosis. However, since the synthesis of clotting factors requires vitamin K, its lack in a normal liver can result in inadequate production. Deficiency of the vitamin might be the result of malnutrition, but since the microorganisms that normally populate the colon produce some vitamin K, dietary deficiencies must be quite severe to overcome their contribution. On the other hand, antibiotic therapy, with moxalactam in particular, can suppress these organisms and reduce the availability of vitamin K. Lack of vitamin K could also follow the various intestinal disorders in which absorption is affected. Note, too, that since vitamin K is lipid-soluble, its absorption is bile-dependent. This means that obstruction of the bile ducts, or liver damage that compromises bile synthesis, can produce a shortage of vitamin K and reduced clotting factor production (fig. 7.16).

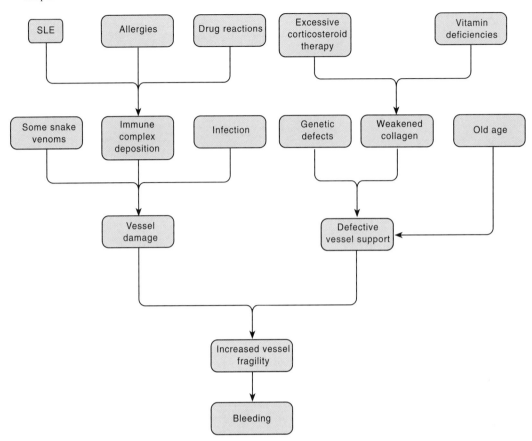

Figure 7.17   **Small Vessel Fragility.** Factors contributing to the vascular fragility that causes bleeding.

Disseminated Intravascular Coagulation (DIC) Disseminated intravascular coagulation can also reduce the level of available clotting factors. The same mechanism that affects platelets is involved. Generalized coagulation can so dramatically deplete clotting factors that their number is inadequate to meet hemostatic demands, resulting in excessive bleeding.

Anticoagulant Therapy Therapy to counter excessive blood coagulation may be complicated by bleeding in up to one-third of patients. Severe hemorrhage is not usual, but bleeding into the GI lumen, as well as skin ecchymoses and hematomas, commonly occur. Patients undergoing anticoagulant therapy require continuous monitoring for signs of bleeding. Invasive procedures involving potential blood loss are usually deferred, if possible. Heparin and **warfarin** are commonly used anticoagulants. Information on their modes of action and some other therapeutic uses can be found in table 8.1. Hypocoagulation etiology is summarized in figure 7.16.

Small Vessel Fragility

Bleeding from small blood vessels (the **microvasculature**) typically produces petechiae or purpura in the skin and GI mucosa. Involvement of glomerular capillaries produces petechiae in the kidney and may also result in blood loss to the urine (**hematuria**). As a group, these conditions are re-ferred to as the **vascular purpura.** Strictly speaking, these conditions might be treated in a later chapter dealing with blood vessel abnormalities, but since bleeding is the chief problem arising from fine vessel fragility, they are grouped with the true hemorrhagic disorders. Overall, the vascular weakness that characterizes these conditions derives from two sources: vascular damage or defective vessel support.

Vascular Damage Damage to the fine arterioles, capillaries, and venules of the microvasculature produces a vasculitis that may involve immune-mediated damage by neutrophils (see frustrated phagocytosis in chapter 1). Immune complex deposition in the fine vessels is associated with various immune diseases—for example, systemic lupus erythematosus (SLE), various allergies or drug reactions, or the idiopathic Henoch-Schönlein purpura (see chapter 3 case study). Vasculitis might also be the result of direct damage to the vessels by the toxins of infectious microorganisms or the venoms of certain snakes. In either case, vessel injury results in weakness and small hemorrhage into the surrounding tissue (fig. 7.17).

Defective Vascular Support The microvasculature is braced by a supporting architecture of connective tissue. This enables its fine vessels to better withstand the pressure of the blood they carry. Deterioration of the perivascular support system can compromise this function, producing vascular rupture and microhemorrhage.

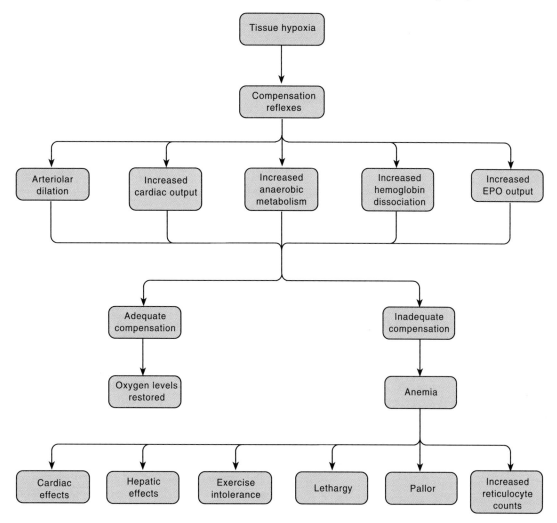

Figure 7.18   **Anemia.** The problem of anemia emerges when compensations cannot restore oxygen levels to meet tissue demands.

In some cases, connective tissue weakness is due to a hereditary defect, as in **hereditary hemorrhagic telangiectasis** (telangiectasis is dilation of fine vessels) or Marfan's syndrome. More commonly, acquired mechanisms underlie the problem. In scurvy, a dietary lack of vitamin C interferes with collagen synthesis, and in Cushing's disease, hypersecretion of corticosteroids induces the breakdown of protein, which weakens vascular supporting tissues.

Connective tissues also deteriorate with advancing age. The lessening of vascular support in the elderly causes **senile purpura.** In this condition, the vessels of the hands, wrists, upper arms, and calves are principally affected. The threat of serious blood loss in this condition is minimal.

ERYTHROCYTE DISORDERS

Problems involving erythrocytes arise if their numbers are excessive or inadequate. If numbers are excessive, the condition is known as **polycythemia.** When hemoglobin levels or erythrocyte numbers are decreased, oxygen transport is compromised and the condition of **anemia** results.

Anemia

Anemia is usually indicated by a hemoglobin level that falls below the lower limit of its normal range: 14–18 g/dl for males and 12–16 g/dl for females. The low hemoglobin levels cause a decline in the blood's oxygen transport capacity, which in turn triggers various physiologic compensations. Arteriolar dilation, accompanied by an increased cardiac output, provides for increased blood flow. A shift to anaerobic metabolism reduces oxygen consumption and indirectly promotes the dissociation of oxygen from hemoglobin. Also, increased renal secretion of erythropoietin stimulates the marrow to increase erythropoiesis and speed RBC production.

If these compensations are unable to restore oxygen delivery, and hemoglobin levels fall to 7–8 g/dl, signs and symptoms of hypoxia emerge. **Pallor** (paleness) is common, as are weakness, lethargy, and exercise intolerance. In severe cases, tissues especially sensitive to hypoxia may be affected, with abnormal cardiac rhythms and hepatic necrosis the result. Related metabolic defects may also produce fatty change in the heart and liver (fig. 7.18).

When anemia is suspected, it is usual to assess red cell numbers and size by means of red cell counts—the **hematocrit**—and tests of the **mean corpuscular volume** (MCV). The hematocrit is the volume of cells expressed as a percentage of total blood volume. Since red cells dominate in the blood, in practice the hematocrit value is taken to be a measure of erythrocyte volume (normal: 45%). Information relating to the blood's oxygen transport capacity comes from testing hemoglobin levels and the **mean corpuscular hemoglobin concentration** (MCHC). The MCV and MCHC tests provide a classification based on red cell size and hemoglobin content. Erythrocytes of normal volume are said to be **normocytic,** while those with an increased and decreased volume (higher and lower MCV values) are **macrocytic** and **microcytic,** respectively. Erythrocytes with a normal hemoglobin content are described as **normochromic,** those with excess hemoglobin (elevated MCHC) as **hyperchromic,** and those with a hemoglobin deficiency (low MCHC) as **hypochromic** (table 7.3).

Reticulocyte counts are also useful in the assessment of anemia. Hypoxia triggers an increased renal secretion of erythropoietin to stimulate a compensating increase in marrow activity. The marrow responds by rapidly moving immature reticulocytes into the circulation. This response provides an insight into the underlying pathophysiology of the anemia. When the anemia is caused by increased red cell destruction, a compensating rise in the reticulocyte count occurs. However, when it is caused by the marrow's inability to produce adequate red cell numbers in the first place, the increased erythropoietin will have no effect. Since the marrow can't meet normal demands for red cells, it can hardly be expected to increase its output, and so reticulocyte counts are lower than normal.

With this background, we can move to consider the etiology of anemia. As previously indicated, the condition is caused either by abnormally high red cell losses or by failure of the marrow to maintain production while normal red cell clearance continues. We will examine the latter case first.

Impaired Erythrocyte Production: Marrow Defects

Anemia is sometimes caused by abnormalities in the stem cells or in progenitors of the various hemopoietic cell lines (fig. 7.1). In such conditions, the defect can be localized in the developmental sequence by analyzing the circulating formed elements. For example, if only red cells are deficient, the defect can be ascribed to one of the progenitors in the red cell line. A rare disease called **pure red cell aplasia** (PRCA) is caused by an abnormality of this type. By contrast, if all formed elements are deficient (**pancytopenia**), the abnormality must occur earlier in the developmental sequence. In some cases, it is due to specific marrow suppressants associated with infections, chemotherapy, radiation, or drug reactions, but many cases are idiopathic.

A common example of a pancytopenic disorder is **aplastic anemia.** In this condition, all the normal formed-

Table 7.3	Terminology Used in Laboratory Red Cell Assessment	
	Volume	**Hemoglobin Content**
Normal	Normocytic	Normochromic
Increased	Macrocytic) (higher MCV	Hyperchromic (higher MCHC)
Decreased	Microcytic (lower MCV)	Hypochromic (lower MCHC)

element precursors are greatly reduced. Fat cells proliferate to replace them and dominate the marrow. Although anemia is a significant problem, bleeding due to thrombocytopenia and infections from depressed white cell numbers are important secondary features. In severe cases, mortality can be quite high; especially threatening is the aplastic anemia that can accompany viral hepatitis. Therapy may require a bone marrow transplant. An underlying autoimmune mechanism may be implicated in the large number of idiopathic cases, since immune suppression therapy has been used with some success.

Impaired Erythrocyte Production: Deficiencies

Deficiencies of substances essential to erythropoiesis may arise either from inadequate supply or from excessive losses. The red cells produced in these deficiency states demonstrate size and staining properties that are useful in diagnosis. The principal deficiencies that interfere with erythropoiesis are described in the following sections.

Iron Deficiency Iron deficiency anemia is a common condition throughout the world. The essential problem is an iron level too low to satisfy marrow demand. Recall that the marrow must produce 25 billion red cells each day. These replace the dysfunctional cells that are cleared from the blood by the spleen, marrow, and liver.

As aging erythrocytes are destroyed, the iron from their hemoglobin is efficiently recycled and used to synthesize new hemoglobin. However, small amounts—1–2 mg daily—are lost in urine and feces, and from the skin via perspiration and sloughing of its superficial layer. These losses must be made up from dietary intake. In women, an additional average daily iron loss of 1 mg can be attributed to menstrual blood flow (fig. 7.19). Most women do not compensate by increasing their dietary intake and are in a marginal iron deficiency state. Because of this, they are more vulnerable to any additional factor that predisposes to iron deficiency.

Although iron is widely available in meat, liver, eggs, nuts, legumes, and beans, the iron in animal products is contained in heme, which is much more easily absorbed. The uptake of iron derived from plant sources depends on

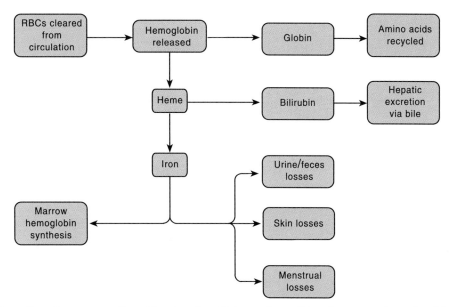

Figure 7.19 **Iron Recycling.** Because recycling of iron is quite efficient, only small iron losses must be replaced from the diet.

processing by gastric acid, which promotes the formation of soluble complexes of iron and other dietary components. These complexes remain soluble in the small intestine, favoring iron absorption. For this reason, patients who have had a total gastrectomy (stomach removal) may require iron supplementation to offset the reduced iron absorption rate that results from lack of gastric processing.

Absorbed iron is stored locally in the intestinal epithelium, in the liver, and in macrophages widely dispersed throughout the body. As iron intake is reduced or losses are increased, these stores of iron can be drawn upon to replenish supplies to the marrow. Eventually, however, the stored iron may be depleted, and if the underlying imbalance is not corrected, signs and symptoms of anemia emerge.

Iron deficiency anemia may result from an inadequate supply of iron to the marrow, which in turn may be due either to an inadequate diet or to absorption disorders (see chapter 13). These causes are not common in developed countries. Far more frequently, iron deficiency anemia develops in adults as the result of blood loss, usually from gastrointestinal bleeding. Such bleeding can be sufficient to deplete iron, but not severe enough to reveal its presence by any noticeable change in stool coloration. If bleeding is prolonged, a chronic anemia may result. In cases in which heavy menstrual flow is unrecognized as abnormal, increased losses can also produce a chronic iron deficiency anemia.

In iron deficiency anemia, the erythrocytes produced by the marrow are small (microcytic) and deficient in hemoglobin (hypochromic). Once the condition is established, these defects are reflected in low MCV and MCHC values.

Vitamin B$_{12}$ Deficiency Vitamin B$_{12}$ is required for normal DNA synthesis. When it is lacking, mitosis in the marrow progenitor lines is suppressed and a pancytopenia re-

Focus on Iron Deficiency Anemia and Pregnancy

Pregnancy can produce anemia because of the considerable transfer of iron from mother to infant during pregnancy and subsequent nursing. If pregnancies are closely spaced, the chance of developing an iron deficiency anemia increases, since there may not be enough time between them for replenishment of maternal iron stores. You might expect that the cessation of menstruation during pregnancy would compensate for losses to the infant. Unfortunately, however, blood loss associated with the delivery of the child offsets those gains.

sults. There is no impairment of RNA or protein synthesis, so cell growth proceeds, but because cell division can't occur, marrow precursors remain enlarged. These **megaloblasts** give rise to the descriptive term **megaloblastic anemia.** Because the erythrocytes that reach the circulation are also enlarged, a macrocytic, normochromic anemia results, with an increased MCV and a normal MCHC. The anemia is compounded by the fact that the enlarged red cells are more quickly cleared from the circulation.

Vitamin B$_{12}$ is also known as **cobalamin.** It is not synthesized in our tissues, so we rely on the dietary intake of meat, liver, seafood, and dairy products to supply our needs. The small daily requirement of 1 μg is easily satisfied by most diets, and an added protection comes from body stores of 2–5 mg. This is enough to meet demand for years, should intake fall to zero. Only strictest dietary

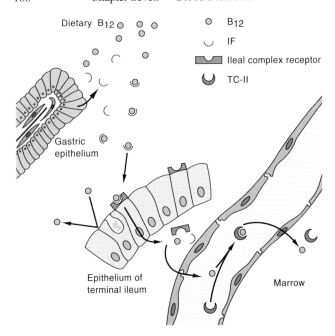

Dietary B₁₂

B₁₂
IF
Ileal complex receptor
TC-II

Gastric
epithelium

Epithelium of
terminal ileum

Marrow

Figure 7.20 **Vitamin B₁₂ Absorption.** The vitamin combines with IF in the proximal small intestine. Complex receptors in the distal ileum promote absorption. Uncomplexed B₁₂ is not absorbed. TC-II carries the vitamin in the plasma. It is split off in the marrow, releasing B₁₂ for its role in hemopoiesis. The inital binding of cobalamin by R-binder is not shown.

avoidance of meat and dairy products for several years could pose the threat of anemia from inadequate supplies of vitamin B₁₂.

Much more commonly, the lack of cobalamin is due to its inadequate absorption from the intestinal lumen. When released from food by digestion in the stomach, cobalamin is in a form that is not readily absorbed. A component of saliva, **R-binder,** takes up dietary cobalamin after it is split from food by pepsin in the acidic environment of the stomach. The R-binder/cobalamin complex then passes to the intestine where pancreatic enzymes release the cobalamin. The vitamin then binds to **intrinsic factor** (IF). This glycoprotein is a product of the gastric epithelium and is critical to the process. When complexed with cobalamin, IF is able to bind to specific receptors in the distal ileum. This is the key—only after binding can the vitamin B₁₂ be absorbed. Following absorption, the cobalamin is released from IF and is taken up by a plasma transport protein called **transcobalamin II** (TC-II). The vitamin travels in the blood complexed with TC-II until it is taken up by the marrow, or by other cells with high mitotic rates that require it (fig. 7.20).

In **autoimmune chronic gastritis,** vitamin B₁₂ absorption is hindered by a lack of IF. The cause is an autoimmune attack on both IF and the parietal cells that produce it. The reasons underlying this immune defect are unknown. The megaloblastic anemia associated with the IF deficiency in autoimmune chronic gastritis is known as **pernicious anemia.** Gastric resection, usually to remove a carcinoma,

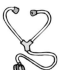

Focus on Deficiencies in Dependent Populations

Most of the deficiencies that lead to anemia are the result of special circumstances such as surgery, excessive losses, or autoimmune mechanisms rather than from pure lack of dietary input. Apart from these cases, many North American deficiency problems arise in vulnerable population: those who depend on others for care, and, in particular, for their diet. Even though key nutrients are readily available, children, the elderly, and the institutionalized may be at risk. If caretakers are too poor, ignorant, or indifferent to adequately provide, their dependents suffer. Alcoholics and drug addicts are a special case in that they have little regard for their own nutrition and anyone who depends on them for support is likely to fare no better.

can also reduce or eliminate IF availability, but the term *pernicious anemia* is reserved for the condition wherein deficiency arises with the stomach essentially intact.

Intestinal malabsorption states (see chapter 13) may also affect cobalamin absorption, as can resection of the ileum. More rarely, abnormal bacterial growth in the intestine or a tapeworm (from undercooked fish) can consume vitamin B₁₂ to a degree that limits its availability for absorption.

Since cobalamin is initially taken up by salivary R-binder and then passed to IF in the intestine, any chronic digestive disorder that interferes with the process can lead to reduced vitamin B₁₂ absorption. Specifically, apart from the IF already noted, salivary secretion of R-binder, gastric secretion of acid or pepsin, and normal pancreatic secretions are required. (Don't overlook the significance of the word "chronic" in the first sentence of this paragraph. Remember that we store more than a 3-year supply of vitamin B₁₂ in the liver, so any such digestive disturbance must be sustained for anemia to emerge.)

Many patients who suffer a cobalamin deficiency anemia also experience some degree of neuropathy. The central or peripheral nervous system, or both, may be affected. Symptom severity is often not linked to the degree of anemia. Loss of myelin due to altered lipid metabolism indirectly linked to the vitamin B₁₂ deficiency is the underlying cause of the neuropathy.

Folic Acid Deficiency Lack of **folic acid** (or **folate,** its salt) produces a megaloblastic anemia that is very similar to that seen in the cobalamin deficiency state. The cells of both marrow and peripheral blood are similar, so diagnosis must be made on the basis of depressed levels of folate in serum. No neuropathy is associated with folate deficiencies.

The dietary sources of folate—meat, eggs, leafy vegetables—are readily available, so pure dietary deficiency states are rare in developed countries. Fad diets, or overcooking,

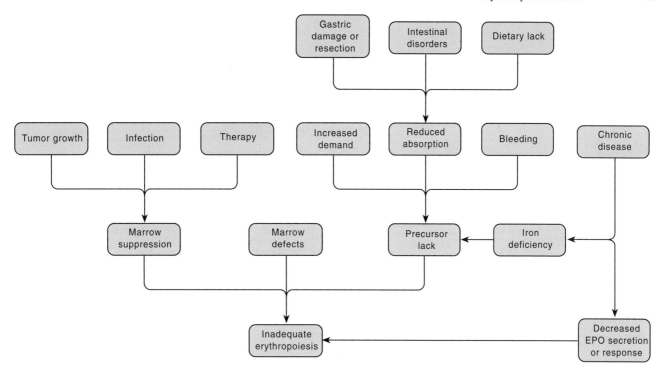

Figure 7.21   **Compromised Red Cell Production.** There are many factors that may contribute to reduced erythropoiesis.

which breaks down heat-sensitive folate, may produce a deficiency, but body stores provide a five-month period of tolerance for deviations from proven dietary practice.

As you might expect, intestinal resection or disease can interfere with folate absorption. In fact, in such cases, deficiencies of folic acid, cobalamin, and iron can all contribute to anemia.

Folate deficiency can also be the result of high-demand states. Examples of these are pregnancy, infant growth spurts, prolonged marrow overactivity to compensate for chronic blood loss, and rapid consumption by rapidly growing malignancies.

Impaired Erythrocyte Production: Anemia of Chronic Disease

A variety of long-term, often systemic disease conditions can lead to mild, nonprogressive anemia. In such cases, the marrow is intact and total body levels of key nutrients are normal. Infections and chronic inflammations are often involved, with anemia developing by various mechanisms. In some cases, the mechanism is a reduced red cell survival time. For some reason in chronic disease states, normal erythrocytes are prematurely removed from the blood by macrophages. In other cases, the mechanism involves erythropoietin (EPO); either marrow precursors become less responsive to it or secretion is inadequate. Since EPO is secreted by the kidney, lack of secretion is typical in chronic and severe renal disease. Iron deficiency is another reason for anemia in chronic diseases. The problem seems to arise

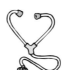

Focus on Folic Acid Deficiency in Tumor Therapy

Some tumor therapy side effects are related to folic acid. Not only do malignant tumors consume more folic acid, but some antitumor chemotherapeutic agents work by interfering with the tumor's utilization of folate, in order to slow or stop its growth. The effect can't be limited to the tumor cells, so a critical lack of folic acid may arise in normal tissues already facing a deficiency from the tumor's high folate consumption.

because, although total body iron reserves are adequate, macrophage stores can't be drawn on quickly enough to meet demand.

The marrow-suppression effects of malignant tumors were described in chapter 6. We can summarize here by saying that nonmarrow malignancies seem to produce anemia by suppressing the marrow. The likely mechanism is the tumor's production of marrow suppressants that reach the marrow by way of the blood. The various factors that can interfere with normal erythropoiesis are summarized in figure 7.21.

Hemolytic Anemia

As we have seen, circulating erythrocyte numbers are the result of the balance between production and clearance.

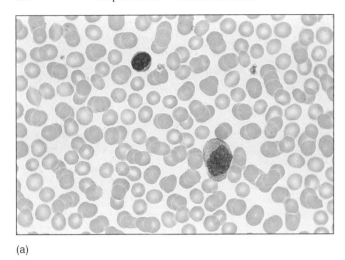

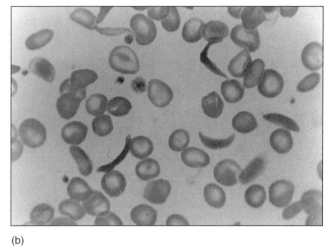

(a)   (b)

Figure 7.22   **Sickle Cell Anemia.** (*a*) Normal blood, for comparison with (*b*) the abnormal cell shapes that occur in sickle cell anemia.

Having considered failure of the marrow to maintain adequate red cell output, we can now turn to the destruction of erythrocytes—**hemolysis,** in particular—and to those anemias that result from the destruction of defective red cells.

Intrinsic Hemolytic Anemia

Intrinsic hemolytic anemia derives principally from hereditary defects that promote hemolysis. These are relatively rare disorders involving flawed erythrocyte enzyme systems, defective RBC membranes, or abnormal hemoglobins. The **hemoglobinopathies** are most important, and are represented by two distinct conditions: sickle cell anemia and thalassemia.

Sickle Cell Anemia In this condition, erythrocytes contain an abnormal hemoglobin, **HbS,** as opposed to the normal **HbA.** Under certain conditions, HbS polymerizes to form long, insoluble filaments. These distort the cell, which assumes a less-flexible crescent shape resembling a sickle (fig. 7.22). Such cells are much more likely to be cleared from the blood by marrow and spleen macrophages. The typical life span of a sickled cell is 20 days, as opposed to the normal cell's 120 days. Sickled cells also tend to become trapped in the microcirculation, where they can obstruct flow and threaten ischemic injury. Either mechanism reduces cell numbers to produce a chronic anemia. The clinical course of sickle cell anemia is quite variable. Most people experience a chronic anemia that produces some degree of weakness. Sufferers are also subject to **sickle crisis:** episodes of acute sickling that block blood flow, posing the threat of widespread ischemic organ damage. The deep pain of these attacks is linked to bone necrosis caused by occlusion of small blood vessels within bone. Sickle crisis can be triggered by hypoxemia, acidosis, or other conditions, such as pregnancy or cold weather, where the causative link is less clear. Although the disease was previously quite threatening, improved therapeutics enable many sufferers to reach maturity.

A benign condition called **sickle cell trait** is determined by the presence of one defective gene, instead of the two present in the full-blown anemia disorder. Affected individuals suffer few complications but there is increased risk of splenic damage in conditions of hypoxemia that favor sickling. Although those with sickle cell trait are essentially normal, they are carriers. This means that two sickle cell trait parents can each contribute a defective gene to a single child who would then develop sickle cell anemia.

Blacks of African origin are the population most affected by sickle cell anemia; incidence is about 0.2%. Other groups affected to a lesser degree originate in Saudi Arabia, India, and in areas near the eastern Mediterranean. The defective allele can be detected, and screening programs have been helpful in providing information and counseling applicable to mate selection and family planning.

Thalassemia The thalassemias are a group of genetic disorders that also involve hemoglobin defects. The most common thalassemias, beta-thalassemias, arise from defective production of the beta-globin component of hemoglobin. The result of impaired hemoglobin synthesis is a microcytic, hypochromic anemia. Beta-globin normally joins to alpha-globin, but when the beta protein is lacking, alpha-globin accumulates and causes destructive membrane effects (fig. 7.23). Not only does the membrane damage cause rapid clearance of red cells from the blood, but before leaving the marrow the defective RBCs in some way suppress mitosis in stem cells so that red cell production falls.

Thalassemia major (Cooley's anemia) is a gravely threatening disease that requires a continuous regimen of transfusions. Sufferers carry two defective genes and are said to be homozygous. **Thalassemia minor** is a milder form of the diseases that occurs in heterozygotes (those who have only one defective gene). It is well tolerated and essentially asymptomatic. These conditions are more prevalent in ethnic groups with origins in countries bordering the Mediterranean.

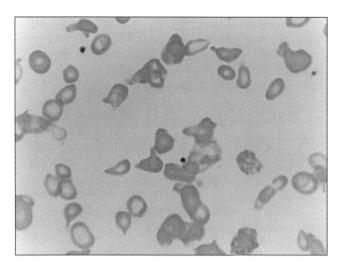

Figure 7.23   **Thalassemia.** Reduced erythrocyte numbers in thalassemia. Compare with normal blood shown in figure 7.22.

Paroxysmal Nocturnal Hemoglobinuria (PNH) This rare condition arises as a genetic defect that occurs in marrow precursors rather than in the sufferer's parents' genes. The abnormality involves a membrane defect that is passed on to daughter cells in the erythrocyte maturation sequence, but cannot be transmitted to the affected person's offspring.

The defect involves genes that normally enable the membrane to resist autoimmune damage. Their level of activity makes the affected cells highly vulnerable to immune-mediated lysis. The disease is characterized by a chronic anemia as well as episodes of hemolysis that occur at night. The hemoglobin that is released from the ruptured red cells is excreted by the kidneys and is detectable in the urine.

Extrinsic Hemolytic Anemias

In these conditions, hemolysis is the result of damaging influences that affect genetically normal erythrocytes. The problem arises outside the red cell, causing surface changes that promote clearance by spleen and marrow macrophages. Alternatively, the cells might be so damaged that they rupture in the blood.

Immune Hemolysis The essential problem in immune hemolysis is the binding of antibodies to red cell surface antigens. This results in more rapid clearance of RBCs from the blood, on the basis of an altered cell surface, or rupture of the RBCs via complement activation (see chapter 5). In normal circumstances, antibodies against red cell surface antigens are not present, but they may be formed in cases of immune incompatibility between a mother and her fetus or as a result of a blood transfusion. Previously, the D (Rh) antigen was most often involved in maternal-fetal incompatibilities, but with the emergence of effective therapy, the antigens of the ABO system are now more prominent contributors (this matter is also treated in chapter 5). Because there is good awareness of the risks of transfusion incompatibility, careful preliminary testing is done to avoid hemolytic reactions involving A, B, and Rh antigens.

Table 7.4	Conditions Involving Immune-Mediated Hemolysis

Autoimmune hemolytic anemia
Warm antibody autoimmune hemolytic anemia
Cold antibody autoimmune hemolytic anemia
Drug-mediated hemolytic anemias
Paroxysmal cold hemoglobinuria*

*This rare condition is associated with syphilis and other infections. It should not be confused with paroxysmal nocturnal hemoglobinuria, a genetic condition.

Table 7.5	Therapeutic Agents Known to Have Some Degree of Hemolytic Effect via Immune Mechanisms

Amino salicylic acid	Cephalosporin
Chlorpropamide	Cisplatin
Isoniazid	Levodopa
Mefenamic acid	Methyldopa
Penicillins	Phenacetin
Quinidine	Quinine
Rifampin	Stibophen
Sulfonamides	Sulfonylureas
Tolbutamide	

In the examples just cited, antigens from one individual interact with antibodies from another individual, but other immune hemolytic conditions involve autoimmunity. In these **autoimmune hemolytic anemias,** an individual's immune system produces antibodies against its own self-antigens. About half of such anemias arise in association with some identifiable disease, but the remainder are idiopathic. The anemias associated with various tumors, infections, and inflammatory conditions are caused by immune-related red cell destruction. Examples of these conditions are provided in table 7.4, where the terms **warm antibody** and **cold antibody** refer to the laboratory incubation temperatures at which the antibodies maximally combine with antigen.

Some therapeutic drugs are able to induce immune destruction of red cells. By direct or indirect means, the drug comes to be bound at the cell surface, causing lysis while in the circulating blood or in the spleen. Some agents known to elicit these effects are listed in table 7.5. Large drug doses or pronounced patient sensitivities are usually involved.

Mechanical Hemolysis Trauma, or physical injury, can disrupt red cells, distorting and tearing them as they are forced through small vessels that are misshapen or blocked by platelets and fibrin. As erythrocytes traverse vascular or cardiac passages, they may encounter trauma

Table 7.6	Drugs Causing Hemolysis through the Production of Injurious Intracellular Free Radicals (Peroxide, Superoxide)

Dapsone
Nitroglycerine
Phenacetin
Primaquine
Sodium perchlorate
Sulfasalazine
Vitamin K analogues

due to a variety of causes. Certain, especially older, artificial cardiac valves are known to physically damage erythrocytes. In **disseminated intravascular coagulation** (DIC), platelet plug and fibrin deposits in small vessels present obstacles to the passage of red cells. As they are forced through the narrowed lumina, they are distorted and damaged by the abnormal surfaces. As a result, fragments of erythrocytes are sheared off, releasing bizarrely shaped membrane remnants in the circulation. Various other factors may produce mechanical hemolysis, such as cardiac structural defects, damaged valves, dialysis, and heart-lung machine pumps. These rarely have clinical significance.

Miscellaneous Hemolytic Anemias   Certain drugs can damage erythrocytes by forming destructive free radicals that damage hemoglobin or the red cell membrane (table 7.6). Snakebite toxins, infectious agents, or various other substances encountered in the environment can disrupt red cells in various ways that promote their more rapid clearance from the blood.

Hypersplenism

Excessive splenic clearance of formed elements from the blood is called **hypersplenism.** It is seen in conditions of splenomegaly most commonly as a result of cirrhotic congestion of the hepatic portal circulation (see chapter 14). The mechanism of red cell loss is based on the cells isolation in the spleen where they are deprived of the steady supply of glucose necessary for their anaerobic energy metabolism. Leukopenia and thrombocytopenia may be present to varying degrees in association with the anemia that accompanies hypersplenism.

In some cases, therapeutic resolution of the condition producing the hypersplenism does not resolve the problem. To avoid chronic anemia problems, the spleen may be surgically removed without serious, long-term functional deficit. The broad array of factors that can produce hemolysis is presented in figure 7.24.

Polycythemia

Polycythemia is the condition of increased red cell concentration in the blood. It may be due to an increase in red cell numbers (with normal plasma volume), **absolute polycythemia,** or to normal red cell numbers suspended in a reduced plasma volume (**relative polycythemia**). The condition produces elevations of **packed cell volume** (PCV), the hematocrit, and the hemoglobin level.

Absolute Polycythemia

This condition involves an overproduction of erythrocytes by the marrow. If marrow activity is increased in response to elevated renal output of erythropoietin (EPO), the polycythemic condition is said to be secondary. **Secondary polycythemias** may arise as a normal physiologic response to the tissue hypoxia that is present in certain lung or heart conditions that interfere with normal blood oxygenation. High-altitude exposure has a similar effect. If there is no physiologic requirement, but EPO secretion is increased, a tumor is usually involved. Renal tumors may secrete excessive EPO, or nonrenal tumors, able to secrete EPO-like substances, may be the source of the marrow stimulus. In some cases, restricted renal blood flow will produce renal hypoxia and activate EPO secretion.

Heavy smokers may also suffer a secondary polycythemia. Inhaling products of combustion delivers significant levels of carbon monoxide (CO) to the blood. CO has a tendency to bind with hemoglobin that is over 200 times that of oxygen. When CO is present in a heavy smoker's blood, oxygen delivery is compromised, and hypoxic renal sensors respond with increased EPO secretion (fig. 7.2).

In **primary absolute polycythemia,** marrow stem cell lines proliferate without an increased EPO stimulus. This condition is, in effect, a benign tumor of the marrow, with red cell proliferation dominating over platelet or white cell production. In such cases, the normal or elevated tissue supply of oxygen suppresses EPO secretion.

Another myeloproliferative condition is referred to as **polycythemia vera** or sometimes **polycythemia rubra vera.** It is characterized by a thickened blood, which flows more sluggishly through small vessels and predisposes to coagulation within them, especially in the kidneys, spleen, and liver. Deprivation of nutrients and tissue destruction follow blockage of the vessels. Males in their 60s to 80s are most likely to be affected by this idiopathic disease.

Relative Polycythemia   In these conditions, hematocrit values are increased but total red cell numbers are normal. The plasma deficiency that produces this state may be the result of generalized dehydration, extensive skin burns, or pronounced diarrhea or diuresis.

Two other conditions that involve a relative polycythemia have only poorly understood reasons for low plasma volume. One is **smoker's polycythemia,** to which heavy smoking contributes in some way; the other is **stress polycythemia,** whose typically hard-driving, male sufferers are also at high risk of heart and brain vascular disease. A summary of etiological factors in pulmonary, secondary, and relative polycythemia is presented in figure 7.25.

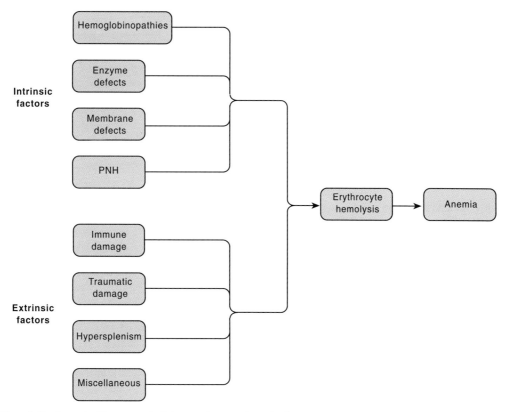

Figure 7.24 **Hemolytic Anemia.** Factors underlying erythrocyte hemolysis.

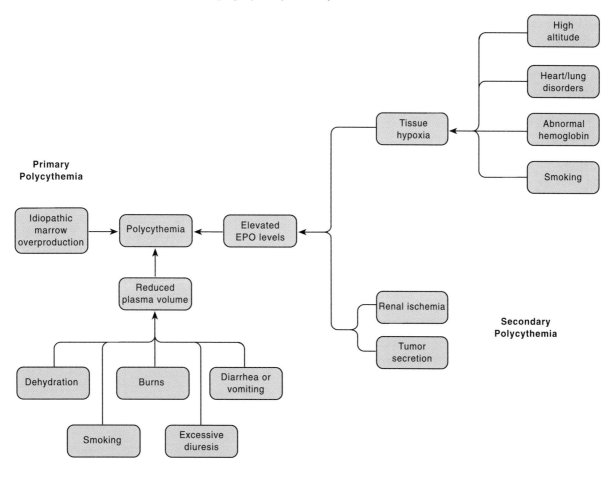

Figure 7.25 **Polycythemia.** Etiological factors in primary, relative, and secondary polycythemia.

LEUKOCYTE DISORDERS

As in the case of red cells, leukocyte numbers in the peripheral blood are determined by the balance between production and destruction. **Leukopenia** is the general deficiency state, while the term **leukocytosis** denotes a nonneoplastic elevation of white cell numbers. The neoplastic proliferation of leukocytes is denoted by the term **leukemia.**

Leukopenia

Most conditions of white cell depletion involve **neutropenia,** although the other granulocytes may be affected as well. The blood's normal range of neutrophil numbers is 1,800–7,200/mm^3. Neutropenia is diagnosed on the basis of sustained counts below 1,800/mm^3. When counts drop to the extremes of 200–300/mm^3, the term **agranulocytosis** is often used to describe the condition.

The usual consequence of neutropenia is an increased risk of infection due to a reduced phagocytosis response. Increased infection rates become significant when neutrophil counts fall to 500/mm^3 and below. The typical signs and symptoms of infection are malaise, fever, weakness, and fatigue. Infections of the oral and pharyngeal mucosa are typically seen in leukopenia. Without timely antibiotic and anti-inflammatory therapy, rapid development of massive systemic infection may occur.

Most neutropenia is the result of inadequate production by a marrow whose functions are suppressed by antitumor therapy involving drugs or radiation. Neutrophil counts decrease with increased dose level, and their lowering is taken into account in the patient's management. In many cases, however, nontumor drugs may have variable marrow-suppression effects, producing neutropenia as an unexpected side effect (table 7.7). A broad variety of other causes can also produce marrow suppression and neutropenia, including marrow replacement by primary or secondary tumor as well as various infections, deficiencies of folic acid or vitamin B$_{12}$ (needed for DNA synthesis in neutrophil precursors), and genetic immune defects. Figure 7.26 summarizes the various etiologies that may operate in neutropenia.

Excessively rapid clearance of neutrophils from the blood can also produce neutropenia. Immune destruction may be involved. Inappropriate immune responses can trigger destruction of neutrophils as part of an underlying autoimmune disorder. Some therapeutic drugs are able to bind to neutrophil membranes, altering them in ways that promote clearance by macrophage phagocytosis. In hypersplenism, neutropenia may result when neutrophils are removed from the blood and destroyed.

Leukocytosis

This condition of elevated leukocyte counts is a functional response to increased demand. Specific white cells may be affected and their increased number linked to their particular defensive role (see table 7.8). Leukocytosis in the context of the inflammatory response is described in chapter 2.

Table 7.7	Selected Agents That May Suppress the Marrow to Produce Neutropenia

Alkylating Agents

Cyclophosphamide
Melphalan

Analgesics*

Phenacetin
Phenylbutazone

Antibiotics*

Ampicillin
Chloramphenicol

Anticonvulsants*

Phenytoin
Trimethadione

Antihistamines*

Tripelennamine

Antimetabolites

Mercaptopurine
Methotrexate

Thyroid Antagonists*

Methimazole
Polypropylthiouracil

X-irradiation

*Indicates agents whose neutropenia effects are unpredictable.

 Checkpoint 7.2

The general principle bears repeating. The number of red cells, white cells, and platelets in the blood essentially depends on two factors. One is their rate of production; the other is their rate of clearance from the blood. Either may increase or decrease, altering the number in the circulation.

Leukemia

Primary malignant tumors of leukocyte precursors in the marrow are called **leukemias.** They do not produce discrete tumor masses but instead are characterized by proliferation in the marrow. In most cases (65%), cells showing varying

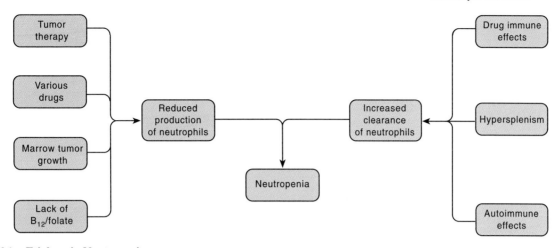

Figure 7.26   **Etiology in Neutropenia.**

Table 7.8	Specific Leukocytoses and Their Principal Associated Conditions

Polymorphonuclear Leukocytosis (neutrophilia)

Acute inflammations

Basophilic Leukocytosis (basophilia)

Myeloproliferative disorders
Lung malignancies

Eosinophilic Leukocytosis (eosinophilia)

Allergic disorders (hay fever, asthma, drug reactions)
Parasite/fungus infection
Sarcoidosis
Skin disorders

Monocytosis

Collagen vascular disease (systemic lupus erythematosus, rheumatoid arthritis)
Chronic infections (TB, brucellosis)
Intestinal inflammations (Crohn's disease, ulcerative colitis)

Lymphocytosis

Acute viral infections
Chronic infections (TB, brucellosis)

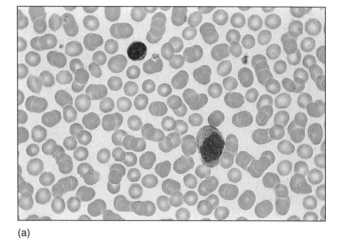

(a)

(b)

Figure 7.27   **Leukemia.** Blood smears showing (*a*) normal blood and (*b*) leukemia.

degrees of differentiation spill over into the blood to increase circulating cell numbers, and it is then that the term "leukemia" is used (fig. 7.27). In the cases where proliferation is confined to the marrow, the term **aleukemic leukemia** is employed.

Pathogenesis

The production of excessive numbers of cells in the leukocyte differentiation line arises because cells retain the ability to divide instead of losing it as they mature and differentiate. The result is a large number of dividing cells, which expand at the expense of normal marrow. In late stages of the disease, the entire marrow volume may be replaced by tumor cells.

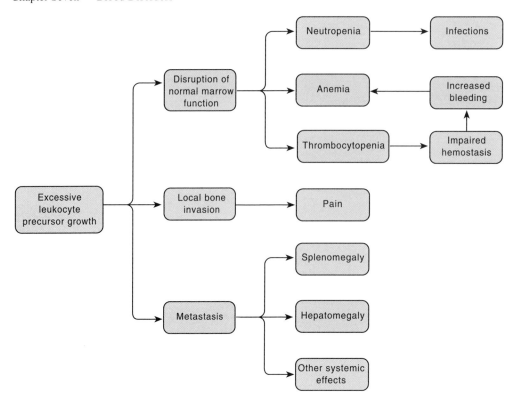

Figure 7.28   **The Principal Consequences of Leukemia.**

One consequence of marrow loss is severe neutropenia, or agranulocytosis, and the pronounced susceptibility to infection it produces. Another is anemia, as red cell production falls. It is compounded by the blood loss resulting from failure of normal hemostasis, which is in turn the result of the thrombocytopenia that follows the marrow's reduced platelet production. As the tumor continues to grow, it may invade to the bone that houses it, causing destruction of bone tissue and bone and joint pain. Metastasis to the spleen, liver, meninges, and lymph nodes is not uncommon and can compromise their function to yield additional systemic complications (fig. 7.28). Secondary growth may enlarge the infiltrated organ to produce hepatomegaly, splenomegaly, and enlarged lymph nodes (lymphadenopathy).

Classification

Leukemias can be classified according to their pattern of progression. They are said to be acute if the onset is abrupt, with more severe signs and symptoms and rapid progression. By contrast, chronic leukemia develops gradually and is associated with milder, less specific early effects—for example, fatigue or weight loss. Acute forms are also characterized by cells that are less well differentiated, while in chronic leukemia, the leukocytes are typically more mature (fig. 7.29).

Further classification is possible in that two different lines of differentiation can be the focus of the disorder. If the precursors of the granulocytes are neoplastic, the dominant marrow cell is a granular descendant. These are the **myeloblastic** or **granulocytic leukemias.** When the lymphocyte line of development is neoplastic, agranular descendants dominate and a **lymphoblastic** or **lymphocytic leukemia** is present. Rare leukemias of plasma cells and monocytes are also known.

Acute Lymphocytic Leukemia (ALL) ALL is predominantly seen in children and adolescents and is the most common malignancy affecting children. Anemias due to inadequate erythropoiesis produce progressive weakness and lack of stamina. Bleeding from thrombocytopenia, susceptibility to infection, bone pain, and cervical lymphadenopathy are also typical. Aggressive combination chemotherapy and the increasing mastery of bone marrow transplants have been quite successful in treating children. The prognosis is less optimistic for adults.

Acute Myeloblastic Leukemia (AML) The prognosis in AML is more optimistic. Intensive therapy achieves remission in other 70% of cases. Many patients suffer a recurrence of symptoms within 18 months. Diagnosis is typically made in those older than age 55.

ALL and AML present clinically similar pictures, so diagnostic certainty depends on analysis of a bone marrow biopsy. ALL patients have characteristic chromosomal abnormalities that can be used in determining a prognosis.

Chronic Lymphocytic Leukemia (CLL) The most common of the leukemias, CLL is typically seen in later life

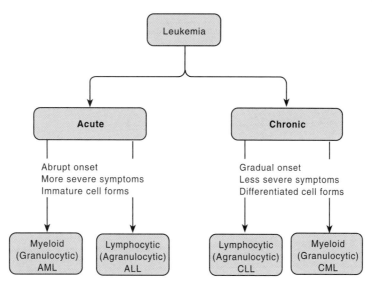

Figure 7.29   **Classification Terminology in Leukemia.**

(above 50 years of age). Its onset is gradual, and the fatigue, weight loss, and anorexia that accompany it are often accepted as being age-related. The cell most typically involved is the B lymphocyte, with extreme cases producing counts as high as 200,000/mm^3. However, these cells are not functional, so a deficiency of the immune system's antibody response results in a predisposition to bacterial infection. Infiltration of lymph nodes is responsible for the lymphadenopathy that is often present in CLL. In many patients, survival is prolonged by a course of chemotherapy.

Chronic Myeloblastic Leukemia (CML) People in the age range from 25 to 60 suffer the peak incidence of CML. In this condition, cells of the granulocyte line can reach counts as high as 100,000/mm^3. Liver and spleen infiltration is marked by symptoms of abdominal heaviness or dragging due to massive splenomegaly. Most sufferers of CML experience a **blast crisis** in the disease's later stage. This is a phase that resembles acute leukemia, with large numbers of immature leukocytes rapidly entering the blood, accelerating the patient's deterioration. Therapeutic intervention has no impact on survival. The presence of a damaged chromosome (#22), known as the **Philadelphia chromosome,** is noted in over 90% of the CML patients.

Lymphomas

Lymphomas are the most common tumor type after carcinomas. They are solid malignant tumors arising in the cells of lymphoid tissue: lymphocytes and their precursors. Their growth produces marrow and lymphoid tissue replacement as well as local effects related to expansion of the tumor mass—for example, invasion into adjacent tissues or compression of nearby organs. Loss of normal lymphoid tissue functions causes immune deficiencies that predispose to infection. Various mechanisms contribute to anemia, and lymphadenopathy is a typical and prominent sign.

Hodgkin's Lymphoma

This condition is also widely known as **Hodgkin's disease** (HD). Although relatively rare, males and blacks experience higher rates of HD. It arises most often in young adults, usually in a single, painless, cervical lymph node. This is followed by spread to adjacent nodes and then more widely dispersed lymphoid organs in a consistent pattern. Splenomegaly and lymphadenopathy are usually present, as are fatigue, wasting, and fever. T-cell immune functions are also usually depressed.

HD has four subtypes based on the cell types that dominate and other histological features. All HD diagnosis is substantiated on the basis of its characteristic marker, the **Reed-Sternberg** (RS) **cell.** This is a large, multinucleate cell with other distinguishing cytologic features (fig. 7.30). Clinical staging in HD is indicated in table 7.9. Therapeutic approach and prognosis are related to the stage of the disease, with younger patients expecting a better outcome than the elderly. Etiology is suspected to involve the interplay between a genetic susceptibility and infection with the Epstein-Barr virus.

Non-Hodgkin's Lymphomas (NHLs)

This group of tumors arises in lymphoid tissue, and its B and T lymphocyte lines in particular. Lymph nodes are the usual primary site, with spread to other nodes and lymphoid organs occurring in a less systematic pattern than is seen in HD. In some cases, following extensive metastasis, cells escape into the blood to mimic leukemia.

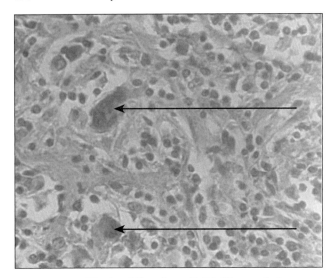

Figure 7.30   **The Reed-Sternberg Cell is Diagnostic for Hodgkin's Disease.** The arrows indicate two R-S cells in this tissue sample from a lymph node biopsy.

This axillary lymph node is typical of the many that were enlarged and heavily infiltrated in a 34-year-old male who finally succumbed to Hodgkin's disease. He had been weak and listless for some time prior to his death because of extensive metastases. This section shows complete loss of lymph node architecture and heavy cellular infiltration throughout the node. The Reed-Sternberg cell is easily distinguished by its size and the presence of several nuclei.

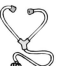

Focus on Complications of Therapy for HD

Note that the radiation chemotherapy used in HD can have suppressing effects on the marrow and immune system. These can complicate the prognosis by adding to the anemia and infection burdens that the patient must bear. In 15% of cases, radiation therapy for HD is implicated in the development of new malignancies.

The classification of the diverse group of lymphoid tumors is complex and has been controversial. The widely used, but not universally accepted, **Working Formulation** shown in table 7.10 combines prognosis data with cytologic features to yield a classification that distinguishes 10 NHLs. Generally, the prognosis in NHL is not as clearly related to its clinical stage as is the case in Hodgkin's lymphoma.

Bone Marrow Transplantation

In conditions where the marrow has been destroyed or replaced by a tumor, marrow transplantation can be effective in restoring marrow functions. In selecting marrow for transplantation, it is essential to avoid incompatibility be-

Table 7.9	The Ann Arbor System of Hodgkin's Disease Staging. More Hopeful Prognosis Is Associated with Lower Stages.

Stage I

Tumor present at a single lymph node region.

Stage II

Tumor present at two or more lymph node regions, all of which are on the same side of the diaphragm.

Stage III

Tumor present at two or more lymph node regions, with involvement on both sides of the diaphragm.

Stage IV

Widespread metastasis to one or more nonlymphatic organs.

Further classification is based on the absence (A) or presence (B) of systemic symptoms (e.g., weight loss, fever). The subscript E indicates invasion to nonlymphatic organs, while the subscript S indicates invasion into the spleen. Stage IIIB would therefore indicate lymph node involvement on both sides of the diaphragm, with systemic symptoms present but no indications of splenic involvement.

Table 7.10	Staging of the Ten Non-Hodgkins Lymphoma Subtypes

Low Grade

Small lymphocytic lymphoma
Follicular lymphoma: small, cleaved cell predominant
Follicular lymphoma: small and large cell types mixed

Intermediate Grade

Follicular lymphoma: large cell type predominant
Diffuse, small, cleaved cell lymphoma
Diffuse, mixed small and large cell lymphoma
Diffuse, large cell lymphoma

High Grade

Large cell, immunoblastic lymphoma
Lymphoblastic lymphoma
Small, noncleaved cell lymphoma

---

tween the donor's and recipient's human leukocyte antigens (see chapter 4). Identical twins or siblings are usually selected.

The procedure begins with removal of marrow from the donor, usually from the hip bones. A volume equal to an ordinary wine bottle, 750 ml, is withdrawn and passed through a screen to free the cells from their stroma supports. The freed cells are then introduced into the recipient via an intravenous injection. The marrow cells circulate and selectively establish in the recipient's marrow. The mechanism involves receptor-mediated adherence to endothelium and marrow stromal elements. Once in place, normal marrow differentiation proceeds.

Of course, where the human leukocyte antigens are other than identical, immune rejection may arise. To increase the likelihood that the transplant will be accepted, the recipient's immune response can be suppressed. As we have noted, this may interfere with erythropoiesis, clotting, and infection defense, so that posttransplant red cell and platelet transfusions may be necessary. In addition, coping with the recipient's infection risk may involve elaborate isolation and special procedures for the handling of food and therapeutic agents.

 Checkpoint 7.3

Recall the number of references to blood transfusions in the previous sections. By now, your keen analytical powers have identified that blood doesn't grow on trees, so perhaps you should consider becoming a blood donor. When people need blood, they usually need it badly and right now. Although a bit more involved, you might also volunteer to have your marrow "typed" and register your availability as a bone marrow donor.

Case Study

A 21-year-old university student went to his Campus Health Center. He complained of feeling weak and tired, experiencing increasing loss of appetite and periodic episodes of diarrhea and constipation. He had lost 30 pounds in the past year and was on a strictly vegetarian diet. He reported that he ate only "whole, natural foods," completely excluding animal products and taking no vitamin or mineral supplements. His goal in adopting this diet was to avoid introducing "toxins" into his body. Recent sensations of burning in his tongue and tingling in his arms had prompted him to seek medical advice.

On examination he appeared pale and emaciated, with normal neurologic signs. When his blood test results were reported, they indicated a megaloblastic anemia with some distortion of red cell shapes. His hemoglobin value was 10 g/dl, the increase in MCV was pronounced, and his serum cobalamin was significantly below normal. With no history of gastric problems, the diagnosis of cobalamin deficiency anemia was made and a regimen of dietary supplementation prescribed. The patient was agreeable to the therapy and his health was soon restored.

Commentary

This classic dietary deficiency condition needs little comment, except to note that the patient's paresthesias (abnormal sensations) were an indication of a worsening condition. Had he ignored the neurological signs, the consequences might have been much more serious.

Although many who embark upon dietary regimens are not as severely affected, this individual interpreted his early signs and symptoms as being caused by the "contaminants" in his food, so he intensified his dietary vigilance, only to compound the problem. However, he readily accepted the recommended supplements of vitamin B_{12}, commenting that he wasn't "stupid, I just want to be healthy." In some extreme cases, there may be resistance to dietary change. In these situations, the diet is seen as integral to a philosophic position or as an indication of one's discipline and worthiness. At any rate, in this case the outcome was a happy one.

Key Concepts

1. Conversion of the fluid blood to a nonflowing gel coagulation is the dominant mechanism that opposes blood loss (p. 171).

2. Blood coagulation depends on the formation of insoluble fibrin filaments via the sequential activation of a cascade of plasma enzymes called clotting factors (pp. 171–172).

3. The extrinsic and intrinsic pathways interact to produce an effective coagulation response (pp. 172–173).

4. An anticoagulation system is balanced against the coagulation system to prevent unnecessary or too

widespread coagulation that might interfere with normal blood flow (pp. 176–178).

5. An inadequate hemostatic response may be the result of decreased platelet numbers, caused by insufficient production, excessive clearance from the blood, or a functional deficit in the platelets themselves (pp. 178–180).

6. An inadequate hemostatic response may be the result of a clotting factor deficiency caused by insufficient hepatic production or by excessive clearance from the blood by widespread coagulation, which depletes CF numbers (pp. 180–184).

7. Bleeding may be caused by a weakness of small blood vessel walls resulting from damage or defective connective tissue support (pp. 184–185).

8. Anemia may result from inadequate red cell production in an abnormal marrow or from a dietary deficiency that limits production by an otherwise normal marrow (pp. 185–189).

9. Red blood cell depletion sufficient to produce anemia may be caused by genetic red cell defects that favor their clearance from the blood by macrophages, by premature membrane rupture due to mechanical or immune-mediated damage, or by excessive splenic clearance (pp. 189–192).

10. Excessive RBC production may result from a benign tumor of red cell precursors or from excessive marrow stimulus by abnormally high levels of EPO or other less clearly understood control factors (pp. 192–193).

11. Neutropenia, and the increased infection risk it produces, is most often the result of therapeutic marrow suppression (p. 194).

12. Leukemia is a primary malignant tumor of leukocyte precursors in the marrow, which typically, although not in every case, spill over into the blood in large numbers (pp. 194–197).

13. Lymphomas are the solid, malignant tumors of lymphocytes and their precursors that arise in lymphoid tissue in lymph nodes and various other sites (pp. 197–198).

14. To augment marrow function, a closely matched donor's marrow may be transplanted into a recipient whose marrow function is critically depressed by tumor growth or other suppressant factors (pp. 198–199).

REVIEW ACTIVITIES

1. Cover the legend in figure 7.3 and identify the following features of the diagram:

RBCs and platelets in lumen	fibrin mesh
subendothelial connective tissue	platelet plug
muscle of vessel wall	RBCs in clot
vessel endothelium and BM	

2. Without reference to the text, lay out a flow chart that illustrates how thrombin contributes to three key components of the blood coagulation response. When you're done, see if your layout tells the same story as figure 7.10. Is there any positive feedback involved? Can you see why this might be usefully applied in the context of hemostasis?

3. Explain how marrow suppression might interfere with disease resistance. Mention at least three blood cell types.

4. Complete the following table.
   Use an asterisk to denote the term that refers to a bruise.

Pattern of Bleeding	Distinguishing Characteristic
Purpura	
Ecchymosis	
Petechia	
Hematoma	

5. Make up a ready reference list, based on the three formed elements and the abnormal conditions involving each, in support of the concept that reduced formed element numbers may derive from inadequate production or excessive clearance from the blood.

6. Check back to figure 7.22 to verify that you can recognize the sickled cells as opposed to the normal RBCs. Also note the RBC shapes in figure 7.23.

7. Is it true that all leukemias are characterized by increased plasma leukocyte counts? Is there a descriptive term that could be included as part of your answer? If you're not clear, look late in the chapter for help.

Hemodynamic Disorders

How should it happen that if you tie the arteries, immediately the parts not only become torpid, and frigid, and look pale, but at length cease even to be nourished?

WILLIAM HARVEY
AN ANATOMICAL DISQUISITION ON THE MOTION OF THE HEART AND BLOOD IN ANIMALS

Hemodynamic disorders arise from interruptions of normal blood flow. As noted in chapter 7, coagulation of the blood limits blood loss when vessel damage occurs. However, if blood coagulation is activated without the threat of blood loss, problems result. These are caused by the formation of a **thrombus** within a vessel by the process of **thrombosis.** Embolism and infarction are the other hemodynamic disorders that may follow thrombosis.

THROMBOSIS

A thrombus is a mass of platelets, red and white blood cells, and fibrin (fig. 8.1). It is different from a clot in three ways. First, a thrombus never forms outside a blood vessel, whereas clots usually do. Second, a thrombus develops from and maintains a point of attachment to a blood vessel's wall. The third difference between a clot and a thrombus lies in the organization of their components. When a clot forms, its fibrin strands entrap formed elements to form a more or less homogeneous mass. By contrast, thrombosis yields a mass in which the blood components are highly organized.

Thrombosis starts at a point where platelets adhere to the vascular wall. As described in chapter 6, platelet adherence occurs at points where the endothelium is irregular or at points where it has been stripped away to expose subendothelial collagen. After initial contact is made, other platelets stick to those first at the scene, forming a mass of fused platelets that adheres firmly to the vessel's inner surface. Platelet activation follows, and the intrinsic coagulation cascade is triggered.

Note that in this instance, there is no vessel injury that threatens blood loss, yet a coagulation cascade is being activated. Normally, thrombin is the agent that stimulates the intrinsic pathway, but in this situation none has been formed. Activation depends on the collagen and other components of the subendothelium that the endothelial injury has exposed to the blood. An inactive clotting factor called **Hageman factor,** or **factor XII,** is activated by this exposure and thrombin and fibrin are produced. But rather than a formless mass of fibrin forming a clot, the blood's motion affects the process and a thrombus results.

The initially formed fibrin deposits on the surface of the platelet plug that lies over the injury site. Where flow is relatively rapid, as in an artery or through a cardiac ventricle, platelets in the blood adhere to the fibrin surface as they arrive at the site. They become activated and further coagulation follows. Additional fibrin deposition results and the next platelets to arrive adhere to the surface. This repeating process yields an alternating series of platelets and fibrin layers known as **lines of Zahn** (fig. 8.2). The process may stop at this point as the flowing blood rapidly removes activated clotting factors to limit fibrin formation. When flow is slower, as in veins or a cardiac atrium, activated clotting factors remain longer and coagulation starts to dominate. The result is an accumulation of coagulated blood massing over the alternating layers of platelets and

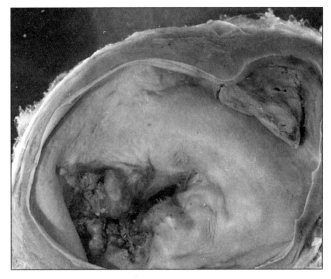

Figure 8.1 **Thrombus.** The damaged valve at left caused sluggish flow through this atrium, a condition favoring formation of the thrombus visible at the upper right.
This view of the floor of the left atrium was obtained from the autopsy of a man whose mitral valve was damaged as a result of an attack of rheumatic fever at the age of 9. Although he tolerated the problem fairly well, by age 39 his condition had started to deteriorate, and his heart ultimately failed when he was 46. The specimen shows the degree to which the mitral valve had been damaged so that its opening and closing were significantly affected. More details of rheumatic fever are presented in chapter 10, but of particular relevance here is the mass tucked into the auricular appendage of the atrium. This is a thrombus that is attached to the atrial endocardium. It probably formed as a result of the obstruction to atrial emptying caused by the damaged valve.

fibrin to form what is known as a **red cap.** The flow of blood over the developing thrombus causes its components to build up in the downstream direction (fig. 8.3). In such a larger thrombus, the region of alternating layers is called the **mixed region.** The pattern of layering is usually less distinct in a venous thrombus because of the slower blood flow that allows more intermixing of platelets and fibrin.

Given the contribution of blood flow to thrombosis, there are implications for postmortem assessment. After somatic death, blood flow stops. This means that clotting factors activated by postmortem tissue changes soon accumulate, causing coagulation of the blood. The clots formed in this way are large, red, gelatinous, and occlusive. This indicates they formed after normal blood flow had stopped. On the other hand, if during an autopsy a coagulated mass is found attached to a vessel's wall, and has a pattern of alternating platelets and fibrin, it is a thrombus and therefore must have formed antemortem (before death) while the blood was still flowing. Sometimes a postmortem clot will not form until the cells have begun to settle out of the blood. The result is a lighter-colored mass that lacks erythrocytes.

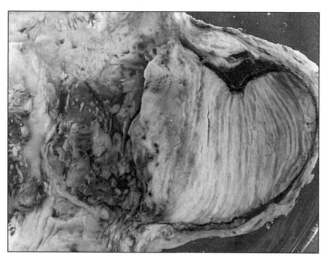

Figure 8.2   **Lines of Zahn.** The alternating deposition of platelets and red cells trapped by fibrin produce the lines of Zahn visible in this arterial thrombus.

This is a section through the aorta of an 87-year-old man who was admitted to hospital following his arrival at the emergency room coughing blood and complaining of back pain. He died suddenly soon after admission. At autopsy he was found to have severe hardening of the arteries, but there were no signs of heart damage. A large aortic aneurysm (bulge) was also discovered. Its wall had weakened and bulged and a large thrombus had formed within it. The lines of Zahn can be clearly seen, as can the lining of the aorta that is badly diseased. The aorta had bulged against the adjacent lung, compressing and penetrating it to produce bleeding into the surrounding tissues and airways. The result was pain and the coughing of blood. The aorta's rupture, at a point not visible in the photograph, was the cause of death.

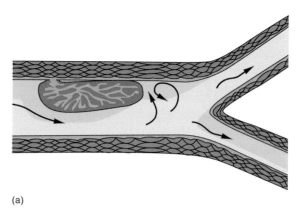

(a)

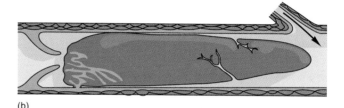

(b)

Figure 8.3   **Arterial and Venous Thrombosis.** (*a*) An arterial thrombus is smaller and denser than (*b*) a venous thrombus. Note the attaching mass of aggregated platelets where each thrombus originated, the lines of Zahn, and the large red cap of the venous thrombus.

Factors Predisposing to Thrombosis

Having considered how thrombi form, let's now turn to the reasons that underlie their development. There are three factors that predispose to thrombus formation: endothelial damage, altered blood flow, and a blood hypercoagulation state.

Endothelial Damage

When a vessel's lining is damaged, endothelial cells may be stripped away or they may draw away from adjacent cells to expose subendothelial collagen. This condition favors platelet adherence, activation, aggregation, and the initiation of thrombosis. A similar change can occur in the cells of the endocardial surface. The endocardium, and cardiac valves in particular, may be damaged by certain bacterial infections. Endocardium may also be affected by damage to the myocardium, which lies immediately deep to it. In either case, platelet adherence is favored by the resulting surface changes.

In the arterial system, two principal mechanisms underlie most endothelial damage. The first involves the normal wear and tear to which the endothelium is subjected.

This is called **hemodynamic stress,** because it is the result of the motion of blood as it is driven through the arterial tree under pressure. During each systolic contraction, the pressure developed causes the arteries to expand and elongate. They then return to their unstretched configuration because of the elastic recoil of their walls. This process is repeated an average of over 70 times per minute. Although the endothelial cells are able to withstand the pressures to which they are exposed, elevation of systemic arterial pressures will increase the level of hemodynamic stress. Thus, any factors that contribute to high blood pressure or **hypertension** will increase endothelial damage and the thrombosis associated with it. The second major source of endothelial damage is the vascular disease called arteriosclerosis, which is described in chapter 9.

In the venous system, endothelia are less commonly damaged, but they are unable to avoid the effects of certain conditions. Some inflammations affect the venous endothelium. For example, the mesenteric veins demonstrate increased thrombosis in appendicitis, perhaps because of irritants carried by the veins from the site of tissue damage. Some tumors also seem to affect venous endothelia. An example is the increased thrombosis of the renal vein in cases of renal carcinoma where endothelial damage may be due to venous drainage of irritating tumor products.

Therapeutic intervention can cause endothelial damage in veins and thus promote **iatrogenic thrombosis.** (Recall that iatrogenic diseases are the result of medical or surgical interventions.) For example, irritation to the endothelium caused by an intravenous needle in long-term fluid administration may induce thrombosis.

Both venous and arterial endothelia are adversely affected by trauma. Thrombosis occurs more frequently following auto accidents, major fractures, falls, or even surgical interventions. In particular, endothelia show an increased predisposition to platelet adherence for periods of up to two weeks after major surgery. Endothelia are also affected by ionizing radiation, high levels of plasma cholesterol, and by components of tobacco smoke.

Flow Abnormalities

Change from the normal pattern of blood flow is the second factor that contributes to thrombosis because it involves increased platelet contact with the endothelium. The two most common hemodynamic changes are reduction in the rate of blood flow (or its complete stoppage—stasis) and turbulence in the blood.

Flow-rate reduction in the arterial system causes a decrease in the axial flow of blood (see chapter 2, fig. 2.8). As a result, platelets in the central column of formed elements move nearer to the vessel wall. This change increases the likelihood of contact, adherence, and thrombosis. There are two principal causes of reduced blood flow rates: cardiac damage, which reduces the heart's pumping capability, and increased blood viscosity. It is obvious that a weakened heart may be unable to maintain normal blood flow in arteries, but the problem may be even greater in the venous system. Because flow is normally slower in veins, any drop in cardiac pumping efficiency can produce significant declines in venous flow that result in thrombosis. When blood viscosity is increased, there is more resistance to flow and, hence, the blood moves more slowly. (By analogy, a mechanical pump moves water more easily than it can move pancake syrup.) Blood viscosity changes can result from increased numbers of formed elements, as in the case of increased white blood cells in leukemia. Alternatively, a dehydrated patient's blood will be more viscous because there is less plasma in which to suspend the normal number of formed elements.

In the venous system, increased blood viscosity reduces the rate of blood flow, but two other factors more often affect venous blood flow. One of these is physical inactivity. Reduction or lack of normal physical activity slows the rate of circulation because of decreased demand by the muscles and, more importantly, because of the loss of skeletal muscle pumping. Peripheral veins, and especially the leg veins, rely on the skeletal muscles to aid blood flow. As muscles contract, they shorten and thicken, compressing the veins that pass over and between them. In conjunction with the veins' internal system of leaflet valves, this massage of

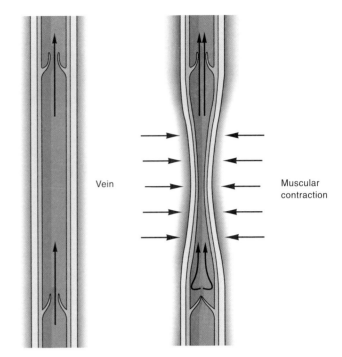

Vein   Muscular contraction

Figure 8.4   **Venous Valves.** Venous blood returning to the heart is assisted by the contraction of adjacent skeletal muscle. In conjunction with venous valves, these contractions produce forward flow and reduce retrograde flow. Inactivity, such as bed rest, compromises this action, causing slower venous flow and favoring thrombosis.

veins by contracting muscle makes a major contribution to venous return from the legs (fig. 8.4).

A second cause of reduced venous blood flow involves a common form of venous pathology. In **varicose veins,** blood flow rates are reduced because of disrupted functioning of the leaflet valves. Venous varices (singular, varix) are regions of the vein wall that become so weakened that they are unable to maintain normal muscular tone. The weakened vein walls sag away from the blood within their lumina to form irregular bulges. As a result, venous pressure drops and the rate of blood flow is reduced. But, significantly, the bulging vein walls prevent opposing valve leaflets from closing. This means loss of the muscle pumping, allowing blood to pool within the veins. This greatly increases the likelihood of platelet contact with endothelia that are quite irregular due to the distortion of the varix wall, so thrombosis is doubly favored. It is therefore not surprising that over 90% of venous thrombi are localized in the superficial veins of the legs. Venous flow rates can be reduced to the point of stasis of the blood, which further predisposes to thrombus formation by greatly favoring the local accumulation of activated clotting factors.

Turbulent, irregular blood flow increases platelet contact with cardiac and vascular linings. Blood normally flows smoothly through open, regular channels. In the heart, damaged valves may present narrowed or otherwise distorted surfaces that cause blood to swirl over their ab-

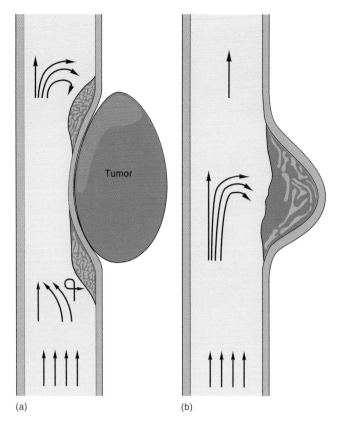

(a)   (b)

Figure 8.5 **Thrombosis in Deformed Vessels.** Deformation of a vessel wall by external compression (*a*) or by changes in the wall itself, such as an aneurysm (*b*), can create turbulent flow and lead to thrombosis.

normal endocardium. Similarly, in cases of congenital cardiac defects, abnormal flow channels in a malformed heart cause turbulence and thrombosis. A thrombus that forms within a cardiac chamber is known as a **mural thrombus.** In blood vessels, typically arteries, turbulence is produced by distortions in a vessel's wall that interfere with smooth flow. One cause of such arterial distortion may be an expanding mass adjacent to the vessel. A tumor or an adjacent organ that is inflamed and swollen can compress the vessel (fig. 8.5*a*). A weakened arterial wall pushed out by arterial pressure forms a pouchlike bulge called an **aneurysm.** Blood flowing past an aneurysm swirls into it, splashing platelets against its stretched endothelium. Thrombosis soon follows (fig. 8.5*b*; see also fig. 8.2). The causes of aneurysm formation are considered in chapter 9.

Blood Hypercoagulation

In situations in which turbulent flow or endothelial damage seem not to be involved, thrombosis is attributed to blood being **hypercoagulable.** In this condition, thrombosis occurs without increased contact between platelets and endothelia. Instead, hypercoagulability of the blood seems to be related to malfunctions in the complex and finely balanced systems that regulate the coagulation and anticoagu-

lation systems. Some of these malfunctions are due to genetic defects that cause an overproduction of coagulation promoters or a lack of coagulation inhibitors. In other cases, immune mechanisms are involved with antibodies against heparin or key plasma proteins indirectly contributing to enhanced coagulation.

In some cases of thrombosis, an underlying reason for the hypercoagulability may be known—for example, the liver's overproduction of clotting factors during pregnancy or, in the elderly, a deficiency of the coagulation inhibitor PG-I$_2$. In other cases, such as in those who are obese or smoke, the reasons remain obscure.

✓ *Checkpoint 8.1*

In looking back over the many factors that predispose to thrombosis, you will appreciate that several may be at work in many of your patients. For example, the hospitalized patient is at greater risk simply due to confinement in bed because of the peripheral pooling of the blood that results. Surgery also favors thrombosis, and so the bedridden, postsurgical patient who may also be an obese smoker is much at risk. As another example, there is little surprise when thrombosis occurs following radiation therapy in a cancer patient who may also have severe arterial disease and varicose veins.

SEQUELAE OF THROMBOSIS

The pathological consequence of some event is the **sequela** of that event. There are several possible sequelae to thrombosis. These are resolution, organization, propagation, infarction, and embolism. The least threat is presented when a thrombus undergoes **resolution.** In resolving the problem, the anticoagulation system overcomes the factors that favor thrombus formation. This means that thrombi that start to form do not all continue to develop. Of thrombi that do form, many are completely broken down or substantially reduced in size so as to lack any significant effects. There are indications that moderate exercise increases thrombus resolution. Cardiopulmonary fitness has been shown to be associated with an increase in the activity of the fibrinolytic system.

Another sequela of thrombosis is **organization.** The process consists of phagocytic digestion of the thrombus two to three days after it forms. Platelets and fibrin are then replaced by fibrous connective tissue. Endothelium forms over the organizing tissue, with the result that the thrombus becomes incorporated into the wall. Small channels often form in a thrombus undergoing organization. The process, termed **recanalization,** allows blood to flow through the obstructing thrombus, reducing ischemia downstream from the thrombus (fig. 8.6).

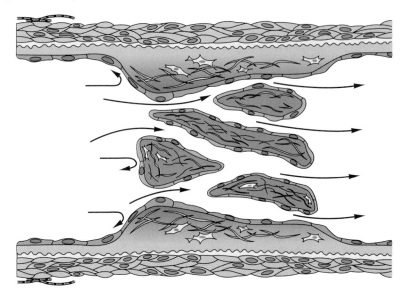

Figure 8.6 **Recanalization of a Thrombus.** This diagram shows a longitudinal section through an organizing thrombus that has occluded the vessel. The newly formed channels lined by endothelium partially restore flow.

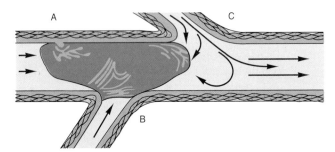

Figure 8.7 **Propagation of a Venous Thrombus.** From an initial site of formation at A, the new deposition of platelets and fibrin from the joining vein at B has extended the process. As thrombosis proceeds, blood from the converging vessel at C continues the extension of the thrombus along the lumen.

Propagation of the thrombus is another possible sequela. In this situation, a thrombus, once formed, enlarges by extending farther along the vessel, usually a vein. In such cases, continued coagulation may produce a red cap that extends for a significant distance within a vein's lumen (see fig. 8.3*b*). In other cases, particularly when one vein converges with another, propagation occurs because the surface of the initially formed thrombus serves as the site for further platelet adherence and further thrombosis (fig. 8.7).

Infarction

A major sequela of thrombosis is **infarction.** This is the process in which an **infarct,** a region of necrosis caused by ischemia, is formed. The ischemia is often caused by a thrombus that narrows or completely occludes the lumen of a vessel. Infarction is most common and most serious in arteries because they directly supply oxygen and various key nutrients. When arterial stenosis (narrowing) occurs, it also reduces waste removal, with toxic effects adding to the tis-

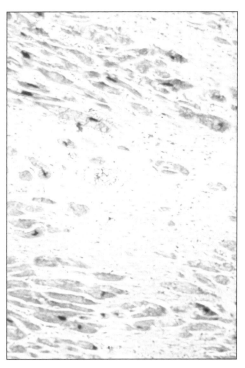

Figure 8.8 **An Infarct in the Myocardium.** The dark nuclei are present in still-living cells at the periphery of the infarct. Other nonnucleated cells are dead but still intact. The central region is scar tissue that has replaced the necrotic muscle tissue.

sue damage as levels of waste products rise. Note that this is a more serious situation than anemia, in which only oxygen delivery is reduced. In such cases, a tissue's shift to anaerobic energy metabolism can limit tissue disruption.

Infarction in most tissues results in the formation of a firm, relatively dry region of coagulation necrosis. After an acute inflammatory response, the necrotic tissue is broken down and replaced by scar tissue (fig. 8.8). In the brain, infarct resolution is quite different. Liquefaction necrosis causes debris-filled fluid to accumulate at the site of infarction. When the debris is cleared, a fluid-filled cavity remains. Fibrosis is limited in the brain, so the cavities are not filled in with scar tissue. Instead, the cavity's size is reduced somewhat by **gliosis,** a proliferation of the neuroglia at the margin of the cavity.

Because of the critical functions they perform, the two most seriously damaging types of infarction are cerebral infarction and myocardial infarction (MI). Most infarction involving the arterial system is caused by thrombosis, but other factors can have the same result. For example, external pressure can narrow or even completely compress an artery. A tumor might affect an adjacent artery in this way. Another common cause of infarction is vascular disease, in which thickening of the vessel wall reduces the size of the lumen.

Venous obstruction as a cause of infarction is much less common because of the vascular pattern of venous drainage. Several drainage vessels, called **collaterals,** usually serve the same area. If one should become occluded, blood can flow through the unobstructed collateral vessels, limiting any interference with blood drainage. Even though infarction can be prevented by venous collaterals, venous drainage from the affected tissues may be reduced. This situation arises in the leg veins and although no actual inflammation may be involved, the term **thrombophlebitis** is used to describe it. In such cases, the reduced drainage produces swelling and pain in the leg as fluid accumulates. The skin overlying the region is also prone to ulceration and infection; further consequences of compromised venous drainage.

Factors Affecting Infarction

We have seen that infarction can lead to serious and potentially fatal consequences, especially when it occurs in the brain or myocardium. However, in other tissues vascular occlusion may have little or no effect. The outcome depends, for the most part, on four factors: (1) the tissue's innate vulnerability to hypoxia; (2) the pattern of its vascular supply; (3) the capacity of the blood to deliver oxygen; and (4) the rate of development of the occlusion.

As described in chapter 1, tissues vary in their ability to tolerate hypoxia. Nervous tissue, in particular, is very sensitive to oxygen deprivation. Even brief periods of brain hypoxia can cause a fatal infarction. In the myocardium, muscle tissue is less sensitive than nervous tissue, but it will succumb to chronic hypoxia. The fibroblasts of the myocardial stroma are much more resistant to low oxygen levels and are thus adapted for work in the repair process that may follow infarction.

The pattern of a tissue's vascular supply is another important influence on the effect of infarction. The essential element is an alternative route by which arterial blood can reach a tissue. The most important factor here is the degree of **anastomosis** the vessels demonstrate. When arteries

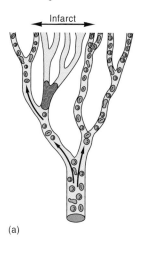

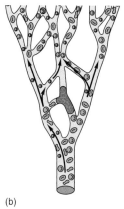

Figure 8.9 **Arterial Anastomosis and Its Consequences.** (*a*) Lack of anastomosis in a tissue makes it more susceptible to ischemia if a vessel is occluded. (*b*) A high degree of anastomosis greatly reduces the risk of ischemia and infarction.

anastomose, they branch and then rejoin. This means, in effect, that the blood can reach a given region by more than one route (fig. 8.9). A tissue with a high degree of anastomosis is more likely to resist the effects of stenosis or occlusion.

An infarct develops more rapidly in an individual whose oxygen delivery capability is already reduced. In such cases, tissues are already partially hypoxic, and less stenosis is required to produce sufficient hypoxia to cause infarction. Such situations exist, for example, in the anemic and in those whose weakened hearts are only marginally able to meet pumping demands.

The rate at which an artery or vein becomes occluded is another factor that affects infarction. The essential mechanism here is the time needed for new collateral vessels to form. These grow out from the existing vessels of an ischemic tissue in a response that can reverse the tissue's oxygen deprivation. Unfortunately, the new vessels can form only slowly, so that only when stenosis and ischemia develop slowly can new collaterals be effective in limiting, or preventing, infarction.

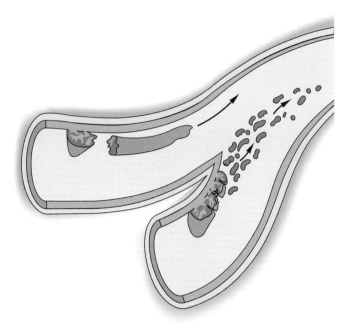

Figure 8.10 **Formation of Thromboemboli.** The gelatinous and easily fragmented red cap of a venous thrombus is a common source of large or multiple small emboli.

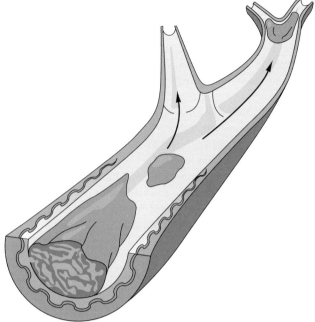

Figure 8.11 **Thromboembolism.** The thromboembolus will lodge at some point in the artery's downstream branches to occlude the vessel.

Embolism

Another important sequela of thrombosis is **embolism.** Embolism is the sudden occlusion of a blood vessel by an **embolus,** an abnormal mass moving with the bloodstream. Anything in a vessel other than the normally fluid blood constitutes an embolus. Interruption of blood flow by embolism is a common cause of infarction.

Thromboembolism

The most common type of embolus is a **thromboembolus,** formed when a thrombus or part of a thrombus breaks away from the vascular wall and is carried off by the moving blood. Emboli originating at arterial or cardiac surfaces consist mainly of fused platelets and fibrin, and are usually smaller and more dense than those formed in the venous system. As a thrombus forms in a vein, its red cap can increase greatly in size as blood coagulation continues. When such a mass becomes detached, a very large embolus results. Alternatively, a large, gelatinous thrombus, tailing downstream in the venous flow, might break up to release several small emboli into the bloodstream (fig. 8.10).

A thromboembolus can become detached from a vascular surface because of normal variations in blood flow. Temporary pressure changes that result from postural changes or exercise could contribute to loosening a thrombus. The resumption of normal activity, after a period of inactivity that favors formation of the thrombus, might also be a factor. Thus, a patient who begins walking after prolonged bed rest runs a higher risk of thromboembolism. Surgery, physiotherapy, or other therapeutic manipulations might also con-

tribute. Another significant factor is the fibrinolytic system, which by fibrin degradation can directly loosen the wall attachments of thrombi. Whatever the cause of thromboembolism, its effects are potentially very serious.

The principal consequence of thromboembolus formation arises when an embolus lodges in a vessel at some distance from its point of formation. Generally, this results in occlusion of the vessel. The site of occlusion and rate of infarction will vary depending on the point in the vascular system at which the thromboembolus first arises.

Arterial Thromboemboli In the arterial system, large vessels branch to form smaller vessels, which in turn branch repeatedly until capillaries with very small diameters are formed. Thus, a thromboembolus in arteries is carried by the blood through successively smaller vessels until, inevitably, it becomes trapped and occlusion occurs (fig. 8.11). Such abrupt occlusion may result in an infarct, whose size depends on the size of the blocked vessel and the degree of arterial anastomosis in the tissue involved. Arterial thromboemboli are most typically formed from cardiac mural thrombi, cardiac valve thrombi, or at sites of aneurysm or arterial disease. Arising from such sites, the emboli are most likely to lodge in the arteries of the lower limbs, kidney, spleen, or brain.

Venous Thromboemboli Throughout the venous system, vessels converge rather than branch. This means that blood flows through increasingly large vessels until it reaches the heart. Thromboemboli that are carried in the systemic venous return, therefore, have little likelihood of occluding a vessel on their way to the heart. However, from the right heart they are pumped into the pulmonary arterial system. As these vessels branch, the emboli ultimately come to an artery through which they cannot pass. Although infarction can result, the effects of the resulting occlusion will tend to be minimized by four factors. One of these is clot retraction. If retraction of thrombus fibrin occurs after it lodges in the pulmonary arterial system, it may reduce the size of the embolus. Such reduction might allow adequate blood to pass through to the dependent tissues beyond. A second factor is the double blood supply of the lung. Its tissue can extract oxygen and nutrients from the blood that comes directly from the heart as well as from the bronchial arteries, which supply the lung independently. Thus, if one source of supply is cut off, the tissues are still supplied by the other. (But note that if a weakened heart, or other factors, reduce arterial blood pressure, bronchial arterial flow may be reduced to the point where it cannot prevent infarction.) A third and quite important factor is the fibrinolytic system. In the lungs, the fibrinolytic system functions at a higher level of activation. This helps to loosen and dissolve thromboemboli that lodge in the pulmonary vessels. Fourth, the fact that many thromboemboli are small will allow occlusion of only minor pulmonary vessels, with correspondingly small effects.

Because of its position in the circulatory system, the lung receives and traps most thromboemboli in its arteries. The factors just described, especially the dual blood supply and increased fibrinolytic activity, make the lung well suited to handle the thromboemboli that are delivered to it. The lung, in effect, acts as a filter that removes thromboemboli before they reach the systemic arteries, preventing them from reaching vessels that might deliver them to the brain or other vital organs. If small, pulmonary thromboemboli produce no signs of symptoms.

However effective it is in coping with thromboemboli, when emboli are large in size or great in number, even the lung will suffer ill effects. These effects can cause partial loss of pulmonary function or even somatic death through large-scale pulmonary infarction and hemorrhage.

The great majority of pulmonary thromboemboli arise in the veins of the leg and contribute to a substantial number of all hospital deaths. When larger emboli occlude pulmonary vessels, upstream blood pressure is increased. This often leads to vessel damage, which causes hemorrhage into the pulmonary tissues. If sufficiently large or numerous arteries are occluded, the resulting back pressure can cause weakening and ultimate failure of the right heart. The danger posed by the massive thromboemboli that can originate in the leg veins is very great. These long, cordlike masses may become trapped at the heart's pulmonary valve or within the pulmonary arteries, shutting off virtually all flow to the lungs. As a result, cardiac output drops below critical levels, and death follows (fig. 8.12).

Not all thromboemboli arising in veins end up in the lung. Those forming in the veins that drain the intestine, stomach, spleen, and other abdominal viscera are carried to the liver (fig. 8.13). They travel in the hepatic portal ves-

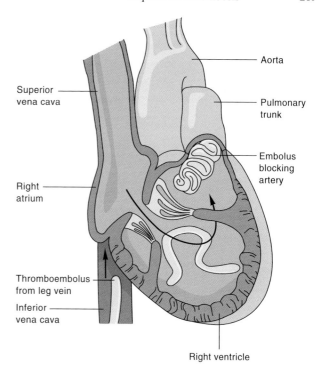

Figure 8.12 **Massive Pulmonary Embolism.** A large gelatinous thromboembolus, the red cap of a leg vein thrombus, has been carried to the right ventricle by the returning blood. It has blocked all pulmonary flow to prevent any oxygenation of the blood.

 Checkpoint 8.2

Just to emphasize the point, an embolus is always trapped when the blood that carries it enters a vessel smaller than the embolus. Therefore, embolism occurs only in arteries. Since veins converge, as an embolus is carried through them it finds itself in larger and larger vessels, so no embolism can occur. The exception is the complex of hepatic portal veins that branch to form smaller vessels within the liver.

sels, which normally carry newly absorbed nutrients to the liver for processing. Because the hepatic artery provides arterial blood directly to the liver, even when emboli obstruct hepatic portal channels, infarction seldom occurs.

Therapy in Thrombosis and Thromboembolism Three approaches are taken in dealing with thrombosis and thromboembolism (fig. 8.14). One involves the use of anticoagulants, which block or otherwise interfere with blood coagulation. The most widely used agent of this type is heparin, which is a potent blocker of thrombin and fibrin formation.

The second therapeutic approach, rather than limiting coagulation activates the fibrinolytic system. Tissue plasminogen activator is used to produce plasmin, which limits

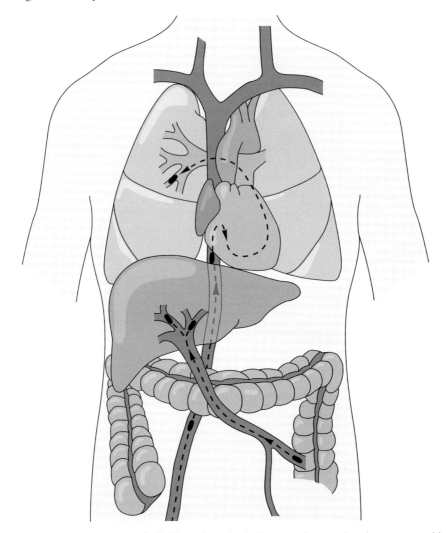

Figure 8.13   **Principal Pathways of Thromboemboli.** Those that arise in the general systemic veins are trapped in the lungs. Those arising in vessels drained by the hepatic portal system will lodge in the liver.

further thrombosis by degrading clotting factors. It is especially effective in that it also breaks down fibrin to clear thromboemboli that have already formed. The designation **rt-PA** is used clinically because the activator is prepared using recombinant DNA technology.

These first two approaches are employed in cases in which there is high risk of thrombosis or when thrombi have already formed. A third, widely used approach seeks to lower the risk of thrombosis over the long term. Prophylactic (preventive) aspirin (ASA) therapy has proven to decrease platelet aggregation and activation. It is effective in those at risk of myocardial infarction, which typically involves thrombotic occlusion of diseased coronary arteries. Particular agents commonly used in these therapeutic approaches are listed in table 8.1.

Fat Emboli

Most fat emboli form when fat-rich, yellow marrow gains access to the blood. They are usually small and form in large numbers. They arise most commonly as a result of long bone

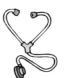

Focus on Leg Vein Thrombosis

Deep vein thrombosis (DVT) of the leg is an important and often serious clinical condition. Although it can present symptoms such as tenderness, edema, and areas of focal discoloration, it often cannot be detected on clinical examination. It is thought that over 90% of pulmonary emboli arise from venous thrombi in the lower extremity. This means a high level of clinical suspicion should be maintained when the predisposing factors for thrombosis are present.

fractures, especially the femur and tibia, usually within 12 to 48 hours of the fracture. Because of their size, they tend to lodge only in smaller arterioles and capillaries. In the lung, this can produce symptoms ranging from mild difficulty with breathing through complete respiratory failure. Because the

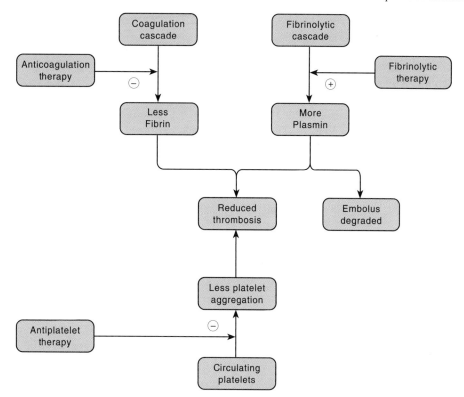

Figure 8.14   **Principal Therapeutic Approaches to Thrombosis and Embolism.** Anticoagulation and antiplatelet therapies limit coagulation and thrombosis. Fibrinolytic therapy based on the use of rt-PA promotes the formation of plasmin.

Table 8.1	Principal Pharmaceutical Agents Used in Therapy for Thrombosis and Thromboembolism	

Drug	Action	Comments
Dicumarol Phenprocoumon Warfarin	These three agents suppress the liver's synthesis of several clotting factors.	These chemically related agents are used in the prevention and therapy of chronic venous thrombosis, pulmonary embolism, coronary artery disease, and in cases of blood hypercoagulability.
Heparin	Blocking agent that interferes with the last two steps of the coagulation cascade.	Widely used to prevent coagulation of blood samples and in surgery and dialysis. Also used in acute venous thrombosis, pulmonary embolism, thrombosis in cerebral vessels, coronary artery disease, and myocardial infarction.
Aspirin (ASA)	Inhibition of platelet aggregation.	Used in the prevention of MI in high-risk individuals.
Streptokinase	Promotes fibrinolytic cascade and plasmin formation.	Extracted from bacteria. Used in acute coronary or other arterial occlusion and massive pulmonary embolism.
Urokinase	Same as for streptokinase.	Extracted from nephron tubules. Used similarly to streptokinase.
Alteplase (rt-PA, recombinant tissue plasminogen activator)	Same as for streptokinase.	Localized effects as opposed to the more systemic effects of streptokinase and urokinase.

globules that form fat emboli are compressible, and because the lung vasculature has channels that can by-pass the small capillary beds, smaller fat emboli can pass through the pulmonary microcirculation to reach the systemic arteries. In this way they can reach the skin, where they often cause a diffuse rash of petechial hemorrhages. The principal threat of fat emboli is that they can't pass through small cerebral vessels. They lodge in these vessels and occlude them. The resulting pressure causes vessel damage and numerous small petechial hemorrhages as the blood is lost to the surrounding brain tissue upstream. Downstream, many small infarcts form, threatening coma and death.

Air Emboli

Gases can also enter the blood and travel as emboli. The most common such embolus is air. It can enter the blood when veins are open to the air. This is especially so when surgery, a fractured rib, or knife wounds damage the veins of the thorax, allowing air to be drawn into the blood by respiratory movements. Neck surgery, suicidal lacerations of the jugular veins, or improper administration of intravenous fluids can have the same result.

An air embolus will have significant consequences only if large. A few small bubbles introduced into the blood with an injected drug preparation are soon dispersed in the flowing blood and dissolve to pose little threat. Problems typically arise with air volumes of over 100 ml. The air bubbles involved are initially quite small, but they can merge to form obstructing masses in small capillaries. This situation is particularly threatening in the brain.

If an air embolus is particularly large, 300 ml. or so, a potentially serious situation is presented to the heart. The cardiac pump is designed to handle fluids that are noncompressible. The myocardium pumps by exerting a pressure that ejects the noncompressible blood. When a large air embolus reaches the heart, it is drawn into a ventricle. When the ventricle contracts, pressure increases and the air yields to it, becoming compressed but not moving out of the chamber. When the ventricle relaxes, the air expands. During the following cardiac cycles, compression and expansion are repeated. The result is a healthy ventricle, filled with a froth of blood and air and unable to pump. In the case of a large cardiac air embolus, cardiac output can fall to critical levels. The churning of the bloody foam in the ventricle also damages platelets and predisposes to thrombosis in the blood that does reach the pulmonary arterial system.

The situation of a pump intended for liquids filling with air is called **air lock.** In the case of an air lock caused by an air embolus in the heart, the effect can be countered by achieving a body position in which the right heart is elevated. The air in the heart will rise, allowing blood to pass under it to reach the ventricle. As the blood continues to flow under the air embolus, small quantities of air gradually enter the blood to be harmlessly dispersed.

In circumstances where abrupt reduction of atmospheric pressure occurs, nitrogen gas normally present in the tissues boils out of them into the blood. The presence of

Focus on Fat Embolism and Alcoholism

Fat emboli may arise following traumatic injury to the liver of alcohol abusers. Such livers are typically engorged with fat (see Fatty Change in chapter 1). Physical injury to the liver can release this fat, allowing it to enter the hepatic veins. Once in these vessels, the emboli pose similar risks to those of marrow-derived emboli: lung and brain damage. Sadly, alcoholics are more likely to suffer just such trauma-related liver injury in motor vehicle accidents, falls, or other incidents related to their drinking.

---

nitrogen gas emboli is associated with joint pain and carries the potential for brain damage. This situation is commonly called the **bends.** It occurs in accidental pressure reductions in underwater divers and in other circumstances where air pressure is artificially increased—for example, in air travelers and in tunnel workers breathing compressed air.

Amniotic Fluid Embolism

This is a rare complication of childbirth that can occur during either a spontaneous delivery or cesarean section. The term **amniotic fluid embolism** is somewhat misleading because a fluid itself can't occlude vessels. The occluding agent is actually the infant's cells that are shed into the amniotic fluid. During the delivery, clumps of these cells and membrane debris enter the circulation via tears in the placental membranes or in the uterine or cervical veins. In the blood they are carried to the lungs, where they are trapped in its small vessels. A pronounced compromise of respiratory function follows with severe breathing difficulty accompanied by a dramatic decline of blood oxygenation. More significant is the severe pulmonary edema caused by injury to lung capillaries and disseminated intravascular coagulation (DIC) triggered by procoagulants in the amniotic fluid. The obstruction of blood flow that results is compounded by an accompanying collapse of blood pressure that deprives tissues of adequate blood flow. Coma and seizures linked to reduced blood flow to the brain often follow. The underlying mechanism in the profound drop in blood pressure is thought to involve substances in the amniotic fluid that induce widespread vasodilation. There is much that is unclear in the pathogenesis of this highly lethal condition, which has a mortality rate in excess of 80%.

Foreign Body Embolism

Less commonly, foreign bodies may gain access to the blood and be carried by it to become emboli. An example is a bullet fragment that might enter the blood after tearing through a vessel wall. As with thromboemboli, the site at which it is finally trapped depends on the point where it enters the circulation.

Case Study

While convalescing at home following a work-related foot fracture, a 57-year-old brick layer felt weak and faint, and then suffered a severe episode of labored breathing and crushing pain over his left chest. He was rushed to the hospital, where he complained of dizziness and persistence of his chest pain. On examination, he was found to be pale, with a rapid heart rate, reduced blood pressure, and distended neck veins. His electrocardiogram produced no evidence of myocardial infarction, but signs of some right ventricular strain were present. Auscultation of the left lung revealed a "friction rub" over the left lung. He was also febrile, with a temperature of 38.8° C.

He reported a history of varicose veins and a recent worsening of calf pain while recuperating from his fracture. His left calf was swollen, tender, warm, and edematous. He also stated he had no history of heart trouble and had recently had a general physical examination by his family physician, who declared him to be "in the pink," apart from minor problems such as his varicose veins. His chest pain and breathing difficulties continued and intravenous heparin therapy was instituted on the basis of a presumed pulmonary embolism. Quickly obtained radiographic and radioisotope scan results confirmed a massive occlusive embolism in the left pulmonary artery, blocking all blood flow to the left lung.

In view of this confirmation of the initial tentative diagnosis, vasoconstriction therapy to support his blood pressure was started and a more aggressive anticoagulation regimen was quickly instituted. Because of the threat of further emboli forming in the leg veins, it was decided to insert a filter in the inferior vena cava, but as the patient was being prepared for the procedure, he abruptly developed a sharp pain in his right chest, gasped repeatedly for breath, and died before any intervention could reverse the situation.

Autopsy findings confirmed the complete occlusion of the left pulmonary artery that presumably produced the patient's initial attack. The occluding mass was formed of a coil of gelatinous thrombus. A similar coil was found blocking the right pulmonary artery. It appeared that a long thrombus initially detached from its site of formation in the popliteal vein, reaching the right ventricle. It was then driven into the left pulmonary artery, producing the initial attack. A second, large mass of embolus, presumably from the same leg vein, was found coiled in the right pulmonary artery, where it completely blocked all lung access to the pulmonary vasculature. A small fragment of embolus, wedged within the trabeculae carnae of the right ventricle's floor, testified to the passage of the larger masses through the chamber en route to the lungs.

An infarcted area of the left lung was also found, verifying the friction rub and ECG indications of pulmonary infarction. The infarct was also the likely explanation for the patient's elevated temperature. Examination of the left leg revealed pronounced varices in the deep calf veins and in the popliteal and great saphenous veins, with residual thrombi at several points in the vessels. In this extreme case, the initial massive occlusion induced the ischemic damage, but because the lung is also supplied by the bronchial arteries, infarction in pulmonary embolism is unusual.

Commentary

The patient's rapid heart rate was compensation for the fall in cardiac output produced by the pulmonary occlusion. His chest pain was the result of right ventricular overload from the abrupt increase in resistance that the blocked pulmonary artery presented to it. Distention of the right pulmonary artery, which arose quickly as the blood supply of both lungs was being forced into it, also probably contributed to the pain. Inability to cope with such high demand caused backup of blood into the large veins of the systemic circulation, producing the observed neck vein distention. The friction rub heard over the lung was the result of infarction damage at the lung's surface that roughened the visceral pleura above the infarct. The result was a rubbing sound as it moved against the adjacent parietal pleura.

The procedure to insert a caval filter was to have been done via the jugular vein. Such filters are able to block access of thromboemboli to the lung, at the same time offering no restriction to blood flow. They can be inserted with relative ease, avoiding full-blown surgery, and have been widely and successfully used. Had time permitted, such a filter would probably have spared this patient's life.

Subsequent discussions with the family physician of the deceased revealed that in view of the man's history of varicose veins, he had provided his patient with a series of lower leg maneuvers intended to promote venous flow and counter the tendency to sluggish venous flow in the fractured and immobilized leg. The victim's wife reported that her husband had not bothered with the exercises, nor had he reported or sought medical help for recent episodes of increased pain and swelling in the calf of his fractured limb.

Key Concepts

1. Hemodynamic factors underlie the differences between arterial and venous thrombosis (p. 202).

2. Thrombosis is the result of blood hypercoagulation states and conditions that favor platelet adherence to endothelia: endothelial damage and irregular, turbulent blood flow (pp. 203–205).

3. Once formed, a thrombus may resolve, or it may enlarge to narrow or completely occlude a blood vessel, raising the threat of infarction (pp. 205–206).

4. An infarct may result from thrombosis, vascular compression, or various vascular diseases that increase wall thickness at the expense of the lumen (pp. 206–207).

5. Infarction depends on a tissue's vulnerability to hypoxia, its pattern of vascular supply, the blood's oxygen delivery capacity, and the rate at which tissue deprivation develops (p. 207).

6. A thromboembolus may be formed from a thrombus, producing an infarct by the mechanism of embolism (p. 208).

7. Once formed, a thromboembolus lodges in the next branching vascular bed to which the blood delivers it (pp. 208–209).

8. In cases of thrombosis, therapeutic intervention is based on anticoagulants that inhibit thrombosis, agents that inhibit platelet aggregation, and those that promote fibrinolysis (pp. 209–210).

9. Emboli of marrow-derived adipose tissue, air, cells accumulated from amniotic fluid, or foreign bodies may be carried in the blood to disrupt blood flow at various points in the cardiovascular system (pp. 210–212).

REVIEW ACTIVITIES

1. Use the information on page 202 to make up a comparison table highlighting the difference between a clot and a thrombus.

2. A handy study aid would be a master list of all the factors that predispose to thrombosis. All the information you need is on pages 203–205.

3. Check all the photos and diagrams in this chapter. How many show lines of Zahn? (The authors count six.)

4. Complete the following table.

Embolus	Origin	Likely Embolism Site
Fat	Leg fracture	
Thrombus	Renal artery	
Thrombus	Leg vein	
Air	Rib fracture	
Thrombus	Arm vein	
Amniotic cells	Placenta	
Thrombus	Mesenteric vein	
Bullet fragment	Femoral vein	

Chapter

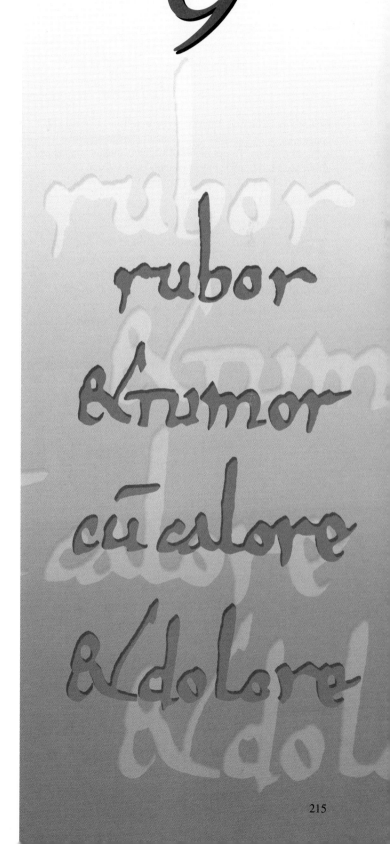

Vascular Disorders

A man is as old as his arteries.

THOMAS SYDENHAM
OBSERVATIONES MEDIC

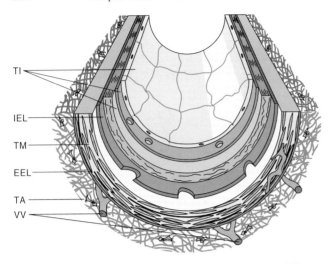

Figure 9.1 **Normal Arterial Structure.** Tunica intima (TI) consists of an endothelium, its basement membrane, and a layer of connective tissue. Tunica media (TM), consisting of muscle and elastic tissue, is bounded by the internal and external elastic laminae (IEL, EEL). The vasa vasorum (VV) supply tunica adventitia (TA) and the outer TM.

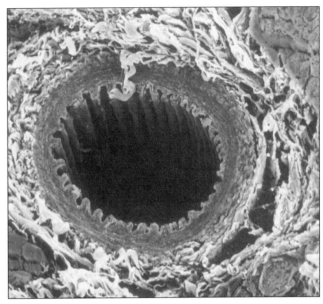

Figure 9.2 **Artery Wall.** In this electron micrograph of a small artery, the collagen fibers of tunica adventitia can be seen merging with those of the connective tissue that supports the vessel. Tunica media is the dense middle region of the wall. Tunica intima is the paler infolded region that lines the lumen.

Disorders of the arteries represent a major source of disease and death in North America. Vein disorders present a much smaller threat to mortality, but they are still responsible for significant clinical disease. Any consideration of these conditions must make reference to various features of arterial and venous structure. The following sections provide the essentials for those who might need a review.

VASCULAR STRUCTURE

Blood flows away from the heart in the system of branching arteries. The lumen that carries the blood is enclosed within the arterial wall, which has three layers, or coats (fig. 9.1).

The innermost is called **tunica intima** (the Latin term *tunica* means covering, or coat). It consists of a single layer of flattened endothelial cells, which line the lumen and provide the smooth surface over which the blood flows. Beneath the endothelial surface is a **basement membrane** of glycoprotein. The third part of the intima is a layer of loosely organized fibrous connective tissue in which are found widely dispersed smooth muscle cells and white blood cells. The middle layer of the arterial wall, **tunica media,** is separated from the intima by a thin, strong mesh of elastic connective tissue, the **internal elastic lamina.** Tunica media is the thickest part of the arterial wall. It consists of elastic connective tissue and circularly oriented smooth muscle tissue combined to form a strong, yet flexible and elastic midwall region. In larger arteries, elastic tissue is the dominant component of the tunica media, whereas smaller vessels have much more smooth muscle. **Tunica adventitia** (*adventitia* means "from afar") is the outermost of the three wall coats. It is separated from tunica media by another elastic mesh called the **external**

elastic lamina. This means the media has an elastic lamina on both intimal and adventitial surfaces. Tunica adventitia is a protective layer of loosely organized fibrous connective tissue (fig. 9.2).

In small arteries, cells of the wall are directly supplied with nutrients by diffusion from luminal blood into the wall. In the larger arteries diffusion can supply only the intima and inner part of the media. The remaining part of the wall is supplied by its own system of small blood vessels, the **vasa vasorum.** These are the vessels' vessels, which deliver blood to capillary networks within the large arterial wall, supplying its external layers.

With aging, arteries undergo a characteristic and generalized pattern of change. In the intima, connective tissue and lipid content increase, as does the number of smooth muscle cells. This process can cause the intima to become as thick as the media by the sixth decade of life. These changes accompany an overall dilation and lengthening of some larger arteries due to a loss of elastic tissue from their walls. This causes them to assume a more irregular, winding configuration. As time passes, the arterial wall becomes more rigid, causing more resistance to arterial pressure pulses. As well, the size of the lumen is reduced, increasing the predisposition to downstream ischemia. As collagen increases and elastic tissue and muscle are lost, the walls of the arteries become more rigid. Because of the wall rigidity, some consider these changes to be a form of disease. However, since the process is virtually universal, it seems more reasonable to consider these changes to be the result of normal aging rather than arising from some pathological process.

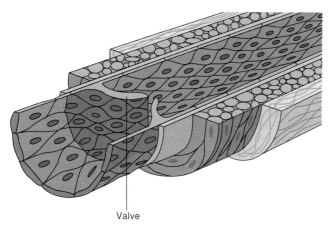

Valve

Figure 9.3 **Vein Structure.** In this view into the interior of a vein, valves, formed of endothelium-lined leaflets, can be seen projecting into the lumen. This arrangement allows blood to flow toward the heart and prevents backflow. Note the thinner media.

In contrast to the typical artery described earlier, most veins have a thinner wall and a larger lumen. In most veins, except for the largest, the elastic laminae are not present and tunica intima has a thinner connective tissue layer deep to the endothelium. Tunica media is also thinner, with its muscle and elastic tissues less uniformly distributed. Veins in the limbs are modified by the presence of leaflet valves. These are formed by foldings of the intima that project into the lumen (fig. 9.3; see also fig. 8.4) to prevent backflow and promote the return of blood to the heart.

 Checkpoint 9.1

Note the terminology shift in regard to vessel wall layers. On initial use, the full term is used, e.g., tunica intima. Once the context is established, since the *tunica* element is the same for all three layers and adds no further information, it can be dropped.

ARTERIAL DISEASE

Most arterial disease involves changes in the vessel wall that reduce its elasticity and flexibility. This is the process of **sclerosis;** the layperson's "hardening of the arteries." This condition was formerly known as *arteriosclerosis,* but that term has fallen into disuse in that it is too general and conveys insufficient meaning to distinguish among the three principal types of arterial disease. These can be distinguished on the basis of the type of artery affected, the part of the wall involved, and the nature of the abnormality that produces the sclerosis. The three conditions are the relatively rare **medial calcific sclerosis,** the more common **hypertensive vascular disease,** and the very widespread **atherosclerosis.**

Medial Calcific Sclerosis

Medial calcific sclerosis, an uncommon and idiopathic condition, is also called **Mönckeberg's sclerosis.** It typically involves the medium-sized arteries of the limbs and genitalia in those past 50 years of age. The condition is characterized by focal calcification of tunica media at sites where its muscle tissue has degenerated. The regions of calcification may be irregular or ringlike, producing a characteristic pattern in radiographs. Calcium deposition also produces focal hardening that may be palpable in superficial vessels, but because such deposition produces no narrowing of the lumen, it is unusual for it to produce clinical disease.

Hypertensive Vascular Disease

This is the condition in which arteriolar walls undergo changes in association with **systemic hypertension.** Since arterioles are principally involved, the term **arteriolosclerosis** is also used to describe it. The arteriole's intima and media thicken due to the accumulation of plasma proteins and the overproduction of basement membrane and extracellular matrix material. This is an example of the hyaline change described in chapter 1; hence, its name **hyaline arteriolosclerosis.** Although a prominent feature of systemic hypertension, hyaline arteriolosclerosis is also present in the common endocrine disorder diabetes mellitus and as a sequela of radiation damage, most of which is linked to radiation therapy.

Systemic Hypertension

This is the widespread problem of elevated blood hydrostatic pressure (BHP) in the systemic arterial system—the layperson's "high blood pressure." Use of the term systemic hypertension has value in differentiating this condition from others where abnormally high BHP is confined to the vessels of the lung (**pulmonary hypertension**) or to those of the hepatic portal system (**portal hypertension**). Once context is established, the simpler term hypertension is used.

Currently, diagnosis of hypertension is based on a diastolic pressure in excess of 90 mm Hg or a systolic pressure exceeding 140 mm Hg in men over 50 years of age and 160 mm Hg for all women. These values are associated with an increase in mortality of over 50%. On this basis, 60 million people in North America are estimated to be hypertensive. Since the condition is essentially asymptomatic, as many as one-third of these are thought to be undiagnosed. Various risk factors are associated with an increased likelihood of developing systemic hypertension. Genetics, race, increased age, smoking, obesity, and stress and other ill-defined environmental factors are some of them. Although the precise roles of these factors are poorly understood, they are recognized as playing some direct or indirect part. A genetic component is suggested, in part, by familial incidence patterns and the much higher frequency of occurrence in blacks: double the rate of whites.

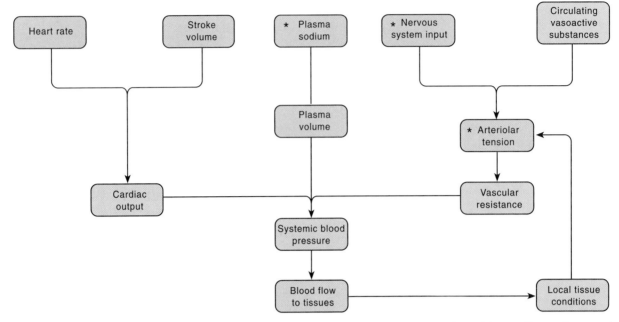

Figure 9.4   **Normal Blood Pressure Regulation.** Asterisks indicate the points where a genetic defect might contribute to hypertension.

Focus on Nitric Oxide: A Role in Hypertension?

Nitric oxide gas (NO) may turn out to be another contributing factor to the hypertension problem. Previously noted for its role as an inflammatory mediator and inhibitor of platelet aggregation, it also appears that NO is an important factor in normal blood pressure regulation. (Before it was clearly identified, it was known as **EDRF: endothelium-derived relaxing factor.**) NO is normally produced by endothelial cells in response to blood flow over their surfaces and causes smooth muscle relax-ation. Increased arterial pressure triggers increased NO production and the resulting dilation eases pressure. The role of NO is seen in animal studies in which suppression of normal NO release is followed by systemic blood pressure elevation. In people with hypertension, there is some loss of NO-induced dilation, but further study is required to determine if the reduced NO activity causes the hypertension. It may be that other factors first elevate the pressure and NO production declines as a result.

Essential Hypertension

Etiology in hypertension is a problem around which much discussion and research is centered. In 90–95% of cases, no specific cause can be identified. This is the condition known as **primary** or **essential hypertension.** It is widely held to be the result of some defect in the complex control mechanisms that have a bearing on systemic blood pressure maintenance. These mechanisms are presented in figure 9.4, where cardiac output and peripheral resistance are indicated as the major determinants of blood pressure. Asterisks indicate those points in the system where a genetic defect may provide some degree of disruption. One of these involves a genetic defect in the kidney's sodium excretion mechanism, which in turn promotes an increase in extracellular fluid volume and cardiac output. The resulting increase in blood flow to the tissues causes local arteriolar constriction responses that increase peripheral resistance and blood pressure.

A second genetic defect may be centered in the membranes of arteriolar smooth muscle. Because the entrance of sodium ions causes the release of the calcium ions that trigger contraction, an inability to expel sodium ions at a normal rate would result in longer periods of elevated calcium levels in the cells. The consequences would be higher wall tension and an increased sensitivity to normal hormonal and neurogenic constriction inputs. These would combine to produce a generally higher level of constriction for a given level of stimulus, causing an elevation of systemic blood pressure.

The third suggested genetic defect involves an exaggerated responsiveness on the part of the autonomic system, so that its constriction inputs to systemic arterioles are excessive. In primary hypertension, there appears to be a complex interplay between these genetic mechanisms and several environmental factors. Obesity, stress, inadequate exercise, and high salt intake are involved, but details of

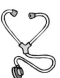

Focus on The Role of Renin in Hypertension

In approximately 35% of cases of essential hypertension, plasma renin levels are abnormal. In **high-renin hypertension** you might expect that excessive renin would promote water retention to produce hypertension. However, since drugs that block renin's effects don't reduce the blood pressure, some other underlying mechanism would seem to be operating. In **low-renin hypertension,** you might think that low renin and, therefore, low angiotensin II levels would lead to water loss and a reduction of blood pressure. Since they don't, the high pressure in these cases may be produced by other, unknown adrenal cortex hormones with water retention effects, or by an excessive arteriolar sensitivity to angiotensin II. In the latter case, the sensitivity would be high enough so that even low levels of angiotensin II could produce hypertension.

---

pathogenesis are unclear. It is speculated that chronic stress might exacerbate arteriolar constriction via increased epinephrine secretion. A high salt intake adds to the burden faced by a genetically defective sodium excretion system.

You can appreciate that there are many possibilities for problems arising in the complex pressure regulation system. Much research is being done to sort out the precise role of each variable, but it has proved to be a difficult and often frustrating challenge.

Secondary Hypertension

In 5–10% of hypertensives, hypertension is **secondary;** that is, some other specific disorder can be identified as the cause of the elevated blood pressure. In most cases, the focus of the problem is the kidney or excessive levels of various hormones. In cases where disease of the renal parenchyma is established, hypertension may be the result of the kidney's failure to excrete sodium and water, to produce more of, or to activate, some unknown vasoconstrictor substance, or to secrete enough of a vasodilator. It may also be that damage to the renal tissue reduces blood flow to the nephrons and activates the **renin-angiotensin system** (RAS).

The RAS is an important mechanism in the regulation of arterial blood pressure (fig. 9.5). It involves the production of angiotensin II, a potent vasoconstrictor that also stimulates aldosterone secretion and therefore sodium and water retention. The system's activation depends on the secretion of renin by the nephron's **juxtaglomerular cells** in response to blood pressure and to sodium levels in the nephron's distal convoluted tubule. (Note: The enzyme here is renin, not rennin, a quite different gastric enzyme.)

Angiotensinogen is the plasma substrate from which renin produces angiotensin I, which is converted to angiotensin II by the angiotensin-converting enzyme (ACE) that is associated with pulmonary endothelial surfaces. If blood pressure or kidney tubule sodium levels fall, increased renin secretion promotes a corrective increase in pressure.

Activation of the RAS is the principal mechanism underlying a second type of kidney-related hypertension called **renovascular hypertension.** It occurs when an intact and functional kidney is supplied by a diseased and stenotic renal artery. The reduced renal blood flow that results triggers increased renin secretion, and hypertension follows.

Excessive levels of certain hormones can also produce secondary hypertension. When the adrenal glands hypersecrete aldosterone, water retention and systemic hypertension result. In Cushing's syndrome (see chapter 17), glucocorticoids are present to excess, but their precise link to hypertension is not clear. About 5% of birth control pill users experience hypertension. Probably the elevated estrogens promote the liver's synthesis of angiotensinogen, which leads to excessive plasma levels of angiotensin II. Not all users of oral contraceptives develop hypertension, however, and it may be that the presence of some additional genetic, environmental, or other factor is necessary before hypertension develops. Any number of other factors may produce a secondary hypertension. Defects in endocrine regulation might be involved through direct or indirect hormonal effects on blood volume or arteriolar constriction. As well, defective neurological regulation of the heart or vessels might also contribute.

Whether primary or secondary, most hypertension steadily progresses and is ultimately fatal unless therapy to control blood pressure intervenes. The condition characterized by a slowly progressive pressure increase is **benign hypertension.** In 1–5% of hypertensives a rapidly progressive **malignant hypertension** develops. This is a serious condition that can be triggered by renal damage from benign hypertension or other causes. The rapid pressure increases in this condition seem to promote endothelial damage in small arterioles, which in turn favors the widespread formation of microthrombi. These contribute to flow restriction and damage to red cells, causing a form of anemia called **microangiopathic hemolytic anemia** (see chapter 7). High pressure in malignant hypertension also produces a pronounced smooth muscle and endothelial proliferation response to produce **hyperplastic arteriolosclerosis** (fig. 9.6). This contrasts with the hyaline arteriolosclerosis typically present in benign hypertension.

Therapy in primary and secondary hypertension seeks reduction of any unfavorable environmental factors combined with one or more antihypertensive drugs. Weight loss through diet and increased exercise and salt restriction are strongly recommended. Drug therapy relies on four major approaches. **Diuretics** are agents that enhance urinary fluid loss to reduce blood volume. **Beta-blockers**

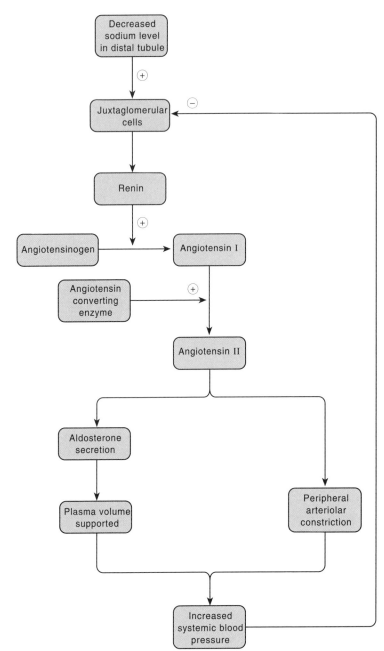

Figure 9.5   **The Renin-Angiotensin System.**

block sympathetic nervous system input to the heart, which causes a reduction of contraction force and a decline in cardiac output that tends to lower blood pressure. **ACE-inhibitors** work by antagonizing the action of the pulmonary angiotensin-converting enzymes that form angiotensin II. By reducing the amount in the circulation, two benefits are achieved. The first is a reduction in systemic vasoconstriction since angiotensin II acts directly on arterioles. The second is more indirect in that angiotensin II also controls aldosterone secretion, which, in turn, regulates renal sodium retention. So when angiotensin II levels fall, more sodium is lost, water follows,

plasma volume is reduced, and pressure declines. The last of these principal therapeutic approaches is directed at the calcium channels involved in arteriolar smooth muscle contraction. **Calcium channel blockers** restrict the availability of calcium in smooth muscle, producing a dilation effect, and in cardiac muscle, causing lower cardiac output. Both effects combine to reduce blood pressure. There are various other vasodilator agents also in use. Note that more than one category of drug is often used to maximize effect while minimizing side effects. The actions of these major therapeutic agents are presented in figure 9.7.

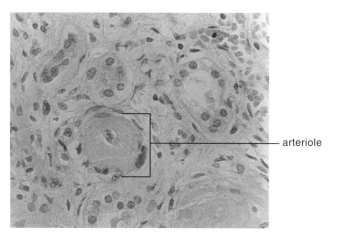

Figure 9.6 **Hyperplastic Arteriolosclerosis.** The arteriole in this micrograph demonstrates the pronounced wall-thickening characteristics of arteriolosclerosis.

This is a microscopic view of the renal cortex in malignant hypertension. The afferent arteriole in the center of the field is greatly thickened and almost completely closes the lumen. The resulting reduction of blood flow is responsible for the damage to glomeruli and tubules that is also apparent. The section is from the kidney of a 40-year-old male. From mild headaches and a somewhat elevated blood pressure of 150/100 at age 38, he progressed to severe headaches, a blood pressure of 225/150, and various CNS effects that combined with his failing kidneys to bring about his death.

Consequences of Systemic Hypertension

Broadly, there are two consequences of systemic hypertension. One is arteriolosclerosis, which, by reducing the arteriole's lumen and its ability to dilate normally, contributes to further hypertension. This mechanism can produce the positive feedback cycling that operates in some malignant hypertension. The second consequence is most significant, in that systemic hypertension is linked to stroke and heart attack because it predisposes to early and severe atherosclerosis, the last of the three types of arteriosclerosis.

☑ *Checkpoint 9.2*

In this matter of antihypertensive therapy, you might reflect for a moment on the research effort involved in finally uncovering the essentials of cardiovascular function and blood pressure control. Then consider the long pursuit of the means to exploit that knowledge in developing and testing the drugs that could affect the system at its key points. Lots of people and lots of money over many years have combined to yield large gains in curtailing the threat of systemic hypertension.

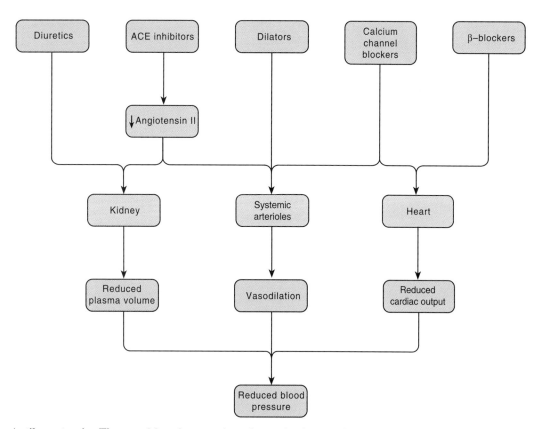

Figure 9.7 **Antihypertensive Therapy.** More than one class of agent is often employed.

Atherosclerosis

Atherosclerosis is by far the most common vascular disease. It accounts for about half of all deaths in North America, and is the underlying disease process in most of the coronary artery disease that causes myocardial infarction and the arterial alterations that produce cerebrovascular accidents. It is the number one killer in economically developed countries worldwide.

Whereas arteriolosclerosis largely affects arterioles, it is the larger arteries that are affected by atherosclerosis. The chief vessels involved, in order of decreasing frequency are the abdominal aorta and common iliacs, coronaries, femoral and popliteal, internal carotids, and the major vessels at the base of the brain (fig. 9.8; see also fig. 20.15c).

Apart from the vessels affected, atherosclerosis can be differentiated from the other types of arterial disease on the basis of its characteristic lesion, the **atheroma** (pl., atheromata) or **atheromatous plaque.** This is a focal thickening of the intima due to the deposition of lipid and connective tissue and the proliferation of cells. The Greek root *athero* means "gruel" or "porridge," and its use in describing this arterial lesion is based on the thick necrotic sludge in the core of the atheroma.

Atheromata are initially distributed in a patchy, scattered pattern in the major arteries, but as the condition progresses, adjacent lesions merge to form larger plaques. The atheroma develops only slowly, gradually enlarging and increasingly protruding into the lumen. Initial intimal thickening can be identified as early as ages 10–20, with subsequent progression producing symptoms as early as age 35. Beyond this age, the atheromata become further enlarged and increasingly irregular. These later changes contribute to an increasing risk of complications, which have potentially devastating effects, especially in males past the age of 40. We will consider these complications after we analyze the pathogenesis of atherosclerosis.

Pathogenesis

Early signs of intimal changes can be found in most individuals, worldwide, after the age of one year. These changes are seen as narrow, pale yellow streaks that run longitudinally along the intima of the aorta. Such visible lines are the result of focal accumulation of macrophages, which enter the intima from the circulating blood. Fat is taken up by these macrophages and is held in their cytoplasm in the form of small globules. The concentration of these swollen cells at this early stage may produce some minor elevation of the intima.

The early formation of these **fatty streaks** seems to be a part of normal development. They remain until about 10 years of age, by which time 10% of the aorta's surface may show streaking (fig. 9.9). At this point a critical distinction arises. In economically undeveloped areas of the world, the streaks remain static or regress, posing no further problem. Where standards of living are high, however, streaks continue to develop into potentially destructive atheromatous plaques.

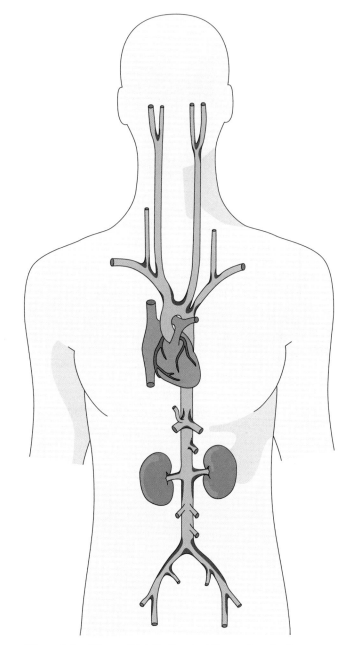

Figure 9.8   **Plaque Distribution in Atherosclerosis.** Common sites of atheroma formation are indicated by heavy shading. Affected brain vessel are not shown.

Study of plaque development (**atherogenesis**) in the coronary arteries indicates that, past 10 years of age, new streaks form and are transformed into plaques by about the age of 30. The process involves the continued entry of macrophages. As some endothelial irregularity accompanies this process, platelets are able to adhere at the site. They and the macrophages release growth factors that promote proliferation of medial smooth muscle cells. Like macrophages, these cells can also take up intimal lipid. As fat accumulates, macrophages and smooth muscle cytoplasm develop a bubbly appearance, microscopically. For this reason they are called **foam cells.** As the years pass, the intima becomes thicker as foam cell numbers increase.

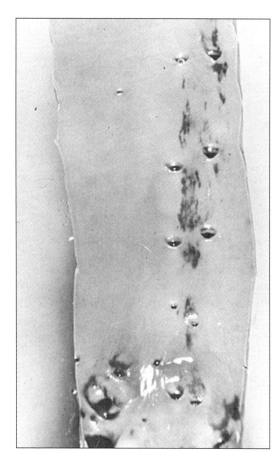

Figure 9.9   Fatty Streaks. A lipid-specific stain has been applied to the surface of the aorta.

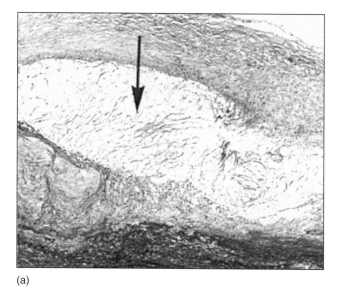

(a)

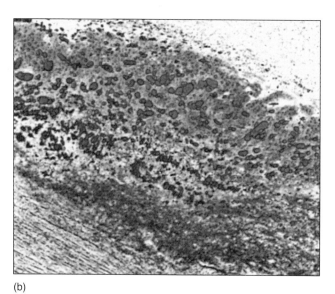

(b)

Figure 9.10   Microscopic View of a Typical Atheroma.
(*a*) The arrow indicates the core of foam cells and lipid-rich debris. Over this central region lies the cellular fibrous cap. (*b*) A stain specific for lipid highlights its accumulation within the atheroma. *This is a section through an atheroma in the aorta of a 65-year-old male who died of pulmonary complications caused by his failing heart. The core of the atheroma contains fat and necrotic debris. The coronary arteries also exhibited extensive atherosclerosis, with some lumina reduced to mere pinpoints. No large infarct was found at autopsy, but many small, diffusely scattered scars were found throughout the myocardium. These produced the myocardial weakness that caused the heart to fail.*

Smooth muscle cells produce collagen and connective tissue matrix material, and the proliferating cells and collagen combine to form a **fibrous cap** just deep to the endothelium (fig. 9.10).

The process continues with the development of one or more of several possible complications. These **complicated lesions** (fig. 9.11) are a major factor in the wall damage that gives rise to the serious consequences of atherosclerosis. The complicating factors are calcification, hemorrhage, medial destruction, and surface ulceration.

As intimal damage is prolonged over months and years, it is accompanied by the deposition of insoluble calcium salts in the intima. This process is called **dystrophic calcification.** It is not restricted to blood vessels but can occur elsewhere in the body—for example, in joints or cerebral infarcts. Calcification can proceed to the point where, in advanced atherosclerosis, cutting through the aorta at autopsy produces an easily audible crunching sound. As the atheroma develops, necrosis in the media elicits a normal revascularization response from the vasa vasorum. The newly formed vessels rupture easily, however, and hemorrhage into the atheroma often results. This causes further damage and enlargement of the lesion. The fibrous cap that forms beneath the endothelium also contributes to destruction of the media. The muscle of the media, which to this point has not been affected by the formation of the atheroma, is dependent on diffusion from the lumen for nutrient supply. The plaque's fibrous cap provides a barrier to diffusing nutrients, causing a reduction of oxygen and nutrient supply that leads to deterioration of the media. Smooth muscle atrophy and destruction of the internal elastic lamina results, producing a gradual weakening of the arterial wall.

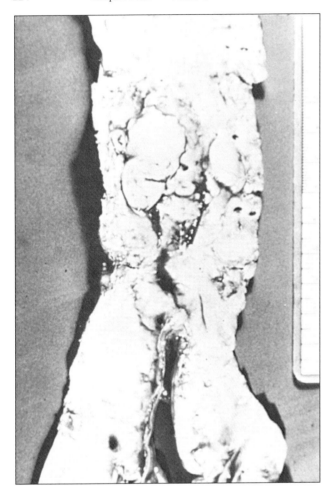

Figure 9.11   **Severe Atherosclerosis.** Complicated lesions of advanced atherosclerosis.

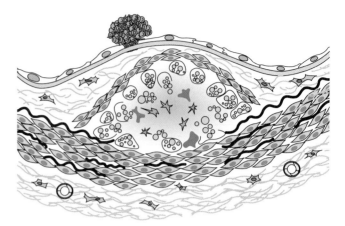

Figure 9.12   **The Complicated Atheroma.** The core of necrotic debris contains free lipid, in part from rupture of foam cells. Note disruption of the internal elastic lamina and the ulcerated endothelium where a thrombus is forming. Dark masses are calcium deposits; pointed masses represent cholesterol crystals.

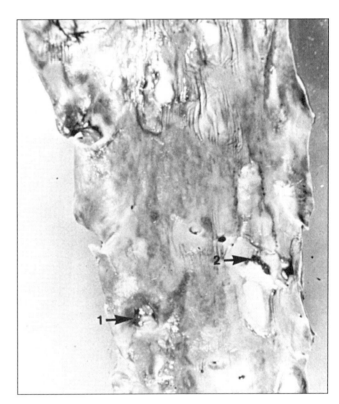

Figure 9.13   **Endothelial Ulceration.** The arrows indicate sites of ulceration in this severely diseased aorta.

As fibrosis, calcification, hemorrhage, and enlargement of the atheroma proceed, its surface is affected (fig. 9.12). Endothelial cells lose their normally firm support as the underlying intima becomes necrotic and softened. As a result, the endothelium becomes damaged or is stripped away, and ulceration at the surface of the atheroma follows (fig. 9.13). This exposes the interior of the atheroma to the blood, allowing either the release of necrotic debris into the blood or further disruption of the wall as blood from the lumen is forced into the lesion.

Note that ulceration of the endothelium also exposes the subendothelial components that can activate the intrinsic coagulation pathway. And remember that platelets will already have begun to adhere to any endothelial irregularities. These two factors combine to favor thrombosis at the surface of the plaque. The risk of arterial thromboembolism is now added to the situation, but thrombosis by itself is even more threatening in the coronary arteries in that they have small lumina to begin with. A thrombus superimposed on an already thickened intima can completely occlude the lumen, producing an often fatal infarct in the myocardium.

Although the many factors involved in atherogenesis are complexly interrelated, the most widely accepted view of the overall process is the **"response to injury" hypothesis.** It is based on many studies carried out over many years and seeks to unify the essential components of the process as described earlier: cell proliferation, lipid deposition, and connective tissue formation. As the name implies, the "response to injury" hypothesis suggests that atheroma formation follows an initial injury to the arterial endothelium. The injury may involve only mild effects, which initially alter endothelial permeability. This change could be followed by increased lipid

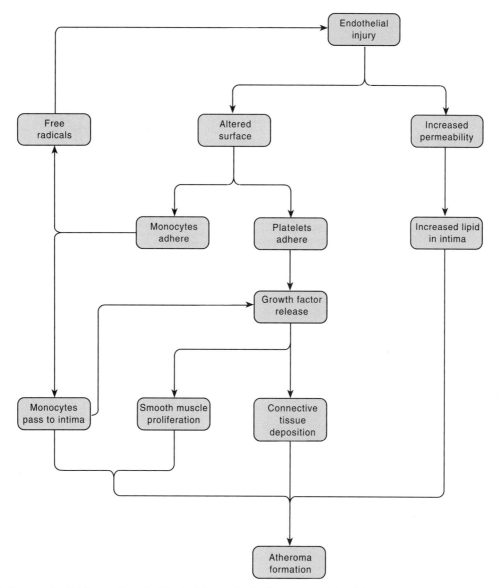

Figure 9.14   **Pathogenesis of Atherosclerosis.** Principal factors in the "response to injury" hypothesis of atherogenesis.

access to the intima. Injured endothelial cells are also known to retract their edges, drawing back from neighboring cells. The retraction exposes the subendothelial tissues, allowing platelet adherence and easier access to the intima for monocytes. These blood cells first adhere and then migrate into the intima, where they are transformed into macrophages. They then proceed to take up lipid, as do smooth muscle cells, to form the foam cells characteristic of atherosclerosis.

A key component to the continued development of the atheroma is cell proliferation. This process is driven by a variety of **growth factors** (GFs) that are released by macrophages and platelets (platelet-derived growth factor, PDGF, has been well studied).

Growth factors were described in chapter 4 in the context of healing. In atherogenesis, they contribute to the enlargement of the atheroma by promoting proliferation of its components. The GFs involved are chemotactic for monocytes, so more are drawn to the site. Their presence can ag-

gravate the situation, since the adhering monocytes can themselves secrete injurious free radicals (superoxides—see chapter 1) that can damage the endothelium and contribute to progression. (We will consider further implications of the effects of free radicals later, in the section on hyperlipidemia.) GFs also promote mitosis of smooth muscle and its deposition of collagen, elastin, and connective tissue matrix material within the atheroma. Figure 9.14 presents an overview of the pathogenesis in atherosclerosis.

Risk Factors in Atherosclerosis

Many long-term and large-scale studies of the incidence of atherosclerosis have identified an association between its progression and various **risk factors.** Generally, the presence of a risk factor increases the likelihood of atherosclerosis, and the presence of two or more significantly increases the probability of earlier and more severe

Table 9.1	Risk Factors in Atherosclerosis
Major Factors	**Secondary or Less Clearly Related Factors**
Hyperlipidemia	Excessive (or no) alcohol use
Genetic predisposition	Obesity
Systemic hypertension	Inadequate exercise
Smoking	Stress
Male gender	
Diabetes mellitus	

complications. The atherosclerosis risk factors are thought to contribute directly or indirectly to the endothelial damage or other components that play a role in the development of atherosclerosis. The most important of these (table 9.1) are the following.

Hyperlipidemia The term **hyperlipidemia** is used to indicate elevated levels of fat in the blood. In the context of atherosclerosis, elevated plasma cholesterol (**hypercholesterolemia**) is generally accepted as a significant risk factor. Although a thorough exploration of lipid metabolism is beyond the scope of this text, an insight into the essentials is necessary to appreciate current thinking and future dietary and therapeutic implications.

Since lipids are not water-soluble, their transport in the plasma requires specific provision for increasing their water solubility. The increase is accomplished by a specialized system of lipid and protein complexes (**lipoproteins**) that also accommodates cellular uptake of the lipids. In essence, the lipoproteins use a coating of phospholipid to surround the lipid that is to be carried in the plasma. The phospholipid molecules are oriented so that their water-soluble ends interact with the plasma's water. The protein-component, called an **apoprotein,** provides for interaction at cell membrane receptors that facilitate cellular uptake of the lipid for metabolism (fig. 9.15). Refer to table 9.2 for the major plasma lipoproteins and their principal functions.

Although study of the plasma lipoproteins has produced a large body of information, much remains unclear about their precise roles in normal metabolism. The most significant information in regard to atherosclerosis has to do with the plasma levels of LDLs and HDLs. Generally, these function in an **endogenous pathway** for cholesterol transport between the liver and the other tissues that metabolize cholesterol. The liver also receives newly absorbed dietary lipid via other lipoprotein complexes in the **exogenous pathway** (fig. 9.16).

In essence, the liver takes up dietary cholesterol from the plasma and uses it to synthesize bile salts. These, along with some free cholesterol, are passed to the intestinal lumen to complete the exogenous pathway. The liver's role in the endogenous pathway involves secreting cholesterol, which is carried by VLDL. Capillary enzymes convert these to LDL, which can be taken up by the tissues that metabolize cholesterol: the adrenal cortex, ovary, and liver. Of the plasma's total cholesterol, 70% or more is carried by LDL. LDL can also be taken up by arterial endothelial cells, with its cholesterol then accumulating in the wall where it is taken up by scavenging macrophages or smooth muscle cells. Any cholesterol not utilized by tissues is carried away by HDL and delivered to the liver, where it is metabolized or lost to the intestine in bile.

Various studies have established that there is a direct relationship between high plasma LDL levels and myocardial infarction caused by atherosclerosis in the coronary arteries. The risk declines, however, when HDL levels increase. If HDL is clearing cholesterol from sites of accumulation in the arterial intima, this would seem to reduce the process of atheroma formation and explain the observed reduction of atherosclerosis.

Research has been slowly uncovering the specific contribution of LDL to atherogenesis. The key appears to be LDL oxidation by free radicals. They are produced, following initial endothelial disruption, by intimal smooth muscle, the endothelial cells themselves, and the macrophages that are drawn to the scene. In its oxidized form, LDL has several effects. It is more rapidly taken up by smooth muscle and macrophages, so lipid is held at the scene and foam cell development favors intimal thickening. Oxidized LDL also stimulates growth factor production, which promotes cell proliferation and connective tissue deposition. Other effects focus on the macrophage. Oxidized LDL is chemotactic for monocytes, attracting them to the site where it also induces modification of the endothelial surface to favor monocyte adherence. Once in the intima, the macrophages that have evolved from the monocytes are held at the scene, again under the influence of oxidized LDL. Beyond these effects is a link to the immune system. Oxidized LDL is antigenic in that it induces antibody production against it. This likely accounts for the lymphocytes and immune complexes known to be present in plaque—another defensive system responding to the initial injury. Lastly, oxidized LDL itself is damaging to the endothelium. This means there is an element of positive feedback cycling in the process of atherogenesis that contributes to its steady progression over the years. All-in-all, the numerous and potent effects of oxidized LDL make it a highly important contributing factor to plaque development (fig. 9.17).

Genetics Having a near relative with atherosclerosis is a significant risk factor. This predisposition is not directly transmitted by a recognizable pattern of inheritance. It may be that different individuals have a genetically determined susceptibility, such as endothelia more prone to injury or some loss of regulatory control of the excretion of cholesterol. Of course, the link may also be the result of shared dietary, exercise, or other family practices that tend toward

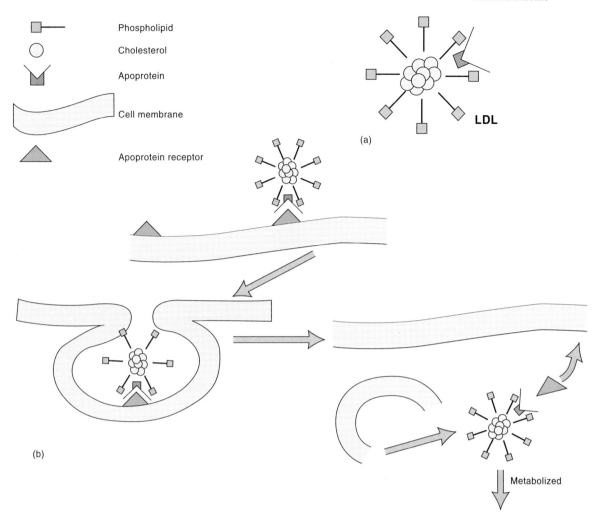

Figure 9.15 **Low-Density Lipoprotein in Cholesterol Transport and Cell Uptake.** (*a*) The cholesterol core of the LDL is enclosed by phospholipids, which shield it from plasma water. (*b*) Binding of the membrane receptor to the apoprotein of the LDL triggers endocytosis. Within the cell, cholesterol is metabolized and the receptor is recycled to the surface.

Table 9.2	Principal Plasma Lipoproteins and Their Major Roles in Lipid Transport
Plasma Lipoprotein	**Function**
Chylomicrons	Formed in the intestinal epithelium from newly absorbed triglyceride and cholesterol; carry lipid to muscle and adipose tissue for utilization or storage.
Very-low-density lipoproteins VLDL	Formed in the liver; carry triglyceride and cholesterol.
Low-density lipoproteins (LDL)	Formed from VLDL; carry cholesterol to various tissues for utilization, also to arteries in which lipid can accumulate.
High-density lipoproteins (HDL)	Take up cholesterol from tissues and carry it to the liver, which excretes it into bile.

greater incidence of atherosclerosis. Another complication is that in some cases, the genetic component might be an inherited tendency toward some other risk factor, such as diabetes mellitus or hypertension.

Apart from these ill-defined cases, there is a group of genetically transmitted diseases that are characterized by high levels of various plasma lipoproteins. They are usually designated by use of the term *familial,* or they may be described with reference to a type, indicated by a Roman numeral that relates to the lipoprotein involved (table 9.3).

An example is the rare genetic disease known as **familial hypercholesterolemia,** which is characterized by

EXOGENOUS PATHWAY

ENDOGENOUS PATHWAY

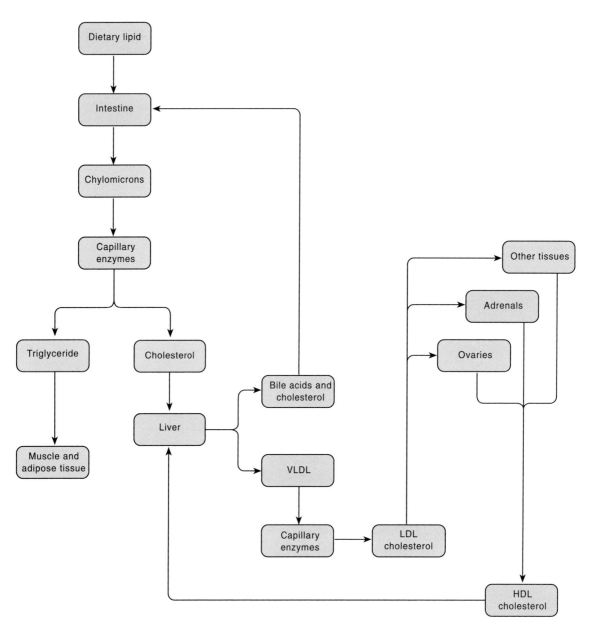

Figure 9.16   **Plasma Lipid Transport.** At the left, the exogenous pathway mediates the dietary intake of lipid and its return to the intestine. In the endogenous pathway, lipid carried by VLDL and LDL is delivered to various tissues, where it is metabolized or returned to the liver by HDL for excretion.

Focus on Diet and Plasma Cholesterol

Many studies have sought to establish that lowering dietary cholesterol intake will result in a lowering of LDL-borne cholesterol. The results of such studies are complicated by the fact that dietary cholesterol is handled by the exogenous pathway. This means that it is only indirectly related to the endogenous pathway.

Results of changing dietary cholesterol are also affected by other processes that seem to adjust cholesterol metabolism

and intestinal absorption, preventing large-scale plasma LDL changes. An example is the case of a healthy, elderly man who, because of a psychological compulsion, ate a normal diet *plus* 20–30 eggs every day. He did this for over 15 years, and suffered no indications of atherosclerosis even though egg yolks are rich in cholesterol. Although his plasma cholesterol levels were elevated somewhat, his body had adapted by absorbing less cholesterol and metabolizing more to bile acids for clearance via the intestine.

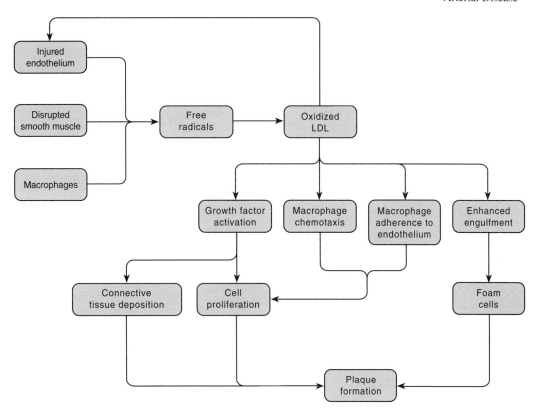

Figure 9.17   **LDL Oxidation and Atherogenesis.** Once oxidized by free radicals, LDL makes multiple contributions to plaque development. Note the positive feedback component that sustains the process.

Table 9.3	Selected Genetic Hyperlipidemias and Their Major Plasma Lipid Elevations

Disease Name	Alternative Designation	Lipoprotein Elevated
Familial hypertriglyceridemia	Type I	VLDL
Familial hypercholesterolemia	Type IIA	LDL
Familial combined hyperlipidemia	Type IIB	LDL/VLDL
Familial type 3 hyperlipoproteinemia	Type III	Chylomicron products

Table 9.4	Drug Utilized in the Treatment of the Hyperlipoproteinemias

Drug	Action
Cholestyramine	Lowers LDLs and serum cholesterol by binding intestinal cholesterol. This promotes more cholesterol utilization, and blood levels fall.
Clofibrate	Reduces synthesis of LDL precursors and endogenous cholesterol formation.
Genfibrozil	Reduces formation of LDL precursors and promotes HDL formation.
Lovastatin	Suppresses the endogenous pathway to cholesterol synthesis.
Nicotinic acid	In large doses, lower both cholesterol and triglycerides in plasma.
Probucol	Reduces endogenous synthesis and absorption of cholesterol and promotes LDL degradation.

defective LDL receptors. When only one defective gene is present, the lack of normal receptor numbers means that less LDL can be taken up by liver, ovary, and adrenal tissues for cholesterol metabolism. The deficiency in uptake causes high LDL levels to be sustained, which in turn causes an accelerated development of atherosclerosis. In such cases, heart attacks may occur as early as age 35. In the even more rare cases (1/1,000,000) where both of an individual's genes are defective, the absence of LDL receptor synthesis produces very high LDL levels and an even earlier onset of AS-related heart attacks, often by age 20.

In treating these familial disorders, as well as selected cases of hyperlipidemia with no genetic cause, dietary cholesterol restriction is augmented by the use of drugs that lower plasma LDL levels (table 9.4). These operate by complexing with cholesterol in the intestine to limit its

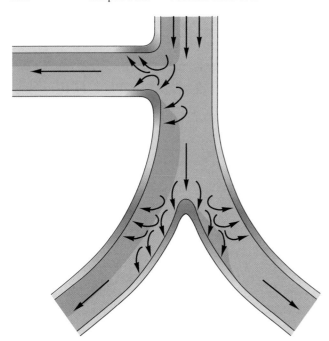

Figure 9.18   **Hemodynamic Stress.** Turbulent blood flow at arterial branch points increases hemodynamic stress and the potential for endothelial damage.

absorption, or by inhibiting endogenous cholesterol synthesis, or by other less understood mechanisms. Some of these drugs have quite unpleasant side effects, and it is often difficult to persuade patients to continue their use long enough to ensure maximum effectiveness.

Hemodynamic Stress   This is the wear and tear to which the endothelia are subjected in coping with arterial blood flow. One source of wear and tear is the pulsing of the blood, which expands and stretches larger arterial walls with every systolic contraction. The second is the stress caused when a rapidly moving column of blood divides at arterial branch points (fig. 9.18). The change in flow direction sets up turbulence and local pressure waves that are damaging to the endothelium. Note that the high-turbulence branch points are also those sites most frequently involved in atheroma formation (see fig. 9.8).

In this context, you can appreciate the observed relation between systemic hypertension and significantly increased atherosclerosis in the coronary arteries. The generally increased blood pressure increases hemodynamic stress and favors endothelial damage. Another risk factor, inadequate exercise, may be related to hemodynamic stress. A sedentary individual has a higher resting heart rate than one who regularly engages in some sustained activity that elevates the heart rate. Brisk walking, running, sustained swimming, squash, racquetball, and cross-country skiing are examples. Although they may promote flexibility and increase strength or coordination, golf, bowling, or weightlifting don't have the same effects in reducing the heart rate.

Focus on Effects of Exercise on Endothelia

A reduction in the heart rate of ten beats per minute can be quickly achieved by a regular program of moderate exercise. This represents an annual decrease of well over 5 million heartbeats, which means over 5 million fewer systolic pressure pulses surging through the arterial tree, a substantial saving in annual wear and tear on the endothelia.

Smoking   The general awareness of the hazards of smoking is usually focused on its role in the etiology of lung cancer. Too few people, however, are aware that it is a major risk factor for atherosclerosis, particularly in the coronary arteries. Evidence continues to accumulate that those who smoke a package of cigarettes daily have a significantly greater likelihood of coronary thrombosis and myocardial infarction. Further, when an acute MI does occur, it is more likely to be fatal in smokers than in non-smokers. Women are also vulnerable, with as much as half their heart disease attributable to smoking. Being a non-smoker who must spend time in the presence of smokers is also risky. Studies show an increased likelihood of death in such cases of **passive smoking.** This is particularly unfortunate in the case of infants and older children of smokers, who have little awareness of the dangers, and few options for avoiding the hazards of their parents' ignorance or indifference. As many as one-third of the several hundred thousand annual deaths from atherosclerosis in North America are due to smoking. From all causes combined, smoking-related deaths exceed 1,000 per day.

Although its role as a major risk factor is clear, the specific mechanisms by which smoking contributes to atherosclerosis are less so. Endothelial injury via hypoxemia may well be involved, since cigarette smoke contains carbon monoxide (CO), which replaces oxygen carried by hemoglobin. Hypoxia may also be atherogenic in that it promotes smooth muscle proliferation and LDL accumulation. The nicotine in cigarettes may contribute by its vasoconstrictive effects, producing myocardial ischemia and hypoxia, or by directly injuring the endothelium. Cigarette smoke also enhances platelet aggregation and so might promote atherogenesis by enhancing the role of platelets and the growth factors they secrete. As well, increased platelet aggregation might underlie the coronary thrombosis that is the major cause of fatal coronary infarction. Perhaps most important of all is the new evidence that tobacco smoke oxidizes LDL. Its central contributions to atherogenesis were noted previously.

The bright spot in the smoking situation is that if smoking is stopped, its effects are reduced. After one to

Focus on Homocysteine: The Newest Risk Factor

Recent research indicates that elevated plasma levels of **homocysteine** are a significant risk factor for atherosclerosis. It was previously recognized that those with a genetic defect that caused plasma homocysteine to rise suffered early and severe atherosclerosis. It now appears that another factor producing high plasma homocysteine is a lack of folic acid and vitamin B. Increasing folate, vitamin B_6, and vitamin B_{12} counters the effect. Deficiencies of these nutrients are common in North America and may be contributing to the high incidence of atherosclerosis.

The specific actions of homocysteine are still being studied, but there is evidence for endothelial damage via free radicals and the promotion of both smooth muscle mitosis and blood coagulation. The latter effect seems based on increased platelet adherence caused by homocysteine's interference with the action of nitric oxide.

---

five years of nonsmoking status, a previous smoker's risk of coronary artery disease returns to normal.

Age and Gender There is firm evidence that one's age and gender have a strong bearing on the development of atherosclerosis: increased age means increased risk. Intimal thickening and sclerosis are common among older people. So any other risk factors that predispose to atherosclerosis operate on vessel walls already thickened and with lumina already narrowed. As well, increased age means that any such factors have had a longer time to superimpose their effects on the aging artery, so that the resulting problems are magnified.

Being male poses a serious risk to the development of atherosclerosis. Males have significantly higher LDL levels and lower HDL levels than do females. Presumably, it is because of this undesirable lipoprotein balance that atherosclerosis occurs more frequently in males. Estrogens appear responsible for the more favorable balance in high HDL and lower LDL levels in females. But note that after menopause, when estrogen's protective effect is lost, atherosclerosis develops rapidly. Once into their sixties, men and women have similar risk of myocardial infarction due to atherosclerosis.

Diabetes Mellitus This condition, more fully considered in chapter 17, is an endocrine derangement that produces early and severe atherosclerosis in its victims. It involves widespread metabolic derangements, but in particular, it causes the plasma's glucose level to be elevated, sometimes considerably (hyperglycemia). The effect is to enhance the addition of sugar units to circulating plasma proteins, by a process called **glycation.** Glycation of LDL is now recognized as contributing to atherosclerosis in diabetics. Glycated LDL easily binds to endothelia and is more aggressively scavenged by intimal macrophages. Other effects are the promotion of connective tissue deposition that enlarges an atheroma and the inactivation of nitric oxide that promotes vasoconstriction. In the small coronary arteries, more narrowing and constriction combine to strongly favor myocardial ischemia and infarction. Even when hyperglycemia is controlled, an increased risk of coronary atherosclerosis is present, likely related to the high LDL/low HDL profile of diabetics. Study of these matters is proceeding, but the problem is a difficult one to unravel because the metabolic effects of diabetes are so widespread.

Miscellaneous Risk Factors The previously described risk factors are those that show the strongest links to increased atherosclerosis. Other factors are implicated, but less strongly and with less information on their underlying mechanisms.

One of these is physical activity. Sedentary individuals are more likely to develop atherosclerosis than those who are more active, particularly in the types of activities described earlier in the context of reducing resting heart rate. Numerous studies have indicated various mechanisms by which exercise and fitness might have beneficial effects, but extracting clear-cut and persuasive evidence is difficult. Generally it appears that increased exercise levels are associated with reduced blood pressure, increased levels of plasma HDL, and lower plasma values of cholesterol, triglyceride, and LDL. The myocardium of strenuously training athletes shows an increased ability to extract oxygen from the blood, the implication being that it is therefore better able to resist ischemia and infarction. Other lines of research show that exercise reduces platelet aggregation, which might limit both atherogenesis and the thrombosis that often accompanies it. As well, some animal studies have suggested that exercise increases collateral circulation and stabilizes myocardial rhythmicity, both of which would allow the heart to cope better with the effects of atherosclerosis.

Obesity is a risk factor for atherosclerosis, but it seems not to operate independently. Its link to increased is atherosclerosis is indirect, through its association with other risk factors such as hypertension, diabetes, hyperlipidemia, and the often sedentary activities of the obese. Note that risk factor effects have been noted only when body weights are 30%, or more, above one's "ideal" weight.

There is a widely held view among medical personnel, as well as the general public, that certain personality types are associated with a reduced ability to handle "stress" and that such individuals are at greater risk of coronary atherosclerosis and MI. Despite careful analysis of the research, it is difficult to draw clear-cut conclusions to support this concept. Part of the problem may lie in the difficulty of clearly characterizing and identifying personality components or in defining "stress" and verifying its presence. It is also difficult to quantify stress levels for the type of analysis from which hard conclusions can be drawn. Stress, however defined, may contribute to heart attacks not by contributing to atherosclerosis, but instead, by the effects of the high levels of epinephrine secreted to help in coping with the stress. High levels of epinephrine can affect the myocardium directly, causing it to become rhythmically unstable. Myocardial contractions can become so uncoordinated that no effective pumping is possible and death follows. This is the condition of **sudden cardiac death** described in chapter 10.

Alcohol is another risk factor for atherosclerosis. Evidence indicates that increased values of plasma HDL are associated with moderate alcohol consumption. Reduced HDL levels are found in those whose alcohol intake is high and, perhaps surprisingly, in those who drink no alcohol at all. No reason for these links have been widely accepted, but there has been some suggestion that the comparatively lower incidence of atherosclerosis in France is linked to the French peoples' high consumption of red wine. Laboratory studies indicate that rather than the wine's alcohol, its tannins and polyphenols can block LDL oxidation. This could be a significant factor in limiting atherosclerosis (fig. 9.17).

Periodically there is some excitement generated by media reports of research that implicates infection as a factor in atherosclerosis. Bacteria, viruses, and yeast organisms (*Chlamydia* species) are examples. Some research has contradicted such findings and, for now, the picture is not at all clear, but if any organism can be shown to disrupt arterial endothelium, it would fit nicely into the overall scheme of atherogenesis.

Risk Factors: A Summary Figure 9.19 indicates the various atherosclerosis risk factors and some of the ways in which they interact. In considering risk factor interactions, note that in many individuals multiple risk factors are present and that their effects aren't simply additive. For example, with three risk factors operating, the risk is not tripled, but actually increases seven-fold. Many sedentary, obese smokers with hypertension are multiplying risks, so that the question becomes less a matter of "if" and more a matter of "when" the consequences of atherosclerosis will take their toll.

In assessing the best risk factor reduction program for one's patients and oneself, one should remember that although age, sex, and genetic makeup can't be changed, the other risk factors can be reduced with significant benefits. Increasing exercise and fitness, therapeutic control of hypertension, elimination of smoking, and reducing but not completely eliminating alcohol consumption can all be expected to reduce the predisposition to atherosclerosis. Di-

Focus on Atherosclerosis; Is It Reversible?

Many studies on this complex issue have yielded a clear answer: maybe. This doesn't mean an affected adult's aorta and coronary arteries can be restored to those of a teenager. Rather, it means that a vigorous program of risk factor reduction can definitely be beneficial. Various studies indicate that with such a program, the progression of atherosclerosis can be arrested and existing plaque can be reduced in size and thickness. Such effects have been seen in studies in which folic acid or B-vitamin deficiencies were corrected. Previously elevated homocysteine levels were restored and early plaques shrank in size. Specifically, foam cell numbers declined, extracellular lipid and necrotic debris were cleared, and the endothelial surface was restored. Of course, well-advanced disease can't be made to quickly disappear, but any risk factor reduction that contributes to some degree of regression may be significant. The best approach is low risk early in life rather than later trying to salvage something of an already deteriorated situation. Of course, any benefit at any age is important because even a small blood flow increase in cerebral and coronary vessels can have a major impact on life expectancy and quality of life.

etary changes may reduce the risk, but this topic has been the subject of many, often conflicting, claims in the medical literature as well as the popular press. Currently, there does not seem to be sufficient evidence to justify dietary extremes that seek to minimize or eliminate cholesterol intake. There is much more support for reducing caloric intake to avoid obesity and to adjust the diet so that less than one-third of its total calories derive from fat. Fat in the diet should be derived less from meats rich in saturated fat (fat that is solid, rather than liquid at room temperature) and more from fish and vegetable oils. Fat eliminated from the diet should be replaced by vegetables, and complex carbohydrates—for example, pasta. Bon appétit!

In concluding this assessment of risk factors in atherosclerosis, note that the past 20 years have seen an encouraging decline in the mortality statistics of coronary atherosclerosis. Much of this decline is due directly to the increased effectiveness of therapy for atherosclerosis and indirectly to better therapeutic control of systemic hypertension. The decline in dietary fat intake and the reduction of smoking have also contributed to the decline in a significant way. Unfortunately, atherosclerosis and its effects remain the major disease threat to North Americans, and further reduction of risk factors, where possible, is a continuing goal.

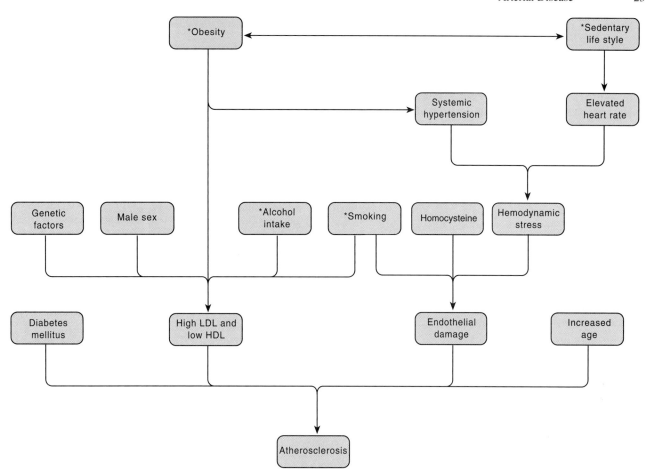

Figure 9.19   **Risk Factors in Atherosclerosis.** The various risk factors that directly or indirectly contribute to atherosclerosis. Note the large amount of overlap and interplay among the risk factors. Asterisks indicate the factors that are avoidable for most people.

Focus on Links between Atherosclerosis and High Iron Levels

The difference in atherosclerosis incidence between males and females may be explained by recent evidence that iron may be a factor. Some research indicates that premenopausal women who require surgical removal of the uterus, leaving ovaries in place to maintain estrogen secretion, suffer more coronary atherosclerosis than other women. The suggestion is that the regular loss of menstrual blood, and the iron it contains in its hemoglobin, keeps iron in most women at a low level that protects them against atherosclerosis. Also supporting this idea is the fact that meat is the source of most dietary iron, and in groups like Seventh Day Adventists, who eat no meat and have correspondingly low iron levels, coronary atherosclerosis rates in males are only half those of meat eaters.

Such provocative observations have been tested in a study of coronary atherosclerosis risk factors that included iron levels in the blood. Close to 2,000 men were monitored over five years and, rather than LDL, it was iron in the blood that seemed to have the largest effect compared with any other single variable. Exactly how iron contributes to the process of atherogenesis is unclear at this early stage, but further research is under way. In the meantime, it might be noted that a male who donates blood three times a year achieves the same iron status as a premenopausal woman. The other benefit, of course, is the often quite significant effect on the person who receives the transfusion.

Sequelae of Atherosclerosis

As atherosclerosis progresses, larger and more numerous plaques form. These changes produce no signs or symptoms until well-advanced, complicated plaques develop. Then stenosis, or narrowing, of the lumen results. Other changes involve damage and deterioration of tunica media. These changes combine to produce an array of sequelae that have devastating effects.

Arterial Stenosis Atherosclerotic stenosis of the major arteries reduces the volume of blood that can be delivered to the dependent tissues downstream. In the aorta, because of its large diameter, stenosis will have only minor effect, but atherosclerotic stenosis of the common iliac and femoral arteries can cause problems in the legs. For example, minor wounds may heal slowly. As atherosclerosis develops, further stenosis may cause skin wounds of the legs to ulcerate, with increasing risk of infection and gangrene. Smaller branches of the aorta may be more seriously affected. The coronary and cerebral arteries are especially significant because of the critical tissues they supply. In either brain or myocardium, the chronic ischemia caused by arterial stenosis can cause a slow, progressive deterioration of function. The memory loss, confusion, and generally reduced mental functions commonly seen in the elderly are, at least in part, reflections of this reduced cerebral blood flow. Stenosis of the renal artery presents a special problem. The resulting renal ischemia activates the renin-angiotensin system, which responds with fluid retention and vasoconstriction. These produce renovascular hypertension, which itself increases the progression of atherosclerosis, which then aggravates the hypertension in a positive feedback cycle. In the heart, reduced blood flow will mean a steadily declining ability of the myocardium to meet its pumping demands. This decline is usually indicated by chest pain at moderate and even low levels of exertion. Chapter 10 considers the myocardial implications of **coronary artery disease** (CAD), also referred to as **ischemic heart disease** (IHD).

Thrombosis and Embolism Further complications in the coronary and cerebral vessels can result from thrombosis. As complicated plaques form, they contribute to thrombosis in two ways. First, because they protrude into the moving blood, they cause blood flow to be irregular and turbulent. This condition, as we have seen, favors the deposition of platelets in and around the plaques. Second, the complicated lesions of advanced atherosclerosis have ulcerated, or otherwise irregular, surfaces to which platelets can readily adhere. In some cases, the loss of endothelial cells from the surfaces of advanced plaques allows platelet access to subendothelial elements that can bind them. The process of thrombosis superimposed on plaques that have already narrowed the lumen of a smaller vessel presents a serious problem. The thrombus may become organized and incorporated into the arterial wall to consolidate the stenosis and ischemia. As organization proceeds, the surface of the thrombus provides a stimulus to further thrombosis, causing still greater reduction of the vessel's lumen. With continuation of this process, the en-

Focus on Downstream Obstruction Effects

Sophisticated imaging techniques and computer systems that model the biophysics of blood flow are providing new insights into the effects of vascular stenosis. One effect is vasodilation. Even when coronary vessels are narrowed as much as 75%, vasodilation from downstream of the narrowed point can provide flow adequate to meet resting levels of demand. Beyond 80% stenosis, compensation limits are reached and downstream blood flow drops abruptly, often producing chest pain at only trivial levels of increased loading.

Another key effect derives from the physics of a liquid flowing past an obstruction. Again, the 80% level of stenosis is critical because at such severe degrees of blockage, high-velocity jets of blood spurt past the obstruction. Such jetting can damage the vessel walls downstream. This would explain the wall weakness and distention often found just beyond points of stenosis.

The turbulence that typically develops around an obstructing mass is another effect of vascular stenosis. The increased forces applied at unusual angles are more likely to dislodge fragments of the obstructing mass: a thrombus or an atherosclerotic plaque.

tire lumen may ultimately be occluded, resulting in cerebral or myocardial infarction. In cases of fatal myocardial infarction, it is thrombosis at an atheroma's surface that usually causes the final coronary occlusion that completely shuts off myocardial flow (fig. 9.20).

Given that thrombosis is favored at plaque surfaces, it follows that the threat of thromboembolism is present. Plaque embolism is also a risk. Larger, complicated plaques may detach intact or may release necrotic debris into the blood. In either case, downstream occlusion of smaller vessels results. This may be a contributing factor in some of the peripheral circulation problems commonly seen in atherosclerosis. Even though the smaller peripheral vessels are not directly affected—that is, no plaques initially form in these vessels—they may be occluded by emboli that originate in larger atheromatous vessels upstream (fig. 9.21). Emboli may also contribute to cerebral dysfunction. As thrombi form at irregular atheromatous surfaces in the carotid arteries, they may release thromboemboli that feed into the brain to occlude many small vessels.

Aneurysm An **aneurysm** is a focal dilation of the wall of an artery or the heart. Most arise in the aorta and its major branches as a result of atherosclerotic wall damage. In practice, this means that males over 50 years of age are the group at highest risk for aortic aneurysms. Some additional, much less frequent, causes of aneurysm are other diseases that involve arterial walls: **cystic medial necrosis** (CMN), **syphilis,** and **rheumatoid arthritis.** Trauma to the aorta or

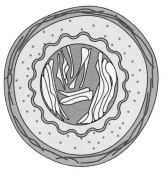

Figure 9.21 **Plaque Embolism.** An embolus, derived from an atherosclerotic plaque, has lodged in a small artery. Note the darker masses of cellular debris, and the lighter areas, which consist of lipid. The lipid masses assume the flattened shapes because they are compressed in the lumen.

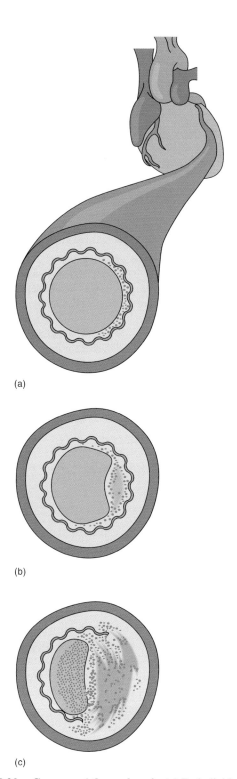

(a)

(b)

(c)

Figure 9.20 **Coronary Atherosclerosis.** (*a*) Early lipid deposition yields a fatty streak: no restriction of flow results. (*b*) Progression has enlarged the lesion at the expense of the lumen. (*c*) A complicated lesion encroaches further into the lumen and has affected the media. A superimposed thrombus occludes the lumen and MI follows.

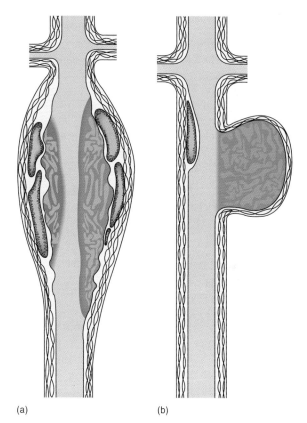

(a)   (b)

Figure 9.22 **Aneurysms.** (*a*) Fusiform aneurysm and (*b*) saccular or berry aneurysm. Note the atheromas and the thrombus that fills the expanded vascular space.

other vessels may also cause aneurysms. These are considered in chapter 24.

When an essentially symmetrical segment of the wall is involved, the aneurysm is said to be **fusiform** (resembling a spindle), while an asymmetric bulging is described as a **saccular aneurysm** (fig. 9.22). Most commonly the aorta and cerebral vessels are affected, with aortic aneurysms able to attain a diameter of up to 20 cm. The small (maximum 1.5 cm) saccular aneurysms that affect certain cerebral vessels are

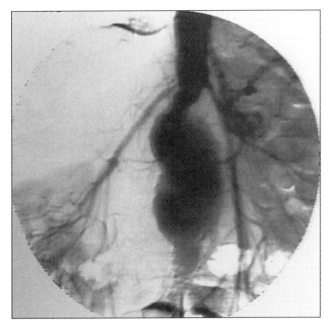

Figure 9.23   **Cerebral Aneurysm.** This aneurysm in a cerebral artery is compressing the nearby brain tissue as arterial pressure pulses surge through it.

This radiograph was obtained in diagnosis of a 72-year-old woman who had been admitted to hospital complaining of a severe headache that had suddenly developed. Soon after her admittance she developed convulsions, lapsed into a coma, and died. In addition to the cerebral aneurysm seen in the X-ray, a sample of cerebrospinal fluid revealed the presence of blood. At autopsy, the ruptured aneurysm was located, as was a large mass of recently coagulated blood in the subarachnoid space at the base of the brain.

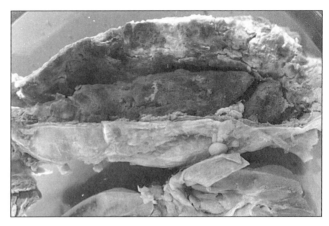

Figure 9.24   **Dissecting Aneurysm.** In this example, atherosclerosis has weakened the wall, allowing blood to separate (dissect) the muscle of the media. The dark coagulated blood is easily identified in the photo. The defect that allowed access to the interior of the wall is at the left.

This is the aorta of a 47-year-old male who had a history of hypertension. He died during a diagnostic procedure aimed at explaining his sudden, tearing chest pain and the loss of sensation and strength in his legs that had followed. The dark mass is coagulated blood that had been driven into the wall at a point weakened by exposure to chronically elevated blood pressure. Blood also dissected the aorta to reach the pericardial sac where it interfered with diastolic filling and reduced cardiac output (see chapter 10—Cardiac tamponade). No evidence of myocardial infarction was found, but there was significant ventricular hypertrophy.

called **berry aneurysms.** These congenital defects are considered in more detail in chapter 20.

The consequences of aneurysm are significant. One of these is thrombosis. Because the aneurysm is a dilated region of a normally symmetrical artery, blood flow is disturbed and turbulence results, predisposing to thrombosis. It is not unusual at autopsy to find the lumen of an aneurysm filled with thrombus showing a characteristic alternation of platelets and fibrin (fig. 9.22). This is the result of turbulently flowing blood depositing platelets, which aggregate. Fibrin forms at the platelets' surface, and further platelet deposition and fibrin formation follow. From such a site, numerous thromboemboli can be released to occlude smaller peripheral vessels downstream. Once formed, an aneurysm may continue to expand, as it is constantly exposed to high arterial blood pressure. This is an especially significant factor in those with hypertension, where the already weakened wall must bear an even greater burden.

A second consequence of an arterial aneurysm is the pulsatile pressure that the expanded wall applies to adjacent structures—for example, the brain (fig. 9.23). In the case of the aorta, this means there is the possibility of complications arising from compression of the esophagus, trachea, or various abdominal structures. Long-term exposure of vertebral bodies to an aortic aneurysm can cause them to atrophy and weaken, causing distortion of the vertebral column.

Ultimately, the bulging wall may weaken to the point where the vessel ruptures with high arterial pressure driving blood into the adjacent tissues. In the aorta or its principal branches, the effect can be fatal, with rapid blood loss quickly compromising flow to the brain and myocardium. Since an aortic aneurysm often produces no signs or symptoms, its often catastrophic rupture may give no warning. In the brain, declining arterial pressure may be less a problem than the immediate effect of rapid hemorrhage into its delicate tissue, confined within the skull. Chapter 23 treats this problem more fully.

The **dissecting aneurysm** is a special case, occurring where tunica media is weakened and the intima torn. This combination allows arterial pressure to force blood through the torn intima and into the media. There, its strong pulses separate (dissect) the media's layers, extending the defect around and along the vessel (fig. 9.24). Such extensions can progress along the aorta's full length and continue into the vessels continuous with it—for example, common carotid, renal, or coronary arteries.

There are three possible consequences from a dissecting aneurysm. One is downstream ischemia as the blood trapped in the wall forces the inner layer into the lumen. Significant interference with blood flow past the site is the

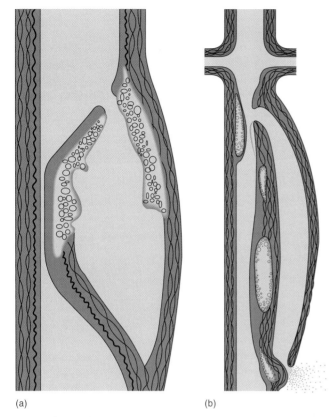

(a)   (b)

Figure 9.25   **Consequences of Aortic Dissection.** (*a*) Blood driven into the wall has torn loose a flaplike section that acts like a valve, blocking flow. (*b*) The wall has given way and ruptured, allowing the escape of arterial blood. Note the atherosclerotic damage at the point where the dissection started.

result (fig. 9.25*a*). A second possibility is that the dissection causes the wall to rupture, with blood rapidly lost through the defect (fig. 9.25*b*). The consequences are similar to those following rupture of other aortic aneurysms. If the aortic wall ruptures near its base, blood escaping the vessel can become trapped in the pericardium. The result is called **cardiac tamponade** and can be fatal (see chapter 10). The third possibility is the disruption of the aortic valve by dissection of the aortic wall adjacent to it.

Most dissecting aneurysms arise in cases of systemic hypertension, where medial damage, attributable to the idiopathic condition cystic medial necrosis, is also present. It is not clear whether both conditions must be present or whether the hypertension causes the medial damage. Given some medial defect, the loss of support at the site would make the intima vulnerable to tearing, especially if blood pressure is elevated. From this start, the process of dissection would then follow.

Although use of the term is well established, describing these defects as aneurysms is not accurate, in that the affected vessel doesn't have the obvious dilation seen in the saccular or fusiform types. Since dissection and bleeding into the vessel wall are the essential features in these cases, the terms **aortic dissection** and **dissecting hematoma** are increasingly encountered. A system for classifying aortic

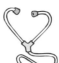

Focus on Vulnerable Vessels

Following corrective procedures to cope with the effects of atherosclerosis in the coronary arteries, the process of atherogenesis seems to speed up. Veins used as grafts in coronary bypass surgery, coronary arteries whose plaque is flattened by the expansion of a narrow balloon catheter (balloon angioplasty), and the normal vessels in a transplanted heart all develop atherosclerosis at an accelerated rate. Rather than the 20–40 years usually involved, the effects of coronary stenosis emerge after only a few years.

 Checkpoint 9.3

You can now appreciate what many laypeople don't. The problem in heart attacks doesn't originate in the heart and the problem in strokes doesn't lie in the brain itself. The real problem is the atherosclerosis that reduces blood flow to these key organs.

dissections is in use. It is based on the site of the dissection: type A when the ascending aorta is involved, with or without extension to the descending aorta, and type B when involvement is limited to the descending aorta.

ARTERIAL INFLAMMATIONS

Arterial inflammation, **arteritis,** is often accompanied by wall damage and some degree of stenosis. It may be confined to the vessels or be one of several complications of a systemic disease. Local irritation from an infection, toxin, or some other irritant may be the cause, but an immune mechanism is usually involved. An example of vascular inflammation in a systemic disorder is **systemic lupus erythematosus** (SLE), described in chapter 5. Other conditions are **polyarteritis nodosa** (PAN) and **thromboangiitis obliterans,** which arises primarily in the veins of young, male smokers.

VEIN DISORDERS

Disorders of the veins are common, but essentially only two are significant and both arise principally in the veins of the leg. These vessels are situated superficially, or travel with the deep supply arteries.

Thrombophlebitis

Thrombophlebitis is the condition of venous inflammation (**phlebitis**) that follows thrombosis. The major sites of occurrence are the deep leg veins.

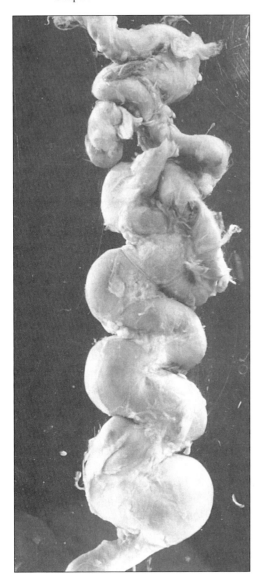

Figure 9.26   **Varicose Vein.** A section of leg vein, with pronounced varices.

This is a length of great saphenous vein resected from the leg of a 50-year-old male. He had had asymptomatic varicose veins since his mid-teens. Three weeks earlier, he had experienced pain and redness above his knee. On admission to hospital, a large varix was found. It was occluded with thrombus at a point above the knee. After its removal, recovery was uneventful.

Thrombophlebitis is usually the result of focal infection, disruptions of blood flow, or hypercoagulation states. Most thrombophlebitis arises in the deep leg veins and poses a significant risk of thromboembolism. The fewer cases that arise in the superficial leg veins present minimal risk of embolism, but can cause discomfort due to the congestion from reduced venous drainage, which arises when the veins communicating to the unaffected deep veins cannot handle the excess volume.

Varicose Veins

In **varicose veins,** the superficial leg veins become dilated and assume a more twisted pattern. Each dilation is a **varix,**

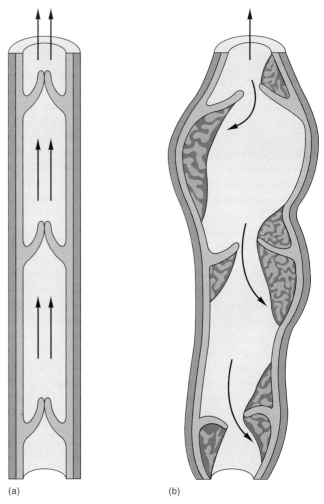

(a)   (b)

Figure 9.27   **Varicose Veins.** Compare the normal vein at left with the varicose vein on the right. The irregular bulging of the varices limits complete valve closure and allows some backflow. Note also the developing thrombi, whose formation is favored by the swirling of blood around the valve leaflets.

and there are usually multiple such varices present (fig. 9.26). These venous deformations are thought to arise as a result of elevated venous pressure. Unable to resist, the walls stretch and dilate. Varicose veins may arise more often in the superficial vessels, probably because they lack the complete support of surrounding muscle that the deep veins enjoy. The leg veins' burden is eased by the presence of leaflet valves that prevent backflow. When varices form and the walls bulge, valve function is compromised, adding to the volume and pressure load the wall must resist (fig. 9.27).

Any factors that increase venous pressure in the legs can contribute to greater loading of the vein walls. Since an upright posture significantly increases venous pressure, those whose normal activities involve chronic and prolonged standing place increased loads on their veins. Any other condition that impedes venous drainage of the legs, such as a thrombus or compression of the communicating abdominal vessels by a tumor, abdominal fat, or a pregnant uterus, will increase venous pressure. The excessive plasma volume produced by a failing heart or kidney disease may also increase the veins' burden. Since many people who suffer these conditions do not develop varices, it may be that an inherited weakness of venous walls is an important underlying factor in the development of varices.

The reduced rates of flow and irregular surfaces that characterize varicose veins predispose to thrombosis, which can reduce flow to aggravate the problem. However, in such cases embolism is quite rare.

Varices in the veins of the rectum and anal canal are called **hemorrhoids.** They are also caused by elevated ve-nous pressure when abdominal factors restrict drainage, particularly in chronic constipation that involves straining to defecate. The high abdominal pressures of pregnancy may also promote hemorrhoid formation.

Esophageal varices may arise in the veins that ac-company the esophagus. These vessels carry some of the blood returning from the abdomen. They may become chronically congested in cases of liver disease, with varices forming as a result. They are considered more fully in chapter 14.

Case Study

While driving with his girlfriend, a 24-year-old man said that he felt "kinda funny and dizzy" and that his vision was blurred. At the woman's insistence, he surrendered the wheel, and she drove to a nearby hospital's emergency department.

The physician on duty examined the man and found him to be in excellent health, but with mildly elevated blood pressure. When questioned about the aroma of alco-hol detected on his breath, the man reported having "only a beer or two," which his girlfriend verified. He was admitted to the hospital for overnight observation.

During the night he complained of feeling ill and hav-ing blurred vision, chest and abdominal pain, and tingling in the feet. His ECG showed tachycardia, and was other-wise grossly abnormal. His legs were cool and no femoral pulse could be found. A CT scan was ordered and revealed a dissecting hematoma of the aorta. He showed signs of cir-culatory shock as he was prepared for emergency surgery.

During the procedure the presence of a 5-cm dissecting hematoma was verified. It was removed and replaced by a Dacron graft. The presence of a somewhat narrowed region of the aorta was also identified distal to the point of dissec-tion, and this region was also removed and replaced. The postoperative period was uneventful and the patient recov-ered fully.

Commentary

The patient's apparent good health, and the indication that he had been drinking, might normally have resulted in his being sent home. In this case, the clinician's decision, based on many years of experience, was vindicated. Had the patient not been under close medical observation, the aorta might have ruptured, threatening his survival.

Microscopic analysis of the excised segment of aorta showed evidence of medial necrosis, probably in response to the abnormally elevated pressures caused by the region of narrowing further along the vessel. It was this damage that weakened the wall, allowing the blood to gain access to it and begin its dissection.

Key Concepts

1. Aging is accompanied by a generalized change in arterial walls that involves increased wall rigidity and thickening (p. 216).

2. The rare condition of medial calcific sclerosis embodies calcification of medium-sized limb arteries, but since no loss of lumen is involved, clinical signs and symptoms seldom arise (p. 217).

3. Arteriolosclerosis involves intimal and medial thickening of arterioles, most typically in association with diabetes mellitus and systemic hypertension (p. 217).

4. A broad range of risk factors predispose to systemic hypertension, but since the condition is essentially asymptomatic, it is often undiagnosed (p. 217).

5. Various genetic defects in the excretion of sodium ion by the kidney, smooth muscle's ability to expel sodium from its interior, and unbalanced autonomic input to arterioles have been suggested as contributing to essential hypertension (pp. 218–219).

6. In secondary hypertension, a specific systemic disorder can be identified as contributing to pressure elevation; usually the disorder involves an endocrine or renal problem (p. 219).

7. If untreated, systemic hypertension is associated with increasing disease occurrence, notably involving vessels or neurological problems, and may take a slowly or rapidly progressive course (pp. 219–221).

8. Atherosclerosis, the major cause of death in North America, is essentially a derangement of the aorta and its major branches and derives from internal thickening caused by its characteristic lesion, the atheroma (p. 222).

9. The atheroma develops progressively with lipid accumulation, cell and connective tissue proliferation, calcification, and surface ulceration that compromise the lumen and weaken the arterial wall (pp. 222–223).

10. The pathogenesis of atherosclerosis is thought to rest on the concept of atheroma formation as a response to injury, with cell proliferation mediated by a variety of

growth factors that are released by platelets and macrophages (pp. 224–225).

11. A broad array of risk factors for atherosclerosis have been identified as directly or indirectly contributing to atherogenesis by promoting endothelial damage or by other less well-defined mechanisms (pp. 225–233).

12. The sequelae of atherosclerosis involve compromised blood flow via arterial stenosis, thrombosis, and embolism or by aneurysm formation, all of which present their greatest threat to the coronary and cerebral circulations (pp. 234–237).

13. A variety of factors such as toxins and infections may activate immune responses that have an irritant effect, producing a focal or systemic arteritis (p. 237).

14. Vein disorders involve inflammation or varicosities, both of which predispose to complications of venous flow and may involve thrombosis (pp. 237–239).

REVIEW ACTIVITIES

1. Study figure 9.12 and identify the following:

   endothelium

   basement membrane

   foam cells

   calcium deposits

   proliferated myointimal cells

   subendothelial connective tissue

   platelet plug

   internal elastic lamina

   vasa vasorum

   If you have trouble, see the relevant text sections and illustrations.

2. Complete the following table of characteristics for the indicated types of arteriosclerosis.

Vessels Affected	Wall Region Affected	Major Cause
Medial calcific sclerosis		
Arteriolosclerosis		
Atherosclerosis		

3. Compare the highlighted regions of figure 9.8 and the sites of turbulent flow in figure 9.18. Now prepare a list that links events in figure 9.18 to sites of atheroma formation in figure 9.8. Be sure to include reference to the general hypothesis that governs atherogenesis.

4. In figure 9.5, use a penciled arrow to indicate an increase in renin secretion. Then follow through the system with other arrows indicating the ultimate effect on systemic blood pressure. Now switch to a red pencil to indicate decreased renin secretion and its consequences. You now have a quick reference diagram for renin's blood pressure effects. (As a quick verification, see figure 9.7 and note the plasma volume effects of ACE-inhibitors.)

5. Draw up a list of key points to use in discouraging tobacco users from smoking. Include some MI and fatality information for pack-a-day users and five mechanisms whereby smoking might contribute to atherosclerosis.

Chapter

10

Cardiac Pathophysiology

Never morning wore
To evening, but some heart did break.

ALFRED, LORD TENNYSON
IN MEMORIAM

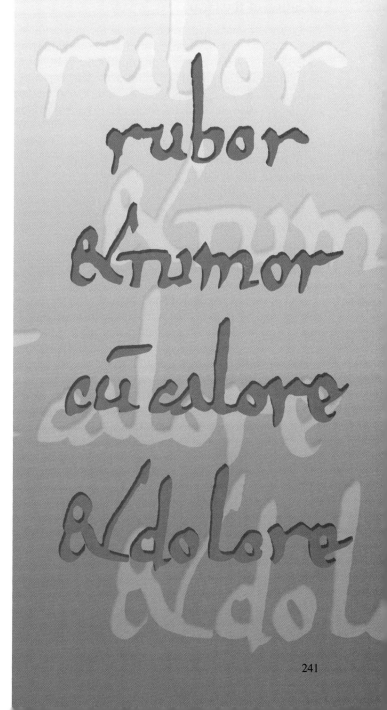

The heart normally functions as a highly effective pump. In a young adult, it is capable of adapting within minutes to dramatic changes in the body's requirement for oxygen, from the 5 liters pumped per minute at rest to perhaps 35 liters during continuous, heavy exercise in a trained athlete (25 liters in an average fit young person). The capacity to meet these pumping requirements depends on the coordinated action of a healthy heart muscle, valves that regulate flow direction, and vessels that facilitate distribution and return of blood. Although diseases may alter or damage different parts of this system, it is the compromise or failure of this essential pumping action that ultimately threatens health. Before turning to cardiac disease details, let us briefly review the working of the normal heart.

THE NORMAL HEART

Location of the Heart

The heart is located within the chest in the mediastinum, the medial cavity of the thorax, with much of its bulk lying posterior to the sternum. About one-third of the heart lies to the right of the midline and two-thirds to the left. Typically, the apex of the heart, which points more or less to the left hip, lies between ribs 4 and 5 when one is lying down on one's left side, and one space lower when one is sitting or standing. In deep inspiration, the apex will descend below the fifth interspace between ribs 5 and 6. The base, which is the point of attachment of the great vessels, is directed toward the right shoulder (fig. 10.1).

The Pericardium

The pericardium is bounded by a substantial and tough outer layer of fibrous connective tissue, the **fibrous pericardium.** It anchors the pericardium to the great veins and arteries at its base, to the sternum anteriorly, and to the diaphragm inferiorly (fig. 10.2) It thus fixes the heart in position as it contracts and relaxes in pumping and provides the cardiac surface with a protective enclosure as well.

Within the fibrous pericardium is a pair of serous membranes. The one lining the inner surface of the fibrous pericardium is the **parietal pericardium,** and the other, which covers the heart's surface, is the **visceral pericardium.** Both secrete a watery fluid that fills the thin space between them, the **pericardial space.** The 15–50 ml of **pericardial fluid** provides lubrication to the serous membrane surfaces to reduce friction as the heart moves during its pumping cycles. The fibrous pericardium and its inner serous lining are known as the **pericardial sac,** while the visceral pericardium is also called the **epicardium** (fig. 10.3).

The Myocardium

The cardiac muscle tissue that forms the walls of the atria and ventricles is the **myocardium.** It is anchored to an internal framework of fibrous connective tissue, sometimes known as the heart's fibrous skeleton. The tissue of the

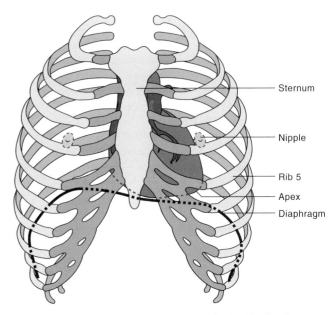

Figure 10.1   **The Position of the Heart in the Mediastinum with Respect to Selected Skeletal Reference Points.**

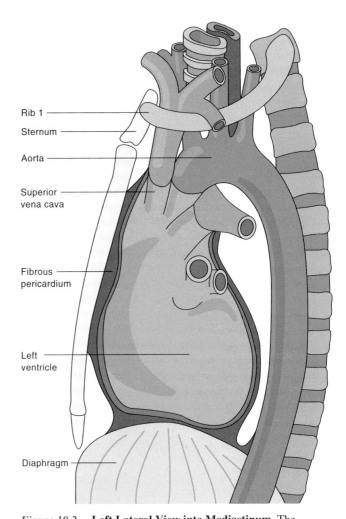

Figure 10.2   **Left Lateral View into Mediastinum.** The attachments of the pericardium to the diaphragm and sternum are clearly visible. Note also the protection provided by the sternum and vertebral column.

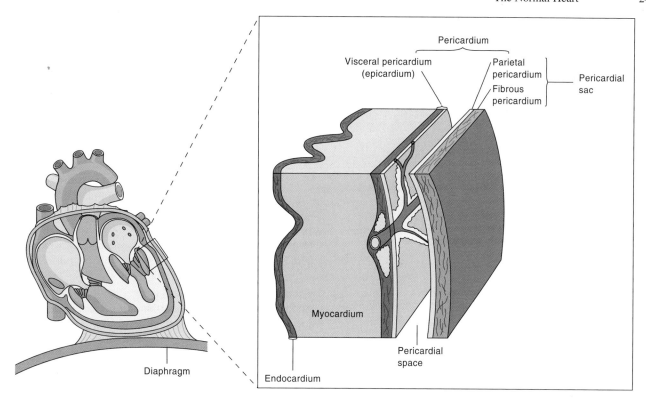

Figure 10.3   Components of the Pericardium and Endocardium and Their Relationship to the Myocardium. Adipose tissue can be seen in the epicardium associated with the vessel.

fibrous skeleton lies on an irregular plane between the atria and ventricles, providing a framework to which myocardial muscle can attach (fig. 10.4). This arrangement provides some distinct mechanical advantages. Bands of longitudinally arranged myocardial cells circle and loop down to form the ventricular walls (fig. 10.5*a*). When these contract, they draw the walls upward in a wringing movement that reduces the ventricular lumen far more for a given shortening of fiber than would a simple parallel arrangement of fibers. The gain in pumping efficiency can be compared to the increase in effect produced by wringing out a wet towel as opposed to just squeezing it.

As well as the encircling of the ventricles just described, there is a continuity and integration of the fibers of the left and right myocardium. Superficial layers circle the right ventricle, wind through the interventricular septum, and then form deep muscle layers in the left ventricle. Superficial layers circling the left ventricle wind backward through the septum and form deep layers in the right ventricle (fig. 10.5*b*). Because of this arrangement, pumping between the two sides is better integrated, but pathology that affects one ventricle is also apt to eventually affect the other.

Chambers of the Heart

The heart consists of two pumps that function synchronously as an integrated unit (fig. 10.6). The right heart acts as a volume pump, propelling blood through the low-resistance vessels of the pulmonary system. The left heart acts as a pressure pump, generating enough pressure to

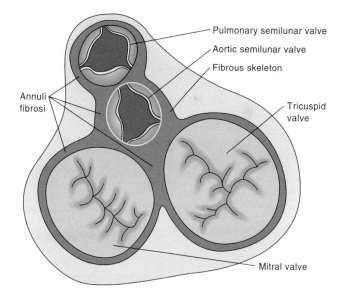

Figure 10.4   Valves Surrounded by Annuli Fibrosi. The fibrous skeleton of the heart is indicated in this diagram by darker pink. Note how the annuli fibrosi form the margins of the flow tracts, providing a strong anchoring for the cardiac valves. This view is from above with anterior to the top. The heart is in ventricular systole, actively pumping blood into the great arteries.

force the blood through the high-resistance vessels of the systemic circulation.

Each pump includes a thin-walled atrium that collects blood returning to the heart. A thin interatrial septum separates the left and right atria. Both atria have small,

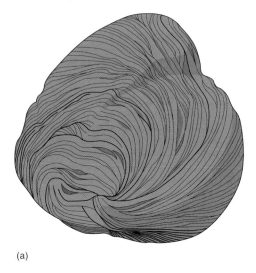

(a)

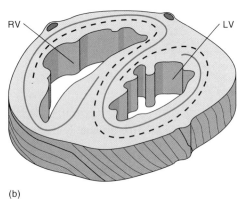

(b)

Figure 10.5 **Myocardial Muscle.** (*a*) The circular swirling of myocardial fibers. (*b*) This section shows the overlapping and continuity of the myocardial muscle sheets.

earlike appendages (auricles) that extend anteriorly. (Note that the terms *atrium* and *auricle* are not interchangeable.) Atrial contraction aids in filling the ventricles. The right atrium receives deoxygenated blood from the inferior vena cava, the superior vena cava, and the heart muscle (the myocardium) via the coronary sinus. The left atrium receives oxygenated blood from the lungs via the four pulmonary veins.

The muscular ventricles compose more than 60% of the mass of the heart and receive most of the coronary blood flow. They are separated by the interventricular septum, which is thick and muscular except near the atrioventricular septum, where it is a thin membrane. (Failure of this membranous septum to form is the most common congenital abnormality of the heart, allowing blood to be shunted from the high-pressure left ventricle into the low-pressure right ventricle.) Blood from the right ventricle is pumped into the pulmonary artery, while blood from the left ventricle is pumped into the aorta. The left ventricular wall is three to four times thicker than the right, reflecting the high workload required to overcome the resistance of the systemic vessels.

The Cardiac Valves

Blood must flow through the vascular system in one direction only. Any change from this flow pattern interferes with oxygenation of the blood and its supply to the tissues, or puts an extra load on the pump. The four cardiac valves are responsible for preventing any backflow in the system. Their structure and position allow blood to move in only the desired forward direction. Valve function in controlling flow of a liquid is illustrated in figure 10.7. This principle applies to the cardiac valves.

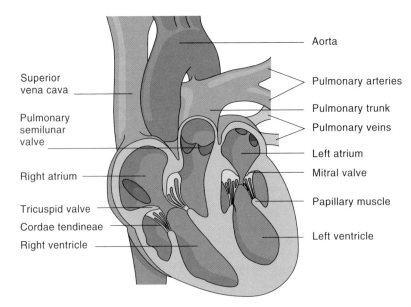

Figure 10.6 **Cardiac Section Showing the Internal Structure of the Heart.** The aortic semilunar valve, at the base of the aorta, is hidden by the pulmonary trunk.

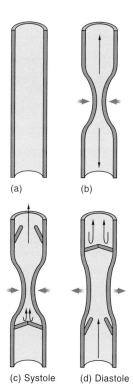

Figure 10.7   **The Principles of Cardiac Valve Function.**
Squeezing the fluid-filled tube (*a,b*) produces flow in both
directions. With valves in place, squeezing drives blood forward
(*c*). When pressure is released, backflow is prevented and more
fluid moves in (*d*) to be pumped during the next cycle.

The four valves are not active structures—that is, they
do not contract or act by themselves to control blood flow.
Their valve function instead depends on their structure and
position within the heart's flow tracts and their passive responses to pressures applied to their surfaces. The delicate
cardiac valve cusps or leaflets are formed of thin layers of
connective tissue covered by endothelium that is continuous with the endocardium (fig. 10.8). When pressure is
greater on one side than the other, the valve moves passively. Depending on the valve's location, pressure causes
the valve leaflet either to move into the flow tract, where it
will contact other valve leaflets and thus block flow, or to
be pushed out of the way to permit forward flow.

The valves of the heart are encircled by tough fibrous
rings of the heart's fibrous skeleton to which the valve
leaflets or cusps are anchored. These rings, the **annuli
fibrosi,** prevent the outlets from the atria and ventricles
from becoming dilated when the myocardium contracts to
force blood through them. When the heart is relaxing, they
form a firm margin or valve seat that makes effective valve
closure possible.

There are two different types of cardiac valve. One
type controls flow between an atrium and its corresponding
ventricle. These are the **atrioventricular valves** (AV
valves). Since the right AV valve has three cusps, it is
known as the **tricuspid** valve. Only two cusps form the left,
or **bicuspid,** AV valve. The bicuspid valve is also known as

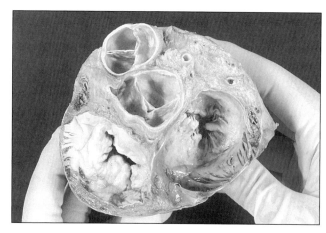

Figure 10.8   **The Cardiac Valves.** See figure 10.4 for details.

the **mitral valve** because when closed, the cusp configuration resembles a miter, the ritual headdress of a bishop.

As the ventricles contract, they generate a pressure that
closes the AV valves. The pressure involved is quite high,
and if unaided, the AV valves could not resist it. They
would be abruptly pushed past their closed position (valve
eversion), allowing blood to be regurgitated back into the
atrium. This does not happen because the AV valves are
tethered by the **chordae tendineae.** As their name suggests,
these are tendonlike cords. Each is attached, at one end, to
the ventricular surface of an AV cusp. The other end is secured to a small protrusion from the ventricular myocardium
called a **papillary muscle** (fig. 10.9). The strong, inelastic
chordae tendineae act as restraints against the ventricle's
high pressure. They are long enough to allow the valve to be
pushed to its full closed position, but not beyond.

Backflow of blood from the arteries into the relaxing
ventricles is prevented by the **semilunar (SL) valves.** Each
valve is composed of three cuplike leaflets that fold against
the vessel walls as the ventricle empties. As the ventricle
begins to relax, blood flow reverses, causing the cusps
to fill and expand and thereby block the lumen. The
pulmonary semilunar valve separates the right ventricle
from the pulmonary artery. The **aortic semilunar valve**
separates the left ventricle from the aorta. In a semilunar
valve, the smaller lumen and the support of the strong annuli fibrosi eliminate the need for the chordae tendineae associated with the AV valves.

The Cardiac Cycle

The sequence of events that composes the repeating, pumping action of the heart is termed the **cardiac cycle.** The portion of the cycle during which the ventricles contract is
termed **systole,** and the remaining interval, when the ventricles are relaxing, is called **diastole.** By convention, unless
specifically indicated, these terms refer to the ventricles. If
the focus is on the period of atrial contraction, atrial systole
needs to be specified.

Left AV valve cusps

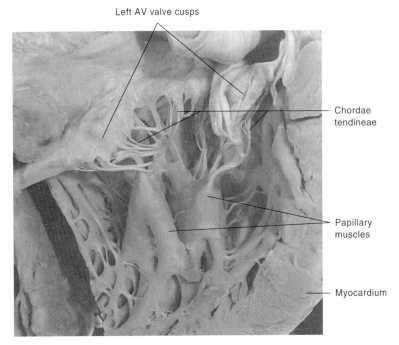

Chordae
tendineae

Papillary
muscles

Myocardium

Figure 10.9   **Valve with Anchoring Structures.** In this sectioned heart it is easy to see the chordae tendineae joining to the margin of the cusps at one end, while their other end is firmly anchored in the myocardium at the protruding papillary muscles. (Note, the papillary muscles are continuous with the myocardium.)

Cardiac Performance

Adequate circulation of blood through the body is achieved by maintaining an appropriate pressure gradient from the arteries through the capillaries to the veins. The arterial pressure is determined, in part, by the rate at which blood is pumped into the arteries and, in part, by the rate at which blood passes from the arterial system into the capillaries and veins. As tissue blood flow requirements change, cardiac pumping is altered to match them.

Each ventricle has a volume of up to 125 ml at the end of its filling period, the **end-diastolic volume** (EDV). During one systolic contraction, the volume of blood pumped from a ventricle is termed the **stroke volume** (SV). Not all the blood in the ventricle is pumped into the arterial system during systole. The volume remaining is termed the **end-systolic volume** (ESV). The percentage of blood pumped from the filled ventricle is the **ejection fraction,** normally about 65–70%. From these definitions it follows that taking the amount of blood in a filled ventricle (EDV) and subtracting the amount remaining after it contracts (ESV) will yield the amount pumped by the ventricle in one contraction (SV). Equation (1) presents this concept more succinctly:

$$SV = EDV - ESV \qquad \text{(Eq. 1)}$$

The ejection fraction can be expressed as in equation (2):

$$\text{Ejection fraction (\%)} = SV/EDV \times 100 \qquad \text{(Eq. 2)}$$

The volume of blood pumped from the left ventricle each minute is called the cardiac output (CO) and is dependent on both the heart rate (HR) and the stroke volume (SV). The relationship is indicated in equation (3):

$$CO \text{ (ml/min)} = HR \text{ (beats/min)} \times SV \text{ (ml/beat)} \qquad \text{(Eq. 3)}$$

A typical resting heart rate is about 70 beats per minute, with a stroke volume of 80 ml. The resting cardiac output in this example is therefore about 5.6 liters per minute.

Heart Rate Control

The heart generates its own regular contraction, which is modified by both nervous and hormonal controls. This intrinsic rhythm, of about 100 beats per minute, results from the spontaneous depolarization of a tiny island of specialized myocardial tissue located in the atrium near the junction with the superior vena cava, and is called the **sinoatrial node** (SA node). This signal is passed through atrial bands of the same specialized (sometimes called conducting) myocardium to the **atrioventricular** (AV) node, embedded in the center of the fibrous skeleton that forms the atrioventricular septum. Here the signal pauses very briefly, allowing the atrial contraction it has initiated to force more blood into the ventricles. Then the signal continues into the ventricles, passing along the conduction pathways (again, specialized myocardial tissue) of the bundle of His, the right and left bundle branches, and the Purkinje fibers to finally reach and activate the working cells of the ventricular myocardium. This depolarization induces ventricular contraction (fig. 10.10).

The capacity for rhythmic depolarization is found throughout the tissues of the SA and AV nodes and conduc-

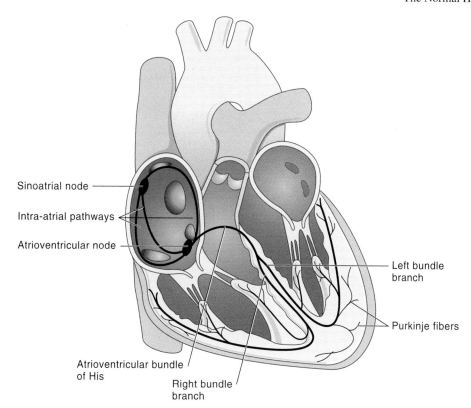

Figure 10.10   **Specialized Myocardium: Pacemaking and Conduction System of the Heart.**

tion pathways. The SA node has the fastest intrinsic rhythm and thereby sets the heart rate. For this reason it is often called the **pacemaker.** A cardiac rhythm that is dependably initiated from the SA node, whatever its rate, is termed a **sinus rhythm.** The term *sinus rhythm* therefore implies normally functioning signal generation and conduction. Certain disease conditions can permit other parts of the conduction system or even parts of the working myocardium to take over signal generation. These abnormally functioning bits of tissue are called **ectopic foci.** Their effect on heart function can range from minor (skipped beats or slightly impaired ventricular filling) to disastrous (ventricular fibrillation, a chaotically disordered ventricular contraction that can be fatal and requires immediate electrical defibrillation and restarting).

The electrochemical events that accompany signal generation and conduction in the specialized myocardium, while critical, are not normally observable on a clinical **ECG** (electrocardiogram, the tracing made of the amplified electrical events in the heart detectable at surface electrodes). However, the depolarization induced in the working myocardium of the atrium, which acts as a signal to contract, is seen as the first (or **P**) wave of the ECG. The second wave form (called the **QRS complex**) derives from ventricular depolarization, while the third (**T**) wave arises during ventricular repolarization (the signal to cease contracting).

The "signal to contract" is expressed in the common myocardial cells (cardiomyocytes) by the sudden influx of

sodium ions. This permits an increase in the intracellular concentration of calcium ions, which, in turn, releases the contractile process. Because the depolarization is conducted in a coordinated direction, the individual electrochemical events are summated into the observable ECG wave forms just noted. The depolarization is sustained for about 0.2 sec. Because this plateau is maintained by the influx of calcium simultaneously, throughout the depolarized myocardium, there is no coordinated directionality and therefore no detectable wave. So the ECG returns to baseline for the S-T segment (fig. 10.11). Ventricular contraction, which is occurring during this period of depolarization from shortly after the beginning of the QRS to the end of the T wave, is principally a biochemical event and is therefore not electrically detectable. By contrast, relaxation of the myocardium *is* electrochemically observable. "Relaxation" is accomplished when the myocardial membrane suddenly becomes permeable to potassium, which is in high intracellular concentration. Potassium outflow returns the cell membrane to resting potential.

For the bulk of the Q-T interval (see fig. 10.11 and the focus box on p. 250), the cardiomyocytes are unresponsive to any further stimulation (the term for this is the **absolute refractory period**). However, during the latter part of the ventricular repolarization (T wave), an intense signal, such as might come from an ectopic focus, may restimulate the myocardial cells. The results of this restimulation could range from a nonfunctional QRS wave in the ECG (an inconsequential

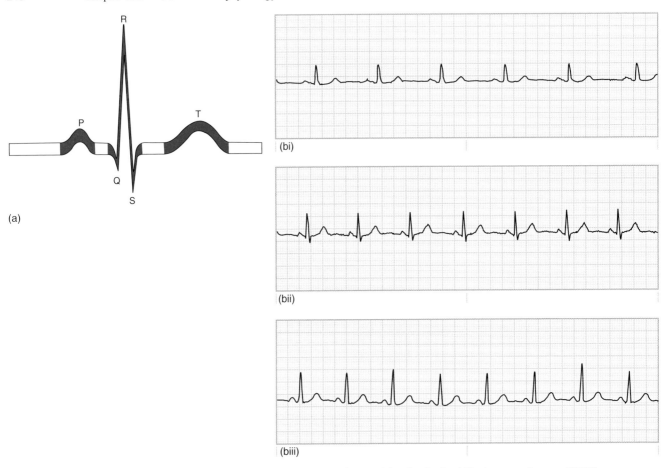

Figure 10.11   **The ECG (Electrocardiogram).** (*a*) Component wave forms of the classic (lead II) electrocardiogram (ECG). (*b*) Examples of regular sinus ECG traces at different heart rates. Each larger box represents 0.2 sec. Therefore, five boxes represent one sec. Knowing that each trace is 6 sec long, can you calculate the heart rate in each case? (Note, these traces have been reduced for economy of space) (Hint: multiply by 10!).

"extra systole") to atrial fibrillation (which interferes with normal heart function) to ventricular fibrillation (fatal unless effectively treated) (see focus box on pp. 250–251).

Any two electrodes placed at some reasonable distance on the surface of the body, especially spanning the chest, will, if amplified and displayed appropriately, show an ECG rhythm. To produce a clinical ECG, electrodes are applied to the wrists and ankles and also to the left chest. The presence, timing, and shapes of the P, QRS, and T waves allow the detection of any deviations from normal sinus rhythm. Tracings of the electrical activity in different combinations of electrodes essentially give different views of the contraction of the ventricles. These can also be used to detect areas of abnormal conduction and possibly areas of infarction. The six "precordial leads" represent the electrical activity evident at electrodes placed on either side of the sternum between ribs 4 and 5 and at four points along the space between ribs 5 and 6 (fifth "interspace") around the left side of the chest. In these positions, they are close to the interventricular septum and most of the wall of the left ventricle. This is usually clinically adequate as most infarcts occur in the left ventricle. Incidentally, the abbreviation EKG is sometimes used, indicative of the original German term *electrokardiogram*.

The heart is continually required to adjust pump-volume to meet altered metabolic demands and adjust pump-pressure to meet altered resistance. It has a simple repertoire of responses to meet these requirements: It can change heart rate and it can alter the force of each contraction (myocardial contractility). The commonly observed resting heart rate of 70 beats per minute is evidence that something must restrain the natural intrinsic rhythm of 100. Parasympathetic neurons reach the SA node of the heart via the vagus nerve. At rest, they release small amounts of acetylcholine, which slows the rate of depolarization of the SA node to 70 bpm. Parasympathetic neurons also innervate the AV node, slowing conduction to the ventricles. Sympathetic neurons innervate the pacemaker and conduction system as well as the ventricular working myocardium. Release of norepinephrine from these neurons or release of epinephrine from the adrenal medulla speeds the rate of depolarization. It also increases the force of each contraction, an issue dealt with in the section on stroke volume control.

The sympathetic nervous system and epinephrine act as cardiac rate accelerators. For this reason, norepinephrine and epinephrine are known as **positive chronotropes.** The parasympathetic nervous system is antagonistic to them, acting as a brake on the heart rate; thus, acetylcholine is a

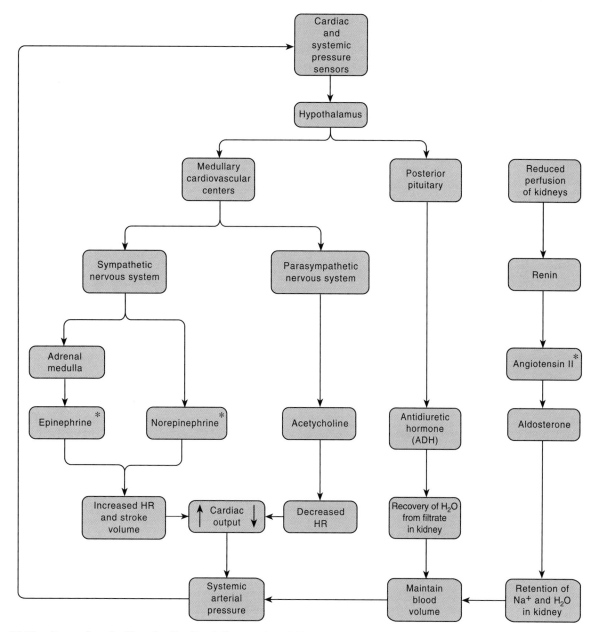

Figure 10.12   **Dynamics of a Negative Feedback System.** Arterial blood pressure depends, in part, on the cardiac output, which is affected by nuclei in the medulla. These monitor systemic pressure and adjust rate of stimulation in the autonomic pathways that supply the heart and influence the release of epinephrine from the adrenal medulla. A sudden drop in blood pressure will trigger the release of ADH from the posterior pituitary with the effect of increasing the reabsorption of water from the filtrate in the kidney that maintains blood volume. A decrease in blood pressure results in impaired perfusion of the kidneys, activating the renin-angiotensin-aldosterone system, resulting in retention of sodium and water which preserves blood volume.

*These hormones also act on arteries and arterioles to increase peripheral resistance (↑ systemic arterial pressure) and on veins and venules to reduce the venous compartment, improving cardiac return and making more blood available to the arterial system and capillaries.

negative chronotrope. The two systems are coordinated by the cardiac centers in the medulla oblongata of the brain stem. Pressure receptors in the right atrium and arterial system form part of a negative feedback system regulating the heart rate and blood pressure (fig. 10.12). Higher brain centers also can influence the heart rate as might be noted in "white coat hypertension."

The autonomic nervous system affects the systemic vasculature in ways that support and complement the ac-

tions it has on the heart. In a situation demanding maintenance of blood pressure or increased cardiac output, the sympathetic release of norepinephrine at the small distribution arterioles ("resistance vessels") induces vasoconstriction. This has the immediate effect of increasing afterload, thereby restoring blood pressure. In conditions of high demand, this conserves the finite volume of blood for the perfusion of active (muscle) tissues. In resting conditions, the venous compartment contains about 60% of the blood.

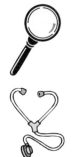

Focus on The ECG: An Introduction to the Basics

Capturing the Signal: Placement of Electrodes

An electrode is in contact with the skin through an electrode gel. Here it can pick up changes in the local electrical charge. A sudden flow of positive sodium ions toward the electrode attracts electrons, producing a positive deflection (depolarization approaching the electrode) while a sudden flow of positive potassium ions away from the electrode repels electrons, producing a negative deflection (repolarization moving away from the electrode). Wires, called "leads," carry these changes to an ECG machine, which amplifies and displays them. Activity in the electrodes can be "viewed" using different combinations called "Leads" (e.g., right arm versus left leg). There are six of these combinations in a clinical ECK and they are called the "Limb Leads." In addition, six electrodes span the left chest and are called "Precordial Leads," giving a total of 12 leads in the clinical ECG.

Limb Leads
("Views" depolarization of myocardium from different perspectives)

Precordial Leads
("Views" interventricular septum and wall of left venticle)

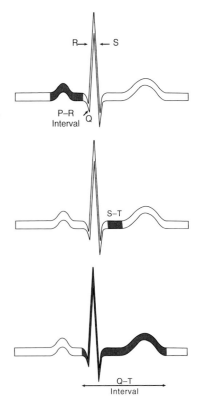

(Lead II, which is illustrated, compares the right arm with the left leg. This produces the "textbook ECG": The wave of depolarization is "viewed" from apex, which emphasizes ion flow in the long axis of the heart. Deflection and the shape of components will appear differently in different leads.)

Steps in "Reading" the ECG

1. **Heart Rate**—Total number of PQRST complexes per minute. Normal resting sinus rhythm ranges between 60–100 bpm (slower = bradycardia; faster = tachycardia; patient's clinical picture, health, and exercise history must be taken into consideration). Count # QRS in 6 sec × 10 = HR (small square, 1 mm = 0.04 sec; large square, 0.5 mm = 0.20 sec). (What were the heart rates shown in fig. 10.11?) If P waves or QRS complexes are occurring independently, do a separate count of each.

2. **Rhythmicity**—Normal rhythm is highly regular (i.e., < 0.06 sec—1.5 small squares) variability in R-R interval. Irregular rhythms range from patterned to completely irregular.

3. **Characteristics of a P Wave**—(assuming regular rhythm). First question in determining if trace is in "sinus rhythm": Is each P wave followed directly by a QRS complex? Additionally, are P waves oriented in appropriate direction, smooth, and regular in occurrence and appearance? When there are more "normal" P waves present than QRS, the regularity and ratio (P-QRS) are informative.

4. **Duration of the P-R Interval** (P-Q Interval)—Second question in determining if trace is in "sinus rhythm": Is the consistent P-R interval between 0.12 and 0.20 sec in duration (three to five small boxes)? Less than 0.12 sec implies that the rhythm is not being triggered by the SA node but by a pacemaker closer to the AV node (not "sinus"). Longer than 0.20 sec implies conduction delay or AV block. Varying P-R intervals are significant.

5. **Characteristics of a QRS Complex**—Normally < 0.12 sec in duration (usually indicating being triggered from the atria via the AV node—i.e., supraventricular). Prolonged (> 0.12 sec) may mean QRS is triggered from a ventricular pacemaker. The shapes of QRS generated from the ventricles are dramatically different from those of atrially generated QRS.

6. **S-T Segment**—Elevation or depression (more usual) of 1 mm in the S-T segment is indicative of myocardial ischemia or infarction (1 mm = 1 mV).

7. **Q-T Interval** (R-T Interval)—Represents the total period of ventricular activation, contraction, and relaxation; varies with heart rate from about 0.4 to 0.3 sec. Prolongation of Q-T interval is a sensitive and specific predictor of myocardial ischemia. Prolonged Q-T interval means the heart is in a longer "relative refractory period" and is vulnerable to a dangerous arrhythmia.

Atrial Fibrillation—No apparent P waves; irregular, rapid (350–400), saw-tooth, small waves; irregular, perhaps accelerated QRS, relatively "normal" shape and duration (< 0.12 sec). Clinical condition will vary. One of most common atrial arrhythmias; may be associated with ventricular fibrillation. (What HR is evident in this ECG trace?)

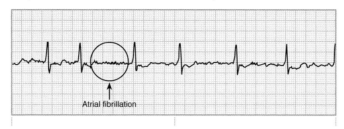

Premature Ventricular Complexes (PVCs)—Regular or irregular interposition of a odd-shaped, perhaps variable, QRS complex without preceding P wave. Variable shape indicates different ectopic foci. May occur without ventricular contraction, so subsequent, delayed QRS produces "thumping" beat as extra blood is expelled. Frequent (six or more per minute) or couplets or salvos of three or more may indicate a worrisome ventricular irritability. Patient's clinical condition is very important to consider.

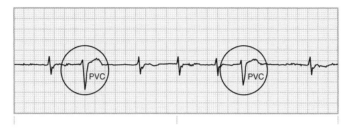

Second-Degree AV Block—ECG trace shows progressively lengthening P-R interval followed by failure of a P wave to elicit a QRS. This illustrates a second-degree AV block, called a Mobitz type I (aka Wenchebach). "Block" varies from Mobitz type I to occasionally missed QRS to regularly missed QRS (Mobitz type II), in which case patient is likely to show some sign of impaired perfusion.

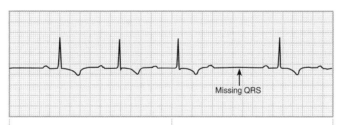

Ventricular Tachycardia—100–250 bpm; P wave is usually not detectable; unrelated to QRS. QRS shape can be highly regular or variable (*torsades de point,* "twisting of the points"). QRS prolonged beyond 0.12 sec is very serious—great potential for progression into ventricular fibrillation. Trace shows V Tach of 260 bpm.

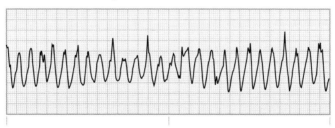

Ventricular Fibrillation—ECG accompanying uncoordinated, pulseless writhing of the ventricles. Death will ensue without cardioversion (defibrillation). Coarse VF will progress into fine VF, which is less responsive to efforts at defibrillation.

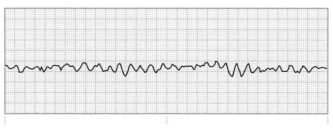

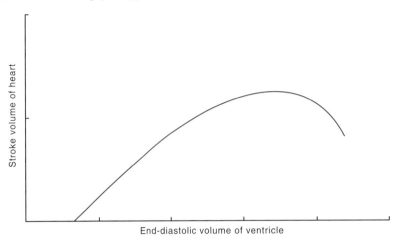

Figure 10.13   **Automatic Accommodation of Cardiac Pumping to the Volume of Blood Supplied.** Starling's law expresses the relation between the end-diastolic volume, which stretches the myocardium, and the resulting force of contraction, which determines the stroke volume.

Sympathetic stimulation of large and small veins can instantly improve cardiac return (increased preload) as well as make an increased volume of blood available for perfusion. The vasoconstriction effect of norepinephrine is also active on resistance vessels in muscle and the heart itself. While this might seem like a biological oversight, the vasoconstriction is overridden by local controls that we will discuss in a moment. So, muscle in general receives less blood, while the specifically active muscles (including the heart) are adequately perfused.

Slower, hormonal compensations also occur to deal with threats to tissue perfusion (fig. 10.12). A gradual drop in blood pressure is accompanied by poorer perfusion of the kidneys, which triggers the release of renin and activation of the renin-angiotensin-aldosterone system. Angiotensin II acts directly on the vasculature, reinforcing the effects of norepinephrine, while aldosterone, released from the adrenal cortex, causes the kidneys to retain sodium and thereby water and blood fluid volume. A sudden drop in blood pressure (or extreme stress) adds the release of ADH (antidiuretic hormone) to the mix, recovering water filtered in the kidneys, thereby retaining body fluid volume. As well, it elicits the sympathetic release of epinephrine from the adrenal medulla, which takes up the vasoconstriction activity of short-acting norepinephrine. These, and other adaptations, will be discussed when we talk about the possible cardiovascular effects of stress and the pathophysiology of congestive heart failure.

Stroke Volume Control

Stroke volume is determined by three main variables: EDV, the resistance of the vascular system to emptying of the ventricle, and the contractility of the myocardium.

The EDV determines the amount of tension applied to the resting myocardium of the fully filled ventricle prior to contraction. For this reason, EDV is sometimes called the **preload.** In turn, the EDV is dependent on the volume of blood available for ventricular filling (the venous return) and the resistance of the ventricle to expansion.

End-diastolic volume and stroke volume are related. The relationship was first demonstrated at the turn of the century by Frank and Starling and is known as **Starling's law of the heart.** Briefly stated, the heart adapts to different preloads by pumping the volume of blood delivered to it. This adjustment occurs automatically, without any external control by nerves or hormones, and is thus termed **autoregulation** or **intrinsic regulation of stroke volume.** The mechanism behind the Frank-Starling effect is a characteristic common to both skeletal and cardiac muscle cells: The force of contraction is greater when the muscle is stretched prior to contraction (fig. 10.13). The degree of stretch of cells in the ventricular wall is determined by the volume of blood delivered to the heart. This means that changes in venous return produce appropriate changes in contraction force that efficiently match preload to contraction force. The essential principle of Starling's law is widely accepted, but its role in normal cardiac output determination is less clear. Intrathoracic pressures vary during breathing, and this leads to unbalanced filling of left and right ventricles as blood pools or is pressed out of the lungs. This imbalance is countered, as described by Starling's law, by an automatic adjustment of stroke volume to EDV. It may play a more significant role in compensating for cardiac dysfunction in the failing heart.

The stroke volume is also determined by the resistance of the arterial system to ventricular emptying. This resistance is called **afterload** and is determined primarily by blood viscosity and the resistance offered by the vascular system itself. Normally, vascular resistance comes principally from the arterioles and precapillary sphincters, whose tension is an important component determining the BP and which function to effectively shunt the fixed volume of blood to the most metabolically active body tissues.

The third major variable influencing stroke volume is **myocardial contractility.** It is defined as the tension that

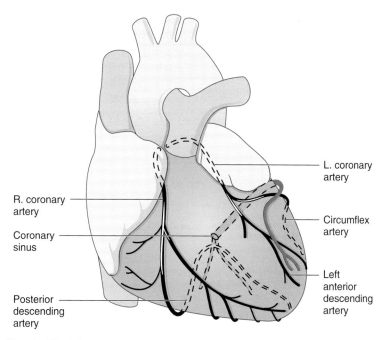

Figure 10.14 **The Cardiac Vessels.** The left coronary artery divides to form the circumflex and anterior descending arteries. The right coronary artery follows the atrioventricular groove and forms the posterior interventricular artery. The cardiac veins join the coronary sinus, which returns blood to the right atrium.

can be developed by the cardiac muscle cell independent of its starting length or tension. Contractility is dependent, in part, on the structural organization of the cell and its metabolic state. Hypoxia and certain toxins decrease myocardial contractility and are termed **negative inotropes.** Other factors, such as digitalis or its derivatives, will increase contractility and are termed **positive inotropes.** In addition, contractility can be increased by sympathetic stimulation and by the hormone epinephrine; so these are also positive inotropes.

Cardiac Perfusion

Cardiac Vessels

The left and right coronary arteries are the first vessels to arise from the aorta. Their openings are situated behind the delicate cusps of the aortic semilunar valves when they are pushed open during ventricular systole. The left coronary artery quickly branches into a left anterior descending artery (LAD), which descends in the anterior groove between the left and right ventricles, and the circumflex artery (CX), which travels in the groove between the left atrium and ventricle. The right coronary artery (RCA) travels in the right atrioventricular groove. The interventricular septum is supplied by the LAD and a corresponding posterior descending artery that usually arises from the RCA. The wall of the left ventricle is supplied from these and the CX (fig. 10.14). Variability occurs in the coronary artery branchings and territories supplied. Drainage is provided through veins that empty into the coronary sinus, which, in turn empties into the right atrium. Some drainage, particularly from the subendocardial tissue of the right atrium and

ventricle, passes from the capillaries into Thebesian veins, which open directly into the heart chambers.

The cardiac arteries must accommodate unique perfusion dynamics. The left ventricle generates significant pressures during systole. This compresses the heart muscle as well as the blood within the left ventricle. So, in contrast to the right ventricle, which follows the expected pattern of increased perfusion during the elevated pressures of systole, 60% of total coronary blood flow takes place through the left coronary artery during diastole. This means, in effect, that the majority of perfusion needs in the left ventricle are met during diastole. The compressive forces differentially affect the subendocardial tissue that lies between the blood and the wringing myocardium. Therefore, it is the left ventricular subendocardial layer that is more vulnerable to ischemia. Partial stenosis of an epicardial artery may produce its first significant ischemia in this region, particularly during exercise or stress, and conditions that have led to ventricular hypertrophy will make this worse. Recall that the interventricular septum contributes a major part of the muscle that forms the left ventricle. If anything, the compressive dynamics are exaggerated in the interventricular septum as there is a longer course for the mid-sized arteries carrying blood from the major branches of the coronary arteries. These larger cardiac arteries travel over the epicardium, not subject to the compressive forces just described. Consequently, they tend to fill maximally during systole and then discharge this blood to the myocardium during low-pressure diastole. This may mean that they are more subject than arteries in the rest of the body to the "wear-and-tear" forces that predispose to atherosclerotic degeneration.

Control of Cardiac Perfusion

Autoregulation ensures that myocardial perfusion is relatively constant, despite changes in the pumping pressure of the heart and the cyclical fluctuations in vessel luminal pressure that occur during the heart beat. Autoregulation involves a reflex adjustment of arterial wall tension to rein in flow at high arterial pressures and relax and permit flow at low arterial pressures, resulting in steady perfusion. Metabolism in the heart is largely aerobic, even at very intense rates of activity. Sustained aerobic metabolism hinges on dynamically matching energy and O_2 demands with their delivery (i.e., perfusion). Most of the adjustment of perfusion in the heart relies on linking blood flow to energy demands as they are reflected in the rate of production of adenosine. You will recall that adenosine triphosphate (ATP) is produced aerobically, particularly in the mitochondria. ATP receives its energy when a phosphate is bound to ADP. That energy is "ferried" to the site of utilization, in this case the actively contracting myofibrils in the cardiomyocyte. There, the phosphate bond is broken and the energy is translated into pumping action. Intensely active myocardium produces higher levels of both ATP and ADP. (Anginal pain, which is associated with ischemia, is triggered by adenosine. The use of adenosine as a vasodilatory drug is often accompanied by the unpleasant side effect of angina.) This adenosine triggers the production of **nitric oxide** (NO), also called **"endothelium-derived relaxing factor"** (EDRF). Nitric oxide, as has been noted when we explained its role in inflammation, is an important locally regulated vasodilator. Diffusing readily in the local tissue, it has an instantaneous and brief (seconds) effect, producing relaxation of vascular smooth muscle with the effect of vasodilation. Other factors will also trigger NO release. Histamine, bradykinin, platelet-derived factors, and fluid sheer stress, which are known to individually elicit NO, would all be produced in a coronary vessel that was initially constricted. Acetylcholine, another factor triggering NO release, would be carried into the heart from actively contracting skeletal muscle, a condition that would demand increased cardiac output.

Endothelin 1 (ET-1), in contrast, is the most powerful vasoconstrictor in the body. It is produced in response to epinephrine, ADH, angiotensin II, and certain inflamma-

tory mediators. The cardiac endothelium possesses **angiotensin-converting enzyme** (ACE), so that angiotensin II (AII) may be produced directly in the heart (most AII is produced through ACE in the pulmonary vasculature). These two substances, NO and ET-1, balance cardiac demand and perfusion. The derangement of these controls in ischemically damaged vasculature is an important pathological mechanism in ischemic heart disease that we will address later.

HEART DISEASE

Death from **heart failure** is the most catastrophic outcome of the disease processes described in this chapter. For a death to be attributed to heart failure, the ventricles must have failed to maintain blood circulation compatible with basic life processes despite adequate venous filling. By this definition, heart failure is a common ultimate cause of death. In practice, if the failure of the pump is indirectly caused by some other disease process—for example, blood loss, acidosis, or widespread cancer—mortality is then attributed to that disease.

Heart failure may be intrinsic to the pump itself. For example, the myocardium may have been weakened by disease or excessive stretching. Other causes might be restrictions to cardiac blood flow that impede filling and pumping, or disturbance of the heart's intrinsic rhythm. On the other hand, the failure might be attributed to factors that place excess demands on the pump—for example, defective valves, or vessels that offer abnormal resistance to blood flow, or excessive pumping demand as in hyperthyroidism, which increases the metabolic/oxygenation demands of the body.

Heart Failure: Terms and Concepts

Acute and Chronic Heart Failure

Before we look at the various sources of heart failure, it will be useful to distinguish between acute and chronic heart failure.

If the heart failure and the processes underlying it develop quickly (a few seconds to a few days), we refer to it as **acute heart failure.** Approximately 35% of individuals suffering acute heart failure succumb to it. Conversely, 65% do not; either spontaneously or with medical intervention, these people survive, with the quality of the remaining heart function dependent on the nature and extent of the cardiac damage. At the other end of the spectrum are chronic conditions that more gradually place an added burden on the individual's heart. When these burdens exceed the capacity of the heart and circulatory system to adapt, the person is said to be experiencing **chronic heart failure.** Individuals with chronic heart failure may experience a sudden deterioration of cardiac function, which threatens them with acute heart failure because of the natural progression of the disease, a failure of therapy, or sudden and excessive cardiac demand (the classic example is shoveling snow). Because the heart and associated vessels are a complex anatomical and func-

 Checkpoint 10.1

The relevance of these details of cardiac blood supply, metabolism, and perfusion control will be clear when we discuss the mechanisms of ischemic heart disease and the medical management of heart failure. In the meantime, what do you think would be the effect of drugs that trigger NO on heart pain (angina) due to poor perfusion? What about chemicals that inhibited ACE activity?

tional system, there are many routes to the end-stage of complete heart failure. Sometimes the function of the entire heart is disrupted, as for example in a sudden arrhythmia. In other cases, one ventricle alone is initially affected.

A variety of terms are used to denote either actual conditions in the heart or hypothetical mechanisms whereby the symptoms and heart failure progress. Bear in mind while you read this material that the most common underlying pathology giving rise to heart failure is ischemic heart disease. This condition will often be expressed as a weakening of the ventricular myocardium, usually that of the left ventricle. Other diseases and other sites and structures may result in chronic heart failure, but left ventricular failure secondary to ischemic heart disease is the most common starting point.

Left-Sided and Right-Sided Heart Failure

The most common pattern of heart failure is for one ventricle, usually the left, to fail first. The left is more often the first to fail because it has a much greater workload, and so is more stressed. It also has the greatest mass and oxygen consumption and is consequently most susceptible to imbalance of O_2 demand over delivery. The pattern of left-sided heart failure includes a number of pulmonary effects, including pulmonary congestion and edema, because the lungs empty into the left heart, which is unable to deliver all that blood to the systemic circulation. As well, decreased perfusion of the kidneys and cerebral hypoxia contribute to the complications of left-sided heart failure. Reduced renal perfusion activates the renin-angiotensin-aldosterone system. Angiotensin II increases peripheral resistance, which puts added strain on an already taxed left ventricle, while aldosterone leads to sodium and water retention, creating a volume overload. Well-advanced chronic heart failure blurs attention and causes irritability, restlessness, and even coma.

Right-sided heart failure often follows left-sided heart failure, but it also occurs independently in primary lung diseases in which the resistance of the lung's vascular bed, and hence the pressure load on the right ventricle, increases dramatically. This situation leads to a classic pattern of signs and symptoms (cor pulmonale) that we will deal with in detail in the section on congestive heart failure. Symptoms include signs of congestion in the capillary beds of the systemic circulation and will include enlargement of the liver (**hepatomegaly**) (see fig. 10.14) and spleen (**splenomegaly**). Congestion of the kidneys affects their perfusion more markedly than the reduced cardiac output that often occurs in left heart failure. The result is increased fluid retention and edema, and impaired clearing (accumulation) of nitrogenous wastes (azotemia). With time, pure right-sided failure will tax the left heart until it, too, is not meeting the challenges of perfusion, and combined heart failure will ensue.

Low-Output and High-Output Heart Failure

In most patients with heart failure, cardiac output is depressed below normal levels. Because the heart is not able to meet normal resting oxygen demands, a clinical pattern of impaired peripheral circulation, due to systemic vasoconstriction, produces cold, pale, and sometimes cyanotic (bluish) extremities—low-output heart failure. On the other hand, some normal or disease states require significant increases in cardiac output to meet very high demand. In these states, the extremities are warm and flushed. If the demand for increased cardiac output outpaces the capacity of the heart to meet it, high-output heart failure will ensue.

Pericardial Disease

Percardial disease manifests itself by the accumulation of fluid in the pericardial space (**pericardial effusion**) and/or inflammation of the pericardium (**pericarditis**). Although there can be pain and discomfort associated with pericarditis, the threat to health occurs when the pumping action of the heart is impeded. The pericardial cavity can fill with up to 2 liters (normal volume 15–50 ml) of serous fluid (**hydropericardium**) or blood (**hemopericardium**) that prevents normal diastolic filling and thereby reduces cardiac output.

Acute Pericarditis

The most frequent clinical form of pericardial disease is acute pericarditis, a nonspecific inflammatory response to a variety of injuries that can be organized into three groups: intrinsic heart disease, disease in adjacent structures, and systemic disorders.

Usually the volume of intrapericardial effusion in acute pericarditis is small (not greater than 200 ml) and with varying fibrin content: **serous, serofibrinous,** or **fibrinous.** The greater the fibrin content, the greater the tendency to roughen the pericardium or form adhesions. This pattern is typical in the acute pericarditis that accompanies rheumatic fever, uremia, myocardial infarction, and immune and viral forms of pericarditis. These usually resolve with no clinically significant sequelae. A **purulent suppurative effusion** is found in bacterial or fungal infections and tends to have more serious consequences (fig. 10.15). There is often fibrous obliteration of the pericardial cavity. Not only do the visceral and parietal membranes adhere to each other, but the fibrous pericardium can adhere to adjacent structures, producing adhesive mediastinopericarditis. This condition disrupts both diastolic and systolic ventricular action, since the heart has to work against the restricting adhesions to surrounding structures.

The classic clinical presentation of acute pericarditis is one of constant chest pain of sudden onset, which worsens on deep inspiration. Pain often lessens when the patient is sitting or leaning forward, because that posture lowers the tension on the pericardium. In 50% of patients, however, chest pain is minor or absent. On auscultation, a faint scratchy sound called a **friction rub** may be heard in systole and diastole as surfaces roughened by the deposition of fibrin from the exudate move over one another. If a large volume of fluid is present, heart sounds are diminished. An electrocardiogram and echocardiogram are needed for a

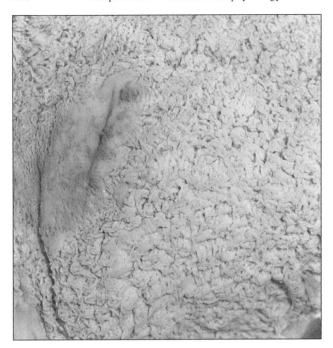

Figure 10.15   **Acute Pericarditis.** In this view of the pericardial surface, a pronounced purulent effusion produces a shaggy appearance.

This cardiac surface is thickly coated with fibrin as the result of an acute pericarditis with a purulent fibrinous effusion. The problem arose in a 57-year-old male who had been overwhelmed by the effects of a malignant lung tumor. He had deferred any medical assistance for his chronic productive cough, loss of voice, and progressive weakness and weight loss. Radiation therapy was unable to significantly reverse his decline, and he died one month later.

A contributing factor to his death was a weakened resistance, which had allowed the establishment of a widespread pneumococcal infection. Acute meningitis resulted, as well as the acute pericarditis that produced the shaggy pattern of fibrin deposition shown here. The surface was heavily infiltrated with polymorphonuclear cells and bacteria.

definitive diagnosis of acute pericarditis. (In echocardiography, also called cardiac ultrasonography, ultrasound is used to image heart structure and study structure and blood flow patterns during the cardiac cycle.) If the volume of fluid is large or the exudate develops quickly, the filling of the ventricles may be impaired because the heart's relaxation is opposed by the high pericardial pressure (the condition called **cardiac tamponade**) and cardiac output will fall. **Pericardiocentesis**—removal of the excess fluid—relieves the pressure on the heart but may have to be repeated if the exudate continues to form. The inflammatory reaction can be therapeutically controlled with salicylate and occasionally corticosteroids, while the pain is controlled by analgesics such as codeine.

Chronic Pericarditis

Acute pericarditis typically resolves, but chronic problems can arise as a complication of healing. When fibrosis is excessive, **chronic constrictive pericarditis** may produce a

diffusely and densely scarred pericardial sac. This sclerosis or hardening of the pericardium means that a nondistensible shell now encases the heart. The reduced elasticity often produces stenosis at the points where veins enter the atria. The resulting restriction of venous return can increase back pressure in the systemic veins, causing hepatomegaly and splenomegaly. Restricted diastolic filling from the limitation of venous return can also combine to reduce cardiac output. Severe cases require surgical removal of both the visceral and parietal layers of the pericardium. This condition is most common as a complication of tuberculous pericarditis, but it is also found as a chronic development in **acute idiopathic pericarditis** (probably viral). In about 50% of cases, the heavily scarred pericardium becomes calcified and can reach a state (called **concretio cordis**) in which the heart appears to be encased in a plaster mold.

Radiation-induced pericarditis is a form of chronic pericarditis that frequently develops after prolonged radiotherapy for Hodgkin's disease, lymphoma, or breast cancer and must be anticipated in these patients. Pericardiocentesis is the common form of management. Uremic pericarditis can develop in patients with chronic renal failure who are not being dialyzed. Why pericarditis develops is unknown, but it promptly disappears upon initiation of dialysis.

Myocarditis

Myocarditis is a condition of inflammatory change in the myocardium. Occasionally, myocarditis presents as focal inflammation of the myocardium (sometimes called primary myocarditis), but usually it is one manifestation of a more general disease process (e.g., rheumatic fever). Myocarditis is usually acute and mild, and followed by a complete recovery. In some cases, however, there can be scattered necrosis of myocardial cells or even heart failure due to extreme weakening of the heart muscle or faulty valve function. The causative agent may be viruses, bacteria, protozoa, parasites, hypersensitivity reactions, trauma, or that diagnostic blind alley—unknown (idiopathic myocarditis).

Viral myocarditis is the most common form, more often affecting infants and young men. Sometimes common exposure in very close living or working environments (e.g., army barracks) has been implicated. Viral forms also are more likely to be restricted to the heart. The Coxsackie B virus is most often implicated, and often there is an associated pericarditis. Changes in the myocardium typically include both fluid exudate and a cellular infiltration. Among otherwise healthy adults, the viral disease is usually mild, with some pericardial pain, weakness, and fatigue. Debilitated or immune-suppressed patients can experience much more serious symptoms and even acute cardiac failure. Fetuses and newborns are also more vulnerable to the effects of viral myocarditis.

The clinical course of myocarditis can be extremely variable. Transient ECG abnormalities may be the only objective sign. Symptoms might include malaise, dyspnea (difficult breathing), low-grade fever, and tachycardia (elevated heart rate). The weakened muscle and fibrous skeleton can allow the AV valve orifices to stretch, a condition leading to mitral or tricuspid valve malfunctions. In most cases, signs and symptoms take one to two months to resolve. In some cases, the problem persists to cause chronic heart failure. Less often, acute heart failure is involved. A chronic form of myocarditis called **Chagas' disease** afflicts up to 30% of the population in certain areas of South America and South Africa. It is caused by an intracellular protozoan called *Trypanosoma cruzi*.

Endocardial Disease: Infective Endocarditis

Untreated **infective endocarditis** (IE) is almost invariably fatal. Even with aggressive and appropriate antibiotic therapy, it still has a mortality range of 30–35%. Bacteria are the most usual infective agents involved in IE, so the disease is sometimes called **bacterial endocarditis.** The more inclusive term, infective endocarditis, is preferable because fungi and rickettsiae are also infective agents that are known to cause endocarditis.

There are two clinically distinct patterns of this disease: **subacute** and **acute infective endocarditis.** One major difference between them is their response to treatment. Subacute IE has a current mortality rate of 5–10%, while that for acute IE runs in the range of 60–80%! The usual cause of death in both is acute or chronic heart failure.

In both subacute and acute IE, the basic lesion is the build-up of a large, easily fragmented infective mass called a **vegetation.** This is essentially a thrombus of tangled fibrin, platelets, and blood cell debris containing masses of bacteria or other microorganisms (fig. 10.16). Especially in acute IE, the bacteria can be effectively isolated in the core of this mass, thus being sheltered from the body's immune system or antibiotics. Vegetations can be as large as several centimeters in diameter, loosely attached, and single or multiple. They usually form at the margins of the affected valve leaflets (the mitral or aortic valve alone, in 80–90% of cases). Valvular infection, especially in acute IE, can cause erosion of the valve leaflet or associated chordae tendineae. This condition leads to impaired valve function and to the major cause of death, heart failure. Vegetations have a tendency to break up, seeding the blood with infective and potentially occlusive emboli. Embolization is more extensive in acute IE, producing petechiae, abscesses, and infarcts. The kidneys are particularly affected, but significant embolic infarction of the brain or heart can also take place.

In **acute infective endocarditis,** a classic pattern of signs and symptoms aids diagnosis. The cardinal signs are a changing heart murmur, high fever, shaking chills, splinter hemorrhages (petechiae visible beneath the fingernails), splenomegaly, anemia, and hematuria (blood in the urine). Preexisting heart disease is uncommon, and the patient often has a preexisting infection. The infective agent is *Staphylococcus aureus* (a particularly virulent and antibiotic-resistant bacterium) in 50% of cases and *Streptococcus* in an additional 35%.

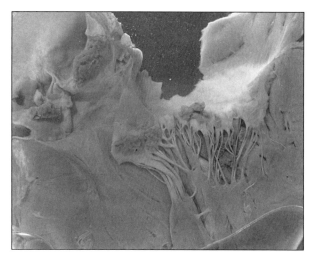

Figure 10.16   Infective Endocarditis. The vegetations on the surface of these valve cusps arose as a result of an infective endocarditis (IE).

Exploratory abdominal surgery was performed on a 72-year-old woman who had chest pains, but no ECG confirmation of infarction. The suspicion was that chronic inflammation of the gall bladder (cholecystitis) might be involved, and the surgery indeed found an enlarged, thick-walled gall bladder, which was removed. Her postoperative course was plagued by a variety of severe complications, including splitting open of her sutured incision, arterial obstruction necessitating a leg amputation, and finally by heart failure, to which she succumbed.

At autopsy her left heart was found to have been damaged by an infective endocarditis. In the specimen, small, crumbly vegetations can be seen. The valve cusps are thickened, as are the chordae tendineae. Microscopic study of the vegetations revealed them to be composed of fibrin, platelets, bacterial masses, and inflammatory cells.

A bacterial infection of the valves appears to develop initially, and this is followed by thrombus formation. The course of the disease is rapid. If untreated, death can occur in two weeks, either from embolism as the loose thrombotic vegetations break up, or from heart failure secondary to mitral or aortic valve dysfunction. Infection and embolic infarction of the kidney contribute to anemia by interfering with renal erythropoietin production and by allowing blood loss to the urine.

Intravenous drug use carries a risk of many infections, including acute IE. In over half of these cases the pattern of vegetation formation is quite unusual: The tricuspid valves alone are affected. Athletes who take injections of psychoactive drugs or performance-enhancing drugs are another growing population of people at risk of developing acute IE.

Typically, the person who develops **subacute infective endocarditis** has a preexisting heart condition (e.g., rheumatic heart disease, congenital defect, valve replacement). A significant number of cases develop after cardiac surgery, particularly in valve replacements. In such cases, prophylactic antibacterial treatment can result in growth of a resistant fungus (e.g., *Candida*), which then becomes the infective agent. Apparently the blood-borne organisms colonize tiny, preexisting thrombi that have developed in areas of turbulence or back eddies in the abnormal heart. Because of this vulnerability, patients with previous cardiac disease are often given prophylactic antibiotic treatment before they undergo procedures (e.g., dental cleaning) that may introduce organisms into the blood. The disease develops slowly (three to six months), often with vague symptoms: low-grade fever, anemia, debilitation, or perhaps only malaise. The spleen is often enlarged, and characteristic hemorrhages of the nailbeds may be observed.

In subacute IE, vegetations develop slowly and are not as damaging to the valves as in acute IE, although some may occur. In the 5–10% of patients who die of subacute IE, death results from chronic heart failure, unless the chordae tendineae rupture or emboli cause myocardial infarction.

Valvular Disease

Valvular diseases of the heart have many causes, but from a functional viewpoint, there are two basic types of malfunction. One is **valvular stenosis,** a narrowing of the valve so that forward flow of blood is restricted. The second is **valvular incompetence** or **insufficiency.** In this case, the valve is unable to close fully; so there is some regurgitation of blood in the backward direction.

It is not uncommon for more than one valve to be affected and for a valve to exhibit both stenosis and insufficiency at the same time. The aortic and mitral valves, subjected to much higher pressure gradients, are more frequently involved than the tricuspid and pulmonary valves.

Valvular Stenosis

When any valve fails to open effectively or is obstructed, blood accumulates in the upstream chambers and vessels. This accumulation, called **congestion,** causes hypertension in the affected vessels. Downstream hypotension is often absent, since compensatory mechanisms maintain an adequate arterial blood pressure. Blood tends to jet through the narrow valve orifice, and the resulting turbulence causes abnormal cardiac sounds called **heart murmurs.** These are often the first diagnostic clue to valve disease. Common causes of stenosis are rheumatic heart disease, infective endocarditis, congenital malformation, calcification of the valve cusps, or an extravalvular obstruction—for example, a tumor or aneurysm.

Mitral Stenosis The most common of all valve diseases, **mitral stenosis** is frequently found in association with other valve disorders. It is one of the typical results of rheumatic heart disease. Adhesion and stiffening of the valve cusps, accompanied by calcification and distortion of the scar tissue formed, all combine to impair filling of the left ventricle (fig. 10.17). The left atrium dilates and hypertrophies, and chronic heart failure may result. Cyanosis and fatigue will occur when the stenosis is severe and compensation cannot sustain downstream pressure and blood flow. (In **cyanosis,** the skin takes on a blue tinge due to insuffi-

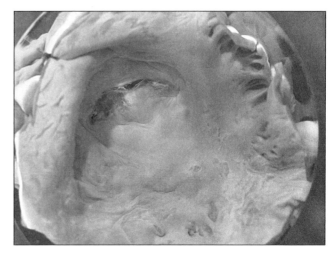

Figure 10.17 **Mitral Stenosis.** This mitral valve (viewed from the left atrium) restricts blood flow between atrium and ventricle because the aperture is narrowed and the thickened valve cusps cannot fully open. The term "fish mouth" is often used to describe the shape of the narrowed valve opening.

This mitral valve shows severe stenosis, probably as a result of an early bout of rheumatic fever. The flow tract to the left ventricle is substantially narrowed, leaving only the small "fish mouth" opening. The restricted blood flow ultimately produced a chronic pattern of heart failure.

The specimen was obtained after the death of a 62-year-old woman who had suffered dyspnea and a long period of declining cardiac function. Her heart was also found to be enlarged, as was her liver, from having to cope with the extra pumping demands placed on it by the stenotic mitral valve. She previously had carcinoma of the breast and a mastectomy, but there was no indication that the tumor contributed to her death.

cient oxygen saturation of the blood's hemoglobin.) Enlargement of the left atrium results in characteristic electrocardiogram and sometimes atrial fibrillation. Impaired swallowing (dysphagia) occurs when the enlarged atrium compresses the esophagus, which lies immediately behind it. Mitral stenosis produces a diastolic murmur, and the stiff valve opens with a snapping sound. In advanced disease, right heart failure can ensue, and the cardiac output will be reduced and unable to meet varied demands. Surgical valve replacement is often necessary.

Aortic Stenosis Another common valve disorder, **aortic stenosis,** is usually due to either valve damage or obstruction caused by atherosclerosis, rheumatic scarring of the valve cusps, or calcification of a congenitally malformed valve.

The increased resistance to ventricular emptying (a greater afterload) seen in aortic stenosis results in left ventricular **dilation** and **hypertrophy.** Since aortic stenosis is usually progressive, the left ventricle ultimately fails. The myocardial hypertrophy is necessary to overcome the resistance offered by the narrowed valve, but it makes the heart susceptible to ischemic injury and angina by increasing its workload and oxygen demand. Dizziness, **syncope** (fainting), fatigue, and skin pallor all reflect the decline in cardiac output. The pulse pressure is also reduced. Since, at least early in the disease, left ventricular hypertrophy can compensate for the stenosis, backup of blood into the lungs and pulmonary congestion are observed only when the condition is quite severe. Auscultation reveals a systolic murmur from blood jetting through the constriction as the ventricle contracts.

Tricuspid and Pulmonary Stenosis Right-sided valve disorders are uncommon, particularly alone. Tricuspid and pulmonary stenosis both produce symptoms of right heart failure, which is due to the loads imposed on it when it tries to pump through narrowed valves. The heart sounds resemble those of the corresponding valve disorder on the left side but vary in location and intensity. Some common causes of valvular stenosis are presented in table 10.1A.

 Checkpoint 10.2

Before we leave this section, go back to figure 10.17. This woman's mitral valve stenosis was related to (caused, in fact) three symptoms: dyspnea, cardiac hypertrophy, and hepatomegaly. The "heart enlargement" is pretty much explained. You have to read a little closer for the reason for her difficulty in getting a satisfactory breath. The swollen liver is another step removed. We will later deal with this directly, but in the meantime, what is *your* explanation?

Valvular Insufficiency/Incompetence

In disorders of valvular insufficiency or incompetence, the valve fails to prevent reverse flow, and a portion of the ejected blood leaks back (regurgitates) into the upstream chamber. Typically, 40–50% of the ejected volume regurgitates, but in severe cases the proportion can reach 80–90%. Since the stroke volume of the ventricle can increase by an amount that approximates the volume regurgitated, the cardiac output is maintained. However, if the condition progresses, the heart is, at some point, overloaded by the excess volume that can't be cleared from it. The ventricle will then dilate without a significant increase in wall thickness. Ultimately, signs of dilatation and ventricular failure become evident, but the disease may go undiagnosed for many years.

Mitral Insufficiency Eversion of damaged mitral valve cusps is frequently the reason for mitral insufficiency. The eversion may be due to rupture of the papillary muscle following a left ventricular infarct, or to rupture of the chordae tendineae in rheumatic heart disease or bacterial endocarditis. The eversion means that the valve cusp can fold back, allowing reverse flow into the atrium. Valve closure may also be impaired when scar tissue formation and contraction thickens, distorts, and misaligns the valve cusps or

Table 10.1	**Conditions Associated with Valve Malfunction**

A. Valvular Stenosis

All Valves (rarely pulmonary semilunar valve)

Rheumatic heart disease
Congenital malformations

Aortic Semilunar

Valve calcification

Pulmonary Semilunar Valve

Tetralogy of Fallot
Carcinoid syndrome (metastatic cancer involving neuroendocrine cells secreting serotonin, bradykinin, neuropeptide K, and substance P)

Tricuspid Valve

Carcinoid syndrome

B. Valvular Insufficiency (Regurgitation)

All Valves (but rarely the pulmonary semilunar valve)

Rheumatic heart disease (valve destruction)
Congestive heart failure (dilated annuli)
Syphilis
Infectious endocarditis
Congenital malformations

Aortic Regurgitation

Chest trauma (steering wheel injury)
Marfan's syndrome
Annulus fibrosus (ankylosing spondilitis, rheumatic arthritis)

Mitral Regurgitation

Ruptured papillary muscle (MI)
Ruptured chordae tendineae (infection, MI)
Floppy valve syndrome

Tricuspid Regurgitation

Carcinoid syndrome (see above)

shortens the chordae tendineae. Blood flows back into the left atrium during ventricular contraction and the resulting turbulence is heard as a systolic murmur.

A surprising 5% of adults have an abnormality of one or both valve cusps and associated chordae tendineae that allows the mitral valve to prolapse into the atrium (**floppy valve** or **Barlow's syndrome**). This usually produces only interesting auscultatory sounds, but can, on occasion, give rise to serious insufficiency and other problems.

With mitral insufficiency, the atrium fills with blood normally returning from the lungs but also with blood regurgitating from the ventricle. The result is an increased pressure in the atrium, which backs up into the lungs to produce congestion, pulmonary hypertension, and an array of related lung signs. The increased atrial pressure also causes the atrium to dilate, as it is chronically stretched by the increased volumes that it can't adequately eject. The stroke volume increases so that the volume of blood ejected into the aorta is close to normal. The electrocardiogram usually indicates evidence of left ventricular hypertrophy, atrial enlargement, and arrhythmia. Echocardiology is the diagnostic technique of choice.

Aortic Insufficiency Perforated valve cusps, which may result from infection or inflammation, and impairment of valve closure by scar tissue are two major causes of aortic insufficiency. Blood regurgitates into the ventricle during diastole, sometimes causing the mitral valve or septal wall to quiver. A diastolic murmur is heard, and the rapidly falling aortic pressure is responsible for a strong, bounding pulse that reflects an increased pulse pressure. Syncope, dizziness, pounding headaches, weakness, and fatigue are common symptoms of the altered hemodynamics in aortic insufficiency, along with the typical signs and symptoms of left heart failure.

Tricuspid and Pulmonary Insufficiency Like stenosis, insufficiency of valves of the right heart is relatively infrequent, except in combination with other valve defects. Isolated tricuspid or pulmonary valve disorders are usually the result of congenital malformation, although they may also be due to the infective endocarditis that occurs in intravenous drug users.

As is the situation with the corresponding left heart valves, tricuspid insufficiency and pulmonary stenosis are characterized by systolic murmurs; tricuspid stenosis and pulmonary insufficiency produce diastolic murmurs. All produce the characteristic symptoms of right heart failure. Ironically, failure of both right and left heart together diminishes the severity of pulmonary edema, since blood does not accumulate in the pulmonary vasculature. Some common causes of valvular insufficiency are presented in table 10.1B.

Rheumatic Heart Disease

Rheumatic heart disease (RHD) is a potential complication of a more generalized condition called **rheumatic fever** (RF). This is an inflammatory disease that affects a variety of tissues in widespread sites in the body. Painful joints are the major complaint in probably three-quarters of the patients, but the heart, skin, serosa, blood vessels, and lungs are commonly affected as well. The majority (90%) of patients have their first attack of RF when they are young (5–15 years of age). Boys and girls are equally affected. The great majority have suffered a streptococcal pharyngitis ("strep throat") one to four weeks before the emergence of rheumatic fever. In the heart, the focus of its effects can be the pericardial sac, the myocardium, the endocardium, the valves, or all four. Impairment of cardiac function can be acute, but the most typical pattern involves

valvular damage that can ultimately lead to congestive heart failure and death.

The name rheumatic fever is derived from the joint pain that often accompanies the disease. (Incidentally, the term **rheumatism** was formerly applied to various conditions involving painful joints, but with increased awareness of the etiology and pathogenesis of these conditions, the older, more general term has been replaced by specific names that differentiate particular diseases. Degenerative joint disease and ankylosing spondylitis are examples of current terms describing conditions that might have previously been known as rheumatism.) The symptoms of rheumatic fever may be sudden and intense, with fever, sore or swollen joints, and tachycardia, or they may be mild, with low-grade fever and malaise. Diagnosis can be challenging, since none of the clinical or laboratory features is specific to rheumatic fever. The diagnostic criteria for RF are presented in table 10.2.

Etiology and Pathogenesis

Although certain features of the etiology of RF are clear at this point, the underlying pathological mechanisms are still in question. Only a small proportion (3–5%) of those who have pharyngitis due to infection with any strain of group A beta-hemolytic streptococci will go on to develop RF. The antibodies produced to streptococcal antigens have an affinity for a wide variety of body tissues, including joint connective tissue and tissues of the heart. In certain individuals, this antibody cross-reaction progresses dramatically. It is triggered by the streptococcal infection but then becomes self-perpetuating. At this point, the signs and symptoms of rheumatic fever emerge. Once an acute case of RF has occurred, subsequent streptococcal infections are quite likely to stimulate further bouts of RF. Treatment of the acute rheumatic fever is based on penicillin, to eliminate the infecting bacteria, and anti-inflammatory agents, principally aspirin or corticosteroids (e.g., prednisone).

The chain of events in the pathogenesis of RF probably involves binding of antibodies to body tissues, which triggers damaging responses. Damaged cells may release histamine and activate kinins, triggering an inflammatory response that promotes the arrival of more macrophages and neutrophils. These cells, and perhaps T lymphocytes, produce further damage, activate complement, and produce fever.

Rheumatic heart disease arises when the cardiac effects of RF threaten to become serious. The heart is affected in about one-third of initial attacks of RF. In younger patients, there is more likelihood of cardiac involvement. Although the transient symptoms associated with other sites can be troublesome, when the heart is implicated severe damage can occur, particularly to the valves.

In acute RHD, the valves become red, thickened, and swollen. On the leaflet surfaces directly exposed to forward blood flow, especially where they meet in closure, tiny (1–2 mm) wartlike vegetations form. These **verrucae** might

Table 10.2 The Jones Criteria for Diagnosis of RF. These criteria are commonly employed in combination, because isolated signs or symptoms might also arise in a variety of other conditions. The presence of two major criteria, or of one major and two minor criteria, together with evidence of an earlier streptococcal infection, is taken as highly suggestive of RF.

Major Criteria

Carditis (as indicated by cardiac indicators—e.g., congestive heart failure, cardiomegaly, heart murmurs, pericarditis)
Chorea (central nervous system disorder involving muscle weakness, motor and emotional disorders)
Erythema marginatum (a characteristic skin rash)
Polyarthritis
Skin nodules

Minor Criteria

Characteristic ECG changes
Joint pain
Previous RF or rheumatic heart disease (often indicated by *Streptococcus*-related antibodies)
Pyrexia (fever)
Nosebleeds

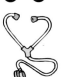

Focus on Aschoff Bodies and RHD

Microscopic examination of affected heart tissue during the active inflammatory phase of RF reveals the presence of **Aschoff bodies.** These consist of a central area of fibrinous material—swollen collagen fibrils, perhaps fibrin and plasma proteins—surrounded by a rim of macrophages (Anitschkow cells) and large, multinucleated cells called **Aschoff cells.** The presence of Aschoff bodies is diagnostic for RHD. It should be noted that these lesions are sterile; most researchers believe that the heart itself is not attacked by the streptococci.

develop through erosion of the soft, inflamed endocardial surface (see fig. 10.16). The subsequent organization of the sites of inflammatory damage can produce valvular stenosis or incompetence, or both (see fig. 10.17). The mitral valve is almost always involved and is the sole site of serious lesion in 50% of cases. This stenosis impedes the flow of blood from the atrium and generates a characteristic heart murmur, as well as producing congestion in the lungs and right heart that can progress to chronic heart failure. On the other hand, the valvular damage can result in incompetence, with regurgitation into the atrium. In this case, assuming mitral damage, the left ventricle hypertrophies in compensation for the lowered efficiency of pumping. As noted, the mitral valve, perhaps because of greater wear and tear, is almost always involved.

In about 50% of cases, the aortic semilunar valve is also damaged. Extensive involvement of other valves is less common. Damage to valves and the chordae tendineae, as well as thrombosis in enlarged atria, embolism, and pulmonary complications may all play a part in the emerging picture of chronic heart failure, the most usual cause of death in RHD. The pathogenesis of RHD is presented in figure 10.18.

Effective antibiotic treatment of streptococcal infections has cut the incidence of rheumatic fever and heart disease by about 70% in the last 50 years, by cutting short this disruption of healthy immunological response. However, in underdeveloped countries, RHD is still a major health problem, accounting for 25–40% of all heart disease.

Ischemic Heart Disease

Coronary Artery Disease (CAD)

Coronary artery disease (CAD), also called **atherosclerotic heart disease** (ASHD), is the cardiac result of the progression of systemic atherosclerosis. This pathology, described in chapter 9, tends to be confined to the aorta and its major branches, including the coronary arteries. In the section on cardiac vessels, we suggested that the large coronary vessels are the focus of vascular dynamics that subject them to particular "wear and tear" (the "response to injury" theory presented in chapter 9). Whatever the mechanisms, the coronary arteries are susceptible to atherosclerotic degeneration and the variety of pathological events with which it is associated (atheromatous plaque development, stenosis, thrombosis, vasospasm, intraplaque hemorrhage, erosion, or rupture, vessel occlusion). The effects on the heart may include ischemia, resultant chest pain (angina pectoris), arrhythmias, and myocardial weakness. When the obstruction is prolonged and/or severe, **myocardial infarction** (MI) will occur. At a minimum, this weakens the heart

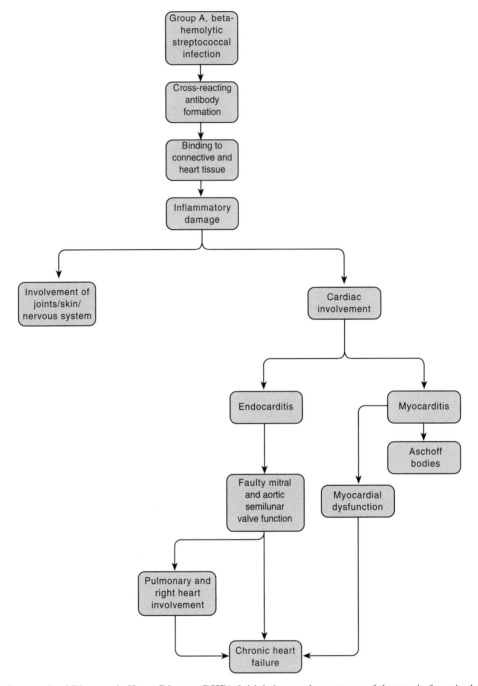

Figure 10.18   **Pathogenesis of Rheumatic Heart Disease (RHD).** Initial signs and symptoms of rheumatic fever in the joints, skin, and nervous system may, over time, evolve to the more serious RHD.

muscle. At worst, the remaining muscle is unable to produce cardiac output compatible with survival and acute heart failure occurs. Further complications of MI, including fatal arrhythmia, will be detailed. Current strategies for CAD treatment are designed to arrest or reverse the atherosclerotic process, reestablish myocardial blood flow, control symptoms, and reduce cardiac workload and oxygen requirements.

Ischemic Heart Disease (IHD)

Ischemic injury of the heart is the most common cause of heart disease and the major cause of death in developed countries. Sudden or progressive loss of coronary blood flow is almost always due to atherosclerosis of the coronary arteries and its complications. (So, in effect, we have a triad of synonyms: CAD, ASHD, and IHD.) Ischemia may be gradual or sudden in onset, depending on the nature of the arterial obstruction.

Chronic ischemia occurs when atherosclerosis and perhaps small, nonocclusive thrombi cause slow but progressive narrowing of the arterial lumen. Gradual narrowing allows time for the myocardial cells to adapt partially to hypoxia and for anastomoses (alternative supply routes) to develop from vessels adjacent to the region of hypoxia. The compensatory mechanisms of vasodilation (autoregulation, NO) are so effective that an occlusion has to progress to 50% of the cross-sectional area (70% of the diameter) before an increase in demand will imbalance perfusion to the extent that function is impaired or angina is produced. With increased occlusion, however, angina will be experienced initially at exertion, but progressively at lower levels of activity. There can be gradual weakening of the myocardium, leading to a decline in cardiac output. Severe stenosis will produce myocardial infarction and **necrosis,** after which damaged cells are replaced by fibrous tissue, making the myocardium weaker and less extensible.

The plaques formed in chronic ischemia tend to be firm with a dense, fibrous cap. An adjacent sandwich of old, consolidated thrombi may be covered by an epithelium. In **acute ischemia,** although the plaque may produce only mild to moderate stenosis, it is more likely to be filled with foam cells and possess a necrotic, lipid-laden core. This sort of plaque is more likely to be invaded by hemorrhage or to rupture, releasing its contents into the vessel lumen. This event triggers coagulation and rapid occlusion of the arterial lumen. This is the classic precipitation of **acute myocardial infarction** (MI) (fig. 10.19).

While the variations in anatomy and vessel distribution mentioned earlier affect the specific portion of the myocardium that will be ischemic due to stenosis of its supply artery, they do not affect the general pattern of atherosclerotic disease in the heart. The plaques will be concentrated in the larger vessels and ischemia will be experienced mostly in the myocardium of the left ventricle, as its metabolic demands are greatest. It is the imbalance between perfusion and demand that produces the ischemia that gives this condition its name. In the healthy heart, the abundance of adenosine would trigger vasodilation to balance the perfusion. The sites of myocardial lesion secondary to ischemic injury are distributed as follows: LAD (40–50%), affecting the anterior interventricular septum, mid-anterior left ventricular wall and much of the apex; CX (15–20%), affecting lateral left ventricular wall except the apex; RCA (30–40%), affecting inferior-posterior wall of left and right ventricle and posterior interventricular septum. Note that most of the injury is confined to the left ventricle and that 55–70% of the disease is in the left coronary artery. Multiple plaques are often seen, resulting in triple bypass surgeries.

Endothelial injury plays an important role in the worsening of the ischemia, whether chronic or acute. The endothelium is the first casualty in the area of the developing atheroma. Its responses will become deranged early in the progression of atherosclerosis. As the atheroma expands

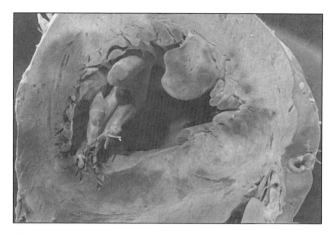

Figure 10.19   **Acute Ischemia.** This section through the ventricular myocardium shows the darkened region of necrosis caused by an occluded coronary artery, which has led to an acute myocardial infarction.

Two days after being driven to the emergency room by his wife, a 60-year-old male died of an acute MI. He had experienced chest pain that radiated to his left arm. He was dyspneic and anxious after being admitted. His pulse was weak and rapid and his skin was cold and "clammy."

Autopsy findings confirmed severe coronary atherosclerosis and a massive, recent MI. In the photograph, the darkened, mottled region of the infarct (C-shaped region filling the left one-third of the field) shows the involvement of the left ventricle and interventricular septum. The infarction also affected the pericardium, producing an acute pericarditis.

and begins interfering with downstream perfusion, small arterioles, capillaries, and venules will be subject to secondary ischemic injury. And while atheromatous plaques develop focally, it is useful to remember that the progression of atherosclerosis is a fairly widespread process within the large and mid-sized arteries, so we might expect the altered responses we will describe for "injured" endothelium to be widespread as well.

Normal endothelium responds to locally generated cues of insufficient perfusion with the release of a variety of vasodilatory chemicals (these were described in detail in the Control of Perfusion section). A normal response of the endothelium to a variety of stimuli associated with a problem of perfusion (e.g., injury, platelet aggregation, stasis and hypoxia, etc.) will be the production and release of prostaglandin I$_2$ (**PGI$_2$, prostacyclin**). This eicosanoid (think back to inflammation and the cyclooxygenase system) is a potent vasodilator and inhibitor of platelet aggregation. Essentially, it functions to flush out the immediate vasculature, which in cases of minor injury is an adaptive response. However, injured endothelium responds to PGI$_2$ with **vasoconstriction**—a response that will worsen ischemia. When serotonin is released from aggregating platelets it produces a similar response: vasodilation in small arterioles in normal tissue, but vasoconstriction in the small arterioles of injured tissue. **NO,** as has been described, has the normal effect of vasodilation. The injured endothelium produces lowered amounts of NO. This not only removes what would be a protective drive for vasodilation, but also induces the release of **endothelin-1** (ET-1), which causes vasoconstriction. To make matters worse, atherosclerosis induces the upregulation ET(B) receptors for endothelin. This increases the effect of the ET-1 that is released and appears to be an important mediator of the predominant vasoconstriction found in the region of the ischemic injury. Chronic ET-1 release also causes hypertrophy and fibrosis of ventricular and vascular tissues, increasing the oxygen demand and reducing the ease of ventricular distension during diastole (reduced "compliance"). It also acts as a proarrhythmic agent, increasing the likelihood of the development of ectopic foci. ET-blockers are being actively investigated for their potential in treating ischemic heart disease.

The response of atherosclerotic vessels to neural regulation also contributes to the pathology. The sense of panic and threat that accompanies angina induces the stress-mediated release of sympathetic norepinephrine and adrenal epinephrine adds to the vasoconstriction. These derangements defy the usual therapeutic approaches to producing protective vasodilation in the area of the stenosis. In addition, the relatively normal endothelium downstream to the plaque is already at maximal dilation to compensate for the relative ischemia the stenosis has induced, so even the response of the downstream healthy myocardium cannot reverse the effects of ischemia. This is why nitroglycerine, which activates the NO system, has relatively little affect on the heart itself but produces most of its beneficial, angina-relieving effect by inducing NO in the peripheral circulation and reducing afterload and, thus, the demands on the heart. The good news is that the vasoconstrictor response of damaged endothelium can be reversed by reductions in serum cholesterol and hypertension, and through aerobic exercise. The deranged response can be reversed.

Pain in Ischemic Heart Disease (IHD)

Typical angina pectoris is chest pain or discomfort arising from transient myocardial ischemia. The mechanism, significantly raised adenosine due to an imbalance of demand over perfusion, has been described. It is typically experienced as retrosternal or precordial pain (the **precordium** is the chest wall overlying the heart), described as constriction, pressure, or heaviness (the person will sometimes make a clenched fist in explanation), often radiating to the left axilla, arm, shoulder, or jaw (fig. 10.20). Radiation to the right side or down the back is not uncommon. It may be experienced as epigastric discomfort (like heartburn) but the radiation is not typically below the diaphragm. Some people will describe the constriction as shortness of breath, but they will want to take a deep breath rather than the quick breathing usually associated with true hypoxia. It is provoked by exertion and stresses that elevate heart rate or blood pressure (emotional upset, cold, eating a large meal), lasts several minutes, and is relieved by rest or nitroglycer-

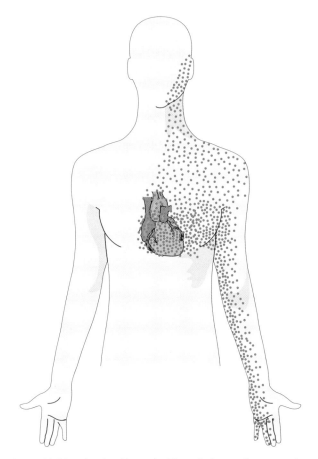

Figure 10.20   **Angina Pectoris.** The pain is usually reported over the chest, with variable patterns of radiation to the arm, shoulder, and jaw.

ine. While simple atherosclerotic stenosis is the principal cause of the ischemia, other factors can play a role in typical angina. Transient platelet clumps from microscopic thrombi in the vicinity of the plaque may temporarily occlude the vessel and can release vasoconstrictive substances. The damaged endothelium can produce vasoconstriction to stimuli that produce vasodilation in healthy vessels (just described). Table 10.3 puts typical angina into perspective. Level III or IV on either scale speaks of very limited capacity. On the other extreme, very intense cardiovascular exertion can produce angina in a heart with perfectly healthy vessels.

Variant angina (sometimes called Prinzmetal's variant angina) is principally ascribed to vasospasm in arteries injured by atherosclerosis. About 15% of people who experience variant angina have no detectable coronary atherosclerotic disease, but in the other 85% the "spontaneous" vasospasm occurs in the vicinity of a fixed atherosclerotic narrowing. Platelet adhesion and microscopic thrombi probably make a contribution to this vasospasm. What differentiates this from typical angina is that it may occur at rest and doesn't respond to nitroglycerine.

Unstable angina is a very serious predictor of the progression of IHD. The symptoms last more than 20 minutes

| Table 10.3 | Two Scales for Rating the Degree of Disability Associated with Cardiovascular Disease |

Canadian Cardiovascular Society Classification of Angina

Class	Activity Provoking Angina	Limits to Normal Activity
I	Prolonged exertion	None
II	Walking > 2 blocks	Slight
III	Walking < 2 blocks	Marked
IV	Minimal or rest	Severe

New York Heart Association Functional Classification of Cardiovascular Disability

Class	Characteristics
I	Cardiac disease that doesn't limit activities.
II	Slight limitation of physical activity; comfortable at rest, ordinary physical activity produces fatigue, palpitations, dyspnea, or angina.
III	Marked limitation of physical activity; comfortable at rest; less than ordinary activity produces symptoms noted in II
IV	Inability to carry on any physical activity without discomfort; symptoms may be present at rest; any physical activity worsens symptoms.

at rest, there has possibly been an onset of new exertional angina within the last two months, or there has been a rapid worsening of a pre-existing angina. ECG changes that parallel the angina are characteristic of unstable angina. ECG signs of ischemia (S-T segment elevation or depression), mitral regurgitation, and pulmonary edema may indicate progression to MI. There is direct progression to MI in about 10% of patients and 5% die subsequently. The progress in understanding and care of patients with unstable angina is illustrated in the fact that this group, given the care available in the 1950s and 1960s, had an MI rate of 40–50% and a mortality rate of 20–30%.

Sudden Cardiac Death This condition is responsible for over 60% of all deaths due to IHD (over 460,000 in North America per year). Typically, the victim suffers a fatal arrhythmia produced by myocardial ischemia. The difference between this condition and myocardial infarction is that we can't assume that there has been any tissue infarction. There may well be postmortem evidence of atherosclerosis, some degeneration of the myocardium, or some previous MI. In sudden cardiac death (SCD), the event inducing the ischemia that causes the arrhythmia could be increased exertion, vasospasm, occlusion of a coronary artery by platelet aggregation and thrombosis (an atherosclerotic plaque may have ruptured, spewing its thrombogenic contents into the lumen), or blood may have hemorrhaged into a plaque, causing it to expand. With younger victims, the causes of sudden cardiac death may include myocarditis, mitral valve prolapse, the sudden failure of adaptation to a congenital structural or coronary arterial anomaly, or valvular disease, perhaps associated with endocarditis. For many, sudden cardiac death is the first indicator of IHD.

In a study by the American Centers for Disease Control (CDC) 63.4% of heart disease deaths were defined as SCDs in 1999. Most (46.9%) of those SCDs occurred outside the

Focus on Cocaine Use and Sudden Cardiac Death

The recreational use of cocaine has produced an epidemic of MI and sudden cardiac death. Cocaine (especially in combination with cigarette smoking) induces a transitory coronary artery constriction. At the same time, it is likely that the user will be aroused and physically active, which will increase myocardial oxygen demand. Added to this is cocaine's tendency to induce disturbances in cardiac rhythm (e.g., ectopic foci or conduction abnormalities). Cocaine may do this by enhancing the effects of epinephrine, norepinephrine, and dopamine, substances normally released in stress or situations requiring increased cardiac output. If the user has a preexisting, probably undiagnosed, atherosclerotic occlusion, either of cocaine's effects could be potentially fatal, producing an MI and/or a serious arrhythmia. The vasoconstriction and rhythm disruption are apparently severe enough for a healthy young person to experience a fatal arrhythmia during cocaine use.

hospital while the remainder (16.5%) occurred in the emergency room or were pronounced dead upon arrival. Women were more likely (51.9% vs. 41.7%) than men to die before reaching the hospital. While the highest percentage of SCD by state was almost 73%, the low in Hawaii (57.1%) was still close to the average. Effective recognition of both the uncommon symptoms of heart attack (breaking out in a cold sweat, nausea, light-headedness) and those that are more common (chest pain or discomfort, pain or discomfort in one or both arms or in the back, neck, jaw, or stomach, and shortness of breath) should result in earlier recognition and treatment, less heart damage, and fewer deaths.

Acute Myocardial Infarction As noted, the precipitating event in acute MI involves the disruption of a mid-sized atheromatous plaque: hemorrhage into the plaque, rupture or fissuring, erosion of the endothelial surface of the plaque. The exposed collagen and thrombogenic contents rapidly induce platelet aggregation and thrombosis, and the release of potent vasoconstrictors (including thromboxane A_2 and serotonin). Within minutes, the entire lumen is filled with thrombus and complete ischemia evolves in the downstream tissues. In a minority (10%) of cases, no thrombus is evident postmortem. These cases are explained by arterial vasospasm, perhaps with associated platelet adhesion and microscopic thrombus formation and embolization; some cases remain "unexplained."

The clinical presentation is varied. About two-thirds of patients have experienced a worsening or change of pattern in pre-existing angina or the onset of new angina. Perhaps one-quarter have very mild symptoms or no symptoms at all (the MI is identified by enzyme/protein blood analysis). About one-quarter have chest pain that mimics heartburn. An equal proportion have chest pain (aching or stabbing pain in the chest, jaw and neck, left arm, or back) that defies the conventional medical wisdom that if they can point to it, it isn't MI. The remaining one-quarter have read the textbook and present with "classic" MI pain: severe chest pain, described as an intense, crushing substernal or precordial pain, often radiating to the left shoulder, arm, or jaw, accompanied by sweating, breathlessness, and anxiety. One thing is common in this varied presentation of pain: it is not relieved by rest or vasodilators.

Nausea and vomiting commonly occur, along with characteristic indicators of a falling cardiac output. A history of angina is common. An electrocardiogram is often the first diagnostic procedure to yield results, permitting an assessment of the location and severity of the infarct and the nature of any arrhythmia that develops. After admission to hospital, continuous ECG monitoring is essential because life-threatening arrhythmias may occur at any time in the first few days after infarction. Serum enzyme assay is used to assess cellular injury. **Creatine kinase** (CK), formerly known as creatine phosphokinase (CPK), and **lactic dehydrogenase** (LDH) are both released from the injured muscle. In the absence of further infarction, CK peaks in about 24 hours and LDH in 48–72 hours after injury. Neither enzyme is specific for myocardial damage, but their elevation in the presence of other cardiac signs and symptoms, without evidence of other muscle damage, can be presumed to indicate an MI. Only a more precise assessment of the plasma to determine the presence of **CK-MB** and **LDH1** can be definitive, in that these **isoenzymes** (enzyme sub-types) are found in greater concentration in cardiac muscle.

The measurement of the cardiac-specific polypeptide **troponin** has recently become the best-available marker of myocardial injury. There are three subunits of the cardiac troponin complex (which associates with actin and enables actin-myosin interaction during Ca^{2+} influx and contraction). They are named after their functions: cTnI inhibits actin-myosin, cTnT binds to tropomyosin, and cTnC is the calcium-binding component. Within three to six hours of cardiac (severe ischemic) injury, **cTnI** can be detected in the blood. Levels peak at 24–48 hours, and then stay elevated for seven to ten days. The combination of cardiac specificity, early release, and then persistence (to confirm a suspected MI that occured before admission) makes cTnI an excellent marker of acute MI. All of these markers take some time (hours) to appear in the blood, so treatment may have to proceed before MI is confirmed.

Therapy in Ischemic Heart Disease

The anatomical variability alluded to in our description of the distribution of the major coronary arteries, while not relevant to the development of atherosclerosis or the usual regions experiencing ischemia, *is* of significance when bypass surgery or angioplasty is contemplated. **Coronary by-pass** is provided when pieces of the saphenous vein harvested from the leg are reversed (recall the presence of valves in veins) and sutured in above and below a known site of atherosclerotic stenosis. Alternatively, sections of the internal mammary artery or Teflon material can be used. In **percutaneous transluminal coronary angioplasty** (PTCA), a catheter is inserted into the coronary artery and a balloon is inflated, compressing the atheroma and stretching the vessel media. So-called "rescue PTCA" is performed if the MI is very recent. If effective perfusion can be restored within 90 minutes, much of the injured myocardium can be saved. **Stents,** which are coils that are treated to impede overgrowth, may be placed in the lumen widened by angioplasty. Restenosis is relatively common following PTCA but the procedure is considered a very useful tool in dealing with stenosis. These procedures are more effective if performed as an MI preventative in vessels where significant stenosis has been identified.

Endothelium that is compressed and damaged during angioplasty is rapidly regenerated, while thrombosis triggered by the exposed basement membrane collagen is controlled by anticoagulant therapy. Currently, the immediate administration of t-PA (tissue plasminogen activator, see chapter 7), either systemically or via catheter to the area of thrombosis, is proving very effective in reversing occlusion and avoiding or limiting infarction. If a race is on to save myocardium threatened by a recent MI and the facilities exist, PCTA is generally preferred over t-PA as offering the best hope (t-PA can take 90 minutes to clear a thrombus, which is an additional 90 minutes of ischemia).

If the prolonged ischemia has weakened the myocardium beyond its capacity to maintain adequate perfusion, first aid can be effectively delivered through the use of an **intra-aortic balloon pump.** This assists the weakened myocardium and may provide the essential perfusion necessary to save myocardium, which, if the heart were left to its own resources, would be lost.

There are many experimental procedures being investigated to recover the normal delivery of blood in the ischemic myocardium. One of the more interesting involves the transfection of genes responsible for angiogenesis into the ischemic myocardium of patients who have such widespread atherosclerosis that conventional angioplasty and by-pass are either not options or options that have been applied to their full extent. Early trials are showing promising results, with functional recovery and presumably effective revascularization. These approaches will be interesting to watch.

There is an array of pharmacological agents beyond those just mentioned for acute care that play a very important role in managing the patient with ischemic heart disease. As some of these are the same as are used for the treatment of chronic heart disease, we will postpone their discussion.

Sequelae of Acute MI

Presuming the patient survives the initial attack, damaged muscle is destroyed and replaced by scar tissue. The healing phase is fraught with hazards that can complicate recovery and threaten the patient's life.

Arrhythmias The most serious arrhythmia is **ventricular fibrillation.** It is usually fatal, since it can be eliminated only with specialized procedures and equipment. Fibrillation involves complete lack of synchronization in the contraction of the myocardial fibers. The myocardial cells are active, but they produce only quivering instead of forceful rhythmic contractions. In this situation, pumping stops and cardiac output fails. Unless a defibrillation procedure is successful within minutes, brain cells will be irreversibly damaged by anoxia. **Defibrillation** (or **cardioversion**) involves delivering an electric shock to the wildly contracting myocardium. The intent is to depolarize all of the myocardial cells momentarily. This change may allow a normal sinus rhythm to be reestablished and normal pumping to be restored. Ventricular fibrillation and other less severe dysrythmias are typically controlled and prevented with antiarrhythmic drugs. If there is a persistent problem restoring normal rhythmicity, a pacemaker may be inserted. These can be set to intervene in a variety of dysrhythmias, only intervening when sinus rhythm fails. They can also be designed to sense ventricular fibrillation or states likely to progress to fibrillation (ventricular tachycardia and torsades de point) and intervene with instant cardioversion.

Cardiogenic Shock Cardiogenic shock (see chapter 12) is the consequence of large infarcts and severe dysrhythmias that decrease cardiac output below the level required to perfuse the tissues adequately. Tissues vulnerable to hypoxia are compromised, and compensatory mechanisms may provide additional stress.

Thrombosis Thrombosis is triggered by activating factors released from injured myocardial tissues. Thrombi may form in the heart over the site of injury or where blood pools in weakly contracting chambers. With cardiac output reduced by injury and the patient's immobility, venous stasis and thrombosis occur. Thrombi in the contracting heart

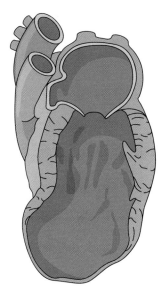

Figure 10.21   **Ventricular Aneurysm.** This section through the heart shows a prominently bulging ventricular aneurysm. Note the thinness of the myocardium, which raises the risk that the aneurysm will rupture.

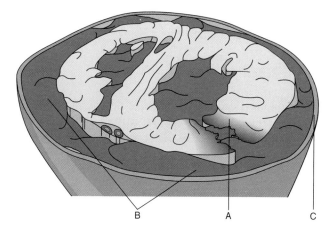

Figure 10.22   **Tamponade Due to Ventricular Rupture.** In this diagram, the pericardial space is filled with coagulated blood from a ventricular rupture. The external pressure increase compresses the heart, restricting its ability to fill adequately during diastole.

and veins of newly ambulatory patients are prone to the production of emboli.

Rupture The necrotic myocardium of the infarct is slowly cleared by phagocytic cells prior to the formation of scar tissue. Typically, around seven to ten days after an infarct occurs, the dead muscle gradually softens (**myomalacia cordis**) and the wall is susceptible to rupture. An infarct of the ventricular wall tends to cause **ventricular aneurysm** (fig. 10.21). If the aneurysm ruptures it causes blood to fill the pericardial sac. Compression caused by pressure from the distended sac (tamponade) impedes filling of the ventricle, and death ensues (fig. 10.22). Infarction of the interventricular septum may lead to rupture into the right ventricle; combined ventricular failure then rapidly develops. In the region of the papillary muscles of the left ventricle,

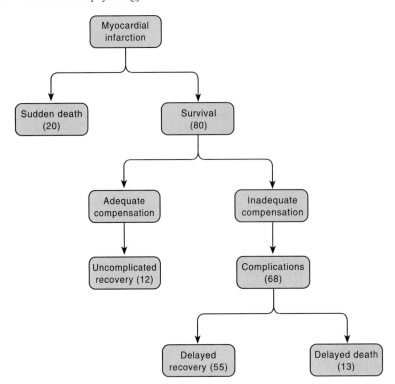

Figure 10.23   **The Prognosis for a Representative 100 Myocardial Infarction Patients.**

infarction may lead to separation of the muscle from the ventricular wall. The muscle, attached by chordae tendineae to the AV valve, flails about in the left atrium and ventricle, producing sudden and severe mitral insufficiency. Left heart failure follows, and without rapid surgical intervention, the patient dies.

Healing of Infarcted Tissue   If the person survives the acute MI, the infarcted area will heal. Necrotic myocardial cells will be replaced by dense fibrous connective tissue (scarring). This area cannot, of course, contribute to pumping except to maintain the integrity of the ventricular wall. In cases of large infarcts, this will seriously impair pumping despite compensatory hypertrophy of remaining, relatively healthy myocardium. Areas of scarring are nonconductive and may show up on an ECG by lessening the signal picked up over that area of the heart on the chest leads of an ECG. By interfering with normal conduction pathways, the scar may also produce a symptomatic ECG.

Prognosis in Myocardial Infarction   The serious nature of MI can be seen in the fact that only 12% of those affected experience uncomplicated recovery. The situation shows signs of improving, however, as better means of postinfarction management are developed. These are based on carefully regulated exercise programs that can increase myocar-

dial capabilities to meet and even exceed preinfarction performance. Also, drugs can be administered immediately post-MI to limit reperfusion injury. Acute MI is suddenly fatal in over 20% of cases, usually from massive myocardial destruction or severe arrhythmia. Here, too, there is improvement in prognosis as cardiopulmonary resuscitation (CPR) skills are increasingly developed in medical personnel and in the general population.

Of those in whom MI is not immediately fatal, 13% will die later from related problems such as arrhythmias, myocardial rupture, or thromboembolism. Thrombosis is, of course, favored by both the reduced cardiac output of the weakened heart, which causes reduced blood flow rates and lack of mobility in the patient recovering from the MI. In well over half of MI cases, neither fatality nor uncomplicated recovery occurs. In these cases, some factor arising out of the initial infarction event weakens the heart. It can still maintain a cardiac output adequate for survival, but undesirable chronic effects develop as well. These progress over a period of months or even years until ultimately the heart fails to maintain a minimal output. A variety of physiological compensations are brought to bear, but they may further complicate the situation rather than resolving it (fig. 10.23). This type of chronic heart failure is called congestive heart failure and is the focus of the next section.

We have seen that atherosclerosis is the most common, but certainly not the only, cause of either acute or chronic heart failure. We have also seen that the problems directly associated with myocardial ischemia (hypofunction, fibrosis, infarction, arrythmia, etc.) are complicated by a derangement of normal responses to impaired perfusion in injured heart tissue. A clear understanding of these processes and the normal compensations and controls that adjust cardiac, vascular, and kidney responses to blood pressure and perfusion requirements will make this next section quite straightforward.

CONGESTIVE HEART FAILURE

Ischemic heart disease is only one of many heart, respiratory, or vascular diseases that can create circulation demands that outpace the heart's ability to respond. In such circumstances, the heart and cardiovascular system can be pushed into a state of progressively decreasing capacity called **chronic heart failure.** In this slowly developing condition, cardiac output is unable to respond adequately to tissue demands.

There are four broad consequences of chronic cardiac failure. One is the backup of blood in the vessels upstream from the heart because the heart can't maintain forward blood flow. This excess of blood in the upstream vessels is called **congestion.** It in turn causes hypertension and edema in the congested tissues (fig. 10.24). Indeed, since congestion is the classic sign of the chronically failing heart, the condition is more typically known as **congestive heart failure** (CHF). The second consequence of longer-term cardiac failure is the activation of an array of circulatory compensations that normally maintain adequate blood flow to the tissues. Some of the characteristic signs and symptoms in CHF derive from these compensations—for example, a rapid pulse rate. Third, when physiological mechanisms are unable to compensate, cardiac output declines. As a result, systemic hypoxia may produce a generalized weakness and tendency to fatigue. In severe cases, cyanosis may be present. Generally, although cardiac output may be adequate at rest, demand for increases in cardiac output cannot be fully met. A fourth consequence, reached when cardiac output is ultimately unable to supply the major organ systems adequately, is death.

Etiology of Congestive Heart Failure

The chronic inability to pump its preload may be the result of the heart's reduced pumping capability or of increased afterload. In the first case, the fault may lie in the myocardium itself or in certain physical factors that interfere with pumping. These etiological factors in CHF are considered in the following sections.

Myocardial Weakness

Most commonly, the myocardium is weakened by ischemia related to atherosclerosis (AS) and its stenosis of the coronary arteries. When stenosis reaches 50–70%, only resting myocardial oxygen demand can be met. As AS progresses, myocardial fibers undergo hypoxic injury and necrosis. They are replaced by fibrous connective tissue, causing a steady deterioration in myocardial pumping capacity and a reduction in venticular compliance. The ventricle becomes stiffer, which impairs diastolic filling and puts added demands on the associated atrium as well as creating a back pressure.

Another cause of myocardial ischemia is thrombosis in the coronary arteries. The injured endothelium lying over an atherosclerotic plaque may induce thrombus formation, further reducing blood flow and damaging the myocardium. Recent studies have also shown that subsequent to platelet adhesion at endothelial surfaces, a sequence of chemical activations, already described, triggers constriction of the coronary vessels. This vasospasm is thought to be a factor in patients who develop MI, even though their coronary vessels show little atherosclerotic involvement.

In addition to weakness caused by ischemia, the myocardium may be directly affected by other factors—for example, myocarditis or the cardiomyopathies described in a later section, Cardiomyopathies.

Restrictions to Pumping

Even when the myocardium is undamaged and adequately supplied with oxygen, the heart may be unable to cope with its preload because of physical factors that restrict its pumping. Cardiac valve malfunction is one such factor. As we described earlier in this chapter, incompetent valves, which cannot tightly close, will allow backward flow in the heart or pulmonary circulation. When valves are unable to open widely, reduced blood flow through the heart may cause cardiac output to fall.

Internal obstructions may interfere with the free flow of blood through the heart. These may arise as a result of inborn malformations of the cardiac flow tracts or vessels. Such congenital malformations are described in more detail in a separate section, Congenital Heart Defects. Another internal obstruction might be a mass (e.g., a thrombus or tumor) present within a cardiac chamber. By occupying a portion of a chamber's volume, this mass reduces the chamber's blood capacity, in addition to interfering with the free flow of blood through the chamber. The most common cardiac tumor (accounting for 35–50% of all primary

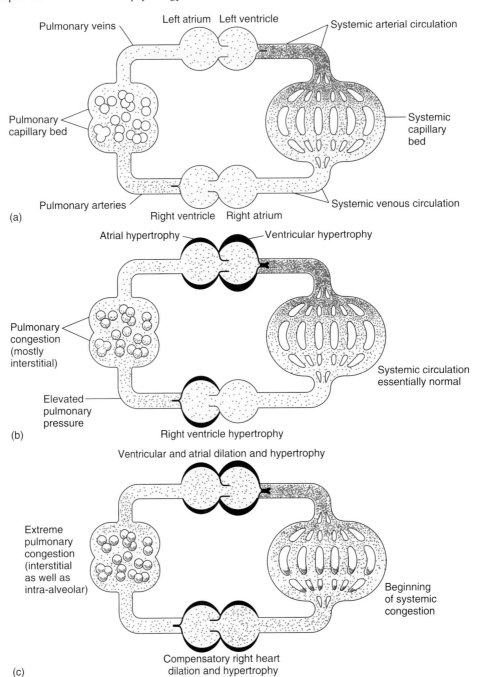

Figure 10.24 **Chronic Heart Failure.** (*a*) **The relationship between the heart's two pumps: the lungs and the systemic circulation.** This figure shows the heart in ventricular diastole, the state in which the pressure gradients have their most significant impact. Pressure is indicated by the density of dots, so it is clear that the role of the left ventricle is to generate the high pressures required for pushing blood through the systemic circulation. The chamber sizes and wall thickness indicate "normal" rather than realistic dimensions. (*b*) **Early response to a stenosed (insufficient) aortic semilunar valve.** Vascular compensations and left ventricular hypertrophy maintain systemic diastolic pressure (*a* and *b*), but impaired emptying of the left ventricle "backs up" blood into the left atrium (hypertrophied) and the pulmonary circulation (producing congestion). (*c*) **Late response.** Now the left ventricle is beginning to "fail" (cardiac output drops, circulatory pressures are not maintained). Backup into the pulmonary circulation has led to compensatory hypertrophy in the right ventricle. Eventual combined heart failure will ensue if no effective intervention (e.g., valve replacement) takes place. In this figure, systemic venous congestion is just beginning to occur.

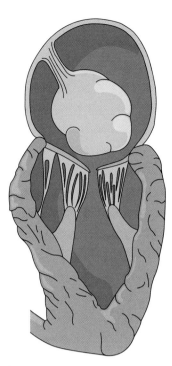

Figure 10.25   **Myxoma.** The atrial tumor is positioned to act like a ball valve. The normal movement of blood causes it to move on its stalk to block flow to the ventricle. Blockage is also favored by atrial contraction, which moves the tumor toward the ventricle.

Table 10.4	Causes of Restriction to Cardiac Pumping

Valve defects

Stenosis
Regurgitation

Congenital malformations

Obstructing mass

Tumor
Thrombus

Dysrhythmia

Pericarditis

Chronic constrictive pericarditis
Pericardial effusion

Cardiac tamponade

cardiac tumors) is a **myxoma,** a tumor of endothelial origin usually (75%) found in the left atrium, but occurring less often in the other chambers. This may form on a slender stalk (a pedunculated myxoma), allowing it to move to and fro within a chamber with changes in blood movements, often moving in and out of a valve orifice and obstructing blood flow or damaging valve structures (fig. 10.25). These "wrecking balls" can occlude the mitral valve, causing instant death, or can be the site of thromboembolus formation. About one-third of people with a cardiac myxoma experience metastasis (embolization) to the brain with disastrous results. On the other hand, surgical resection is usually a successful treatment where metastasis has not occured.

Pumping may also be restricted by cardiac dysrhythmias. In such cases, ischemia, infarction, or other factors may initially interfere with the cardiac conduction system. Alternatively, electrolyte imbalances or chemical toxins can alter the myocardium's electrical stability. Whatever the cause, the resulting rate and/or rhythm abnormalities can seriously compromise cardiac output.

The pericardium is also a potential source of restriction to cardiac pumping. As we described earlier, changes to the pericardial surfaces involving fibrin deposition (as may occur in lupus) or adhesions can severely limit cardiac activity. Also, the accumulation of fluid, be it a pericardial effusion or blood, can produce significant external pressures (cardiac tamponade) that compromise cardiac filling (see fig. 10.22). The factors that can restrict cardiac pumping are presented in table 10.4.

Increased Afterload

An inability to maintain cardiac output may also result from overload. When the myocardium is constantly exposed to high physical demand, the strain may ultimately overwhelm it, with the result that contractility and stroke volume steadily decline. This decline is seen most commonly when cardiac afterload is increased. The right ventricle faces such a situation in certain lung diseases where vascular damage causes pulmonary hypertension. (See the Cor Pulmonale section later in this chapter.) In systemic hypertension, chronically elevated blood pressure presents an increased resistance that the left ventricle must overcome to maintain adequate cardiac output. This is the case in essential hypertension as well as the hypertension associated with obesity. In the case of valve disease or congenital defects in the cardiac outflow tracts, valves, pulmonary trunk, or aorta, the ventricle's afterload may also be excessive.

Excessive cardiac workload may complicate preexisting CHF even when afterload is relatively low. This situation arises in high-demand states, where elevated tissue metabolism increases demand for blood flow via reflex cardiac stimulation. The resulting chronic increases in heart rate and contractility can progressively exhaust the already weakened myocardium, hastening its ultimate failure. One high-demand state that may contribute to CHF is chronic anemia, where even resting tissues are deprived of adequate oxygen delivery. Another is thyrotoxicosis, in which excessive thyroid secretion elevates systemic metabolism to levels requiring extraordinary blood supply. In such cases, cardiac output may be well above normal as the already failing heart labors to satisfy a chronic high demand for its output.

In summary, a variety of etiologies can produce a chronic and progressive decline in the heart's pumping

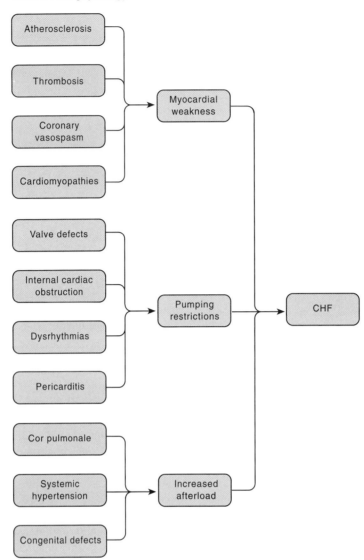

Figure 10.26   **Etiological Factors in Congestive Heart Failure.**

capability. They affect the heart by weakening the my-ocardium either directly, as in the case of ischemia or infec-tion, or indirectly by increasing afterload. On the other hand, internal obstructions or factors external to the heart may interfere with its contraction or rhythm. In either case, in the absence of intervention, the ability of the heart to re-spond to demands progressively declines until failure of the pump is complete (fig. 10.26).

Pathogenesis of Congestive Heart Failure

CHF presents an excellent demonstration of the relation-ship between a functional abnormality and its related pat-tern of signs and symptoms. In considering the pathogene-sis of CHF, two factors are significant. One is the essential problem of the heart's inability to clear itself of the blood delivered to it. The second is the comparatively long time over which signs and symptoms develop. In the following analysis, mitral stenosis is used as an example of a condi-

tion that produces the characteristic signs and symptoms of CHF. These are weakness and fatigue, pulmonary conges-tion and edema, dyspnea, cardiomegaly, systemic conges-tion and edema, hepatomegaly, and splenomegaly.

Stenosis of the mitral valve is often the result of fibro-sis and calcification. The hardened, thicker valve cusps can't fully open, and the flow tract between left atrium and left ventricle is reduced in size. Stenosis interferes with ventricular filling and causes a decline in stroke volume and cardiac output. As the stenosis increases, cardiac output may even fail to meet demand at rest. Weakness, quickness to fatigue, and fainting may result.

Upstream from the narrowed mitral valve, the effects are more extensively felt. Blood that can't easily clear the atrioventricular flow tract backs up into the right atrium and then into the lungs (see fig. 10.24). This **pulmonary congestion** produces pulmonary hypertension, with pres-sures sometimes rising to three to five times above normal. (This is to be distinguished from the pulmonary hyperten-

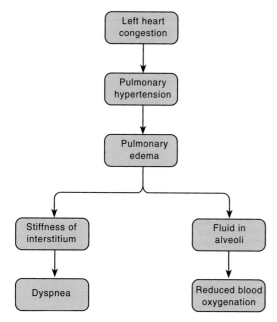

Figure 10.27   **The Problem of Pulmonary Edema Is an Important Aspect of Chronic Left Heart Failure.**

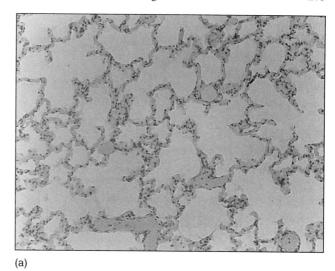

(a)

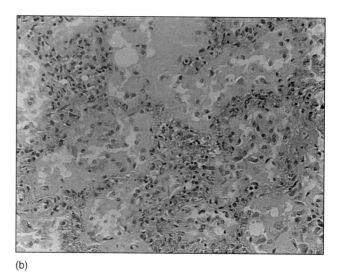

(b)

Figure 10.28   **Pulmonary Congestion in CHF.** (*a*) Normal alveoli. (*b*) Lung in CHF with fluid filling the alveoli. Numerous phagocytic cells are also present.

sion that occurs in hypoventilation of the lung.) The high pressures cause an accumulation of fluid in the lung interstitium: **pulmonary edema** (fig. 10.27). Edema causes a stiffening of the lungs; they become firm and less elastic. As the condition progresses, higher pressures force fluid from the pulmonary tissues into alveolar air spaces (fig. 10.28). This process reduces the surface available for diffusion and leads to airway obstruction as fluid accumulates in the alveoli and bronchioles.

Both airway obstruction and the loss of normal lung elasticity contribute to another problem—difficulty of breathing, or **dyspnea.** Dyspnea in heart failure may be intensified when lying down. This condition is called **orthopnea,** and seems to result from an increased loading of the failing heart as the reclining position favors movement of blood from the legs and abdomen to the heart. The additional burden causes more pulmonary congestion, edema, and increased respiratory difficulty. Orthopnea is quickly relieved by elevating the head and shoulders. Severe bouts of dyspnea also often occur at night in CHF patients. However, this condition of **paroxysmal nocturnal dyspnea** is not quickly relieved by assuming an upright posture; as much as 30 minutes in an upright position may be required for breathing to become easier. Although the underlying mechanism is not well understood, it appears that partial depression of the brain's respiration and cardiac centers during sleep contributes to the problem.

In addition to breathing difficulties, pulmonary hypertension can cause aneurysms in small pulmonary vessels. These may rupture to yield small areas of hemorrhage in the lungs. Pulmonary hypertension and congestion predispose to secondary infection; bronchopneumonia is a common complication of CHF.

Further progression of CHF involves the backup of blood into the right heart (fig. 10.24*c*). This means an increase in the right heart's preload—another burden that is added to the increased afterload presented by the elevated pressures in the pulmonary vessels. The right ventricle responds, as does the similarly congested left atrium, with hypertrophy that increases their strength and enables them to compensate with an increased stroke volume. The result is an enlarged heart, the **cardiomegaly** that characterizes the chronically failing heart. We will deal with another aspect of cardiomegaly, cardiac dilatation, in the Myocardial Compensations section later in this chapter.

As right heart congestion develops, blood returning to it from systemic veins confronts a high resistance, and systemic venous congestion results. This is evident in the swelling of the major superficial veins, especially the internal jugulars, that is often observed in CHF patients. Elevated systemic venous pressure is also reflected in

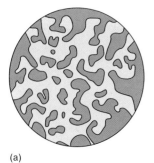
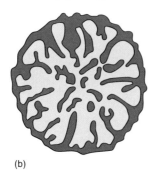

(a)   (b)

Figure 10.29 **Hepatic Congestion and "Nutmeg Liver."**
(*a*) The characteristic microscopic pattern of liver damage caused
by hepatic congestion. It resembles a slice through a whole
nutmeg (*b*), hence the descriptive term nutmeg liver. In (*a*), the
dark regions represent islands of surviving cells at a distance from
the congested vessels. The cells near the vessels are damaged and
appear pale.

increased capillary pressures, which cause systemic edema.
As tissue fluid accumulates, it tends to percolate through
the tissue spaces following the pull of gravity. It collects at
low points, such as the ankles, when the person is sitting or
standing, producing the condition of **dependent edema.**

Beyond widespread systemic edema, venous congestion has significant effects in the liver and, in some cases,
the spleen, which drains into it. Hepatic congestion arises
when the hepatic vein is unable to empty into the congested
inferior vena cava. The resulting blood accumulation in the
liver causes it to enlarge—the condition of **hepatomegaly.**
In the hepatic sinusoids, hepatic congestion produces high
pressures that can damage hepatocytes or cause hemorrhage as the vessels rupture. Pressure damages those cells
that are adjacent to the congested vessels, while tissues further removed from the vessels are unaffected. These retain
their normal dark color. Damaged tissue is lighter in color,
providing a contrasting pattern that resembles the coloration of a nutmeg; hence, the descriptive term **nutmeg
liver** (fig. 10.29).

Hepatic portal system hypertension may cause back
pressure, which leads to congestion in the spleen. The resulting **splenomegaly** is associated with severe and advanced CHF. In such cases, the effects of congestion may
also be seen in a reduced intestinal absorption as drainage
from the congested mesenteric veins is impeded by hepatic
congestion. The major elements of pathogenesis in CHF are
presented in figure 10.30. This explanation has focused on
the blockage of flow to the left ventricle, a case of pure mitral stenosis. In this relatively rare circumstance, the left
ventricle has no increased pumping demand and therefore
doesn't hypertrophy or dilate. More often there is a different problem or mixture of problems—for example, mitral
regurgitation, or aortic stenosis, or regurgitation on their
own, or combined mitral stenosis and regurgitation. In
these cases the left ventricle will undergo hypertrophy
and/or or dilation. These will add to the cardiomegaly noted
in pure mitral stenosis. Focal ischemia or infarct may lead

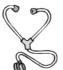

Focus on Heart Failure in Infants

Newborns and young infants with heart failure
present a special diagnosis challenge, since
many of the characteristic signs and symptoms are different
from those seen in adults or may be confused with those of
lung disease.

Common features of heart failure in infants include:

- repeated pulmonary infections
- excessive sweating
- feeding difficulties
- failure to grow and gain weight
- rapid breathing
- facial edema (versus peripheral edema)

Respiratory distress, experienced as in the adult, may be
expressed as flaring of the nostrils, grunting, and retraction of
the ribs (i.e., depression of the rib cage) rather than the labored
elevation of the rib cage seen in adults. When the diaphragm
of an infant is very forcefully depressed, the relatively flexible
rib cage collapses. These children will tend to become cyanotic when crying because of the added demands this action
places on their compromised heart function. On the other
hand, the infant whose primary problem is compromised lung
function will tend to become pinker while crying because of
improved ventilation of the lungs.

to compensatory hypertrophy in the rest of the relatively
normal myocardium.

In summary, the dominant clinical pattern in CHF can
be seen to arise from the pulmonary and systemic congestion
that follows the heart's failure to deal effectively with its preload. Most often, right heart failure follows left heart failure,
as in the preceding example. A similar pathogenesis may result from heart failure that originates in the right heart.

Cor Pulmonale   Numerous diseases of the lung or associated structures such as the rib cage or diaphragm produce
alterations of the lung tissue and vasculature that directly or
indirectly cause pulmonary hypertension. The resulting increase in the right heart's afterload causes hypertrophy and
dilatation in the right ventricle. Right heart enlargement
that arises as a result of impaired ventilation of the lungs is
called **cor pulmonale.** Its effects typically produce CHF
without left heart involvement. Chronic bronchitis and emphysema most often cause cor pulmonale, but a large number of other lung diseases may also give rise to this condition, which is responsible for 10–30% of North American
hospital admissions for CHF (table 10.5).

There are two essential mechanisms underlying the
pulmonary hypertension that causes cor pulmonale. The
first is damage or reduction in the number of pulmonary
vessels, which, because it forces blood through fewer vessels, causes congestion and hypertension. The second is a

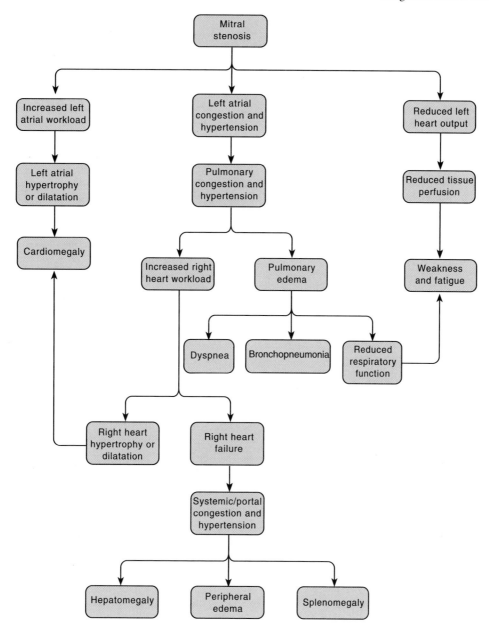

Figure 10.30 **Pathogenesis of Congestive Heart Failure (CHF).** In this example, a narrowed left atrioventricular valve (mitral stenosis) produces a chronic condition that compromises downstream blood supply and generates upstream congestion, which in turn gives rise to an often seen pattern of cardiac, pulmonary, and systemic complications.

Table 10.5	Conditions Causing Cor Pulmonale

Pulmonary embolism
Pulmonary fibrosis
Chronic bronchitis*
Emphysema*
Idiopathic pulmonary hypertension[†]
Disorders involving reduced air flow (e.g., distortions of the vertebral column like kyphoscoliosis, obesity, or muscle weakness)

*These may be present to varying degrees in the clinical syndrome known as chronic obstructive lung disease (COLD).
[†]This condition is rare.

reflex vasoconstriction of pulmonary arterioles in response to the hypoxia, hypercapnia (excessive carbon dioxide), and acidosis that often accompany lung disease. These conditions are discussed more fully in chapter 12.

Physiological Compensations in Congestive Heart Failure

Myocardial Compensations

The failing myocardium has two responses that enable it to better cope with its pumping task. One is triggered by the increased EDV that occurs when the heart fails to maintain an adequate ejection fraction. The larger EDV stretches the myocardium to induce a more forceful contraction, an

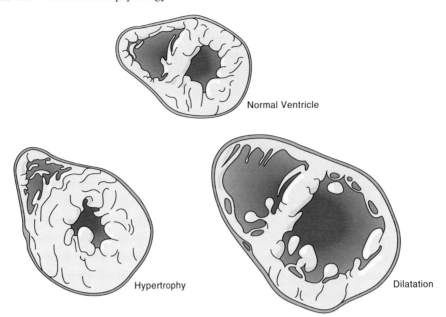

Normal Ventricle

Hypertrophy

Dilatation

Figure 10.31   **Myocardial Compensations.** The distinction between dilatation and hypertrophy can be easily seen in these cardiac sections.

application of Starling's law. This response provides increases in stroke volume that support cardiac output and limit congestion. However, as the myocardium must chronically cope with excessive volume, the increased stretching involved becomes disruptive to its tissues. The myocardium becomes thinner and less elastic, and normal tone is reduced; this is called **myocardial dilatation.** It contributes to the cardiomegaly seen in CHF. Thus, the cost of maintaining an adequate stroke volume is contraction under conditions of increasing myocardial dilatation. As dilatation increases, the myocardium's ability to develop adequate contraction force is reduced. This is the stage of decompensation indicated by the downward sloping portion to the right in the Starling curve (see fig. 10.13).

The second myocardial compensation is hypertrophy. In confronting a greater afterload, myocardial cells quickly respond by enlarging. They synthesize new contractile proteins and thus increase overall myocardial thickness and strength. Formation of additional supporting connective tissue accompanies this enlargement of the myocardium. Hypertrophy, like dilatation, can contribute to cardiomegaly (fig. 10.31). Increased muscle mass also increases myocardial demand for oxygen, further taxing blood supply in the ischemic heart.

Nervous System Compensations

Several compensations involving sympathetic nervous system reflexes are activated by declining cardiac output and systemic blood pressure. In response, sympathetic input to the SA node causes elevation of the heart rate. At the same time, sympathetic stimulation to the myocardium promotes a positive inotropic response, increasing stroke volume. Both responses increase cardiac output and, hence, blood

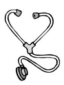

Focus on Normal versus Abnormal Compensation

It is important to recognize that hypertrophy also occurs in a normal heart that is regularly subjected to high demand, as in laborers or those who regularly pursue some form of athletics or fitness training. In such cases, the heart's weight can double. With such a strengthened myocardium, stroke volume increases to the degree that resting cardiac output can be maintained at lower heart rates. The savings in hemodynamic stress may reduce the risk of atherosclerosis and ischemic heart disease. In CHF, cardiac weight can triple. Also note that CHF may involve both increased EDV and increased afterload. In such cases, both hypertrophy and dilatation can contribute to cardiac enlargement. For example, the increased afterload problem of the hypertensive may induce an adaptive hypertrophy. As well, the elevated blood pressures may damage the coronary endothelium, predisposing to coronary atherosclerosis and a weakened myocardium. This in turn leads to a reduction of the ejection fraction, increases in EDV, and, in time, cardiac dilatation.

pressure. Sympathetic stimulation also causes vasoconstriction in systemic arterioles. This conserves the reduced cardiac output for perfusion of essential organs. It also increases peripheral resistance, supporting systemic blood pressure but increasing afterload. The vasoconstriction reflex reduces blood flow to the skin's surface. This means that less heat reaches the skin and so the evaporation of per-

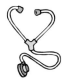

Focus on Digitalis Toxicity

When cardiac glycosides are used, drug dosage must be calculated carefully, because they have an extremely narrow margin of safety. There is very little difference between a therapeutic and a toxic dose. Studies indicate that as many as 20% of patients taking digitalis show some form of toxic response.

Prominent among the effects of digitalis overdose are cardiac arrhythmias. Spontaneous depolarization (automaticity) is increased, leading to ectopic beats, tachycardia, and fibrillation. The conduction rate may decrease, particularly at the AV node, and varying degrees of heart block may result. There are characteristic ECG changes that aid in the diagnosis of digitalis toxicity. The ECG of the digitalized patient on a cardiac monitor should be examined frequently and carefully, since potentially fatal arrhythmias may be the first signs of digitalis toxicity.

Nausea, vomiting, and diarrhea are the gastrointestinal manifestations of glycoside toxicity. Neurologic symptoms include headache, anorexia, dizziness, and visual disturbances, particularly in color perception.

Although simple overdose is the most common cause of digitalis toxicity, several factors increase the sensitivity of the heart to digitalis doses that would otherwise be acceptable. A low plasma and intracellular potassium concentration (hypokalemia) markedly increases the risk of toxicity. Since the glycosides may be prescribed in combination with diuretics, which promote renal potassium loss, great care must be taken to maintain a proper potassium balance. Acidosis also provokes intracellular potassium depletion (see chapter 16). Hypokalemia and acidosis are both caused or aggravated by diarrhea.

---

spiration fluid is reduced. The result is the cold, "clammy" skin of the CHF patient in a state of "compensation."

Renal Compensation

Recall from chapter 9 and earlier in this chapter our discussion of the renin-angiotensin system (RAS). When cardiac output falls in CHF, renal blood flow is reduced. In response, the kidney increases its secretion of the enzyme **renin.** This favors formation of a plasma protein called **angiotensin I,** which is converted to its active form, **angiotensin II,** as it passes through the lungs. When activated, angiotensin II stimulates secretion of aldosterone, the principal mineral corticoid of the adrenal cortex. Aldosterone stimulates renal retention of sodium ion, and water is increasingly retained by the kidney. This effect in turn causes an increase in plasma volume, which contributes to maintaining blood pressure in compensation for a reduced cardiac output. However, this compensation attempt also complicates the situation, since the extra plasma volume also contributes to congestion, already a major problem in CHF. In this case, the compensation attempt hinders more than it helps.

Another renal compensation response is based on **atriopeptin** or **atrial natriuretic factor** (ANF). It is released from the atrial myocardium in response to atrial tachycardia or distention. As its name implies, it induces sodium loss via the kidney. This loss results in diuresis that reduces fluid volume and, therefore, cardiac workload. Renin secretion and release of ADH (antidiuretic hormone) are both suppressed by ANF, a factor that further contributes to renal water loss. Another benefit derives from ANF's vasodilation effects, which reduce cardiac workload. Why this potent substance is unable to counter the antagonistic effects of enhanced renin secretion in CHF is unclear. Its effects are being analyzed for potential therapeutic

application. Physiological compensations in CHF are summarized in figure 10.32.

Ultimately, the chronic progression of CHF overcomes available compensations, with total heart failure the result. This outcome can be delayed by therapeutic intervention.

Therapy in Heart Failure

In CHF it is sometimes possible to eliminate the cause of the heart's reduced pumping ability. Surgical replacement of defective valves or correction of certain arrhythmias with electronic pacemakers are two, often successful, examples. The use of coronary by-pass surgery, angioplasty, and t-PA has already been mentioned in the context of treating acute ischemia. These procedures can also be used to support or limit injury to the failing heart. Often, however, it is not possible to eliminate the cause of CHF, and therapy must be directed toward increasing the heart's ability to maintain its output.

A major thrust of therapy in CHF is aimed at strengthening the myocardium while reducing afterload. This is achieved by various pharmaceutical agents with enhanced myocardial inotropic effects. Various of these agents as well as those that promote diuresis are described in the following section.

Principles of Cardiac Pharmacology

A wide variety of drugs influence the performance of the heart. They do so by modulating the electrical and mechanical events of the cardiac cycle or the regulatory systems that influence cardiac output. Cardiac drugs can be classified in various ways, but clinically, only six types are typically encountered: drugs that reduce the susceptibility to thrombus formation, and drugs with chronotropic, inotropic, diuretic, antiarrhythmic, or vasodilation effects.

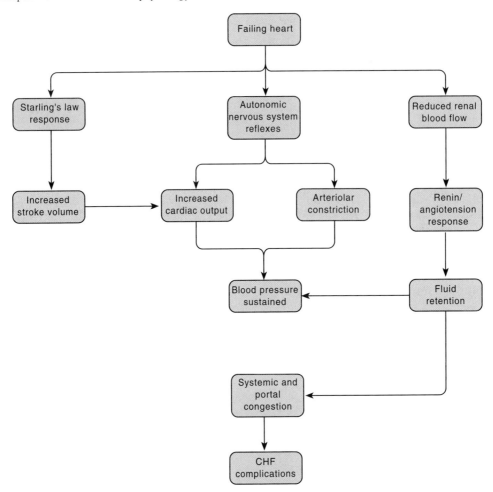

Figure 10.32   **Compensations in CHF.** Physiologic compensations for a failing heart may be able to maintain adequate blood pressure to meet a reduced level of demand, but complications may be introduced by the fluid retention responses.

Drugs that alter the susceptibility to thrombus formation fall into antiplatelet agents and anticoagulants. Aspirin, a classic antiplatelet drug, blocks thromboxane synthesis in platelets. Another antiplatelet drug, clopidogrel, prevents the ADP activation of platelets. Warfarin, an anticoagulant, interferes with the progression of the coagulation cascade by activating "antithrombins." Typically, antiplatelets are taken to reduce the progression of atherosclerosis, where platelets play a key role. Anticoagulants, like warfarin, are used where coagulation may be the central problem (as in the case of thrombus formation in atrial fibrillation).

Chronotropic drugs alter the heart rate. Positive chronotropic agents increase heart rate, while negative chronotropic agents decrease it. **Inotropic drugs** alter myocardial contractility and therefore stroke volume. Positive inotropic drugs increase contractility; negative inotropic drugs decrease it. **Digitalis** and its derivatives **digoxin** and **digitoxin** are widely used positive inotropic agents. **Diuretics** indirectly affect the heart by promoting urinary fluid loss. This limits volume overload and reduces edema. **Antiarrhythmics** alter the electrical properties of the myocardial cells to restore normal rate and rhythm, and **vasodilators** relax smooth muscle in arterioles. Some agents have the most effect in the coronary vessels, increasing myocardial blood

flow. Others dilate systemic arterioles to decrease afterload. This effect eases myocardial workload and reduces angina.

Because the effects of these clinically important groups overlap, they are organized in a different order in the following section.

Cardiac Glycosides Digitalis and its derivatives form a group of drugs, termed **cardiac glycosides,** that are widely used to treat the failing heart. Although they affect the heart and vasculature in several different ways, their principal action is to augment the inotropic response of the myocardium by raising stroke volume and cardiac output. When the inotropic effect is enhanced, an increased contraction force is obtained at lower degrees of myocardial distention. This means less myocardial strain and an improved ability to meet increased demand (fig. 10.33).

The cardiac glycosides increase contractility by raising the intracellular concentration of calcium ions. In fact, it seems that all drugs with a positive inotropic effect function in this way. At the same time, they act as positive chronotropes. This tendency to increase heart rate, which would increase the oxygen demand of an already compromised myocardium, is offset by other effects. The increase in cardiac output achieved by effective use of digitalis

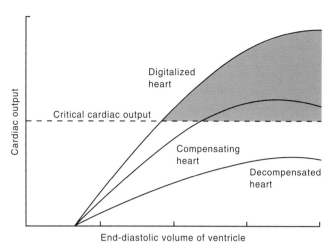

Figure 10.33 **Effect of Cardiac Glycosides.** The inotropic effect of digitalis provides more cardiac output for smaller degrees of myocardial stretch. This alteration provides some additional capacity to cope in higher-demand conditions. See figure 10.13.

raises the arterial blood pressure, tissue perfusion, and venous return. There is thus a reflex decline in sympathetic nervous system output, causing arteriolar and venous vasodilation and a decline in heart rate, in spite of the direct increase in automaticity that digitalis produces. This is a good example of a normal homeostatic regulatory response.

Diuretics In response to declining cardiac output and arterial blood pressure in congestive heart failure, the renin-angiotensin-aldosterone pathway induces fluid retention. This is of value to the degree that it raises blood volume, venous return, and stroke volume. However, excess fluid retention causes edema and injurious overdilation of the ventricles, which in turn reduces the ejection fraction and stroke volume. Salt restriction in the diet can reduce sodium levels and promote water loss. Diuretic agents can be used to further stimulate urinary water loss in an effort to ease the heart's fluid volume burden.

The multitude of diuretics can be divided into four major groups as shown in table 10.6. Most operate on the renal tubules by interfering with the reabsorption of

Table 10.6	Major Classes of Diuretics and Some Specific Agents That Might Be Encountered Clinically. (Other types of diuretics antagonize the action of aldosterone and so promote diuresis. These agents also reduce the secretion of fluid into the eye, and so are more often used to reduce the increased pressure in glaucoma.)

Osmotic Diuretics

These indirectly promote sodium loss and diuresis by increasing filtrate concentration.

| Mannitol | Urea |
| Isosorbide | Glycerine |

Loop Diuretics

These reduce sodium, chloride, and other electrolyte reabsorption, which decreases water reabsorption to induce diuresis.

| Bumetanide | Ethacrynate sodium |
| Ethacrynic acid | Furosemide |

Thiazide Diuretics

These increase the loss of sodium and chloride, which promotes water loss.

Bendroflumethiazide	Benthiazide
Chlorothiazide	Cyclothiazide
Hydrochlorothiazide	Hydroflumethiazide
Methyclothiazide	Polythiazide
Trichloromethiazide	

Aldosterone Antagonists

These oppose the action of aldosterone, so sodium and water loss increase while potassium is retained. These are known as "potassium-sparing" diuretics.

Amiloride
Spironolactone
Triamterene

Carbonic Anhydrase Inhibitors

Inhibition of this key enzyme indirectly induces water loss by limiting bicarbonate reabsorption and hydrogen ion secretion.

| Acetazolamide | Acetazolamide sodium |
| Dichlorphenamide | Methazolamide |

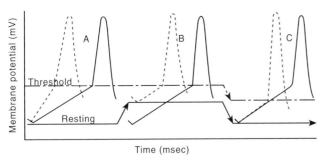

Figure 10.34 **Possible Mechanisms Underlying the Acceleration of the Myogenic Rhythm Employed by Various Positive Chronotropic Agents.** Solid curves represent a slower reference rhythm. In curve A, influx of positive ions is increased. The distance from rest to threshold is decreased in curve B by raising resting potential and in curve C by lowering the threshold. Most antiarrhythmics have the opposite effect (slowing myogenic rhythm) by the reversal of any combination of these mechanisms.

sodium, chloride, and various other ions. This in turn reduces the osmotic reabsorption of water, and urinary water loss is increased. The major problem encountered with diuretic use is electrolyte imbalance, particularly hypokalemia. This is usually handled by using a diuretic that causes potassium loss in combination with one that counters this effect by retaining potassium, such as aldactone. These problems are explored in more detail in chapter 16.

Antiarrhythmic Drugs An arrhythmia is an abnormality in the cardiac rate or rhythm caused by an abnormal origin of cardiac impulses, or a defect in cardiac conduction. These abnormalities are the consequence of altered myocardial depolarization (automaticity), faulty conduction pathways, or a combination of both. Normally the specialized conducting cells of the heart exhibit spontaneous activity, generating the myogenic rhythm. The rate of firing of these cells is dependent on three factors: the inflow of sodium and/or calcium or the outflow of potassium, the resting potential, and the threshold potential. Lowering the threshold, raising the resting potential, and increasing sodium or calcium influx, for example, all cause the myocardium to reach threshold sooner and accelerate the myogenic rhythm.

Figure 10.34 illustrates these effects. In the figure, the solid curve provides a reference. The broken-line curves show the effects and changes caused by more rapid sodium inflow (curve A), raised resting potential (curve B), and a lowered threshold potential (curve C). These effects are primarily elicited by digitalis and the catecholamines (norepinephrine and epinephrine). Atropine achieves its accelerating effects by blocking the inhibiting effects of parasympathetic stimulation on the heart rate.

In contrast, various antiarrhythmic drugs slow the myogenic rhythm. Some interfere with sodium availability, while others block calcium flow through calcium channels in the cell membranes. Various antiarrhythmic agents are listed in table 10.7.

Table 10.7	Drugs That Influence the Myogenic Rhythm
Drugs That Increase the Heart Rate	**Drugs That Decrease the Heart Rate**
Epinephrine	Digitalis (indirect effect)
Norepinephrine	Quinidine
Atropine	Procainamide
	Lidocaine
	Propranolol
	Disopyramide

Drugs Used for Treatment of Angina Pectoris As we have noted, angina is the characteristic crushing chest pain associated with myocardial hypoxia. The pain can occur at rest but is usually triggered by exercise, emotion, or physiological stress. It represents an imbalance between oxygen demand and supply to local areas of the myocardium. The underlying cause in the vast majority of cases is ischemia from coronary atherosclerosis. Oxygen demand is proportional to cardiac workload; thus the approach to therapy is two-pronged: to increase the blood supply and to decrease myocardial workload and the heart's oxygen demand.

Although coronary blood flow is almost entirely regulated by local control mechanisms that in the poorly perfused myocardium are working at maximum, some drugs are used to interfere with the effect of circulating or locally produced vasoconstrictors. **ACE inhibitors** (angiotensin-converting enzyme inhibitors) are an excellent example. These (ramipril is an example) interfere with the conversion of angiotensin I into the vasoactive substance angiotensin II. The enzymes that are blocked are resident in both the pulmonary and cardiovascular endothelium. Besides reducing the concentration of a major vasoconstrictor (AII), ACE inhibitors disrupt one of the harmful compensations of congestive heart disease—aldosterone-mediated sodium and water (volume) retention. Reduction of cardiac workload is an alternative strategy, and it is achieved by the use of three types of drugs: beta-blockers, peripheral-vasodilating nitrates, and calcium-channel blockers. These drugs are often used in combination.

Propranolol and nadolol are both drugs that block the beta receptors that mediate the effects of the sympathetic nervous system on the heart. Thus, the heart rate and contractility of the myocardium are reduced and the blood pressure falls. Since beta-blockers also induce bronchospasm, they are not appropriate for patients with asthma and should be used cautiously for patients with any respiratory disease.

Nitrates and other vasodilators induce NO release from vessels and thereby reduce arterial resistance. This reduces venous return, stroke volume, and cardiac output,

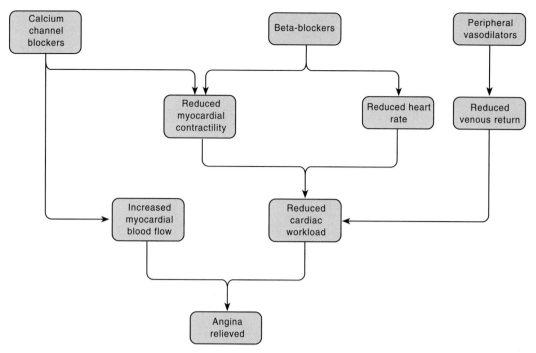

Figure 10.35   **Relief of Angina Pectoris.** This is achieved by the use of agents that either reduce cardiac workload or increase myocardial blood flow. With a better balance between work demand and blood supply, angina is alleviated.

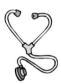

Focus on Breaking Therapy

An often unexpected, yet common, cause of heart failure is the inappropriate withdrawal of therapy. This often occurs when digitalis, or another agent, is effective in alleviating symptoms. Too often, patients will reduce the prescribed dosage, without informing their physicians. Alternatively, frustration with sodium or other dietary restrictions may induce binges of excess intake, often on vacations or special occasions. Either can trigger a severe and potentially fatal episode of cardiac decompensation.

and thereby the workload and oxygen demand of the heart. **Nitroglycerin** and related compounds act in the same way.

Calcium antagonists such as **verapamil, nifedipine,** and **diltiazem** are examples of calcium-channel blockers that inhibit calcium influx into myocardial and vascular smooth muscle cells. This means they have the dual effect of reducing contractility and promoting coronary artery vasodilation; that is, they simultaneously reduce cardiac workload and increase blood flow to the myocardium. The actions of some common agents used in treating angina pectoris are summarized in figure 10.35.

STRESS AND HEART DISEASE

The concern is often raised that stress may predispose people to cardiovascular disease or exaggerate the effect of other risk factors on heart disease. There is a rich history of

research establishing the **general adaptation syndrome** (GAS). Animals undergoing prolonged experimental exposure to a variety of physical and psychosocial "stressors" experience catastrophic and nonspecific systemic effects, including cardiovascular disease. The "stressors" in these experiments were largely manipulations of the environment (cold, heat, sustained immersion, overcrowding, isolation) but also included elements of the animals' ability to interact with or control their environment. This GAS model is compelling enough in our stress-conscious world that it has been widely adopted as an explanatory model within nursing and allied health programs. This is despite the fact that studies with human populations do not usually demonstrate the kind of direct relationship between "stress" and heart disease or other health problems that we have widely come to accept exists for recognized risk factors like smoking, high fat/cholesterol diet, lack of exercise, or uncontrolled chronic hypertension. You may have the sense that "orthodox" risk factors incrementally contribute to illness and that they are supported by unambiguous research findings. It should be remembered that risk factors are just that: they increase our likelihood of experiencing a disorder to a degree that is only "predictable" on a population basis. We all know of people who break all the "risk factor" rules and live to be 90. On the other hand, the research to clearly establish a "risk factor" is difficult to perform with human subjects because of ethical and logistical problems. Longitudinal research, which is the only type that is relevant in the area of risk factors, is expensive, time consuming, and hinges on asking the right questions at the outset. While such work has been done in the area of many cardiovascular risk factors (the Framingham study is classic)

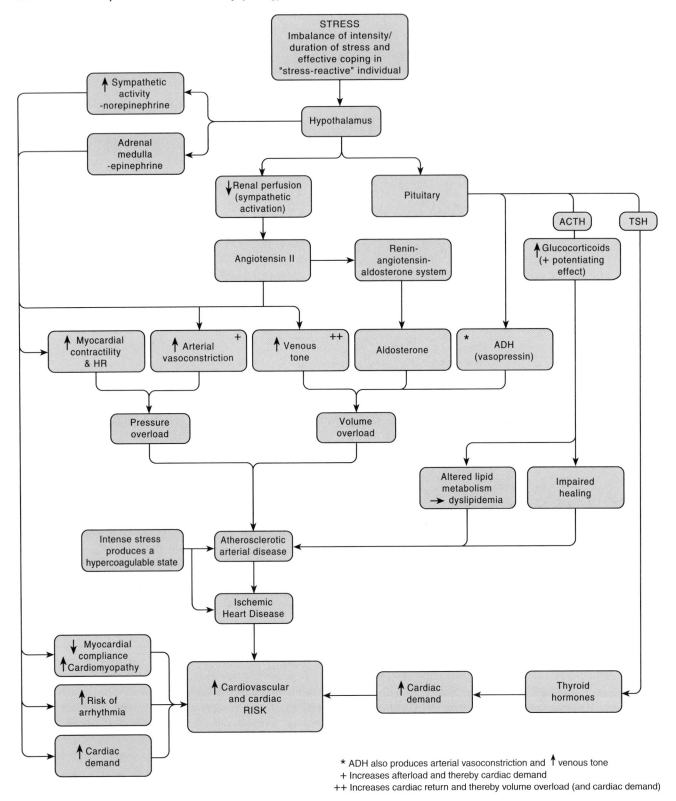

Figure 10.36   **Stress.** Mechanisms of stress can predispose to, or worsen, heart disease.

"stress" has not received this attention. The basis for a stress–cardiac/cardiovascular interaction is founded on the well-established physiology adapting blood pressure, cardiac output, peripheral resistance, venous tone, and blood volume to meet demands on the cardiovascular system. In a stressful situation, the system trigger is threat rather than a drop in blood pressure or volume, which we established earlier as the relevant cue to preserve blood pressure and critical tissue perfusion. It is our opinion that intense and persistent psychosocial stress constitutes a significant risk to cardiovascular health. We present this simply as a framework within which to organize the available information.

This text is not the proper forum for building a tight operational definition for "stress." We have suggested a loose context in the lead-in box in figure 10.36. This figure pulls together physiological adaptations to intense stress and links them to the factors that we have identified as propelling chronic heart failure—namely, pressure and volume overload. Most of this information is familiar to you from previous chapters. Some bits will be new or need focusing. While the activation glucocorticoid release from the adrenal medulla by adrenocorticotropic hormone (ACTH) functions principally to mobilize energy to meet a challenge, it has four effects of relevance to heart disease. (1) Cortisol, the principal glucocorticoid, slows wound healing, probably by breaking down collagen and impairing phagocyte function. This may have a role in repair of the endothelial injuries that characterize atherosclerosis. (2) While mobilizing glucose (gluconeogenesis), cortisol inhibits its uptake by cells. This induces a shift to fat metabolism with a resultant rise in circulating low-density lipoproteins and ketone bodies, which contributes to dyslipidemia that may propel atherosclerosis. (3) There is evidence that posttraumatic stress disorder is associated with increased sensitivity of glucocorticoid receptors—stress makes one more vulnerable to stress. (4) The potential for inducing cardiomyopathy is one of the concerns in prescribing glucocorticoids and may be an effect of stress-related cortisol. Of course, with all these tentative linkages, the dose level at which cardiac or cardiovascular problems are seen is very important but not clearly established.

Two of the hormones identified are only associated with stress when it is sudden and intense: ADH and thyroxine. This spurt of ADH may cause a brief increase in fluid volume and, hence, volume overload by inappropriately retaining water by reabsorption from the distal tubules and collecting ducts in the kidneys. Thyroid hormones will elevate basal metabolic rate, which has the effect of burning off more energy than would otherwise be the case. This may be great if you want to lose weight, but it places an additional burden on the heart to deliver the oxygen and nutrients necessary to sustain this elevated BMR. In a compromised heart, this can have disastrous effects. Along with thyroxine, insulin is secreted briefly. Rats exposed to social stress have been shown to develop insulin-resistant diabetes, another illness that induces abnormal lipid metabolism that may be a factor contributing to atherosclerosis.

You will note that figure 10.36 says that intense stress produces a hypercoagulable state. This is based on studies that related intense stress to increases in thrombin and increased fibrin turnover. Again, this is a small piece, but it may contribute to the development or progression of atherosclerosis. Microthrombi, as you will recall from chapter 8, are involved in the pathogenesis of atherosclerotic disease.

Besides their well-recognized roles in cardiac and vascular responses to increased CV demand, epinephrine and norepinephrine have been linked to heart disease. Chronic stress has been related to the development of arrhythmias, decreased ventricular compliance (the ventricles don't relax as completely, impeding diastolic filling), and cardiomyopathy. Epinephrine is considered a likely factor. For a person with reduced cardiac function, epinephrine, administered with a dose of stress, is to be avoided because of the increased oxygen demand it creates with increased heart rate and pumping force. While the flow chart in figure 10.36 may seem compelling, remember that each of these linkages to heart disease is relatively weak and individual effects may not be summative. But to put this in context, if you review the long history of research and social-political activity framed on the one side by the U.S. Surgeon General's first major report on smoking in 1964, and on the other by Surgeon General Everett Koop's scathing report in 1989, you will get an appreciation of how pieces of research that are tentative individually can be compounded to make a final, inexorable case.

CARDIOMYOPATHIES

The **cardiomyopathies** are those noninflammatory conditions that cause impaired myocardial function and are unrelated to the more common causes of heart failure: coronary artery disease, valve dysfunction, hypertension, or congenital defects. Because the cardiomyopathies are diverse, their classification takes two approaches.

Etiology is the basis for one approach, with two categories identified. In **primary cardiomyopathy,** two criteria are applied. First, the myocardium, rather than valves or the pericardium, is the focus of damage, and second, etiology is unknown or unrelated to some other systemic disease. In **secondary cardiomyopathy,** the direct cause of damage can be identified or at least seen to be the result of some systemic disorder—for example, uremia or Cushing's syndrome. The secondary cardiomyopathies may be further categorized on the basis of etiology, with infiltrative, toxic, and other categories recognized. However, since over half of cardiomyopathies are idiopathic, the etiological approach to classification is less useful than one based on functional abnormalities.

From a functional viewpoint, the cardiomyopathies are divided into three groups. **Dilated (congestive) cardiomyopathy** is characterized by pronounced dilation and failure of the ventricle. In **hypertrophic cardiomyopathy,** the major feature is ventricular hypertrophy, which is so pronounced that it reduces ventricular volume and obstructs outflow from the heart. The third type, **restrictive cardiomyopathy,** has

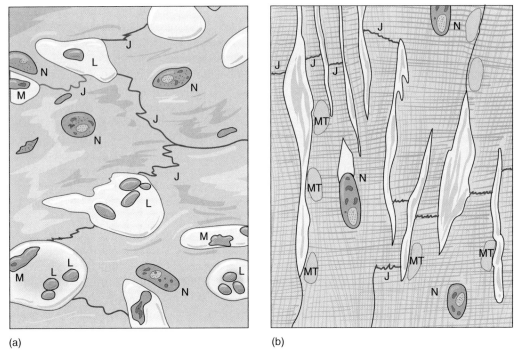

(a)   (b)

Figure 10.37   **Hypertrophic Cardiomyopathy.** (*a*) The characteristic pattern of myocardial tissue is clearly evident in this diagram of hypertrophic cardiomyopathy. Cardiac muscle cell nuclei are apparent (N), cells are swollen, intercellular junctions (J) and intracellular organization of myofibrils are indistinct, spaces between cells are infiltrated with lymphocytes (L) and macrophages (M). (*b*) Normal tissue for comparison (MT—mitochondria).

the key feature of a stiffened ventricular wall, which is only poorly distensible.

Although we will describe these groups separately, note that some degree of overlap exists between them.

Dilated Cardiomyopathy

Diffuse myocardial injury that impairs contractility is the underlying abnormality in dilated cardiomyopathy. As a result of the impairment, the ejection fraction typically falls to 40% or less (55–78% is normal), while end-systolic volume and end-diastolic volume increase, producing a chronic stretching of the myocardium. This causes damage, scarring, thinning, and dilation of the ventricles. Some hypertrophy is often present as well, accounting for observed increases in the heart's weight, which in extremes can double to reach 700 g.

With diminished contractility, signs and symptoms of heart failure appear, but since the right ventricle is also failing, the pulmonary vessels are partially protected from hypertension and edema. Onset of symptoms is usually gradual, but an inexorably downhill course is typical as the ejection fraction and cardiac output continue to fall, in spite of cardiac compensations. Prognosis is quite variable, with many patients surviving for years, while others with acute and severe (fulminant) attacks may die within weeks of diagnosis.

Since etiology in dilated cardiomyopathy is usually unknown, therapy cannot be directed at a specific cause. Instead, a general treatment for patients with heart failure is instituted. The usual regimen seeks to maintain stroke vol-

ume by means of cardiac glycosides and to limit fluid accumulation and edema by means of salt restriction and diuretics. Anticoagulant therapy is also frequently employed, since a reduced ejection fraction predisposes to intravascular and intraventricular thrombosis. Vasodilators may also be used to lower peripheral resistance and reduce cardiac workload.

Alcohol is the major cause of nonischemic dilated cardiomyopathy. It is seen primarily in males aged 30–55, where consumption of alcoholic beverages is heavy for 10 years or longer.

Hypertrophic Cardiomyopathy

Etiology in hypertrophic cardiomyopathy is usually poorly identified, but most cases have a genetic component. The dominant feature is focal, asymmetric hypertrophy of the myocardium. Microscopically, the myocardial tissue can be seen to be disorganized, with shortened, nonparallel cell arrangements and fibrosis. Intracellular organization of myofibrils is also distorted (fig. 10.37).

Hypertrophy is often asymmetric, with the septum enlarging disproportionately, sometimes enough to impede left ventricular emptying and aortic valve function. When either of these features dominates, descriptive terminology is employed: **asymmetric septal hypertrophy** (ASH) in the first case and **idiopathic hypertrophic subaortic stenosis** (IHSS) in the second. If outflow obstruction dominates the functional disruption, the term **hypertrophic obstructive cardiomyopathy** (HOCM) is employed.

The congestive heart failure that develops in these patients generally arises from three problems: obstruction of ventricular outflow, mitral insufficiency, or **reduced ventricular compliance** (the ventricle stiffens). The ejection fraction is often elevated, although in severe disease the end-diastolic volume is reduced by the enlarged and encroaching myocardium. Although surgery may repair valve dysfunction, pharmacotherapy is more commonly employed.

Restrictive Cardiomyopathy

The least common type of cardiomyopathy is characterized by the deposition of amyloid, glycogen, or mucopolysaccharide in the myocardium. Such infiltration is typically accompanied by fibrosis and is the result of an inherited metabolic disease. The rare primary tumors of the heart and more common metastatic tumors may also be responsible for the infiltration.

Typically, heart failure in restrictive cardiomyopathy occurs because of loss of resilience and contractility in the myocardium. Falling values of EDV, SV, and cardiac output are typically present. Pharmacological therapy is usually unable to restore cardiac output, and death ultimately occurs from arrhythmia or congestive heart failure.

CONGENITAL HEART DEFECTS

Congenital heart disease develops as a result of malformations in the heart and includes, by convention, defects in the great vessels. Congenital cardiac defects are present in under 1% of live births, with a greater proportion found in stillborn infants; cardiac defects presumably contribute to the increased prenatal mortality. Generally, the mechanisms underlying these abnormalities are the persistence of normal fetal blood channels into extrauterine life and faulty embryologic development during the third through eighth weeks of gestation.

Complex interactions between genetic and environmental factors appear to be responsible for most congenital cardiac defects. Those in which hereditary factors predominate will often be found in association with other genetic conditions such as DiGeorge syndrome, osteogenesis imperfecta, trisomy 21 (Down's syndrome), trisomy 13, trisomy 18, and Turner's syndrome. Environmental factors known to be involved during pregnancy are maternal rubella (German measles) or other infections, certain drugs, (e.g., lithium), and maternal alcohol abuse. However, with that said, it should be noted that currently over 90% of congenital cardiac disease is idiopathic. Severe, complex cardiac abnormalities are a significant cause of neonatal death or require surgery in infancy. If untreated, survivors typically face a declining course of congestive heart failure.

The structural abnormalities present in these conditions divert blood through the heart and pulmonary circulation to other than normal passages. For example, blood flow may be diverted from the pulmonary circulation to the systemic circulation to produce a **right-to-left shunt.** In such cases,

Table 10.8	Incidence of Congenital Cardiac Defects as a Percentage of All Such Abnormalities. Various studies of the incidence of these conditions yield values that fall within the indicated range. The incidence of congenital cardiac defects is estimated at less than 1% of all live births.

Ventricular septal defect (VSD)	20±5%
Atrial septal defect (ASD)	12±2%
Patent ductus arteriosus (PDA)	15±5%
Tetralogy of Fallot	10±5%
Aortic coarctation	6±1%

blood is poorly oxygenated, often to the degree that cyanosis results. Cyanosis starts to develop when hemoglobin saturation falls below 65%, and may be accompanied by polycythemia. This excess of red blood cells results from the response to systemic hypoxia. A hematocrit of 60% is typical in polycythemia (45% is normal). In a **left-to-right shunt,** blood flow is diverted from the systemic circulation to the lungs, producing congestion in the pulmonary vessels.

Abnormal flow of blood through malformed cardiac or great vessel passages often produces unusual sounds called heart murmurs. These are often early signs of the presence of congenital cardiac defects.

The incidence of congenital defects in the heart is indicated in table 10.8. Those with most clinical significance are the following.

Ventricular Septal Defects (VSD)

Although they are the most common cardiac malformation of infancy, **ventricular septal defects** are rare in adults because they either close spontaneously or result in a high rate of infant mortality. Only small defects (less than 1 cm in diameter) are compatible with survival beyond childhood. These are usually the result of a failure to close the membranous portion of the interventricular septum, which lies adjacent to the floor of the atria (fig. 10.38). The pathogenesis is predictable. Blood is driven from the higher-pressure left ventricle to the lower-pressure right ventricle, producing a loud murmur during systole. The resulting right heart overload increases pulmonary congestion, causing hypertension, dyspnea, fatigue, and a susceptibility to pulmonary infections. If the condition is prolonged for months and years, hypertension in the pulmonary vascular bed can lead to sclerosis, raised pulmonary resistance, and shunt reversal in late stages (fig. 10.39). Right-sided congestive heart failure is the usual end-stage of the unrepaired defect.

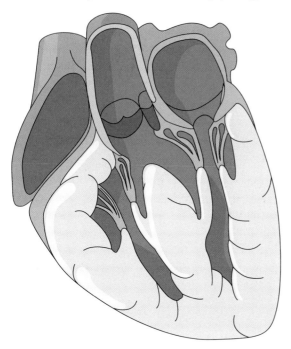

Figure 10.38   **Ventricular Septal Defects.** In this typical case, the thin membranous portion of the interventricular septum has failed to close the opening between the ventricles. Extreme compensatory hypertrophy of the right ventricle is observed.

Atrial Septal Defects (ASD)

Atrial septal defects often arise as the result of an abnormal fusing of the interatrial septum during embryonic development. They may also arise when the **foramen ovale** (fig. 10.40) fails to close. During fetal life, the foramen ovale provides a direct route to the left heart atrium, bypassing the nonfunctioning lungs. Normally this passage closes during the early postnatal period.

Atrial septal defects are often not diagnosed or treated in childhood and therefore represent a significant group among adults with congenital heart disease. The opening in the septum allows blood to be shunted from the left atrium to the right atrium. Increased right heart volume increases flow through the pulmonary valve, causing a systolic murmur. Another finding on auscultation is a characteristic alteration of the second heart sound.

Fatigue, pulmonary congestion, dyspnea, and frequent upper respiratory tract infections are common findings in severe left-to-right shunting, although many young victims are asymptomatic. With increasing age, the chronic overcirculation of blood through the lungs causes pulmonary sclerosis. Later in the course, pulmonary arterial pressure increases and the left-to-right shunt declines, becomes variable, and finally reverses (see fig. 10.39). This puts a great burden on the right heart, and right heart failure is a likely outcome. As pulmonary blood flow diminishes and blood by-passes the lungs, cyanosis, fatigue, and fainting spells develop. Surgical repair is a safe and effective procedure, but is usually not done if shunt reversal has occurred.

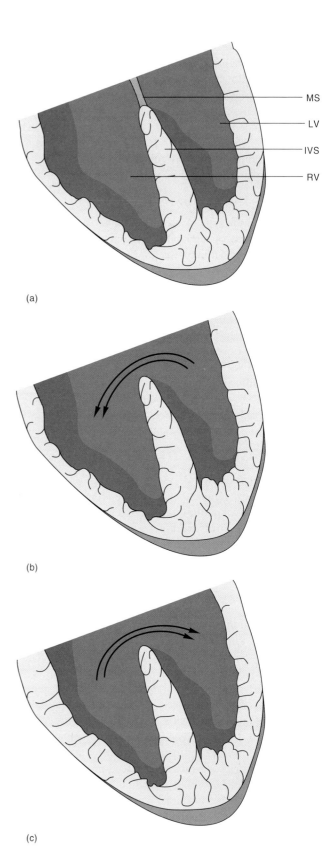

(a)

(b)

(c)

Figure 10.39   **"Shunt Reversal."** (*a*) The normal isolation of the right ventricle (RV) from the left ventricle (LV). The interventricular septum (IVS) is muscular except for the membranous section (MS). (*b*) In cases where lack of closure allows communication between ventricles, left-to-right shunting results. (*c*) Later, with lung damage, the shunt reverses.

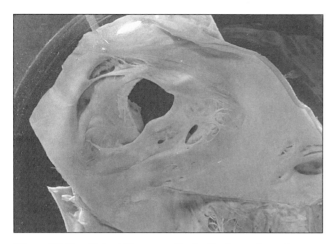

Figure 10.40 **Patent Foramen Ovale.** During embryonic development, if the normally present foramen ovale does not close, an atrial septal defect results.

This is the heart of a 72-year-old woman, showing a large defect in the atrial septum due to the failure of closure of the foramen ovale. The woman's history included long-standing hypertension and several bouts of heart failure, which she had survived until her last hospital admittance. At that time, a chest X-ray indicated a possible aneurysm in the pulmonary artery, but no definitive clinical diagnosis was made. She soon died of a suspected acute MI.

At autopsy, the atrial septal defect, which had previously escaped detection and which caused the overloading of the right heart and pulmonary trunk, was discovered. This condition explained the X-ray findings and revealed that it was cor pulmonale, rather than a MI, to which the unfortunate woman ultimately succumbed.

Patent Ductus Arteriosus (PDA)

During fetal life, the ductus arteriosus joins the aorta and pulmonary artery, shunting blood from the pulmonary circulation into the systemic vessels to by-pass the nonfunctioning lungs. Following birth, the lungs inflate, pulmonary resistance declines, and blood flow through the duct is reversed. Within hours of birth, the high concentration of dissolved oxygen in the systemic arterial blood and the reversal of flow through the ductus arteriosus cause the duct to become stenotic and finally close.

Persistence of the ductus arteriosus causes chronic shunting of blood from the high-pressure aorta into the low-pressure pulmonary artery (fig. 10.41). This is sustained throughout the cardiac cycle so that a continuous (systolic and diastolic) murmur is evident. The severity of the disorder is proportional to the degree of patency, most children being asymptomatic. Volume overload of the left ventricle, with pulmonary congestion and hypertension, occurs in severe cases. When present over many years, pulmonary sclerosis develops, raising pulmonary arterial pressure and reversing flow. Pressure overload on the right heart eventually causes right-sided congestive heart failure. When the condition is diagnosed before shunt reversal has occurred, surgical correction is the treatment of choice.

Coarctation of the Aorta

Coarctation of the aorta is a congenital narrowing (fig. 10.42*a*) that primarily occurs in males and exists in two quite distinct forms, based on the position of the coarctation with respect to the ductus arteriosus. In both types, there is a large pressure gradient across the coarctation, producing downstream hypotension and upstream hypertension.

Preductal, or **infantile, coarctation** occurs at a point proximal to the ductus arteriosus, which remains open following birth since pressure in the distal aorta is insufficient to reverse flow and initiate duct closure (fig. 10.42). Left ventricular failure follows, as a result of the increased resistance to flow offered by the narrowed aorta. This produces symptoms of left heart failure. Also, volume overload of the right ventricle develops, since part of the ejected blood is shunted into the aorta. Cyanosis, dyspnea, and heart failure are all observed. Death may follow unless surgical intervention is prompt.

Postductal coarctation usually arises distal to the left subclavian artery and is compatible with survival to maturity—hence, the designation **adult-type coarctation.** The characteristic high pressure in the aortic arch leads to the normal postpartum flow reversal in the ductus arteriosus, which closes in the usual way. Some relief of the distal hypotension and ischemia is achieved by way of a multitude of collateral vessels that develop to by-pass the point of coarctation, particularly branches of the subclavian and intercostal arteries. This adaptation permits survival to middle age. There is hypertension in the head and upper limbs, and hypotension in the lower limbs and abdomen. Left ventricular hypertrophy is evident, and left heart failure may ultimately occur if surgical repair is not performed. The young individual may suffer aneurysm, thrombosis, or rupture of cerebral vessels or of an aortic aneurysm.

Tetralogy of Fallot

In the condition known as tetralogy of Fallot, four structural abnormalities are present. They include a ventricular septal defect, pulmonary stenosis, and an aorta that is shifted to the right (dextroposed aorta) to lie over the right as well as the left ventricle. The fourth component, right ventricular hypertrophy, is not a malformation but rather the adaptation of the right ventricle to the high afterload presented by a narrowed pulmonary outflow tract. The fourth element of this condition was first described by a French physician, E. A. Fallot. Of those persons affected, 40% have one or more additional cardiac defects. In over 20% of cases, abnormalities in other organs are also present.

Right-to-left shunting occurs in this complex malformation as the narrowed entrance to the pulmonary trunk diverts blood through the septal defect into the left ventricle. When a lesser degree of stenosis is present, pulmonary blood flow may be sufficient to prevent cyanosis, but more typically, cyanosis is present at birth or develops within the first year of life.

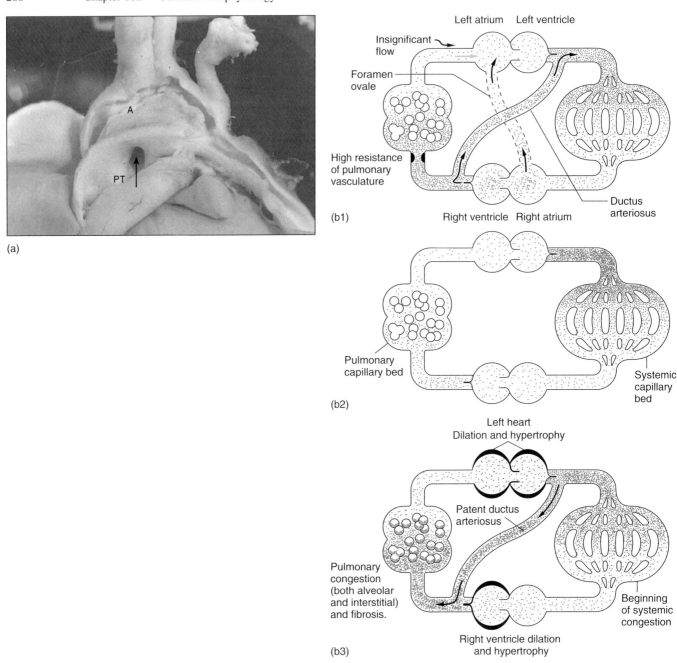

Figure 10.41   **Patent Ductus Arteriosus.** (*a*) The arrow shows the connecting link between the aorta (A) and the pulmonary trunk (PT) that failed to close off after birth. (*b*) Schematic representation of the relation between the aorta and pulmonary trunk, and of the cardiac and pulmonary overloading that results when the fetal vessel (ductus arteriosus) is retained. (*b1*) The fetal circulation. The foramen ovale passes most blood from the right atrium to the left atrium. The ductus arteriosus shunts most right ventricular output to the aorta and thence to the systemic circulation. Both result in relatively little pulmonary circulation in the fetus. (*b2*) Normal postpartum circulation. The foramen ovale and ductus arteriosus are closed off; thus, they are not contributing to circulation. (*b3*) The ductus arteriosus that served to shunt blood from the right heart, by-passing the nonfunctional and high-resistance fetal lungs, to the systemic (and umbilical) circulation, is now shunting blood in the opposite direction.

A temporary by-pass vessel between a systemic artery and the pulmonary artery may be surgically introduced in the infant's first year. This allows sufficient oxygenation to sustain growth and development to later childhood, when a complete surgical correction of the defect is better tolerated.

Without surgical intervention, the outlook is bleak, with death occurring in infancy or early childhood. Various complications beyond systemic hypoxia contribute to the decline: cardia arrhythmias, infective endocarditis, coagulation disorders, and cerebral abscess or infarction, among others.

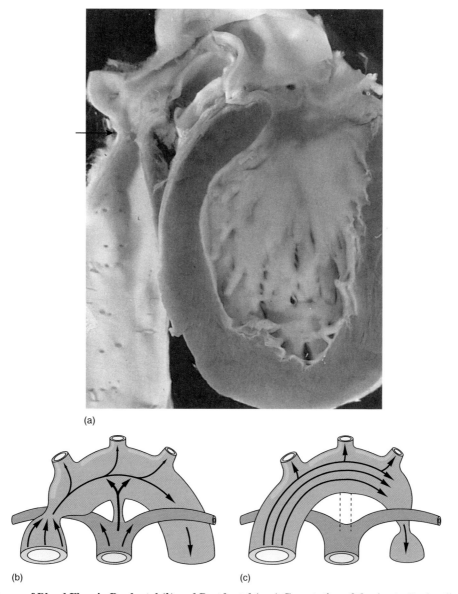

(a)

(b)   (c)

Figure 10.42 **Patterns of Blood Flow in Preductal (*b*) and Postductal (*a, c*) Coarctation of the Aorta.** Broken lines
(*c*) indicate site of ductus arteriosus. Note how the position of the point of coarctation has implications for the cranial circulation.
(In (*a*), the left ventricle is being viewed from the right side.)

*In this photo, a coarctation at the base of the aortic arch can be seen. It was responsible for the early death of an infant, caused by the
inability of the heart to drive blood past the coarctation. As the photo shows, the lumen of the aorta was extremely narrow, offering high
resistance that even the markedly hypertrophied ventricle could not overcome.*

*Additional evidence of high ventricular pressure can be seen in the thickness of the endocardium, which had adapted to the abnormal
pressures to which it was subjected. Also note an additional congenital defect: a bicuspid aortic valve.*

CARDIAC DISEASE:
IMPACT ON MORTALITY

We have chosen to organize our discussion of heart disease
to parallel our treatment of basic cardiac anatomy. This ordering, however, does not reflect the relative incidence with
which you will encounter specific heart diseases. The incidence in clinical populations will, of course, vary immensely: In infant cardiac wards, for example, you may see
a much higher proportion of congenital heart disease, while
in respiratory wards you will more commonly encounter
cor pulmonale associated with chronic lung disease. Mortality statistics give us a more balanced way of ranking the
significance of competing pathologies. On this basis, cardiac disease is the major killer in industrialized societies,
responsible for perhaps 35% of all deaths. Of those deaths,
the vast majority (about 85%) are attributable to atherosclerosis and ischemic heart disease.

Although the coronary atherosclerosis progresses
slowly, processes superimposed upon it make its expression

in ischemic heart disease quite variable. Resultant conditions include angina pectoris, sudden cardiac death, myocardial infarction, and chronic ischemic heart disease. The incidence of, and recovery from, IHD have been improving over the past two decades—a function of decreases in coronary atherosclerosis. This in turn is possibly due to improved medical intervention (particularly in the control of the major risk factor systemic hypertension), diet, exercise, and life style. Certainly, an increasing amount of attention is being directed to these factors in efforts to lessen the life-shortening effects of epidemic atherosclerotic disease. A large proportion of the 6–7% of deaths due to cerebrovas-

cular disease is atherosclerotic in origin, as are all of the additional 1% of deaths directly attributable to atherosclerotic degeneration of the aorta, renal, or other systemic, noncerebral arteries.

Of fatal cardiac disease, 85% is caused by IHD. What of the remaining 15%? Five specific diseases account for almost half of this number. Hypertensive heart disease gives rise to about 2%, while rheumatic heart disease, congenital heart disease, infective endocarditis, and cor pulmonale account for about 1% each. The remainder, a wide variety of specific diseases, can be grouped effectively into pericardial, myocardial, or endocardial valvular diseases.

Case Study I: Acute Heart Failure

A 63-year-old male was admitted to the emergency room (ER) at 9:30 P.M. after suddenly collapsing while reading a newspaper at his home. An emergency inhalator crew found him unconscious and gasping for breath. He was resuscitated with some difficulty and rushed to hospital.

On arrival at the ER he was found to be in ventricular fibrillation. He was successfully defibrillated, and an airway was established by intubation. Oxygen, anticoagulant, and digoxin therapies were promptly instituted. After he was stabilized, he was transferred to the intensive care unit (ICU), where a second defibrillation was required.

He regained consciousness the next morning and could speak, describing a 10-year history of angina and nitroglycerin therapy. His skin was pale and cool, consistent with compensatory peripheral vasoconstriction. He was sweating, restless, and his urinary output was low. BP was 80/60 mm Hg. Blood chemistry studies showed an SGOT level of 300 IU (normal: 6–22) and an LDH level of 900 IU (normal: 90–210). His condition deteriorated and he succumbed at 12:30 P.M. the same day.

At autopsy, six rib fractures were noted, the result of the inhalator crew's resuscitation attempts. The right coro-

nary artery was occluded by a large, gelatinous thrombus. The left anterior descending and circumflex arteries showed signs of severe atherosclerosis and were narrowed to only pinpoint lumina. Extensive recent infarction was noted in the left ventricle, as were areas of old, healed, subendocardial infarction in both ventricles and the septal myocardium.

Commentary
This history is, unfortunately, not unusual. About 20% of acute MI patients die of the initial attack, while others may ultimately succumb to its complications or to subsequent infarction. Serious arrhythmias are common, resulting from direct damage to the conduction system or from more generalized ischemic damage to the myocardium.

Following admission, findings were consistent with acute MI, the low BP and high serum enzymes indicating significant myocardial injury. Low urinary output follows widespread vasoconstriction and fluid retention. Physiological compensations and therapeutic intervention were unable to protect against the devastating loss of functional myocardium.

Case Study II: Congestive Heart Failure

A mentally confused 37-year-old male was admitted to a large hospital's intensive care unit (ICU). He was pale, sweating, and suffered severe dyspnea. He was diagnosed as suffering from right heart failure due to mitral insufficiency, with associated pulmonary and right ventricular congestion and hypertension. His blood pressure measured 110/90 mm Hg, and his heart rate was 120 beats per minute. He had dependent edema and pronounced jugular venous distension, and was mildly jaundiced.

Although he was too ill to provide any history, according to previous records that were obtained, he had suffered nine years previously from rheumatic fever complicated by

bacterial endocarditis. The resulting damage had necessitated surgical replacement of the mitral valve.

During open-heart surgery the patient was supported by cardiopulmonary by-pass. It was found that some of the sutures of the old mitral prosthesis had pulled away from their anchorage, producing an orifice that allowed regurgitation into the left atrium. A new valve was secured in position, and the patient was removed from cardiopulmonary by-pass. A very low cardiac output was in evidence, and BP could not be sustained without cardiopulmonary support, which was therefore resumed. Adrenalin, isoproterenol, and calcium were administered to support myocardial function, but all attempts failed and the patient was finally pronounced dead after two hours on the by-pass apparatus.

At autopsy, the heart was found to be markedly enlarged, particularly the left ventricle. Cardiac weight was 950 g (normal: 375 g). The pericardium showed evidence of previous rheumatic fever damage; it was completely adherent with no detectable pericardial fluid. The myocardium was seen to be seriously weakened by extensive areas of fibrosis and calcification. The coronary vessels were widely patent, with only minor focal indications of early atherosclerotic involvement.

The liver weighed 1,550 g (normal: 1,350 g) and was cirrhotic, with prominent nutmeg patterning. Both spleen and kidneys showed signs of minor infarctions, possibly from thromboemboli. Examination of the brain revealed indications of previous surgery to relieve pressure at the site of an earlier cerebral hemorrhage. Various small infarcts were also observed.

Commentary

This interesting case demonstrates the risks associated with rheumatic heart disease and with valve replacement. Left-sided valve damage is a common result of rheumatic heart disease; pericarditis and myocardial involvement are found less frequently. Following surgery, the patient's condition had improved, but he later suffered a cerebral hemorrhage, presumably related to his anticoagulant therapy, which was instituted to prevent thrombosis and embolism from the surfaces of his mechanical valve prosthesis. He had undergone surgery to relieve the pressure that developed as a sequela of the cerebral hemorrhage. His records indicated that he had also suffered transient attacks of ischemia involving the cerebral vasculature, probably from small thromboemboli. His mental condition had progressively deteriorated following these small emboli. For the preceding two years he had had a steadily declining course of fatigue, exercise intolerance, and exertional dyspnea, characteristic of chronic cardiac decompensation.

Previous cardiac diagnostic procedures, carried out in the referring hospital, had revealed significant mitral regurgitation and a left ventricular end-diastolic pressure of 30 mm Hg (normal: 9–12 mm Hg). This finding indicated a weakened ventricular myocardium, unable to eject its preload, and stretched at the end of diastole into the decompensating portion of the Starling curve. Pulmonary hypertension was severe, with pulmonary arterial pressure of 100/50 mm Hg (normal: 22/8 mm Hg).

Further ECG, radiographic, and laboratory analyses indicated CHF with cardiomegaly, pulmonary hypertension, hepatomegaly, and serious liver dysfunction. Echocardiography indicated left atrial and left ventricular dilation and color flow Doppler studies revealed a regurgitant jet around the valve prosthesis. Although he was a poor candidate, it was determined that surgery offered the only possibility of saving this unfortunate patient.

Thrombosis and embolism are persistent problems with valve prostheses, but, as the cerebral hemorrhage and small hemorrhagic brain infarcts illustrate, preventive anticoagulant therapy also has its hazards. The failing heart produced the classic features of left-sided CHF, with blood backing up through the lungs and liver. The prosthetic valve failure and volume overload of the left ventricle was complicated by the rheumatic myocardial injury, which could not be relieved by surgery.

Key Concepts

1. Heart failure implies that the heart is not pumping sufficient blood to meet normal demands. Acute heart failure develops quickly, while the conditions that underlie chronic heart failure progress more slowly (pp. 254–255).

2. The most common underlying pathology giving rise to either acute or chronic heart failure is ischemic heart disease affecting the left ventricle (p. 254).

3. Anything that interferes with the pumping capacity of the heart can lead to acute or chronic heart failure. This includes conditions that restrict its filling, impair valve efficiency, weaken the muscle, disturb its coordinated rhythm, or present abnormal resistance to the blood pumped (p. 255).

4. A less common cause of heart failure is any condition, such as extreme anemia, that places excessive pumping demands on the heart (p. 255).

5. Pericarditis can present problems in two ways: The accumulated fluid can restrict the heart and impair filling, or alternatively it can produce adhesions that restrain heart movement (pp. 255–256).

6. Inflammatory disease of the heart muscle (myocarditis) is usually acute and mild, although chronic conditions can be very debilitating and rare acute cases can weaken the heart sufficiently to produce acute heart failure (pp. 256–257).

7. Acute infective endocarditis, which can cause valvular degeneration and throw off infective emboli that damage kidney, brain, or heart, is lethal in a significant proportion of cases (pp. 257–258).

8. Stenosis of heart valves (commonly the mitral and aortic) increases the resistance to blood movement and leads to compensatory hypertrophy and potential chronic heart failure (pp. 258–259).

9. An improperly closing valve (valvular insufficiency or incompetence) allows the partial return of already pumped blood, adding to the volume the heart must pump to maintain adequate perfusion (pp. 259–260).

10. Rheumatic heart disease results when a cross-reacting antibody binds to valve leaflets and initiates inflammatory degradation that may produce both stenosis and insufficiency (pp. 260–261).

11. Atherosclerosis of the coronary arteries and superimposed thrombosis causes ischemia, which may produce pain, focal or diffuse infarction, or a life-threatening arrhythmia (p. 261).

12. Suddenly impaired local circulation or increased cardiac demand can precipitate acute myocardial infarction, which may cause death, predispose to many short-term complications, or set the stage for chronic heart failure (p. 263).

13. Changes in the response of endothelium in the region of the atheroma and downstream, secondary to ischemia, contribute to the pathogenesis of ischemic heart disease (pp. 263–264).

14. A wide variety of cardiac, vascular, hematological, and respiratory conditions can create excessive demands on the heart or impair its function and push it into a state of progressively decreasing capacity called chronic or congestive heart failure (CHF) (p. 269).

15. A decrease in the pumping capacity of the heart, so that it fails to clear the blood delivered to it, leads to congestion of upstream vessels and tissues and elicits a variety of compensatory mechanisms, the normal

16. function of which is to sustain perfusion (pp. 272–273).

16. Normal adaptations to increased cardiac demand (e.g., dilatation, hypertrophy, increased heart rate and force of contraction, retention of plasma fluid volume) extract relatively increased performance from the failing heart but also contribute to the pathophysiology of CHF (pp. 275–277).

17. Pharmacological agents can improve the performance of the failing heart by increasing its force of contraction, relieving the volume overload, stabilizing its rhythm, or reducing the resistance to pumped blood (pp. 277–281).

18. A variety of independent and interacting factors could play roles in the development of heart disease resulting from exposure of vulnerable individuals to intense or prolonged stress (pp. 281–283).

19. The term *cardiomyopathy* applies to a diverse collection of noninflammatory disorders of the myocardium that impair pumping by weakening the muscle or interfering with filling or outflow (pp. 283–285).

20. Congenital heart defects result from malformations or the persistence of normal fetal blood channels and impair the pumping of blood or its appropriate routing (pp. 285–289).

REVIEW ACTIVITIES

1. Lay out a flow chart that indicates the cause-effect relationships that develop in the pathogenesis of congestive heart failure. Start on the premise that an area of atherosclerotic artery has developed a thrombus that caused infarction of a substantial area of the left ventricular wall.

2. Assume that a clinical instructor has asked how a patient's body was compensating for congestive heart failure, and prepare a response.

3. Explain the use of diuretics and salt restriction for the patient in activity 2.

4. List the possible outcomes of myocardial infarction. When are the crisis points in the recovery from a myocardial infarction, and to what are they related?

5. Explain how left heart failure might become combined heart failure.

6. Differentiate the various types of angina.

7. Explain the role of deranged local control of perfusion in chronic ischemic heart disease.

8. Using figure 10.18 as your guide, describe and explain the development of rheumatic heart disease.

9. Cover all of figure 10.35 except for the top line and then construct your own flow chart to explain the actions of these agents (i.e. calcium-channel blockers, beta blockers etc.).

10. Figure 10.26 summarizes the etiologic factors in congestive heart failure. Cover the column on the left-hand side and generate it on your own with appropriate explanations.

Chapter

11

Circulatory Shock

Yet who would have thought the old man to have had so much blood in him?

WILLIAM SHAKESPEARE
MACBETH

rubor

&tumor

cū calore

&dolore

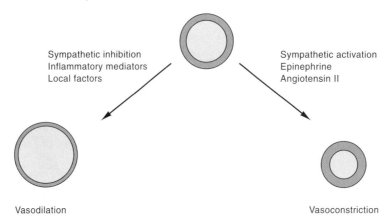

Sympathetic inhibition
Inflammatory mediators
Local factors

Sympathetic activation
Epinephrine
Angiotensin II

Vasodilation

Vasoconstriction

Figure 11.1   **Arteriolar Tension.** Factors that play a role in determining the wall tension of systemic arterioles.

The condition of **circulatory shock** is an acute and serious one. It involves a rapidly developing fall in blood pressure that significantly reduces blood flow to tissues.

To understand the pathogenesis of shock, it will be helpful to review the essential factors that determine blood flow in the cardiovascular system.

NORMAL BLOOD FLOW

To maintain normal homeostatic balance, tissues depend on an adequate blood flow reaching the **microcirculation.** This term describes the extensive networks of capillaries that pass among the cells of almost all tissues, including the arterioles that supply them and the venules that drain them. The capillaries are especially significant in that their thin walls allow for the movement of nutrients and wastes between tissues and the blood. It is only in the capillaries that vascular walls are adapted to accommodate the passage of fluid, nutrient, and waste molecules between the blood and tissue spaces. When blood adequately perfuses the microcirculation, nutrient supply and waste removal are consistent with normal function. When perfusion declines, the tissue's life is threatened.

Adequate blood flow in the microcirculation depends on **arterial blood pressure.** This is the driving force that moves blood through the body's vessels. Three factors combine to determine blood pressure. One is cardiac output—the blood that is pumped by the heart into the systemic circulation. The second factor is the plasma that fills the vascular spaces. The third is the degree of constriction produced by arteriolar smooth muscle tension. Both cardiac pumping and vessel wall tension are regulated by the autonomic nervous system—its sympathetic and parasympathetic branches provide input to the heart; there is only sympathetic input to arterioles. Circulating vasoconstrictors, principally epinephrine and angiotensin II, are also important in regulating systemic arteriolar tension (fig. 11.1).

MECHANISMS OF CIRCULATORY SHOCK

Systemic blood pressure is determined by the relationship of three key elements: the heart's pumping, arteriolar constriction, and blood volume. In circulatory shock, this normally balanced relationship is abruptly thrown out of equilibrium. Although many etiologies are involved, only three basic patterns of pathogenesis contribute to the development of shock. One of these is cardiac malfunction, which causes cardiac output to decline. With less blood pumped into the vascular system, pressure drops, and the result is **cardiogenic shock.** Rapid loss of blood from the circulatory system can cause a rapid fall in blood pressure. Shock due to such lack of circulating blood volume is **hypovolemic shock.** The third type of shock is caused by changes in the vascular system. **Vascular shock** results from widespread dilation of the systemic arterioles. In dilating, arteriolar muscle tension eases and the walls draw away from the blood within them. This change causes pressure to fall, often abruptly (fig. 11.2). The vessels of the abdominal viscera, the **splanchnic circulation,** are especially significant in vascular shock. Because they are so numerous and their capacity is so large, their dilation can cause significant drops in pressure.

Primary Shock

Any given case of circulatory shock will usually be the result of one of these three basic mechanisms. But two or even three may contribute to the overall loss of pressure. A good example is **primary shock,** which is also known as **neurogenic shock.** This condition usually passes quickly and is followed by rapid recovery. In primary shock, rapidly falling blood pressure sharply reduces cerebral blood flow, causing loss of consciousness. This is fainting, or **syncope.** Emotional trauma, intense pain, or other threateningly vivid experiences (for some, merely the sight of

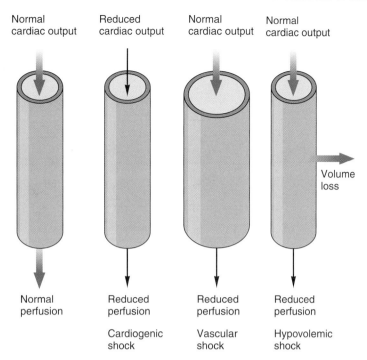

Normal
cardiac output

Reduced
cardiac output

Normal
cardiac output

Normal
cardiac output

Volume
loss

Normal
perfusion

Reduced
perfusion

Reduced
perfusion

Reduced
perfusion

Cardiogenic
shock

Vascular
shock

Hypovolemic
shock

Figure 11.2 **Patterns of Circulatory Shock.** At left, normal cardiac function, arteriolar tension, and plasmal volume combine to produce normal tissue perfusion. As each of these variables is compromised, shock may result.

blood) can result in altered nervous system output to the vessels and heart. (The term *neurogenic shock* refers to this nervous system involvement.) The result is vasodilation and a fall in cardiac output, which combine to reduce blood pressure. Note also that when the blood enters dilated arteriolar networks, flow rates are greatly reduced and blood tends to move only sluggishly through veins. This holding of blood in peripheral vessels is called **peripheral pooling.** It reduces the systemic venous return, which can in turn cause further reduction of cardiac output.

In primary shock, then, we have cardiogenic and vascular components both contributing to an abrupt fall in blood pressure. Insufficient cerebral flow follows, and the affected individual experiences a feeling of light-headedness and then loses consciousness. It is this loss of consciousness that interrupts the emotional stimulus to the autonomic centers that control heart and vessel activity. As a result, normal cardiac output and vasoconstriction are restored.

Neurogenic shock can be more serious when other than emotional factors are involved. In the case of brain damage or **central nervous system** (CNS) **depression** from drugs such as barbiturates or anesthetics, neural output to the heart and vessels may be inadequate to maintain BHP. If the spinal cord is injured, or in cases of excessive spinal anesthesia, normal autonomic output from the brain may be blocked and prevented from reaching the heart and vessels. Reduced cardiac output and vasodilation combine, causing the blood pressure to fall (fig. 11.3).

In primary shock, the onset of signs and symptoms is immediate. Most shock, however, is characterized by signs and symptoms that are slower to develop. This more common type is called **secondary shock.** It can develop from a wide variety of etiological factors, but all involve the three essential patterns of pathogenesis already described. These can now be considered in greater detail.

Cardiogenic Shock

Cardiac malfunction leading to a decline of cardiac output is the basis of cardiogenic shock. Its most common cause is failure of the left ventricle due to myocardial infarction (MI). In many cases of MI, loss of myocardial function is limited, so that cardiac output is adequate to meet resting tissue demands. In over 10% of all MI cases, however, loss of myocardium is substantial, and these demands cannot be met. When 40% or more of the myocardium is lost, cardiogenic shock results. In over 80% of such cases, death will follow in spite of therapeutic intervention.

Although MI is the most common cause of cardiogenic shock, several other etiologies that produce a relatively rapid failure of the myocardium may be involved. These were discussed in chapter 10 as factors contributing to acute heart failure. The relatively rare cardiomyopathies or certain bacterial toxins (e.g., diphtheria toxin) can weaken the myocardium. Other circulating substances, such as narcotic drugs or excessively high levels of potassium ion, can also depress cardiac function.

Cardiogenic shock may develop even though the myocardium is undamaged. This might be caused by a thrombus within the heart that obstructs blood flow through it, or

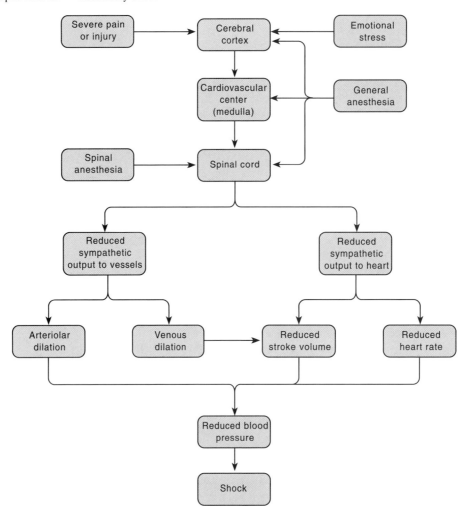

Figure 11.3   **Neurogenic Shock.** Note that both cardiac and vascular mechanisms play a contributing role.

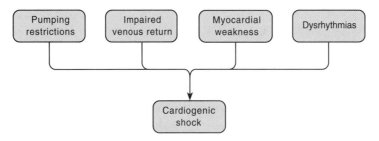

Figure 11.4   **Principal Causes of Cardiogenic Shock.**

by cardiac tamponade in which the heart is compressed so that it can't adequately refill after emptying (see chapter 10). Factors that block the blood's return to the heart can also lead to cardiogenic shock when they develop rapidly. For example, in cardiac tamponade the venae cavae may also be compressed so that venous return and cardiac output quickly fall. Compression of the venae cavae is also a factor in **tension pneumothorax.** In this condition, rising pressure in the pleural space can cause lung collapse and vena cava compression that blocks venous return.

Another way that blood flow to the heart can be restricted involves the pulmonary circulation. Very large thromboemboli can completely block blood flow through one or both lungs. This causes a profound drop in the blood volume reaching the left heart and an abrupt collapse of cardiac output.

Various patterns of cardiac dysrhythmia can also cause significant reduction in cardiac output so that shock develops. Whatever the etiology, a sharply reduced cardiac output is the significant event of cardiogenic shock. Figure 11.4 summarizes the etiology of cardiogenic shock.

Hypovolemic Shock

Hypovolemic shock is the condition arising from inadequate circulating blood volume. Most hypovolemic shock is **hemorrhagic shock.** That is, shock caused by severe bleeding, often following massive trauma. Blood escaping the body's vascular channels is usually easily seen, and quick intervention can often prevent shock from developing. However, intervention may be delayed, or bleeding may occur without visible blood loss, as in the cases of hemorrhage into body cavities, muscle groups, or the GI tract. For example, blood lost into the abdominal cavity following rupture of the aorta or into the muscle mass surrounding a fractured femur can result in serious drops in blood pressure. In some cases, hypovolemic shock may arise without the loss of whole blood from the vessels. Examples are fluid losses due to vascular changes that can accompany severe inflammation, to skin burns, or to dehydration from inadequate fluid intake, pronounced perspiration, or prolonged vomiting and diarrhea.

Shock may also be caused by large-scale fluid loss into the tissues across intact capillary walls. Such fluid losses may be the result of an abrupt obstruction in the venous system—from extensive and severe thromboembolism, for example. The obstruction prevents normal drainage of the microcirculation, and congestion and increased blood pressure result. The elevated pressure can rapidly drive substantial volumes of fluid into the tissue spaces. The result is **hypovolemia,** a reduction of circulating blood volume. A similar result follows damage to capillaries, usually from trauma, anoxia, or immune causes. When a capillary wall is damaged, its permeability increases, allowing the escape of fluid to the tissues. In either case, although total body fluid volume is not reduced, the volume of blood circulating in the vessels is. Shock follows, as venous return falls to levels that cannot sustain adequate cardiac output. Such increased capillary permeability can complicate hemorrhagic shock, since both often accompany massive trauma.

Shock may also be caused by extensive skin burns, where fluid loss can be substantial. The greatest losses occur in **third-degree burns,** in which both epidermis and dermis are lost. (**First-degree burns** are mild and involve only the epidermis, which can quickly regenerate; **second-degree burns** are more severe because they involve epidermal loss as well as some dermal damage.) Two factors contribute to fluid loss at burned surfaces. One is a pronounced inflammatory response in the severely damaged tissue. Large-scale exudate formation follows when large volumes of fluid rapidly leave the vascular spaces. Also, because blood vessels damaged by burns tend to lose protein, tissue osmotic pressure increases, drawing further fluid from the vessels by osmosis. The second fluid loss factor in burns is the loss of the body's protective surface lining. The skin normally prevents loss of tissue fluid by evaporation to the surrounding dry air. When the skin is lost, evaporation to the surrounding air can be considerable (fig. 11.5). So great is this loss in third-degree burns, that when over 15% of the

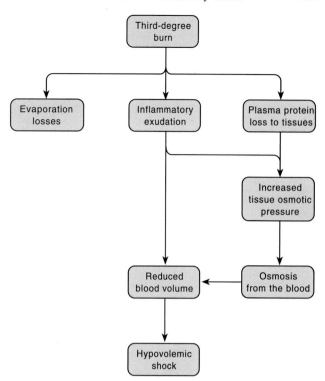

Figure 11.5 **Burns and Shock.** Severe burns present the risk of fluid loss and hypovolemic shock.

body's surface is involved, therapy must first be directed to preventing shock. Only then can attention be directed to the burned tissues.

In dehydration, substantial water is lost from the body. The result is a drop in plasma volume followed by a fall in blood pressure. When the dehydration is severe, hypovolemic shock can result. Sustained vomiting or diarrhea can lead to large losses of body water. Children are especially susceptible to this type of dehydration. Dehydration can also result from kidney disease. For example, in one type of kidney disease, large amounts of protein are lost into the urine. This in turn causes large urinary water losses, plasma volume reduction, and the potential for shock. In another type of disease, the kidney may be unable to regulate electrolyte levels properly. The resulting electrolyte imbalance can also cause large water losses (see chapter 16). Even prolonged and intense exertion in warm temperatures can lead to such large perspiration losses that shock from dehydration is a threat.

Hypovolemic shock develops on the basis of a reduction in circulating blood volume. However, any such losses will have much more severe effects if they occur over a short time span. Although much information on the effects of hemorrhage has been derived from studies using dogs or other animals, similar patterns are assumed to apply to the human. At one extreme, 10% of the body's approximately 5-liter blood volume can be lost, even abruptly, with minimal effect. At the other extreme, rapid loss of 50% of the blood is almost invariably fatal. Between these, the time

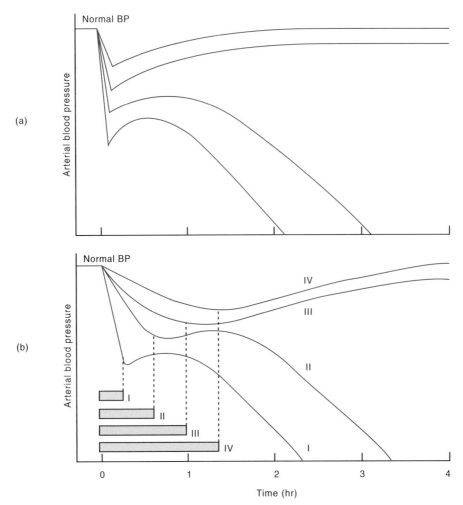

Figure 11.6   **Hypovolemic Shock.** (*a*) In the face of small volume and pressure declines, compensations can restore pressure. If losses are large, no recovery may be possible. (*b*) Outcomes of the same fluid volume lost over different time periods. Slow losses (III, IV) allow compensations to take effect and restore BHP. Rapid loss (I, II) of the same volume is fatal.

Source: Modified from A. C. Guyton, *Textbook of Medical Physiology,* 5th edition, 1971, W. B. Saunders, Philadelphia.

factor becomes more significant. The rapid loss of only 20% of blood volume will pose a greater threat than the gradual loss of 35% or even more (fig. 11.6). The reason for these different effects has to do with physiological compensations that are activated by a falling blood pressure. These are explained in detail following a description of vascular shock.

Vascular Shock

In vascular shock, rapid and widespread vasodilation expands vascular capacity. The result is a decrease in blood pressure. This means that even though no blood is lost, the relationship between the normal blood volume and the vascular space has been thrown out of balance. In this situation of **relative hypovolemia,** the existing blood volume is unable to adequately fill the enlarged vascular space. The result is a fall in blood pressure and a decline in venous return to the heart. As the heart receives less blood to pump, cardiac output can fall to reduce pressure even further.

The most common type of vascular shock is **septic shock,** in which falling pressure is the result of widespread

peripheral microcirculation effects. These are triggered by components of bacterial cell walls, usually Gram-negative bacilli, with other organisms involved less commonly. In a typical low-level infection, the inflammatory response is able to clear the invading bacteria with little systemic effect beyond the usual fever and malaise. With severe infection, as in bacterial peritonitis, the situation can rapidly become far more serious. In such case, the problem is the large-scale phagocytic destruction of bacteria that releases significant quantities of lipopolysaccharide material, typically called **endotoxin.** This material forms complexes with a binding protein that enables the complex to interact with circulating monocytes and macrophages in tissues. This causes the cells to release large quantities of TNF-α and other mediators that combine to produce the devastating effects that make septic shock so threatening. An important effect is arteriolar vasodilation, which causes blood pressure to fall. Beyond this, the mediators directly and indirectly cause widespread endothelial damage that greatly increases vessel permeability, allowing large volumes of plasma to escape to the tissue spaces. This is the problem of hypovolemia now superimposed on the dilation problem. The other prominent effect of

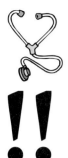

Focus on Blood Donation and Hypovolemic Shock

In considering the matter of hypovolemia, you may have wondered about the risk of shock to blood donors. Of course, you would quickly recognize that since knowledgeable people oversee the donor process, it can't be very dangerous. Two factors operate to reduce the risk. First, only a small volume is withdrawn: 450 ml. This is referred to as one unit. Second, blood is withdrawn over a period of 10–15 minutes. At this rate, blood loss is well tolerated and no shock is likely to develop. Recall the point made earlier: 10% of one's blood volume can be lost, even abruptly, without ill effect. On the basis of our total of 5 liters of blood, this works out to 500 ml, so the one unit withdrawn is even less than this well-tolerated level. Note also that the lost volume is readily restored in a day or two, although red cell replacement may not be achieved for six to eight weeks. For this reason, blood donations can only be done after a 56-day interval. Even with the care taken in withdrawing blood, a small percentage of people may experience some light-headedness or become faint. These effects are largely based on psychogenic factors—the fainting being a benign and transient episode of primary shock.

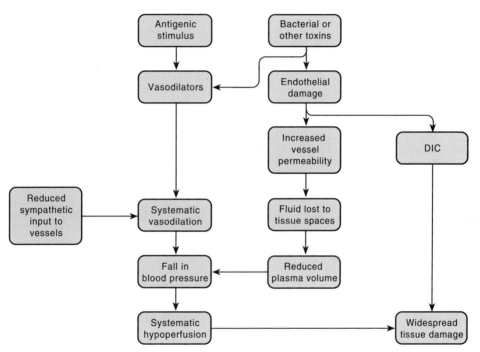

Figure 11.7   **Pathogenesis of Vascular Shock.** The nervous system's involvement (at left) is a component of primary shock. Note how hypovolemia may be an added complication. DIC: disseminated intravascular coagulation.

extensive endothelial damage is widespread blood coagulation triggered by exposure of the subendothelium. The falling arterial pressure also contributes, since sluggish microcirculation flow favors platelet aggregation and the accumulation of activated clotting factors. These various factors now combine their effects, resulting in disseminated intravascular coagulation (DIC), with tiny vessels throughout the system becoming blocked by masses of platelets and fibrin. Numerous destructive effects on multiple organs follow to compound the situation. Given this, you will not be surprised that septic shock has a very high mortality, accounting for over 100,000 fatalities annually.

When circulating vasodilators are toxins of nonbacterial origin, the term **toxic shock** is used. Such toxins may be released from damaged tissues or they may reach high levels when damage to the liver reduces its ability to clear toxins from the blood.

Another type of vascular shock is **anaphylactic shock.** It involves an immune response following a second exposure to a foreign antigen. The antigens react with sensitized cells, causing the widespread release of histamine and other vasodilators. Insect bites, blood transfusions, and some therapeutic or diagnostic agents can trigger the response. Anaphylactic shock presents significant risks, because it can develop with dramatic speed and intensity.

The significant vasodilation component of primary shock has already been described. The pathogenesis of vascular shock is summarized in figure 11.7.

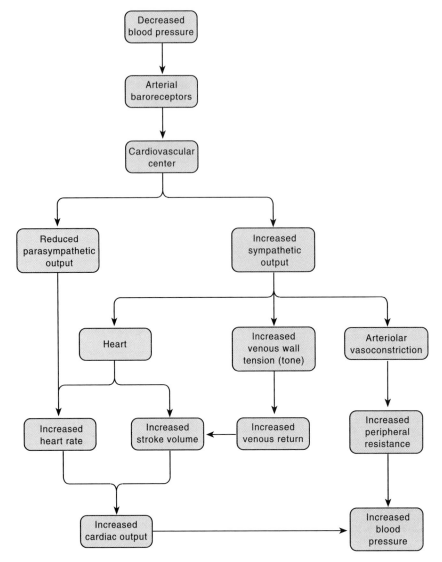

Figure 11.8   **Reflex Control of Blood Pressure.** These responses counter the development of circulatory shock.

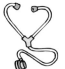 **☑ *Checkpoint 11.1***

In considering the role of endothelial damage in septic shock, were you tempted to pause to reflect on the larger issue of the vascular endothelium? Good. While pondering, you likely recalled your first exposure to this tissue simply as the passive liner of the vessel's interior surface. By this point in our studies, we've found more and more important functions of this vital tissue. Consider its role in binding phagocytes in inflammation, binding tumor cells as a factor in metastasis, and its numerous other direct and indirect procoagulation and anticoagulation functions. Then there is the endothelial contribution to promoting vasodilation by its secretion of nitric oxide. Endothelial membranes are also involved in the uptake of the lipoprotein complexes that play such an important role in atherosclerosis. And this is only a partial list. All-in-all, this is quite an impressive tissue whose importance is often overlooked.

Focus on Distributive Shock

You may encounter use of the term **distributive shock** in some clinical settings. It is essentially the same as vascular shock, but with a different focus. Rather than emphasizing the essential vascular mechanism that produces the problem, it emphasizes the inappropriate distribution of blood in peripheral tissues: the peripheral pooling that reduces venous return and lowers cardiac output. You are likely to meet the term in cases of anaphylactic, septic, and neurogenic shock—the most frequently encountered types of vascular shock.

COMPENSATION IN SHOCK

In response to falling blood pressure, several reflex compensations are triggered. These reflexes are part of the cardiovascular regulatory mechanism that is based on the principles of negative feedback control (chapter 3). They include baroreceptor reflexes, which support cardiac function and vasoconstriction, and renal fluid retention.

The cardiovascular system has pressure-sensitive receptors (**baroreceptors**) distributed throughout the body. Some are located in the arch of the aorta. A second concentration of baroreceptors called the **carotid sinus** is found near the division of the common carotid artery. From these sites baroreceptors send blood pressure-related information to the medulla oblongata, where integration for blood pressure regulation occurs. These medullary integrating centers are collectively described as the **cardiovascular center.** Output from this center elicits a pattern of responses that appropriately adjust blood pressure. Through control of heart rate, stroke volume, and arteriolar constriction, pressure is maintained at its set point (Fig. 11.8).

The cardiovascular reflexes function to adjust blood pressure during normal activities—for example, during exercise or when changing from a reclining to an upright posture. They are also available when circulatory shock develops, and can greatly reduce its threat. It has been estimated that these reflexes approximately double the volume of blood loss that can be tolerated before hypovolemic shock develops (fig. 11.6*b*).

In cases of extreme pressure reduction, to about half of normal levels, the cardiovascular center's neurons are directly affected by ischemia and the hypoxia it produces. In response, the cardiovascular center produces an intense outpouring of sympathetic stimulation in an emergency attempt to raise pressure and avoid serious anoxic damage. This is known as the **central nervous system ischemic response.**

There are other compensations that can counter the effects of shock. As blood pressure falls, the pressure balance across capillary walls between the blood and tissues is disturbed. Since the blood's hydrostatic pressure is the major factor in moving fluid into the tissue spaces, when BHP is reduced, less tissue fluid is formed. With less fluid leaving the vessels, BHP falls less rapidly. A lower BHP also promotes the drawing of more tissue fluid into the blood from the tissue spaces. The additional fluid raises plasma volume and supports systemic arterial pressure.

The kidney is also involved in shock compensation. Because of falling BHP and the compensating vasoconstriction that follows, blood flow to the kidney is reduced in shock. The kidney's response is based on the renin-angiotensin system. When it is activated, blood levels of angiotensin II are increased. This most potent of the endogenous vasoconstrictors supports the CNS reflexes that maintain blood pressure by vasoconstriction. In addition, angiotensin II stimulates aldosterone secretion by the adrenal cortex. This steroid hormone promotes renal sodium retention, which in turn results in more water retention by the kidney. Retention of water maintains plasma volume, with favorable effects on BHP (fig. 11.9). There is a more detailed explanation of the renin-angiotensin system in chapter 9.

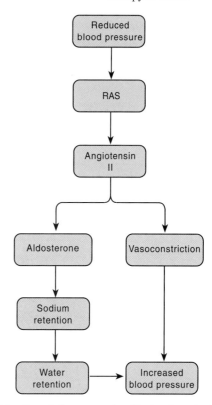

Figure 11.9   **Renal Compensation Mechanisms in Shock.** RAS: renin-angiotensin system.

THERAPY IN SHOCK

Therapeutic intervention in shock must first restore adequate levels of blood flow to dependent tissues. Then, attempts to eliminate the cause of shock and to cope with its secondary effects can be made. In hypovolemic shock, the lost blood volume must be replaced to restore pressure and blood flow. Whole blood, plasma, or plasma substitutes may be used in such cases.

Various drug therapies are also useful in shock. They are especially beneficial in correcting unfavorable vascular dilation states. For example, in neurogenic or vascular shock, where vasodilation is an underlying cause, a vasoconstrictor might be used. On the other hand, in cardiogenic shock, vasoconstriction reflexes may place an increased burden of afterload on a heart that is already experiencing difficulty in maintaining cardiac output. In such cases, administration of **isoproterenol** is of benefit because it increases heart rate and myocardial contractility while at the same time reducing afterload by inducing systemic vasodilation. The increases in cardiac output produced by the drug cause an elevation of blood pressure that outweighs any pressure reduction produced by the vasodilation. Alternatively, vasoconstrictors may be used to augment pressure if further flow reduction in dermal and splanchnic capillaries will not result in tissue damage. There are many drugs available and most have multiple sites of action; therefore, great care is taken in selecting and administering an appropriate vasoactive agent to avoid

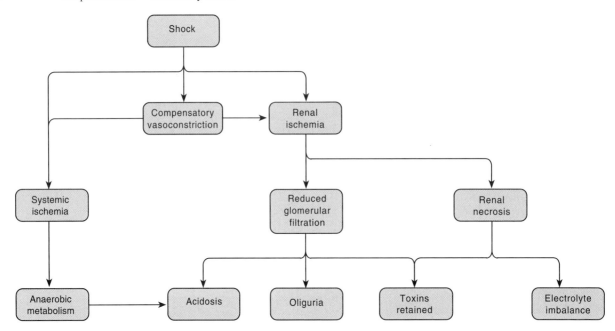

Figure 11.10   **Renal Failure in Circulatory Shock.** Once pressure falls, renal function is compromised with consequences that produce additional, potentially grave disruptions.

aggravating the situation instead of helping it. For the same reason, it is important to establish the cause of shock before a therapeutic course is selected.

Elimination of the cause of shock may be difficult in cardiogenic shock, because infarction is often extensive and because of the acute onset of the attack. In the case of cardiac tamponade, some surgical correction may be possible. Antibiotic therapy can sometimes eliminate the bacteria responsible for septic shock, but the time required for achieving adequate control is usually too long to save the situation. In general, hypovolemic shock has a better prognosis than does cardiogenic or septic shock because of the speed and relative ease with which fluid replacement therapy can be instituted. Apart from any neuronal or myocardial damage, the effects of shock are usually reversible once intervention restores blood pressure and tissue perfusion is stabilized.

SYSTEMIC EFFECTS OF SHOCK

As blood pressure falls, many organs suffer the effects of hypoperfusion. As the situation deteriorates, this may be aggravated by DIC, which can further compromise already reduced blood flow. There is a generalized muscular weakness and drop in body temperature as metabolism is slowed for lack of adequate supply of fuel molecules. Although reflexes tend to sustain brain flow, restlessness and confusion may indicate that the compensations are unable to fully cope.

Lung involvement is typical in shock because alveolar epithelia and underlying vessels are vulnerable, especially in septic and cardiogenic shock. When damaged lung capillaries become highly permeable, large volumes of fluid escape to accumulate in the pulmonary interstitium. Res-

piratory function is severely compromised as a result. This is the condition known as **adult respiratory distress syndrome,** which is more fully described in chapter 12. In the context of shock, the condition is called **shock lung.**

Anoxic damage to the kidney is also quite common in shock, causing acute renal failure as nephron losses mount. The result is a characteristic drop in urine output—oliguria. The damaged kidney also tends to retain substances it would normally excrete and to lose substances it would normally retain. This means that beyond the additional damage caused by retained toxins, many tissues will be disrupted by the kidneys' inability to maintain body fluid homeostasis. Acid retention is a particularly pressing problem in that systemic hypoxia causes many tissues to shift to anaerobic energy metabolism, which, unfortunately, generates additional acid products. Note that the usual compensation for such developing **acidosis** is increased exhalation of CO_2, which indirectly reduces acid levels. But in shock, the lung is itself damaged and is unable to help the situation (pH disturbances are discussed in chapter 16). Figure 11.10 summarizes the major renal effects that accompany severe shock.

Another site of hypoperfusion damage is the G-I tract, where mucosae are vulnerable to necrosis. Of course, the accompanying hemorrhage aggravates any preexisting hypovolemia. The liver and heart can also be damaged in shock. The liver's functions are so numerous that its failure has many serious consequences. The heart, if not initially involved, may suffer secondary damage, causing it to weaken and reduce its output. As you can see, the multi-organ damage seen in circulatory shock produces an expanding and interlocking set of problems that progresses from one level of dysfunction to another. This tendency to the progressive involvement of more and more organs is responsible for the high mortality associated with circulatory shock.

PROGRESSION IN SHOCK

Circulatory shock has the potential for progressing through three stages. The first is **nonprogressive shock,** in which a combination of physiological compensations and therapy may overcome the process and lead to recovery. The second stage is **progressive shock,** which is characterized by tissue hypoperfusion and organ damage. In the third stage, **irreversible shock,** organ and tissue damage is so severe that death is inevitable, even though aggressive therapy restores blood pressure.

The stages of circulatory shock lie on a continuum and the lines of demarcation between them may be difficult to distinguish in clinical situations. The three stages are described separately in the discussion that follows to better focus on the distinguishing characteristics of each.

Nonprogressive Shock

In **nonprogressive shock,** reflex compensatory mechanisms are activated and blood pressure and microcirculation flow are restored. As a result, tissues return to their normal functional status. If available, therapeutic intervention (e.g., fluid replacement) may contribute the restoration of blood pressure. In those tissues damaged by hypoxia, adequate flow is available to meet the demands of regeneration and repair. Secondary problems of acidosis, lung disruption, and renal disturbances are relieved by the restoration of blood flow and corrective therapy.

Progressive Shock

The situation in **progressive shock** is potentially much more serious. In this situation, microcirculation flow progressively declines because of the high degree of pressure loss, inadequate reflex compensation, or the lack of therapeutic intervention. The result is hypoxic cell injury to the vital organs. This leads to the initiation of positive feedback cycling, which increases the damage and decreases the likelihood of effective compensation.

Depression of cardiac function is an important feature of progressive shock and is due to a number of factors.

First, with falling blood pressure, the coronary circulation may be compromised, with the myocardium becoming ischemic, damaged, and weakened. This condition leads to a reduction of cardiac output, further declines in pressure, then further declines in myocardial perfusion, and so on. A second factor involves the cardiovascular center in the medulla. With hypoperfusion of the hypoxia-sensitive brain, cardiovascular center function may be depressed, causing reduced sympathetic stimulus to the heart and systemic arterioles. The result is a further fall in blood pressure, reduced brain perfusion, more hypoxia in the medulla, and continued positive feedback cycling. A third factor in progression occurs in the intestine. When hypoperfusion causes bowel damage, normally resident bacteria may escape to enter the circulation. As they are cleared from the circulation, endotoxin is released. This adds the additional dimension of septic shock to the already declining situation and contributes to the cycle of low blood pressure that reduces perfusion. Continuation of the positive feedback cycling causes rapid deterioration of an already serious situation (fig. 11.11).

Another major problem in progressive shock is peripheral pooling, which reduces venous return to the heart. There are a number of causes of this accumulation of blood in the peripheral veins. With a persistent cellular oxygen deficit, a shift to anaerobic metabolism produces a lactic acidosis, which affects arterioles. The chronic acidity interferes with their normal vasoconstriction responses and they dilate, allowing blood to accumulate in veins. Peripheral pooling is also favored by the reduced sympathetic nervous system output from the hypoxic cardiovascular center. Such input is a major factor in sustaining the vasoconstriction that normally promotes rapid blood flow.

Vasodilation and pooling may also result from functional deterioration of the vessels themselves. Compensatory constriction demands greatly exaggerate the vessels' workload at a time when their own nutritional needs are compromised by reduced blood flow. Fatigue may then limit the ability of vascular smooth muscle to maintain tension, with consequent vasodilation and pooling. As discussed previously, there are other factors that may contribute to vasodilation—for example, bacterial toxins in septic shock.

The combination of cardiac suppression and peripheral pooling produces a deteriorating pattern of diminished cardiac output, which is driven by the positive feedback cycling characteristic of progressive shock. The various contributing factors are summarized in figure 11.12.

Progressive shock may also develop from other causes, either cardiac or vascular. When blood flow rates decline, for whatever reason, risk of intravascular thrombosis is increased. Some bacterial endotoxins also stimulate thrombosis. In shock, DIC may develop, especially in septic shock as described earlier, causing further reduction in blood flow or even complete stasis. In addition, bacterial toxins or toxins released from necrotic tissues can damage capillary endothelia, greatly increasing their fluid permeability. Large-scale losses of fluid to the tissue spaces result, followed by

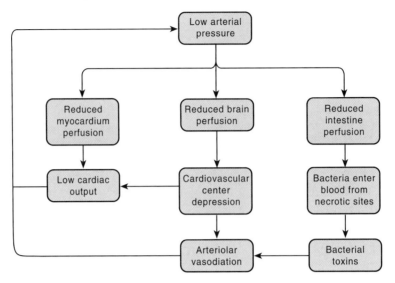

Figure 11.11   **Positive Feedback Cycling in Progressive Shock.**

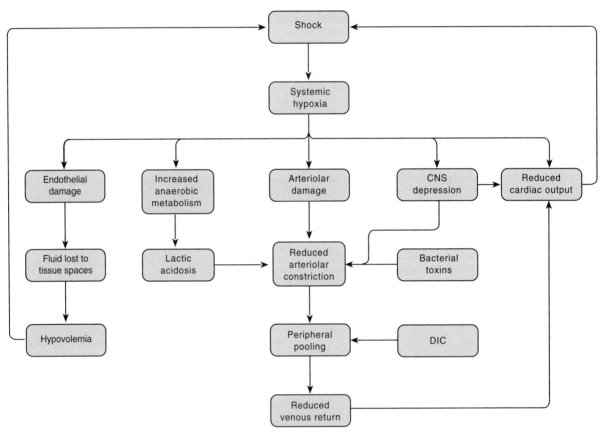

Figure 11.12   **Progressive Shock.** A summary of the essential derangements that characterize progressive shock. Note the characteristic positive feedback component.

great reductions in circulating plasma volume, venous return, cardiac output, blood pressure, and further downward spiraling of circulatory function.

Irreversible Shock

When shock is acute and severe, or when prolonged without therapeutic support, such positive feedback cycles may be impossible to interrupt. Unless therapeutic intervention is applied quickly and aggressively, the prognosis is poor. In fact, beyond a certain level of anoxic and toxic damage, even restoration of normal blood pressure by fluid replacement or other therapy cannot prevent the patient's death. This is the situation of **irreversible shock.** That a given shock victim is at the point of irreversible damage is impossible to determine. Therefore, therapy is always maintained vigorously until either shock progression is arrested or the patient dies (fig. 11.13).

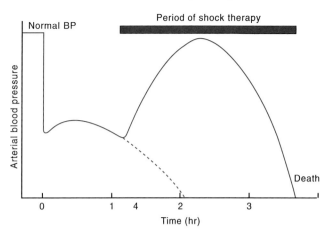

Figure 11.13 **Irreversible Shock.** The loss of arterial pressure causes damage from which recovery is ultimately impossible, even though therapy may temporarily restore BHP. The rise in pressure during the first hour is due to reflex compensations.

Case Study

A 66-year-old male arrived by ambulance at a hospital's emergency room on IV fluids and oxygen. He had collapsed at work after complaining of heartburn over a 30-minute period. His wife had accompanied the ambulance and was able to provide some medical history to the effect that although the man had been in generally good health, he had been experiencing heartburn and dull pains in his chest and left shoulder over the past few weeks.

On examination, the ER physicians found him to be confused and lethargic, with pale, cool, "clammy" skin. His pulse was "thready"—that is, rapid and weak—and his respiration rate was elevated. The ambulance crew's blood pressure report of "70/unrecordable" was verified in the ER. A tentative diagnosis of MI and cardiogenic shock was made.

IV lines and ECG monitoring were quickly established, after which the patient almost immediately lost consciousness, with the ECG indicating ventricular fibrillation.

Cardiac stimulant drugs and defibrillation were unable to reverse the arrythmia, and the patient died.

Commentary

In this all too typical case, cardiogenic shock due to MI quickly overwhelmed the victim before supportive therapy could reverse the process. The low arterial pressure noted in the ambulance had compromised cerebral flow to induce the patient's loss of consciousness. The pulse, respiration, and skin signs all testified to a marshalling of the sympathetic nervous system's reflexes in the face of rapidly declining arterial pressure.

At autopsy, a massive left ventricular infarct was found, as were coronary arteries showing evidence of severe atherosclerosis. Fibrillation in such cases is common, as the widespread destruction of cardiac tissue so disrupts conduction that effective, coordinated contraction is impossible.

Key Concepts

1. Circulatory shock is the result of the cardiovascular system's inability to maintain blood flow adequate to meet tissue requirements (p. 294).

2. Although specific etiologies are numerous, only three essential mechanisms of shock are involved: cardiac malfunction, which causes cardiogenic shock; inadequate blood volume, which causes hypovolemic shock; and widespread vasodilation, which causes vascular shock (p. 294).

3. In primary shock, a neurogenic mechanism produces both cardiac and vascular alterations that combine to produce a critical fall in arterial blood pressure (p. 294).

4. Primary shock may arise as a result of emotional trauma or some compromise of CNS function that interferes with normal output to the heart and arterioles (pp. 294–295).

5. Although myocardial infarction is the most common cause of cardiogenic shock, many other factors may contribute to the heart's inability to maintain adequate output (pp. 295–296).

6. Hypovolemic shock is produced by the direct and rapid loss of blood, or by various indirect means such as burns or kidney malfunction (pp. 297–298).

7. The widespread vasodilation that characterizes vascular shock may be triggered by bacterial endotoxins, by other chemical vasodilators, or by immune or neurogenic mechanisms (pp. 298–299).

8. Various physiological compensations are activated in the face of falling blood pressure (pp. 300–301).

9. Therapy in shock first addresses the problem of restoring adequate blood flow, then seeks to eliminate the cause of shock and deal with its secondary effects (pp. 301–302).

10. Progression in shock is based on positive feedback cycling in which the effects of hypoperfusion cause declines in pressure, more severe consequences, further pressure drops, and still more pronounced effects, etc. (pp. 303–304).

11. Progression in shock may be prevented by physiological compensations and therapy, but if cardiovascular structures malfunction because of ischemia, shock may progress to cause severe organ damage that may be fatal (pp. 303–305).

REVIEW ACTIVITIES

1. Using CS (cardiogenic shock), HS (hypovolemic shock), or VS (vascular shock), categorize each of the following specific shock types. Note that some types might fall into two categories.

Septic shock	Toxic shock	Neurogenic shock
Primary shock	Burn shock	Distributive shock
Anaphylactic shock		Hemorrhagic shock

2. Complete the following table by using ST (short term) or LT (long term) to indicate the time over which each of the cardiovascular compensations is likely to have an effect when BHP declines.

Increased heart rate

Increased myocardial contraction strength

Arteriolar constriction

CNS ischemic response

RAS-mediated water retention

Increased venous tone

3. Cover the legend in figure 11.11. Pick any starting point and from it, follow the process through successive steps. Once you start the sequence, can you stop? What kind of feedback is involved? Is it the same type that operates in the body's temperature regulation system, described in chapter 3? Is this relevant to progression in shock? Why?

4. In the case study, explain why the patient's heart rate was elevated and why his skin was pale and cool. Assess this case of shock in terms of progression: Was it progressive or nonprogressive, reversible or irreversible?

Respiratory Pathophysiology

Oft fetchying of the winde, declares a sicknesse of the lungus.

THOMAS WILSON
LOGIKE

rubor

et tumor

cū calore

et dolore

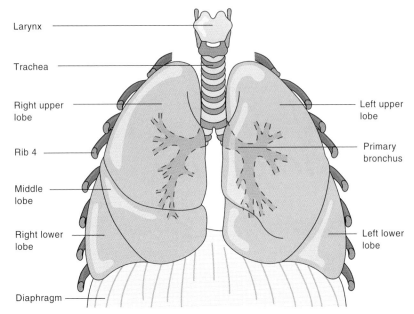

Figure 12.1   **The Lungs.** Note that the right lung has three lobes, while the left lung has two.

Disordered respiratory function can have serious and even lethal consequences. It also accounts for the usually less serious, but widespread, misery associated with the common cold and the numerous other minor respiratory infections that plague humankind. Before we consider respiratory pathophysiology, it will be helpful to review the normal structure and function of the respiratory system.

ANATOMY AND PHYSIOLOGY

The Lungs

The paired lungs occupy the pleural cavities, which lie within the larger thoracic cavity. Each lung has a superior extreme, the **apex,** which lies opposite its **base.** The concave base accommodates the superior thrust of the diaphragm on which it rests. The region of the lung's medial surface where blood vessels and bronchi enter the lung is called the **hilum** (or hilus). The cluster of blood vessels, lymphatic vessels, and bronchi entering at the hilum is the **root** of the lung. Each lung is separated into subdivisions, called **lobes,** by fissures that penetrate deep into the pulmonary mass. A single fissure in the left lung yields a superior and inferior lobe, while two fissures in the right lung give rise to superior, middle, and inferior lobes (fig. 12.1).

Associated with the lungs is a system of membranes called the pleural membranes, or **pleurae.** The pleurae are sheets of squamous epithelial cells that rest on a supporting bed of collagenous and elastic connective tissue. These are serous membranes, which secrete a watery fluid that coats their surfaces. They are arranged so that one part of the pleural membrane, the **visceral pleura,** covers the lungs' surfaces, while the other part, the **parietal pleura,** folds back to line the inner surface of the thoracic cavity. The

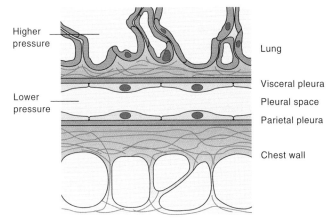

Figure 12.2   **The Pleurae.** The visceral pleura is adherent to the surface of the lung, while the parietal pleura is attached to the thoracic wall. The thin pleural space between them contains the pleural fluid. Pressure in the pleural space is lower than atmospheric pressure, allowing the lung to expand against the chest wall.

pleural fluid is found in the **pleural space** between the two pleurae (fig. 12.2). In this way, during respiration, the surfaces of lungs glide over a film of fluid as they move against the thoracic wall.

Pressure in the pleural space is lower than air pressure in the lungs' airways. This causes stretching of the lungs, expanding them to fill the pleural cavities. This expansion must overcome the lungs' tendency to remain in their smaller, unstretched state. Two factors contribute to this tendency. One is the presence of the lungs' elastic connective tissue, which resists being stretched. After it is stretched, it returns to its original length, much like a rubber balloon returns to its smaller size after its air escapes. The second factor is the surface tension that is present at the

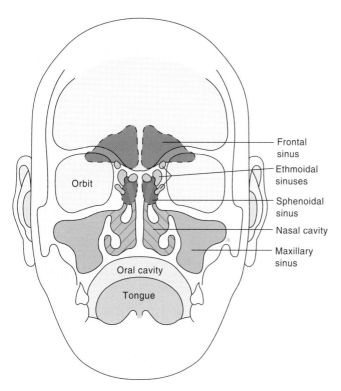

Figure 12.3   **Paranasal Sinuses.** The ethmoid sinuses consist of several small, interconnected air spaces that lie anterior to the sphenoid sinuses.

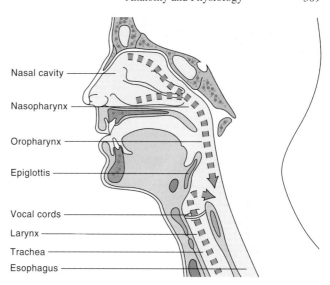

Figure 12.4   **The Nasal Cavity and Pharynx.** Mucus and trapped particles are swept from the airways by cilia to the oropharynx for swallowing.

inner alveolar surfaces. This is the result of the thin fluid layer that coats their surfaces. Alveolar surface tension is normally quite low because of the presence of **pulmonary surfactant.** This phospholipid is secreted by the specialized type II alveolar cells (see fig. 12.6). Both surface tension and the lungs' elasticity must be overcome to keep the lungs fully expanded against the thoracic wall. The same forces must be overcome to produce an inhalation.

Respiratory Airways

Air is delivered to the alveoli of each lung by the upper and lower respiratory passages, or airways. These communicate directly with the atmospheric air. Inhaled air first enters the upper respiratory passages: the nasal cavities and then the **pharynx.** Communicating with the nasal fossae are the **paranasal sinuses.** These are air spaces that protrude from each nasal cavity into the adjacent facial and cranial bones. They take their names from the bones in which they lie: the maxillary, sphenoidal, ethmoidal, and frontal sinuses (fig. 12.3). The pharynx is the muscular tube that is continuous with the nasal cavities, the mouth, and the lower respiratory passages, which consist of the larynx, the trachea, and the bronchi.

The **larynx** lies at the base of the pharynx. It is structured of several cartilage pieces that provide sufficient strength and rigidity to prevent its collapse. Positioned in the throat, the larynx is subjected to the twisting and folding that accompanies head movement. Without a rigid wall,

such movement could interfere with air flow through the larynx. The vocal cords are situated within the larynx. Their vibration produces the basic sound that is modified by the tongue, lips, and sinuses in voice production (fig. 12.4).

The **trachea** emerges at the inferior end of the larynx. It is a hollow tube formed of incomplete cartilage ring segments, some of which branch. These are stacked and held in place by fibrous and elastic connective tissues to yield a tubular structure with a characteristic segmented appearance (fig. 12.5). At about the midpoint of the mediastinum, the trachea divides to form the two **primary bronchi.** Each primary bronchus conducts air to a complex of smaller bronchi, which repeatedly branch within the lung to form the **bronchial tree.**

Like the trachea, the bronchi have walls containing cartilage segments that allow them to resist collapse. As their branching continues, many small **bronchioles** are formed, the largest of which have a diameter of about 1 mm. Bronchioles have no cartilage in their walls, but instead contain smooth muscle tissue. The elasticity of the adjacent lung tissues exerts a tension on their external surfaces that prevents their collapse.

The smallest bronchioles are called terminal bronchioles. They branch to form still finer ducts, which have periodic bulges where the wall becomes very thin. Pulmonary capillaries associate with these, and some exchange of carbon dioxide and oxygen occurs across the wall. For this reason, these airways are called **respiratory bronchioles.** From their smallest branches, air passes into **alveolar ducts,** which have a succession of thin-walled, alveoluslike bulges forming their walls. Each alveolar duct delivers air to a small number of **alveolar sacs.** These dead-end pouches form the termination of the respiratory passages. They are formed of many **alveoli** (singular: *alveolus*), which present the large surface across which the blood gases diffuse

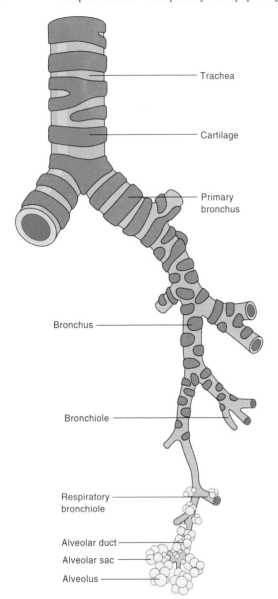

Figure 12.5 **Lower Respiratory Passages.** The bronchial tree branches to form the distal airways, where respiratory gas exchange occurs.

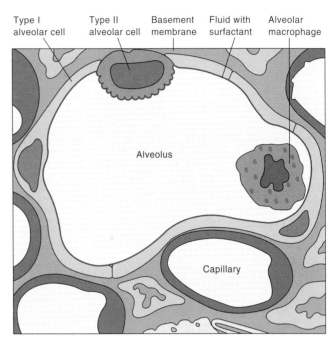

Figure 12.6   **The Respiratory Membrane.** The endothelium and basement membrane of the capillary lie adjacent to the epithelium of the alveolus, with only a thin layer of elastic lung tissue between them. Most alveolar cells are type I pneumocytes. The type II cell is the source of pulmonary surfactant. An alveolar macrophage is also shown.

(fig. 12.6). The lungs have an average of about 400 million alveoli, with a total surface area of about 75 m^2.

The term **acinus** is used to describe the functional unit of the lung. It consists of the airways and alveoli supplied by each terminal bronchiole: the respiratory bronchioles, alveolar ducts, and alveolar sacs. In normal lungs, three to five acini are supported by thin sheets of connective tissue. Each of these is known as a **lobule.**

Both the upper and lower respiratory passages are lined by mucous membrane. It consists of an epithelium supported by a layer of connective tissue, which in turn is limited by a thin layer of smooth muscle, the **muscularis mucosa.** In the bronchioles, this muscle layer can alter the airway's diameter by changing tension. The mucosal epithelium, with only few exceptions, is a protective pseudo-stratified type. It has cilia that project into the mucous layer present at its luminal surface. Mucus is secreted by the specialized goblet cells of the epithelium and by glands in the submucosa. These glands also secrete a serous fluid and so are called **seromucous glands.**

Respiratory Movements

At rest, air is moved into the lungs and then expelled. The approximately 500 ml of air moved in this way is called the **tidal volume.** Inhalation is achieved by contracting the inspiratory muscles—mainly the **diaphragm,** with a small contribution from the **internal intercostal muscles.** Their contraction produces a taller and wider thoracic cavity by lowering its floor (the diaphragm) and elevating the ribs. As the walls of the cavity expand to these positions, the adhesion of the pleurae causes the lungs to be drawn into an expanded configuration. Because pulmonary tissue is attached to the walls of the lungs' airways, expansion of the lung causes the airways to expand as well. The result is an increase in the total volume of the pulmonary airways. This in turn causes a drop in pressure within them. As pressure falls below atmospheric levels, air is pushed into the lungs. Relaxation of the inspiratory muscles and the recoil of the lungs' elastic tissues return thoracic dimensions to normal. This reduction of volume raises air pressure within the pulmonary airways, and air is forced from the lungs. Note that, at rest, exhalation is passive; that is, it requires no muscle contractions.

The usual rate of respiration is in the range of 10–18 breaths per minute. When increased **ventilation** (the total volume of air moving through the airways each minute) is required, both rate and depth of respiration are usually increased. These changes are the result of output from centers in the pons and medulla oblongata. In response, the respiratory muscles contract more often and more forcefully, producing a greater volume of air flow. To expel such increased volumes, active expiration is required, and the abdominal muscles are called upon. In tensing, they increase abdominal pressure, which causes the abdominal viscera to push the diaphragm past its rest position. The external intercostal muscles are also employed. As they contract, the ribs are depressed beyond their rest position. Both these movements further decrease thoracic volume to increase exhalation pressure. When lung disease makes breathing especially difficult, even the sternomastoids and those muscles that straighten the vertebral column are brought into use to increase the force of inspiration. To meet the high ventilation demand of vigorous exercise, energy expenditure to contract the respiratory muscles can approach 3% of the body's total output.

Oxygen and Carbon Dioxide Exchange

The respiratory system's principal contribution to overall somatic function is the exchange of carbon dioxide (CO_2) and oxygen (O_2) between the blood and atmospheric air. This exchange is accomplished in the lungs, where pulmonary capillaries are in intimate contact with the linings of the lung's terminal air spaces, the alveoli. Each alveolus has a wall, or septum, formed by a thin epithelial cell and its **basement membrane** (BM) (see fig. 12.6). The pulmonary capillary walls are formed of a thin endothelium, also with basement membrane on its tissue surface. Where the alveolar wall and capillary wall are in contact, their basement membranes merge to form a single layer. This arrangement provides only a thin (0.5 μm) layer of cytoplasm and basement membrane between capillary blood and alveolar air. This layer is the **respiratory membrane,** across which exchange of oxygen and carbon dioxide occurs.

The dominant cells of the alveolar wall are the **type I pneumocytes.** These cannot divide and if damaged are replaced by division of **type II pneumocytes.** In this way, the type II cells act as a reserve cell source, in addition to secreting pulmonary surfactant. Imbedded in the lungs' intercellular material is the connective tissue that produces the lungs' elasticity. Macrophages are also present, roaming over alveolar surfaces to take up particles that might interfere with normal respiratory function.

After returning to the right heart from the systemic circulation, blood is pumped to the lungs and reaches the pulmonary capillaries. These provide a large surface area that matches the large surface presented by the alveoli. Blood in the pulmonary vessels carries carbon dioxide produced by systemic cells as a by-product of their energy metabolism. It contains about 100 times the carbon dioxide of arterial blood.

In the blood, carbon dioxide is transported in three forms. About 25% is combined with hemoglobin (Hb) in erythrocytes; not with the heme group where oxygen binds, but with the protein portion of the molecule: globin. This means that carbon dioxide and oxygen do not compete for the same bond sites on the hemoglobin molecule; both carbon dioxide and oxygen are simultaneously carried by hemoglobin. About 65% of carbon dioxide is present in the form of bicarbonate ion (HCO_3^-) derived from carbonic acid (H_2CO_3). Carbonic acid is formed from water and carbon dioxide, which combine within the erythrocyte in a reaction catalyzed by the enzyme **carbonic anhydrase.** As the carbonic acid is formed, it dissociates to yield bicarbonate ion and hydrogen ion by the formula:

$$CO_2 + H_2O \rightleftharpoons H_2CO_3 \rightleftharpoons H^+ + HCO_3^-$$

This is the carbonic acid equilibrium. As carbon dioxide enters red blood cells from the systemic tissue spaces, the equilibrium shifts to the right to produce bicarbonate ion (fig. 12.7). As this ion accumulates, a concentration gradient is established between the red cell and the plasma. This gradient favors the diffusion of the bicarbonate ion into the plasma, where it remains until it reaches the pulmonary capillaries.

A small amount (about 10%) of the blood's carbon dioxide is carried as a gas, directly dissolved in the plasma's water. As a dissolved gas, it contributes to the total pressure exerted by all of the gas molecules dissolved in the plasma (others are nitrogen and oxygen). The portion of the total pressure contributed by the carbon dioxide is called the **partial pressure** of carbon dioxide. This is usually written PCO_2.

As carbon dioxide enters the blood in systemic capillaries, oxygen diffuses from the blood to the tissue spaces. Some of this oxygen was carried in the blood as a dissolved gas, producing a certain partial pressure of oxygen (PO_2). Only a small amount (1–2%) of all the blood's oxygen travels in this way, however. Most is carried in the erythrocyte, bound to the iron atom found in each of the four heme groups of hemoglobin. This combined form is **oxyhemoglobin** (HbO_2). The oxygen-hemoglobin equilibrium can be expressed as follows:

$$O_2 + Hb \rightleftharpoons HbO_2$$

(It should be understood that Hb is an abbreviation and not a chemical symbol.) In the tissues, cells consume oxygen and a lowered tissue PO_2 results. This change favors the diffusion of oxygen from the plasma and red blood cells into the tissues. As a result, red blood cell PO_2 falls, causing the hemoglobin equilibrium to shift to the left. This shift releases oxygen, making it available for diffusion to the tissues (fig. 12.7).

The relative partial pressures of carbon dioxide and oxygen between blood and air favor diffusion of oxygen into the blood and of carbon dioxide into the alveolar air. As a result, plasma PCO_2 falls, favoring the release of hemoglobin's carbon dioxide. Shifting of the carbonic acid

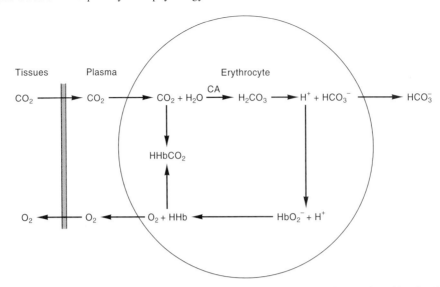

Figure 12.7   **Gas Exchange in Tissues.** Hydrogen ion is produced from the dissociation of carbonic acid. It is taken up by oxyhemoglobin, which promotes oxygen release. This frees the oxygen to diffuse into the tissues where it is needed. Note that hemoglobin also combines with carbon dioxide. CA: carbonic anhydrase.

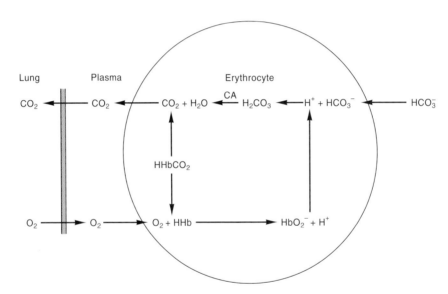

Figure 12.8   **Gas Exchange in the Lungs.** The delivery of CO_2 to the lung for excretion and the uptake of oxygen from the alveolus. CA: carbonic anhydrase.

equilibrium to the left is also favored by a lower PCO_2, so that additional CO_2 is formed, followed by its diffusion into the adjacent alveolus. Similarly, the arrival in the blood of newly diffused oxygen elevates the red blood cell's PO_2. This increase in PO_2 drives the hemoglobin equilibrium to the right, and oxyhemoglobin is formed. In this way, the blood is continually cleared of its carbon dioxide burden at the same time that it takes up needed oxygen (fig. 12.8).

Respiratory Defense Mechanisms

Because microorganisms and other particles are drawn into the airways with each inhalation, there is great potential for airway irritation and damage. We respond with an array of

defense mechanisms that resist the threat. These mechanisms also provide for adjusting the temperature and humidity of the air to which the delicate alveolar epithelium will be exposed.

The mucous membrane of the respiratory airways has a well-developed blood supply. This means that air, which is normally cooler than the lungs, and whose humidity may be quite low, is warmed and moisturized as blood heat and moisture pass to it from mucosal surfaces.

The mucous coating of the respiratory passages also plays an important role in preventing particles from reaching the distal airways. Inhaled particles pass over the mucous-covered surface and stick to it. The cilia of the pseudostratified epithelium beat rhythmically to move the

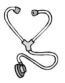

Focus on Mucosal Damage in Tracheostomy

The value of the warming and moisturizing of inhaled air can be appreciated in patients who have had a **tracheostomy.** In this procedure, an opening into the trachea is made to allow air to by-pass an obstruction that lies in the pharynx or larynx, above the site of the tracheostomy (box fig. 12.1). The procedure permits air to be drawn directly into the lower airways without the benefit of exposure to the moisturizing and warming mucosae of the upper respiratory passages. As a result, long-term tracheostomy patients have a much greater risk of damage to their bronchial mucosal surfaces and of subsequently developing chronic bronchitis (described later in this chapter in the Chronic Bronchitis section).

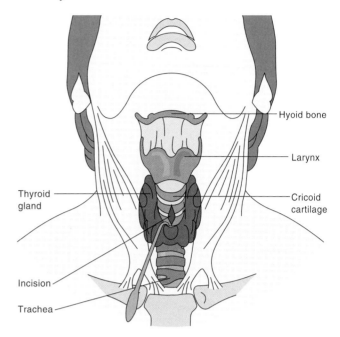

Box Figure 12.1 **Tracheostomy.** A tracheostomy involves an incision in the trachea that provides an alternative airway when an obstruction arises in the pharynx or larynx.

particle-laden **mucus blanket** down toward the oropharynx from the upper passages, and up toward the oropharynx from the lower passages (see fig. 12.4). At the pharynx, the mucus and particles are swallowed and broken down by gastric acid.

The branching pattern of the bronchial tree is another factor that contributes to the process of particle clearing. At each branch point, air flow becomes turbulent, increasing its contact with airway mucus. It has been estimated that inhaled air passes an average of 16 branchings of the airways before reaching the respiratory bronchioles.

Larger particles are initially trapped by the nasal hairs and upper respiratory surfaces, while medium-sized particles deposit on bronchial surfaces. These are cleared by the action of the epithelium's cilia. The smallest particles that reach the alveoli are cleared by macrophages. If the inhaled particles are bacteria, they are killed. If nonliving particles, they may be broken down or remain intact within the macrophage. Following phagocytosis of alveolar particles, the macrophages and the particles they carry may be picked up by the moving mucus blanket, or they may enter the lymph to be carried to the region's lymph nodes.

Macrophages, surfactant, and free particles are known to move from alveoli to the edges of the moving mucus blanket where they are easily picked up for clearance. The mechanisms underlying these movements are poorly understood, but surface tension and pressure gradients may be

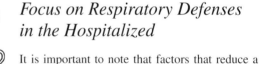

Focus on Respiratory Defenses in the Hospitalized

It is important to note that factors that reduce a patient's respiratory air flow may compromise particle clearance and predispose to infection. In many hospitalized people, restricted lung movement and ventilation may arise due to positioning, constricting bandages, central nervous system depression, or coma. The high rate of pneumonia in hospitalized patients is due, in large part, to impaired ventilation that leads to reduced clearance.

involved. Whatever the precise mechanisms, they are adversely affected by hypoventilation.

In addition to its function in particle clearance, the mucus blanket of the respiratory passages contains various secretions that have antibacterial (lysosome and lactoferrin) and antiviral functions (interferon). Complement (C') is present to augment anti-infection inflammatory responses. The immune system is also active in the lung, with pulmonary secretions containing specific antibodies against bacteria and viruses (fig. 12.9).

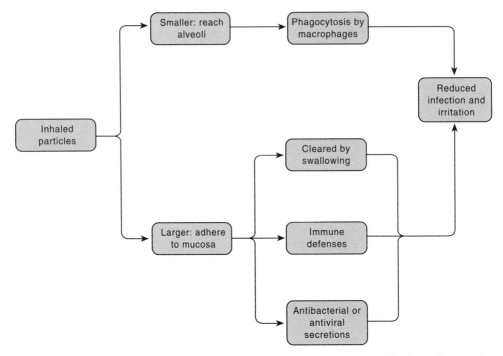

Figure 12.9   **Airway Defenses.** The defensive mechanisms that are arrayed against inhaled particles in respiratory airways.

RESPIRATORY DISEASE

Since the respiratory system provides for the exchange of carbon dioxide and oxygen between blood and air, it should be clear that respiratory function will be compro-mised by inadequate blood flow to the pulmonary capillar-ies (**hypoperfusion**) or inadequate air flow to the alveoli (**hypoventilation**).

The following sections consider how pulmonary em-bolism or heart failure can contribute to hypoperfusion of the lungs. Also discussed are the airway obstruction and the pulmonary or other disorders that limit normal lung ex-pansion, in the context of their ability to compromise ven-tilation (fig. 12.10).

Before turning to these major patterns of respiratory pathophysiology, it will be useful to consider the principal signs and symptoms associated with respiratory disease and various pulmonary function tests.

Signs and Symptoms

Cough

Cough is a common sign associated with respiratory disor-ders. This is a reflex response that attempts to clear the lower respiratory passages by the abrupt and forceful ex-pulsion of air. It is effective when particulate matter, such as food, accidentally enters the respiratory airways. It is most commonly found in lung disease when mucus or other fluids accumulate in the lower airways. Such accu-mulations may result from inflammation of the lung parenchyma or from increased secretion in response to mu-cosal irritation. Irritation might arise from the inhalation of irritants or from intrinsic sources of mucosal disruptions—for example, a tumor that invades a bronchial wall. Fluid may also accumulate as a result of excessive blood hydro-static pressure in the pulmonary capillaries. This causes pulmonary edema, with excess tissue fluid passing into the adjacent airways.

When cough is successful in raising fluid to the phar-ynx, from where it can be cleared by swallowing or **expec-toration** (spitting), it is described as **productive cough.** The fluid so produced is called **sputum.** Production of a

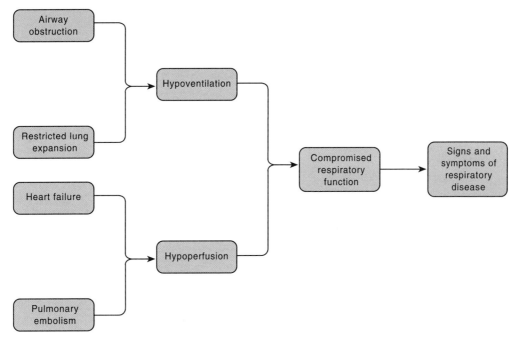

Figure 12.10 **Respiratory Insufficiency.** The essential disruptions that produce respiratory disease.

bloody sputum is called **hemoptysis.** It usually involves only small amounts of blood loss. Although the loss of blood in sputum is not threatening, it may indicate serious pulmonary disease. If sputum is purulent, an infection in the lung or airways is usually indicated. Cough that is not productive of sputum is called dry, **nonproductive,** or **hacking,** cough.

Dyspnea

A second common symptom of lung disease is **dyspnea.** This is the shortness of breath reported by patients who experience the need for greater respiratory effort at a given level of physical activity. It ranges from mild discomfort during exertion to extreme difficulty in breathing even at rest. In such cases, all the respiratory muscles may be required to exchange only the small tidal volume.

Dyspnea may result from airway obstruction. In such cases, greater force is necessary to produce adequate ventilation. The wheezing sound associated with many obstructive conditions is the result of air being forced through airways narrowed by constriction or fluid accumulation. Another common cause of dyspnea is the stiffness of pulmonary tissues present in many lung diseases. Such stiffness means that the lung's **compliance** is reduced. Compliance of the lung refers to the amount the lung tissues will expand in response to a given inspiratory effort. If, because of changes in the lung tissue, a normal inspiratory pressure produces a reduced lung expansion, then the lung is said to have decreased compliance.

Cyanosis

Cyanosis is a third sign of respiratory malfunction. It is the condition in which the blood contains large quantities of reduced (unoxygenated) hemoglobin. As a result, the blood has a dark red-blue color, which produces a characteristic bluish appearance in the skin. (The effect is masked in those with heavier skin pigmentation, but it may be visible in the whites of the eyes or mucous membranes, which are not pigmented.)

Most cyanosis arises because of peripheral vasoconstriction. The result is reduced flow, which allows hemoglobin to yield up more of its oxygen to the tissues, thus producing venous blood with a high level of reduced hemoglobin. This is called **peripheral cyanosis.**

Central cyanosis involves inadequate blood oxygenation, which can arise because of an abnormality of the respiratory membrane or from a mismatch between air flow and blood flow. This mismatch is described in terms of a change in the ventilation (V) to perfusion (Q) ratio. A larger V/Q ratio is produced, for example, in the case of pulmonary thromboembolism, where blood flow through a region of the lung is reduced. Various causes of hypoventilation, such as airway obstruction, will cause the V/Q ratio to decrease with the same result: inadequate blood oxygenation and clinically detectable central cyanosis when reduced hemoglobin levels reach 5 g/dl (fig. 12.11).

Pulmonary Function Tests

A variety of laboratory studies of pulmonary function are useful in diagnosing respiratory disorders, determining

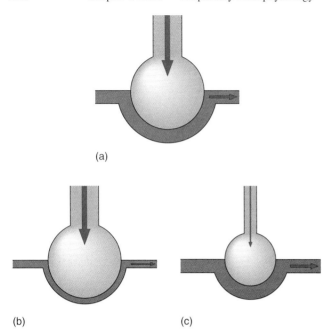

(a)

(b)   (c)

Figure 12.11   **Ventilation to Perfusion Ratio.** (*a*) Normal ventilation and perfusion of the lungs permits adequate gaseous exchange. Hypoxia is threatened if perfusion is impaired, increasing V/Q (*b*) or if ventilation is impaired and V/Q is lowered (*c*).

Table 12.1	Selected Pulmonary Function Tests and Their Application in the Assessment of Respiratory Function
Test	**Variables Measured**
Spirometry	One-second forced expiratory volume (FEV_1)
	Vital capacity
Diffusing capacity	CO uptake as an indication of respiratory membrane functioning
Arterial blood gases	Arterial PO_2, PCO_2, pH as indications of respiratory function
Lung elasticity (compliance)	Lungs' elastic properties, relevant in emphysema and restrictive disease
Lung volumes	Residual volume (RV) and total lung capacity (TLC) used as indicators of obstructive or restrictive disease

their severity, and monitoring the response to therapy. The most commonly used pulmonary function test employs **spirometry** to assess air flow versus time in a forced exhalation from maximally inflated lungs. This is a convenient method of assessing airway obstruction, indicated by a reduction in the volume of air exhaled during the first second of the test: **one-second forced expiratory volume** (FEV_1). The maximum exhaled volume is the **vital capacity** (VC). A low VC indicates airway obstruction or restricted lung expansion.

Tests of **diffusing capacity** use uptake of carbon monoxide (CO) to indicate the status of the respiratory membrane. In combination with other pulmonary function tests, diffusing capacity is applied to the diagnosis of interstitial fibrosis and in differentiating emphysema from chronic bronchitis and asthma.

Arterial blood gas studies provide information on blood levels of oxygenated carbon dioxide and of arterial blood pH. In particular, alterations in the V/Q will produce lower values of PO_2, while elevated arterial PCO_2 indicates reduced alveolar ventilation.

Less commonly employed are tests for **lung elasticity** (compliance) in assessing the lungs' ability to expand and recoil normally. **Lung volume** tests provide information on the ability of the respiratory system to ventilate the pulmonary airways normally. In particular, alterations in the **residual volume** (RV) and **total lung capacity** (TLC) are useful in the diagnosis of hypoventilation problems (fig. 12.12). The major pulmonary function tests are listed in table 12.1.

HYPOPERFUSION

The major factor that limits perfusion of pulmonary capillary beds is pulmonary hypertension, which can result from left heart failure, thromboembolism, or hypoventilation. These were described in earlier chapters, but will be briefly treated here in the context of their impact upon the V/Q and respiratory function.

Heart Failure

When the acutely or chronically failing left heart is unable to cope with its preload, pulmonary congestion and hypertension cause reduced blood flow as the higher pressure in the lungs' vessels offers increasing resistance to the right heart's pumping efforts. If pulmonary hypertension is chronic, progressive thickening of the media and intima may result, causing stenosis and reduced vascular elasticity. The increased mitosis caused by tissue growth factors released from pressure-damaged endothelia or activated platelets is thought to play a role in the medial hyperplasia that characterizes this condition. Of course, the narrowed vessels further increase pulmonary blood pressure to aggravate the existing hypertension, and a progressive deterioration that can lead to cor pulmonale (see chapter 10). In severe cases, vascular wall necrosis and pulmonary hemorrhage are present. Cardiac obstructions—for example, mitral stenosis—are typical causes of severe pulmonary hypertension. Of course, in the case of right heart

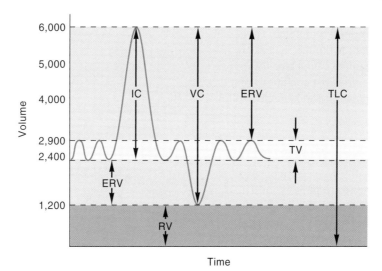

Figure 12.12   **Lung Volumes in Milliliters.** A subject, breathing into a respirometer, is asked to breathe normally, inhale as deeply as possible, and then exhale. After a normal breath, the subject is asked to exhale as much as possible and then breathe normally. TV: Tidal volume; exchanged during resting breathing. ERV: Expiratory reserve volume; exhaled below TV. RV: Residual volume; cannot be voluntarily exhaled. IRV: Inspiratory reserve volume; maximum inhalation above TV. IC: Inspiratory capacity after tidal volume exhalation. VC: Ventilatory capacity, the total volume voluntarily exchanged. TLC: Total lung capacity.

failure, reduced pulmonary blood flow is due to the inability of the heart to maintain an adequate output.

Thromboembolism

Whereas a failing heart may produce hypoperfusion of the lungs, if the pulmonary vessels are blocked first, heart failure may follow. When more than half of the lungs' vessels are occluded by thromboemboli, the resistance offered to the right heart becomes overwhelming and heart failure results.

Most thromboemboli arise in the deep veins of the calf or thigh. As they lodge in the pulmonary vessels, flow is blocked to a degree determined by their size and number. Pulmonary thromboembolism is typically accompanied by some degree of pulmonary hypertension. Two mechanisms are involved. One is the blocking of a vessel by the embolus, which causes higher pressures upstream from the occlusion. The second involves the release of vasoconstrictors from platelets that are activated when they contact and adhere to the surface of the embolus (fig. 12.13). Depending on the degree to which blood flow is reduced in pulmonary thromboembolism, an increased V/Q, as well as varying degrees of dyspnea, **tachypnea** (elevated respiratory rate), and PO_2 reduction may follow.

Infarction following pulmonary embolism is uncommon because of the presence of links between the pulmonary circulation's vessels and the bronchial arteries that supply the bronchial tree. Following pulmonary embolism, flow from the bronchial arteries to an area of ischemia is usually adequate to prevent infarction, although V/Q increases may still arise. Of course, when a thromboembolus is large enough to completely block the pulmonary trunk, all respiratory function ceases, brain oxygen is depleted, and death follows.

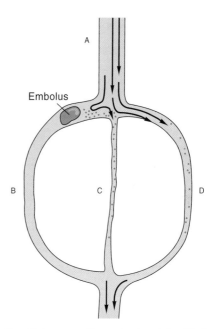

Figure 12.13   **Pulmonary Hypertension After Embolism.** Activated platelets at the surface of the embolus release constrictors that narrow vessels C and D. Congestion and hypertension in vessel A result. Reduced flow through B, C, and D produces a smaller V/Q.

Reduced Ventilation

In hypoventilation states, there is a reflex vasoconstriction response by the pulmonary arterioles. This is a useful response in normal circumstances, where regions of transient hypoventilation can be matched with regions of reduced flow. However, when ventilation is chronically reduced, the resulting vasoconstriction produces pulmonary hypertension, which offers an increased load to the right heart, producing pulmonary hypoperfusion to complicate the existing hypoventilation problem. The principal conditions that can give rise to reduced ventilation are the focus of the following sections.

HYPOVENTILATION

In addition to hypoperfusion, the second principal mechanism that commonly contributes to respiratory insufficiency is reduced air flow: hypoventilation. In this condition, a normal pulmonary blood flow is delivered to underventilated alveoli so that carbon dioxide can't be adequately cleared from the blood and not enough oxygen can enter it. This effect of a larger V/Q ratio is called **shunting,** because it produces the same effect that would result if blood were bypassing, or shunting, the lungs. As figure 12.10 indicates, pulmonary air flow may be reduced by factors that restrict normal lung expansion and by those that obstruct the airways. We will first consider the obstruction problems.

Obstructive Lung Disease

Upper respiratory inflammation produces increased mucus and serous fluid secretion by the mucous membranes that line the nasal fossae and pharynx. Usually this is in response to viral infection, but inhaled irritants are often involved. Although annoying, the excessive fluid at mucosal surfaces presents no threat. A more serious situation arises, however, when the virus or irritant gains access to the lower respiratory passages. In the larynx, trachea, and bronchial tree, excessive mucus and fluid can obstruct air flow. Acute inflammations of these respiratory passages (e.g., laryngitis and bronchitis) will usually resolve without significant functional loss. Coughing tends to clear excess secretions, and body defenses will usually cope with the damaging agent. Cough is especially important in unblocking these passages, because the infectious agent or irritant may interfere with the action of cilia and alveolar macrophages. The loss of clearing may also allow bacteria to become established. Bacterial infections usually develop secondary to viral infections in the lower respiratory passages. In addition to viral and bacterial infections, acute bronchitis may result from exposure to irritant fumes from solvents, acids, ammonia, or industrial pollutants.

Lung airway obstruction typically produces hypoventilation, essentially due to reduced expiration, which is indicated by smaller FEV_1 values. Outflow is restricted by reduced airway size, the presence of excessive secretions, or by a reduction of the lung's elastic recoil that reduces expiration pressure. The principal pulmonary obstructive conditions are asthma, emphysema, and chronic bronchitis.

Chronic Bronchitis

Chronic bronchitis is the most common chronic obstructive disease in the Western world, with peak incidence in males

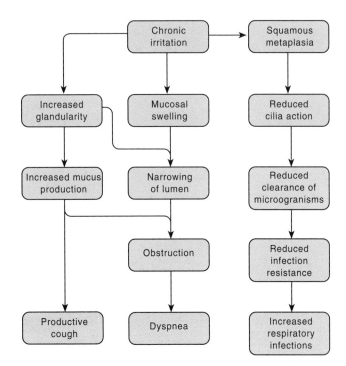

Figure 12.14 **Pathogenesis of Chronic Bronchitis.** Effects of chronic irritation on the bronchial mucous membrane in chronic bronchitis.

over the age of 45. To distinguish this condition from a recurrent acute inflammation, it is usually diagnosed on the basis of two consecutive years in which a productive cough is present for three months. The cough is an attempt to clear sputum formed in response to chronic irritation of the respiratory mucous membranes.

The dominant factor in the etiology of chronic bronchitis is cigarette smoking. Although exposure to air pollutants may produce some acute exacerbation of existing chronic bronchitis, even long-term inhalation of industrial pollutants does not seem to produce CB in nonsmokers. After ten or more years of heavy smoking, the characteristic pattern of productive cough, dyspnea, and increased respiratory infections becomes established. Sputum production can exceed 2 oz daily, with pus or blood present when infection develops.

Pathogenesis in chronic bronchitis reflects the mucous membranes' response to long-term irritant exposure (fig. 12.14). Inflammatory hyperemia and exudate cause thickening of the mucosa, as does hypertrophy and hyperplasia of its mucus-secreting glands (fig. 12.15).

Metaplasia of the bronchial epithelium also develops. The resulting loss of cilia favors mucus accumulation and reduced clearance of particles and microorganisms. This factor, coupled with increased mucus secretion that can plug smaller airways, contributes to an increased incidence of acute respiratory infections that complicate the underlying chronic bronchitis.

In advanced chronic bronchitis, hypoventilation produces hypoxemia and **hypercapnia** (CO_2 excess). These in turn trigger a pulmonary vasoconstriction reflex (described

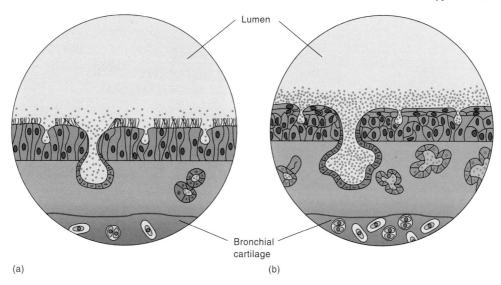

Figure 12.15   **Chronic Bronchitis.** (*a*) Normal respiratory mucous membrane. (*b*) The mucous membrane in chronic bronchitis. Note the increased number of glands and the inflammatory swelling in the submucosa, metaplasia and excessive mucus at the surface.

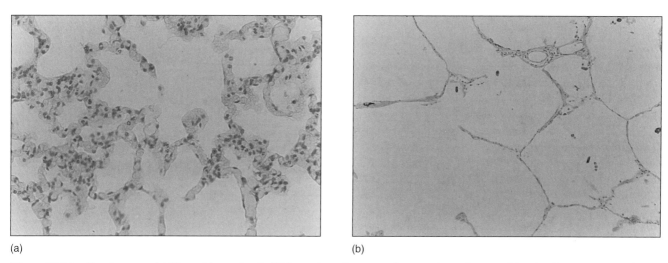

Figure 12.16   **Emphysema.** (*a*) Normal lung alveoli. (*b*) Loss of respiratory surface area in emphysema. The alveolar sacs are greatly enlarged and many septa have been lost.

earlier, in the thromboembolism section) that elevates pulmonary pressure to increase the right heart's workload. Chronic hypoxemia also increases renal secretion of erythropoietin (EPO), to which the marrow responds with increased red cell production—hence, the higher hematocrit values seen in chronic bronchitis. Unfortunately, this response is usually ineffective in that the obstructed airways prevent sufficient oxygen from reaching the alveoli, no matter how many red cells are there to receive it. An added complication is that the increased blood viscosity caused by high red cell numbers tends to produce more sluggish blood flow and a tendency to thrombosis.

Pulmonary Emphysema

Pulmonary emphysema is a lung disease characterized by abnormal enlargement of the lungs' airways, beyond the level of the terminal bronchioles. Enlargement is due to the destruction of alveolar septa. As septal damage progresses, adjacent, already distended airways merge to form even

☑ *Checkpoint 12.2*

As noted earlier, the common, upper respiratory viral inflammations aren't usually threatening—we suffer through them until our immune system catches up to clear the viruses. The situation may be very different in the case of young children, however. The small size of their upper airways means that inflammatory swelling can significantly reduce air flow and serious hypoventilation can result.

more extensively enlarged sacs, which contrast markedly with the precisely ordered structure of normal lung parenchyma (fig. 12.16). The term **bulla** is applied to air spaces that enlarge to diameters above 1 cm (fig. 12.17). Loss of alveolar septa means there is less surface area

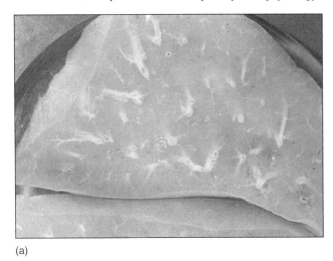

(a)

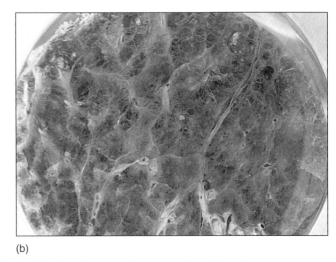

(b)

Figure 12.17   **Emphysema.** (*a*) A normal lung in section. (*b*) A similar section through an emphysematous lung. Note the numerous bullae.

The marked emphysema apparent in this lung was the reason that a 59-year-old man led the life of a "respiratory cripple" in his last years. Although this heavy smoker coughed little, he experienced years of progressively increasing dyspnea and falling FEV$_1$ values. The lungs were enlarged, obscuring the heart over the midline. At autopsy, lung damage was found to be severe, with numerous bullae, especially in the upper 75% of the lungs.

available for gas exchange. The septa also contain the elastic connective tissue that drives the lungs' recoil after an inhalation. In emphysema this is greatly reduced and exhalation is more difficult.

The obstructive effects of emphysema also follow from the loss of alveolar septa. The elastic connective tissue in the septa of air-filled alveoli applies tension to the walls of the smaller airways. This outward pull (called **lateral traction**) keeps the airways open during an exhalation, allowing adequate outflow of air. With the destruction of the alveolar walls, support for the small airways is lost and they collapse during exhalation, obstructing outflow (fig. 12.18).

Pathogenesis in emphysema is based on an exaggerated destruction of alveolar septa that is linked to a normal plasma constituent called **alpha$_1$-antitrypsin** (α_1-AT). It functions to antagonize the action of the enzyme **serine elastase,** which degrades elastic tissue in the walls of the alveoli. Serine elastase is released in the lung by PMNs and macrophages responding to injury caused by minor infections or inhaled irritants. Normally, alpha$_1$-antitrypsin reduces the damage caused by the elastase. This, combined with the production of replacement connective tissue, normally limits septal losses to low levels that are well tolerated. Estimates put normal septal losses at about 0.5% per year during adult life.

In most smokers, no acceleration of this process is seen, but in a smaller subset of the group, septal losses mount, so that declining FEV$_1$ values emerge after 10 or 20 years of smoking. The components of cigarette smoke affect the process in three ways: by (1) blocking the action of alpha$_1$-antitrypsin, (2) causing damage that draws more elastase-releasing phagocytes to the lungs, and (3) promoting excessive elastase release by phagocytes (fig. 12.19).

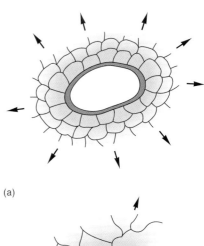

(a)

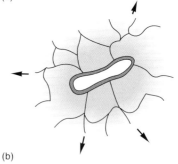

(b)

Figure 12.18   **Loss of Lateral Traction in Emphysema.**
(*a*) The normal arrangement of alveolar septa produces tension (arrows) that maintains airway dilation, particularly during exhalation. (*b*) Loss of septal elastic tissue allows the airways to collapse. See figure 12.16*b*.

Alpha$_1$-antitrypsin is also called α_1-proteinase inhibitor. This more general term is applied in the context of its role as one of the group of acute-phase reactants (see p. 43). Their levels in plasma are increased in conditions of acute inflammation, tumors, bacterial infections, and burns.

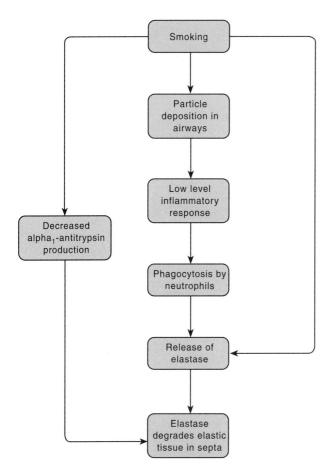

Figure 12.19   Pathogenesis of Emphysema. Although there are some cases caused by hereditary alpha$_1$-antitrypsin deficiency, most emphysema can be linked to the effects of smoking. Note that smoking not only activates the inflammatory response and promotes elastase release, which destroy the septa, but inhibits the response that protects them.

The classification of emphysema uses terminology that refers to the lung's acini or its lobules. When only the proximal respiratory bronchioles are involved, the terms **centriacinar** or **centrilobular** are used. When the emphysematous changes are distributed over both proximal and distal airways, the terms **panacinar** or **panlobular** are used (fig. 12.20). Note that these designations can be made only on the basis of surgically removed lung tissue, often related to lung cancer, or at autopsy. Although the terms are commonly encountered, the different emphysema types cannot be distinguished clinically.

Small Airway Disease

Nonrespiratory bronchioles with diameters less than 2 mm are also known to be damaged by tobacco smoke. They initially exhibit mild inflammatory changes that may induce some degree of fibrosis in the airway wall. Progression intensifies the changes, with obstruction of air flow developing from lumen reduction by fibrosis in the airway walls. Bronchiolar constriction responses to inflammatory media-

Focus on Emphysema in Nonsmokers

A severe panlobular emphysema can develop in people who have never smoked. This might seem puzzling until you consider that such individuals have a genetically determined lack of α_1-antitrypsin. They are unable to release it from the liver cells that produce it. As a result, normal elastase action is unopposed and septal losses progress until emphysema emerges.

---

tors might also play a role, as might the dilution of surfactant by inflammatory exudate. Although this condition is actually **bronchiolitis,** the term **small airway disease** has found wide acceptance. In the case of many smokers, the early effects of small airway disease are present, but since the small airways are so numerous, any early narrowing has little impact on FEV$_1$ values. Since at this early stage no other symptoms are present, smoking and its irritant effects usually continue. By the time full-blown chronic bronchitis and/or emphysema develops, falling FEV$_1$ values are attributed to the obstructive mechanisms previously described. It appears that small airway disease represents the early, and often unrecognized, beginning of the airway changes that progress to later, severe airway obstruction.

Even nonsmokers may develop small airway disease if chronically exposed to smoke-filled environments. Sensitive pulmonary function tests can identify small airway changes in those inhaling "secondhand smoke." There may be small consolation in being a nonsmoker if it is necessary to spend much time with smoking companions in smoke-filled environments. Consider, in particular, the risks to the children who are subjected to breathing the products of their parents' addiction.

Chronic Airway Obstruction

In many cases, the clinical picture of pulmonary obstruction presented by many patients does not allow a definitive diagnosis. Elements of chronic bronchitis and emphysema are often both present, and although difficult to accurately assess, it can be assumed that some degree of small airway involvement is also present. It is likely that a subsequent autopsy will confirm the degree to which each of these conditions may have contributed to the patient's respiratory difficulties. To deal with this situation, several terms have been proposed that recognize that both obstructive conditions may well be present and contributing to long-term airway obstruction. Two of these are **chronic obstructive lung disease** (COLD) and **chronic obstructive pulmonary disease** (COPD). Recently the term **chronic airway obstruction** (CAO) has become widely used, with a variation also proposed: **chronic airway limitation** (CAL). It

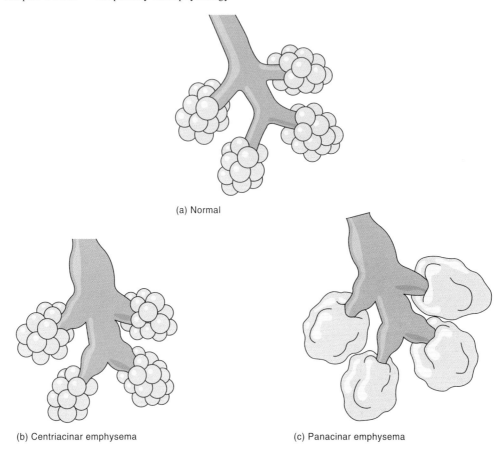

(a) Normal

(b) Centriacinar emphysema

(c) Panacinar emphysema

Figure 12.20   **Lung Changes in Emphysema.** (*a*) Distal airways in normal lung. (*b*) The more proximal, central airways are affected in centriacinar emphysema, while in panacinar emphysema (*c*), the more distal airways are primarily involved.

may be some time before the clear favorite emerges, so you should recognize that, essentially, they all describe the same condition.

A typical CAO patient initially presents with a degree of dyspnea and exercise intolerance that has finally prompted the seeking of medical attention. A history of heavy smoking and some degree of chronic cough and sputum production are usually reported. Slowly progressing exertional dyspnea is usually attributed to increasing age or lack of physical fitness to explain not seeking medical assistance. By the time that severe dyspnea develops, irreversible lung damage has likely produced progressive bouts of respiratory insufficiency and its complications.

The degree to which chronic bronchitis or emphysema is present in a given individual determines the emergence of signs and symptoms; so a wide range of clinical variability is characteristic of CAO. Common clinical usage recognizes two designations that characterize the CAO patient. In Type A, emphysema is dominant, and the typical sufferer is a male who breathes rapidly and with difficulty, pursing the lips in working to force expiration against collapsing airways. The Type A patient is usually thin and gaunt and often has an enlarged "barrel chest"; the result of hyperinflating the lungs to reduce airway collapse. In contrast, the Type B patient has a productive cough and the systemic edema that reflects his right heart failure. The

Table 12.2	Patterns of Clinical Presentation in CAO
Type A	**Type B**
Dyspnea	Productive cough; copious sputum
Exercise intolerance	Systemic edema
Expiratory wheezing	Superimposed respiratory infections
Near normal PO_2 and PCO_2	Hypoxia, hypercapnia
Normal hematocrit	Increased hematocrit (in response to hypoxia)
Mild pulmonary hypertension	Pulmonary hypertension
Lung hyperinflation	Right heart failure

combination of hypoventilation and heart failure produces a characteristic cyanosis. Type B patients exhibit little hyperventilation, even though their PCO_2 is elevated. This seems to be the fault of some defect of respiratory control, perhaps due to the system becoming desensitized to a chronically elevated PCO_2. Table 12.2 shows the key features

Focus on Prognosis for Smokers with CAO

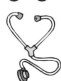

The FEV$_1$ of a 25-year-old nonsmoker decreases 25% by age 75. Those who start smoking at age 25 and develop CAO reach the same FEV$_1$ values at age 50. With continued smoking, progressive deterioration leads to the experience of breathlessness after only light exertion by age 55. By age 60, the typical CAO victim is breathless even at rest and can be expected to face respiratory failure and death before age 65.

In those who stop smoking, lost function cannot be restored, but the rate of FEV$_1$ decline returns to normal. Cessation of smoking at age 45 delays respiratory disability to age 75. Even stopping the use of cigarettes after the onset of respiratory disability can "buy" five additional years of life.

 ## Checkpoint 12.3

The Type A and Type B designations in CAO have some unfortunate, irreverent terminology associated with them. Because of their good oxygenation and pursed-lip breathing, Type A patients are described as "pink puffers." The characteristic cyanosis and blocky body type of the Type B patient attract the designation "blue bloater." These terms are widely established and usually used only among medical staff who are feeling whimsical, and never within earshot of patients or their families.

usually present in Types A and B. Note that many CAO patients will present a clinical picture that blends these two patterns.

Both Type A and Type B categories are based on a common history of heavy, long-term cigarette use that terminates in CAO. The reasons for the differing patterns of pulmonary damage that produce a Type A or Type B patient are ultimately determined by the smoker's genetic makeup.

The incidence of CAO is high, accounting annually for over 1,500,000 cases in North America. Its contribution to loss of working days is second only to that of heart disease. CAO also has an important effect on the sufferer's ability to cope with many everyday demands. Lack of tolerance for exertion is often so pronounced that sufferers can justifiably be described as respiratory cripples.

Therapy in CAO Since CAO causes irreversible destructive effects in lung tissues, therapy can only seek to avoid further damage and to cope with the respiratory consequences of the particular combination of chronic bronchitis

and emphysema found in a given patient. Cessation of smoking is paramount and can prevent further pulmonary damage and reduce cough and sputum production (see the Focus box "Prognosis for Smokers with CAO"). Greatest benefits are seen in earlier, less advanced cases. Beyond this, a regimen of therapy will typically involve oxygen therapy to cope with hypoxemia, and various combinations of pharmaceutical agents depending on a given patient's condition. Many benefits are derived from bronchodilator therapy, corticosteroids, antibiotics, and, when right heart failure develops, diuretics and vasodilators.

Bronchial Asthma

Asthma sufferers are subject to acute episodes of bronchial obstruction. For this reason, bronchial asthma may represent a component of a given patient's overall CAO problems. Although it is far less frequently involved than chronic bronchitis or emphysema, its potential contribution to CAO cannot be overlooked. Also note that many asthmatics have some degree of chronic bronchial obstruction on which acute attacks are superimposed. The significant feature of asthma that sets it apart from chronic bronchitis and emphysema is its reversibility. Following an attack of dyspnea, extended periods of essentially normal respiratory function are typical.

The major airway events in an acute asthma attack are bronchiolar constriction, mucus hypersecretion, and inflammatory swelling (fig. 12.21). These obstruct air flow, principally during expiration, to produce dyspnea, bouts of often severe cough, and a wheezing exhalation, the result of air forced through constricted, edematous, and mucus-filled airways. Attacks are usually of one to two hours' duration, but they may be more severe and continue for days and even weeks.

Two fundamental processes underlie the disturbances seen in asthma. One is based on an inappropriate immune response, while the other involves neural mechanisms. These are explored in the following sections.

Immune Mediation At work here is an immune hypersensitivity response mediated by antibodies (IgE) that form in response to airborne allergens (see chapter 5). Usually pollen, animal danders, household dusts, or insect excretions are involved. Once formed, the antibodies bind to airway mucosal surfaces, mast cells, and basophils. Subsequent exposure to the allergen produces a dramatic mast cell response (fig. 12.22). They degranulate explosively, releasing an array of chemical mediators that induce bronchospasm, pronounced mucus secretion, and increased capillary permeability. The IgE binding also affects autonomic neurons, which release acetylcholine to add to the bronchoconstriction problem. Table 12.3 lists various mediators known to be involved in extrinsic asthma. Their precise contributions have yet to be definitely determined. It is also significant that people with immune-mediated asthma often have a family history of the disorder.

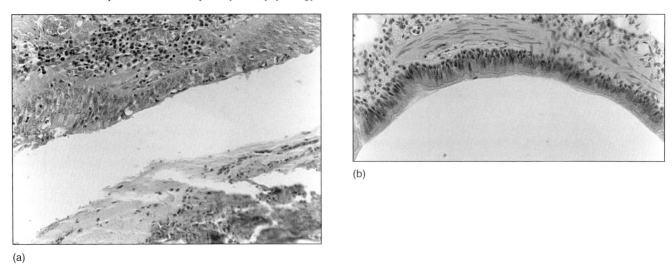

(a)

Figure 12.21 **Asthma.** (*a*) In this micrograph of a section through the airway of an asthmatic, the lower region is thick mucus containing epithelial debris and inflammatory cells. Note how the mucus narrows the lumen. Inflammatory cells can be seen crowding into the subepithelial regions of the bronchial wall in the top part of the micrograph. (*b*) Normal wall for comparison.

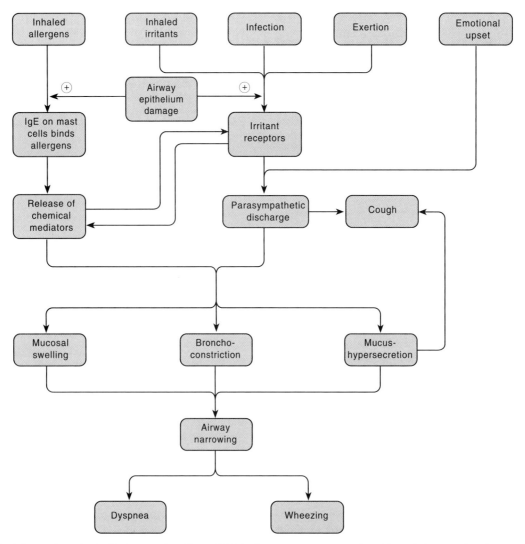

Figure 12.22 **Mechanisms in the Pathogenesis of Bronchial Asthma.** Note the enhancing effect of airway epithelium damage, which increases access to both irritant receptors and IgE.

Table 12.3	Mediators of the Extrinsic Asthma Response. As their precise roles are determined, therapeutic antagonism of these agents may prove beneficial.

Acetylcholine (Ach)
Bradykinin
Eosinophil chemotactic factor of anaphylaxis (ECFa)
Histamine
Interleukins
Leukotrienes
Neutrophil chemotactic factor (NCF)
Platelet-activating factor (PAF)
Prostaglandin D_2 (PGD$_2$)
Thromboxane (TxA$_2$)

Focus on Eosinophils in Asthma

In asthma, the role of the eosinophil, drawn to the site of mast cell degranulation by chemotactic agents, is beginning to be better understood. The eosinophil releases substances that promote further mast cell degranulation in a positive feedback loop. This may explain, in part, the rapidity with which the immune-mediated asthmatic attack develops. Eosinophils also release substances that are toxic to epithelium. These toxins may damage the respiratory epithelium, allowing inhaled allergens to trigger mast cell degranulation more easily.

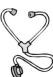

Focus on Some Cautions for Bronchodilator Use

Recent approaches to therapy have focused on the inflammatory component of asthma. The vascular leakiness that contributes to mucosal swelling and airway lumen reduction plays an important role in the asthmatic's reduced ventilation capacity. Bronchodilators and constriction antagonists bring relatively rapid results and so have been accepted widely, but there are some problems with their long-term use. Moreover, in spite of their extensive use, chronic asthma incidence and severity seem to be increasing.

It has been suggested that bronchoconstriction reflexes are a normal means of restricting irritant and antigen access to the lower airways. Therefore, long-term bronchodilator therapy may actually expose the lower airways to a greater irritant burden and more pronounced and chronic symptoms. By contrast, longer-term benefits have been identified in therapy based on inhalation of anti-inflammatory agents, especially corticosteroids and cromolyn sodium. By reducing mucosal edema, over the long term, these agents seem to promote a mucosal state better able to tolerate an acute asthma attack. On the basis of preliminary studies, side effects at therapeutic doses appear not to be significant.

Neural Mediation Bronchial asthma may arise without immune system involvement. In these cases, disordered autonomic control is the principal factor in producing muscle constriction, mucus hypersecretion, and increased vessel permeability. The mechanism responsible may be based on abnormal autonomic receptors in bronchial smooth muscle and mucus glands, or on hyperactive irritant receptors in airway mucous membranes. These receptors are sensitive to a variety of irritants that are commonly found at respiratory surfaces. For example, asthma attacks are known to be induced by air pollutants, a broad range of particles associated with occupational exposure, infections, and physical exertion. The high ventilation associated with exercise seems to affect the airway receptors by excessively cooling the mucosal surface.

Beyond these stimuli that seem to affect irritant receptors directly, various other factors are able to induce asthma attacks. For example, some individuals are particularly sensitive to therapeutic agents, in particular, aspirin, other NSAIDs, or the ACE-inhibitors used in hypertension and congestive heart failure. The underlying mechanism seems to be based on drug action that blocks formation of specific mediators to produce a therapeutic benefit, while at the same time favoring production of mediators that cause the asthma response (see fig. 2.15, which shows that NSAID's blocking of the cyclooxygenase pathway may favor the lipooxygenase pathway with increased formation of vasoconstrictors). A few asthma sufferers (only about 5%) react to the sulphite compounds that are widely used as food preservatives. In some people, emotional distress can precipitate an asthma attack, presumably via autonomic pathways that induce bronchoconstriction. Whether the stress-related stimulus is excessive or the airways are particularly sensitive to normal stimulation is not known.

Most asthmatics exhibit responses mediated by both immune and neural mechanisms. There are interactions between the two that might explain this. For example, some inflammatory mediators released by mast cells can affect airway irritant receptors. Conversely, stimulation of some autonomic airway receptors can trigger the release of mediators by mast cells. By such links, activation of one mechanism may trigger the other to produce the exaggerated responses that are seen in the acute asthma attack. An additional factor that contributes is damage to airway epithelium. Anything that disrupts its integrity may allow more intense stimulation of irritant receptors and provide easier access for allergens to mucosal mast cells (fig. 12.22).

For reasons that are unclear, 25–50% of children who suffer from asthma experience no symptoms after

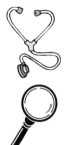

Focus on The Role of Ion Transport in CF

It appears that abnormal membrane transport of chloride and sodium ions produces a critical reduction of mucus water content, causing its high viscosity. Recently, the CF gene, which codes for a particular protein involved in ion transport, has been identified. This discovery opens the door to earlier, more reliable diagnosis, better insight into the underlying pathogenesis of CF, improved therapy, and a potential cure.

It may be possible to employ genetic engineering techniques to produce a functional CF gene. It could be introduced to the respiratory epithelium by linking the gene to the nucleic acid of a virus. Inhalation of the virus would allow it to enter the epithelial cells, delivering the needed genetic information. This approach may not be in place tomorrow, but it is a possibility for the future.

---

adolescence. This may reflect some increased stability in their autonomic or immune systems that accompanies maturity.

It is not difficult to appreciate how a given individual might confront more than one factor capable of inducing an asthma attack. A worker doing heavy labor in an environment of industrial fumes and a cigarette smoking co-worker might need to open containers of some allergenic substance to which the workers had been previously exposed and sensitized. An emotional component might be superimposed if one of the workers had just received a layoff notice. Furthermore, once an attack is under way, the emotional stress of not being able to ventilate adequately can aggravate the situation and introduce a vicious circle of positive feedback cycling.

Therapy for Asthma Therapy seeks to eliminate exposure to the allergen or other inhaled stimulant to interrupt induction of the response. Attempts to counter airway narrowing are based on bronchodilators and agents that oppose autonomic vasoconstriction. When infection is involved, or a threatened complication, appropriate antibiotics are used. A potential complication can arise from the prolonged inhalation of bronchodilators. These may have irritant effects on the airways and aggravate the problem. Where emotional upset is a factor, sedatives may be indicated. The patient's confidence in the attending medical personnel is also an important factor in reducing anxiety.

Status Asthmaticus This condition results when a prolonged and severe asthmatic attack does not respond to therapy. It may continue over days and even weeks, compromising ventilation to produce pronounced cyanosis. It is a life-threatening condition. Aggressive therapy often reverses the airway blockage, but several days may be required to fully restore ventilation.

In fatal asthma attacks, typical postmortem findings include hyperinflated lungs containing air trapped behind mucus-plugged airways that are narrowed by edema. The mucus is usually thick and often contains remnants of epithelium and inflammatory cells. Increased numbers of goblet cells in the epithelium and bronchial muscle hyperplasia are also characteristic and point to the persistence and severity of the condition.

Cystic Fibrosis (CF)

The disease cystic fibrosis is a systemic condition that involves defective exocrine secretions. Membrane transport abnormalities produce increased viscosity of the secretions of the pancreas, salivary glands, liver, intestine, and lungs. The involvement of the different organs is variable, but the lungs are affected in almost every case, with a particularly viscous mucus obstructing the airways. This viscous property of secretions in CF is the basis for its alternative, but much less frequently used, name, **mucoviscidosis.**

Cystic fibrosis is a genetic (autosomal recessive) disease most commonly arising in Caucasian children of normal parents. Although the parents are themselves normal, they are carriers who each transmit their single defective gene to their offspring. The disease emerges when a single individual receives two abnormal genes.

Sufferers experience an inability to clear the respiratory passages of accumulations of thickened mucus. Airway obstruction reduces ventilation, and inadequate mucus clearance gives rise to a pattern of recurrent respiratory infections that begin in childhood and continue throughout the victims' shortened lives. Repeated bouts of bronchitis and bronchopneumonia cause damage that is followed by fibrosis, causing further loss of respiratory function, pulmonary hypertension, and ultimately cor pulmonale. Many clinicians include cystic fibrosis as an element of chronic airway obstruction, while others regard it as a separate disease entity. Although there is no cure for this disease, therapeutic advances have reduced the respiratory disability of CF sufferers and extended their life span. However, survival beyond age 30 is unusual.

 ✔ Checkpoint 12.4

Let's just pause to reestablish our current position in the overall scheme of respiratory dysfunction. We first noted that respiratory problems arise as the result of a mismatch between blood flow and air flow. Then we saw that blood flow could be reduced by pulmonary emboli or a weakened heart that then affects the lungs. We've just explored the situations that can obstruct airways, causing hypoventilation. Now we turn to the other situation that involves hypoventilation: restrictive lung disease.

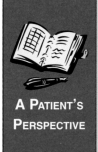

A PATIENT'S PERSPECTIVE

Bronchial Asthma

"This is your breathing . . . ,
if it stops, you stop."
—Patricia High

I've been asthmatic since my teens, but didn't really realize it. I wheezed all the time and had various allergies, so I didn't think much about the wheezing except that that's the way things are. When I had my first bad asthma attack, it was pretty scary. I was wheezing a lot more than normal and couldn't get my breath at all, so I panicked. They rushed me into the hospital and it was all new to me. They seemed to get it under control pretty fast, although I did have to stay in for quite a while. That's when they told me it was asthma, so then afterwards in other attacks, at least I knew what the chest tightness and shortness of breath was all about.

Knowing what I have also makes it easier to understand what the medication is all about. It took me some time to learn the right use of the medications and inhaler. At first I wasn't so well versed on it, and I realize now that I wasn't taking the medications properly because I didn't know how to recognize the signs when I was getting into trouble. I wasn't in control of the situation, but I am now. To begin with I was very out of control, and I feel safer now that I've been asthmatic for so long now and I know what my disease is and how my medications work. I'm tuned in to how I'll feel if the medications are wrong. I also have a peak flowmeter that is really useful to me. I really rely on it so that I can find out if I'm getting out of control.

Then too, going back a few years, my daily activity was pretty limited; I wasn't able to do anything without being out of breath. I'd be at home, sitting, being short of breath. I wouldn't even get dressed, thinking I'll take my medication and it's going to get better. But it didn't improve and then maybe a day or so later I'd be in the hospital. Now I'm able to do mobility exercises and I'm on an outpatient program where we have group maintenance. We monitor ourselves with our pulse and our exercises. We do mobility exercises and are supervised by a nurse. The important thing for me, even if I don't feel up to going, is the social aspect. It's like a family.

I can do some things, like go for a walk to the store, or the laundry (if my husband carries it down stairs) but I have to plan ahead and make sure I have my inhaler with me. With me I go day by day; that's my rule in life now. Lately there's been more good days than bad, so that's a positive and that's what I've got to look forward to.

It's still scary though. Fear is the most upsetting psychological part of asthma. I mean this is your breathing . . . , if it stops, you stop. And when it starts to get hard to breathe, you can't help wondering if this might be the time it gets to be more than you can deal with. That's scary. Then there's the pain because you can't breathe and you get a lot of muscle pain in the back and front. You also have to be able to identify when you have an infection. You do it yourself by checking your phlegm, so you have to know your own body—it's all part of getting educated about your condition. I'm feeling pretty good because I'm pretty much in control.

Restrictive Lung Disease

In this major category of pulmonary dysfunction, the essential problem is restricted expansion of the lungs (see fig. 12.10). Reduced lung expansion may be the result of changes in the **pulmonary interstitium**—that is, the lung tissue itself, as opposed to its airways. This condition can be described as **intrinsic restriction.** The other factors that limit lung expansion produce **extrinsic restriction.** These involve abnormalities in the system, external to the lungs, that generates the respiratory movements. In either case, sufferers exhibit a decreased total lung capacity as a result of their inability to expand the lungs fully.

Extrinsic Restriction

Normal ventilation not only requires unobstructed airways, but also depends on a normally structured and intact thoracic framework that is expanded by sufficiently strong muscular contractions triggered by an appropriate neural input from the brain stem. Derangements in any of these components can compromise ventilation (fig. 12.23).

Defective Thoracic Framework Congenital malformations or trauma can alter the thoracic skeleton and interfere with normal lung expansion. Deformities of the spinal column are **kyphosis,** an anterior displacement of the thoracic vertebrae causing "rounding" of the shoulders, and **scoliosis,** a pronounced lateral curvature of the spine. When both are present, the column is rotated and bent laterally: **kyphoscoliosis.** Most often, these conditions are idiopathic and produce a diminished vital capacity, reduced total lung capacity, and impaired ventilation. They are described more fully in chapter 18.

Trauma can damage the thoracic cage to compromise ventilation. Pain associated with bone fractures can significantly inhibit inspiration. In auto accidents, when an unrestrained driver is thrown against the steering wheel, rib fractures on both sides of the sternum may result. As a consequence, the anterior segment of the thoracic wall is

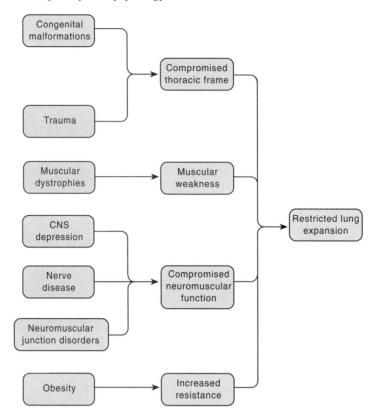

Figure 12.23   **Etiology in Extrinsic Restrictive Lung Disease.**

detached from its supports and floats freely on the chest's surface. On inspiration, the floating segment is drawn inward, and on expiration, it is pushed outward. (These movements are described as paradoxical respiration; see fig. 24.17.) The result is diminished chest expansion and reduced ventilation.

Respiratory Muscle Weakness This term covers several relatively rare conditions that have a genetic cause or are idiopathic. They are usually referred to as one or another type of **muscular dystrophy.** The weakened respiratory muscles are unable to generate sufficient chest expansion and diaphragm depression to sustain adequate ventilation. It is not unusual to have respiratory difficulties emerge as first indications of such an abnormality.

Neural and Neuromuscular Defects These problems may be the result of faulty output from the brain stem's respiratory control centers or of defects in the neural pathways from brain stem to respiratory muscles. At the neuromuscular junction, the neurotransmitter or receptor may be the focus of the problem.

Damage to the brain stem or CNS depression may result in an inadequate stimulus to the respiratory musculature. Direct brain stem injury or compression from increased intracranial pressure following cranial trauma or surgery may be involved. CNS depression may be caused by accidental or suicidal drug overdoses, excessive anesthesia, and, rarely, epileptic seizures.

Neural pathways from brain stem respiratory centers pass to the spinal cord, so injury in the high cervical region, where they leave the cord, can depress ventilation. Otherwise, various nerve disorders (neuropathies) may produce sufficient interference with conduction to compromise ventilation. In **poliomyelitis,** viral damage to the motor neurons that supply the respiratory muscles can be life-threatening. Motor neurons are also involved in **amyotrophic lateral sclerosis** (ALS), known as **Lou Gehrig's disease** after the famous baseball player who died from its effects. In this fatal disease, respiratory failure often develops in its later stages. In **Guillain-Barré syndrome,** acute respiratory failure is a common result of faulty stimulus to the respiratory muscles. Demyelination of the motor neurons causes faulty nerve conduction in this rare disease.

The neuromuscular junction, between the respiratory motor neurons and the respiratory muscles it supplies, is another potential site for the development of hypoventilation problems. In **botulism,** caused by the extremely potent toxin of a bacterium (*Clostridium botulinum*), respiratory failure from paralysis of the respiratory muscles is a common cause of death. The toxin blocks the release of acetylcholine (ACh) from motor nerve endings. Without the stimulation of ACh, respiratory muscles can't contract. The other side of the neuromuscular junction is involved in **myasthenia gravis.** In this disease, the ACh receptors are damaged by an autoimmune mechanism. A completely normal brain stem, conduction paths, and strong, intact muscles are present, but loss of the minute ACh receptors can sufficiently compromise ventilation to produce respiratory failure.

Increased Resistance to Expansion This problem may arise in extreme obesity. Excessive accumulations of thoracic wall fat, particularly in females with large breast fat deposits, can restrict thoracic expansion. Increased abdominal pressure from large masses of abdominal fat or accumulations of fluid (see ascites in chapter 14) may also offer resistance to depression of the diaphragm. If pronounced and prolonged, these resistance factors can exceed the ability of skeletal muscles to adapt by hypertrophy, and hypoventilation results.

Intrinsic Restriction

Various lung disorders produce alterations whose dominant effects are seen in the pulmonary interstitium. These disorders are grouped under the title **interstitial lung disease** (ILD). They involve the supporting connective tissue framework of the lung. This tissue consists of collagen and elastic fibers imbedded in extracellular ground substance, with small numbers of scattered fibroblasts, smooth muscle cells, and macrophages also present. The elasticity of the interstitium is a significant factor in the lung's expansibility and recoil in normal respiration.

In intrinsic restrictive lung disease, diffuse changes in the pulmonary interstitium produce stiffening of the lung and reduced compliance. This means that the lung's normal expansibility is affected, so that it takes more inspiratory effort to produce the same degree of expansion. Reduced lung compliance is the cause of the reduced total lung capacity (TLC) that is characteristic of intrinsic restrictive lung disease. Low compliance is also associated with increased recoil of the lung's interstitium. Greater recoil contributes to the expiratory drive in exhalation.

Dyspnea and a reduced tidal volume typically accompany intrinsic restrictive disease. **Tachypnea** (rapid and shallow breathing) is also present, as a compensation to maintain ventilation. The rapid breathing is especially pronounced during exertion, producing hyperventilation that exaggerates carbon dioxide clearance.

Cough is common in ILD and may be present without other signs of respiratory disease. It is typically nonproductive and may be the result of interstitial changes affecting airway irritant receptors. Productive cough is associated with more acute damage to the interstitium, where accumulating exudate and mucus may require clearance to avoid airway obstruction.

Restrictive lung disease typically arises in one of two forms. One is usually acute or subacute, and can quickly produce respiratory failure and death. It is characterized by pulmonary edema, which produces a pattern of signs and symptoms called **adult respiratory distress syndrome** (ARDS). The second form of restrictive disease in the lung involves long-term changes in the pulmonary interstitium.

This condition is called **chronic intrinsic restrictive lung disease** (CIRLD).

ARDS: Pulmonary Edema The acute development of the severe pulmonary edema that characterizes ARDS is the result of damage to pulmonary capillaries that causes them to become highly permeable. As a result, water, electrolytes, and protein pass from the blood to the pulmonary tissues. When the pulmonary capillaries are severely damaged, even erythrocytes may escape. As this protein-rich exudate forms, compliance is reduced. With increasing interstitial pressures, alveolar epithelia are damaged and the exudate is forced into the alveoli to further compromise respiratory function. The pattern of signs and symptoms produced by these changes is known as ARDS: adult respiratory distress syndrome. (The designation "adult" distinguishes this condition from the surfactant deficiency state that may arise in the newborn, see the section on NRDS later in this chapter.)

Onset of ARDS typically follows some injurious event, usually after a period varying from a few hours to two days in which no respiratory disorder is apparent. In some cases, early respiratory difficulties may be masked by other, nonrespiratory effects of the injury. Tachypnea, dyspnea, and cyanosis then emerge, with the threat of rapid progression to complete respiratory failure. Mortality in ARDS is high—generally, over 50%, and approaching 90% in the elderly. In those who survive, some degree of permanent respiratory dysfunction is usual.

Pathogenesis in ARDS involves intrinsic restriction from the presence of nondistensible fluid filling the interstitial spaces. The loss of compliance is complicated by the dilution or washing away of pulmonary surfactant by exudate passing to alveolar surfaces. The reduction in surfactant increases surface tension, which means that increased effort is required to achieve inspiration. Fluid in the interstitium also presents an obstacle to diffusion, so that oxygenation of the blood is also reduced. Carbon dioxide levels are less affected, since the higher water solubility of carbon dioxide means that more of it can be carried to the alveoli for exhalation, even though less oxygen is entering the blood.

The presence of fluid in the alveoli also leads to loss of respiratory surface and reduced airway volume. The result is a lowered V/Q ratio, causing shunting, which contributes to the cyanosis associated with ARDS. The situation is aggravated by a layer of hyaline membrane that can line the respiratory surfaces extending as far as the respiratory bronchioles. In addition to fibrin, hyaline membranes contain plasma proteins and cellular and basement membrane debris. If a severe ARDS attack is not fatal, it is often followed by fibrosis in the interstitium, which can lead to chronic loss of compliance (fig. 12.24).

ARDS can result from a broad array of injuries, all affecting the integrity of the pulmonary capillaries. In many cases, the cause of damage to capillary endothelia is unknown. Trauma, biological toxins from infectious agents, or inhaled irritants may be involved either directly

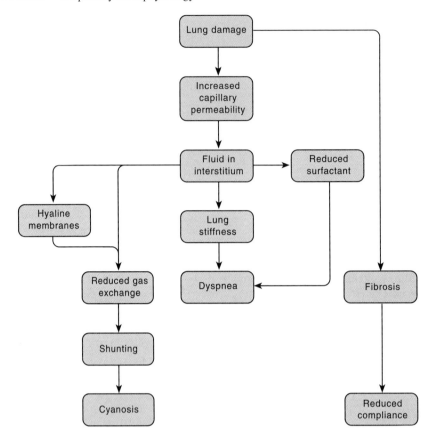

Figure 12.24   **Pathogenesis of ARDS.**

or indirectly, alone or in combination. A most common cause of ARDS is circulatory shock (see chapter 11). The characteristic pulmonary changes associated with ARDS in circulatory shock are collectively called **shock lung.** Trauma is also capable of producing ARDS, either directly, by effects at the thoracic wall that can bruise the underlying lung, or indirectly, via the central nervous system. In severe CNS injury, a pronounced vasoconstriction response greatly increases pulmonary blood pressures. This forces fluid into the pulmonary interstitium, causes capillary endothelial damage, and increases capillary permeability (fig. 12.25).

Infection may produce ARDS when severe. **Pneumonia** is a common example. This condition is an acute inflammation of the lung parenchyma that is normally reversible. Viral pneumonia is most common and most likely to produce ARDS. Bacterial pneumonia may follow an initial viral attack. Most bacterial pneumonia is caused by organisms of the genus *Pneumococcus,* although pneumonia resulting from many other bacteria is also common. (The rare but notorious **legionnaire's disease** involves ARDS that follows bacterial infection.) Pneumonia may also develop without infection. When gastric contents are inhaled, their acidity induces a pronounced inflammatory response that can produce ARDS. Usually such **aspiration pneumonia** is associated with the aspiration of vomitus while unconscious. For example, aspiration pneumonia may follow

general anesthesia or may occur during an alcoholic stupor. Mortality associated with aspiration pneumonia is high.

In disseminated intravascular coagulation (DIC—see chapter 7), multiple sites of microcirculation coagulation damage endothelia and increase permeability. At the same time, thrombi obstructing the capillaries produce increased BHP. This additional pressure adds to fluid losses through the more permeable capillaries to favor the development of ARDS. Near-drowning can also produce ARDS. In such cases, the exposure of the lungs to seawater or freshwater presumably causes damage via pronounced osmotic water movement.

Pulmonary capillary endothelium is also subject to damage from toxins or irritants that are inhaled or bloodborne. Inhalation of smoke, from fires as opposed to tobacco, or toxic fumes can induce ARDS, as can prolonged inhalation of therapeutically enriched oxygen mixtures. Oxygen toxicity is related to the production of oxygen-derived free radicals, which damage endothelia.

Blood-borne irritants may arrive at the lungs from an inflamed pancreas that is releasing its digestive enzymes. In fat embolism, pulmonary enzymes produce injurious degradation products from the breakdown of the emboli. Since fat emboli are usually numerous, lung capillary damage can be extensive. The blood may also bring additional fluid to the lung to produce pulmonary hypertension, apart from the problem of a failing left heart. If IV fluid administration

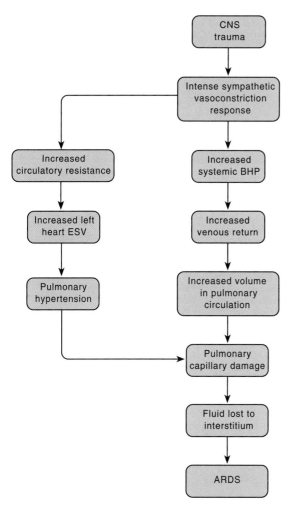

Figure 12.25 **CNS Trauma in the Etiology of ARDS.**

Focus on Some Aspects of Drowning

Although drowning fatalities are usually due to water in the lungs, 10–30% of drowning victims have a laryngospasm reflex that blocks water aspiration. In such cases, death is caused by asphyxiation. In near-drowning, aspiration of seawater (hypertonic to plasma) causes osmotic water flow from the plasma to the alveoli. The rapid loss of blood volume that follows poses the threat of hypovolemic shock. If freshwater (hypotonic to plasma) is aspirated, it moves by osmosis into the plasma and then into RBCs. The large water inflow can quickly produce widespread rupture of cells, releasing sufficient K^+ to cause cardiac arrhythmias.

leads to overloading of the pulmonary vasculature, damage from congestion and hypertension can occur. This is particularly dangerous in patients with renal damage and a reduced capacity for urinary water loss (diuresis). The etiology of ARDS is summarized in figure 12.26.

Although there are numerous etiological factors in ARDS, insights into the role of a common underlying mechanism are emerging. Although not insignificant, the initial capillary damage from whatever source would not, by itself, produce the clinical picture seen in ARDS. The problem lies in the inflammatory macrophages and PMNs that respond to the initial injury. These cells release mediators that draw more cells into the response. They then release free radicals and destructive enzymes. In some cases, especially infection, the complement system is activated. The result is a dramatic escalation of the damage to capillary and alveolar epithelium that allows the rapid loss of fluid and protein seen in ARDS.

Whatever the cause, treatment of ARDS requires immediate relief of hypoxemia, usually with oxygen inhalation therapy. Ventilation assistance is often provided by a mechanical ventilator that uses positive pressure to keep airways expanded and increase air flow. Attempts to reduce lung fluid loading by the use of diuretics may be effective, but only in the absence of heart failure that might compromise arterial BHP. Even with prompt and aggressive intervention, high mortality can be anticipated.

Chronic Intrinsic Restrictive Lung Disease (CIRLD)

This is the restrictive lung condition that involves long-term changes in the pulmonary interstitium, as opposed to the acutely developing problems of ARDS. In this condition, lung stiffness develops over a long period following initial damage. Because of the resulting infiltration of inflammatory and immune system cells, destruction of the interstitial tissues continues. Also released are chemical mediators that promote a fibrogenic response. Over time, collagen deposition by fibroblasts proceeds at the expense of the normal elastic tissues, causing a progressive loss of compliance.

A broad array of damaging agents can induce chronic restrictive changes in the lung. In most cases, the changes derive from low-level occupational exposure to the irritant over a long time. The irritants may be dust particles, industrial gases or airborne liquid droplets, drugs, or infectious agents. The usual occupational exposure involves irritant levels that are low enough to be tolerated so that work and inhalation continue. If levels are too high, acute effects become intolerable, thus preventing further exposure and long-term damage. Typically, low-level exposures of several months to two years or more are required before progressive cell infiltration and fibrosis produce clinical signs of impaired respiratory function. Because sufferers often adapt to their slowly deteriorating respiration, clinical presentation may well be delayed until significant damage has occurred.

Overall, infection and dust inhalation are the two principal categories in the etiology of CIRLD. A third, miscellaneous category serves as a catchall for the large number of its diverse and less common causes.

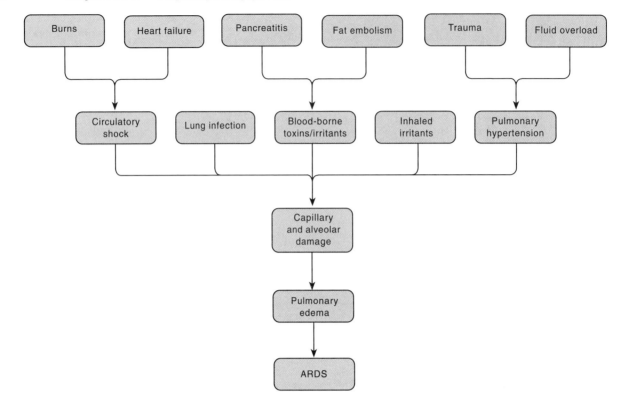

Figure 12.26   **Etiological Factors in ARDS.**

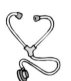

Focus on Oxygen Therapy and ARDS

Oxygen therapy for correction of hypoxia and cyanosis is indicated in ARDS. However, since extended inhalation therapy can itself damage the respiratory membrane, careful monitoring of patient responses is necessary. Prolonged inhalation of air with a 40% oxygen content is usually not harmful, but in ARDS, higher oxygen levels may be necessary to reestablish adequate arterial PO_2 values. The danger is a vicious circle of oxygen therapy to cope with lung damage, which causes further damage, necessitating more oxygen therapy.

Table 12.4	Selected Pneumoconioses and the Inhaled Agents That Are Implicated in Their Etiology

Disease	Agent
Asbestosis	Asbestos
Aspergillosis	Fungal spores of *Aspergillus* species
Berylliosis	Beryllium
Bird-breeder's lung	Ill-defined bird antigens
Coalworker's lung	Carbon dust
Farmer's lung	Molds in hay or grain
Silicosis	Silicon
Welder's lung	Iron oxide

Pneumoconioses These are conditions of chronic restrictive lung disease caused by inhalation of irritant dusts or droplets. Most involve prolonged occupational dust inhalation in mining or secondary industrial processing. Levels of dust inhalation gradually overwhelm the airways' clearance defenses, resulting in particle accumulation in the alveoli and interstitium. The pattern of damage and fibrosis that follows particle deposition varies with the physical, chemical, and antigenic properties of each type of dust, but all are characterized by inflammatory and/or immune cell infiltration, fibroblast proliferation, and fibrosis. Specific terminology is applied to describe a particular pneumoconiosis when the damaging dust component is known. For example, **asbestosis** is used when asbestos crystals are involved, and **silicosis** when the retained dust is sand, which consists of silica. Where the inhaled irritant is unknown, reference is typically made to the occupation in which exposure occurs (table 12.4). The most common pneumoconioses follow prolonged inhalation of coal dust, dusts containing silica or silicates, and dust that contains asbestos. Although specific differences in pathogenesis exist, there are broad similarities between advanced coalworker's pneumoconiosis, silicosis, and asbestosis.

Typically, early fibrosis develops at foci of particle deposition to form nodules of fibrous tissue. A more diffuse

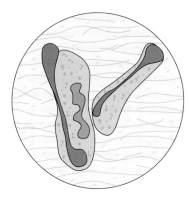

Figure 12.27   **Asbestosis.** In this microscopic field, two distinctively shaped asbestos bodies are represented by the club-shaped dark masses. The pale, surrounding structures are phagocytes attempting to engulf and degrade the asbestos bodies. Such efforts inevitably fail.

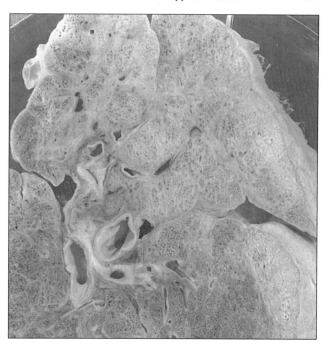

Figure 12.28   **Idiopathic Pulmonary Fibrosis.** Compare with the normal surface in figure 12.17a.
This is the lung of a heroin addict who died of respiratory failure at age 34. Pronounced pulmonary fibrosis can be seen throughout the specimen. Severe dyspnea and a productive cough had confined her to her home for the previous year. On admission to the hospital she looked old and emaciated, had markedly reduced ventilation, and a left pneumothorax. At autopsy, evidence of her addiction history was apparent in fibrotic arm veins damaged by excessive injection injury, suicidal scars at the wrists, and systemic foreign body granulomas and fibrosis, which were induced by the deposition of talc used by her heroin suppliers to dilute the drug.

fibrosis, lacking nodules, is characteristic of asbestosis, as is the presence of **asbestos bodies.** These are crystals coated with protein and iron, often club-shaped (fig. 12.27). As fibrosis continues, nodules may enlarge to reach several centimeters in diameter. This condition is called **progressive massive fibrosis.** It is a complication seen most often in silicosis and severe coalworkers' pneumoconiosis. Other, less common pneumoconioses may involve granulomatous inflammation in the lung. An example is **berylliosis,** which involves granuloma formation in response to retention of dust containing particles of the metal beryllium.

Pneumoconiosis is often asymptomatic for many years. With increased particle retention and fibrosis, dyspnea may develop progressively as lung compliance is reduced. Cough is also characteristic and may be productive or not, depending on the particle involved. Those suffering from pneumoconiosis are also at increased risk of respiratory infection because of the enormous demand placed on airway clearance mechanisms. Susceptibility to the effects of dust inhalation is widely variable, so that workers exposed to an identical particle burden may suffer significant debility on the one hand and be asymptomatic on the other. The differences may be explained, in part, on the basis of individual variations in the immune system's response to a particular retained particle. Smoking is a common additional risk factor.

Infection   CIRLD may follow infection, with fibrosis the response to the presence of the infectious agent, its products, or the products of tissue damage. Bacteria, viruses, and fungi have all been implicated in the etiology of CIRLD. Even the common and usually benign influenza virus may be a causative factor when it is followed by pneumonia. The organisms induce a chronic inflammatory response that may involve a diffuse or granulomatous pattern of cell infiltration and fibrosis. (See the Lung Infection section later in this chapter.)

Miscellaneous Etiologies   Some infectious agents, their spores, and a wide variety of inhaled organic dusts induce an allergic response in the lung. The result is a widespread cellular infiltration, with granuloma formation throughout followed by diffuse fibrosis. Such a condition is described as **hypersensitivity pneumonitis** or **extrinsic allergic alveolitis.** Many animal and plant antigens are known to induce this response. Exposure often occurs as the result of long-term, low-level inhalation of the antigen while doing farmwork.

Therapeutic agents may induce chronic fibrosis and lung restriction. Radiation and various antitumor drugs may damage normal lung tissues and trigger the progression to interstitial infiltration and fibrosis. Various other drugs are known to have similar capabilities in susceptible individuals.

Idiopathic Pulmonary Fibrosis (IPF)   This is a condition involving immune complex deposition with some evidence that an autoimmune mechanism is involved. If this explanation is validated, the condition may be renamed, but for now the term "idiopathic" is retained. Males from 30 to 50 years of age are predominantly affected by slow progression and loss of interstitium, with steadily worsening dyspnea and hypoxemia (fig. 12.28). Another idiopathic condition, **sarcoidosis,** involves widespread granuloma

Table 12.5	Principal Types of CIRLD, Based on Etiology

Drug-induced CIRLD
Hypersensitivity pneumonitis
Infectious and postinfectious CIRLD
Inhalation of irritant gases
Pneumoconiosis
Radiation pneumonia
Sarcoidosis*
Collagen vascular diseases*
Eosinophilic granulomas*

Asterisks indicate systemic disorders that may be associated with CIRLD.

formation, usually favoring the lungs. Interstitial fibrosis typically follows long-term granulomatous damage, complicated by lymphocyte and macrophage mediated interstitial damage.

In **Goodpasture's syndrome,** an autoimmune defect causes antibody formation against lung and kidney basement membranes. The result is a condition involving both a type of glomerulonephritis (see chapter 15) and a pattern of pulmonary damage causing interstitial hemorrhage and varying degrees of fibrosis. Although a serious complication, pulmonary dysfunction is usually overshadowed by more rapidly developing kidney failure. Goodpasture's syndrome predominates in young males and is a particular example of a more general category of disorder known as **diffuse pulmonary hemorrhage.** CIRLD etiologies are summarized in table 12.5.

Therapy in CIRLD Therapeutic options in cases of CIRLD are relatively limited because of the essentially nonreversible nature of its interstitial damage. Recall that alveolar epithelium can regenerate only if its basement membrane and adjacent extracellular matrix are intact. In most CIRLD, this is not the case and only scarring can replace the damaged tissue.

If an irritant is known to be inhaled or a therapeutic agent is suspected, stopping exposure is the first step. This is not possible where the agent is unknown, so treatment of such conditions as IPF or sarcoidosis is much more difficult. In some cases, steroidal anti-inflammatory agents, such as prednisone, can limit the damage caused by inflammatory cells. However, this treatment does not eliminate the underlying cause of the inflammation, and the ultimate interstitial losses are only delayed. Overall, there is much disagreement on the modes and actions of anti-inflammatory drugs for CIRLD.

LUNG INFECTION

Lung infections are a major cause of death in North America. The lungs' exposure to large volumes of inhaled air makes them vulnerable to potent, airborne infectious agents

that can overwhelm or elude defenses. This is particularly true in the elderly, whose airway defenses are less vigorous, and in those whose immune systems are suppressed. Immune suppression may arise as an indirect effect of tumor therapy, or may be therapeutically induced to prevent transplant rejection. In the case of AIDS, one infecting organism (HIV) suppresses the immune system, allowing other organisms to establish a secondary infection.

Bacterial infections, now much less common because of their susceptibility to antibiotics, typically cause an acute inflammatory response that is characterized by exudate formation centered in the alveoli. Subsequent infiltration by inflammatory cells produces a solidification of the affected area called **consolidation.** By contrast, viral damage draws inflammatory cells to the interstitium. In both cases, the pattern of acute inflammation is termed pneumonia, although **pneumonitis** is increasingly employed to describe the viral disease.

Two forms of pneumonia are worth noting. One is a type of bronchopneumonia caused by an obscure organism first studied as a result of an outbreak of severe respiratory symptoms at an American Legion convention in a major U.S. city. Some fatalities due to ARDS occurred. The organism has since been named *Legionella pneumophilia.* It seems to propagate in warm, standing water in air conditioning or heating systems, from which it periodically escapes to produce scattered outbreaks. Hospitals and nursing homes are particularly dangerous locations, as many occupants have compromised infection resistance.

The second pneumonia is caused by the protozoan *Pneumocystis carinii.* Usually this organism can't overcome normal resistance mechanisms. However, if the immune system is suppressed, the organism can become established in the lungs, with lethal consequences. Those most at risk are AIDS sufferers and transplant recipients whose immune system has been suppressed to reduce rejection of an implanted donor's organ. Various other agents may infect the lung. The most important of these are listed in table 12.6.

The terms **lobar pneumonia** and **bronchopneumonia** attempt to describe bacterial infections that are limited to a lung lobe or that originate in the bronchioles. Because there often is overlap and lack of a clear distinction, the terms have limited clinical relevance.

RESPIRATORY FAILURE

Given the lungs' primary function of oxygenating the blood and clearing it of carbon dioxide, the inability to perform these tasks constitutes respiratory failure. Whether it arises by an acute mechanism, as in pulmonary embolism or ARDS, or as the result of a long period of progressive hypoventilation from airway obstruction or restrictive disease, the inability to maintain adequate pulmonary function presents a serious threat. Dyspnea is virtually always present, but it may be difficult to identify the slight increases in breathing effort that indicate respiratory failure, since they

Table 12.6   Selected Organisms Implicated in Pneumonia

Bacteria

Escherichia coli
Group A beta-hemolytic streptococci
Hemophilus influenzae
Klebsiella pneumoniae
Pseudomonas species
Staphylococcus aureus
Streptococcus pneumoniae (pneumococcus)

Viruses

Adenovirus
Influenza virus
Measles virus
Varicella

Rickettsiae

Coxiella burnetii

Mycobacteria

Mycobacteria tuberculosis

Chlamydia

Chlamydiae psittaci

---

are often superimposed on the chronic dyspnea that is present in various respiratory disorders. Since nervous tissue is highly oxygen-dependent, CNS signs and symptoms will also emerge in respiratory failure. Memory loss, visual impairment, and drowsiness are typical. Headache may be present as a result of the increased intracranial pressure that follows cerebral vasodilation in response to hypoxemia.

Two principal patterns are recognized, one in which arterial hypoxemia is the dominant feature and one in which arterial hypoxemia is accompanied by hypercapnia (elevated carbon dioxide).

Hypoxic Respiratory Failure

This condition is present when PO_2 falls to, or below, 60 mm Hg. It is typically seen in chronic bronchitis and emphysema, in lung consolidation due to bacterial infection, in lung collapse (see the Atelectasis and Pneumothorax sections later in this chapter), or in pulmonary hypertension. High V/Q values due to intracardiac right-to-left shunting or pulmonary embolism are also able to lower PO_2 critically. This is also a result in ARDS.

Initially, hypoxemia produces headache and nervous agitation, which is soon followed by a decline in mental activity and by confusion. With progressive lowering of PO_2 values, more widespread tissue damage and loss of consciousness can be expected. In the event of brain stem hy-

poxia, CNS output to the heart and systemic arterioles can produce circulatory shock. Hypoxic renal damage, and the loss of homeostatic balance and waste accumulation that follow, complicate the problem.

Hypoxic-Hypercapnic Respiratory Failure

When arterial PCO_2, normally at 40 mm Hg, exceeds 45 mm Hg, the condition is described as hypercapnia. Most often, obstructive conditions produce this form of respiratory failure, as may hypoventilation from CNS, thoracic cage, or neuromuscular abnormalities. Attempts to compensate include an increased heart rate and vasodilation, which produce a warm, moist skin. CNS effects produce muscular tremors, drowsiness, and, at extremes, coma. Hypercapnia also produces an acidosis in the body fluids via the plasma bicarbonate equilibrium.

The pathogenesis of respiratory failure is presented in figure 12.29. The acid-base imbalances related to respiratory failure are considered in chapter 16.

MISCELLANEOUS PULMONARY CONDITIONS

Atelectasis

Atelectasis is the collapse of a portion of the lung. It is usually associated with bronchial obstruction. Following airway blockage, over a period of several hours, the air in alveolar sacs is absorbed into the blood. If the obstructed airway prevents new air from replacing the absorbed air, pressure in the isolated area drops and the affected region collapses (fig. 12.30). If the affected region is small, the collapse will probably be asymptomatic, but if large, the perfusing blood neither receives oxygen nor loses carbon dioxide. The various obstructive diseases of the lung may all produce atelectasis, as may aspiration of a foreign body that lodges in a bronchus.

Obstruction may also stem from a tumor's growth within an airway, or by a tumor or other factors compressing the airway from without. The latter condition is called **compression atelectasis.** A very common form of atelectasis follows surgery. **Postsurgical atelectasis** seems to result from anesthesia effects, which cause obstruction by increasing mucus secretion. Atelectasis is also often associated with ARDS. It is assumed that whatever factor produces the altered capillary permeability also, in some way, depresses surfactant production or release. The resulting increase of surface tension causes collapse of the small terminal airways, the condition known as **microatelectasis.**

Bronchiectasis

In **bronchiectasis,** the medium- to small-sized bronchi are abnormally dilated because of contracture in the scar tissue that replaces damaged muscle and connective tissue in their

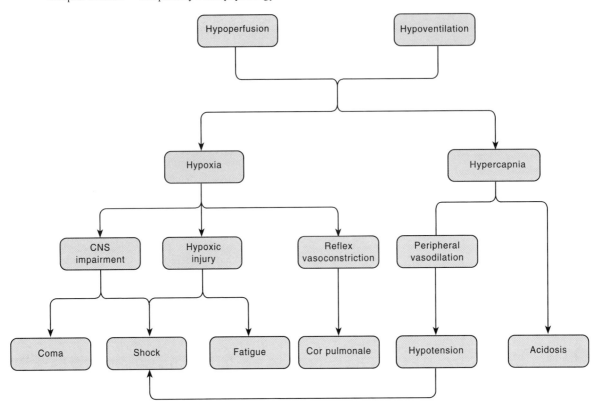

Figure 12.29   **Respiratory Failure.** Lack of oxygen and carbon dioxide retention can produce serious consequences.

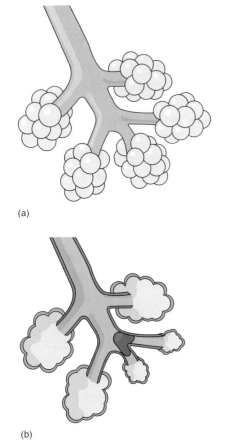

(a)

(b)

Figure 12.30   **Atelectasis.** In this case, an aspirated object has obstructed an airway. Air trapped beyond the blockage has been absorbed by the blood, causing the isolated region to collapse.

walls (fig. 12.31). In some cases, the cause is congenital, but in most cases, damage is secondary to necrosis associated with recurrent infection. After damage, the respiratory epithelium is lost or replaced by a stratified squamous epithelium. The dilated bronchi are unable to clear secretions, so obstruction and cough result. The inability to clear secretions also predisposes to further infection, purulent sputum, and further bronchial damage. Hemoptysis is a common sign in bronchiectasis. It is probably the result of damage associated with the severe paroxysms of coughing that may accompany this disorder. Production of sputum is quite pronounced in bronchiectasis and may exceed 500 ml per day.

Pneumothorax

In **pneumothorax,** collapse of the lung follows the entrance of atmospheric air into the pleural space. The air removes the normal pressure gradient that provides for the expansion of the lungs against the thoracic wall. As a result, the elastic recoil of the lung draws it into a collapsed configuration.

Pneumothorax may result from trauma, as when a fractured rib, sharp object, or bullet lacerates the parietal pleura, or it may occur secondary to thoracic surgery (fig. 12.32). Most commonly, it occurs accidentally, as a result of a medical procedure such as aspiration (suction) of fluid from the pleural space (see pleural effusion in the following section) or a lung biopsy. Pneumothorax is also associated with emphysema when enlarging bullae form near the surface of the lung. With destruction of lung surface tis-

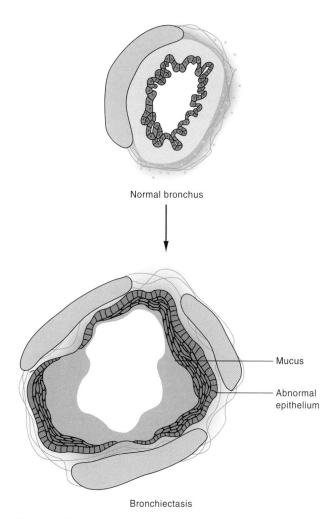

Normal bronchus

Mucus

Abnormal
epithelium

Bronchiectasis

Figure 12.31 **Bronchiectasis.** Abnormal dilation of small airways is accompanied by replacement of normal epithelium by a stratified squamous epithelium. Excessive secretions, which cannot be cleared by compromised clearance mechanisms, accumulate to cause airway obstruction.

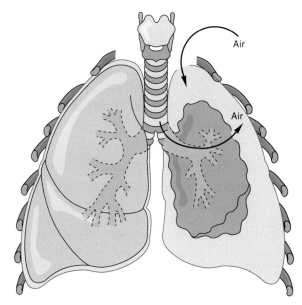

Air

Air

Figure 12.32 **Pneumothorax.** The lung collapses as air enters the pleural cavity. The combination of lung elasticity and surface tension causes the collapse when pleural and airway pressures equalize. The arrows indicate two access routes to the pleural space, from within the lung and through the thoracic wall.

tion is called **tension pneumothorax.** It is a serious condition requiring prompt intervention, since compression of the opposite lung that is caused by the shifted mediastinal structures can compromise the only remaining source of respiratory function. Tension pneumothorax is considered in more detail in the context of thoracic trauma in chapter 24.

Pleurisy

Pleurisy is the same as **pleuritis**—that is, inflammation of the pleurae. Like pneumothorax, pleurisy is not a disease in itself but is the result of some other abnormality. Usually this is an infection in the adjacent lung parenchyma, but thoracic trauma or an invading tumor might also be at fault. In some cases, inflammatory exudate is minimal, so the description **dry pleurisy** is used. More typically, significant exudate accumulates between the pleurae. This is termed **pleural effusion.**

The presence of a substantial effusion may produce sufficient pressure on the adjacent lung tissue to cause compression atelectasis. It may also restrict lung movements in respiration, causing dyspnea and outright pain, especially on coughing. The underlying mechanism involves the parietal pleura, which is particularly pain sensitive. Pressure waves generated by coughing and transmitted through the pleural exudate to the parietal pleura. The accumulated fluid may be reabsorbed as the underlying cause subsides, as in the case of infection. In other cases, as in tumor invasion of the pleurae, excess fluid may be therapeutically drawn off by aspiration. If the pleural effusion contains pus, the condition is **pleural empyema;** the presence of blood in the pleural space is called **hemothorax.**

sue, the visceral pleura may be the only barrier separating the pleural space and the atmospheric air in the airways. With rupture of the visceral pleura, air enters the pleural space and lung collapse follows. Pneumothorax is also common in interstitial lung disease. Tumor invasion might penetrate the visceral pleura to produce pneumothorax. In some cases, especially in males 20–40 years of age, pneumothorax occurs without a known cause. This is **spontaneous pneumothorax.** It may result from rupture at the lung's apical surface. This is usually due to undiscovered lung disease, or because of some partial airway obstruction that produces terminal airway hyperinflation.

In pneumothorax, the defect that allows air to enter the pleural space usually closes as the lung collapses. With subsequent healing of the defect, the lung reexpands. In some cases, however, the atmospheric air in the pleural space does not rapidly reabsorb. The result is an additional volume of thoracic air at atmospheric pressure that shifts the mediastinal organs to the lower pressure side. This condi-

Neonatal Respiratory Distress Syndrome

Neonatal respiratory distress syndrome (NRDS), also known as **respiratory disease of the newborn** (RDN), is seen in a significant number of infants who are premature, whether by spontaneous delivery or by cesarean section. Also, full-term infants of diabetic mothers are at greater risk of NRDS. Affected infants suffer from extreme dyspnea that develops with first breathing, or normal respiration may occur for several hours before the onset of the dyspnea. Breathing difficulty is the result of a lack of pulmonary surfactant. It appears that a critical mark of the lung's maturity is its production of pulmonary surfactant. If the child is delivered before this maturity is achieved, alveolar surface tension becomes a significant force that interferes with respiration in two ways. First, high surface tension means that a greater effort is required to achieve inspiration. This produces dyspnea and chronic fatigue, as a larger portion of total energy output is required just to breathe. The second problem arises during expiration. When increased surface tension combines with the normal forces that reduce alveolar volume, the result is collapse of the terminal airways when alveolar air pressure is exceeded. Because of this, during each inspiration, collapsed airways must be reinflated. Atelectasis occurs when inspiratory effort can't reinflate them.

In NRDS, alveolar surfaces are lined by a characteristic coating. It consists of a protein-rich fluid that is drawn out of the lung's interstitium by the increased surface tension. Also present is necrotic debris, the result of hypoxic tissue damage. This lining of the alveolar surface is called a hyaline membrane. For this reason, NRDS is often described as **hyaline membrane disease.** Because hyaline membranes greatly slow diffusion, and because increasingly widespread atelectasis reduces the surface available to diffusion, hypoxemia and hypercapnia result. Formerly, death often followed in a matter of hours or days because of acute respiratory failure, with mortality rates in the range of 20–30%. Recently, improvements in oxygen administration and ventilation techniques have improved the prognosis in NRDS. In particular, the more effective use of pulmonary surfactant therapy has brought a significant reduction in mortality for NRDS infants.

The necessary oxygen therapy in NRDS introduces the risk of oxygen toxicity, with particular effects in the eyes and lungs. Retinal capillary endothelium is particularly sensitive to oxygen, responding to it with increased apoptosis. After therapy is discontinued, the endothelia respond with excessive proliferation, causing loss of retinal sensitivity. This is referred to as **retrolental fibroplasia.** Lung tissue is also sensitive to oxygen damage, with airway disruption and fibrosis characteristics, producing the condition known as **bronchopulmonary dysplasia.**

LUNG TUMORS

Primary malignant lung tumors are the most common of all tumors and are highly lethal. They are responsible for more deaths than any other tumor. Highest incidence is found in males between 50 and 60 years of age. This is about four times the rate in women, but the incidence in females is steadily rising. Lung cancer fatalities in women exceed breast cancer fatalities. It is widely accepted that the single most significant etiological factor in pulmonary malignancies is cigarette smoking. The rising incidence of primary lung cancer in women is probably a reflection of their increased use of tobacco. Those chronically exposed to airborne industrial contaminants show a higher incidence of primary lung cancer, and those who also smoke have a higher incidence still. It may be that air pollutants are promoters that increase the carcinogenic effects of initiators in tobacco smoke (see chapter 5). The effect is also seen in asbestosis. Nonsmokers with asbestosis have a low incidence of lung cancer. Smokers with asbestosis have incidence rates higher than smokers who have no asbestosis involvement.

Over 90% of primary lung cancer develops in the mucous membranes of the larger bronchi. It is therefore called **bronchogenic carcinoma.** The most common form is **squamous cell carcinoma,** which produces characteristic whorled masses of keratin. Another form consists of small, highly anaplastic cells that resemble oat grains. This tumor is called a **small cell** or **oat cell carcinoma.** It metastasizes early, and by the time of diagnosis is likely to have spread to multiple secondary sites. Small cell carcinoma and the squamous cell type are the tumors most strongly associated with smoking. They are also the most lethal forms. An adenocarcinoma may also arise in the mucus glands of the bronchial mucous membrane. This is the form most common in women.

The impact of cigarette smoking on the bronchi and lungs is reflected in a continuum of effect that can be seen in young smokers. Bronchial irritation results in mucosal inflammatory changes accompanied by hyperplasia in the epithelium. Inflammatory exudate produces pulmonary edema accompanied by fibrosis, particularly in the small airways. Epithelial changes also involve loss of cilia. These early airway changes cause productive cough and an increase in respiratory infections in the smoker. As time passes and cigarette smoking increases (the usual pattern), bronchial damage increases, with chronic bronchitis and emphysema much more likely to develop. Mucosal epithelia thicken as chronic irritation produces early hypertrophy and later hyperplasia, metaplasia, and all too frequently, neoplasia.

As the tumor enlarges, a typical early sign is cough. This is unremarkable, however, because cough is a way of life among heavy smokers, those most at risk of lung cancer. Hemoptysis is often the first indication that the situation is serious. The tumor mass usually invades the bronchial

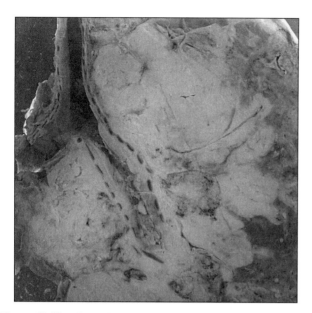

Figure 12.33   **Bronchogenic Carcinoma.** The white tumor tissue can easily be identified in contrast to the darker lung tissue. Note that the tumor originated in the bronchial epithelium and invaded the wall, gaining access to the lung parenchyma. Segments of bronchial cartilage can still be identified, delineating the boundaries of the airway.

X-rays had revealed a lesion in the right upper lobe of a 60-year-old male. He had refused therapy and was readmitted some time later with severe dyspnea and marked jugular distention. He died soon thereafter. Autopsy revealed a tumor in the right lung that had invaded extensively. It had spread from its site of origin in the bronchus and penetrated into the lung and beyond to the pericardium. Metastasis was widespread, involving the liver, adrenals, stomach, bone, and brain.

wall. As it grows around the airway's circumference, greater and greater obstruction to air flow occurs (see fig. 12.33). With complete obstruction, atelectasis distal to the blockage is common. Another result of infiltration of the bronchial wall is bronchiectasis from damage that causes airway dilatation. There is also an increased likelihood of lung abcess formation as infection resistance is further eroded.

Bronchogenic carcinoma tends to spread as a large, irregularly expanding mass rather than by narrow invasions into the lungs' parenchyma. Such spread may produce focal compression and atelectasis in the adjacent parenchyma. Collapse occurs when external pressure from the tumor exceeds the pressure of air within the terminal airways. About half of all lung tumors originate at the lung's root and, therefore, often invade the mediastinum, where the pericardium or heart may become involved, introducing the possibility of pericarditis and cardiac arrhythmias. More peripheral tumors may invade to the thoracic cavity's wall. Pain is experienced in such cases, because the parietal pleura is much more sensitive to painful stimuli than are the visceral pleura and lung parenchyma. Irritation of the pleurae by an invading tumor often produces substantial pleural effusion. The effects of primary lung tumors are summarized in figure 12.34.

Prognosis in primary lung cancer is poor. Metastasis is frequent and widespread, typically involving the brain, lymph nodes, bone, and liver.

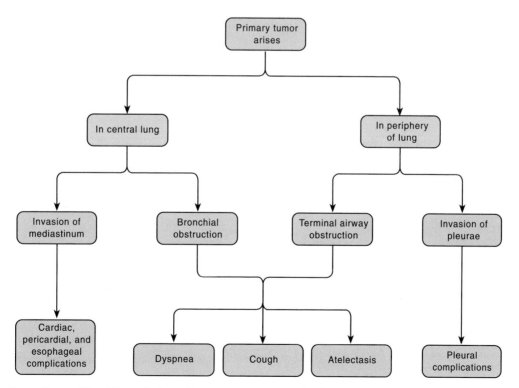

Figure 12.34   **Lung Cancer.** The effects of primary lung tumors may vary with the location of the tumor.

Case Study

A general practitioner was visited by a 50-year-old male who was worried by a shortness of breath that had developed over the previous month. He indicated that he had had a recent "cold" with a cough, which had since improved. On questioning by the doctor, he indicated that he smoked two packs of cigarettes each day and had developed a "smoker's cough" in the last five years. He replied to further inquiries that for the past two years he had experienced some difficulty breathing while climbing stairs and in similar demand situations. When pressed, he further revealed that his "smoker's cough" was sometimes productive of a thick and occasionally colored sputum, and that every winter he tended to develop what his previous doctors had called bronchitis. He was quick to point out that the prescribed antibiotics were able to deal with the problem quite effectively.

On examination, he appeared normal with no apparent cyanosis. Lung auscultation revealed slight wheezing on expiration. Spirometry revealed a depressed FEV_1, while a chest X-ray and complete blood count proved normal.

On the basis of these findings, a diagnosis of early COPD was made. Antibiotic therapy was started to control any residual infection, along with a bronchodilator to ease the patient's breathing. The patient was also urged to stop smoking and to return for periodic reassessment. He failed to return and no follow-up was possible.

Commentary

This patient is all too typical of the long-term, heavy smoker. Note that he had to be persistently questioned to obtain the full story of his condition. The history and FEV_1 results were strongly indicative of his problem, the blood counts established no anemia, and the radiograph was useful in establishing that no significant infection was present.

The fact that bronchodilation was able to improve, if only somewhat, the patient's FEV_1 values indicates some degree of reversibility. With appropriate monitoring, therapy for recurring infections, and support for the patient's efforts to stop smoking, the progression can be slowed, but not avoided.

The patient's failure to return was not unusual in that many smokers require a great deal of time to come to grips with the need to break their addiction. Of course, while the necessary resolve is being mustered, the disease is progressing.

Key Concepts

1. Cough, dyspnea, and cyanosis are the typical signs and symptoms that accompany various respiratory disorders (pp. 314–315).

2. Various studies of pulmonary function are employed in the diagnosis of respiratory disorders, the determination of their severity, and the monitoring of the disease's response to therapy (pp. 315–316).

3. Compromised respiratory function may be the result of hypoperfusion of the pulmonary vasculature due to heart failure, thromboembolism, or the reflex vasoconstriction triggered by hypoventilation (pp. 316–318).

4. Pulmonary shunting is the result of a decreased ventilation to perfusion ratio caused by hypoventilation, which is in turn caused by airway obstruction or restriction of lung expansion (p. 318).

5. Airway obstruction is characterized by reduced ventilation caused by smaller airway size, accumulated secretions, or loss of pulmonary elastic recoil (p. 318).

6. The long-term inhalation of irritants, most commonly cigarette smoke, is the stimulus to the inflammation, hypersecretion, and mucus gland hyperplasia typical of chronic bronchitis (pp. 318–319).

7. The distinguishing features of pulmonary emphysema are bronchiolar stenosis, alveolar enlargement, and septal loss, which reduce respiratory surface and pulmonary perfusion (pp. 319–320).

8. An essential component of the pathogenesis of emphysema is the role of cigarette smoke in inhibiting the action of alpha$_1$-antitrypsin (p. 320).

9. The term chronic airway obstruction (CAO) has clinical descriptive value for those obstructive conditions in which elements of chronic bronchitis, emphysema, or bronchial asthma combine to an extent that may be difficult to determine for a given patient (pp. 321–323).

10. The essential elements of a bronchial asthma attack—bronchiolar constriction, mucus hypersecretion, and inflammation—usually involve interplay between allergic and neural mechanisms. (pp. 323–326).

11. Hypoventilation may be caused by extrinsic factors that restrict lung expansion: a defective thoracic framework, insufficient respiratory muscle strength, or faulty neural input from the brain stem (pp. 327–328).

12. Intrinsic restriction of the lung involves diffuse changes in the pulmonary interstitium that produce stiffness and reduced compliance, which may emerge in an acute form, ARDS, or a chronic form, CIRLD (p. 329).

13. The principal feature of ARDS is acute pulmonary edema from capillary damage, which might arise from many etiologies (pp. 329–331).

14. Most CIRLD is due to long-term, low-level occupational exposure to inhaled irritants, producing inflammatory and immune-mediated damage that is superimposed on the effects of particle accumulation (pp. 331–334).

15. In respiratory failure, the clinical picture may be dominated by either hypoxia or hypoxia and hypercapnia (pp. 334–335).

16. Absorption of air by a portion of a lung isolated by airway blockage can lower pressure sufficiently to allow the lung portion to collapse, producing atelectasis (p. 335).

17. Collapse of an entire lung (pneumothorax) results when atmospheric air gains access to the pleural space, eliminating the pressure gradient that provides for the lung's expansion against the thoracic wall (pp. 336–337).

18. A premature infant's lack of pulmonary surfactant can produce a life-threatening combination of dyspnea, atelectasis, and hyaline membrane formation called neonatal respiratory distress syndrome (p. 338).

19. Bronchogenic carcinoma is the principal primary malignant lung tumor, whose poor prognosis is due to its frequent and extensive metastasis to vital tissues (pp. 338–339).

REVIEW ACTIVITIES

1. In figure 12.5, use a pencil to encircle the area that contains an acinus. (The acinus is not completely shown in the diagram.) The key can be found on p. 310.

2. Rough out a flow chart that indicates the difference in the fate of inhaled particles, based on their size. Indicate the specific fates and, when you're through, compare with figure 12.9 to see how well you did.

3. State how the V/Q ratios in figure 12.11*b,c* would compare with normal. See page 315 if you have any uncertainty in answering. Now get more practice by similarly assessing figure 12.13, points A, B, and C. The legend may offer help if you need it.

4. Cover the legend in figure 12.15. Of *a* and *b,* which is normal? Can you identify each factor that differs between *a* and *b* and relate it to the etiology and pathogenesis of chronic bronchitis? If you can't, refer to pages 318–319.

5. List the respiratory disorders mentioned in this chapter that are identified as being caused or complicated by smoking. For each, indicate the essential mechanism involved.

6. Complete the following table.

Key Characteristic	Respiratory Condition
Airway dilation	
Lung portion collapses	
Airway clearance reflex (sign)	
High blood level of reduced hemoglobin	
Inadequate pulmonary surfactant	
Entire lung collapses	
Allergy triggers	
Pleural effusion	
Difficulty breathing (sign)	

7. Jot down the principal differences in the effects a primary malignant lung tumor produces when it originates in a primary bronchus as opposed to when it originates in a peripheral airway. Don't overlook pain as one effect. Include any effects that might arise regardless of the site of the tumor's origin. A certain flow chart will be useful if you aren't certain your jottings are complete and accurate.

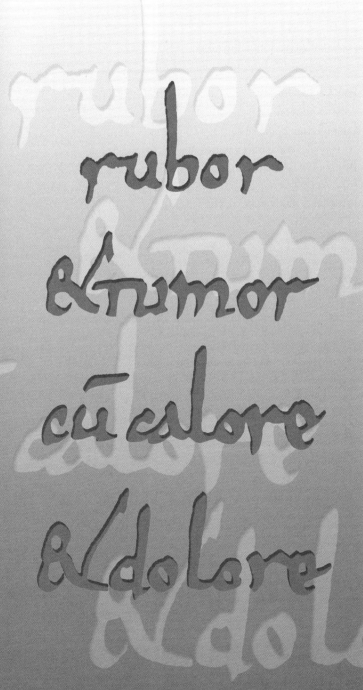

Chapter

13

Gastrointestinal Pathophysiology

A mannerly belly is a great part of a man's liberty.

MICHEL DE MONTAIGNE
ESSAYS

Digestion and the absorption of nutrients that follows it occur in the **alimentary canal,** which extends from the mouth to the anus. This chapter will not deal with diseases of the mouth, and will follow the common usage of the term gastrointestinal (GI). That is, although the usage is not strictly accurate, gastrointestinal will be taken to include the esophagus along with the stomach and intestines.

ANATOMY AND PHYSIOLOGY

The fundamental task we face in obtaining nutrients is moving them from the body's exterior to its internal compartments. Nutrients present in the lumen of the GI tract are considered external to these compartments, since the alimentary canal is open to the exterior at its two ends. This concept may not be obvious because of the manner in which the rest of the body is ingeniously folded around the GI lumen, but it is an important one (fig. 13.1). It means that digestion occurs outside the body, and that the crucial event that provides access to the nutrients is absorption. Absorption involves the passage of nutrients from the lumen through the membranes of the epithelial cells that line it, and then to the blood and lymph for distribution to appropriate sites of utilization or storage.

Most absorption occurs in the small intestine. It is particularly well adapted for this purpose, as it presents to the lumen the enormous surface area required for efficient absorption. Two major factors that contribute to the small intestine's large surface area are its length and the configuration of its internal lining. The small intestine (or small bowel—the terms are used interchangeably) is quite long. Its 9 feet (2.6 m) repeatedly folds back on itself to fit within the shorter abdominal cavity. Its proximal portion, the **duodenum,** receives the stomach's contents and passes them to its midportion, the **jejunum.** The **ileum** is the distal segment of the small bowel. It joins to the **cecum,** the inferior portion of the large bowel, or **colon.**

✓ *Checkpoint 13.1*

You may encounter descriptions of the small intestine that refer to its length as being 6 m. While this is accurate, it is often not explained that such a length can only be achieved after normal tension in its smooth muscle has eased. At autopsy, the small intestine can be drawn out to a length of about 6 m (20 ft), but during normal activity, the wall's muscle tension draws the intestine into shorter lengths: duodenum—20 cm (8 in); jejunum—2.4 m (8 ft); ileum—3.6 m (12 ft). It probably doesn't matter which number you use, as long as you understand the difference, and use the numbers in a way that doesn't introduce any ambiguity or confusion.

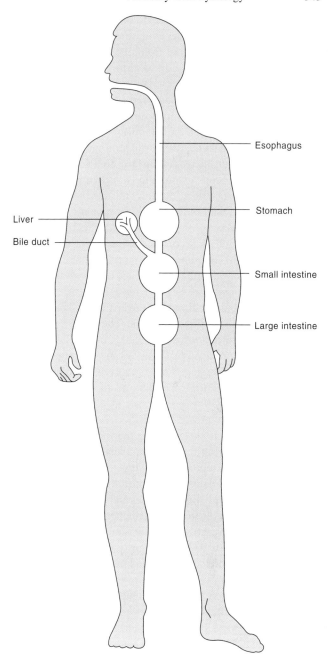

Figure 13.1   The Alimentary Canal. The lumen of the alimentary canal (GI tract) is an external space. In this schematic diagram, the tract has been simplified to illustrate this important concept.

The small intestine—in fact, the entire alimentary canal—has its internal surface lined by a **mucous membrane** or **mucosa.** This consists of an epithelium resting on a cushion of loosely organized fibrous connective tissue, under which lies a thin layer of smooth muscle. For most of its length, the epithelium is only one cell thick, to accommodate nutrient absorption. The thicker stratified epithelium in the mouth and esophagus is better adapted to protection. Specialized cells of the epithelium and glands beneath it in the **submucosa** (the layer of fibrous connective tissues that supports the mucosa) secrete mucus onto the epithelial surface. This viscous, protein-containing fluid acts as a protective covering and lubricant that promotes easy passage of **chyme** from one part of the canal to the next. (Chyme is the preferred term for the contents of the stomach and small intestine. With the addition of various secreted substances and the start of digestion, the contents of the stomach and small bowel are quite different from the food that entered the mouth.)

In the small intestine, three structural modifications are present that provide increased surface area for absorption. In the first, the mucous membrane is thrown into a pattern of circular folds. In effect, the internal mucous membrane is longer than the wall of the small bowel and must be collapsed into a folded configuration in order to fit the intestine's shorter length. A second modification of the mucosa involves the **villi.** Thousands of these tiny, mucosal projections protrude into the lumen to greatly increase absorptive surface. A third and very large increase in surface area derives from the **microvilli,** which cover the luminal surface of each epithelial cell in the villus. These are extremely fine, hairlike projections of the cell's membrane across which nutrients are absorbed (fig. 13.2). The small intestine's length and its mucosal configuration combine to provide an absorptive surface estimated to be in excess of 3,000 square feet (279 m^2).

Digestion is the processing of food that converts it into the molecular forms that are capable of being absorbed. Most food is in the form of macromolecules, which cannot cross the mucosal epithelium. Digestion reduces these macromolecules to their simpler, absorbable subunits. The process of **chemical digestion** depends on enzymes that catalyze a sequence of several small chemical changes. The products of these reactions are the simpler molecules that can be readily absorbed. The digestive fluids needed for this process are produced by the mucosal epithelium and by glands whose secretions are poured into the alimentary canal's lumen. Such secretions contain not only enzymes but also other substances that contribute to digestion. Since the salivary glands, liver, and pancreas are situated apart from the canal, long ducts are needed to deliver their secretions to the lumen.

A significant amount of digestive activity is devoted to reducing the physical size of food particles, because chemical digestion is more efficient if food particle size is small. This **physical digestion** of food has three components: mastication, secretion, and alimentary wall motility. In chewing, or **mastication,** the tongue and cheeks position food so the teeth can tear and crush it. Secretion involves the movement of digestive fluids into the lumen to promote physical breakdown of the food. For example, water is secreted into the mouth, stomach, and small intestine to loosen, soften, and dissolve food components. Acid is secreted into the stomach to disrupt the connective tissues binding the cells of the plant and animal tissues in food. The acid also kills bacteria, activates gastric enzymes, and prepares protein for chemical digestion. Bile, which is secreted by the liver, is delivered to the duodenum by way of

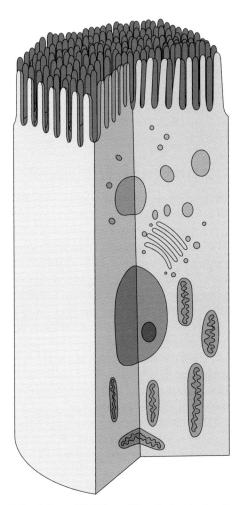

Figure 13.2   **Microvilli.** Microvilli at the luminal surface of the intestinal epithelium greatly increase the surface area where absorption may take place.

a duct system. The bile salts it contains act to convert large fat globules to large numbers of tiny globules. This process, called **emulsification,** is a physical change that greatly increases the surface area available to fat-splitting enzymes. The third component of physical digestion involves the activity of the GI wall. In it are two layers of smooth muscle. In one the muscle fibers are arranged longitudinally and in the other they are circumferentially arranged. Unlike the rest of the alimentary canal, the stomach has a third, partial layer, which contributes to the vigorous contractions that churn and mix chyme with the water, acid, and enzyme secretions of the stomach. Mastication, secretion, and gastric churning combine to yield the small particle size required for efficient enzyme functioning.

The process of digestion requires that food in the alimentary canal be moved through its lumen at an appropriate rate. The canal wall's smooth muscle layers achieve this by a series of coordinated, rhythmic contractions called **peristalsis.** This pattern of contractions provides the required direction and rate of motion along the length of the alimentary canal. Generally, the direction of peristalsis is from the esophagus toward the anus, but in the small intestine short, retrograde

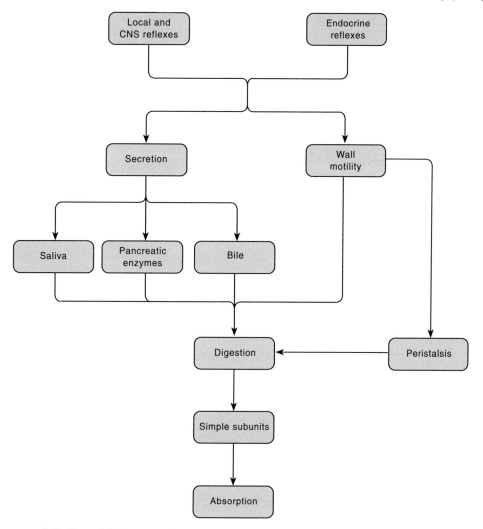

Figure 13.3   **Summary of the Essential Elements of Digestion.** Control of secretion and muscle contraction is mediated by nervous and endocrine reflexes.

movements ensure adequate mixing of chyme with digestive fluids, as well as increasing the time available for digestion.

Throughout the alimentary canal, the process of digestion is regulated to provide close coordination between secretory and muscular activity. Nervous reflexes are involved, some confined to the canal and others involving the central nervous system. At times of stress or emotional disturbances, input from the central nervous system (CNS) can adversely affect the functioning of the system. The endocrine system is also involved in the regulation of digestion. Hormones secreted by glands in the stomach and small bowel contribute to the responses needed to meet changing digestive requirements. These essentials are summarized in figure 13.3.

GI PATHOPHYSIOLOGY

Much hospitalization in North America involves the digestive system: the alimentary canal and its associated glands. In this chapter we consider those disorders that principally involve the GI tract. Although there is a fairly large number of these disorders, their effects produce only a relatively small number of GI manifestations. Each of these will be considered in the sections that follow.

Expulsion from the GI Tract

Expulsion of the GI contents, by vomiting or diarrhea, is a common indicator of tract irritation or malfunction. Although the expulsion episodes are typically of short duration, producing minimal disturbance and resolving promptly, severe or prolonged bouts can have serious systemic consequences.

Vomiting

In expelling the gastric contents, close coordination of several interrelated processes is required. Pallor and increased salivary output precede vomiting as a result of altered CNS output. Peristaltic contractions in the stomach and small intestine stop, and the pyloric sphincter, between the stomach and duodenum, closes. Access to adjacent airways is cut off as the glottis, the larynx's opening to the lower respiratory passages, is closed and the soft palate moves back to tightly seal off the posterior openings into the nasal passages. In this way, expulsion is limited to only a single path.

Following these preparations, an abrupt increase of abdominal pressure develops as the diaphragm, the intercostal muscles, and the muscles of the abdominal wall contract. (The fairly common experience of soreness in the abdominal muscles following a vigorous bout of vomiting testifies to their forceful contribution to the process.) The mounting pressure is applied to the stomach and adds to that produced by its own contractions. The result is a high pressure that is applied to the closed gastroesophageal sphincter, causing it to open and allowing gastric contents to be forced into the esophagus, past the opened hypopharyngeal sphincter at the top of the esophagus, and into the mouth. This process clears the vomited material, the **vomitus,** from the tract. The occasional presence of bile in vomitus is evidence of the small intestine's participation in vigorous vomiting episodes. Contraction of its proximal portion can generate sufficient pressure to drive bile through the pyloric sphincter into the stomach.

The sequence of responses just described is the result of nervous output from an integrating center for the vomiting reflex, located in the medulla oblongata. This **vomiting center** initiates the vomiting reflexes in response to input from sensitive receptor cells in the walls of the GI tract, abdominal viscera, or other parts of the nervous system. Irritating substances from chemical or biological sources, inflammatory changes in the mucosa, or distortion of the canal—usually small bowel distention—typically induce the vomiting reflex. **Nausea,** the awareness of the tendency or need to vomit, occurs because activity in the vomiting center is being signaled to the cerebral cortex.

The vomiting center also receives input from another part of the brain nearby called the **chemoreceptor trigger zone** (CTZ). This area has a rich blood supply and is highly sensitive to certain circulating chemicals that stimulate the CTZ and, in turn, the vomiting center. Some of these are substances released from tissues damaged by bacterial infection or ionizing radiation. Activity in the chemotactic trigger zone may also result from exposure to circulating therapeutic drugs administered for conditions unrelated to GI problems. This is the reason for the nausea and vomiting side effects associated with the use of certain drugs. Various neurological disturbances are also associated with vomiting, as they directly or indirectly affect the vomiting center or the CTZ. Such conditions as meningitis, cerebral ischemia, and increased intracranial pressure are examples. The CTZ also receives input from the inner ear structures involved with the maintenance of somatic equilibrium. In sensitive individuals, visual and other activities associated with the motions of air, sea, or land travel can cause these inner ear structures to activate the CTZ, resulting in the nausea and vomiting of motion sickness.

In certain individuals, merely the aroma or sight of vomitus or the sensations evoked by the memory of a previous episode of vomiting may induce the response. A case in point is the author, who has been aware of a distinct abdominal queasiness while researching and writing this material. Psychological disturbances can also produce chronic vomiting—for example, where there is some compulsive fear of poisoning, or where the mere thought of eating can induce nausea. The latter case is typical of **anorexia nervosa,** a potentially grave condition deriving from an obsession with weight loss. Figure 13.4 summarizes the elements of the vomiting response.

Most vomiting is a direct approach to clearing the upper GI tract of irritants. Usually, as the offending material is expelled, normal functions are quickly restored. Complications may arise, however, in the case of chronic vomiting, especially in children. Loss of fluid in such cases may lead to dehydration, and loss of needed electrolytes may lead to potentially severe fluid and electrolyte imbalances. Chronic vomiting may also lead to deficiencies of essential nutrients, especially vitamins. Another source of complications is frequent or particularly vigorous vomiting that occurs without full relaxation of the esophagus. In such cases, the mucosa may tear, with subsequent bleeding into the lumen and the vomitus. The **Mallory-Weiss syndrome** involves such gastric and esophageal bleeding. It results from lacerations of the mucosa caused by paroxysms of retching associated with chronic alcohol abuse and with the period following general anesthesia. The lack of esophageal relaxation seems linked to the effects of the alcohol and anesthetic on the vomiting center.

With loss of consciousness, CNS reflex coordination may be sufficiently depressed to produce faulty vomiting responses. If the stomach's contents are expelled to the oropharynx while the glottis remains open, aspiration of vomitus may result (see fig. 12.4). The potential consequences are pulmonary damage or complete blockage of the respiratory passages. Those in an alcoholic stupor or those recovering from surgical anesthesia are particularly at risk.

Diarrhea

The large bowel functions to complete the absorption process by removing up to 900 ml of water and various salts from the colon's lumen daily. This process prepares the contents of the colon (the **feces**) for expulsion from the alimentary canal. The colon's smooth muscle undergoes two to three periods of vigorous peristalsis per day. One of these may fill the rectum, stimulating pressure receptors there. In response, the spinal cord activates the defecation reflex, and fecal matter is expelled. There is wide variation in the frequency of defecation among normal individuals, from as few as two per week to as many as three per day.

Diarrhea is usually defined in terms of increased fecal fluidity, but increased volume of feces or frequency of defecation in a given individual may also indicate an abnor-

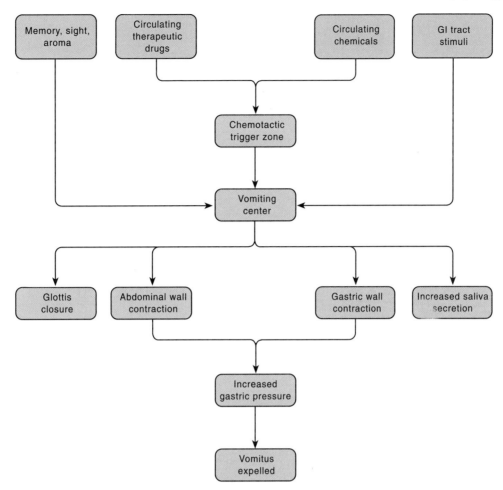

Figure 13.4 **Mechanisms Underlying the Vomiting Reflexes.** Local GI stimuli, circulating therapeutic drug, or other chemicals, as well as sensory and memory inputs can all induce the response.

✓ *Checkpoint 13.2*

The wide range of normal defecation frequency surprises most people. Keep it in mind when dealing with patients and resist the quite natural tendency to accept your own frequency as normal and any deviations from it as constipation or diarrhea.

mality. The essential cause of diarrhea is increased colonic fluid volume, which, by producing distention, activates the defecation reflex. Greater colonic distention will also lead to increased frequency of the response.

Fluid accumulates in the intestinal lumen by three distinct mechanisms. One is an active secretion process, while the second involves osmosis. The third mechanism is based on faulty intestinal or colonic water absorption.

Secretion The secretion of water into the intestinal lumen is a common response to irritation. In some cases, bacterial toxins, in particular from *Vibrio cholerae* and *Escherichia coli,* and irritation from laxatives or unabsorbed fatty acids are known to produce an intestinal secretion response. The movement of fluid to the lumen promotes distention, and the resulting defecation would seem a beneficial response in that irritants are initially diluted and then evacuated from the tract. In other cases, patients who undergo removal of all, or part, of the ileum are unable to reabsorb bile salts, since the ileum is the principal site for their uptake for recycling via the liver (this is the enterohepatic circulation of bile salts). As a result, abnormally large amounts of these irritant salts are present to elicit a secretion response. Also, certain GI tumors stimulate intestinal secretion by direct or indirect means that are not well understood. In these cases, the related bouts of diarrhea can be quite intense.

Osmosis Osmotic flow of water to the lumen depends on high luminal osmotic pressures. These are the result of increased particle concentrations, which are usually caused by faulty digestion, impaired particle absorption, or an increased intake of indigestible or unabsorbable molecules. Digestive problems may arise from a lack of bile or the

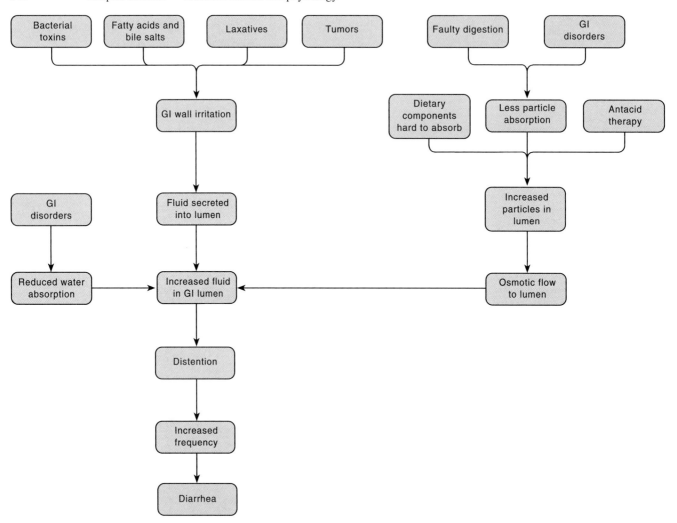

Figure 13.5   **Factors Contributing to Diarrhea.**

enzymes needed to degrade food macromolecules to their absorbable subunits. As a consequence, the particles remain in the lumen and raise its osmotic pressure.

The slowing of intestinal motility favors bacterial growth, which is normally inhibited. As they proliferate, the bacteria metabolize luminal nutrients to produce greater numbers of product molecules. These increase osmotic pressure and water is drawn into the lumen. Diarrhea results, even though no toxic or infectious damage is involved. Impaired absorption of digestion products has the same effect: an increased luminal osmotic pressure, which draws water from the intestinal mucosa.

Increased dietary or therapeutic intake can also raise lumen osmotic pressure. Diets rich in legumes and carbohydrates have a high content of indigestible elements and can produce diarrhea. Also, patients undergoing antacid therapy to reduce gastric hyperacidity may ingest preparations with high concentrations of poorly absorbed ions, such as magnesium. Therapy based on these preparations often produces an osmosis-mediated diarrhea as a side effect.

Impaired Water Absorption Certain diseases of the intestine and colon reduce the mucosa's permeability to water and therefore impede water absorption. This effect is significant in light of the approximately 2 liters of dietary fluid ingested daily and the addition of 8 liters of digestive fluids secreted into the lumen each day. Since normal daily fecal loss is only about 400 ml, the small intestine and colon must absorb 9,600 ml daily. Thus, a reduction of water absorption can readily generate significant intestinal fluid volume and diarrhea. Various malabsorption syndromes that produce such problems are described in the Malabsorption section later in this chapter.

Alcohol and certain classes of therapeutic agents can produce diarrhea as a side effect. Antibiotics and antitumor agents are the principal drugs involved. They may act either to irritate the intestine, promoting fluid secretion, or to interfere with water absorption. The various factors predisposing to diarrhea are summarized in figure 13.5.

Of course, **laxatives**—agents that promote defecation— might also cause diarrhea. These are normally administered

Focus on Mechanisms of Laxative Action

Insights into the mechanisms that increase intestinal fluid volume to cause diarrhea can be applied to promoting bowel evacuation in cases of constipation. Four laxative mechanisms are currently employed by various agents. Some add water-binding materials to the GI tract to prevent water absorption. The objective is to maintain sufficient colonic water volume to increase distention and thus stimulate the defecation reflex. An example of such a **bulk-forming agent** is methylcellulose. Other laxatives rely on an **osmotic** or **saline** mechanism to draw water from the mucosa by using high ion concentrations to produce high luminal osmotic pressure. Because of its low absorption by intestinal epithelium, magnesium ion is often used in osmotic laxatives as their principal active agent. A third laxative category contains **irritant** or **stimulant** agents. These irritate the intestinal mucosa to promote secretion and enhance distention. Where longer periods of constipation have increased colonic water absorption, a hardened and difficult-to-evacuate fecal mass may result. In such cases, a member of the fourth laxative category, a **stool-softening** agent, such as **docusate potassium,** may be used. It acts as an emulsifying agent to promote the mixture of water and fecal fat. This action softens the stool and provides for easier evacuation.

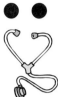

Focus on Laxative Abuse

In some cases of chronic diarrhea for which no cause can be found, laxative abuse may be a hidden factor. Excessive and concealed laxative use has been identified in people, usually young women, who have eating disorders and who try to reduce their weight by inducing diarrhea. Another group of abusers, for less clear but presumably psychogenic reasons, includes people who work in medically related jobs. Women also predominate in this group, whose members' ages range from 20–50.

Diagnosis of laxative overuse can be made on the basis of stool ion concentrations, which are altered by the laxative. This analysis can be particularly important in undiagnosed chronic diarrhea in children, where an abusive parent is forcing the child to ingest a laxative when one is not needed.

to counter **constipation** (difficulty in defecation), which may be due to altered intestinal motility (see the Irritable Bowel Syndrome section) or to faulty rectal reflexes. Whatever the cause of the constipation, excessive laxative use can produce diarrhea in those particularly sensitive to their effects (see the Focus box on laxative action).

The principal consequences of diarrhea are water loss, leading to dehydration, and acidosis, due to the loss of alkaline bicarbonate ions. These are particularly threatening in the very young, the elderly, and those already weakened by disease or other debilitating factors.

Dehydration and acidosis are less likely to occur in acute diarrhea, which typically resolves without intervention. They are more likely to arise in cases of liver or pancreatic dysfunction, intestinal resection, or severe mucosal damage where diarrhea becomes chronic. If diarrhea is severe or chronic, therapeutic agents that inhibit motility in the intestines, reduce frequency, and promote fluid absorption are employed. Typical antidiarrheal agents are preparations of **loperamide** and **paregoric.**

Irritable Bowel Syndrome This condition, also known as **spastic colon,** is involved in as many as half of the GI problems for which people seek medical consultation. It is characterized by a varying symptom mix that may include abdominal discomfort or pronounced cramping, fatigue,

and constipation, alternating with diarrhea. The diarrhea typically involves increased frequency and urgency of defecation, even though stool volume is low. A higher than normal mucus content is also characteristic of the stool in the irritable bowel syndrome.

Diarrhea in this condition appears to be the result of increased intestinal motility, which reduces the time available for adequate fluid absorption. Loss of peristaltic coordination may produce cramping when a peristaltic wave in one part of the colon drives fecal material toward another part that is constricted.

The mechanism underlying the irritable bowel syndrome is not clearly understood. The lack of peristaltic coordination noted earlier may indicate an underlying neurogenic etiology. No structural defect in the colon wall or its mucosa has been identified. Speculation on possible links to insufficient dietary fiber or personality type as factors in the irritable bowel syndrome have not been substantiated.

Gastrointestinal Inflammation

Acute inflammation in the GI tract is quite common. Most is a response to local injury or irritation that produces the expected inflammatory symptoms and signs: congestion and exudate formation in the mucosa, along with pain and redness. As healing follows, there is usually little problem with epithelial regeneration, but scarring in the submucosa may be followed by stricture in the GI tract. The result is a narrowing of the lumen that impedes normal motility.

Esophagitis

Most inflammation in the alimentary canal occurs in the stomach and intestines. The esophagus is less commonly

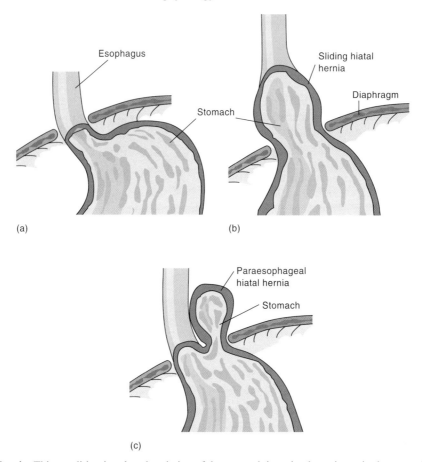

Figure 13.6 **Hiatal Hernia.** This condition involves herniation of the stomach into the thoracic cavity by way of the esophageal hiatus. (*a*) Normal. (*b*) Sliding hernia. (*c*) Paraesophageal hernia. This type may progressively enlarge.

involved, but it can be irritated by the reflux of gastric contents. The intense acidity of gastric juice is the major factor in such irritation, because the esophageal mucosa lacks the gastric adaptations that provide acid tolerance. The resulting **reflux esophagitis** is associated with epigastric pain, usually described as a dull or burning ache that may radiate to the neck. This sensation is commonly known as **heartburn.** A wide variety of commonly encountered agents can induce a lowering of tension in the region of the gastroesophageal junction known as the **lower esophageal sphincter** (LES). This change allows gastric pressures to drive acidic chyme into the esophagus. CNS depressants such as valium or morphine can reduce normal input to the LES, and certain foods (e.g., chocolate or fats) and alcohol and smoking are also known to elicit this response.

Reflux esophagitis is common in pregnant women and the obese and is linked to the increased abdominal mass in these conditions. The resulting increase in abdominal pressure, combined with gastric pressure, exceeds the resistance offered by the lower esophageal sphincter and gastric reflux follows. Most sufferers of reflux esophagitis have a **sliding hiatal hernia.** In this condition, a segment of the stomach herniates (projects from its normal cavity) into the thoracic cavity through an enlarged or loosened **esophageal hiatus**—the opening in the diaphragm through which the

esophagus passes into the abdominal cavity. A less common type is the **paraesophageal** or **rolling hiatal hernia** (fig. 13.6). Both conditions are idiopathic.

Acute esophagitis may also be the result of damage that follows esophageal infection—for example, by a fungus, *Candida albicans,* by herpes simplex virus, or from irradiation for thoracic tumors. Less common, but much more severe, is the esophagitis that follows accidental or suicidal ingestion of corrosive liquids such as strong acids or lye. As you might expect in such cases, the potential for scarring and stricture is high, but even chronic, severe reflux esophagitis may result in stricture that makes swallowing difficult **(dysphagia).**

Inflammations of the Stomach and Intestines

In the stomach and intestines, various irritants can provoke mild inflammations of short duration. Many are idiopathic. These conditions are termed gastritis, enteritis, gastroenteritis, enterocolitis, or colitis, depending on the part of the tract that is affected. Most such inflammations are the result of ingested irritants of biological or chemical origin, which often trigger vomiting and diarrhea. Damage is usually minimal, with rapid healing of mucosal damage.

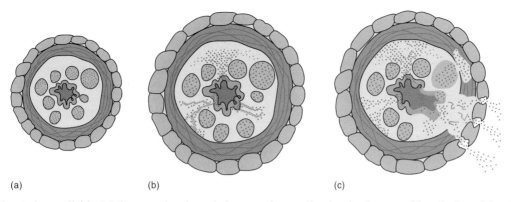

(a)   (b)   (c)

Figure 13.7   **Acute Appendicitis.** (*a*) Cross section through the normal appendix, showing lumen and lymphatic nodules. (*b*) Acute appendicitis, showing swelling and bacterial proliferation. Ischemic injury may follow. (*c*) Necrosis from hypoxia or bacteria toxins may result in perforation of the wall, allowing bacteria and debris to spill into the abdominal cavity.

Most chronic gastritis seems linked to damage caused by a particular bacterium. **Helicobacter pylori** colonizes the surface of the gastric epithelium below its mucus layer. While unable to penetrate deeply, the organism is adapted to resist gastric acid and thrives at the epithelial surface. It induces an infiltration of PMNs and over time, metaplasia in the epithelium that may predispose to gastric carcinoma. Symptoms usually present as nonspecific **dyspepsia.** This is the GI disturbance that is characterized by pain, gas, nausea, and loss of appetite commonly known as "indigestion." H. pylori infection increases with age, with as many as half of those age 60 infected, although many of these are asymptomatic or have only low-level symptoms. The role of this organism in ulceration of the stomach and intestine is described later in this chapter in the Ulceration section.

A particular form of chronic gastritis is caused by an autoimmune attack on the mucosa. It is called **autoimmune chronic gastritis** and is implicated in pernicious anemia (see chapter 7).

The gastric mucosa is especially sensitive to alcohol, aspirin (ASA), and other nonsteroidal anti-inflammatory drugs (NSAIDs). Chronic ingesters of such substances may suffer from acute gastritis combined with bleeding erosions of the mucosa, a condition called **acute erosive gastritis.** The loss of mucosal surface in these cases is superficial. More severe erosions of the GI mucosa are considered in the Ulceration section later in this chapter.

Sufferers of chronic pain or non-GI inflammatory conditions—rheumatoid arthritics, for example—may become dependent on ASA or NSAID use and suffer significant gastric mucosal disruption, which raises the threat of chronic bleeding. (Note that although ASA has anti-inflammatory effects, and therefore can be grouped with the NSAIDs [e.g., ibuprofen or indomethacin], it is separately identified here because much of its use is based primarily on its analgesic properties.) Individuals who suffer dyspepsia as a result of alcohol abuse often seek to correct the discomfort with aspirin. Of course, this only compounds the problem by adding to the mucosal damage already caused by previous alcohol ingestion.

Appendicitis

The vermiform appendix is a potential site of inflammation. This 8–10 cm long structure is a slender extension of the cecum containing nodules of lymphoid tissue in its submucosa (fig. 13.7*a*). Acute inflammation of the appendix can occur at any age, but the highest incidence is in the range of ages 10–20. It is the most common cause of abdominal surgery in children.

The pathogenesis of acute appendicitis involves obstruction of its narrow lumen, which appears to establish conditions favoring resident bacterial growth. (fig. 13.7*b*). This seems to be the key initiating event in appendicitis because mucous secretion continues behind the obstruction and its accumulation causes luminal pressure to increase. Small mucosal veins yield to this pressure and their collapse blocks the inflow of blood, causing mucosal damage followed by swelling and pain. The initial damage may be relatively minor but as inflammation develops, pressure in the swelling appendix, trapped in its peritoneal wrapping, rises higher, causing collapse of even larger vessels. With oxygen levels continuing to fall, the growth of anaerobic bacteria is favored. Their proliferation and digestion of necrotic appendiceal tissue produce the gangrene that is characteristic of the later stages of acute appendicitis (fig. 13.8).

Initially, the pain of acute appendicitis is relatively mild and poorly localized. Rather than the lower right quadrant of the abdomen, it is referred to the midline in the epigastric or umbilical regions. With continued swelling, the appendix presses against the adjacent abdominal wall and its sensitive parietal peritoneum. This causes the pain to become more intense and sharply focused (see the Focus box).

The obstruction that starts the inflammatory response in appendicitis is is often a hardened mass of fecal material called a **fecalith.** External compression by a tumor or other mass—for example, an abscess or blockage by a gallstone or intestinal parasites, such as pinworms—may also be implicated. Where no obstructing factor can be identified, it is thought that a transient viral infection might cause enlargement of the lymphoid nodules in the appendix, restricting

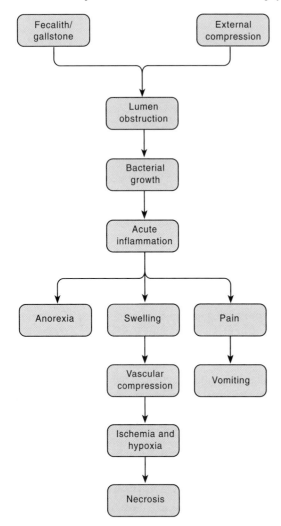

Figure 13.8   **Pathogenesis of Acute Appendicitis.**

Focus on Rebound Tenderness

Because of the pattern of innervation in abdominal organs, when damaged, they produce pain that is felt as an aching or gnawing sensation in the region of the midline, regardless of the organ's actual location. Patients experiencing such pain are often restless, constantly changing position to ease their discomfort.

The parietal peritoneum lines the inner surface of the abdominal wall. When an inflamed organ disturbs the parietal peritoneum, causing it to become inflamed, the peritoneum's rich nerve supply generates much more intense pain that is localized over the affected organ. Because of the peritoneum's sensitivity, any motion exaggerates the pain. In these cases, patients resist any movement, lying rigidly in their beds.

Palpation (using touch in an examination) of the abdomen to identify any abnormalities can verify peritoneal involvement. The fingers gradually apply pressure at the abdominal wall, then are quickly removed. An experience of sharp pain as the wall rebounds verifies that the peritoneum is involved. This phenomenon is known as **rebound tenderness.**

---

the lumen and fostering bacterial proliferation. Signs and symptoms of the viral infection might be mild or completely unnoticed, so the appendicitis that emerges has no apparent cause.

A major risk in appendicitis is that the damaged appendix wall will weaken and perforate, allowing the lumen's bacteria-laden contents to spill onto adjacent peritoneal surfaces (fig. 13.7c).

Peritonitis

The **peritoneum** is an extensive serous membrane system in the abdominal cavity. Its parietal layer lines the inner walls of the cavity, whereas its visceral layer is adherent to the surfaces of most abdominal organs. The smooth peritoneal surfaces are coated with a thin film of protective lubricating fluid. Its presence greatly reduces friction between the viscera, and between them and the cavity's wall, during peristaltic and other normal movements. In addition, the peritoneum supports the viscera and aids in maintaining their relative positions within the abdomen. The sheets of

peritoneum also carry blood, lymphatic vessels, and nerves to and from the intestines.

The irritants that induce peritonitis are usually bacterial or chemical and may be endogenous or exogenous. A ruptured appendix or colon wall may be the source of bacteria, while damage to the gall bladder or pancreas, or the duct systems that drain them, can release highly irritant bile salts or enzymes onto adjacent peritoneal surfaces. Penetrating wounds of the abdomen, sexually transmitted bacteria, or surgical procedures are the usual source of exogenous irritants.

Peritonitis typically produces the syndrome of acute pain onset, fever, and vomiting that is called the **acute abdomen.** It is also typical in cases of acute appendicitis, cholecystitis (gall bladder inflammation), GI wall perforation, and various other abdominal disorders.

In the more common case of an endogenous irritant, pathogenesis in peritonitis involves peritoneal inflammation, with formation of a fibrinous exudate at the site of irritation. A fibrin mesh, which is continuous between peritoneum and the adjacent organ, walls off the inflamed area, isolating the irritants from the rest of the abdominal organs.

In some cases, an abscess will form at the site if clearance of exudate and pus is delayed. In other cases, post-inflammatory scarring produces adhesions that can compromise normal intestinal motility. If stricture follows healing, obstruction of normal movement within the lumen is likely. In the case of peritonitis resulting from colon perforation, the inflammation following fecal contamination may be complicated by abscess formation and perforation of the wall of an adjacent pelvic structure. This complication may

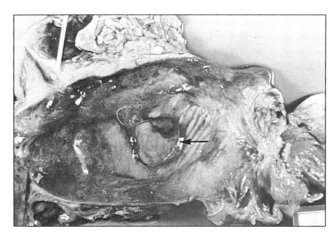

Figure 13.9 **Fistula.** A fistula (arrow) allows communication between the colon and the vagina.

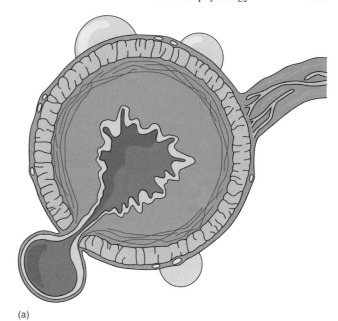

(a)

result in fibrosis that joins the two adjacent organs in such a way that a passage forms between their normally separate lumina. Such a passage is called a **fistula.** The same term applies when the perforated organ's lumen communicates with another surface or cavity instead of another organ's lumen (fig. 13.9).

When fistulae form, problems arise because substances normally confined to one site may well produce irritation or infection when they contact vulnerable surfaces that are unable to resist their effects. Bile is particularly irritating to tissues other than the gall bladder or bile duct linings, and it is not difficult to appreciate the irritation and infection threat when colon contents pass through a fistula connecting with the urinary bladder, small intestine, or vagina.

Following perforation of a GI organ, irritation of the peritoneum may not remain localized. More widespread involvement is called **generalized peritonitis** and presents the potential for more serious consequences. Since the peritoneal membranes are continuous throughout the abdominopelvic cavity, irritants and infectious agents exposed to them can produce extensive damage. Some of the irritants and toxins involved in peritonitis may be absorbed from peritoneal surfaces. Once in the blood, they can cause various systemic complications such as fever, septicemia, and vascular shock. Mortality in generalized peritonitis is high if the leaking perforation can't be closed. The elderly and debilitated are particularly at risk.

Diverticulitis

Diverticula are thought to be present in as much as one-third of the population of economically well-developed nations, usually in people over age 50. Each **diverticulum** is a pouchlike sac of mucosa that protrudes through the wall of the large intestine (fig. 13.10). The presence of diverticula is described by the term **diverticulosis.** Most diverticula form in the sigmoid colon, but more proximal regions may also be involved. In many cases diverticula are asymptomatic,

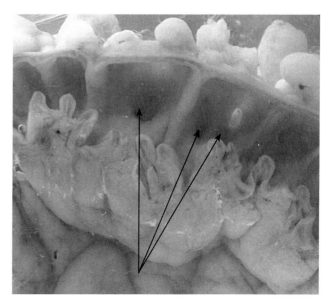

(b)

Figure 13.10 **Diverticulosis.** (*a*) Diverticula are flask-shaped sacs of mucosa that project through the muscular layers of the intestine, usually the colon. (*b*) Numerous colon diverticula can be seen as the rounded masses projecting from this sectioned length of colon. The arrows indicate the openings of the diverticula, which communicate to the bowel lumen.

This colon segment was removed from the abdomen of a 58-year-old man who had suffered years of intermittent bouts of pain, fever, and vomiting. On one such occasion, swelling in the lower left abdominal quadrant was pronounced, and a radiographic study revealed extensive diverticular disease in the sigmoid colon. The patient elected to have the affected segment of bowel removed, and he was no longer troubled. The specimen shown here has been cut on its long axis to reveal the openings into several diverticula. The resection was done during a period of remission, so no signs of inflammation are apparent.

Focus on Caution with High-Fiber Diets

Of course, it doesn't necessarily follow that if a little is good, more must be better. In those seeking a high degree of immediate protection against diverticulosis, a sudden change to a high-fiber diet can induce rectal gas accumulation and frequent, forceful, even explosive episodes of diarrhea. As in most things, a gradual change in fiber intake, with monitoring of any ill effects, is the wise course.

---

but some produce abdominal pain, less intense abdominal discomfort, and constipation.

Pathogenesis in diverticulosis is linked to age and stool volume. In those people whose diets include sufficient indigestible residues—collectively referred to as fiber—fecal volume is high and readily triggers defecation. A high-fiber diet also reduces time spent in the colon, which in turn limits water absorption. The result is a moister, more easily evacuated stool. By contrast, the low-fiber diet produces less colonic peristalsis and thus promotes water absorption. The smaller, dryer stool may then require more forceful colonic contractions, which raise pressures and promote formation of diverticula. In older people, many years of consuming low-fiber foods produces changes in the colon's wall. Its diameter becomes smaller, exaggerating abdominal pressure to favor diverticula formation.

A peculiarity of colon wall structure allows formation of diverticula. When luminal pressure is high, the mucosa is squeezed through the inner muscle layer at points where blood vessels and nerves pass through it. Since the external colon muscle is formed of three narrow strips rather than a continuous layer, the protruding mucosa can pass easily between them to form the diverticulum.

In support of the relationship between intraluminal pressure and diverticulosis, the problem is much less common in countries where high-fiber diets, based on cereal grains and vegetables are the norm. In striking contrast is the incidence in countries where refined carbohydrate and meat form a high proportion of the diet. Vegetarians have a much lower incidence of diverticulosis; and in animals that eat only vegetable matter, the problem is unknown, even though they have points of weakness in their colon walls similar to those in humans.

A few scattered diverticula may be present in diverticulosis, or there may be over a hundred. In about 15% of affected individuals, fecal matter becomes impacted in the diverticula to form fecaliths. Irritation and bacterial damage to the wall may follow to produce **diverticulitis.** In these cases, lower left quadrant abdominal pain, fever, and episodes of diarrhea or constipation, or both, are characteristic.

A major threat of diverticulitis is bleeding, because the inflamed diverticulum can affect the blood vessels that accompany it as it protrudes through the colon's wall. Another risk is necrosis of the wall of the diverticulum, followed by its perforation. The resulting spill of colon contents onto adjacent organ surfaces presents the risk of peritonitis and formation of fistulae to adjacent organs. Furthermore, fibrosis following successive bouts of diverticulitis may cause stenosis of the colon, obstructing free passage through it.

The presence of diverticulosis is often unnoticed, and because, after an episode of diverticulitis, the condition may again become asymptomatic, it is often difficult to determine the status of the situation in a given patient. For this reason, the term **diverticular disease** is increasingly used. It implies the condition of diverticulosis and the possibility of periods of diverticular inflammation, without the need to select a term of uncertain clinical precision.

Inflammatory Bowel Disease

The designation **inflammatory bowel disease** (IBD) includes two conditions that have certain underlying features in common. Both **Crohn's disease** and **ulcerative colitis** are inflammatory diseases with no known cause and a well-established pattern of familial incidence. Both conditions involve abdominal cramping, diarrhea, and fever. The two bowel disorders also occur in similar populations: whites, especially Jews of European extraction, with onset in early adulthood. Many investigations have pursued the cause of Crohn's disease and ulcerative colitis, but without definitive results. A genetic predisposition is involved, with some evidence of an immune mechanism contributing to the process. Although specifics are few, the general mechanism seems based on luminal factors that induce an inadequately regulated immune response. This is followed by the long-term infiltration of PMNs that cause the mucosal damage. Apart from these broad similarities, the following specific differences in pathogenesis and clinical course are known.

Crohn's Disease (CD) In this condition, granuloma formation and sometimes more diffuse cellular infiltrations produce mucosal swelling and erosion of the mucosal surface, often producing a linear pattern of ulceration. Fibrosis in the submucosa and hypertrophy of muscle layers often contribute to intestinal stenosis. As these changes affect a given section of the colon or small intestine, adjacent areas may remain uninvolved—hence, the alternate designation **regional enteritis.** Symptoms are quite variable among those affected, with intervals of pain and diarrhea separated by asymptomatic periods of remission, which usually last weeks to months and, in some cases, years. A pattern of chronic recurrence, producing progressive weight loss and anemia from inadequate absorption of iron or vitamin B_{12}, is common in Crohn's disease. Reduced red cell production may also be caused by a folate lack, secondary to food intake reduction caused by an accompanying anorexia. Although most CD affects the colon, it may arise in any part of the alimentary wall.

Ulcerative Colitis (UC) In this condition, blood in the stool often accompanies diarrhea and abdominal pain. As in Crohn's disease, bouts of remission separate the attacks, but onset is usually more abrupt with more severe signs and symptoms. Among sufferers, 85% have mild or moderate symptoms, but 15% have a much more threatening **fulminant** or **severe ulcerative colitis.** Fluid and electrolyte losses can be serious in this condition, as can hemorrhage, which poses the threat of hypovolemic shock. The mortality rate in this condition is 15%.

Ulcerative colitis is limited to the colon and is characterized by a diffuse involvement confined to the mucosa. Inflammatory swelling, redness, and cellular infiltration are typical, but the mucosal surface also displays a progressive loss of epithelium (fig. 13.11). This surface erosion, or ulceration, begins in deep epithelial folds where foci of purulent necrosis arise. These abscesses enlarge and merge with adjacent abscesses to produce extensive mucosal ulceration. Over the course of the disease, inflammation in the mucosa takes on a more cellular characteristic typical of a chronic inflammatory response. A comparison of relevant aspects of Crohn's disease and ulcerative colitis is presented in table 13.1.

Complications and Therapy The two conditions that contribute to IBD have similar complications, which are related to weakening and perforation of the wall of the bowel. The potential consequences are peritonitis and fistula formation. Scarring during periods of remission may produce intestinal stricture, more so with Crohn's disease than ulcerative colitis. Systemic effects include eye and joint inflammation, liver damage, and cancer. The increased cancer rate is more significant in cases of ulcerative colitis that are of prolonged duration and generalized colon involvement. The cancer risk in Crohn's disease is above normal, but smaller than in ulcerative colitis (see table 13.1).

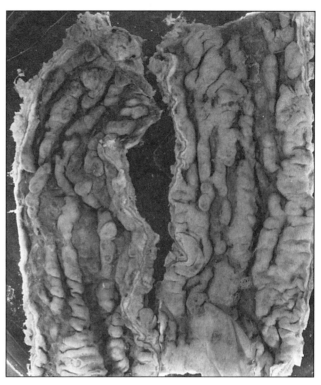

Figure 13.11 **Ulcerative Colitis.** These colon segments show a thickened wall with longitudinal ridges in the mucosae. Between the ridges are depressions of ulcerated mucosa.

A 13-year-old girl suffered from ulcerative colitis and had a long history of diarrhea, bleeding, and pain. Therapy had been ineffective, and because she was having trouble avoiding malnutrition, the affected segments of her colon and rectum were surgically removed. Her condition improved and she gained weight, although the postsurgical period was complicated by various intestinal disturbances. The colon segments shown here have elongated ridges of thickened wall separated by linear troughs of ulcerated mucosa. Various regions of fibrosis are also present, with some sites of acute inflammation. No indications of malignancy were found.

Table 13.1   Comparison of Selected Characteristics of Ulcerative Colitis versus Crohn's Disease

Characteristic	Ulcerative Colitis	Crohn's Disease
Inflammation type	Acute/chronic mix; no granulomas	Chronic; granulomas present
Site of lesion	Confined to mucosa	Mucosa with wall penetration
Affected bowel	Colon only	Usually terminal ileum
Pattern of onset	Often acute, severe	Low level, slow to develop
Ulceration pattern	Irregular and superficial	Linear and penetrating
Stool	Watery; blood and mucus typical	Watery; blood uncommon
Complications are similar except:	More anemia and hemorrhage	More malabsorption and stricture
Lesion distribution	Diffuse; more uniform mucosal involvement	Unaffected segments between areas of involvement
Association with cancer	Approx. 5% when disease is active more than 20 years	Approx. 1%

Therapy in IBD involves easing symptoms with antidiarrheal drugs and attempts to limit the disease with anti-inflammatory and immunosuppresive agents. Since there is no known way to undermine the unknown causative mechanism, surgical resection of an affected bowel segment or the entire colon may be necessary in severe cases or if cancer indications arise. Removal of a segment of bowel is often followed by recurrence and exacerbation of symptoms in the remaining sections.

Previously, it was thought that psychological or emotional stress contributed to IBD. Currently, stress is not thought to be causal, but it may intensify signs and symptoms in some ulcerative colitis sufferers.

Ulceration

As indicated at the beginning of this chapter, the process of digestion, which produces the nutrient forms that we can absorb, occurs outside the body in the external space that is the GI lumen (see fig. 13.1). One benefit that derives from this arrangement is the opportunity to use harsh acid and potent enzymes to degrade the large molecules that make up most of our food. Isolating acids and enzymes in the lumen of the tract means that the body fluids and tissues are not disrupted by the extreme conditions tolerated by the GI mucosa's epithelial lining. For example, at its most acidic, the H^+ concentration of gastric juice is about 3 million times that of plasma.

To tolerate such conditions, the stomach and small intestine have an array of protective mechanisms. One is the mucus blanket that coats their epithelial surfaces. Protein and bicarbonate components of this lining are able to reduce acidity so that the immediate epithelial cell environment is much less acidic. Secondly, adjacent epithelial cells are joined by specialized membrane structures called **tight junctions.** These effectively block the diffusion of hydrogen ions back into the submucosa. This is particularly important, given the enormous concentration gradient favoring diffusion of H^+ from the lumen across the mucosa's epithelium. Another factor is the continual sloughing of epithelial cells into the lumen. Any damage the cells do sustain presents little problem, as the injured cells are soon lost and replaced with new, resistant cells.

Taken together, these defenses allow the GI's lining epithelium to stand up to the acid and enzyme challenge it normally confronts. If it is weakened or if the challenge is intensified, the surface epithelium may be overwhelmed. Undefended subepithelial tissues then become exposed to the acid and enzymes, which can digest them as they normally do food. The result is an ulcer (fig. 13.12).

Peptic Ulcers

Since the protein-digesting enzyme pepsin is involved in production of this common ulcer, the term **peptic ulcer** is applied to distinguish it from the other, much less common GI ulcers. For example, the mucosal ulceration that occurs

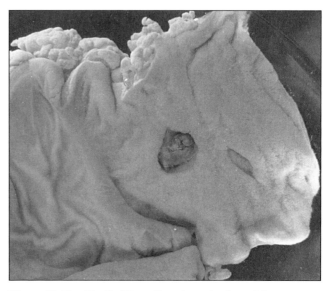

Figure 13.12   **Peptic Ulceration.** A peptic ulcer of the duodenum. Two ulcers are visible in this specimen. The smaller appears to have been healing, but the larger one had eroded an artery, causing massive blood loss.
This segment of duodenum shows the large peptic ulcer that was responsible for the death of an 11-year-old boy. The ulcer had eroded an artery in its base, causing bleeding and hypovolemic shock, which proved fatal. At autopsy, the stomach was found to contain 1.5 liters of blood. The child had an unfortunate history of a lymphoid tumor, which had been effectively treated, as well as liver cirrhosis, which developed from a case of hepatitis B that he had contracted while living in the Orient. These conditions were apparently unrelated to the development of the peptic ulcer.

in ulcerative colitis and Crohn's disease derives from a disease process within the mucosa, as opposed to the peptic ulcer, in which erosion proceeds from the surface.

Peptic ulcers may arise throughout the esophagus, stomach, and small intestine—that is, those sites subjected to the action of the acid and pepsin of the gastric juice. In the esophagus, they are uncommon, but may occur in patients with chronic reflux of gastric juice. They are also much less likely to occur in the jejunum or ileum, most (98%) arising in the stomach and duodenum. They typically arise singly; only 20% of cases involve multiple sites. The size of a peptic ulcer ranges between 1 and 3 cm. Its margin is usually smooth, as opposed to the more irregular pattern seen in ulcers caused by surface disruption from tumors.

The relatively high incidence of peptic ulceration has prompted much examination of its etiology and pathogenesis. Although new insights continue, there still is no definitive description of the process that accounts for all the elements known to play some direct or indirect part in it. Previously, the most widely held view of ulcerogenesis proposed that the less common gastric ulcers were the result of some compromise in mucosal defense mechanisms. Duodenal ulceration was thought to arise because a normal mucosa was exposed to excess gastric juice as a result of gastric hypersecretion and/or too rapid gastric emptying.

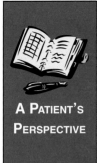

Ulcerative Colitis

". . . every day is a gift"
—Cathy McGee

I have a mild to moderate form of ulcerative colitis. A description of the physical symptoms of ulcerative colitis involves a variety of experiences. Each person might describe it differently, but I can only report how it affects me. When my ulcerative colitis is active, it is a lot like having the flu. It can have a gradual beginning, with just a bit of stomach cramping or the occasional urge to hurry to the bathroom, or it can be more violent, with severe bouts of diarrhea and vomiting. If it progresses without treatment, there is the possibility of blood being present, which can be very scary! Fatigue and exhaustion are constant companions as your body fights to get better, and sometimes a liquid diet to "rest" the bowel as well as bed rest are necessary. So far I have avoided a hospital stay, but that sometimes can't be avoided in severe bouts when the risk of dehydration is present. Eye and joint involvement, an increased likelihood of kidney stones etc. are all part of the struggle in dealing with my disease.

Having ulcerative colitis means, among other things, having more frequent bowel movements, so the bathroom and everything associated with it, quickly becomes a focal point of your life. Your entire day must be planned around the proximity of bathrooms. How exciting, not to mention a boost to your self-image . . . (not really!). Daily experience involves getting up early to "sort yourself out" before work, knowing the location of public washrooms on any outing, and watching what and when you eat.

Over the years you have to deal with lost opportunities for education, fear of making new relationships because they may not withstand the difficult days of your condition, fewer chances to travel, camp out, or just stay over with friends. These are then kinds of things you mourn as having to miss to some degree.

Although a struggle, there are some ways to fight back. Like many with a medical condition, I spend more time, effort, and dollars trying to maintain the best possible health. Extra rest, medication, vitamins, and proper nutrition on a somewhat restricted diet are all part of the battle. Sometimes, when the condition is active, there are bonus treatments like suppositories and retention enemas . . . ugh! There have been several new medications and treatments available in recent years, and as is the case in so many conditions, early and accurate diagnosis is necessary for therapy to be most effective. That's where colonoscopies come in. They are not very pleasant, but are excellent diagnostic aids. They also offer an opportunity for biopsies because of the risk of colon cancer.

Other ways of coping are important to those of us with ulcerative colitis. Most important of these is being able to share your feelings with similarly afflicted people in a support group: those who really understand. A sense of humor is also important, as is relying on the support of family and friends, especially on those really "down" days. Above all hope for the future is of the greatest importance. With hope you feel every day is a gift, another day closer to improved therapies and, ultimately, closer to a cure.

Currently, it is thought that it is more probable that hypersecretion alone is unlikely to produce peptic ulceration, and that impaired defenses permit acid to erode the epithelium.

Impaired Defenses The number of factors known to compromise mucosal defenses against acid and pepsin is growing. The dominant factor is the role of the widely occurring bacterium *Helicobacter pylori*. This organism is thought to predispose to gastric mucosa ulceration by inducing a gastritis that weakens its defenses. The link between peptic ulcers and gastritis induced by *Helicobacter pylori* is quite strong, but in many cases the organism is present in those without ulcers. This finding suggests that other factors may contribute to the breakdown of mucosal defenses and that *Helicobacter pylori* infection may enhance their effects.

A second important factor that predisposes to the weakening of mucosal defenses is the effect of NSAIDs such as aspirin, indomethacin, and phenylbutazone. These widely used agents are known to cause damage and bleeding in the gastric and duodenal mucosae. Superficial erosion of these surfaces exposes deeper layers to acid and pepsin to promote peptic ulceration. NSAIDs also have relevant systemic effects in inhibiting prostaglandin synthesis, because certain prostaglandins contribute to mucosal defenses by promoting secretion of mucus and acid-neutralizing bicarbonate and by maintaining local blood flow.

Gastric Hypersecretion In many patients who suffer from duodenal ulcers, hyperplasia of acid-producing **parietal cells** and pepsin-secreting **chief cells** is typical. In addition, the same patients often demonstrate an exaggerated secretion response to normal levels of stimulus. The excessive gastric wall motility also seen in many such cases increases duodenal exposure to gastric juice. Cigarette smoking is known to be strongly associated with peptic ulcers and seems to operate in two ways that are related. Smoking stimulates gastric acid secretion and inhibits pancreatic production of the bicarbonate ion that neutralizes acid in the small intestine.

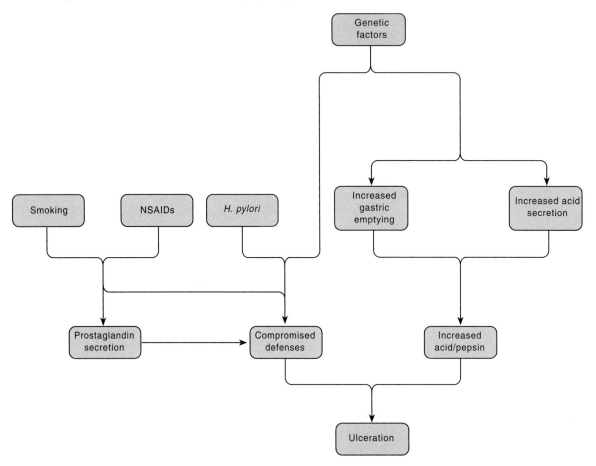

Figure 13.13 **Pathogenesis of Peptic Ulcer Formation.** It should be emphasized that the various contributing factors are more likely to operate in combination than in isolation.

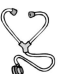

Focus on Spicy Food and Gastric Irritation

Direct viewing of the interior of the digestive tract can be achieved with an **endoscope,** a tubular instrument that is passed through the mouth and esophagus to reach the stomach or duodenum. In experiments to assess the gastric and duodenal effects of various foods and aspirin, subjects were given bland and spicy meals, and a meal with aspirin. The effects on the mucosa were then viewed with an endoscope. The results showed that 11 of 12 subjects suffered no irritation when they ate either bland or spicy (jalapeño peppers, pepperoni) foods. Even when ground jalapeño peppers were inserted into the stomach and placed directly on its lining, no irritation resulted. However, in 11 of the 12 subjects, a bland meal (steak and potatoes) containing aspirin produced pronounced irritation and multiple erosions in the stomach's mucosa.

Those who feel they are under physical or emotional stress also suffer from increased acid secretion.

Since there is a familial tendency to peptic ulceration, genetics likely play a role. The parietal and chief cell hyperplasia that causes hypersecretion is probably genetically determined, and a genetic mucosal vulnerability may also be involved. Similarly, smoking may have an impact in compromising mucosal defenses, as it is known to reduce blood flow and prostaglandin synthesis. The association between peptic ulcers and high alcohol consumption is likely based on alcohol's irritation of the gastric epithelium.

In summary, the pathogenesis of peptic ulcers involves various factors whose effects combine to compromise gastroduodenal defenses. The effects of acid and pepsin can then produce the ulcer, even at normal levels and especially, when acid is hypersecreted. (fig. 13.13).

Incidence and Complications Adult males in the industrialized Western nations who have other family members with peptic ulcers represent the high-risk population. Middle age and beyond are the years of greatest risk, and the male-to-female preponderance is 2 to 1 or even 3 to 1. There is also some evidence suggesting more peptic ulcers in those with hepatic cirrhosis, obstructive lung disorders, and rheumatoid arthritis.

Ulcer sufferers complain of 15 to 60-minute periods of gnawing or burning pain over the **epigastrium,** the central and superior surface of the abdomen. Food intake has varying effects on ulcer pain, which is often dependent on the ulcer's location. Sufferers of duodenal ulceration often report pain onset 30–45 minutes after a meal, with later food intake offering relief. Presumably the initial ingestion of food triggers a secretion response that brings on the pain, then subsequent food intake absorbs the gastric acid to reduce irritation. Many who suffer from gastric ulcers report anorexia and vomiting and often experience weight loss as a result. Food often increases bouts of epigastric pain in these individuals. Aspirin has the effect of intensifying the epigastric ache, presumably through its blocking of prostoglandin formation.

In uncomplicated peptic ulcer disease, patients are otherwise normal. The condition is chronic, and episodes of recurrence are separated by varying time intervals. Most peptic ulcers are resolved by healing that involves epithelial, but not glandular, regeneration and scarring in the submucosa and deeper layers. Healing is typically slower in the stomach because of its high acid levels.

Complications are uncommon, but 20% of patients suffer ulcer-related bleeding. Normally only small blood loss occurs, but if the ulcer penetrates deeply enough to erode an artery, severe bleeding and circulatory shock may result. Seriously bleeding peptic ulcers have a mortality of about 10%.

Perforation of the stomach or duodenal wall may also occur, introducing the threat of peritonitis. Involvement of the nearby pancreas can also induce acute pancreatitis (see chapter 14). Mortality is high if perforation occurs, particularly with involvement of the gastric wall.

Gastric obstruction may also complicate peptic ulcer disease. The obstruction typically involves the gastric outlet at the pylorus, where ulcers may induce muscle spasm or hypertrophy. Healing may also contribute to obstruction if stricture follows scarring.

Therapy in Peptic Ulcer Disease With recognition of the role of *H. pylori* in peptic ulceration, antibiotic therapy has come into wider use. Relief from the ulcer often follows eradication of the organism. Effective therapeutic support for antibiotic therapy involves the diet and control of acid secretion. The assumption is that if acidity is reduced and irritants are avoided, healing will follow. Previously, ulcer patients were advised to eat bland diets and consume milk or cream regularly. In fact, this regimen is unnecessary (indeed, milk products may stimulate acid secretion), and any diet that does not aggravate ulcer pain is acceptable. Usually, patients soon recognize the irritation and pain associated with coffee, any acid stimulus, or casual NSAID use, and restrict their intake.

Table 13.2	Some Side Effects Associated with the Use of Selected H_2 Receptor Antagonists
Agent	**Side Effects**
Cimetidine	Mental confusion, diarrhea, hepatitis, pancreatitis, impotence
Famotidine	Headache, insomnia, diarrhea, constipation, anorexia, impotence
Ranitidine	Headache, dizziness, cardiac arrhythmias, diarrhea, constipation, hepatitis

In reducing acid levels to limit ulceration and promote healing, two approaches are taken. In one, antacids are used to neutralize existing acid. Many low-cost and effective agents are available; hence, this is the most widely used therapy. An increasingly popular second approach suppresses acid secretion by interfering with a normal histamine stimulus to the parietal cells. Antihistamine drugs that belong to a class called **H_2-receptor antagonists** are employed in this task. The more common antihistamines affect the H_1 receptors that histamine activates to promote vascular and bronchial constriction, but histamine also activates H_2 receptors. This group of receptors stimulates acid secretion in the stomach. H_2-receptor antagonists selectively inhibit this and reduce gastric acidity, allowing more rapid ulcer healing. Note that in some individuals these agents can produce significant side effects (table 13.2).

In severe cases of chronic ulceration that resists therapy, surgery may be indicated. Surgery may involve sectioning the vagus nerve by which the CNS stimulus to acid secretion reaches the stomach. This procedure is now used less frequently, since H_2 blocker therapy can achieve smaller benefits with less risk and cost. In extreme cases, surgical removal of the affected portion of the stomach may be required.

Stress Ulcers

These gastric ulcers may represent a form of severe, acute gastritis. The term **stress ulcers** relates to their occurrence in response to a wide variety of acute systemic stresses. They are usually multiple and smaller than peptic ulcers. They arise following severe trauma—for example, automobile accidents, falls or crushing injuries, CNS damage, or extensive skin burns. Serious illness, generally, can also induce stress ulcers, as can bacterial infections that spread through the blood (septicemia). Cardiovascular shock, in relation to these conditions or due to other causes, also promotes the development of stress ulcers.

Mucosal disruption in stress ulcers is linked to mucosal ischemia that develops secondary to a widespread

Table 13.3   Major Causes of Upper and Lower Gastrointestinal Bleeding

	Cause	Incidence
Upper GI bleeding	Erosive gastritis/duodenitis	$9x$
	Duodenal peptic ulcer	$7x$
	Esophageal varices	$5x$
	Peptic/gastric ulcer	$4x$
	Mallory-Weiss laceration	$2x$
	Carcinoma	x
Lower GI bleeding	Colon cancer	$8x$
	Benign polyps	$4x$
	Diverticulitis	$2x$
	Inflammatory bowel disease	x

Relative incidence is expressed in terms of a base unit, x, which has an approximate value of 3%.
The level of the duodenum is the commonly used line of demarcation between the upper and lower regions of the GI tract.

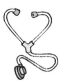

Focus on Meckel's Diverticulum

Meckel's diverticulum is a congenital malformation of the ileum consisting of an elongated (up to 6 cm) pouch. It occurs in only about 1–2% of the population and is clinically insignificant except for the few cases in which it undergoes peptic ulceration and perforates.

vasoconstriction response or to hypotension related to circulatory shock. The reduced mucosal blood flow weakens defenses or damages the mucosa, and gastric acid is able to produce widespread surface erosions.

Typically, stress ulcers are asymptomatic and present minimal difficulties, especially in the context of the generally severe systemic conditions with which they are associated. Mild bleeding may occur, but only rarely is hemorrhage a problem. Perforation of the wall is also rare, but when it does occur, the duodenum is the usual site.

Gastrointestinal Bleeding

Blood loss into the GI lumen may be indicated by the presence of blood in vomitus or feces. The vomiting of blood (**hematemesis**) is typically associated with gastric or esophageal bleeding. Gastric ulceration, peptic or otherwise, may be the source of the blood. It might also originate at a laceration of the gastroesophageal junction, as in the Mallory-Weiss syndrome described earlier, in the Vomiting section.

When blood spends some time in the stomach before being vomited, gastric acid and enzymes alter it, producing a dark, granular material resembling coffee grounds. Blood lost directly into the small intestine, or reaching it from a gastric lesion, is similarly darkened. It affects the stool, producing a darker, tarlike coloration. This condition is called **melena.** Bleeding peptic ulcers are the most common cause of such blood loss into the stomach and small intestine.

Bleeding from the colon's wall usually appears bright red in the stool, since the blood is not exposed to acid or enzymes to any significant degree. Diverticulitis is the common cause of colonic hemorrhage. Of course, at all levels of the GI tract, surface erosion by a benign or malignant tumor can produce bleeding. Table 13.3 indicates the relative frequency of the principal sources of upper and lower GI blood loss.

In cases of GI bleeding, the source is often difficult to determine. Assessment of the patient's stool or vomitus may provide information based on coloration and the obvious presence of blood, but these can be confusing. For example, when blood is lost rapidly from an upper GI site, it may be darkened only slightly, so that when seen in the stool it suggests colonic bleeding.

Long-term bleeding of smaller quantities of blood may not be detected in the stool on casual inspection by the affected person. The presence of a low-grade anemia may be evidence of the slow bleeding, and confirmation can be had by laboratory analysis of a stool sample to detect **occult** (hidden) **blood.** At the other extreme, acute hemorrhage may be so severe that it is immediately life-threatening, requiring emergency treatment to avoid circulatory shock.

Therapy for episodes of acute GI bleeding is not usually necessary, since it tends to be self-limiting. If the bleeding is acute and severe, fluid replacement therapy to restore and stabilize blood volume and to counter hypovolemic shock may be necessary. Beyond such an immediate threat, therapy must be directed to the underlying problem.

Obstruction

Restriction or blockage of the movement of chyme along the GI tract is referred to as **ileus.** If a physical blockage is responsible, the condition is usually described as a mechanical obstruction, or mechanical ileus. If peristalsis stops, it is described as adynamic ileus.

Mechanical Obstruction

Mechanical blockage of the GI tract may result from an internally obstructing mass (e.g., a swallowed foreign object or colon tumor), from compression or distortion of the bowel (usually the small intestine), or from a congenital malformation. Although uncommon, a congenitally narrowed or closed esophagus can present an obstruction to the swallowing of food, and **congenital pyloric stenosis** (narrowing of the stomach's opening to the duodenum) may limit gastric emptying. Surgery in early childhood is usually necessary to cope with such inborn obstructive malformations.

A malignant tumor or benign polyp may physically block the GI lumen (see fig. 6.24b). Most such growths occur in the colon as adenomas or carcinomas of the sigmoid colon and rectum. Tumors that metastasize to the colon may also mechanically obstruct its lumen. Swallowed foreign objects that can act as obstructions are highly varied. Virtually any object that fits into the mouth and resists breakdown by gastric acid has the potential for obstructing the tract. Children are particularly at risk. Tangles of roundworms or other parasites, though not swallowed, can also be considered as obstructing foreign objects. The obstruction of the esophagus by dilated veins is described in relation to cirrhosis of the liver in chapter 14.

Various abnormalities can produce obstructive distortion or compression of the GI tract, with the small intestine often involved. The most common is herniation of a loop of small intestine through the abdominal wall. This condition is usually seen at points where the scrotum is continuous with the abdominal cavity (the inguinal canal), at the umbilicus, or at weakened surgical scars. In uncomplicated herniation, the loop of bowel may be easily drawn back into the abdominal cavity (reduced). If reduction is not promptly achieved, compression of the loop of intestine at the point of herniation can obstruct the passage of chyme (fig. 13.14). (Note that hiatal hernia, described earlier, does not usually produce obstruction effects.) Beyond its obstructive effects, if compression at the point of herniation is severe enough to collapse the vessels that supply and drain the herniated loop, **strangulation** of the bowel results. In such cases, the resulting ischemic injury can produce necrosis and gangrene, adding the risk of perforation and peritonitis to the problems associated with bowel obstruction.

Healing complications following bouts of peritonitis or abdominal surgery can also produce bowel obstruction. Most often involved are adhesions that form between abdominal organs and the abdominal wall. If a loop of bowel is joined to the wall by an adhesion, it may kink to form a narrowed point (fig. 13.15a). Adhesions can also contribute to obstruction by abnormally isolating regions in which an adjacent bowel loop may then become trapped (fig. 13.15b).

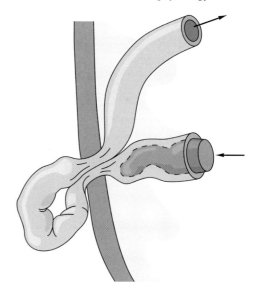

Figure 13.14   Obstruction from Herniation. Herniation of a loop of small intestine through a weak spot in the abdominal wall. In such cases, if strangulation occurs, the complications of ischemic injury may be added to those of obstruction.

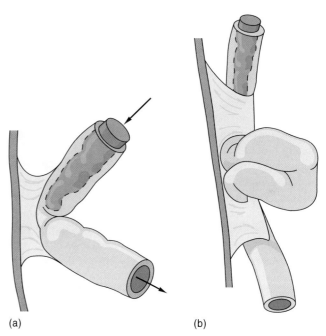

(a)   (b)

Figure 13.15   Adhesion Complications. Obstruction can follow adhesion formation. (a) An adhesion causes a kink that narrows the lumen. (b) Adhesions between a bowel loop and the abdominal wall form an opening in which another loop can become trapped and compressed.

Another complication of healing ulcers, or of intestinal surgery, is contracture of fibrous tissue at the site of healing, which can produce a stricture that obstructs the bowel (fig. 13.16).

In North America, most GI tract obstructions are caused by herniation, adhesions, or primary tumors. Much less frequently, **volvulus** is involved. In this condition, a

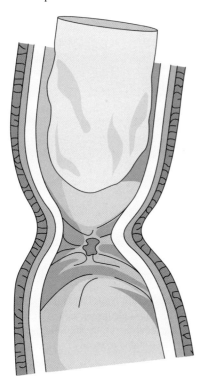

Figure 13.16 **Stricture of the Intestine.** Contracture of scar tissue at the site of a healing peptic ulcer has produced this obstruction. Inflammation, trauma, or tumors may all produce stricture.

loop of large or small intestine rotates around its supporting mesentery, compressing the lumen, which becomes completely blocked at the point of twisting (fig. 13.17). More importantly, the twisting compresses the arteries and veins in the mesentery. Strangulation and the risk of necrosis and perforation are typical consequences.

An even less common bowel obstruction problem is **intussusception.** The problem here is the telescoping of a segment of small intestine into the immediately distal portion of the bowel. This condition may arise at the ileocecal junction, where the ileum projects into the cecum, or at sites where a polyp or other mass is present within the lumen. The essential mechanism is based on peristaltic contractions that force the mass, and the wall from which it projects, into the immediately distal intestinal segment. As peristalsis continues, the segment's mesentery is dragged along. The compression of a bowel segment within an adjacent section of intestine blocks its lumen. Involvement of the mesentery threatens compression of its vessels to introduce the risk of infarction and gangrene (fig. 13.18).

Adynamic Ileus

This is a functional GI tract disorder that involves a loss of motility in the intestines. Two types are usually identified: **paralytic ileus** and **vascular ileus.**

Paralytic ileus involves a neurogenic reflex that halts normal intestinal motility. It is triggered by various abdom-

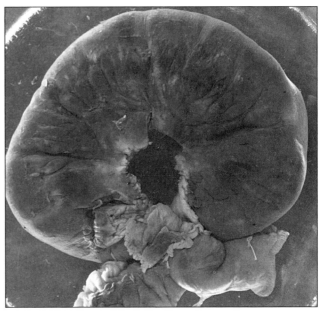

Figure 13.17 **Volvulus.** Twisting of a loop of intestine and its mesentery has caused an obstruction. The segment isolated by the twist is distended and darkened in comparison to the lighter sections adjacent to the twist.

An elderly male came to a hospital emergency room complaining that he had awakened at night with intense abdominal cramping pain. There were no signs of an acute abdomen, but he vomited once following his admission. Blood studies revealed no indication of infection; however, an enema showed the presence of blood in the stool. His symptoms intensified and an exploratory abdominal operation (laparotomy) was performed. It revealed the 12-in loop of bowel shown here. The segment had become twisted, and was swollen, thick-walled, and hemorrhagic, with the outer surface covered in a fibrinous exudate. Bowel segments adjacent to the volvulus had a normal appearance. With resection of the damaged section, recovery was uneventful.

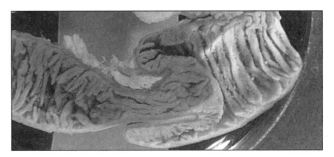

Figure 13.18 **Intussusception.** A section through the region where a segment of small intestine has been drawn, by peristalsis, (from the left) into the immediately adjacent distal segment (on the right).

An abrupt episode of abdominal distention, severe cramping pain, and vomiting was diagnosed as intestinal obstruction and an emergency laparotomy was performed. The section of small intestine shown here was found. The intussusception had compressed the veins of the bowel and its mesentery, causing congestion, hemorrhage, and the risk of gangrene. The situation could not be corrected by drawing out the affected region to straighten it, and it had to be removed.

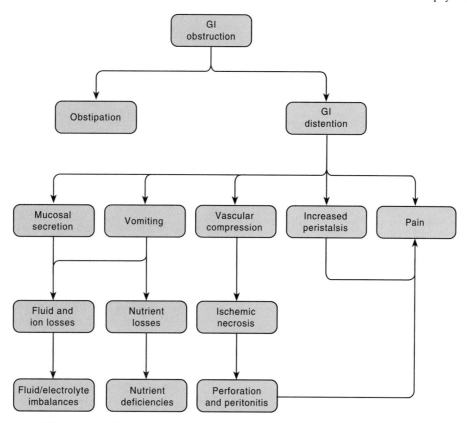

Figure 13.19   **Sequelae of Obstruction.** The potential derangements that can arise as a consequence of GI obstruction.

inal stimuli such as pain, peritonitis, appendicitis, trauma, or acute distention of an abdominal organ. Paralytic ileus also frequently accompanies certain systemic conditions such as infections or renal disease, and those involving electrolyte imbalances, especially potassium deficiencies.

In vascular ileus, the failure to sustain normal motility is due to a compromised blood supply. Thrombosis, atherosclerosis, or compression of the mesenteric vessels that supply the intestines is usually the underlying cause. Beyond the immediate problem of focal loss of motility, this condition carries the risk of infection, necrosis, and gangrene.

Sequelae of Obstruction

GI obstruction is associated with four clinical features that may vary with the degree of obstruction and its location: vomiting, abdominal distention, pain, and **obstipation** (lack of fecal or gas evacuation, due to obstruction).

Vomiting is the response to obstruction in the upper GI tract, especially from stricture at sites of gastric or duodenal peptic ulcer healing. The vomiting reflex is triggered by distention as food accumulates proximal to the point of obstruction. Vomiting in such cases is often persistent, with large volumes of undigested food expelled from the tract. When the blockage is in the proximal small intestine, its contents may reflux back to the stomach, with bile appearing in the vomitus. The consequences of persistent vomiting are as would be expected: fluid loss leading to dehydra-

tion, electrolyte imbalance as needed ions are lost in the vomitus, and the loss of nutrients.

When obstruction occurs in the lower GI tract, vomiting is less able to clear backed-up lumen contents. The consequence is intestinal distention, as parts of the GI tract proximal to the obstruction dilate to accommodate the increased volume. Obvious abdominal bloating results, as does cramping pain from the pronounced peristaltic waves that drive the lumen's contents to the point of blockage. The pain can be quite severe, with peak intensity associated with waves of peristaltic contraction.

With progressively increasing intestinal distention and no intervention, bouts of severe vomiting may occur even when the obstruction is situated in the distal small bowel or colon. In these cases, backup of lumen contents prevents small intestine and gastric emptying, and the severity of the resultant vomiting may yield fecal material in the vomitus.

In cases of colon obstruction, stasis favors bacterial proliferation and thereby increases the possibility of bowel necrosis, perforation, peritonitis and more widespread infection. The sequelae of GI obstruction are presented in figure 13.19.

Malabsorption

The problem of inadequate absorption of nutrients, **malabsorption,** may be generalized, affecting most nutrients, or it may be specific to a particular nutrient—for example,

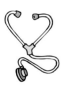

Focus on Paralytic Ileus and Bowel Sounds

The intestinal response to the trauma of abdominal surgery, or to associated general anesthesia, is paralytic ileus. It usually lasts for two to three days, and then normal bowel motility patterns are spontaneously restored. The restoration of bowel activity is accompanied by characteristic bubbling and gurgling sounds that can be easily detected with a stethoscope. A delay in the return of normal bowel sounds may indicate a complication. In cases of mechanical bowel obstruction, bowel sounds are typically intensified as chyme is forced past the blockage by strong peristaltic waves.

---

vitamin B_{12}. Malabsorption conditions may be mild and of short duration, or more severe and chronic. They are the result of three essential defects: of digestion, of absorption, and of transit across the intestinal mucosa.

Defective Digestion

Since absorption requires that the digestion process convert nutrients to molecules that can be easily absorbed, it is clear that interference with digestion will lead to malabsorption. Most commonly, defective digestion is due to lack of pancreatic enzymes or bile, in severe pancreas or liver failure, respectively. Obstruction of the bile or pancreatic ducts produces similar effects. Bile insufficiency may also arise following surgical resection of the ileum, the site of bile salt absorption and recycling via the liver, or in conditions involving bacterial overgrowth in the small intestine. Factors that impede normal intestinal motion, such as an obstruction or paralytic ileus, can have this effect. Bacterial metabolism alters bile salts and makes them much less likely to be recycled, thus producing a bile deficiency. They can also enhance osmotic water movement to the intestinal lumen to produce diarrhea.

Defective digestion might also be due to a resection of part of the stomach and/or small intestine and the surgical rejoining of the remaining structures. The resulting problems are caused by inadequate digestive processing by the resected regions and by the loss of their normal contribution to the feedback control mechanisms that regulate the process.

Defective Absorption

The small intestine's major adaptations to absorption are its very large surface area and its epithelial transport and enzyme systems. Any interference with these compromises the absorptive capabilities of the small bowel, and malabsorption results.

Loss of surface area may be due to resection of an intestinal tumor or to extensive intestinal trauma. Specific disease states may also reduce surface area by damaging or infiltrating the mucosa. Relatively mild and transient malabsorption may accompany enteritis from whatever cause. The following are conditions in which the results of malabsorption are clinically prominent.

Most clinically significant malabsorption problems in North America involve **gluten-sensitive enteropathy** (GSE), also known as **celiac sprue** or **celiac disease.** The underlying problem is immune-mediated damage to intestinal epithelia that results in loss of villi and compromised absorption. Those affected react to gluten, the protein component of wheat, rye, and barley. The reason for this sensitivity to gluten seems to have a genetic component and a link to early childhood viral infection. It may be that components of the virus to which the immune system responds have a structural similarity to gluten, so after the usually subclinical infection, exposure to dietary gluten triggers the immune system's attack on the epithelial cells involved in its absorption. The genetic role is unclear and may involve susceptibility to an immune system defect or to the viral infection. Elimination of gluten from the diet gradually restores intestinal structure, and more normal absorption soon follows. Sufferers of celiac sprue have an increased incidence of a particular tumor: **primary intestinal lymphoma.**

Tropical sprue also produces flattening of the villi, but in this condition an infection is the cause. Most tropical sprue responds well to antibiotic therapy. As the name implies, this disease occurs primarily in the tropics.

Mucosal surface loss due to inflammatory cell infiltration is responsible for the malabsorption associated with Crohn's disease, described earlier, and **Whipple's disease,** a rare, systemic infectious condition characterized by mucosal infiltration by bacteria-filled macrophages. Malabsorption may also be caused by absent or defective membrane enzyme systems, which compromise digestion (usually genetic defects involving the intestinal disaccharidases lactase, sucrase, or maltase.) These are relatively rare conditions, as are the genetic defects that produce malabsorption as a result of loss of membrane transport systems specific to carbohydrate or amino acid absorption.

Transit Defects

Even if digestion and absorption occur, transport of absorbed nutrients via lymph and blood to systemic utilization sites is still required. Any conditions that compromise this transit will cause a deficiency, as if absorption had not occurred. For this reason, such conditions are regarded as malabsorption syndromes. Two examples of diseases that compromise lymph flow, and therefore transit of lipids, are Whipple's disease and **lymphangiectasia.** In Whipple's disease, the pronounced macrophage infiltration of the mucosa compresses its lacteals and other small lymphatics to obstruct lymph flow. In lymphangiectasia, lymph obstruc-

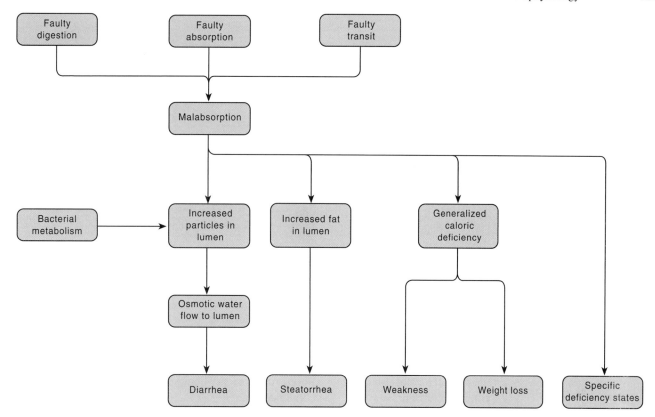

Figure 13.20   **Pathogenesis of GI Malabsorption.**

tion is due to lymph channels that are narrowed or closed. This rare condition is idiopathic.

Another genetic defect reduces lipid transit from the intestinal epithelium because of the lack of beta-lipoproteins. Without these, chylomicrons cannot be formed and absorbed fat is confined to the epithelial cells, which become engorged. This rare condition is called **abetalipoproteinemia.**

Sequelae of Malabsorption

The signs and symptoms associated with malabsorption states reflect the deficiencies that such states produce and the intestinal disturbances that are often present. In generalized malabsorption states, an overall caloric deficiency typically produces weakness, weight loss, fatigue, and variable anorexia. Particular deficiencies may give rise to specific systemic problems, such as coagulation disorders resulting from a lack of vitamin K, anemia resulting from a vitamin B$_{12}$ deficiency, or abnormal muscle function resulting from a lack of calcium.

Steatorrhea, excessive fat in the stool, is often seen in malabsorption states. The excess of fat is due, in part, to its lack of uptake from the intestinal lumen, but to another reason if digestion is defective. In such cases, lack of adequate caloric intake triggers an increased appetite, which brings more fat-containing food into the lumen, and it passes to the colon undigested and unabsorbed. If malabsorption is due to an intestinal defect, anorexia is more often present, and steatorrhea may be characterized by

large volumes of foul-smelling feces that float because of their intestinal gas content. A patient's first indication of a problem may be difficulty in flushing bulky, floating stools from the toilet.

Diarrhea is often present in malabsorption states. It may be the direct result of inadequate water absorption or the indirect result of the underlying malabsorption. When lumen solute concentration is high, osmotic water movement into the lumen follows. Such concentration increases may be due to the accumulation of nutrient molecules that can't be absorbed, or to products of bacterial action, if stasis fosters their proliferation. During digestion, much albumin, a small and plentiful plasma protein, is secreted into the intestinal lumen; but if it can't be digested and reabsorbed, it contributes to the lumen's osmotic pressure and aggravates the predisposition to diarrhea. These factors are summarized in figure 13.20.

Gastrointestinal Tumors

The most common tumors of the GI tract are carcinomas, arising, in order of frequency, in the colon, stomach, esophagus, and small intestine. Their typical effects are pain, obstruction, and bleeding where tumor growth breaks through the mucosal surface. Metastasis by blood and lymph is common but may be delayed, so early detection is important.

Benign adenomas are also common in the GI tract, principally in the stomach and colon. Such growths may be broad-based or may project into the lumen, supported by a

✓ *Checkpoint 13.3*

In many GI conditions, peristaltic hyperactivity, excessive gas or fluid volume, or various distortions of the tract produce easily detectable sounds as the GI wall propels and churns its contents. The term *bowel sounds* is most often used to describe these rumblings and splashings (see the Focus box that refers to the restoration of bowel sounds in paralytic ileus). In more formal medical writings, you may well encounter the equivalent term **borborygmus** (plural, *borborygmi*) instead of the term "bowel sounds." Both terms have the same meaning. If you don't come across the formal term in your reading, it can at least serve as a useful addition to your cocktail party conversation grab-bag.

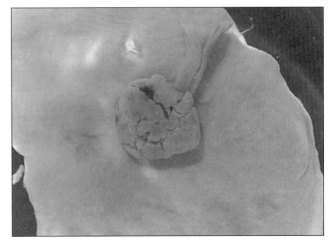

Figure 13.21   A Pedunculated Adenoma of the Colon. This polyp was found at the autopsy of an elderly man who had died of the cumulative effects of a colon carcinoma that had metastasized extensively, especially affecting the lungs and liver. The pedunculated adenoma shown here was found in the colon. Although, the adenoma was benign, it may well be that the fatal carcinoma developed from such a small, innocent-appearing mass.

stalk—a **pedunculated polyp** (fig. 13.21). Benign pedunculated tumors have a predisposition to bleeding. In the colon, an adenoma may have fingerlike extensions that resemble intestinal villi. This is a **villous adenoma.**

In some adenomatous polyps of the colon, malignant cells may arise. Their more rapid growth dominates to produce an invasive adenocarcinoma. It is thought that most colon cancers arise in this way. Currently, improved technique and instrumentation provides for easy and safe polyp removal in a **colonoscopy.** No surgical access through the abdominal wall is required for this procedure, which is routinely used to remove colon polyps. The term **hyperplastic**

polyp refers to the benign colon polyp that does not become malignant.

A rare genetic defect of the colon involves multiple adenomatous polyps associated with a high risk of colon carcinoma. This condition is known as **familial polyposis coli** (FPC). The problem of multiple polyp growth in the colon may not emerge until as late as age 30, with an average of 1,000 polyps present in those affected. The risk of cancer is sufficiently strong that complete resection of the colon may be necessary in FPC.

Case Study

A hospital emergency room received a 23-year-old male with complaints of severe diarrhea, abdominal cramping, nausea, and "just not feeling too good." He reported that similar symptoms had been present for the past ten days, but the intensity of the current bout of symptoms had frightened him and he felt the ER was a better choice than his regular doctor.

His history revealed no significant previous illness except for a similar, milder GI attack six months prior, as well as periodic episodes of mild diarrhea, which he diagnosed as "allergies to all the stuff they put in food these days," but for which he'd sought no medical help. His temperature was mildly elevated (37.9°), he had a slight tachycardia, and his blood pressure was normal. His right lower quadrant was tender on palpation, and rebound tenderness was present. Bowel sounds were normal. Blood tests indicated a reduced hemoglobin of 11 g/dl and an increased WBC count.

The young man was admitted with a possible diagnosis of acute appendicitis. A general surgeon agreed with the diagnosis and the patient was scheduled for surgery.

During the operation the appendix appeared only mildly hyperemic and no other abnormalities were noted, except for some mild swelling in a few mesenteric lymph nodes. A routine appendectomy was performed, and the patient's recovery was uneventful. Subsequent microscopic study revealed the appendix to have been normal. The patient was discharged after three days.

After six weeks he reported to his GP that his symptoms had returned after going back to his normal solid food diet. He also complained of feeling fatigued and reported weight loss since the operation. He was examined and found to be tender in the lower right quadrant as before. A rectal examination revealed additional sensitivity, and blood was noted in the stool.

Blood tests showed WBC counts increased and Hb decreased (9 g/dl) with respect to their previous levels. Urinalysis and blood tests were normal, and blood and urine cultures for bacteria and parasites were negative. A lower GI radiographic study revealed a normal ileal lumen except for a 6-cm segment that demonstrated pronounced stenosis.

On the basis of these observations, a tentative diagnosis of Crohn's disease was made, and the patient was referred to a gastroenterologist. Following an endoscopic study of the ileum, she confirmed the diagnosis and prescribed prednisone in a tapering dose for six weeks. This regimen proved successful in alleviating the acute symptoms.

Over the next two years the patient experienced several repetitions of the same signs and symptoms, with periodic hospitalizations during which he was fed by an intravenous line to rest the bowel. This total parenteral nutrition (TPN) increasingly frustrated the patient, who opted for surgical resection of the affected ileal segment. He was advised of the likelihood of recurrence, but accepted the risk and proceeded with the surgery.

At operation the affected bowel segment was respected and the adjacent edges of the normal ileum were joined (an end-to-end anastomosis). Postoperative recovery was uneventful, and the patient was discharged. Follow-ups at 3, 6, 9, and 12 months found him well and without symptoms.

Commentary

This is an example of the difficulties present in the assessment of abdominal signs and symptoms. Had the patient noticed his rectal bleeding, the appendectomy might have been avoided, but the small quantity of blood involved was easily missed. The dangers associated with perforation in acute appendicitis justify appendectomy on what may seem inadequate evidence, but the general opinion among surgeons is that if a high percentage of removed appendices aren't later found to be normal, surgery is being delayed too long.

Initial diagnostic testing in acute abdominal attacks seeks to establish the absence of infection before other diagnoses are considered—hence, the blood and urine studies and stool cultures. The episodes of exacerbation and remission illustrated in this case are unfortunately typical of Crohn's disease. The sufferer must avoid any irritation to the intestine that might trigger further episodes, but often there is no apparent reason for a renewed attack.

Key Concepts

1. Vomiting and diarrhea expel excessive or irritating GI contents and are usually minimally disruptive, unless prolonged or severe, in which case serious systemic consequences may result (p. 345).

2. Various factors other than GI wall irritation can induce vomiting by means of the effects of circulating substances on the chemoreceptor trigger zone (pp. 345–346).

3. Acute inflammation of the GI mucosa is common, usually only moderately disruptive, and readily healed, although serious postinflammation complications may arise in some cases (pp. 349–351).

4. The pathogenesis of acute appendicitis often involves obstruction by a fecalith, which promotes bacterial growth and the threat of gangrene and wall rupture (pp. 351–352).

5. Rupture of an abdominal organ is a common cause of peritonitis, which can in turn give rise to abscess formation, perforation, fistulae, or generalized peritonitis, with its threat of widespread and serious damage (pp. 352–353).

6. Diverticulosis is relatively common and may be asymptomatic, but in diverticulitis, pain, bleeding, or constipation may result. If the walls of the diverticula are irritated, inflammation and rupture may give rise to peritonitis (pp. 353–354).

7. Although of essentially different pathogenesis, Crohn's disease and ulcerative colitis are both characterized by abdominal cramping, diarrhea, and fever, causing them to be included together under the clinical designation inflammatory bowel disease (IBD) (p. 354).

8. The GI wall's defenses against the lumen's acid and enzymes may be weakened to allow formation of a peptic ulcer, usually in the stomach or duodenum (pp. 356–357).

9. The bacterium *Helicobacter pylori* directly or indirectly contributes to the weakening of GI mucosal defenses in most peptic ulcer formation (p. 357).

10. Bleeding into the GI lumen is often revealed in vomitus or feces, but the precise site of the wall damage may be difficult to determine without special diagnostic procedures, such as endoscopy (p. 360).

11. Interference with peristalsis may be the result of mechanical blockage of the GI tract by an internally obstructing mass, external compression, or a congenital malformation (pp. 360–362).

12. Consequences similar to those produced by mechanical obstruction may be the result of a cessation of tract motility that is due to neurogenic disturbances or compromised blood supply (pp. 362–365).

13. GI obstruction is associated with four clinical features determined by the location and degree of obstruction: vomiting, abdominal distention, pain, and obstipation (p. 363).

14. Malabsorption arises principally from defects of digestion, absorption, or nutrient transit from the intestinal mucosa, and may be generalized or specific to a particular nutrient (pp. 363–365).

15. GI tumors may produce pain, obstruction, or bleeding, and, if malignant, may metastasize by both blood and lymph (p. 365).

REVIEW ACTIVITIES

1. Explain why, in eliciting the vomiting reflex, the CTZ's blood supply is more important than its nervous input, and why the opposite case is true for the medulla's vomiting center.

2. Construct a flow chart that ends with the words "Bowel Evacuation." Have it begin with four types of laxative, and include the essential features of the action of each.

3. Refer to pages 349–356 to compile a list of irritants known to cause GI inflammation.

4. Having been told that IBD is involved, and given a single clinical feature to go on, as listed here, determine in each case whether the disease is more likely to be ulcerative colitis or Crohn's disease.

Clinical Feature	UC/Crohn's?
Superficial mucosal ulceration	_____
Only colon involved	_____
Acute onset	_____
Affected and normal regions in same bowel segment	_____
No blood in stool	_____
Granulomas present	_____

5. Test your knowledge of GI ulceration by listing the key points of its pathogenesis. (Don't forget to mention *H. pylori.*) Check figure 13.13 to be sure you've left nothing important off your list.

6. Your aunt Harriet phones to say that she lost the dietary suggestions her doctor gave her after her peptic ulcer was diagnosed. She wants to know if a soothing glass of milk before bed would be a good idea. She also wonders how her prescribed H_2-receptor antagonist works. Decide how you should respond to each question.

7. Make up a ready reference chart showing specific causes of malabsorption and its specific sequelae.

Chapter

14

Hepatobiliary and Pancreatic Pathophysiology

All seems infected that the infected spy,
As all looks yellow to the jaundiced eye.

ALEXANDER POPE
AN ESSAY ON CRITICISM

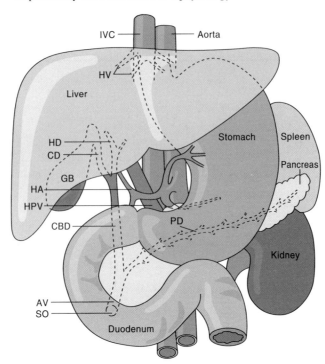

Figure 14.1   **The Hepatobiliary System.** The liver receives blood via the hepatic artery (HA) and the hepatic portal vein (HPV), which drains the GI tract. Blood leaves the liver via the hepatic veins (HV) to reach the inferior vena cava (IVC). The hepatic duct (HD) and cystic duct (CD) form the common bile duct (CBD), which carries bile from the liver and gall bladder (GB). Other structures to note: hepatic duct (HD), cystic duct (CD), pancreatic duct (PD), ampulla of Vater (AV), sphincter of Oddi (SO).

The liver and pancreas are the principal accessory organs of the digestive system. For this reason, and because pancreatic disorders can cause hepatic disturbances, and vice versa, the two organs are considered together in this chapter, beginning with the liver.

The hepatocyte's remarkable metabolic capabilities make a vital contribution to several of the body's critical functions. Damage to the liver or its associated bile system causes a wide variety of physiological disturbances. These may be short-lived and relatively benign, or so serious as to be life-threatening. In either case, such large numbers of people suffer from the effects of some form of liver failure that it constitutes a major medical threat. Before discussing the pathogenesis of the different forms of liver failure, we'll first describe normal liver structure and function.

STRUCTURE OF THE LIVER AND BILE SYSTEM

The liver is situated in the superior extreme of the right abdominal quadrant. It is the largest of the body's internal organs, contributing about 2% of body weight. It consists of two principal lobes: a large right lobe and a much smaller left lobe, which extends somewhat beyond the midline. Liver cells utilize their elaborate metabolic capabilities to chemically alter various of the substances they take up from the blood. Large metabolic capacity is therefore consistent with the enormous volume of blood that flows

through the liver: 1.5 liters per minute, the equivalent of about 2,000 liters per day. The liver has a dual blood supply involving both the arterial and the venous systems. The hepatic artery (fig. 14.1) provides about one-third of total hepatic flow. (The hepatic artery is a branch of the celiac artery, which in turn arises from the aorta.) The remaining two-thirds of the liver's blood flow comes to it by way of the hepatic portal vein, a large vein that receives blood from the veins that drain the spleen, pancreas, stomach, and intestines. This arrangement provides for the direct delivery to the liver of newly absorbed nutrients instead of their being dispersed in the general circulation. This quick access to substances absorbed from the intestine provides for their prompt and efficient metabolism. The portal blood also provides over 50% of the liver's oxygen supply. After passing through the liver, blood is returned to the inferior vena cava (IVC) by the hepatic veins. These usually consist of two or three larger and several smaller vessels.

Within the liver, blood passes from the portal vein's branches to a complex of fine blood channels called **sinusoids.** These are thin-walled vessels like capillaries, but they are somewhat larger and more permeable. The hepatic artery's branches also supply arterial blood to the sinusoids, where it mixes with portal venous blood. After flowing through the sinusoids, blood enters the central veins, which deliver blood to the hepatic veins and then to the inferior vena cava (fig. 14.2). Adjacent to the sinusoids are rows of hepatocytes, each having one surface directly

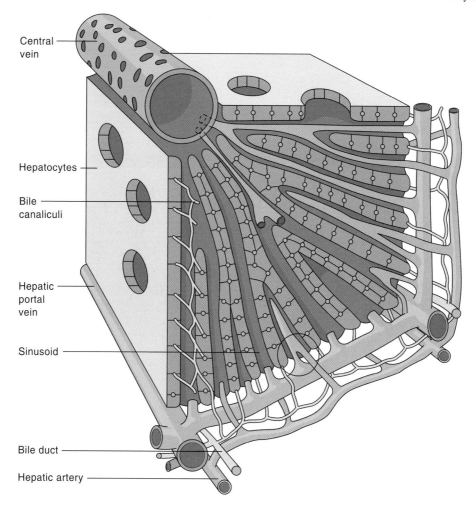

Central vein

Hepatocytes

Bile canaliculi

Hepatic portal vein

Sinusoid

Bile duct

Hepatic artery

Figure 14.2 **Liver Histology.** Plates of hepatocytes lie parallel to the hepatic sinusoids. These fine vessels carry a mixture of blood from the hepatic portal vein and the hepatic artery. The circle indicates the point where the two blood sources join to supply the sinusoid. Hepatocytes pass bile into the tiny bile canaliculi and then to the larger bile ducts.

abutting the thin space that surrounds the sinusoid walls (fig. 14.3). This arrangement allows the hepatocytes to absorb from, or secrete into, the sinusoidal blood directly. In this way, substances arriving via the portal vein can pass from the sinusoids to the liver cells, where their metabolism proceeds. Products of metabolism can then be secreted into the sinusoids for distribution with the blood that reaches the IVC via the central and hepatic veins.

Specialized phagocytes called **Kupffer cells** (fig. 14.3) are found in the liver's sinusoids. These cells can expand to bulge into or cross the sinusoids' lumen. In this way they increase their contact with the blood and with any potentially threatening particles carried in it. The Kupffer cells make an important protective contribution in removing antigen-antibody complexes, colonic bacteria, or tissue debris that finds its way into the portal blood.

The liver's major secretion, bile, is drained from it in a separate system of ducts that isolates bile from the blood. Instead, hepatocytes secrete bile into **bile canaliculi.** These fine ducts originate between adjacent liver cells and con-

verge to form larger ducts, which ultimately deliver bile to the small intestine.

The converging system of bile ducts drains the right and left lobes of the liver into the **hepatic duct.** A short distance below the liver the hepatic duct is intersected by the **cystic duct,** which communicates with the **gall bladder.** (The term *gall* refers to bile and is no longer in common usage.) The cystic duct and hepatic duct join to form the **common bile duct** (CBD), which proceeds to the duodenum and then passes through the duodenal wall to open into the intestinal lumen. The **pancreatic duct,** draining the digestive secretions of the pancreas, also joins the duodenum in this region, the **hepatopancreatic ampulla (ampulla of Vater)** designated AV in figure 14.1. The passage of bile into the duodenum is controlled by the **sphincter of Oddi,** located at the distal end of the ampulla of Vater (see fig. 14.1).

When the sphincter is closed, bile secreted by the liver backs up into the duct system and then into the gall bladder. The gall bladder can store about 50 ml of bile until such

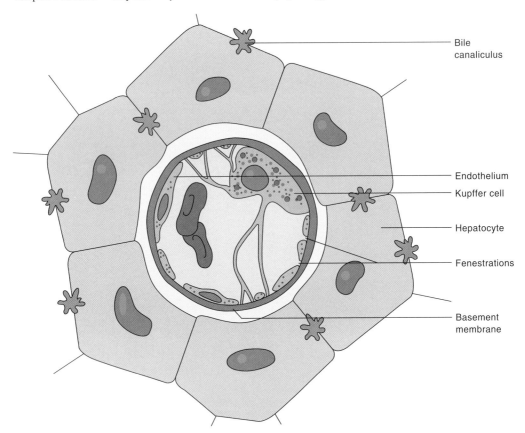

Bile
canaliculus

Endothelium
Kupffer cell

Hepatocyte

Fenestrations

Basement
membrane

Figure 14.3   **Cross-Sectional View of a Hepatic Sinusoid.** A Kupffer cell's cytoplasmic extensions span the lumen of the sinusoid. This increases exposure to the blood to enhance the cell's phagocytic activity. The endothelium of the sinusoid is fenestrated (perforated) to permit rapid exchange between hepatocytes and the blood. The bile canaliculi between adjacent hepatocytes receive bile and carry it to the hepatic duct.

time as it is required in the small intestine. When fat arrives at the duodenum from the stomach, it indirectly stimulates the gall bladder to contract and the sphincter of Oddi to relax. Normal duodenal peristalsis will also draw small amounts of bile into the duodenum. The gall bladder empties in this way in about one hour. The gall bladder is also able to concentrate bile by removing nonessential electrolytes and water. This process allows for the storage of increased quantities of the active ingredients of bile, the bile salts.

FUNCTIONS OF THE LIVER AND BILE SYSTEM

Bile Secretion

The secretion of bile is a major hepatic function. From 800 to 1,000 ml of bile are secreted each day to supply the needed for fat digestion and absorption. The liver synthesizes two major bile acids, **cholic** and **chenodeoxycholic acids,** and secretes their sodium and potassium salts into the bile ducts. In the intestine, the bile salts perform two essential functions in the digestion of fat. First, they emulsify it. This means they work to prevent the small fat globules, formed by mechanical digestion, from coalescing to form

larger globules. Small fat globules tend to merge to form larger globules, separating from the watery chyme in the same way that the oil and vinegar in a salad dressing separate after standing. Emulsification keeps the globules small, thus maintaining the large surface area that favors the efficient action of digestive lipases.

The second function of bile has to do with the absorption of the products of fat digestion: fatty acids, monoglycerides, and fat-soluble vitamins. Bile salts combine with them in a way that makes them water-soluble. They remain in this soluble form until they contact the small intestine's epithelium. There the bile salts release their lipids to dissolve in the membrane, allowing their absorption. After releasing the lipids, the bile salts complex with other products of lipid digestion to repeat the process. This sequence continues until the bile salts are themselves reabsorbed at the distal ileum. In this way, about 80% of the bile salts are retained for recycling by the liver. The circulation of the bile salts from the intestine to the liver to the bile and then back to the intestine is called the **enterohepatic** circulation. Bile salts may be cycled through it five to ten times per day. This efficient use of the bile salts means that the liver must synthesize only the amount needed to replace the small quantity lost in the feces (fig. 14.4).

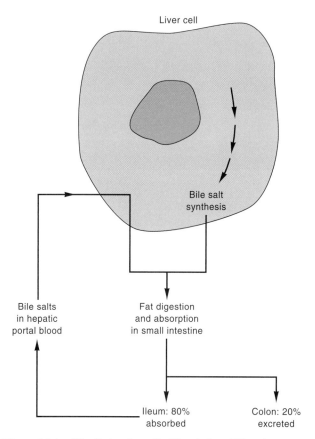

Liver cell

Bile salt
synthesis

Bile salts
in hepatic
portal blood

Fat digestion
and absorption
in small intestine

Ileum: 80%
absorbed

Colon: 20%
excreted

Figure 14.4   **The Enterohepatic Circulation.** Bile salts
circulate between the small intestine and the liver: an efficient
recycling mechanism.

Bile is also important as the vehicle of **bilirubin** excretion. Bilirubin is a product of hemoglobin degradation and is toxic if allowed to accumulate. It is formed primarily in the spleen, where most aging erythrocytes are removed from the circulation. There, hemoglobin is degraded to form heme and the protein globin. The globin is metabolized to release its amino acids, and the heme is first converted into **biliverdin** and then into the yellow-brown pigment bilirubin. Lesser amounts of bilirubin are also formed in the marrow and liver. From the spleen and marrow, bilirubin is carried to the liver by the plasma protein albumin. There it is picked up by hepatocytes and chemically modified by the addition of two molecules of glucuronic acid. This process is called **conjugation.** Its product is bilirubin diglucuronide or, more simply, conjugated bilirubin (CB).

There are two significant consequences of the bilirubin conjugation. One is that CB is much less toxic than unconjugated bilirubin (UCB). The other is that CB is water-soluble and UCB is not. (This is why albumin is needed to transport UCB in the plasma.) By converting bilirubin to a water-soluble form, the liver facilitates its incorporation into bile for the purpose of excretion. Some bilirubin is converted to a sulfate, which is also water-soluble. The excretion of bilirubin in bile is one of the few cases in which

the alimentary canal is used for excretion. Because the intestine's lumen is an external space, and because the bile duct system directly communicates with it, at the moment bile enters a bile canaliculus, it is technically outside the body and has been excreted (see fig. 14.1). In this way, bilirubin is cleared from the blood and prevented from accumulating in the body tissues. On reaching the colon, bilirubin is converted by bacterial action to **urobilinogen** and then to the darkly colored **urobilin** pigments that are responsible for the color of feces. Bilinogens are also absorbed from the colon and carried to the liver, where they are again secreted into bile. Small amounts are also excreted by the kidney into the urine (fig. 14.5).

Metabolic Functions

The liver makes major contributions to the metabolism of carbohydrate, lipid, and protein. Its cells contain the many specialized enzymes needed to accomplish these complex metabolic tasks. In lipid metabolism, the liver takes up fatty acids delivered to it from fat stores around the body. About one-half is converted to lipoprotein and returned to the blood for transport back to adipose tissue. The remaining half is used in a variety of metabolic pathways—for example, the synthesis of **cholesterol.** This steroid lipid serves as a precursor of the steroid hormones and the bile salts. It is also found in cell membranes. Cholesterol made in the liver is also present in bile. It is normally kept in water solution by the action of the bile salts, aided by a phospholipid, **lecithin,** that is synthesized by the liver from triglyceride. The liver can also synthesize fat from carbohydrate and protein when these are present in oversupply. The resulting fat is then stored against future demand (fig. 14.6).

In the metabolism of carbohydrate, the role of the liver is vital because the simple sugar glucose is the principal fuel of energy metabolism. As newly absorbed glucose enters the blood after a meal, the liver converts much of it to a storage form, **glycogen.** This process is called **glycogenesis.** Later, as glucose is utilized, the liver degrades glycogen to glucose and moves it into the blood to support its glucose level. This process is called **glycogenolysis.** When necessary, the liver can synthesize glucose from amino acid precursors by a process termed **gluconeogenesis.**

Protein metabolism in the liver includes the **deamination** of amino acids. In this process, the amino group is removed from an amino acid, leaving a carbon-containing molecule that can be used in various synthetic pathways—for example, in glucose synthesis or energy metabolism. The amino groups produced by deamination are used by the liver to make **urea,** which is then excreted by the kidney. The liver also uses ammonia absorbed from the colon, where it is formed by bacteria, to synthesize urea. In addition, hepatocytes synthesize most of the plasma proteins and the protein clotting factors of the blood's coagulation system. Also produced in the liver are some proteins of the fibrinolytic system.

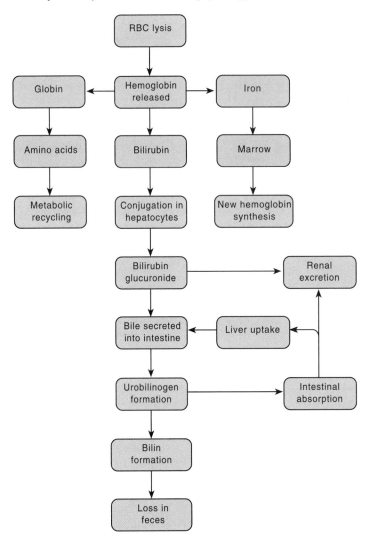

Figure 14.5   **Bilirubin Excretion.** The fate of hemoglobin after its release from RBCs lysed in the spleen, marrow, and liver.

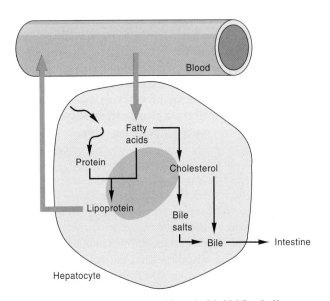

Figure 14.6   **Some Important Hepatic Lipid Metabolism Pathways.** Fatty acids from the blood are metabolized in the production of bile salts or in other pathways not shown. Combination of lipid and protein synthesized within the cell (curved arrows) forms lipoprotein. Only in this form can unmetabolized fat be cleared from the cell.

Detoxification

The liver cells' smooth endoplasmic reticulum contains an array of enzymes that chemically alter certain substances so that they can be cleared from the blood, especially hormones and exogenous substances. In the case of circulating hormones, the benefit of their inactivation by liver enzymes is that new secretion is required to replace them. This requirement allows for the closely regulated secretion that provides fine hormonal control of various body functions. The hormones of the pancreas, adrenal cortex, and thyroid gland are inactivated by enzymatic degradation in the liver.

The process of enzymatic degradation (or **catabolism**) is called **detoxification** when exogenous substances are involved. Drugs, harmful chemicals, and biological toxins can be cleared from the blood in this way, providing an early defense against potentially threatening substances. The process is similar to that seen in preparing bilirubin for excretion. The drug or chemical is metabolically altered and the product converted to conjugated forms that are water-soluble. This makes them suitable for renal excretion (fig. 14.7). The liver's blood supply arrangement has significance for detoxification in that toxins or chemicals ab-

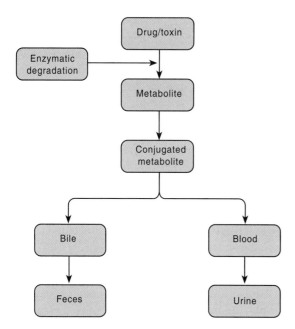

Figure 14.7   Hepatic Detoxification of Drugs and Toxins.

Table 14.1	Principal Liver Functions
Detoxification of toxins/drugs	Synthesis of plasma proteins
Vitamin storage	Hormone inactivation
Clotting factor synthesis	Protein/lipid metabolism
Glycogen formation/storage	Urea production
Phagocytosis	Bile production

Liver damage may affect any of these to a greater or lesser degree, depending on the severity of the injury, the nature of the injury, and other variables.

sorbed from the GI tract are carried directly to the liver. The liver clears the blood of a certain fraction of the toxic chemical during each passage through its sinusoids. This arrangement greatly reduces the amount to which the systemic tissues are exposed.

Liver detoxification enzymes may not be present at all times. However, the presence of a toxin or drug causes the liver cell to produce the enzymes needed to eliminate the drug or toxin. This process is called **enzyme induction** and is nonspecific; that is, the enzymes formed can catabolize more toxins than the one that first induced their formation.

Vitamin and Nutrient Storage

Hepatocytes contribute to metabolism by storing several needed nutrient substances. These can't be synthesized; so the diet must supply them. When available amounts are more than are required, the liver stores them. If supplies should decline at some later time, the liver releases its stored nutrients for use. The quantities stored are usually adequate to meet the body's needs for periods of weeks to months. The important vitamins stored by the liver's cells are vitamins A, B_{12}, D, and K. Other nutrients stored are glycogen, triglycerides, riboflavin, nicotinamide, copper, and iron. The liver's major metabolic functions are presented in table 14.1.

LIVER FAILURE

Because it receives the direct venous drainage of the stomach and the intestines, the liver is subject to substantial threat. This threat takes the form of absorbed microorganisms, their products, and any toxic chemicals or drugs absorbed from the intestine. To cope with this situation, the liver brings two powerful defenses to bear. One is its enormous reserve capacity: the liver is estimated to use only

10% of its cells in meeting normal, day-to-day requirements. The other defense is the liver's highly developed regenerative capacity, which can produce large amounts of functional cells to replace those lost to injury. However, any advantages gained by these hepatic capabilities may be offset by the fact that a disease process may be well advanced before sufficient liver tissue is destroyed to produce significant signs and symptoms. This means that, aside from some acute infections or focal trauma, much liver disease involves diffuse damage that affects large amounts of liver tissue before signs and symptoms emerge. The result is often chronic and severe disease, because a long period of tissue destruction may overwhelm the liver's reserve and regeneration capacities. The major sequelae of liver disease that are commonly seen, regardless of etiology, are considered in the following sections.

Jaundice

Hyperbilirubinemia is the condition in which bilirubin levels in the blood are elevated above the normal range of 0.3–1 mg/dl. In **jaundice,** a yellow-brown color becomes visible in the skin and the sclera of the eye when the bilirubin level in the blood exceeds 2 mg/dl. In liver failure, jaundice is almost always present and serves as an easily observed sign of some disturbance in the liver or bile system. (**Icterus** is an older, less commonly used term that refers to the discoloration of the sclerae seen in jaundice.) Jaundice may be the result of one or more of three problems that can arise in the liver and bile (hepatobiliary) system. One is excessive lysis of red blood cells, which are normally the source of most bilirubin. (Some bilirubin, about 20% of the total, is produced from other heme-containing proteins—for example, myoglobin and heme-containing enzymes.) Another is a breakdown in the liver's ability to conjugate or excrete bilirubin. The third problem is obstruction of the bile duct system.

Hemolytic Jaundice

Jaundice resulting from excessive erythrocyte lysis is called **hemolytic jaundice.** The rupture of red cells is followed by the release of hemoglobin. Hemolysis may arise because of red cell membrane abnormalities of the type described in the Hemolytic Anemia section of chapter 7. Significant amounts of hemoglobin may also be released when large hematomas are broken down.

Whatever etiology produces the hemolysis, the large amounts of bilirubin released overwhelm the liver's conjugation and excretion capacity. Initially, the liver can cope because of its large reserve. During this early stage, the urine will be darker because increased hepatic bilirubin excretion produces larger quantities of bilinogens in the intestine. Increased amounts then enter the enterohepatic circulation and, as a result, more are excreted via the kidney. When the liver reaches the point at which its excretory capacity is exceeded, bilirubin levels in the blood and tissues rise. Because liver conjugation and excretion are operating at maximum, the bilirubin that appears in the blood and tissues will be the more toxic, unconjugated form. This can pose a special threat to newborns since their blood-brain barrier is unable to prevent higher levels of UCB from gaining access to the brain and threatening serious damage. This condition is called **kernicterus.** Renal excretion of bilirubin can't increase to compensate because the kidney can excrete only the conjugated diglucuronide form of bilirubin, and only when it is present in high plasma concentrations.

Hepatocellular Jaundice

A second type of jaundice results from a failure of the liver cell to take up or to conjugate bilirubin. This type is called **hepatocellular jaundice.** It is the most common type of jaundice seen clinically, usually in association with viral hepatitis (see the Hepatitis section later in this chapter). Faulty hepatic uptake of bilirubin is sometimes at fault, but failure to conjugate bilirubin is a more common problem. It may result from damage to liver cells caused by infection, tumors, therapeutic drugs (e.g., steroids), or toxic chemicals. In some cases, a genetic lack of the conjugating enzymes is the underlying problem.

A mild and transient form of hepatocellular jaundice is often seen in the newborn. Because the liver conjugation enzymes and excretion systems may not be functional for the first 7–14 postnatal days, hemolysis of the newborn's RBCs releases more bilirubin than can be excreted by the immature liver cells. A mild jaundice results, but it soon passes as the liver matures and is better able to cope with normal dilirubin excretion demand. This condition is quite common and is known as **neonatal jaundice.**

Cholestatic Jaundice

The essential feature in this condition is the failure of bile to drain normally from the liver. Such **cholestasis** may be caused by hepatocyte damage that interferes with the cell's ability to excrete conjugated bilirubin. More commonly, bile duct obstruction is at fault, thus, the term **obstructive jaundice** is often used to describe this condition.

With reduced bile clearance from the liver, bilirubin and bile salts accumulate, first in the liver and then in the blood. The bilirubin initially entering the blood is CB, but later UCB uptake by hepatocytes is reduced as well, causing a hyperbilirubinemia characterized by both CB and UCB. As the blood carries bile salts to peripheral tissues, they can produce an intense itching sensation in the skin called **pruritus.** In hepatocellular and cholestatic jaundice, bile flow to the intestine is reduced. The resulting lack of urobilinogens produces lighter colored feces that become gray when obstruction is complete. In such cases, urinary urobilinogens are also lacking. Microscopic studies of liver affected by cholestatic jaundice may show dilated bile canaliculi with leakage of bile into the surrounding tissues. These bile accumulations are known as **bile lakes.** The damaged bile canaliculi and duct cells release alkaline phosphatase, which can be detected in the blood to aid in diagnosis.

Obstruction of the bile ducts may be caused by abnormalities inside or outside the liver. **Intrahepatic obstruction** occurs when viral or other infections, or drugs, damage the liver. Swelling follows injury, as in the case of fatty liver, or because of infiltration by inflammatory cells. As a result, the fine intrahepatic bile canaliculi are compressed, reducing or completely stopping bile flow. In **extrahepatic obstruction,** mechanical blockage of the bile ducts is involved—for example, a carcinoma of the bile duct epithelium or an externally compressing tumor. Inflammation or neoplasia of the adjacent pancreas might also be involved, since swelling can compress the hepatopancreatic ampulla to block bile flow. A common cause of extrahepatic obstruction is inflammation of the bile ducts, **cholangitis.** Other causes are accumulating pus from a bacterial infection and bile duct stricture associated with postinfection repair of the ducts. Obstructive jaundice is also commonly caused by gallstones, which can lodge in the ducts. Details of their formation are discussed later in the Cholelithiasis section.

In **biliary atresia,** obstruction is the result of congenitally deficient bile ducts that are inadequate to drain bile from the liver. The atresia, or absence, of ducts may be intrahepatic or extrahepatic and presents serious risks of progressive irritation and necrosis from accumulating bile salts. The consequences are fibrosis and cirrhosis (discussed later in the Cirrhosis of the Liver section), and the affected child is unlikely to survive. Although quite rare, the cases often gain attention via the news media, where pleas for a liver donor are often made. Transplantation offers the only hope of a cure.

The various causes of jaundice are summarized in figure 14.8.

Malabsorption

Because of its role in digestion and absorption, liver damage may be accompanied by malabsorption. Following cholestasis, malabsorption of fat often occurs. With the loss

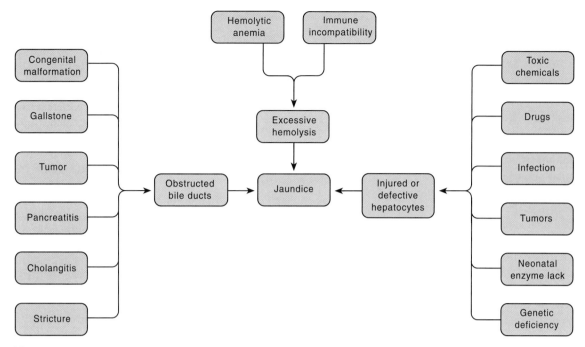

Figure 14.8   **Jaundice.** Principal etiologies in hemolytic, hepatocellular, and obstructive jaundice.

of bile salts, fat emulsification and absorption are diminished, falling to about half of normal levels. This is one factor in the weight loss and steatorrhea that characterize chronic liver failure.

Abnormal blood coagulation is another problem indirectly related to malabsorption. Vitamin K is required for normal hepatic synthesis of various plasma clotting factors. Because vitamin K is fat-soluble, it is dependent on bile salts for its absorption. When liver damage interferes with bile secretion, or when cholestasis prevents its reaching the duodenum, vitamin K levels may be depressed.

Disordered Hepatic Metabolism

When hepatocytes are damaged, their numerous metabolic functions may be disrupted. A few cells, or many, may be affected to differing degrees, with systemic effects producing a variety of signs and symptoms. For example, the overall effects of chronically depressed hepatic metabolism are generalized weakness and weight loss. On the other hand, more specific effects are seen when a particular hepatic function is affected. For example, the blood coagulation abnormalities that result from malabsorption of vitamin K are enhanced by defects in the liver's synthesis of clotting factors. With protein synthesis depressed, a deficiency of albumin gives rise to hypoalbuminemia. Lack of albumin reduces blood osmotic pressure, with peripheral edema the result. As fluid accumulates in the tissue spaces, a finger's pressure on the skin produces a pit that only slowly returns to normal. For this reason, the condition is called **pitting edema.** The pit results because the excess tissue fluids can move only slowly through the tissue spaces to refill the depression produced by the finger's pressure.

Another sequela of hepatic injury is called **hepatic encephalopathy.** It is characterized by a series of neurological abnormalities thought to be related to the failing liver's altered protein metabolism. Although deamination continues with amino groups split from amino acids, the damaged liver can't synthesize enough urea to clear them. They accumulate as ammonia, which has toxic CNS effects that cause the encephalopathy. Some substances that are normally inactivated by the liver produce disruptive neurotransmitter effects, while others contribute to the problem in ways that are not understood. Mild forms may produce only a passing sluggishness or lethargy. More severe expressions involve disorientation and coma. In severe liver failure, hepatic encephalopathy produces a characteristic flapping tremor of the hand when the arm is extended—called **asterixis.** Usually the prognosis is less favorable if hepatic encephalopathy develops in acute liver damage rather than in chronic cases.

Injury that prevents hepatic lipoprotein synthesis leads to altered lipid metabolism. As discussed in chapter 1, such injury disrupts the normal exchange of fat and lipoprotein between the liver adipose tissue stores around the body, and fat accumulates in the liver cells. This fatty liver condition is reversible, but if damage is severe or chronic, the cells may not survive.

With depression of the liver's chemical and drug detoxification function, the effects of a given toxin may be exaggerated since the damaged liver is less effective in clearing it. Similarly, therapeutic drug doses may require adjustment;

because less drug is inactivated by a damaged liver, greater effects are produced by a smaller than normal dosage.

Another type of metabolic effect involves hormone inactivation. As this hepatic function diminishes, higher levels of circulating hormones may result if feedback controls can't compensate. For example, in male alcoholics, liver damage appears to interfere with inactivation of the small amounts of estrogens produced by the adrenal cortex. The result is the exposure of the tissues to estrogen levels that produce **feminization: gynecomastia** (breast enlargement) and testicular atrophy. Faulty hepatic estrogen inactivation is also thought to contribute to the elevated level of circulating estrogen that causes dilation of the palmar arterioles, producing a characteristic reddening: **palmar erythema.** The increased incidence of peptic ulcer in association with liver damage may similarly be the result of reduced hepatic inactivation of the hormone gastrin. Higher levels of gastrin in the blood lead to excessive stimulation of the stomach's parietal cells, and therefore to oversecretion of acid and a tendency to ulceration.

Renal failure may follow liver failure. This condition, known as the **hepatorenal syndrome,** usually arises late in the course of severe liver disease and indicates a poor prognosis. Although its pathogenesis is not well understood, it is possible that elevated levels of circulating vasoconstrictors, normally destroyed in the liver, damage the kidney by interfering with its blood flow. Although the kidney is functionally impaired, a renal biopsy reveals no structural changes; indeed, such kidneys have been successfully donated in transplant procedures. Normal function follows restoration of an adequate blood supply.

With this survey of the typical sequelae of liver damage as a foundation, we can now consider the principal patterns of pathogenesis that produce them.

HEPATITIS

Viral infections and exposure to toxic chemicals commonly cause liver damage sufficient to produce at least some disruption of function. The result is an inflammatory response in the liver, called **hepatitis.** Two forms of hepatitis, acute and chronic, are recognized. Although the "-itis" suffix implies certain inflammatory changes in the liver, they are not typical of the usual acute inflammatory response. For example, in acute hepatitis, there is little fluid exudate, and lymphocytes are characteristically present, dominating over macrophages and neutrophils.

Acute hepatitis is often caused by viruses, but toxic chemicals are also damaging. The result is moderate injury with scattered areas of necrosis and regenerating hepatic parenchyma. The liver is swollen and may be discolored by bile that damaged cells can't pass to the bile canaliculi, or that can't clear canaliculi that are compressed by the swollen hepatocytes. The victim feels weak and fatigued and typically experiences nausea, anorexia, fever, and jaundice. Various hepatic functions are sufficiently depressed to produce abnormal diagnostic test results. The typical course

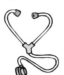

Focus on HAV in Day Care Centers

The risk that children may develop hepatitis A from contact at day care centers seems to be increasing. The increase is due, in part, to the more widespread use of day care centers at the same time that there is increasing use of cloth diapers because of environmental concerns. A recent study of children in day care centers showed that cloth diapers, even when doubled, were more likely to allow fecal leakage, significantly increasing contamination of the hands of the children who wear them. Increased infections in the day care population were found, as communal toys and other surfaces were soon contaminated. The study showed that disposable paper diapers were better able to reduce contamination and the incidence of infection.

of the disease involves a four- to six-week period of symptoms, followed by restoration of normal functions and complete recovery.

In a small percentage of acute hepatitis cases, hepatic damage is extreme and death may follow the initial attack in a matter of days or weeks. This pattern of hepatic damage is called **massive liver necrosis** or **fulminant hepatitis.** It may arise in a type of viral hepatitis, but toxic damage from various drugs or chemicals may produce the same extensive damage. When acute hepatitis produces massive liver necrosis, most hepatic functioning is disrupted, and prognosis is poor, with mortality rates exceeding 70%. Hepatic encephalopathy commonly accompanies massive liver necrosis.

Viral Hepatitis

Most viral hepatitis is produced by a group of viruses that specifically attack the liver. These are grouped in a separate category from the various other viruses that can incidentally affect the liver as part of a systemic infection; Epstein-Barr virus, herpes virus, adenovirus, enterovirus, and cytomegalovirus are examples. Essentials of the principal hepatitis viruses and their related conditions follow.

Hepatitis A Virus (HAV)

This virus is the cause of hepatitis A, an acute and usually mild condition that resolves with minimal therapeutic intervention. It has a relatively short (three to six weeks) **incubation period**—that is, the time during which the infection is proceeding without producing signs or symptoms. As the viruses become established in the liver, they pass with bile to the intestine, where they contaminate the feces. As a result, the organisms typically are spread by contact where hygiene is poor or by a contaminated water supply. This mode of transmission is described by the term **fecal-oral.** Shellfish, such as clams and oysters, may be contaminated by sewage to become a source of infection in human populations. Hepatitis A is often involved in epidemic outbreaks that are confined to a closed population, such as on naval vessels or at boarding schools. Only a few viruses are present in body fluids, so spread of HAV via saliva, urine, or semen is quite unlikely. A normal immune response clears the virus and provides lifelong immunity against further infection. Many people achieve such protection following childhood exposure to the virus that produces only a mild, essentially asymptomatic infection. Although the term hepatitis A is now widely accepted as standard, you may still encounter the previous term for this condition, **infectious hepatitis.**

Hepatitis B Virus (HBV)

The hepatitis B virus is the causative agent of hepatitis B, a potentially more serious condition than hepatitis A. HBV, sometimes known as the **Dane particle,** has an antigenic surface coat that surrounds its infective core. The core contains a DNA strand, a core protein, and an accompanying enzyme. These enable the virus to infect hepatocytes and proliferate inside them. Infected cells produce the viral surface coat to great excess and it spills over into the blood, where it can be detected on the basis of its antigenic properties. It bears the designation HB_SAg (hepatitis B surface antigen) (fig. 14.9). The core protein is also antigenic and is termed $HB_cAg.$

HBV is present in all body fluids and even in the fluids present at wound sites—for example, pus or inflammatory exudate. Any exchange of such fluids between individuals can give rise to infection. This means the virus can spread through blood transfusion or, more commonly, via contaminated needles shared by drug abusers or in medical accidents such as needle pricks. This blood transmission is the reason that hepatitis B was previously known as **serum hepatitis.** Sexual contact can also lead to infection as can transmission from a mother to her infant during the birthing process (vertical transmission). Note that there is no HBV in feces. Although these routes of spread are well established, approximately 30% of hepatitis B infections are of unknown origin.

Detection of HB_SAg can be used to verify HBV infection and is the basis for screening donors of blood to be used in transfusions. Although the viral coat is not itself infective, finding HB_SAg is taken as evidence of HBV infection. Screening of blood donors has greatly reduced transmission via transfusion, but high risks remain for medical personnel who can't avoid blood contact and for illicit drug users who use contaminated needles.

Signs and symptoms in hepatitis B are usually more severe than those of hepatitis A, but in many cases they are mild and may not develop at all. Infected hepatocytes present HB_SAg and HB_cAg at their membrane surfaces where

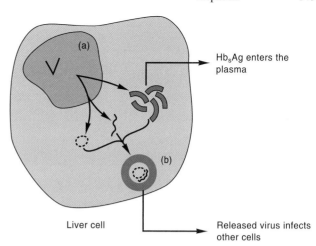

Figure 14.9   Hepatitis B. (*a*) Viral nucleic acid (v) generates production of HB_SAg, other proteins, and more viral nucleic acid. (*b*) Assembly of new virus. Excess HB_SAg spills over into the plasma.

they elicit the immune response, which destroys the infected cells and the viruses they contain. In most people, the signs and symptoms subside after four to six weeks and a long-lasting immunity to reinfection is achieved. In about 1% of acute hepatitis cases, a defective immune response allows large-scale damage that results in a fatal fulminant hepatitis. Hepatitis B also presents the possibility of progression to a chronic condition (described later in the Chronic Hepatitis section).

Hepatitis D Virus (HDV)

The HDV virus is an incomplete viral particle that is also known as the **delta agent.** It is defective in that it is incapable of infecting on its own; it can infect only if it is coated with HB_SAG. This means HDV infects only when an HBV infection is already underway and producing the HB_SAG it needs. (That is why it is discussed here before the discussion of hepatitis C, which is considered next.) When a chronic hepatitis B sufferer has a superimposed HDV infection, it is usually more severe and more likely to result in massive liver necrosis—perhaps 5–7% of victims. It is relatively difficult to transmit, so casual contact with an infected person is unlikely to produce disease. The biggest threat is HDV-bearing blood passing from one drug abuser to another by a shared needle. Homosexual males are also at greater risk of infection. The key factor is the higher incidence of HBV infection in these subgroups. Because the HBV infection rate in medical personnel is low, hepatitis following accidental HDV exposure is uncommon in this group.

Hepatitis C Virus (HCV)

The vast majority of HCV transmission is by way of the blood. Prior to its identification and the establishment of screening procedures, HCV was responsible for 95% of posttransfusion hepatitis. HCV appears to be more difficult

Table 14.2   A Comparison of Some Key Characteristics of Hepatitis A, Hepatitis B, Hepatitis C, and Hepatitis D

Characteristic	Hepatitis A	Hepatitis B	Hepatitis C	Hepatitis D
Mode of transmission	Fecal-oral	Skin* or venereal	Skin,* idiopathic	Skin,* or venereal
Time to postinfection symptoms	3–6 weeks	6–16 weeks	5–10 weeks	6–16 wks
Carrier state	No	Yes	Yes	Only in relation to HBV infection
Chronic hepatitis	No	Up to 10% of cases	Frequent	Only in relation to HBV infection
Association with hepatocarcinoma	No	Yes	Yes	No
Mortality	Negligible	Up to 1.5%	High	Higher than hepatitis B

*Most often via contaminated intravenous needles.

Focus on Hepatitis without Needles or Sex

Significant numbers of those positive for HCV have never had a transfusion or any exposure via sexual contact; nor do they use illicit drugs. Obviously, they pick up the virus in some way, but it is difficult to establish a source. Many such cases are never satisfactorily explained.

One study in Europe identified local outbreaks of hepatitis C that were traced to barbers who unknowingly used contaminated razors to shave their customers.

to transmit than HBV, so the repeated exposures of drug abusers places them at risk. Sexual transmission does occur, particularly among homosexuals. Note also that 20% of infected heterosexuals pass the virus to their spouses. Mother-child transmission does occur but is uncommon. Apart from these recognized modes of transmission, 40% of hepatitis C cases are idiopathic (see focus box).

An initial bout of hepatitis C confers no lasting immunity, so repeated infections may occur, especially in high-risk populations. About half of those infected have an uneventful recovery, but the other half suffer a slowly progressive, chronic disease. Like hepatitis B, liver damage in hepatitis C occurs not by the direct action of the virus, but from an immune system attack on infected cells. The key distinguishing features of the major hepatitis viruses are presented in table 14.2.

Other Hepatitis Viruses

Hepatitis E virus (HEV) is not usually encountered in North America. It is responsible for epidemics of acute hepatitis in developing countries, in which outbreaks have been linked to fecal-oral transmission. The essential underlying cause is the lack of infrastructure to effectively provide clean water and sewage treatment. The clinical course

is similar to that of hepatitis A. There is no progression to chronic hepatitis. Pregnant women are particularly at risk, with mortality rates that may exceed 15% following massive liver necrosis.

When donated blood is analyzed, 1–2% is found to be positive for hepatitis G virus (HGV). This hepatitis virus presents an interesting situation in that it may not actually cause hepatitis. Although the virus is present in blood, and can be transmitted by it, it is still not known whether it has any damaging effect on liver cells. Since it may not actually produce disease, the term *hepatitis G* may be inaccurate. Research to clarify the situation continues.

The Carrier State

A subset of hepatitis B sufferers are unable to completely eliminate HBV particles. This is due to their inability to mount an adequate immune response. In these individuals, the infection persists, in some cases with minimal signs of liver derangement and in other cases with no indication of abnormality. Such **carriers** present a constant hazard in that, without realizing it, they remain capable of spreading the disease, sometimes for many years. The problem of identifying carriers is difficult, because in many cases the initial acute attack of hepatitis may be mild enough to be overlooked or passed off as a brief period of "feeling under the weather."

Although the carrier state does not exist in hepatitis A, it is well established for both hepatitis B and C. There are estimated to be 300,000 HBV carriers worldwide and, in North America, over 1% of people with no symptoms harbor the HCV. This represents a large pool of infection, especially with an increasing population mobility producing greater numbers of contacts and, therefore, higher infection risk. Carrier incidence is high among homosexuals, intravenous drug users, and infants born of HBV-positive mothers.

Chronic Hepatitis

A large majority of acute hepatitis cases resolve without complication. However, in up to 10% of cases, the disease

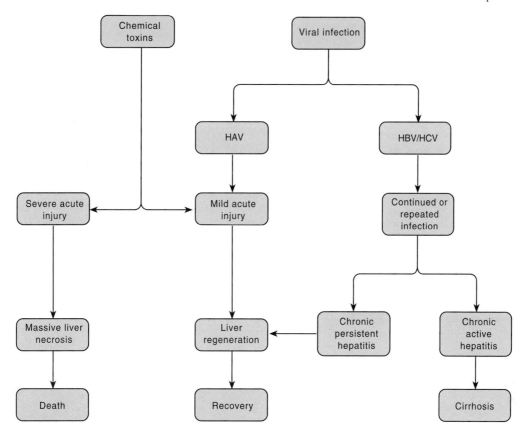

Figure 14.10 **Pathogenesis of Acute and Chronic Hepatitis.** Note that although not indicated in this diagram, some viral infections can induce massive liver necrosis.

persists beyond six months and enters a chronic phase that may last for many months or years. Viruses or drugs may be responsible for the initial acute attack, but a large number of chronic hepatitis cases are idiopathic. Where the causative agent of chronic hepatitis is identified, it is usually HCV.

In chronic hepatitis, two forms are traditionally recognized. **Chronic persistent hepatitis** (CPH) is characterized by a long period of limited hepatic necrosis and only minor symptoms such as mild fatigue or, in some cases, no symptoms at all. Hepatic regeneration is able to replace damaged parenchyma so that functional losses do not occur. Resolution after a few years is typical. Therapy is usually not indicated, but information on the risks of spreading infection to others should be provided to the patient.

Chronic active hepatitis (CAH) is a more threatening progressive condition that may follow acute attacks of hepatitis B or C. Some cases of CAH may be the result of a chronic persistent hepatitis that is complicated by an HBV infection on which an HDV infection is superimposed. The signs and symptoms of CAH are quite variable and may be so mild that the condition is confused with CPH. On the other hand, intermittent bouts of abdominal pain, jaundice, anorexia, splenomegaly, or encephalopathy may be quite severe. Various derangements of the GI tract, pericardium and heart, pleurae and kidneys may also accompany CAH. In this condition the mortality rate can be

as high as 50% five years after diagnosis, as parenchymal regeneration is unable to keep pace with necrosis. Scarring and the development of liver cirrhosis follow. Chronic hepatitis due to HBV and HCV is associated with an increased risk of hepatocarcinoma.

The pathogenesis of acute and chronic hepatitis is summarized in figure 14.10.

Drug and Chemical Hepatitis

A large variety of chemicals, some of which are used therapeutically, are known to have hepatotoxic effects. These effects may be acute or chronic and will vary in intensity from mild, subclinical injury to massive liver necrosis.

Many chemical agents known to be directly hepatotoxic are not available to the general public, or access to them is strictly controlled. Of course, in the case of a therapeutic drug, unequivocal hepatotoxicity would prevent it being approved for use. More problematic are agents that produce **idiosyncratic** reactions—that is, reactions that are unpredictable because individuals vary in their susceptibility to damaging effects. Note that acetaminophen is hepatotoxic in higher doses. This effect is amplified by alcohol ingestion. The alcoholic using acetaminophen to combat alcohol-related gastritis pain is particularly vulnerable. Table 14.3 lists various hepatotoxic agents that may produce acute hepatitis. Note also that any of these can

Table 14.3   Selected Drugs and Chemicals Known to Have Hepatotoxic Effects

	Category	Examples
Direct Toxicity	Industrial chemicals	Carbon tetrachloride, vinyl chloride, benzene, and related compounds
	Plant toxins	Mushroom toxins *(Amanita)*
	Analgesic	Acetaminophen
Unpredictable Toxicity	Anesthetics	Halothane, methoxyflurane
	Antibiotics	Isoniazid, rifampin, sulfonamides
	Anticonvulsants	Diphenylhydantoin
	Street drug	Methylenedioxymetamphetamine (MDMA—"ecstasy")
	NSAIDs	Phenylbutazone
	Oral contraceptives	All, as a class
	Tranquilizers	Phenothiazines

produce massive liver necrosis in susceptible individuals. Of particular note is the fatal effect of suicidal overdoses of acetominophen and the hepatotoxicity of a street drug commonly known as "ecstasy."

Drug-induced bouts of acute hepatitis have no characteristics by which they can be distinguished from acute viral hepatitis. The patient's history may provide a clue, and rapid recovery when a chemical or exposure to drug is stopped is usually taken as confirmation of its role in causation.

CIRRHOSIS OF THE LIVER

Long-term necrosis caused by infection (10–15%), drug or other chemical damage, from alcohol in particular (60–70%), or by extrahepatic bile obstruction can eventually overwhelm the liver's regeneration capacity. In response to such chronic destruction of liver parenchyma, numerous infiltrating inflammatory cells stimulate fibrosis. The resulting scarring becomes increasingly prominent until sheets of fibrous repair tissue form throughout the liver (fig. 14.11). These are diffusely distributed, isolating areas of hepatocytes that retain their regenerative capacity. Such foci of regeneration are called nodules, and are readily apparent at the affected liver's surface (fig. 14.12). This condition of nodularity and fibrosis is called **cirrhosis.** Since differing patterns of parenchymal loss and scarring can produce smaller nodules (<3 mm) or larger ones (up to several centimeters), you may encounter references to **micronodular** or **macronodular** cirrhosis; however, the size of the nodules has no bearing on the clinical presentation of the disease or its course.

Cirrhosis is a nonspecific end-stage toward which various pathogenetic sequences converge. Its signs and symptoms are variable, reflecting differing degrees of functional

 Checkpoint 14.1

One of the metabolic derangements associated with a cirrhotic and failing liver is its inability to adequately break down certain sulfur-containing compounds produced by intestinal bacteria. These compounds are aromatic and can be detected in the affected person's breath—the condition referred to as **fetor hepaticus.** Sources disagree in their descriptions of the aroma (e.g., "sweet-sour," "musty," "mousy"). If you should encounter this aroma, see which description you agree with. Or will you come up with a better one?

loss and typically involving jaundice, wasting, blood coagulation disorders, gynecomastia and testicular atrophy in males, and plasma protein deficiencies—hypoalbuminemia in particular. As well, various indications of a deranged intrahepatic vasculature may be present. In some cases, however, parenchymal regeneration may be just able to compensate for necrosis, so that only minimal symptoms, or even none, are present. The consequence is a slowly progressing destruction of liver cells that goes unnoticed until it reaches the point at which adequate function can't be sustained. Continued necrosis then depletes functional reserves so rapidly that complete liver failure can't be avoided. In some cases, death from other causes comes before the liver is overwhelmed, and "silent" cirrhosis is discovered as an incidental finding at autopsy.

The clinical presentation in cirrhosis derives from its two principal consequences: portal hypertension and hepatic dysfunction. These are described next.

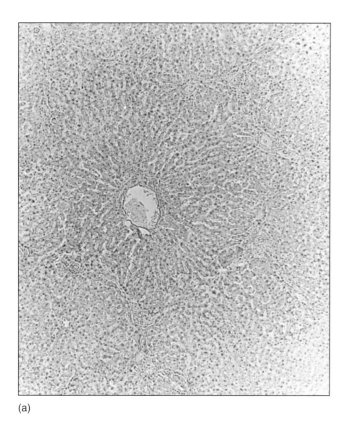

(a)

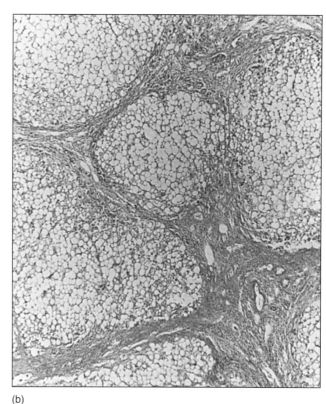

(b)

Figure 14.11   **Cirrhosis.** Micrographs of (*a*) normal and (*b*) cirrhotic liver. Note the bands of fibrous tissue and regenerating parenchyma that are characteristic of cirrhosis.

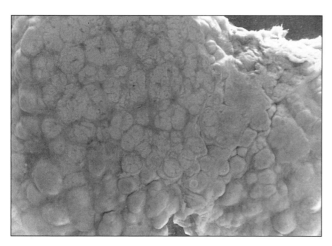

Figure 14.12   **Cirrhosis of the Liver.** The large, rounded masses are foci of regeneration. Contracture in the scar tissue that separates them has drawn in the fibrous bands to produce pronounced irregularity at the hepatic surface.

Portal Hypertension

The **hepatic portal vein** drains the intestines, stomach, pancreas, and spleen and carries their blood to the liver. Increased blood pressure in this system, **portal hypertension,** is the result of restricted flow of blood through the liver to the hepatic veins and then to the inferior vena cava (IVC). Although portal hypertension may be caused by thrombosis or by compression of the inferior vena cava, hepatic, or portal veins, in most cases it is a consequence of liver cirrhosis.

Two factors seem principally responsible for the liver changes that induce elevated portal system pressures: vascular compression and increased arterial loading. In cirrhosis, both regenerating nodules and scar tissue deposition occur at the expense of the fine sinusoids and intrahepatic venules, compressing them and increasing their resistance to flow. The resulting portal congestion elevates portal pressures. Arterial loading is the result of an increased flow through the hepatic artery that accompanies cirrhosis for unknown reasons. This flow increases the volume with which the sinusoids and venules must cope and adds to an already increased vascular congestion. The principal consequences of portal hypertension are the result of reduced blood flow through the liver and the effects of elevated pressure in the hepatic portal system.

Hepatic Shunting

With less blood flowing through the cirrhotic liver, its remaining functional cells have reduced access to the blood, compromising their detoxification activities. It's as if the blood is by-passing the liver (shunting). As a result, toxins are more concentrated in the blood and are more likely to produce damaging effects. Of particular significance is the ammonia produced from the breakdown of amino acids. Its

Table 14.4   Typical Patterns of Laboratory Results in Cirrhosis

Analysis	Comment
Bilirubin	Elevated due to hepatocyte damage; very high in biliary cirrhosis
Serum albumin	Low values because of low production by the damaged liver
Prothrombin time	Increased due to lack of clotting factor synthesis by the damaged liver
ALT and AST	Alanine amino transferase and aspartate amino transferase values are typically elevated because damaged hepatocyte membranes allow their escape.
ALP	Levels of the enzyme alkaline phosphatase are very high in biliary cirrhosis.

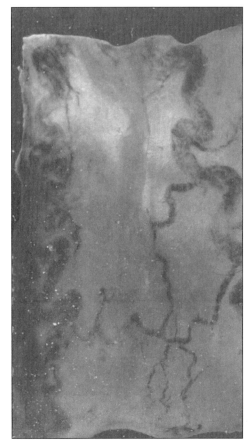

Figure 14.13   **Esophageal Varices.** In this view of the esophageal mucosa, the enlarged and tortuous varices of the esophageal veins can be clearly seen.
This specimen is from the esophagus of a male cirrhosis victim. The esophageal varices ruptured, causing catastrophic blood loss that proved to be fatal. He had been a very heavy drinker for 20 of his middle years and had been hospitalized for the last three years of his life. He suffered severe lower limb edema and pronounced ascites. Repeated abdominal taps were necessary to reduce his abdominal distention, often yielding as much as 4 liters of fluid.

normal incorporation into urea in the liver is reduced in cases of portal hypertension. Instead of being excreted as urea, the ammonia remains in the blood, causing an increased risk of hepatic encephalopathy. Of course, the steady loss of hepatocytes that produced the cirrhosis in the first place continues. This leads to a progressive deterioration in various already existing hepatic dysfunctions: hypocoagulation, hypoalbuminemia, and so on (table 14.4).

Pressure Effects

Congested hepatic blood vessels offer high resistance to the blood in the portal system that is moving toward the liver. This condition results in the diversion of blood into lower-resistance collateral vessels that link the portal vessels to other venous channels. These collaterals normally carry only limited volumes of blood, but when portal pressure rises, they are forced to accommodate additional blood to deliver to the inferior vena cava, by-passing the high resistance liver. For example, some of these collaterals travel in the abdominal wall to converge on the umbilical vein. As they become engorged with the diverted blood, the dilated veins are easily visible at the abdominal surface (fig. 14.14). Similar engorgement of the veins of the anal and rectal mucosae is responsible for the **hemorrhoids** that often accompany portal hypertension.

Of particular significance are the collaterals that accompany the esophagus, because they are thin-walled and have little surrounding connective tissue support. As they receive increasing portal flow and their pressure rises, focal dilatations called **esophageal varices** may form. (These are analogous to the varices seen in superficial leg veins.) Because they cause the mucosa to protrude into the esophageal lumen (fig. 14.13), esophageal varices are subject to trauma as food is swallowed, and they may be ex-

posed to the reflux of gastric juice. The precise mechanism is not understood, but trauma, gastric juice, and the high pressure within the varices probably combine to produce the erosions, rupture, and bleeding that make esophageal varices a serious complication of cirrhosis.

Usually without symptoms until they rupture, esophageal varices can produce sudden, large-scale blood loss whose origin in the esophagus may be difficult to identify. Hematemesis is a common accompanying sign, and bleeding may be prolonged because of a faulty coagulation response since the cirrhotic liver can't maintain adequate clotting factor production. Bleeding of esophageal varices is a serious condition, with mortality approaching 60% in those whose initial indication of damage is an episode of hemorrhage. Subsequent bleeds and continuing liver failure contribute to the poor prognosis.

Therapy for bleeding esophageal varices may rely on compression of the bleeding veins from inside the esopha-

*Focus on Rubber Rings
to Stop the Bleeding*

The technique of endoscopic variceal ligation is increasingly used to effectively cope with bleeding esophageal varices. The ligation, or tying off, is accomplished with small rubber rings that are positioned with an endoscope that is introduced into the esophagus. The scope expands the rubber ring so that a region of mucosa that contains a bleeding varix can be drawn through it. The ring is then released. This applies firm pressure to the base of the isolated pouch of mucosa, cutting off its blood supply. In a short time the tissue above the ring that contains the weakened vein becomes necrotic and sloughs into the lumen. By this time the tissue below the ring has undergone fibrosis, strengthening the site to limit further bleeding.

gus by a balloon device inserted into its lumen. Alternatively, an agent that promotes a pronounced fibrosis response (a **sclerosing agent**) may be directly injected, via an endoscope, at the point of bleeding. This procedure has significant side effects and is being replaced by a technique that uses rubber rings to tie off the dilated and weakened esophageal vessels (see Focus box). In extreme cases, pressure in the esophageal veins may be relieved surgically by the introduction of a by-pass that carries blood to a point in the systemic venous return. This is an emergency procedure and has a high mortality rate.

Portal hypertension produces two other major complications of cirrhosis: ascites and splenomegaly. **Ascites** is the condition of fluid accumulation in the peritoneal cavity. It can be quite pronounced, leading to significant abdominal distention, which in turn can compromise breathing and compress the abdominal viscera (fig. 14.14). The ascites fluid derives from the plasma and "sweats" off hepatic and intestinal surfaces because of the increased BHP in the sinusoids and capillary beds of the liver and intestines. Also contributing is reduced hepatic albumin production, which lowers blood osmotic pressure and reduces the return of fluid to the blood from the tissues of the portal system. A third factor is the backup of blood in the portal system vessels. This reduces venous return to the heart, which, in turn, can trigger sodium and water retention reflexes that add to the already exaggerated fluid burden.

A serious complication of ascites is **spontaneous bacterial peritonitis.** By mechanisms unknown, but presumably related to high vascular pressures, intestinal organisms gain access to the peritoneal cavity. In it they find the ascites fluid, a medium that readily supports their rapid proliferation, and peritonitis follows. This is another complication of cirrhosis that can be immediately fatal.

In cirrhosis **splenomegaly,** enlargement of the spleen results from portal hypertension. The veins that drain the

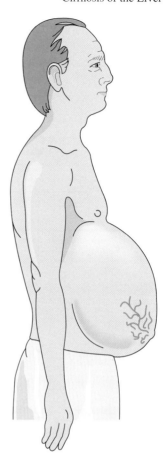

Figure 14.14   Ascites. This drawing shows the degree of abdominal distention often seen in ascites.

spleen empty into the hepatic portal system, and when its vessels are congested, the splenic vessels become congested in turn. The resulting size can produce spleen weights of up to 1,000 g, over seven times normal. Splenomegaly is often accompanied by hypersplenism. In this condition, formed elements of the blood are increasingly taken up and held by the enlarged spleen. Hypersplenism can produce thrombocytopenia, exaggerating any preexisting cirrhotic coagulation defects. Anemia may also develop, as erythrocytes held in the spleen add to circulatory red cell losses caused by bleeding from esophageal varices or other sites. The sequelae of liver cirrhosis are presented in figure 14.15.

Alcoholic Cirrhosis

Most cirrhosis involves an alcohol abuse etiology, with 15% of alcoholics becoming cirrhotic after ten years of high alcohol intake—at least one pint of spirits per day. Alcoholism is the single most common cause of hospitalization for liver derangements in North America.

The mechanism of alcohol toxicity involves the production of high levels of metabolites that have damaging effects. One of these is the asymptomatic fatty degeneration that typically precedes irreversible alcoholic liver damage (fig. 14.16). Such fatty degeneration can produce liver

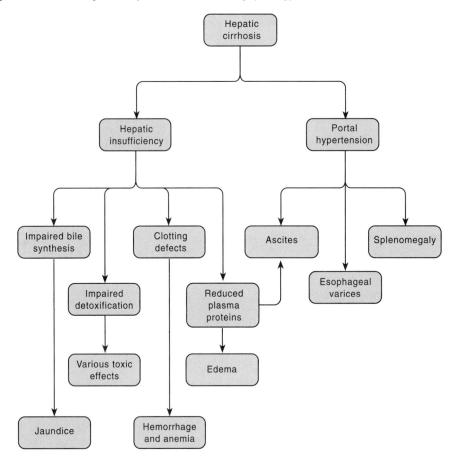

Figure 14.15   **Sequelae of Hepatic Cirrhosis.**

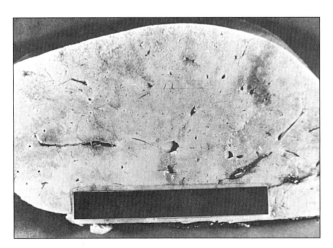

Figure 14.16   **Fatty Change in the Liver.** Note the swollen appearance of this section through a liver severely damaged by chronic alcohol abuse. Only traces of the normal dark liver coloration remain because fat, much of it extracellular at this late stage, has largely replaced functional parenchyma.

In sectioning this liver, it was noted to be heavy, and was greasy to the touch from the additional pound of accumulated fat it contained (weight 1,980 gm, normal 1,550 gm). The autopsy revealed no evidence of cirrhosis or esophageal varices. Although this degree of fatty change is extreme, the immediate cause of death of this 45-year-old male alcoholic was pneumonia. He had a history of many years of alcohol abuse and was generally debilitated.

enlargements as much as two to three times normal. Alcohol also gives rise to the formation of damaging free radicals and induces activation of enzyme systems that produce toxic products. The result is damage and disruption of a variety of cell structures and the infiltration of inflammatory cells that also contribute to liver damage as they release their lysosomal enzymes.

As alcohol abuse persists, chronic damage is followed by cirrhotic scarring and continued tissue destruction that ultimately produces a decrease in liver size. In the alcoholic, steadily declining liver function is typically exaggerated by binges of alcohol intake, which can produce acute alcoholic hepatitis. This insult may overwhelm the already damaged liver and cause complete hepatic failure and death.

Once cirrhosis is established and alcohol intake is not reduced, the likelihood of death within five years from liver failure or ruptured esophageal varices exceeds 60%. Most alcoholic cirrhosis is seen between the ages of 40 and 65 in males, whereas in females, the highest incidence occurs between 30 and 45 years of age. The pathogenesis of alcoholic liver damage is presented in figure 14.17.

Other Cirrhoses

After alcoholic cirrhosis, the second most common type is known as **postnecrotic cirrhosis.** It is the most common

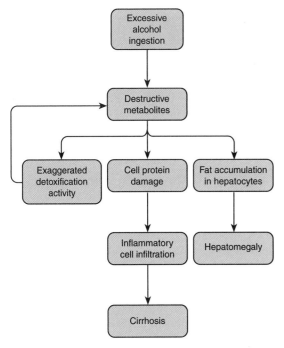

Figure 14.17   **Pathogenesis of Alcoholic Liver Damage.**

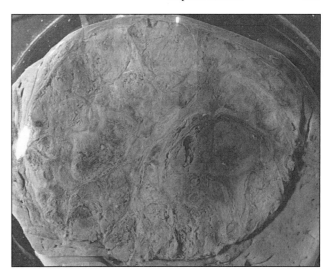

Figure 14.18   **Hepatocellular Carcinoma.** The large tumor mass is easily distinguished from the normal liver visible at the lower right of the photo. Note the large area of necrosis.
This portion of liver contains a very large hepatocellular tumor. The mass was soft and fragile compared with normal liver. Its cells retained the ability to form bile, which imparted a greenish tinge to the tumor. The mass was removed from a 15-year-old girl who died of a hemorrhage into her peritoneal cavity after the tumor broke through the liver's surface. The child had refused food and ran a fever three months preceding this terminal event. Lung metastases were found at autopsy.

type of cirrhosis worldwide, but the high consumption of alcohol in North America distorts the overall incidence figures. The term *postnecrotic* is misleading, but has unfortunately been retained in describing this condition. As must by now be apparent, all cirrhosis follows chronic hepatic necrosis, so the term offers no descriptive advantage. However, common usage reserves the term for the severe cirrhosis that follows the fulminant necrosis linked to toxic or viral damage, most often the result of chronic hepatitis B or C. In fact, postnecrotic cirrhosis is the end-stage condition toward which CAH progresses.

In another type, biliary cirrhosis, two forms are recognized. **Primary biliary cirrhosis** arises most often in middle-aged females. It appears to involve chronic auto-immune destruction of the intrahepatic bile ducts, progressing to cirrhosis. There is no way to reverse the process, and liver transplantation may offer the only therapeutic option. **Secondary biliary cirrhosis** is the result of a chronic extrahepatic obstruction that allows bile to accumulate within the liver. The result is inflammation, necrosis, and fibrosis.

HEPATIC TUMORS

The liver supports metastatic growth, and the vast majority of hepatic tumors are secondary growths, usually originating in the colon, breast, stomach, or lung. Multiple tumor emboli typically establish several metastatic foci in the liver, with their location reflecting the path taken through hepatic vessels. In advanced stages, secondary tumors may produce pronounced liver enlargement. Approximately one-third of all malignant tumors growing in the liver are secondary (see fig. 6.12).

 Checkpoint 14.2

Congratulations if you noticed an inconsistency in the use of the term *hepatoma* for a malignant tumor. As we noted in chapter 6, the suffix "oma" denotes a benign tumor. Unfortunately, misuse of the term is well established and you are likely to encounter it. Don't be misled when you do—the tumor is, indeed, malignant.

By comparison, primary hepatic tumors are rare. If benign, such as the **liver cell adenoma** or **bile duct adenoma,** they are well tolerated and seldom produce liver enlargement. The incidence of liver cell adenoma is low but seems linked to the use of birth control pills. The hormones in these pills seem, in some way, to favor the development or growth of liver cell adenomas. When growing near the liver's surface, these tumors can break through it to produce serious hemorrhage into the abdominal cavity.

Malignant tumors arise from two different hepatic cell types. The most common (80%) is the **hepatocellular carcinoma,** or **hepatoma,** which derives from the hepatocyte (fig. 14.18). These are rare in North America but are more frequently encountered in parts of Africa, Japan, and Southeast Asia. These regions have high HBV infection rates and large numbers of HBV carriers. It is thought that since the virus is known to associate with the hepatocyte's DNA, it may also be able to induce the neoplastic transformation that yields the malignancy. Of primary hepatic malignancies, 20% originate in bile duct epithelium, forming a scirrhous tumor termed **cholangiocarcinoma.** In North America, hepatocarcinoma often develops in association with chronic hepatitis and alcoholic or other cirrhoses.

CHOLELITHIASIS

Hospitalization in North America is often the result of complications arising from the presence of a stone in the bile ducts. Such stones usually form in the gall bladder; for this reason, they are called **gallstones.** Gallstone formation is a common occurrence, with autopsy studies indicating their presence in approximately 15% of adults, most of whom have no indication of their presence. Peak occurrence is seen in obese females who are past the age of 40. The process of gallstone formation is called **cholelithiasis.**

The major constituents of normal bile are water, various inorganic ions, bile salts, cholesterol, lecithin, and conjugated bilirubin. Since cholesterol is a lipid, it has low water solubility. However, bile salts and lecithin combine with cholesterol to form large, water-soluble complexes. When a change in bile permits low-solubility bile components to come out of the solution, they are said to precipitate out of the bile. As they do, they form small crystals on the gall bladder's mucosal surface. Over time, these enlarge to produce grossly visible stones that may exceed 1 cm in diameter. Several or many stones commonly form instead of only one or two (fig. 14.19). In North America, 80–90% of gallstones are formed mostly of precipitated cholesterol. The remainder are predominantly composed of calcium bilirubinate, the calcium salt of the heme-derived pigment bilirubin. These stones are known as **pigment stones.**

The key event in the pathogenesis of cholelithiasis is bile cholesterol reaching a level that exceeds the bile's ability to dissolve it. The situation can arise because of an excess of cholesterol, or from a deficiency of the bile salts needed to maintain cholesterol solubility. In addition, high levels of cholesterol are irritating to the gall bladder mucosa, causing surface changes that predispose to cholesterol precipitation. Mucosal irritation also stimulates mucous secretion, which can interfere with normal gall bladder emptying, another factor that favors precipitation.

Several risk factors are known to involve cholesterol hypersecretion: increased age, obesity, pregnancy, gender, ethnicity, hypercholesterolemia, and high-calorie diets are most significant. Lowered secretion of bile salts may arise because of a genetic defect that reduces bile salt synthesis, but more commonly, intestinal malabsorption of bile salts is involved. Recall the enterohepatic circulation that returns bile salts to the liver from the intestine. Crohn's disease, cystic fibrosis, and ileal resection are examples of conditions that can compromise absorption of bile salts.

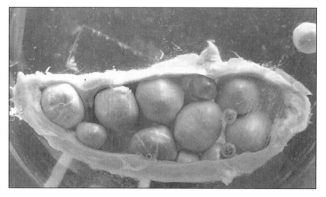

Figure 14.19   Gallstones. This gall bladder is filled with gallstones, whose principal constituent is cholesterol.
This is the gall bladder of a 56-year-old woman. It was removed after a severe attack of right upper quadrant abdominal pain. She reported that prior to the attack she had experienced six years of indigestion and flatulence, particularly after eating fatty foods. The gall bladder was nonfunctional, with its mucosa atrophied and its wall thickened and scarred from working against its stony contents. The pearly stones that fill the lumen are composed largely of cholesterol.

Cholecystitis (inflammation of the gall bladder) may contribute to stone formation by providing an irritated mucosal surface that is hypersecreting mucus, but most often the presence of a stone that has entered a bile duct causes the inflammation. In some cases, it's hard to know whether the stone or the inflammation came first. Also, any factor that impedes gall bladder emptying, such as a swollen pancreas that blocks access to the duodenum, or a tumor that compresses a bile duct, may also contribute to the process. For all that, many cases of gallstone formation are idiopathic in that the precise contribution of the various factors remains unclear. Postinflammatory scarring in the gall bladder reduces the ability to concentrate the bile and may be lost altogether. In chronic cholecystitis, long-term exposure of the mucosa to stone irritation may necessitate removal of the gall bladder.

In the less common **pigment stones,** their high-calcium bilirubinate contents is linked to excessive hemolysis as is seen in sickle-cell anemia or the thalassemias. The large-scale rupture of erythrocytes releases more bilirubin than the bile can dissolve, and precipitation results.

In many cases, the presence of stones in the gall bladder produces no symptoms; in fact, many are first discovered in examinations of the abdomen for reasons unrelated to their presence. The major complications of cholelithiasis are caused by the movement of a stone into the bile ducts, where it obstructs bile flow. Once a stone has lodged in a duct, pain soon follows. As the bile duct muscle contracts, its mucosa presses on the stone's surface, producing pain that is known as **biliary colic.** It often presents as intense episodes of epigastric pain that can radiate to the back or shoulder with accompanying nausea and vomiting. In other cases, it is described as having a more aching character.

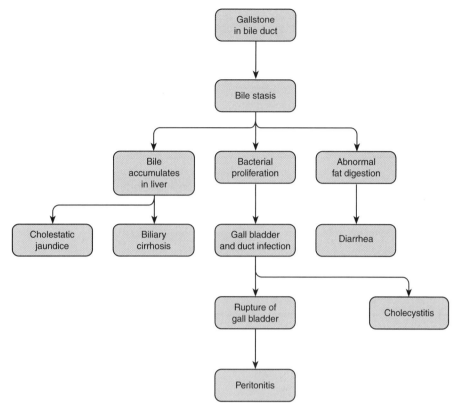

Figure 14.20   **Sequelae of Bile Duct Obstruction.**

 ✓ *Checkpoint 14.3*

It was noted earlier that the presence of asymptomatic gallstones may be uncovered during examinations of the abdomen for unrelated problems. You might be surprised to learn that radiographs aren't usually involved. The cholesterol that dominates most gallstones doesn't block the X-rays, and so the stones won't be visible in the X-ray image. Although there may be a tiny calcium salt in the core of a cholesterol stone, it is typically too small to be seen in medical radiographs.

If the blockage is not corrected, cholestatic jaundice may also develop as a consequence of bile flow obstruction. Lack of normal bile flow can also favor ascent of bacteria from the intestine to the biliary system. Inflammation in the ducts and gall bladder then follows from bacterial activity, as well as from irritation by the obstructing stone. Bacterial damage and compression of gall bladder vessels may contribute to necrosis of its wall and raise the threat of rupture and peritonitis (fig. 14.20). Of course, an obstructed bile duct means less bile in the intestine and reduced fat digestion and absorption. In the colon, bacteria degrade some of the unabsorbed fat, forming products that draw water

Focus on Gallstones as a Side Effect

Because of the link between high serum lipid levels and coronary atherosclerosis (see chapter 9), drug therapy to lower those levels has become more common. As a rule, pharmaceuticals are employed only when dietary control of hyperlipidemia is unsuccessful or when lipid levels are extremely high. The agents involved are generally directed at cholesterol and the serum lipoproteins that carry it. Two such drugs, clofibrate and gemfibrozil, have cholelithiasis as a potential side effect, particularly after long-term use. Although the exact mechanism of action is not fully understood, their use in some way directly or indirectly affects bile composition or the gall bladder mucosa, to increase the likelihood of stone formation.

---

into the lumen. This can cause significant water and electrolyte depletion which further complicates the situation.

The usual therapy for gallstones that obstruct the duct system is surgical removal. However, surgical risk may be high because of a patient's advanced age (a common problem) or because of a reduced clotting response that is caused by depressed hepatic synthesis of clotting factors. In

Table 14.5	Common Liver Function Tests Used to Assess Liver Damage

Test	Comments
Blood	
Serum bilirubin	Both CB and UCB are elevated in hepatitis. In obstructive jaundice, CB is higher than UCB; in hemolytic jaundice, UCB is higher.
Serum albumin	Depressed in chronic hepatitis and cirrhosis.
Serum enzymes Alkaline phosphatase (ALP) 5′-nucleotidase Gamma-glutamyl transpeptidase (GGT) Aspartate transaminase (AST) Alanine aminotransferase (ALT)	These enzymes are released from a damaged liver. They are assessed to differentiate among the various causes of liver damage.
Urine	
Bilirubin	CB present in hepatitis and obstructive jaundice.

such cases, an alternative treatment is the long-term administration of bile acids to dissolve existing cholesterol stones and prevent the formation of others. Another alternative is to fragment the stones with ultrasound energy, because the small pieces that result are more easily passed to the intestine for evacuation.

DIAGNOSTIC TESTS FOR LIVER FAILURE

Blood and Urine Tests

The usual approach to the diagnosis of liver disease is an evaluation of the blood and urine. Abnormally high or low levels of substances derived from normal hepatic functions are taken as an indication of liver damage. The level of serum bilirubin is a commonly used diagnostic indicator. Because it is possible not only to determine the total bilirubin but also to distinguish between CB and UCB, serum bilirubin analysis yields some information as to the specific nature of the malfunction. For example, in hepatitis, plasma levels of both CB and UCB are elevated because damaged hepatocytes cannot adequately conjugate bilirubin. This produces the rise in UCB. At the same time, hepatocytes are less able to clear the conjugated bilirubin they have produced, so CB levels also increase. In obstructive jaundice, CB is dominant because the liver cells are able to conjugate bilirubin, but the blocked bile ducts prevent its passage to the intestine. In hemolytic jaundice, the liver's capacity to handle bilirubin conjugation is overwhelmed, so UCB levels are higher than those of CB.

Urinalysis for the presence of CB is also of diagnostic value, because the kidney will excrete CB only when its plasma level is abnormally high. This is the case in hepatitis and obstructive jaundice. Note that even when CB levels are quite high, UCB levels will be normal. This is because unconjugated bilirubin is tightly bound to albumin and can't pass into the urine.

The liver's protein metabolism functions can also be assessed to gain insight into the functional status of the liver. Such assessment is most significant in chronic hepatic parenchymal disease—for example, chronic hepatitis or cirrhosis. The most common indicator in such cases is hypoalbuminemia due to impaired hepatic albumin synthesis.

Like other necrotic tissues, necrotic hepatic tissue releases certain characteristic enzymes whose presence in plasma can be taken as an indication of liver damage. The principal enzymes are included in Table 14.5 along with some other liver function tests.

Imaging

Radiation imaging plays a role in diagnosing liver damage. Scanning the liver to assess its uptake of radioisotopes is useful in localizing hepatic tumors. The focus of increased uptake indicates a primary tumor. An area of decreased uptake indicates a secondary growth, since it lacks the phagocytic cells needed for uptake of the isotope. Because only about 25% of gallstones contain calcium, most of them can't be visualized in X-ray studies. For this reason, ultrasound or computerized tomography (CT) scans are much more accurate in assessing their presence and location.

Biopsy

Sometimes it is helpful to obtain a sample of liver tissue for microscopic study. The procedure used is a **needle biopsy,** in which a hollow needle is passed through the abdominal wall into the liver and then withdrawn. The tissue in the needle is then removed for examination. Although the procedure is not safe if hypocoagulation is a problem, it is useful in diagnosis of hepatomegaly and jaundice, and in monitoring liver transplants for rejection. It is also an important means of assessing the status of a hepatic tumor. The serious complications associated with the procedure are peritonitis, from bile leakage, and hemorrhage.

LIVER TRANSPLANTATION

This procedure is becoming increasingly successful as suitable recipients are better defined and more carefully selected, and as rejection suppression techniques are refined. In the latter case, continually evolving immunosuppressive agents are an important factor. Candidates for a liver transplant are those who suffer massive liver damage or whose bile duct system is malformed from birth (biliary atresia).

The transplantation procedure involves surgical removal of the diseased organ. This may prove more difficult if the organ is badly scarred or if blood coagulation is compromised by the damaged liver's inability to sustain normal production of clotting factors. Cadaver livers are usually used. Prior to the procedure, the donor liver is thoroughly flushed to clear the donor's blood, and the organ is quickly cooled. The cooling depresses metabolic activity, allowing the liver to tolerate anoxia for up to eight hours. Without cooling, the entire procedure would have to be completed within about one hour. During transplantation, the recipient's blood supply is connected to the donor liver and the bile duct is joined to the duodenum. A bile drain to the abdominal surface may be used to reduce bile irritation during healing at the duct sutures. The entire procedure is usually completed in under ten hours.

The "new" liver starts metabolic activity as its temperature and blood flow are restored. Improvement in the patient's condition soon follows, as previously deficient liver functions are reestablished. Monitoring of progress is based on blood tests and needle biopsies to detect any sign of rejection. Liver transplantation has a high success rate, with only 5–10% of cases failing. Complications of the procedure include thrombosis in the hepatic artery and portal veins and in newly sutured bile ducts, which may leak irritating bile onto adjacent peritoneal surfaces. Stricture in the bile ducts may also contribute to bile stasis. As many liver recipients are weak and undernourished, they are also more susceptible to posttransplant infections. Various immunosuppressive agents carry the risk of side effects that include renal damage, neurological and psychiatric derangements, systemic hypertension, as well as skin and pancreas problems.

Should rejection occur, another transplant procedure is required. In such cases, the situation is critical because only minimal time—two or three days—may be available for locating another donor.

PANCREATIC PATHOPHYSIOLOGY

Apart from some quite rare developmental abnormalities, only two disease processes affect the pancreas: inflammation and neoplasia. Although these disorders are uncommon, when they do arise they can have severe conse-

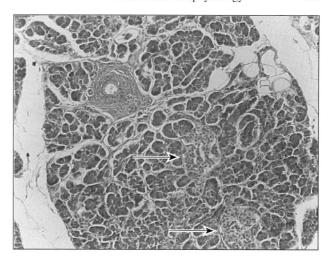

Figure 14.21 **The Pancreas.** A typical section of normal pancreas, showing the darkly stained exocrine cells with lighter islets of Langerhans (arrows) interspersed among them. A duct can be seen at the upper left, supported by the gland's connective tissue.

quences. This chapter will consider only derangements of the exocrine component of the pancreas. Its endocrine disorders are described in chapter 17. Before we consider pancreatic pathophysiology, a review of the normal pancreas will be useful.

Anatomy and Physiology of the Pancreas

The pancreas is positioned with its **head** lying in the curve of the duodenum and its tapered **tail** lying against the hilus of the spleen (see fig. 14.1). The intervening central portion is the **body.** Its parenchyma is dominated by exocrine tissue, which secretes a collection of approximately 20 digestive enzymes (fig. 14.21). These enzymes are delivered to the small intestine by a duct system that terminates at the hepatopancreatic ampulla, alongside the common bile duct. The pancreatic duct cells secrete an alkaline secretion of concentrated bicarbonate, which neutralizes acid arriving in the duodenum from the stomach. Nervous and hormonal mechanisms control the daily secretion of 1,500 to 3,000 ml of pancreatic juice. Also present in the pancreas are islands of endocrine tissue known as the islets of Langerhans. Their pathophysiology is described in chapter 17.

Pancreatitis

The inflammatory response to damage of the exocrine pancreas takes two forms: an acute pancreatitis, which can be life-threatening, and a chronic form involving recurring acute episodes.

Acute Pancreatitis

This condition typically presents with midepigastric or back pain. Nausea and vomiting may accompany the pain, and although fever is sometimes present, an underlying

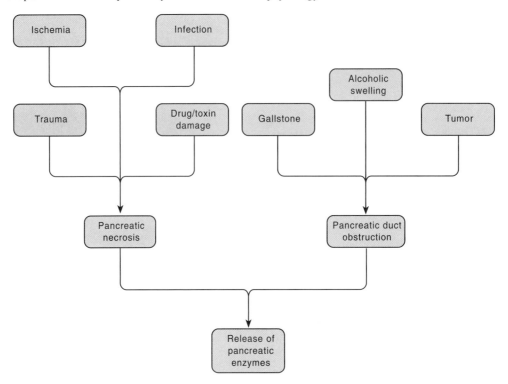

Figure 14.22   **Acute Pancreatitis.** Principal factors that cause the release of pancreatic enzymes to produce acute pancreatitis.

infection is rarely involved. Many attacks are relatively mild, involve no pancreatic necrosis, and resolve without intervention. More severe attacks are characterized by a more intense, radiating pain, pancreatic necrosis, and extensive local hemorrhage. Vascular shock, renal failure, and ARDS may also arise to profoundly threaten the victim. Survivors may develop cysts filled with necrotic debris, blood degradation products, and pancreatic enzymes. These can enlarge to compress the adjacent duodenum and, in particular, the hepatopancreatic ampulla.

Etiology in acute pancreatitis has been much studied, but exact mechanisms have yet to be determined. In considering the problem, there are three key factors. First, under normal circumstances the potent proteolytic and lipolytic enzymes of the pancreas are isolated from pancreatic tissue. They are held within pancreatic cells as inactive **proenzymes,** in the cisternae of the ER and Golgi complex, until secretion. They are activated only after they leave the cells to enter the fine pancreatic ductules. Second, the digestion of pancreatic tissue and blood vessels by the gland's own enzymes is the underlying cause of the necrosis and hemorrhage that characterize severe attacks. Third, most acute pancreatitis is seen in alcohol abusers and in association with cholelithiasis.

On the basis of these three factors, anything that limits normal drainage of the ducts would seem to favor the enzymes gaining access to the normally protected pancreatic tissue (fig. 14.22). Sources of obstruction, or at least restriction of flow, might be gallstones or an adjacent tumor, or they

might be alcohol-related. Bouts of alcohol intake are known to have an irritant effect on the duodenal mucosa and can produce inflammatory swelling at the sphincter of Oddi, limiting drainage of pancreatic juice from the ducts. At the same time, alcohol has an indirect stimulating effect on pancreatic secretion. As a result, additional enzymes enter the ducts at a time when drainage is limited, and thus there is a greater likelihood that enzymes will escape to the adjacent pancreatic tissue. In cases linked to cholelithiasis, an obstructing gallstone may favor the retrograde movement of bile into the pancreas. Its irritant effect on the duct lining may then allow the escape of activated enzymes to the tissues.

In the rare cases of acute pancreatitis not linked to alcohol or cholelithiasis, damage to the pancreas by various means may involve release and activation of its digestive enzymes and the destruction of pancreatic tissue (fig. 14.23). For example, tissue damage from trauma, ischemia, an infection, or some chemical agent may induce an attack of acute pancreatitis. Some therapeutic agents are also known to be potentially damaging to the pancreas—for example, corticosteroids, thiazides, and furosemide. In some cases of idiopathic pancreatitis, a link to gallstones has been identified (see Focus box).

Pathogenesis of acute pancreatitis is based upon the effects of enzyme release and tissue and vessel destruction. Pancreatic lipases digest fat stored within the pancreas and fat adjacent to it. The enzymes produce fatty acids from triglycerides, which then react with plasma cations to form pale masses of necrotic fat (fig. 14.24). The calcium and

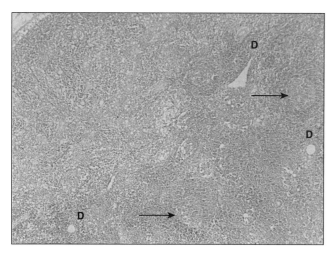

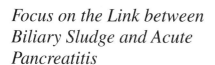

Figure 14.23 **Acute Pancreatitis.** Compare with the slide of the normal pancreas in figure 14.21. Organization has been enormously disrupted. Two circular islets (arrows) can still be faintly seen, as can a few ducts (D). The acinar cells have been greatly damaged; their debris and large numbers of inflammatory cells dominate the site.

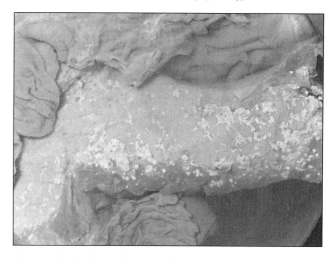

Figure 14.24 **Acute Pancreatitis.** Pale areas of soapy necrosis are visible at the surface of the swollen gland.
A 60-year-old male developed a severe infection as he was convalescing from surgery for a cardiac valve replacement. He then experienced bouts of increasingly severe abdominal pain and died during attempts to diagnose and treat these complications. The pancreas shown here was found to be severely necrotic and heavily damaged by the infecting organisms and inflammatory cells. Although most acute pancreatitis is related to alcohol abuse, there was none in this patient's history.

Focus on the Link between Biliary Sludge and Acute Pancreatitis

Many sufferers of acute pancreatitis have biliary sludge at the root of the problem. Analysis of the bile in such patients reveals the presence of numerous tiny gallstones. The difficulty in detecting this "sludge" of fine stones cause them to be overlooked, but the link between their presence and an increased incidence of acute pancreatitis is now established.

Exactly how the process of **microlithiasis** that produces the sludge might contribute to pancreatic damage is not clear. Backup of pancreatic juice into the pancreas might occur because the sludge blocks its flow or from effects on the sphincter of Oddi that controls access to the duodenum. Removal of the gall bladder or therapy that limits gallstone formation reduces the frequency of acute pancreatitis attacks.

Focus on a Bit of History

In noting the soapy consistency of the necrotic fat formed in acute pancreatitis, recall how early settlers made soap from animal fat and lye. The animal fat was a source of triglyceride, while the lye, which is concentrated sodium hydroxide, was a source of sodium ions. When combined, the two ingredients formed sodium salts of the fatty acids: soap.

magnesium salts of fatty acids have a soapy consistency (see Focus box). In extreme cases, the uptake of calcium ions by fatty acids can deplete plasma calcium levels and produce peripheral muscle hyperactivity.

In an attack of acute pancreatitis, the combined effect of extensive inflammatory exudate formation and hemorrhage can lead to hypovolemic shock. Renal ischemia and renal failure may follow in extreme cases. In cases where ARDS develops, it seems to be because pancreatic enzymes are carried by the blood to the lungs, where they damage susceptible pulmonary capillaries. Digestive disruptions

and malabsorption may also arise because of the lack of adequate pancreatic secretions (fig. 14.25). Acute pancreatitis has a mortality rate of about 5%.

Chronic pancreatitis is a condition that seems to involve repeated moderate attacks of acute pancreatitis. Successive episodes produce a progressive loss of functional parenchyma, which is replaced by scar tissue. The situation is complicated by calcified masses forming in the pancreatic ducts. With progressive loss of pancreatic tissue, islet cells are also destroyed and diabetes mellitus may develop. The high-risk population is composed of males who suffer an initial alcohol-related attack and who continue to indulge (i.e., chronic alcoholics), and those with persistent and severe cholelithiasis.

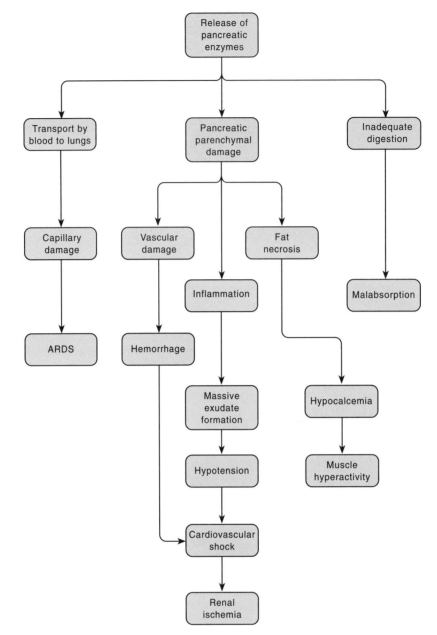

Figure 14.25   **Pathogenesis of Acute Pancreatitis.**

Pancreatic Tumors

The benign pancreatic **cystadenoma** is a rare condition that arises principally in women in their middle to later years. The tumors may take the form of multiple small masses containing mucous-filled cysts.

By contrast, malignant **carcinoma of the pancreas** is a much more common and threatening disease, which is increasing in frequency in North America. Some correlation with smoking, heavy alcohol use, and high caloric intake has been identified but there is little agreement on their pre-

cise role. Most of such tumors arise from pancreatic duct cells, and although most appear late in life, emergence in the 20s is not unusual.

Prognosis in this condition is very poor, with approximately 90% of victims dying within the first year after diagnosis. Pancreatic carcinoma has its devastating effects because of early and widespread metastasis. This seems based, in part, on its location, which has elaborate venous and lymphatic drainage that provides readily accessible metastasis routes.

Case Study

At a general physical examination for his insurance company, a 55-year-old businessman mentioned that over the past year he had lost about 6 pounds, experienced some loss of appetite, and had some vague bowel and bladder problems. These had not particularly alarmed him, since they didn't suggest any heart disease, and he had attributed them to his age. He reported that he was a nonsmoker, exercised little, used no drugs, and was a "social" drinker.

On examination he appeared generally well, but with a slight pallor. Some borderline palmar erythema (redness) was noted, and there were several spider angiomata (singular: angioma) on his chest and abdomen (see Commentary). There was a slight abdominal fullness and the just palpable margin of the liver was smooth and nontender. Asterixis was not present, and other neurological findings were normal.

The palmar erythema, spider angiomata, and slightly enlarged liver suggested liver damage, so the physician questioned the man further on his drinking habits. He again reiterated that he was "just a social drinker," but when pressed to be more specific, his typical drinking pattern proved to be one or two cocktails at lunch, three or four drinks with office associates after work, and a drink or two before dinner. He admitted that at dinner, since his "wife didn't much like wine" he drank most of a bottle of dinner wine. He also was in the habit of having "a little brandy at night" before retiring. His weekend "social" drinking was increased even above this weekday intake, but he insisted that he was never drunk, never craved alcohol, and was not an alcoholic.

Blood tests revealed a hemoglobin level of 10 g/dl, with normal values for BUN and creatinine. Liver function tests were generally abnormal, and his prothrombin time (PTT) was delayed. Serum levels of gamma-glutamyl transpeptidase (GGT) and alkaline phosphatase were both elevated.

On the basis of these findings the patient was referred to a gastroenterologist, who agreed with the probable diagnosis of liver cirrhosis. A liver biopsy was performed and confirmed the characteristic pattern of cirrhotic liver damage.

The patient was advised that there was no treatment for this condition, but a regimen of abstention from alcohol and a balanced and nutritious diet, supplemented by vitamins and iron, might help prevent further decline in his liver's functional capacity. He was also given information on contacting Alcoholics Anonymous and asked to come back for a follow-up, but he never returned.

Commentary

Although sometimes present, jaundice more often appears later in the course of cirrhosis. Spider angiomata are isolated arterioles that dilate and appear as focal red points with tiny radiations. They are often present in women, especially during pregnancy, but they are abnormal in men. Both these and the vasodilation that produces reddening of the palms are linked to liver damage in men by mechanisms that are obscure, but that may involve a damaged liver's reduced inactivation of adrenocortical estrogen. These signs, coupled with the indications of liver enlargement, were sufficient to establish some doubt about the patient's claims to only moderate drinking.

The elevation of both GGT and alkaline phosphatase, while not specific for liver disease, are strongly indicative when there is no evidence of the cardiac, renal, or pulmonary disorders that might also produce elevation of these enzymes. An increased PTT is attributed to the liver's inadequate synthesis of clotting factors and the low hemoglobin level to reduced absorption of the iron needed for normal erythropoiesis.

Although there was no further contact with this patient, and no evidence that he didn't adhere to the prescribed regimen, his failure to return for any follow-up was not surprising. Many who abuse alcohol have great difficulty in coping with their addiction, and the likelihood that the complications of cirrhosis will progress to liver failure is unfortunately high.

Key Concepts

1. The liver's immediate exposure to potential damage from newly absorbed microorganisms or toxins is countered by a large functional reserve and a highly developed capacity to regenerate damaged cells (p. 375).

2. Jaundice, the accumulation of bile pigments, may be caused by excessive red cell lysis, injury to liver cells, or obstructions that reduce clearance of bile from the liver (pp. 375–376).

3. Liver damage produces a variety of systemic signs and symptoms reflecting the disruption of one or more of the liver's numerous metabolic functions (pp. 377–378).

4. Acute hepatitis is the liver's response to moderate injury from viruses or toxins, which produces a characteristic pattern of nausea, anorexia, fever, and jaundice (p. 378).

5. While HAV typically produces a relatively mild and self-limiting acute hepatitis, HBV infection is more serious in its potential for spread through sexual contact and exposure to blood or saliva (pp. 378–379).

6. HBV and HCV are associated with an often undiagnosed carrier state, which presents a constant threat of transmission to the noninfected population (pp. 379–380).

7. Some acute hepatitis sufferers progress to chronic hepatitis, with the disease taking either a relatively mild course or a form that can be life-threatening (pp. 380–381).

8. Chronic or severe injury that overwhelms the liver's regenerative capacity causes cirrhosis, which is characterized by scattered areas of focal regeneration separated by sheets of scar tissue (p. 382).

9. Cirrhotic changes in the liver's architecture cause congestion and hypertension in the hepatic portal vessels, producing a variety of complications, some of which may be life-threatening (pp. 383–385).

10. Alcohol abuse is the single most important factor contributing to hepatic cirrhosis in North America (pp. 385–386).

11. Primary liver tumors are rare, but tissue-specific factors and the liver's large blood flow make the liver a site that greatly favors secondary tumor growth (pp. 387–388).

12. Alterations in bile composition can trigger the formation of insoluble gallstones, which are typically composed of cholesterol and other bile constituents (p. 388).

13. Most cholelithiasis involves formation of cholesterol gallstones whose formation is linked to hypersecretion of cholesterol into bile, or to an inadequate production of the bile salts that keep cholesterol dissolved in the bile (p. 388).

14. The major threat of cholelithiasis is obstruction of the bile ducts, which may lead to jaundice, and irritation of the duct or gall bladder walls, presenting the threat of rupture and peritonitis (pp. 388–389).

15. Various diagnostic tests are based on analysis of the plasma or urine for evidence of disrupted hepatic function, on imaging techniques that can localize tumors or gallstones, or on needle biopsy for the direct study of hepatic tissue (pp. 390–391).

16. Liver transplants to save those with severely damaged tissue are increasingly successful, provided that immune rejection of the implant can be avoided (p. 391).

17. Obstruction of pancreatic flow caused by alcohol-related inflammation, gallstones, or tumors can produce attacks of acute pancreatitis from the destructive effects of pancreatic enzymes on the tissue of the pancreas (pp. 391–394).

REVIEW ACTIVITIES

1. For each of the following conditions, indicate the liver-related problem that contributes to it.

   Jaundice

   Hepatic encephalopathy

   Hypoalbuminemia

   Pruritus

   Hypocoagulation

   Steatorrhea

   Kernicterus

   Gynecomastia

2. Explain why the terms *infectious hepatitis* and *serum hepatitis* are potentially misleading. With that as a warm-up, explain (in at least three ways) how hepatitis A and hepatitis B differ. Then point out the meaning of CAH and CPH and the essential differences between them.

3. Examine figure 14.11. Is the section shown in (*b*) normal? Why are the cells in (*b*) swollen with lipids? What term describes this condition? What are the dark bands that pass through (*b*)? Why are they there? What consequences outside the liver often result from this condition?

4. Make a photocopy of figure 14.15. Cut out the boxes and drop them into a container. Then pick out the boxes at random and arrange them in logical fashion to indicate the sequelae of hepatic cirrhosis. Tape them down when you're sure, and draw the appropriate connecting arrows. Now check against the original to verify.

5. Cover the Comments column of table 14.5. Now, for each blood or urine test, quickly jot down whether the analyzed substance will be increased or decreased, and why. Uncover the Comments column. How did you do? Try this again tomorrow.

6. Look at figure 14.3. Note the position of the bile canaliculi. How do you think they'd be affected by damage to hepatocytes that might cause them to swell? What is the name of the condition in which these bile channels do not develop normally? What can be done for infants born with such a liver defect?

7. Without first checking figures 14.22 and 14.25, list the principal causes of acute pancreatitis. Then name four body organs likely to be affected by the release of pancreatic enzymes from a damaged pancreas.

8. Referring to figure 14.1, speculate on how two conditions described in this chapter might arise from a tumor growing in the vicinity of the ampulla of Vater.

Renal Pathophysiology

What is man, when you come to think about him, but a minutely set, ingenious machine for turning with infinite artfulness, the red wine of Shiraz into urine?

ISAK DINESEN
SEVEN GOTHIC TALES

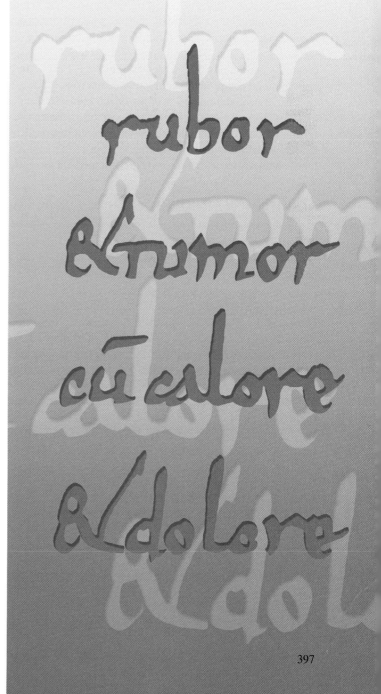

THE NORMAL KIDNEY

A principal function of the kidney is excretion. This process involves the removal of certain substances from the blood and their passage to the body's exterior. Such substances are either toxic or potentially so; hence, the kidney's ability to reduce their levels in the blood is an important one. Because of their toxicity, the nitrogen-containing products of protein metabolism—urea, creatinine, and uric acid—are especially significant in renal excretion. Hydrogen ion and several other potentially troublesome substances are also excreted.

A second important kidney function is homeostatic. That is, the kidney modifies the plasma to achieve a state wherein each plasma constituent is at a level that provides for optimal cell functioning. In addition, the kidney is indirectly able to provide homeostatic regulation by means of its secretion of renin and erythropoietin. Release of renin into the blood causes a series of responses that affect plasma volume both directly by the formation of a vasoactive substance, angiotensin II, and indirectly by renin's effects on sodium ion. The hormone erythropoietin is also secreted by the kidney and serves as a means of regulating normal blood cell production in red bone marrow.

The essential structure features of the kidney are indicated in figure 15.1. These structures are often used in referring to renal disease, which may be centered in a particular section of the kidney. Note the position of the nephron tubule with respect to the renal cortex and medulla.

The Nephron: Structure

Renal functions derive from the functional unit of the kidney, the **nephron.** Approximately 1 million of these are present in each kidney. The nephron has two distinct components: a tubule and its associated blood vessels.

The nephron tubule is an elongated, hollow duct with walls that are one cell thick. One end is modified to form a cup-shaped enlargement, **Bowman's capsule,** whose hollow interior communicates directly with the lumen of the rest of the tubule. Two parts of the tubule are thrown into twists and folds, and between them a characteristic loop is formed as a straight-running portion of the tubule folds back on itself. These are the proximal and distal convoluted tubules and the loop of Henle, respectively (fig. 15.2).

The nephron's vasculature consists of two capillary beds and their associated arterioles and venules. The first capillary bed is the glomerulus. It rests in the cup-shaped hollow of Bowman's capsule with its capillaries' walls in intimate contact with the epithelial cells of the capsule (fig. 15.3). These cells, called **podocytes,** provide points of attachment and support for the glomerular vessels. Blood flows to the kidney via the renal artery, by means of tiny **foot processes** (see fig. 15.6) whose branches ultimately deliver blood to the glomerulus by means of the **afferent arteriole.** Blood then drains from the glomerulus, not by

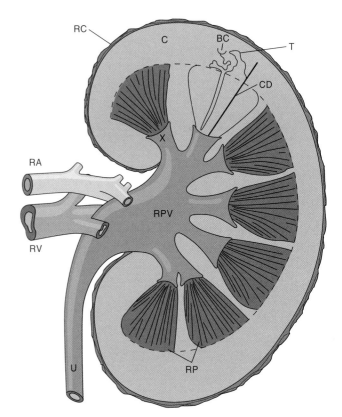

Figure 15.1   **Normal Renal Anatomy.** Indicated structures are the renal capsule (RC), the cortex (C), renal pyramids (RP), the renal artery (RA), and renal vein (RV). The renal medulla contains the renal pyramids and lies deep to the broken line. Also indicated are the ureter (U), the renal pelvis (RPV), and a calyx (X). An enlarged nephron tubule (T) with Bowman's capsule (BC) is shown in relation to the cortex and a renal pyramid. The tubule is joined to a collecting duct (CD).

the expected venule, but instead by another arteriole called the **efferent arteriole.** This vessel carries blood from the glomerulus to a second, larger capillary network that surrounds the nephron tubule: the **peritubular capillaries.** From these vessels, blood moves into the veins that drain the nephron and ultimately into the renal vein (fig. 15.4).

The Nephron: Function

The essential task of the nephron is modifying the blood delivered to it so that the blood will have fewer toxic products and a composition otherwise adjusted to meet homeostatic requirements. How does this modification of the blood occur?

The ability of the nephron to alter the blood's composition is based on three processes. In combination they provide for the removal of waste products and for homeostatic regulation. The first of these processes is **glomerular filtration.** This filtration of the blood involves no removal of waste or toxic products, but is instead the physical separation of the blood's formed elements and its plasma proteins from the

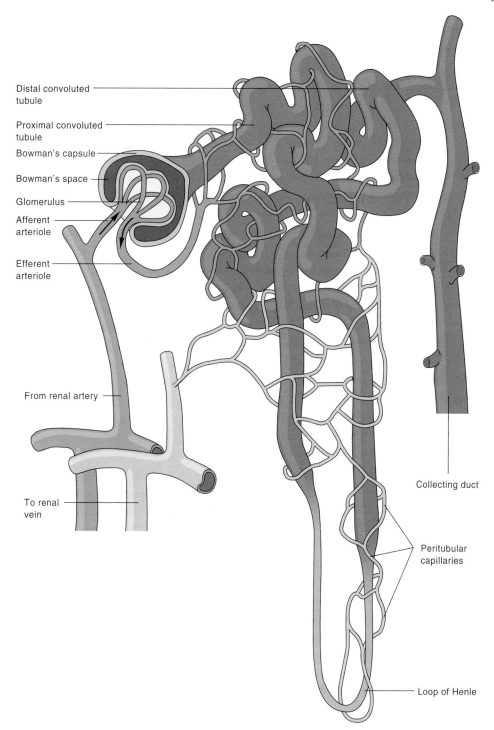

Distal convoluted
tubule

Proximal convoluted
tubule

Bowman's capsule

Bowman's space

Glomerulus

Afferent
arteriole

Efferent
arteriole

From renal artery

To renal
vein

Collecting duct

Peritubular
capillaries

Loop of Henle

Figure 15.2   **The Structure of the Nephron.**

fluid component of the blood. This separation occurs in the glomerulus as a result of blood pressure applied to the **filtration membrane.** This structure is a filter consisting of the glomerular endothelial cells, their basement membranes (BMs), and the podocytes of the epithelium of Bowman's capsule whose **pedicels** interlock to form narrow slits. This arrangement allows water, and the small molecules dissolved in it, to move from the glomerular capillary into

the lumen of Bowman's capsule (**Bowman's space**) (see fig. 15.3). This fluid product of the filtration process is called **glomerular filtrate.** The rate of filtration in both kidneys, over 24 hours, is the **glomerular filtration rate** (GFR). It has a normal value of about 180 liters per day.

Following the formation of a filtrate, some further action is required, because if left to itself, filtrate will pass along the tubule to the kidney's collecting system, the urinary bladder,

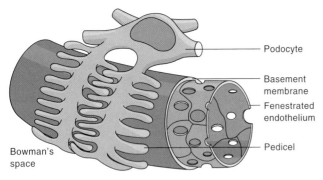

Figure 15.3 **Glomerular Fine Structure.** Fluid from the lumen of the glomerular capillary passes through the perforations (fenestrations) in the endothelium, the basement membrane, and the narrow slits formed by the podocyte's foot processes (pedicels) to arrive in Bowman's space.

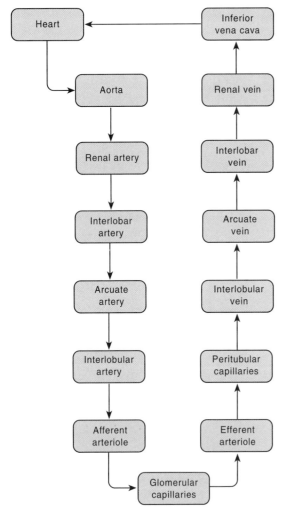

Figure 15.4 **Renal Blood Flow.** The sequence of blood flow through the renal vasculature. In essence, blood entering the kidney is directed to a nephron. After processing by the nephron, blood is returned to the general circulation.

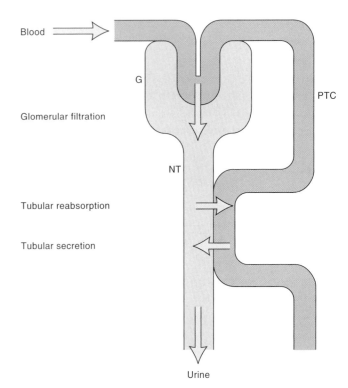

Figure 15.5 **Nephron Function.** Essential mechanisms of nephron blood processing involved in urine production. G: glomerulus, NT: nephron tubule, PTC: peritubular capillaries.

and finally to the body's exterior. This means that anything in the glomerular blood is inside the body and anything in the tubule is outside; there is no middle ground. In effect, following filtration, our body fluid and its many valuable components are at risk of being lost.

To cope with this situation, the nephron employs the second principal mechanism of renal function: **selective reabsorption.** By this process, substances in filtrate pass from the nephron's lumen back into the blood of the peritubular capillaries, and their loss is prevented. They have been reabsorbed and, hence, retained for the body's use (fig. 15.5). Note, however, that not all of the constituents of filtrate are reabsorbed. Some remain in the lumen and are excreted. Thus, there is a selection process involved in reabsorption. It is based, essentially, on the relative permeability of the tubule wall to the various filtrate constituents. Some substances pass to the peritubular spaces by simple diffusion through the tubule wall, whereas others are carried by specific membrane transport systems.

With certain substances, the nephron employs a third mechanism to adjust the composition of filtrate. It is called **tubular secretion,** and involves the movement of substances from the blood of the peritubular capillaries into the tubule lumen (fig. 15.5). These substances are excreted in the urine. (The term *tubular secretion* is defined in the context of excretion into the lumen and should not be confused with the more general concept of secretion, where the substance that

Checkpoint 15.1

To quickly review, consider the following. If given the task of removing impurities from the blood, most of us would try to find some way of filtering them out and discarding them. That works in a standard engineering context, but note the clever nephron's approach. After glomerular filtration, *everything* in the plasma—except the formed elements and plasma proteins—has been discarded. (Remember: The tubule lumen is an outside space and everything in it is headed for the urine.) With selective reabsorption, the nephron now takes things back, but only the "good stuff"—only things that are needed; wastes are left "out there" to be lost in the urine. An indirect but highly effective approach.

passes from a cell serves some useful purpose.) As in the case of selective reabsorption, a system of simple diffusion and specific membrane transport mechanisms is involved, the latter in particular. Filtration, reabsorption, and tubular secretion rates vary based on the body's overall need to excrete or retain various substances. In this way, these nephron processes combine to provide the kidney's excretory and homeostatic functions.

Urine Production

It should be apparent from the preceding discussion that the excretion of a particular constituent of the blood plasma is determined by its ability to be filtered, the degree to which it is reabsorbed, and the amount of it, if any, that is added to the nephron lumen by tubular secretion mechanisms. All such excreted substances are passed to the urinary bladder for elimination in the form of urine. Urine is therefore derived from the blood plasma and contains anything that has been filtered and/or secreted but not reabsorbed. Some of these urine constituents are toxic if allowed to reach high levels in the tissues. Others are present in the urine because their levels exceed homeostatic requirements. For example, water, sodium ion, and bicarbonate ion are not in themselves toxic. However, if their respective levels are not precisely maintained, serious problems can arise. Normally, any such substances present in urine represent amounts in excess of those required for homeostatic balance. Table 15.1 compares the composition of the blood, nephron filtrate, and urine. It shows that blood and filtrate composition differ only in the filtrate's almost complete lack of formed elements and plasma proteins. In comparing the filtrate and urine, it can be seen that all substances not toxic or present to excess in filtrate remain in the tubule to form urine.

Table 15.1   Comparative Composition of Renal Fluids

Blood	Filtrate	Urine
Formed elements	Trace	Trace
H_2O	H_2O	
H_2O_E	H_2O_E	H_2O_E
Plasma proteins	Trace	Trace
Na^+	Na^+	
Na^+_E	Na^+_E	Na^+_E
K^+	K^+	
K^+_E	K^+_E	K^+_E
HCO_3^-	HCO_3^-	
$HCO_3^-_E$	$HCO_3^-_E$	$HCO_3^-_E$
Glucose	Glucose	
Amino acids	Amino acids	
H^+		
H^+_E	H^+_E	H^+_E
Urea	Urea	Urea
Creatinine	Creatinine	Creatinine
Uric acid	Uric acid	Uric acid
Cl^-	Cl^-	
Cl^-_E	Cl^-_E	Cl_E
Mg^{++}	Mg^{++}	
Mg^{++}_E	Mg^{++}_E	Mg^{++}_E
NH_3	NH_3	
NH_{3E}	$NH_4^+_E$	$NH_4^+_E$

The subscript E indicates a quantity in excess of the homeostatic optimum. These are excreted in the urine with metabolic wastes such as urea, uric acid, and creatinine, and others not indicated in the table. Essential filtrate components are retained by reabsorption from filtrate. (NH_3 is converted to NH_4^+ in the nephron tubule.) The essential similarity of plasma and filtrate reflects the nonspecific nature of the filtration process. Urine composition is determined by the tubule cells as they process filtrate by means of selective reabsorption and tubular secretion.

RENAL DISEASE

Renal disease typically involves some degree of waste retention or of fluid and electrolyte imbalance. Several etiologies and patterns of pathogenesis are recognized as contributing to loss of nephron function. In many cases, this loss is reversible, but nephrons may be permanently lost. The large number of nephrons in the kidney seems to allow for a wide safety margin, and as more and more losses occur, existing nephrons can increase in size, enabling them to process more filtrate. This hypertrophy response can't compensate completely, however, and functional deterioration continues, with lost nephrons being replaced by scarring. Initially, malfunction may derive from a problem in the nephron itself or from infections that arise in the urinary tract or collecting system and then spread to the tissues of the renal medulla. Either situation may quickly resolve, but if the problem persists, it can involve the permanent loss of entire nephrons.

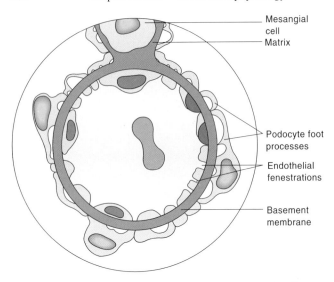

Mesangial cell

Matrix

Podocyte foot processes

Endothelial fenestrations

Basement membrane

Figure 15.6   **Cross Section Through a Glomerular Capillary.** The drawing shows its fenestrated endothelium, podocytes, and their foot processes (pedicels). Note that mesangial cells are present in a matrix that is continuous with the basement membrane of the capillary.

Glomerular Disorders

The process of glomerular filtration provides the fluid that tubule cells modify to produce urine. It follows, then, that any change in the glomerular components that make up the filtration membrane will have an effect on the filtration process. Most often, this is the loss of needed substances.

Impaired filtration is the common element in a broad range of kidney disorders. Before we turn to the details of these conditions, it will be useful to analyze figure 15.6, which presents a simplified section through a single glomerular capillary loop supported by podocyte foot processes. Note the supporting mesangial cells and their intercellular matrix, which is continuous with the capillary basement membrane. The mesangial cells are important to glomerular function. They are contractile and, by altering their tension, they can affect blood flow in glomerular capillaries. They also secrete the matrix substance and basement membranes that contribute to the support of the glomerulus. These mesangial elements are not shown in figure 15.3.

In normal filtration, fluid passes from the glomerular capillary lumen through the endothelial fenestrations, the basement membrane, and the slits formed by the pedicels. Therefore, any disease process that alters or distorts any of these components will have an effect on filtration. The conditions that will be described shortly are examples involving loss of pedicels, and immune-mediated BM damage that affects glomerular function. Proliferation of endothelial, mesangial, or Bowman's capsule cells may also occur to obstruct blood flow, filtrate flow, or both.

Terminology

A complex terminology has arisen around the various glomerular disorders, reflecting the focus of the clinician, histologist, and pathologist. Glomerular disorders are usu-

ally grouped under the term **glomerulonephritis** (GN), even though some glomerular disease lacks a clearly inflammatory component. More precise usage is emerging, but traditional usage is difficult to change.

From the clinician's perspective, GN is described as acute, rapidly progressive, or chronic. **Acute GN** is typically benign and relatively quick to resolve, whereas **rapidly progressive GN** is a swiftly advancing disorder that can lead to death in a matter of a few months. **Chronic GN** is a long-term disease that may take years or decades to run its course.

From the pathologist's point of view, the distribution of the glomerular lesions throughout the cortical tissue might well be significant, and the terminology will reflect this fact. **Diffuse GN** involves most or all glomeruli, whereas in **focal GN** only some of the glomeruli are abnormal. The term **segmental GN** indicates that some capillary loops in a given glomerulus are involved while others are unaffected.

Study of the histology of glomerular disease gives rise to still other terms differentiating three types of glomerular change. In **minimal change** disease, little histological alteration is seen except for changes in the pedicels' tiny foot processes. Ordinary lab microscopes don't show the detail, but electron microscopy reveals flattening and fusion of adjacent foot processes. Although the abnormality is histologically minimal, the defect can certainly give rise to clinical disease. This is one of the conditions often grouped with GN, even though it lacks an inflammatory component.

The term **proliferative** is applied to those cases of glomerulonephritis that involve an increase in some glomerular component. Thus, the cells of Bowman's capsule, mesangial cells, or the endothelia of glomerular capillaries might proliferate (fig. 15.7b). The effect is restriction of blood flow through the glomerulus, causing impaired filtration.

Of course, with more than one glomerular change present, terminology becomes more complex. For example, both cellular proliferation and basement membrane thickening may be present. In such cases, the term **membranoproliferative GN** is appropriate, if cumbersome. Terminology can be further complicated by adding information regarding the distribution of the lesions, as in **diffuse proliferative GN.**

However you may encounter these terms, if you recognize their patterns of use, and also the user's frame of reference, you will have insight into the essential nature of the glomerular abnormality.

Pathogenesis of Glomerulonephritis

The central feature in the pathogenesis of most glomerulonephritis is immune-mediated damage to the glomerulus. In a few cases, T cells contribute to the problem, as in minimal-change GN. More often (70% of cases), immune complexes are involved. Their presence triggers the activation of complement and the infiltration of inflammatory phagocytes. These, along with glomerular mesangial cells, engulf

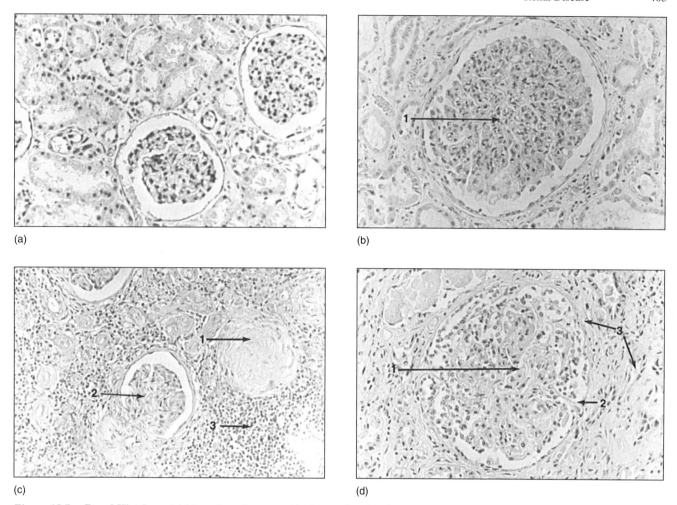

(a)

(b)

(c)

(d)

Figure 15.7   **Renal Histology.** (*a*) Normal renal cortex with glomeruli and various tubule sections. (*b*) In proliferative glomerulonephritis, the increased number and size of the glomerular components gives rise to the congested appearance of this glomerulus. (1). (*c*) Chronic pyelonephritis. Some glomeruli are normal (2), while others have been replaced by scar tissue (1). Tubular necrosis is extensive and numerous inflammatory cells have infiltrated (3). (*d*) Chronic glomerulonephritis. Glomeruli are enlarged and exhibit some hyalinization (1). Proliferation of glomerular and capsular cells has almost obliterated Bowman's space (2). Tubules are atrophied and there is extensive scarring (3).

the complexes, but as they do, they release destructive proteases and free radicals that damage the glomerulus. Inflammatory mediators from disturbed mesangial cells also contribute to the process. The damage exposes basement membrane, favoring platelet aggregation and the formation of microthrombi.

In chronic GN, the prolonged course of the disease seems related to the enormous reserve capacity of the kidneys. Low-level glomerular malfunction may go unnoticed as damage proceeds, since the undamaged nephrons are able to provide essentially normal function. Unfortunately, the emergence of signs and symptoms is an indication that the reserve nephrons have been destroyed, and there is no possibility of regeneration. Another factor in chronic GN is the defensive clearing of complexes after their deposition. Infiltrating inflammatory cells and phagocytosis by mesangial cells can perform this job to a degree, delaying complex deposition. However, continued deposition exceeds their scavenging capacity, ultimately giving rise to glomerular destruction (fig. 15.7*d*).

Focus on Histological Staining and GN Diagnosis

Special histological staining techniques can demonstrate the difference between the deposition of immune complexes that are preformed in the plasma and anti-BM antibody that reacts with the BM. When the uncomplexed antibody is exposed to the BM, it can bind to it all along its surface to produce a uniform, linear staining pattern. The preformed complexes, by contrast, produce a granular appearance as they are trapped at their points of filtration, forming nonuniform clumps. This difference can be useful in diagnosis when tissue from a renal biopsy is specially stained, and you may encounter references to the staining pattern in lab reports.

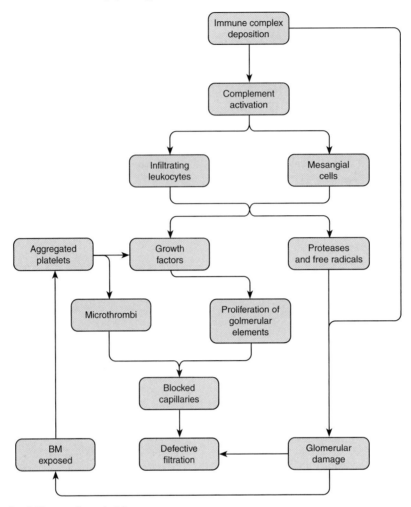

Figure 15.8   **Pathogenesis of Glomerulonephritis.**

In proliferative GN, the specific mechanisms that bring about the increased production of endothelial, epithelial, or mesangial components of the glomerulus and Bowman's capsule are not clearly understood. Growth factors secreted by mesangial cells, infiltrating leukocytes, or aggregated platelets appear to be involved (fig. 15.8)

Having noted the role of immune complexes in the pathogenesis of glomerulonephritis, let us consider how it is that these complexes come to be present in the first place.

In most cases of glomerulonephritis, antibody is formed and then binds to antigens that are circulating in the plasma. The resulting complexes become trapped in glomeruli, activating the mechanisms that produce the range of damage and proliferation responses that characterize GN (fig. 15.9).

Some specific infectious agents are the sources of the antigens involved in the development of GN, with signs and symptoms usually emerging some weeks after the infection subsides. Certain bacteria of the genus *Streptococcus* and the hepatitis B and C viruses are examples. Many cases of chronic glomerulonephritis are the result

of recurring infections, with each attack generating new waves of immune complexes that yield further glomerular damage. Each recurrence adds to the number of destroyed glomeruli, and over months and years, the kidney is overwhelmed.

In certain conditions, endogenous antigens are involved. For example, some tumors, notably lung carcinoma, shed antigens into the blood that form complexes with circulating antibody. In systemic lupus erythematosus (SLE, described in chapter 5), the antinuclear antibodies that characterize the disease can also contribute to immune complex formation. In many cases, the initiating antigen remains unidentified, so the term *idiopathic* is still encountered in reference to the etiology of much glomerulonephritis.

The second mechanism involves an autoimmune defect in which the immune system produces antibody against the glomerular basement membrane (fig. 15.10). This occurs infrequently. It is the underlying defect in **Goodpasture's syndrome,** in which circulating antibody also attacks pulmonary capillary basement membrane, allowing blood to reach the sputum (hemoptysis).

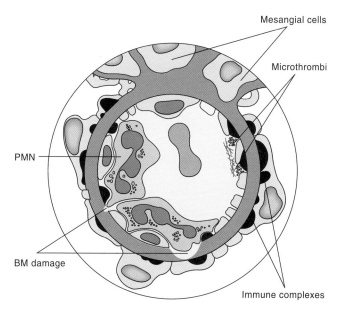

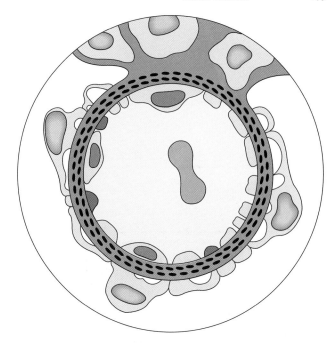

Figure 15.9   **Glomerular Derangements in Glomerulonephritis.** Dark-antigen/antibody complexes are trapped in the glomerulus, producing a granular appearance in microscopic studies. PMNs are disrupting the BM, and fibrin deposition is also under way. Proliferation of mesangial cells, their supporting matrix, and the basement membrane are also present. Compare with figure 15.6.

Figure 15.10   **Glomerulonephritis.** Interaction of circulating antibody and glomerular basement membrane antigen produces a pattern of deposition that appears linear in microscope preparations. Compare with figure 15.6.

Sequelae of Glomerular Change

Whatever the source of the immune complexes, damage to the glomerulus yields a predictable pattern of glomerular malfunction. Essentially, defective filtration retains substances normally lost and allows the escape of plasma constituents that are normally retained. Of the many different glomerular disorders, most develop toward one of two clinical patterns: the **nephrotic syndrome** and the **nephritic syndrome.**

Nephrotic Syndrome   This is the clinical condition that is characterized by large-scale **proteinuria,** and by hypoalbuminemia, systemic edema, and hyperlipidemia. The proteinuria is caused by the inability of the damaged glomeruli to retain protein. Because they are small, the albumins are the first to pass a defective filtration membrane and, once they are in the tubule, they overwhelm its limited capacity for protein reabsorption. As damage progresses, other larger proteins are also lost to exaggerate the proteinuria.

The hypoalbuminemia that results from protein loss to the urine is also the key to the systemic edema of the nephrotic syndrome. This is because the albumins are not only small, but are also the most numerous of the plasma proteins. This means that they are a major determinant of the blood's osmotic pressure. As hypoalbuminemia develops following glomerular damage, blood osmotic pressure falls and tissue fluid that would normally be drawn into the blood remains in the tissue spaces, causing sytemic edema.

The condition is aggravated by the kidney's reflex fluid retention response in the face of declining filtration. The result is a rise in fluid volume that boosts blood pressure, forcing more fluid into the tissue spaces to exaggerate the edema problem.

The hyperlipidemia of the nephrotic syndrome is based on an increased hepatic synthesis of lipoprotein in response to low plasma protein levels. An increased tendency to blood coagulation is another aspect of the nephrotic syndrome that can produce systemic effects. It seems to be caused by the urinary loss of protein anticoagulants. Protein loss in more severe GN may involve immune globulins and elements of the complement system. This explains the increased susceptibility to infection that may complicate the nephrotic syndrome. Figure 15.11 summarizes the pathogenesis of the nephrotic syndrome.

Minimal-change GN commonly produces the nephrotic syndrome in children. It is also seen in **focal-segmental nephrosclerosis,** an idiopathic glomerular disease characterized by glomerular hyalinization. Its pathogenesis is linked to HIV infection, heroin addiction, extreme obesity, and sickle-cell anemia. The precise relation between these conditions and the nephrotic syndrome is unclear, although hypoxic damage to the glomerulus may be a factor in sickle-cell disease.

Nephritic Syndrome   In this condition, the clinical picture is dominated by inflammatory damage that restricts glomerular filtration and allows erythrocytes to escape to the urine

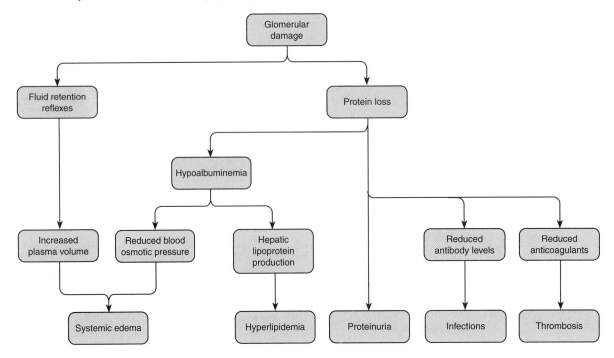

Figure 15.11   **Nephrotic Syndrome.** Large-scale protein loss and its consequences characterize the nephrotic syndrome.

Focus on Mechanisms Underlying the Nephrotic and Nephritic Syndromes

You may be wondering how glomerular damage that allows red cells to escape from the blood (as in the nephritic syndrome) wouldn't, at the same time, allow large-scale losses of the plasma proteins, which are much smaller. The explanation has to do with a specialized property of the glomerular BM. Its components carry negative charges, which repel the negative charges on plasma proteins. In the nephrotic syndrome, BM damage disrupts these charges. No longer repelled, protein can more easily escape while the larger red cells remain in the blood. Over the extensive glomerular BM surface, protein loss by this mechanism can be significant.

In the nephritic syndrome, capillary endothelial damage is associated with cellular proliferation. These changes may generate pressures that can expel erythrocytes at points where the endothelium gives way. This would occur only at certain points, allowing red cell loss but limiting protein escape because the BM and its negative repulsive charges remain essentially intact.

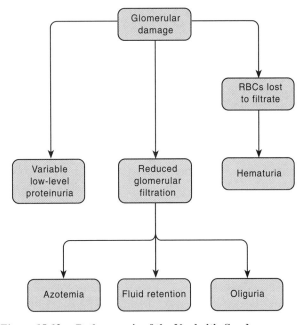

Figure 15.12   **Pathogenesis of the Nephritic Syndrome.** Although fluid retention and some protein loss occur in the nephritic syndrome, edema does not usually develop.

(hematuria). The decreased filtration causes reduced urinary output (**oliguria**), systemic hypertension, and the accumulation of nitrogenous wastes in the blood (**azotemia**). The lack of filtration explains the azotemia, since waste products won't reach the urine if they aren't filtered into the tubule. Reduced filtration also explains the systemic hypertension—

it is the kidney's attempt to compensate for lower filtration by retaining fluid as a means of increasing plasma volume. In normal circumstances, boosting plasma volume is a useful way to increase blood pressure, but, of course, circumstances here aren't normal and the added problem of high blood pressure just complicates the situation. In the nephritic syndrome, glomerular damage may also allow protein loss, but this is a variable occurrence and the amounts are less than in the nephrotic syndrome (fig. 15.12).

Checkpoint 15.2

A physician's reference might describe ten or more types of glomerulonephritis, each with its own particular pattern of glomerular disruption. The details of histological change and pathogenesis for each type are beyond the scope of this text. Just remember that whatever specific GN condition you encounter, the patient is likely to present the signs and symptoms of either the nephrotic syndrome or the nephritic syndrome. And just to make life interesting, many GN cases will have a clinical picture that has elements of both (e.g., urine containing high levels of protein *and* blood).

The low level of filtration in the nephritic syndrome places less demand on tubule cells and they atrophy in response. Ultimately, lost nephrons are replaced by scarring. The nephritic syndrome is also commonly associated with postinfection GN. HIV and HCV are most often implicated in North America, while streptococcal infections dominate in other parts of the world. In some cases, rapidly progressive GN produces an acute and severe nephritic syndrome that does not respond to therapy. Complete renal failure is the result.

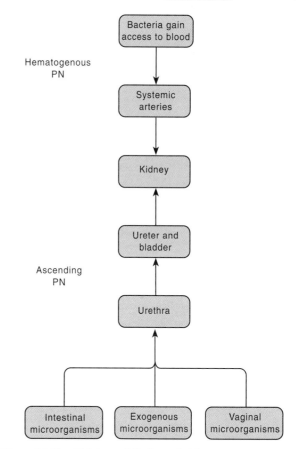

Figure 15.13   **Etiology of Pyelonephritis.**

Tubulointerstitial Disorders

The renal medulla contains the straight-running arms of Henle's loop and the collecting ducts that receive processed filtrate from the nephrons. The remaining medullary tissues, consisting of a supporting intercellular matrix and the peritubular capillaries, are referred to as the renal interstitium. In glomerular disease, the clinical presentation is based on defective filtration. The tubulointerstitial disorders are characterized by faulty tubule processing. Usually, the consequences are water and sodium loss and the retention of acid. There are two principal forms of tubulointerstitial disease: **pyelonephritis** and **interstitial nephritis.**

Pyelonephritis

Pyelonephritis (PN) is an inflammatory condition of the renal interstitium that also affects the calyces and pelvis of the collecting system. Glomeruli are not normally affected, or are only minimally so, unless the condition is prolonged. Bacterial infections are the usual cause of such inflammation, although viral or other agents may be involved. Pyelonephritis is the most common renal disease, the kidneys' involvement deriving from the frequent occurrence of urinary tract infections in the adult. Chronic PN is the second most common source of renal failure, next to chronic glomerulonephritis.

PN may be **hematogenous,** with blood-borne bacteria from an infected site being carried to the kidney. In such cases, the typical result is abscess formation and necrosis in the renal cortex. Subsequent spread to lower parts of the urinary tract distinguishes descending PN from the much more common cases (over 90%) of ascending PN, in which bacteria reach the kidney from lower parts of the urinary tract. These are often of fecal origin (e.g., *Escherichia coli, Proteus,* and *Enterococcus* species), but vaginal and exogenous organisms are also commonly involved (fig. 15.13). Females have a higher incidence of ascending PN, which is probably due to the shorter length of the female urethra. A longer urethra and the antibacterial properties of prostate secretions favor a lower incidence in the male up to the age of about 40. With increasing age, enlargement of the prostate may limit complete emptying of the bladder, causing increased infections.

Pathogenesis

Normally the urine and the urinary tract are sterile, excepting the distal urethra. With normal flushing of the urinary tract by the usual pattern of urine flow, bacteria cannot proliferate. If bladder emptying is incomplete, the remaining urine may serve as a growth medium for urethral bacteria. Bladder abnormalities that involve inadequate urine expulsion pressures or blockage of urine outflow are the main sources of incomplete bladder emptying. Factors contributing to obstruction of the urinary tract are kidney

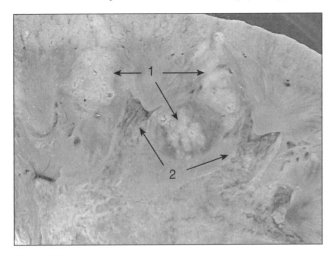

Figure 15.14   **Pyelonenephritis.** In this section of a kidney demonstrating pyelonephritis, abscesses are easily seen as pale areas. (1). The surfaces of the renal pelvis and calyces are inflamed (2) and the entire kidney is swollen.
This is the kidney of an elderly man who was admitted to hospital with seizures. He was unable to convey any elements of his medical history that might aid in diagnosis, and he was admitted in the hope that antiseizure medication would stabilize him. His urinary incontinence was assumed to be related to his seizures, and when a urinary catheter was inserted, his prostate was found to be enlarged. Although his seizure activity subsided somewhat, he soon became feverish and his urine became cloudy and odorous. Culture revealed E. coli *to be the contaminant. In spite of antibiotic therapy, the infection quickly became systemic and he died. Autopsy revealed acute bilateral pyelonephritis, probably from an ascending infection that had become established as a result of urinary obstruction.*

stones (see the section on urinary calculi), prostate enlargement in the male, pregnancy (involving increased pelvic pressure), pelvic inflammations related to disease or trauma, and tumors.

In some children, a congenital malformation of the joining of the ureters to the bladder allows backflow of urine from the bladder to the ureters during urination. The condition, known as **vesicoureteral reflux,** is associated with an increased incidence of pyelonephritis.

Two types of PN, acute and chronic, can be distinguished on the basis of the duration and severity of their signs and symptoms.

Acute Pyelonephritis   Acute PN is a common, comparatively mild condition of primarily bacterial etiology, ranking as the second most common infectious disease, after infections of the respiratory system. It involves inflammation of renal tissues, which can lead to suppuration and necrosis as well as bleeding in the mucous membrane of the adjacent collecting system (fig. 15.14). Acute PN may involve one or both kidneys and is characterized by sudden onset accompanied by pain, chills, and fever, **pyuria** (pus in the urine), and **bacteriuria,** although the latter is not always

observed. This acute form of the disease is typically mild and self-limiting, but overwhelming infections can lead to necrosis of the renal medulla, which is followed by renal failure. Although treatment with antibiotics is normally successful, recurrent infection is common.

Chronic Pyelonephritis   The devastating pattern of development in chronic PN consists of a slow, long-term deterioration of renal function that is often asymptomatic until substantial renal damage has occurred. As in the case of glomerulonephritis, this leads to loss of functional parenchyma, which is replaced by scar tissue (see fig. 15.7c). Onset of the disease is often insidious, with signs and symptoms indicating a progressive deterioration of renal function. Pain, fever, systemic hypertension, and potassium retention may be involved to varying degrees. Grossly, the surface of the kidney shows evidence of scarring where infection has destroyed the medulla and, often, the adjacent cortex. Vesicoureteral reflux is a major factor in chronic pyelonephritis, as is obstruction of the urinary tract. Where urinary obstruction is involved, long-term back pressure produces dilation of the collecting system and proximal ureter. In a significant number of cases, chronic PN results in renal failure, necessitating dialysis or kidney transplantation.

Interstitial Nephritis

This term denotes the tubulointerstitial disorders that have an etiology other than infection. The principal damaging agents are therapeutic drugs, other exogenous toxins, or endogenous substances that are toxic to the interstitium. One aspect of this problem is the large volume of blood that circulates through the kidneys. Although they represent only about 0.5% of the body's weight, the kidneys receive 20% of the resting cardiac output. As a result, the entire plasma volume circulates through the kidneys about 60 times a day. This means the renal tissues have a great deal of exposure to any plasma toxin.

A number of antibiotic and analgesic preparations, as well as lithium salts and the increasingly used immunosuppressant cyclosporine, are implicated in interstitial nephritis. Note, in particular, that chronic pain sufferers such as rheumatoid arthritics or those with low back pain have a significant risk of nephrotoxic damage from their long-term analgesic ingestion. As well, derangements that increase plasma levels of calcium and uric acid, (e.g., gout and polycythemia) or that decrease potassium levels have roles in its etiology. Lead, mercury, and cadmium poisoning can produce interstitial nephritis, but less frequently.

Selected nephrotoxins are presented in table 15.2. Signs and symptoms of interstitial nephritis reflect evidence of varying degrees of tubular malfunction. Additional effects based on hypersensitivity reaction to the drug may also develop: fever, skin rashes, hematuria.

Table 15.2	Selected Nephrotoxins

Metals

Mercury compounds	Cadmium
Arsenic	Copper
Uranium	

Organic Solvents

Carbon tetrachloride	Tetrachloroethylene
Methanol	Ethylene glycol (automobile antifreeze)

Therapeutic Agents

Antibiotics

Ampicillin	Penicillin
Methicillin	Sulfonamides
Tetracycline	Streptomycin

Analgesics

Aspirin (ASA)	Acetaminophen

Various Diuretics and NSAIDS

Insecticides

Chlorinated hydrocarbons	Biphenyl compounds

Miscellaneous

Carbon monoxide	Cresol
Mushroom poisons	Mannitol

 Checkpoint 15.3

Before going on, let's do a brief check on matters to this point. In GN, damage is focused in the glomerulus, with disrupted filtration the principal result. In the tubulointerstitial diseases, damage is centered in the medulla, causing faulty tubule function. Problems arising in one region can affect the other, especially in late stages of severe disease.

Renal Vascular Disorders

Many vascular disorders have prominent renal effects even though, for the most part, the renal vessels are themselves not abnormal. For example, atherosclerotic narrowing of the aorta and renal artery can produce renal ischemia that affects kidney function. Emboli from an atherosclerotic aorta may cause diffuse cortical damage. Similar damage is also seen in circulatory shock, where falling BHP is the cause of ischemia.

Other systemic disorders have effects on the renal vasculature. In diabetes mellitus, the glomerular capillaries are affected (see chapter 17). In systemic hypertension, the renal arterioles undergo thickening, the condition referred to in chapter 9 as arteriolosclerosis. In the context of the kidney, this arteriolar thickening is known as **nephrosclerosis.** It typically results in renal ischemia and scattered areas of atrophy and necrosis.

The two types of systemic hypertension produce different patterns of nephrosclerosis. In **benign nephrosclerosis,** the damage is usually mild, with minimal polyuria or filtration abnormalities and little risk of renal failure. As we indicated in chapter 9, the biggest risk in benign hypertension is its related cardiac and cerebrovascular morbidity.

The renal vascular problems associated with malignant hypertension, **malignant nephrosclerosis,** are much more likely to lead to serious complications and renal failure. Details are not clear, but an essential mechanism in this condition is renal arteriolar wall damage, which may be caused by the pressures associated with pre-existing benign nephrosclerosis. Fibrinogen seeps into the wall at these sites and, aided by adhering platelets, fibrin forms within the arteriolar wall. Growth factors from platelets and other cells also stimulate proliferation of wall smooth muscle. These factors combine to produce pronounced thickening of the wall, corresponding loss of lumen, and severe ischemia. In response, the renin-angiotensin system is activated, triggering fluid-retention reflexes that increase the already elevated blood pressure. Cycles of further ischemia and pressure rises continue, exaggerating the problem. Another consequence of diffuse coagulation within the narrowed arterioles is trauma to red blood cells. As they are driven over fibrin deposits, their membranes are damaged. The damaged erythrocytes are cleared from the circulation faster than they can be replaced, and a **microangiopathic hemolytic anemia** develops.

With the increased kidney damage associated with malignant nephrosclerosis, renal dysfunction gives rise to hematuria, proteinuria, and decreased acid and waste excretion. If untreated, it will steadily progress to complete renal failure, often within one year. Therapeutic intervention to lower blood pressure can greatly reduce mortality.

URINARY CALCULI

The process of **nephrolithiasis,** or **urolithiasis,** involves the formation of insoluble stones, or **calculi,** in the urinary tract. A calculus usually forms in a single kidney. Once formed, it may remain in the renal pelvis or pass to the ureter and then to the urinary bladder. Often it will lodge in the tract to obstruct urine flow.

Most urolithiasis presents only minor problems, because stones that remain in the kidney are well tolerated, and others may be unknowingly passed in the urine. Thus, although the incidence of calculi seen at autopsy is relatively high (1 in 100), the incidence of hospitalization for

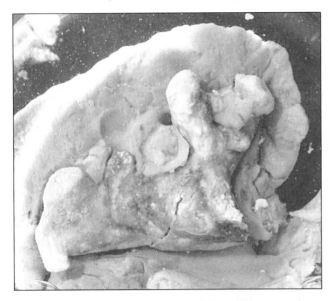

Figure 15.15 **Staghorn Calculus.** This large kidney stone is, essentially, a cast of the renal pelvis and calyces. It resembles a deer's antler.

This staghorn calculus was an incidental autopsy finding in a middle-aged male who died of an acute MI. In this view, the loss of renal cortex and medulla is apparent. The pelvis is filled with the stone, which sends rough projections into the calyces. In addition to the stone, microscopic studies confirmed the presence of tubular atrophy and scarring consistent with chronic pyelonephritis.

urolithiasis is quite low (1 in 1,000). The disorder is three times more likely to occur in males than in females, with peak incidence at 20–30 years of age.

Calculi vary in size and number. One or several stones may form, ranging in size from the microscopic to those with diameters of several centimeters. They may have smoothly rounded or polygonal shapes, or their surfaces may be jagged and rough. When a large calculus forms in the renal pelvis with extension into the calyces, the resulting shape resembles a deer antler and is referred to as a *staghorn calculus* (fig. 15.15). Most calculi are composed of crystals of inorganic ions. Many different ions have been found in calculi, with composition generally reflecting pathogenesis. Most commonly involved are calcium, oxalate, phosphate, and urate ions.

Stone formation is usually associated with an increased urine concentration of the ions found in the stone. The change in concentration most often derives from increased renal excretion, but might also involve a diminished urine volume, as in dehydration states. Even when urine concentration is normal, changes in urinary acidity can lead to stone formation. For example, a lowered urine pH favors precipitation of uric acid, while a more alkaline urine predisposes to phosphate stone formation.

Etiology in urolithiasis is complex and usually reflects disturbances in the metabolism of the ions involved. Most cases involve **hypercalciuria** (high levels of calcium in the urine), which may be the result of an idiopathic increase in

Focus on Stones That Can Hurt!

As noted earlier, renal colic can be quite severe. In that context, it's not unusual for an emergency vehicle to rush into a hospital, with the driver needing assistance in extracting a person from the floor of the rear of the vehicle. In these cases, it's usually a kidney stone in the ureter that is responsible for the victim's thrashing about in agony.

intestinal calcium absorption, with an attendant increase in the need for calcium excretion. Or, for example, an increased intake of vitamin D in an attempt to prevent osteoporosis may produce the high levels of plasma calcium. In the case of a parathyroid adenoma that hypersecretes parathyroid hormone, hypercalciuria follows the hormone's effect of increasing calcium retention. Again, the excess calcium ion must be excreted by the kidney, and the resulting hypercalciuria may then contribute to stone formation. Not only calcium but other substances, such as oxalate ion, may become incorporated into calculi as a result of the increased urinary excretion that follows increased dietary intake. Urinary tract infections and chronic pyelonephritis also predispose to urolithiasis.

After obstruction of the urinary tract by a stone, urinary stasis and increased back pressure may result. This can lead to destruction of renal parenchyma, a predisposition to secondary infection, and further renal damage.

The presence of a renal stone may often be asymptomatic, but if a large stone enters the ureter, **renal colic** follows. This is pain of an exquisite and excruciating character, originating at the ureter and often radiating to the upper leg. It derives from the periodic waves of ureteral peristalsis that press upon the stone. Chills and fever are often associated with the ureteral passage of a stone, and hematuria often follows, the result of ureteral damage from abrasion of the mucosa.

In cases of unacceptable pain, infection, or bleeding, obstructing calculi that are not passed from the urinary tract may be removed surgically or with instruments introduced into the urinary tract via the urethra. Alternatively, cystoscopes introduced into the ureter or collecting system can be used to break stones mechanically or by ultrasound energy, so that they can be passed in the urine. Once the stones are removed, prognosis is excellent.

If there is no pressing need for surgery, therapy may simply be directed toward reducing the stones to a size easily passed to the bladder for evacuation. Some drugs can cause existing stones to dissolve or can prevent their enlargement. Other drugs can help by reducing excessive excretion or by changing urine pH, which aids in dissolving the stone.

A condition related to urolithiasis, but only about one-tenth as common, is **nephrocalcinosis.** This involves the formation of minute, insoluble calcium deposits in the nephron tubules and collecting ducts. Fine crystals also form at the papillae. Nephrocalcinosis may occur alone or in association with nephrolithiasis.

OVERVIEW OF ETIOLOGY IN RENAL DYSFUNCTION

You may encounter a system that distinguishes different patterns of etiology in renal disorders. It is based on the position of the kidney between the blood that brings waste to it and the tract that drains urine from it. These components are, of course, essential to normal renal functioning, but each can also be a source of potentially damaging agents. Microorganisms can be blood-borne, or they can reach the kidney via the urinary tract. The blood may also deliver antibodies or immune complexes (earlier implicated in glomerular damage) or any number of toxins also previously considered. The situation is further complicated by the high volumes of blood that perfuse the renal vessels, providing high exposure to any damaging agents that might be present. On the other hand, the dependence of renal function on high blood flow rates can be a source of disruption should blood flow be reduced. Figure 15.16 summarizes the essentials.

Given the position of the kidney with respect to its blood supply and the urinary tract, it can be useful to classify renal disease as **prerenal, renal** (sometimes **intrarenal**), or **postrenal.** In essence, this system describes renal problems whose root cause lies in the renal blood supply, the kidney itself, or in the urinary tract, respectively.

Prerenal Disease

The essential problem in prerenal disease is renal ischemia. However it may come about, any reduction of renal blood flow produces a state of inadequate glomerular filtration, with a consequent decline in the kidney's ability to meet the need for homeostatic regulation and excretion. Clinically, this produces a characteristic oliguria and loss of excretory function.

Figure 15.17 indicates the essential ways in which renal ischemia might arise to produce the signs and symptoms of prerenal disease. They should look familiar because they were mentioned earlier in the section on renal vascular disorders. An important one of these is renal artery stenosis. Atherosclerosis, and the thrombosis often associated with it, is the usual cause of the vessel's narrowing.

A second cause of renal ischemia is low systemic blood pressure, which leads to reduced perfusion of the renal vessels. With normal fluctuations in systemic arterial pressure, the kidney arterioles respond to provide a constant glomerular filtration pressure. This process is known as **renal autoregulation.** However, in circulatory shock states, arterial pressure falls below the kidney's compensation capacity, and filtration is compromised. The specific mechanisms underlying the development of circulatory shock were treated

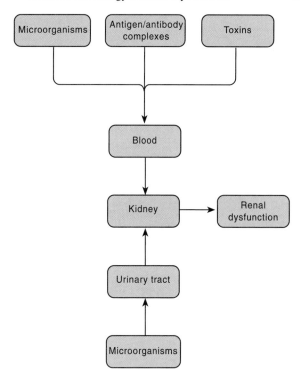

Figure 15.16   **Etiology in Renal Disease.** Pathways to renal damage and dysfunction.

in some detail in chapter 11, so you will quickly recognize the obvious cardiogenic, vascular, and hypovolemic mechanisms as being relevant. In cases of severe renal ischemia, perfusion may be inadequate to maintain renal tissues, and kidney necrosis results. This condition of reduced filtration and renal necrosis is called **shock kidney.**

A third major source of renal ischemia is the nephrosclerosis associated with systemic hypertension (as opposed to hypotension). Various other conditions are also known to reduce renal blood flow—the hepatorenal syndrome mentioned in chapter 14, for example. Most of these conditions are relatively uncommon.

Postrenal Disease

The essential problem in **postrenal disease** is urinary obstruction. With blockage of flow through the urinary tract, back pressure causes urine to accumulate in the kidney. This can compromise excretory function and directly damage renal tissues. Vesicoureteral reflux may be a factor in postrenal disease.

There are two principal sources of urinary tract obstruction. One is the lodging of a kidney stone (or stones) within the ureter or renal pelvis. A second is blockage or compression of the tract by swollen or neoplastic tissues. In males, obstruction arises in the relatively common problem of prostatic hyperplasia, where prostate enlargement directly compresses the urethra.

Before we proceed to the third renal etiology classification, note that in both prerenal and postrenal disease, the kidney is initially able to function normally. That is, a problem

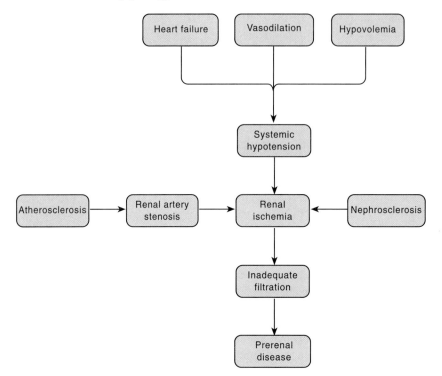

Figure 15.17   **Prerenal Disease.** The causes of the renal ischemia that underlie prerenal disease.

first arises outside the kidney, and altered renal function then follows. In other words, without renal ischemia or urinary tract obstruction, the kidney would function normally.

Renal Disease

Renal, or intrarenal, disease is different from prerenal or postrenal disease in that the problem stems from changes within the kidney itself. The two most common renal disorders are glomerulonephritis and tubulointerstitial disease. Remember that although bacterial infections are the most common causes of these infections, drug and toxic damage can also be significant.

RENAL FAILURE

Renal damage, from whatever source, sooner or later produces signs of renal failure, which may be either acute or chronic. Since both conditions are associated with some degree of uremia, we will consider this topic first.

Uremia

In renal failure, progressive loss of renal function results in the accumulation of waste products whose presence in the blood produces a clinical syndrome called **uremia.** Some of these toxic substances include certain of the products of protein metabolism, but various other accumulating waste products are also involved. When renal excretion drops to about 10% of normal, the signs and symptoms of uremia emerge. These include nausea, vomiting, loss of appetite, and itching in the skin (pruritis).

Fluid and electrolyte imbalances are prominent in uremia and involve water retention and acid-base disturbances. Excessive potassium retention and calcium loss can produce cardiac arrhythmias and cardiac and skeletal muscle weakness. Loss of body weight is common and is related to the anorexia, vomiting, and diarrhea that the uremia toxins induce. The toxins also affect the nervous system, producing a pattern of confusion, apathy, convulsions, and coma called **uremic encephalopathy.** Pericarditis often develops in uremia, but it is unusual for it to interfere with cardiac function. More serious are the blood coagulation problems that result from inhibition of platelet factor 3 (PF-3). They include bleeding at mucosal surfaces or into the pericardial sac or meninges.

The list continues, but suffice it to say that since the accumulating uremia toxins affect cells at a fundamental functional level, almost all organ systems will suffer some degree of derangement in uremia. Usually, by the time uremia develops, the underlying renal disease has progressed too far to be responsive to treatment.

Acute Renal Failure

Rapid, usually reversible decline of renal function is known as **acute renal failure** (ARF). Its dominant feature is a pronounced decline in urinary output **(oliguria),** which may drop to 400 ml/day (25% of normal) or even stop altogether **(anuria).** Many factors can produce rapidly developing oliguria, but they tend to be grouped into three categories: glomerulonephritis, tubulointerstitial disease, and renal ischemia.

Bilateral renal ischemia occurs whenever there is a pronounced drop in the systemic blood pressure. Such circulatory shock can take many forms, the most common of which are the result of surgical or other trauma, hemorrhage, burns, infection, or cardiac damage.

The most common cause of ARF is ischemia or toxic injury, producing a condition called **acute tubular necrosis** (ATN). This condition involves damage to nephron tubules and can be quite severe (fig. 15.18). Regeneration of tubule epithelium and, hence, restoration of function, depends on the degree of damage to the tubule's basement membrane. Nephrotoxins usually damage the basement membrane much less then renal ischemia; hence, the poorer prognosis when renal blood flow is reduced. The toxic agents listed in table 15.2 may be involved in ARF and ATN.

In acute renal failure, oliguria may continue for several weeks, depending on the severity of damage and on tubular regeneration capacity. As restoration of function proceeds, a period of diuresis is usual, as previously retained water is lost to restore fluid balance. The regeneration of tubular epithelium, and the restoration of function that follows, occurs gradually over several weeks. Where damage is severe, or infection or other complications are present, acute renal failure may prove to be fatal.

Chronic Renal Failure

As renal parenchymal damage increases, the declining number of functional nephrons leads inevitably to increased excretory loading on the remaining nephrons and a progressive reduction of function. This is the case following chronic GN or severe PN. In chronic renal failure, effects are irreversible and derangements of homeostatic regulation and excretion are in evidence, but only after nephron losses exceed 50–70% of the total. At this point the consequences of renal insufficiency emerge, and **chronic renal failure** develops. It is characterized by the combination of derangements associated with uremia, which progress toward the condition known as the **end-stage kidney.** Chronic GN or PN is usually the cause, with damage from malignant nephrosclerosis also common. This last condition is typically superimposed on long-standing benign nephrosclerosis.

Excessive water loss dominates during early end-stage disease because the loss of reabsorptive capacity by the tubules is greater than the reduction in filtration at the glomeruli. For example, if the glomerular filtration rate falls 90%, to 18 liters a day, but the tubules can reabsorb only 50% as opposed to their normal 99%, the result is a daily loss of 9 liters, a significant increase over the normal liter and a half. Later, as glomerular function is even further reduced, oliguria or even anuria can result. Urine that is produced is characteristically dilute, usually with a fixed specific gravity, the result of failing tubular concentration mechanisms.

Another condition, called **polycystic kidney disease** (PKD), accounts for up to 10% of chronic renal failure even though its incidence is quite low: only 1 in 1,000. It is

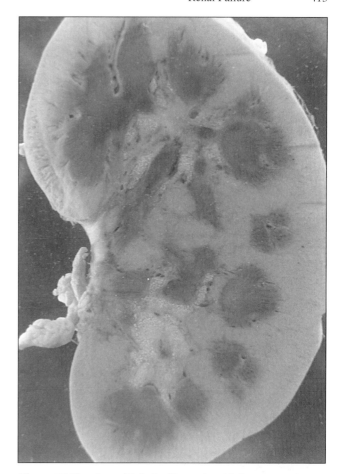

Figure 15.18   Acute Tubular Necrosis. This is an example of acute renal failure. The tubules of the cortex were heavily damaged by exposure to a nephrotoxin, as evidenced by the pale, swollen cortex.

Large-scale kidney and liver damage were responsible for the death of a woman who broke a large bottle of carbon tetrachloride she had been using as a cleaning solvent. She had been cautioned about its hazards, but stubbornly maintained that her mother and grandmother had used it in preference to "modern" cleaners, and furthermore, she was always careful. In cleaning up the spill, she could not avoid heavy fume inhalation and exposure to the skin of her hands and ankles. In bed at night she developed a headache and became drowsy. The next morning she was admitted to the emergency room in a coma and severely oliguric. She died soon after admission. Kidney damage from the solvent produced the swelling, the cortical pallor, and the hyperemia in the medulla seen here. Most damage involved the proximal portions of the tubules, since these are the tubule segments first exposed to the solvent after it is filtered at the glomerulus. These proximal segments lie in the cortex.

a genetic disorder in which the kidneys are filled with multiple fluid-filled cysts, causing them to become hugely distended (see the patient history in the legend for fig. 15.22).

When chronic renal failure gives rise to irreversible and progressive uremia, only aggressive therapeutic intervention can cope with the situation. The two possibilities are dialysis and transplantation.

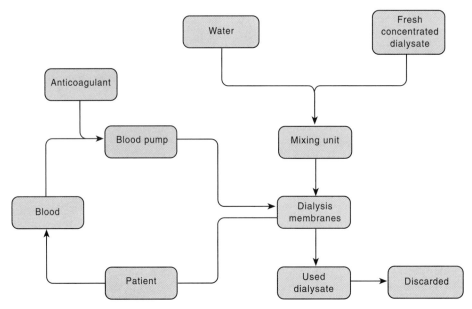

Figure 15.19   **Hemodialysis.** The essential elements of extracorporeal dialysis.

RENAL DIALYSIS

In **renal dialysis,** wastes, uremia toxins, and excess water are cleared from the blood, and electrolyte balance is restored. Two methods are commonly used, both based on establishing favorable concentration gradients between the patient's blood and an appropriately constituted dialysis fluid, the **dialysate.**

Hemodialysis

Hemodialysis involves moving the patient's blood to a device called a **hemodialyzer,** where it flows through a series of fine tubes whose walls are formed of semipermeable membrane. Because the hemodialyzer lies outside the body, this procedure is also called **extracorporeal dialysis.** Surrounding the dialyzer tubes is the dialysate. Its composition favors the diffusion of waste products, toxins, and unwanted electrolytes from the blood into the dialysate and the diffusion of needed substances from the dialysate into the blood.

The dialysis membrane characteristics and the dialysate composition are both critical to successful hemodialysis. The dialysis membrane must have properties that allow water, electrolytes, and small toxin and waste molecules to pass through it. At the same time, it must retain the formed elements, plasma proteins, and other large molecules in the blood.

The dialysate's composition can be varied to meet individual requirements, but its basic composition is such that electrolytes are present in concentrations near to those of normal plasma. As a result, if any plasma ions are present to excess because of faulty renal excretion, the concentration gradients are selected to favor diffusion of those ions out of the blood and into the dialysate. Conversely, if there are

electrolytes that the failing kidney can't retain, the gradients will favor their diffusion from the dialysate into the plasma. Typically, the failing kidney retains sodium and potassium ions while losing calcium ion. Dialysate composition also adjusts chlorine and magnesium ion concentrations.

To maximize removal of waste products, no urea, creatinine, or uric acid is present in dialysate. Thus, there is a high concentration gradient across the dialysis membrane, which ensures maximum diffusion of these unwanted substances out of the blood. Other uremia toxins, whose exact identities are unknown, are also removed by diffusion, since they are not present in the dialysate solution.

Dialysis also attempts to compensate for the kidney's inability to excrete water adequately. It does so by using a pump to raise the pressure under which blood is driven through the dialysis tubes. This elevated pressure directly forces more water out of the blood by filtration. The same effect is achieved in some systems by lowering the pressure in the dialysate through the application of suction.

Since the dialyzer membranes tend to activate the coagulation system, heparin or sodium citrate is used to inhibit clotting. Various therapeutic manipulations, beyond the scope of this text, are employed to deal with the problem of patients who are at risk of bleeding and need all the coagulation they can muster, but who also require dialysis. This situation is not uncommon because, as you may recall, the uremia that necessitates dialysis also interferes with coagulation. Postoperative patients are similarly at risk. The essential elements of extracorporeal dialysis are shown in figure 15.19.

In typical cases, hemodialysis will be repeated several times. To avoid vessel damage from repeated venipuncture, there must be a special means of gaining access to the patient's blood for efficient delivery to and return from the hemodialyzer. The most widely used approach is based on

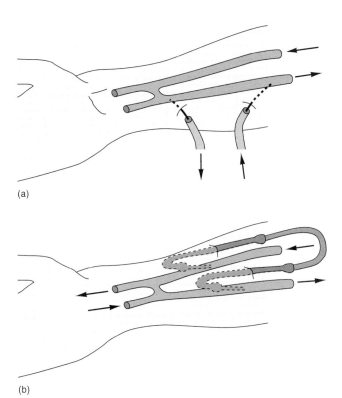

(a)

(b)

Figure 15.20   **Access to the Blood in Hemodialysis.**
(*a*) Arteriovenous fistula. (*b*) External arteriovenous shunt.

the direct surgical joining of an artery of the forearm or leg with its parallel vein, thus creating an **arteriovenous fistula.** This exposes the vein to arterial pressure, and over time it enlarges in response, forming a larger vessel that more easily accommodates venipuncture (fig. 15.20).

Another technique, the **external arteriovenous shunt,** or by-pass, involves exposing an artery and vein in the forearm or leg. Into these parallel vessels are placed rigid cannulae (thin, rigid tubes), which are then passed through the skin, where they are secured with sutures and tape. The arterial cannula is then connected to the venous cannula by a length of flexible tubing (fig. 15.20). Prior to dialysis, the flexible tubing is removed to provide access to arterial blood for the dialyzer, as well as access to a vein for return of the blood after dialysis. The shunt apparatus provides ready access to the blood but is often complicated by infection, clotting, or bleeding as a result of becoming dislodged. For this reason, the external shunt is used only for short-term dialysis.

Peritoneal Dialysis

Compared with hemodialysis, **peritoneal dialysis** is a simpler and easier approach. It uses the peritoneal cavity as a dialysis chamber and the peritoneal membranes as the dialysis membranes. These membranes provide over 2 square meters of surface across which diffusion can occur. A cannula passes the dialysate into the peritoneal cavity by grav-

ity. The dialysate is allowed to remain for a period of four to six hours, during which diffusion and osmosis provide exchange between blood in the peritoneal vessels and the dialysate. The cavity is then cleared of dialysate by means of gravity drainage, and the process is repeated until the desired blood chemistry restoration is achieved.

The term **continuous ambulatory peritoneal dialysis** (CAPD) is increasingly used because it conveys the sense that the patient undergoing peritoneal dialysis is able to remain at home and can pursue some degree of normal activity with less reliance on the medical delivery system. Although CAPD is used less than hemodialysis because of the risk of peritonitis, it has several factors in its favor. It fosters a generally improved morale, avoids coagulation complications, and minimizes the use of expensive equipment. Also, because it is slower than extracorporeal hemodialysis, blood chemistry changes develop gradually. CAPD thus eliminates the more rapid swings associated with hemodialysis, which many uremic and generally debilitated patients have difficulty tolerating.

KIDNEY TRANSPLANTATION

As the function of any organ progressively deteriorates, it becomes apparent that available therapies can only extend the time until its failure is complete. In the case of renal failure, we are fortunate in possessing sophisticated dialysis technology. However, although there is increasing use of CAPD, hemodialysis is still the most widely used dialysis technique. Overall, given the cost, inconvenience, and patient morale problems associated with hemodialysis, transplanting a functional replacement kidney into the ailing recipient is obviously appealing. The advantages of replacing a diseased kidney with a normally functioning organ have long been recognized, but only in the last 20 years has kidney transplantation become a widely available therapeutic option. As the technique has become more widespread, its rate of success has steadily improved.

In transplantation of the kidney, two obstacles must be overcome. One is that of obtaining a replacement kidney. The other is the need to work very quickly to avoid ischemic damage to the organ.

Two sources of kidneys are currently relied upon. The most desirable source is a living donor (LD) closely related to the recipient. A living, unrelated donor or a cadaver donor (CD) may also be used. Because related donors are not always available or able to donate, and living unrelated donors are in short supply, cadaver donors provide about 65% of kidneys for transplantation.

The kidney can tolerate anoxia for up to one hour at body temperature (its **warm ischemic time**). If the organ is quickly cooled to 4° C, the tissue's metabolic demands decrease and its viability can be maintained for up to ten hours (its **cold ischemic time**). Cooling allows more time for preparation of the recipient after the implant becomes available.

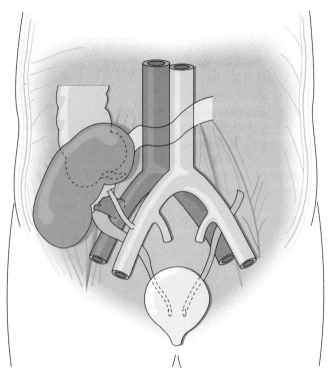

Figure 15.21 **Renal Transplantation.** Typical implantation of a renal transplant.

Implantation

The currently favored site for implantation is different from what one might expect. Instead of being positioned in the space previously occupied by the diseased kidney, the implant is placed in the right iliac fossa. This site is well protected by the innominate bone and the abdominal musculature, but more importantly, it is nearer to the urinary bladder than is the usual kidney location. This is significant because of the ureter's blood supply. Branches of the renal artery supply the proximal parts of the ureter, and these vessels can be retained during the donor's **nephrectomy** (kidney removal). The distal ureter relies more on vessels that can't be retained during nephrectomy, so it is difficult to support in the recipient. Implantation in the iliac fossa allows the shorter proximal ureter, with its better blood supply, to reach the nearby urinary bladder.

The implantation procedure starts with an oblique incision into the right abdominal wall. The iliac arteries and veins are located, and the implant's renal artery and vein are joined to them to establish a renal blood supply. After the blood flow to the implant is restored, urine formation follows, usually within a few minutes in the case of a related living donor. Next, the urinary bladder is opened and a small incision is made in its base to accommodate the attachment of the ureter. The urinary bladder is then closed, and closure of the abdomen completes the procedure (fig. 15.21). The recipient's diseased kidneys are not usually removed after a donor's kidney is implanted.

Care of the recipient after the implantation is similar to that of most postoperative patients. Recipients are able to leave bed on the first postoperative day and to remain up for increasing periods thereafter. Urinary output is closely monitored, because falling urinary output is indicative of the major complication of an implantation—namely, immune rejection of the donor kidney. Cellular and humoral mechanisms may combine to effect rejection, either immediately, where the antigenic match is not sufficiently close, or over a prolonged period.

Immune Rejection

Immune rejection may take one of three forms. In **hyperacute rejection,** urinary output may decline by 90% within minutes to hours after implantation. Failure of renal function is due to the presence of host antibodies against the donor's red cells or renal antigens. The recipient's antibodies may have arisen through previous exposure to antigens by way of a blood transfusion, a previous transplantation, or during a pregnancy in which fetal antigens gained access to the maternal circulation. However the antibodies arise, their presence in the recipient sets the stage for their binding to the endothelial linings of the implanted kidney's blood vessels. This results in the activation of complement and the arrival of phagocytes that strip away the endothelium. This exposes subendothelial tissues, allowing platelets to adhere. Thrombosis and vascular occlusion follow, causing the rapidly developing ischemia and necrosis that overwhelm the implanted kidney. The ability to test recipients to determine their preoperative antibody status has greatly reduced hyperacute rejection in current transplantation practice.

The second pattern of rejection involves both cellular and humoral immune attack and is called **acute rejection.** It typically emerges in the second or third postoperative week and develops rapidly. The recipient's immune system attacks both nephron tubules and arteries in the donated organ. It occurs between the 1st and the 16th postoperative week in the case of an LD. The potential threat extends to two years when a CD is used (fig. 15.22).

Chronic rejection develops over several months. In this case, antibody against the graft binds to the implant's vascular endothelium. The resulting damage disrupts blood flow to produce ischemic injury and irreversible nephron loss.

Immune Suppression

In view of the devastating potential of immune rejection mechanisms, increased success in transplantation depends on therapeutic suppression of the response. This is achieved by the use of chemical immunosuppressant agents, often in combination. Cyclosporine and tacrolimus are widely used in such therapy, especially in combination with drugs with additional immunosuppressive and anti-inflammatory effects, such as prednisone and azathioprine. The goal is the inactivation of those cells of the immune system that mount the immune attack. This approach yields consistently good

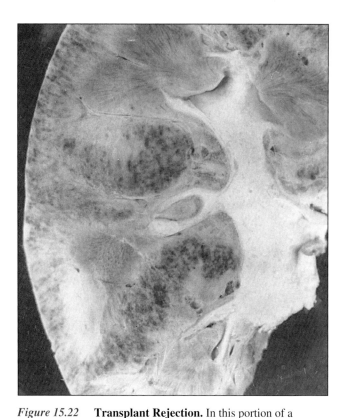

Figure 15.22 **Transplant Rejection.** In this portion of a sectioned renal implant, the organ is generally swollen and edematous. Congestion and small hemorrhages are responsible for the dark mottling of the cortex and medulla.

This is a cadaver donor kidney that was rejected 16 months after implantation. Evidence of immune-mediated vascular damage can be seen in the swollen, edematous organ and in the fine hemorrhages scattered throughout both cortex and medulla. Microscopic study showed degenerated glomeruli and numerous casts in the tubules as evidence of faulty filtration in the glomeruli. The recipient was a 50-year-old man who had polycystic kidneys. After 11 years of hypertension, proteinuria, and hematuria, one kidney was removed. Eighteen months later a suitable cadaver donor kidney became available. The failure of the implant developed rapidly, and uremia and kidney failure could not be prevented.

results, but it carries with it certain hazards, which in some cases are potentially as grave as the renal loss that the immune suppression seeks to prevent.

Apart from the nephrotoxicity of the commonly used immunosuppresants, the major problem associated with immune suppression is infection. This is because the immune system that rejects the implanted kidney is also the principal means of defense against invading microorganisms. When its defensive ability is therapeutically suppressed, the danger of infection increases. It is ironic that the most common cause of death associated with transplantation of the kidney or other organs is not rejection of the transplant but rather infection following immune suppression. A secondary complication of immune suppression involves tumors. It is possible that a renal tumor may be implanted with the donor kidney, but this is less likely than is the de-

velopment of a primary tumor. Immune-suppressed patients are more likely than the normal population to develop leukemia, for example. Of course, the fact that the development of the tumor might take many years before presenting a significant threat must be balanced against the immediate requirement for a new kidney.

Results

The success rate of renal transplantation has steadily increased with improvements in the ability to match donor and recipient antigens and to control the complications of the procedure. Currently, the recipient of a related LD's kidney has a high likelihood of indefinite survival. Improvements in immunosuppression therapy have also increased the success rate of CD implants, so that they currently compare favorably with those of an unrelated LD.

URINARY TRACT TUMORS

Benign renal tumors are fairly common but produce no signs or symptoms and may come to attention only as an incidental postmortem finding. Two malignancies of the kidney are important. **Renal cell carcinoma** (RCC), also known as **renal adenocarcinoma,** is the dominant malignant renal tumor in adults. It makes up almost 90% of all adult kidney cancers. It metastasizes extensively via the blood, especially to lung and bone, before clinical indications warn of its presence. Prognosis is poor unless therapy can be instituted before metastasis occurs. An enlarging renal cell carcinoma is the most frequent cause of inferior vena cava compression by a tumor. Another complication may involve heart failure. A growing tumor can extend along the renal vein and continue up the inferior vena cava to reach the heart. Smoking, obesity, and hypertension are recognized as risk factors in RCC.

Wilms' tumor, also known as **nephroblastoma,** is a common tumor of childhood. It often reaches a large size before its presence is detected in investigating abdominal distention and hematuria in children 2–5 years of age. Intervention involving surgery, radiation, and chemotherapy is usually effective and the prognosis is generally good.

The urinary tract is the site of few benign tumors, but carcinomas do arise in the epithelium of the collecting system and urinary bladder. Obstruction and the risk of pyelonephritis are superimposed on the local damage caused by invasion. Metastasis via the lymphatic system is typical.

ASSESSMENT OF RENAL FUNCTION

A wide range of diagnostic techniques is applied to the assessment of renal functional capacity. Various tests focus on excretion, because the kidney removes unwanted substances from the blood to form urine. High levels of such substances in the blood or low levels in the urine indicate the kidneys' malfunction. The tests described in this section

Table 15.3	Reference Values for Some Commonly Performed Tests of Renal Function

Test	Reference Value
Blood	
Plasma creatinine	0.7–1.5 mg/dl
Blood urea nitrogen (BUN)	8–20 mg/dl
Urine	
Specific gravity	1.025–1.032
Protein	<165 mg/day
Blood cells	0–5/high-power field
Casts	Occasional, hyaline
Bacteria	Urethral organisms only
Clearance Tests	
Creatinine clearance	91–130 ml/min
Urea clearance	60–100 ml/min
Inulin clearance	105–150 ml/min

are used primarily to assess nephron function. Normal values for these tests are indicated in table 15.3.

Blood Tests

Blood is routinely studied to determine its content of toxic substances. Most typically these are the nitrogen-containing products of protein metabolism. If their level in the blood is elevated, renal excretion is assumed to be impaired.

Plasma Creatinine Level

Creatinine is a normal plasma constituent and is derived from the creatine normally found in muscle tissue. Creatinine is toxic and is excreted primarily by the kidney. Under normal circumstances, its level in the blood is quite stable.

Blood Urea Nitrogen Level (BUN)

Urea is synthesized in the liver from nitrogen derived from the metabolism of amino acids. It is excreted only by the kidney. Its level in the blood is expressed in terms of the nitrogen it contains. Values can vary depending on changes in dietary protein or protein metabolism. The blood urea nitrogen (BUN) determination is widely used to screen for renal function.

Elevation of the plasma creatinine or BUN is interpreted as a nonspecific indication of impaired renal function. Because of its stability, the plasma creatinine is regarded as being a more reliable indicator. Neither test can warn of early pathological changes in the kidneys, since creatinine and urea levels are not elevated until damage is severe enough to reduce the kidney's substantial reserve capacity.

Urinalysis

The constituents and characteristics of normal urine are well known. Changes in the makeup of the urine can indicate altered renal function, often with some specificity as to the part of the nephron involved.

Physical Examination of the Urine: Urine Volume and Specific Gravity

Because urine production is a major role of the kidney, an altered urine volume can be taken to reflect altered renal function, assuming normal fluid intake. Urine production normally varies throughout the day, so urinary output is typically monitored over a 24-hour period. An increased urine volume (polyuria) is an indication of the tubules' inability to reabsorb water. This might result from damage to the tubules or from an excessive demand for solute reabsorption. As solutes are left in the tubule, reabsorption is reduced and water loss is increased. Decreased urine volume (oliguria) is associated with nephron damage, as seen, for example, in certain types of glomerulonephritis and pyelonephritis. A complete lack of urinary output (anuria) might result from substantially reduced renal blood flow, urinary tract obstruction, or severe renal damage, especially toxic damage.

In measuring **specific gravity,** a solution's density is compared with that of pure water. Because it is a ratio, the result has no units of measure. In all body fluids, water is the solvent, so in comparing solutions the weight of the solute particles is the major cause of difference. As particle number increases, so does the specific gravity. Specific gravity is thus related to concentration, and because it can be measured more easily, specific gravity is more commonly used in urinalysis than are direct concentration measurements. Specific gravity is used as an indicator of the kidneys' ability to excrete a concentrated urine. Loss of tubular concentrating function will produce urine with a specific gravity equal to that of glomerular filtrate, normally a value of 1.010.

Chemical Examination of the Urine: Protein Levels

Of the small amount of protein filtered, most is reabsorbed. This means that normal levels of urinary protein are quite low. The presence of larger quantities of protein in the urine (proteinuria) is an indication of faulty filtration, since the filtration membrane must be passing protein that it would normally withhold. Albumin, the smallest and most prevalent plasma protein, is found most commonly in the urine, so much so that the terms **albuminuria** and **proteinuria** are often used synonymously. The appearance of more and larger proteins in urine indicates more extensive damage of the filtration membrane. Proteinuria is typically seen in glomerulonephritis and in cases of glomerular damage secondary to pyelonephritis. In the later stages of chronic GN or PN, proteinuria diminishes because scarring reduces nephron numbers so that filtration generally is reduced.

Microscopic Examination of the Urine: Particulate Matter

Information on the number and type of any particles in the urine can provide important insights into the nature of a renal malfunction.

Urine will normally contain very small numbers of both red and white blood cells, as well as some epithelial cells from nephron tubules, the bladder, or the urethra. Erythrocytes gain increased access to the urine when glomerular damage allows the escape of erythrocytes into the nephron tubule. In acute GN, this loss of erythrocytes to the urine is so pronounced that the disease is often called **hemorrhagic GN.** Disruption of other parts of the nephron vasculature or damage to the urinary tract can also allow blood to appear in the urine.

Elevated counts of white blood cells are indicative of an inflammatory process in the kidney or urinary tract. Laboratory reports of urine cell counts will seem to be quite small, but because only a minute volume of urine is examined, even small numbers in a microscope field can represent a large loss of cells in each day of urinary output. For example, the normal urine erythrocyte count of one to two cells per field represents a daily loss of over 100,000 cells.

Casts are tiny, cylindrical masses in the urine that are formed when tubule material coagulates and then dislodges to pass to the urine. Casts form when the tubule secretes a protein into its lumen. This protein may be the only constituent of the cast (the so-called **hyaline cast**), or cells reaching the tubule may embed in the protein, forming more complex casts. Because red and/or white blood cells and/or tubule cells may embed in the protein matrix of the cast, analysis of the cast components may provide indications of diagnostic value. For example, red blood cells in casts are most commonly associated with the glomerular damage of GN. A predominance of white blood cells in casts is seen in PN as well as GN, whereas tubule cells in casts might result from PN, advanced GN, or toxic damage such as from heavy metals. In the nephrotic syndrome, damaged tubule cells are engorged with fat. As these cells are sloughed from the tubule, they may lodge in its lumen to form fatty casts. Whatever the composition of a particular cast, its principal diagnostic significance lies in localizing the problem in the kidney as opposed to other parts of the urinary tract.

Bacteriological Examination of the Urine

Urine is tested for bacteria to establish bacterial involvement in cases of inflammation. Urine produced by the kidney is sterile, as is the normal urinary tract with the exception of the distal urethra. For this reason, normally voided urine is contaminated only by small quantities of urethral bacteria; so elevated bacterial counts indicate infection. The therapy chosen depends, in part, on bacteriological testing to determine the nature of the infecting organism(s). These may travel to the kidney via the blood, but they more commonly enter the urinary bladder, which provides access to the ureters and kidney.

Clearance Tests

Clearance tests are a valuable means of assessing renal function. Essentially they attempt to assess how the nephron handles certain plasma constituents. Each clearance test focuses on a specific substance in the plasma, one that may be normally present, or one that has been injected into the blood for the purpose of the test. The test involves comparing the amount of the substance in the blood with the amount found in the urine. The result provides a measure of the kidneys' ability to remove, or clear, the substance from the blood and, hence, of renal functional capacity. Since the nephron applies different combinations of filtration, reabsorption, and tubular secretion in processing plasma, the different clearance tests can provide information about a specific nephron process that might be abnormal.

Clearance test values are obtained by a calculation that takes into account the concentration of a particular substance in plasma and urine, urine output, and a correction factor for body surface area, since this is related to clearance. Results may be reported in terms of the amount of substance cleared per volume of blood (e.g., milligrams per hundred milliliters) or as a volume of blood cleared of the substance per unit of time (e.g., milliliters per minute).

Creatinine Clearance

Because creatinine is freely filtered at the glomerulus and none is reabsorbed, the amount present in urine reflects the glomerular filtration rate (GFR). There is, however, some tubular secretion of creatinine, so that test results may tend to indicate a somewhat elevated GFR. Test results are regarded as a useful approximation of renal filtration.

Urea Clearance

Renal clearance of urea is also used as an indication of the GFR. Since some urea is reabsorbed from the nephron tubule lumen, the reported value of urea clearance will be approximately 60% of the actual GFR. The normal value of urea clearance is about 60–100 ml/min. Test results are often reported as a percentage of this reference value.

Inulin Clearance

The carbohydrate inulin is not normally present in the blood. After injection it is freely filtered at the glomerulus. Because none is subsequently secreted into the tubule, nor is any reabsorbed, inulin clearance accurately reflects glomerular filtration. The test unfortunately requires rather elaborate and costly procedures, so it is not commonly performed.

Renal Biopsy

Obtaining a sample of kidney tissue for microscopic study is not routinely done. It may, however, prove valuable in cases where an accurate diagnosis of renal malfunction is needed for selection of an appropriate course of therapy. In a renal biopsy, the kidney is localized via X-ray technique in order to identify a point on the skin that overlies the lat-eral margin of the kidney's inferior pole. Next, under local anesthesia, a long needle guide is passed through skin and muscle to reach the kidney. The guide is then removed and the hollow biopsy needle quickly introduced into the track established by the guide. Finally, the tissue obtained is prepared for microscopic study.

Case Study

A 9-year-old Native American boy, living in an isolated village, experienced significant weight gain and some abdominal distention in a period of only two weeks. Also noting his general malaise, his complaints of abdominal discomfort, and traces of blood in his urine, his parents took him to the nearest medical facility, a small cottage hospital.

They reported that he had recently had a bad cold with sore throat, but since it seemed to get better, no medical treatment had been thought necessary. On physical examination, a generalized massive edema was apparent, the abdomen, including the genitalia, being particularly swollen.

Blood tests were done, and blood cell counts, the BUN, and plasma electrolyte and creatinine levels were all essentially normal, with the exception of a positive test for serum antistreptolysin O antibodies and a significant degree of hypoalbuminemia.

Urinalysis revealed severe proteinuria (2.5 g/day) and traces of blood in the urine. Microscopic study indicated the presence of red cell and hemoglobin casts.

A nephrologist at the nearest referral center, who was consulted by phone, said that in view of the child's age, a biopsy need not be done, and that local treatment should be adequate. The boy was hospitalized and prednisone therapy started, with the dose tapering down after two weeks. A supportive low-protein, high-carbohydrate diet was also started, and fluids were restricted.

After ten days the boy experienced a pronounced diuresis and his weight returned to normal. He was released two weeks later with normal blood and urine values, and has since been well.

Commentary

In this case, the presence of antistreptolysin O antibodies indicated a streptococcal infection had preceded the attack of acute glomerulonephritis. The resulting glomerular dysfunction produced the classic complex of proteinuria, hypoalbuminemia, and widespread edema. The anti-inflammatory action of prednisone was able to suppress the process of glomerular damage and prevent any progression.

A more severe attack might have required a renal biopsy to obtain a more precise diagnosis on which to base therapy. In this case, because of the child's age and the relative mildness of his condition, a biopsy proved to be unnecessary.

This case also illustrates the lack of a clear distinction between the nephrotic and nephritic syndromes. A daily urinary loss of 3.5 g of protein is the amount usually taken as defining the nephrotic syndrome. Although the level here was significantly lower, it induced a massive edema. On the other hand, the nephritic syndrome usually involves more prominent hematuria than was detected in this case.

It is also interesting to note that the incidence of severe streptococcal infections is on the rise in North America. This increase appears not to be the result of the past years of antibiotic therapy, which might have allowed only resistant strains to survive. Instead, there is evidence that spontaneous genetic mutations in the organisms have produced streptococcal strains of greater virulence.

Key Concepts

1. Any disease process that compromises glomerular filtration produces signs and symptoms related to renal retention of potentially toxic substances or the loss of needed substances via the urine (p. 401).

2. Immune destruction of glomerular elements is the dominant feature of glomerulonephritis and may involve antibody directed against the glomerular basement membrane or damage caused by the trapping of immune complexes in the glomerulus (pp. 402–403).

3. Immune complexes in the glomerulus induce PMN and macrophage responses that produce glomerular damage via complement activation, the release of enzymes and toxins, fibrin deposition, and scarring (pp. 403–404).

4. In some GN, the pattern of glomerular damage allows the loss of albumins from plasma, producing a syndrome of hypoalbuminemia, proteinuria, and systemic edema known as the nephrotic syndrome (p. 405).

5. Glomerular damage that results in the retention of wastes and water, with some loss of blood to the urine, produces the clinical syndrome of oliguria, azotemia, and hematuria known as the nephritic syndrome (pp. 406–407).

6. Tubulointerstitial disorders are characterized by altered tubule processing, typically producing loss of water and sodium and the retention of acid (p. 407).

7. The most common tubulointerstitial disorder is pyelonephritis, in which infectious agents reach the renal medulla either by ascent from the urinary tract or by transport in the blood from an infection site (p. 407).

8. Acute PN is usually of bacterial origin and readily resolves after a relatively mild illness in which pyuria may be present. Chronic PN is potentially much more threatening, since signs and symptoms may not arise until substantial nephron loss has occurred (pp. 407–408).

9. Interstitial nephritis is the tubulointerstitial disease that is caused by toxic chemicals, among which are therapeutic agents such as some antibiotics and analgesics (p. 408).

10. Various diseases, such as hypertension, diabetes mellitus, and atherosclerosis, may affect the kidneys' functions by their effects on renal vasculature, which lead to renal ischemia (p. 409).

11. Insoluble calculi may form in the kidney, producing pain and urinary obstruction and increasing the risk of infection and renal parenchymal damage (pp. 409–411).

12. A widely used clinical approach to etiology in kidney disorders employs the categories of: renal disease, where the fault lies with the kidney; prerenal disease, in which an initially normal kidney is compromised by ischemia; and postrenal disease, where the normal kidney is affected by urinary obstruction (pp. 411–412).

13. The widespread functional derangements associated with failing kidneys are the result of waste retention and fluid and electrolyte imbalance, which are clinically designated as uremia (p. 412).

14. Toxic nephritis and renal ischemia produce the rapidly progressing decline of renal function called acute renal failure (pp. 412–413).

15. More severe and irreversible nephron loss produces chronic renal failure, which is characterized by more pronounced functional derangements, progressing to uremia (p. 413).

16. Given evidence of renal failure, therapeutic intervention to clear toxins and provide homeostatic adjustments may employ hemodialysis, which uses an external hemodialyzer, or peritoneal dialysis, which infuses dialysate into the peritoneal cavity (pp. 414–415).

17. When a suitable donor kidney is available and immune rejection responses can be suppressed, renal transplantation is the optimal therapeutic choice in cases of irreversible renal failure (pp. 415–417).

18. Assessment of renal function is accomplished by examining the blood and urine for indications of retained wastes, excretion of needed plasma constituents, or homeostatic imbalance (pp. 417–420).

REVIEW ACTIVITIES

1. The longest term in this chapter is membrano/proliferative glomerulo/nephr/itis. For each of the indicated word elements, write out its meaning and briefly relate it to altered kidney function. Consult your medical dictionary if you must.

2. With respect to figure 15.9, answer the following: How did the immune complexes shown trapped in the BM form? Why are PMNs present? How are the PMNs linked to glomerular damage? Check your answers by consulting pages 402–403.

3. Both the nephrotic and the nephritic syndromes may involve oliguria, but oliguria is produced by different mechanisms in each case. If you think about it, you may be able to work out what they are. If not, see figures 15.11 and 15.12.

4. From the information presented on page 410, lay out a handy reference flow chart showing the pathogenesis of urolithiasis. Add the principal sequelae of urolithiasis. Check back to the diagram at least twice before your next exam.

5. With a pad of sticky notes, make ten labels, one each for the elements that contribute to the development of prerenal disease. Stick them to a large sheet of paper and draw connecting arrows. You could put the notes down randomly, but if their positions and the arrows reflect the actual sequence (figure 15.17), the exercise will be more worthwhile.

6. On a blank sheet of paper, draw a vertical line and label it "Dialysis Membrane." Label the space to its left "Blood" and the space to the right "Dialysate." Add large and small symbols on either side to indicate high and low concentrations of metabolic wastes (MW), Na^+, K^+, and Ca^{++}. Now add arrows to indicate the direction of net diffusion of each. Will your arrow directions produce a blood lower in waste Na^+ and K^+ and higher in Ca^{++}? Is this the condition needed for blood returning to the patient? If yes, good! If no, see pages 414–415.

7. Before checking pages 405–407 and the case study commentary, recall the situation in the case study. The young boy's urinalysis indicated a pronounced proteinuria. Of the plasma proteins in the urine, which one would have been most prevalent? Why? The case study also notes that the nephrotic and nephritic syndromes were not clearly separated. Which aspect of the boy's urinalysis pointed toward the nephrotic syndrome and which toward the nephritic syndrome?

Fluid and Electrolyte Imbalances

There is in man the bitter and the salt, the sweet and the acid, the sour and the insipid. . . . These, when all mixed and mingled up in one another, are not apparent, neither do they hurt a man; but when any of them is separate, and stands by itself, then it becomes perceptible and hurts a man.

HIPPOCRATES
ON ANCIENT MEDICINE

rubor

rubor

&tumor

cū calore

&dolore

FLUID AND ELECTROLYTE BASICS

Overall somatic functions are a product of the smoothly co-ordinated activities of the body's various organ systems. These depend on the functioning of the vast numbers of cells that form the tissues of the different organs. Cellular functioning in turn depends on numerous chemical reactions that occur in an environment dominated by water. Water is not only the cells' principal internal constituent, it also bathes their external surfaces and fills the spaces between them. It is not difficult to appreciate, then, that for optimal cell functioning, the quantity and composition of body water, both inside and outside cells, must be carefully controlled. Only when such body fluid homeostasis is achieved can normal functioning occur. When there are imbalances in the body fluids, disease and even death can result.

Body Fluid Compartments

Water contributes about 55% of a typical female's body weight and about 65% of a male's. All water in the body (**total body water,** TBW) is distributed among four separate fluid compartments (fig. 16.1). One compartment contains the **intracellular fluid** (ICF). The ICF consists of all water present within the body's cells. The remaining body water, that found outside the cells, is the **extracellular fluid** (ECF). Of the total body water, 65% is found in cells and 35% in the ECF. Within the ECF are three subcompartments. About 25% of TBW is found between cells, forming the **intercellular fluid,** also referred to as the interstitial fluid. About 8% of TBW is found in the **plasma.** A third, small compartment is also recognized as part of the ECF. This contains the **transcellular fluid,** constituting only about 2% of TBW. It consists of cerebrospinal fluid, glandular secretions, the fluids in the eyes, and in the GI, urinary, and respiratory tracts. Its volume is sufficiently small to leave little impact on overall water distribution, so it is usually excluded from clinical calculations in fluid imbalance cases.

From this description, it should be clear that the boundary between the extracellular fluid and the intracellular fluid is the cell membrane, and that the plasma and interstitial fluid are separated by the capillary wall. Both of these dividing membranes are freely permeable to water, so that it normally moves easily among plasma, the interstitial spaces, and the cells. Much of the water movement that occurs is the normal exchange of fluid between the plasma and interstitium; blood hydrostatic pressure drives water from the blood into the intercellular spaces, and blood osmotic pressure draws it back from the intercellular spaces into the blood. This movement is an example of the **bulk flow** of water. That is, water and any dissolved substances move together from one compartment to another. Bulk flow also occurs as interstitial water moves into lymphatic vessels, which return it to the plasma. In terms of body water compartments, the lymphatic vessels can be thought of as an extension of the blood vessels, because lymphatics

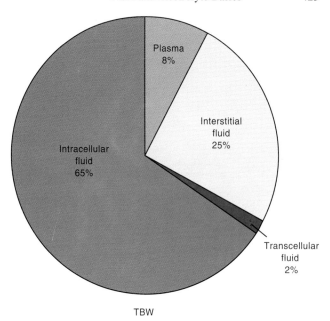

Figure 16.1   Fluid Compartments. Relative size of the body fluid compartments expressed as a percentage of total body water (TBW).

empty lymph directly into the blood. The body's water, therefore, is continually exchanged among plasma, interstitium, cells, and lymph (fig. 16.2). Let us now consider these fluid movements in the context of the balance between overall input and output of fluid and electrolytes.

The Balance Concept

Fluid and electrolyte homeostasis can be viewed in terms of a balance between inputs and outputs. These will change in the course of normal activities, but the optimum amounts of water and electrolytes must still be maintained. This means that if input is increased, a corresponding increase in output is required to balance it. When input matches output in this way, a steady state, or **neutral balance,** is said to exist, or a patient is said to be **in balance.** If input exceeds output for a particular substance, it accumulates and the patient is said to be in **positive balance.** If output exceeds input, a deficit develops, and the patient is said to be in **negative balance.**

Water Balance

Normal physiology involves a continual loss of body water. This water must be replaced, and when water input matches water loss, water balance is achieved. The typical daily balance of water input versus output, averaged over a range of normal variation, is approximately 2,500 ml. The input total is based on drinking 1,300 ml as pure water or in various beverages, with about 900 ml contained in solid food. After ingestion, water is absorbed and enters the ECF. The remaining 300 ml of input is formed as a product of cellular energy metabolism.

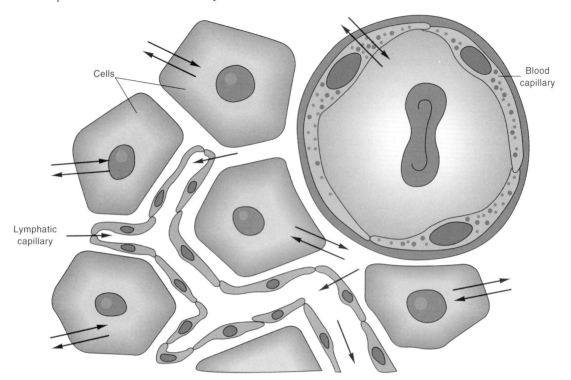

Figure 16.2 **Intercompartment Flow.** Fluid moves freely among the plasma, interstitial spaces, lymph, and cells. Note that fluid moves in only one direction from tissue spaces into the lymphatic capillary.

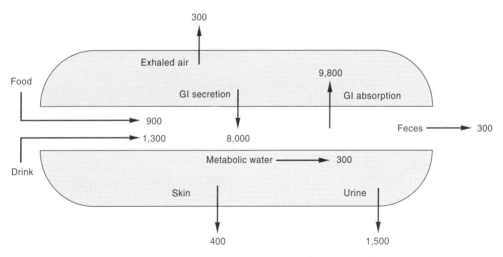

Figure 16.3 **Water Balance.** Principal inputs and outputs that determine normal body water balance. Colored masses represent the body. Central region represents the GI tract. All volumes are in milliliter units per day.

Body water is lost primarily in the urine, which accounts for a daily output of about 1,500 ml. Another 300 ml are lost in feces, and a similar volume leaves the body via the skin. This skin loss occurs as perspiration fluid is moved to the skin's surface by sweat gland ducts, and as tissue fluid slowly percolates to the skin's surface. The remaining 300 ml escape from airway surfaces and are lost in expired air. In addition, approximately 8,000 ml of fluids, containing mostly water, are secreted into the gastrointestinal lumen every day. This, however, is not an output from the body, because almost all is reabsorbed in the small and large intestine (fig. 16.3 and table 16.1).

Electrolyte Concentration

The body's water molecules have numerous molecule-sized particles mixed among them. These are called **solute** particles. They are described as being **dissolved** in the water, which is called the **solvent.** The resulting mixture is a **solution.** Most solutes have a positive or negative charge associated with them. Such solutes are called ions. Their presence in a water solution enables it to conduct an electrical current, which would not flow through pure water. For this reason, such charged particles are called **electrolytes.** Those with a positive charge are called **cations;** those with a negative charge are called **anions.**

Table 16.1	Determination of the Normal Water Steady State

Total Body Input and Output

Input		Output	
Diet	2,200 ml	Exhaled air	300 ml
Metabolism	300 ml	Skin	400 ml
Total	2,500 ml	Feces	300 ml
		Urine	1,500 ml
		Total	2,500 ml

GI Tract Input and Output

Input to Tract		Output from Tract	
Diet	2,200 ml	Absorbed	9,800 ml
Secretions	8,000 ml	Feces	400 ml
Total	10,200 ml	Total	10,200 ml

Although many different solutes are present in the body fluids, relatively few have clinical significance. Of the cations, sodium (Na^+), potassium (K^+), calcium (Ca^{++}), and hydrogen (H^+) ions are most important. The more significant anions are chloride (Cl^-), bicarbonate (HCO_3^-), and phosphate ($PO_4^{\equiv}$). Because protein has a negative charge associated with its constituent amino acids, it also makes a significant contribution to the total anion complement of the body fluids. In this context it is referred to as **proteinate.**

The **concentration** of a solution is based on the ratio of its solute to its solvent. The total of all solutes present can be used to express the overall concentration of the solution. For example, a solution that contains little solute is said to be **dilute** while a **concentrated** solution contains a large amount of solute for its volume. Concentration may also apply to a single solute; a solution may have a certain concentration of Na^+ and a different concentration of K^+. Brackets are used to denote the concentration of a solute. The expression $[Na^+]$, for example, is read "the concentration of sodium ion."

The terms "concentrated" and "dilute" provide only a rough approximation of the solute/solvent ratio. In dealing with fluid and electrolyte balance, it is often necessary to express the exact quantity of solute present in a specified volume of solution. In solution chemistry, the ratio is expressed as the weight of solute present in a liter of solvent. The solute weight is often expressed in terms of **gram molecular weight.** This is the molecular weight of a substance expressed in grams. The term is often shortened to **mole** (M). A liter of solution containing 1 M of a solute is said to be a 1 molar (1M) solution; if the liter of solution contains 2 M of solute, it is a 2 molar (2M) solution. Specifically, since sodium chloride ($NaCl$) has a molecular weight of 58 atomic mass units, a gram molecular weight of $NaCl$

weighs 58 g. A 1.5M solution of $NaCl$ would therefore contain 1.5×58, or 87 g, of the salt in each liter of solution.

Expressing solution concentration in this way has many advantages, but physiologically it is often less appropriate. Another system of expressing concentration is therefore quite common. It is based on the number of **equivalents** (Eq) present in a liter of solution (Eq/L). An equivalent is the weight of a substance that will interact with one equivalent of another substance when the interaction is based on charge. Thus, the number of equivalents is determined by the charge (or valence number). A liter of solution containing 1 Eq of solute is described as a 1 normal (1N) solution. If there were 0.3 Eq present, the concentration would be 0.3N. For example, 1 M of Na^+ in a liter of solution is the same as 1 Eq, since there is a single positive charge on the sodium ion. The same holds for the hydroxide ion (OH^-), with its single negative charge. By contrast, 1 M of Ca^{++} contains 2 Eq, since the calcium ion has a charge of 2. This means that 1 M of Ca^{++} has the potential to react with 2 M of OH^-. By the same logic, 0.5 M of Ca^{++} has the same number of equivalents as 1 mole of OH^-, and they would completely interact on that basis. To summarize, using normality to express concentration puts emphasis on the number of ions that react, rather than on the weight of the solute.

Because the mole and equivalent are inconveniently large for dealing with physiological concentrations, the **milliequivalent** (mEQ, 1/1,000 of an equivalent) and the **millimole** (mM, 1/1,000 of a mole) are more appropriate.

Diffusion

The concentration of ECF electrolytes is the same in the plasma and interstitial fluid compartments because of the ease of fluid motion between the blood and tissue spaces. The only significant exception is proteinate. Because the large plasma proteins can't pass through the capillary walls as easily as water, the interstitial concentration of protein is only about 1/15 that of plasma. For most electrolytes, any change of concentration in either the plasma or interstitial fluid is quickly followed by a compensating shift of electrolytes between them until their concentrations are again equal.

Molecular or ionic movement of this sort in solutions occurs by **diffusion** (fig. 16.4). The frequent and random collision of solute and solvent particles produces a net particle motion down a concentration gradient—that is, from a region of high solute concentration to a region of lower solute concentration—until an equilibrium is established, meaning that the concentrations of the two regions are equal. At equilibrium, diffusion continues, but there is no concentration change because particle movement is equal in both directions.

Movement through cell membranes occurs when small molecules and ions diffuse through membrane pores, when molecules dissolve in membrane lipid, or when a specialized **membrane transport system** (MTS) assists the passage of a specific ion or molecule. Such systems transport

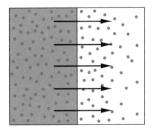

Diffusion down the
concentration gradient

Equilibrium

Figure 16.4 **Diffusion.** Simple diffusion of particles through a permeable membrane. At equilibrium, diffusion continues but rates in both directions are equal, so no net displacement of particles occurs.

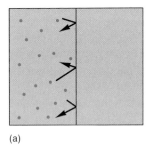

(a)

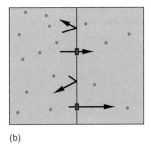

(b)

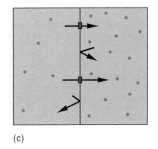

(c)

Figure 16.5 **Membrane Transport.** (*a*) Some ions and larger molecules cannot pass through cell membranes. (*b*) Membrane transport systems (dark boxes) assist in moving such particles through the membrane. (*c*) Active transport, in which the transport system moves particles against the concentration gradient.

molecules whose size or other properties prevent their diffusion through the cell membrane (fig. 16.5). Some transport systems can move a specific ion or molecule from a region where it is in low concentration to one in which its concentration is higher. In other words, the ion or molecule is moved against its concentration gradient. To do this, a cell must expend energy. For this reason, such systems are often called **pumps.** They are said to work by **active transport,** as opposed to passive diffusion, which requires no expenditure of cellular energy.

In contrast to the situation that exists between the plasma and the interstitial fluid, electrolyte concentrations between the intracellular and extracellular compartments are substantially different for some ions (table 16.2). Such differences are the result of two factors. One is the permeability characteristics of the cell membrane, which limit the

Table 16.2   Ion Concentration of the Intracellular (ICF) and Extracellular (ECF) Fluid Compartments

Ion	Concentration	
	ICF	ECF
Sodium	10	140
Potassium	140	4
Chloride	4	104
Bicarbonate	10	24
Biphosphate	100	3
Calcium	1	5

Values are in milliequivalents per liter of water

passage of certain electrolytes. The other is the action of ion pumps in the cell membrane. These produce and maintain an intracellular fluid that has, for example, a much higher concentration of K^+ and a much lower concentration of Na^+ than the ECF.

Osmosis

Not only electrolytes pass through cell membranes. Water freely passes through them by the process of **osmosis.** Osmosis is based on the same molecular collisions that produce diffusion, but the term *osmosis* refers specifically to the motion of water molecules through a membrane.

Osmosis is significant when water can move more easily than solute particles through a membrane that separates solutions with different concentrations. The solution's concentrations are determined by calculating the ratio between the total of all solute particles and the volume of water in which they are dissolved. The particle concentration is expressed in terms of **osmolality,** which describes a solution in terms of the total number of its solute particles per unit volume of water. The unit of osmolality is the **osmole.** It is the concentration of particles produced when 1 M of a solute that does not dissociate in water is added to 1 kg of water. In the case of glucose, therefore, 1 gram dissolved in 1 kg of water produces a solution of 1 osmole. For sodium chloride (NaCl), 2 osmoles are present in 1 kg of water, because NaCl dissociates to yield two particles: a sodium ion and a chloride ion. For potassium phosphate (K_3PO_4), 4 osmoles would be produced, since this molecule splits into three potassium ions and one phosphate ion. Because an osmole is too large a unit for practical use in describing body fluid concentrations, the **milliosmole** (mOsm: 1/1000 osmole) is generally used.

The significance of osmolality as an expression of a solution's concentration lies in its emphasis on particle number. Osmolality is dependent only on the number of particles and not on the particle size. This means that from 1 g of a high-molecular-weight protein that contains few

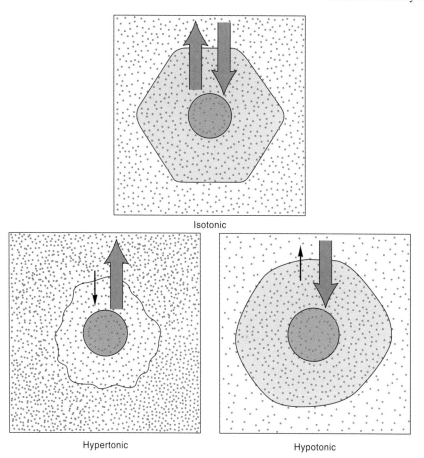

Isotonic

Hypertonic

Hypotonic

Figure 16.6   **Osmosis.** Water movement through cell membranes is indicated by the arrows. When the extracellular fluid (ECF) is isotonic to a cell, no net water displacement occurs even though osmotic flow occurs. If the ECF is hypertonic to the cell, then net osmotic loss from the cell causes cell shrinking. When the ECF is hypotonic to the cell, osmotic inflow exceeds outflow and the cell swells.

particles, there is a much smaller osmotic effect than from 1 g of a low-molecular-weight material that contains many particles. In osmosis, water moves from an area of lower osmolality (lower total solute particle concentration or higher water concentration) to one of higher osmolality (higher total solute particle concentration or lower water concentration).

Under normal circumstances, the intracellular and extracellular compartments have the same osmolality, even though the concentrations of particular ions may vary greatly on either side of the cell's membrane (table 16.2). In this case, the two solutions are said to be **isotonic.** When the ECF has a greater osmolality than that within cells, the ECF is said to be **hypertonic** to the intracellular fluid. When ECF osmolality is less than that of intracellular fluid, the ECF is described as **hypotonic** compared to the intracellular fluid. Note that the concept of osmolality allows expression of overall solute concentration in precise units, whereas the terms *hypertonic* and *hypotonic* provide only comparative information. Cells exposed to hypotonic solutions accumulate water by osmosis and swell. The intracellular pressure may rise to the point at which the cells rupture. Cells exposed to hypertonic solutions lose water by osmosis and shrink (fig. 16.6).

Electrolyte Balance

The level of electrolytes in the body fluids is determined by the balance between their input and their loss. All normal electrolyte input is derived from the diet. The plant and animal tissues, and their derivatives, that make up most well-balanced diets contain all the electrolytes needed to maintain normal cell functions. Losses occur mainly in three ways. First, as perspiration fluid passes to the body surface, it carries with it various electrolytes, which are then lost. Second, substantial quantities of electrolytes are present in the secretions passed into the alimentary canal daily. Most of these are absorbed along the GI tract, but small amounts are not, and these are lost in feces. The third and most important route of electrolyte loss is the urine. Under normal circumstances, urinary losses of electrolytes far exceed losses from the skin and feces. The kidney receives a very large plasma flow from which it can remove and excrete water and various ions to achieve fluid and electrolyte balance.

Renal Regulation of Fluid and Electrolytes

The role of the kidney in fluid and electrolyte balance is vital. On the one hand, the kidney functions to excrete any fluid and/or electrolytes present in excess of homeostatic set points. On the other hand, it can retain fluid and/or electrolytes when they fall below the required level. Note here the importance of dietary input. When an electrolyte deficiency occurs, the kidney can only reduce loss of that electrolyte via the urine. It thus supports the existing level and reduces further losses, but this is still not the same as providing an additional input. In the case of water deficiency, when the body fluids are hypertonic, the thirst drive is activated to stimulate new water input. In the case of electrolytes, however, the situation is different. There is no potassium "thirst" or calcium "hunger" to induce a new electrolyte input; people don't develop a craving for chloride. So when an electrolyte deficiency does exist, if the diet does not make enough of these ions available for uptake from the GI tract, renal retention mechanisms can only delay a worsening of the deficiency state.

The essential nephron mechanisms of filtration, selective reabsorption, and tubular secretion were described in chapter 15. These mechanisms are applied to water and the various body electrolytes to achieve the appropriate balance between loss and retention that is needed to maintain homeostasis. The ability of the nephron to regulate a particular ion depends on the ion's diffusion properties and the membrane transport systems of the nephron's tubular cells, which determine the rates of reabsorption or tubular secretion of that ion. These processes are important to fluid and electrolyte balance because they selectively transport specific ions out of the tubule lumen to retain them, or into it to excrete them. By comparison, filtration is nonspecific. Except for the plasma proteins, the composition of glomerular filtrate and plasma is quite similar (see table 15.1). Following filtration, closely regulated tubule membrane transport systems achieve the precise degree of retention or excretion for each critical molecule in the filtrate. Nephron excretion of the major electrolytes—Na^+, K^+, and Cl^-—has a major impact on water balance.

The high concentration of Na^+ in the ECF (140 mEq/L) means that a large amount will enter the nephron tubule after filtration at the glomerulus. The proximal convoluted tubule reabsorbs about 65% of this Na^+, which accumulates in the peritubular tissue spaces. Cl^- and HCO_3^- passively accompany Na^+ ion, maintaining a balance of positive and negative charges. K^+ is almost completely reabsorbed, but

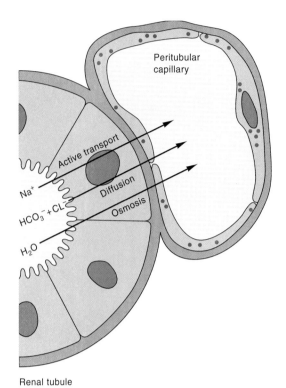

Figure 16.7   Nephron Tubule Reabsorption. Sodium is actively transported from filtrate. Chloride and bicarbonate ions follow the positively charged sodium, maintaining the charge equilibrium. The resulting concentration gradient is responsible for the osmosis that draws water from the tubule into the peritubular capillary.

its low concentration in filtrate produces a smaller effect than that of Na^+, Cl^-, and HCO_3^-. As these ions enter the peritubular spaces, they increase osmotic pressure, and the resulting osmosis causes large volumes of water to be reabsorbed from the tubule. By this mechanism, over 80% of filtrate is returned to the blood in the peritubular capillaries (fig. 16.7). This process provides retention of the greatest portion of Na^+, Cl^-, and water.

Most homeostatic regulation is accomplished in the distal convoluted tubule, even though the bulk of the filtrate is reabsorbed in the proximal tubule. The composition of blood is adjusted by secretion into, and reabsorption from, the fluid in the distal tubules under the influence of several controlling inputs. The adrenocortical hormone **aldosterone** regulates uptake of Na^+ from the tubule lumen. For each Na^+ reabsorbed, one K^+ is secreted into the lumen. Na^+ excretion is also regulated by one or more natriuretic factors, so named because they promote urinary sodium loss, **natriuresis**. The best known of these is **atrial natriuretic factor** (ANF), which is secreted by the atria in response to their distention by increased plasma volume. The increase in ANF increases filtration and blocks sodium reabsorption, producing sodium loss, water loss, and a reduction of circulating plasma volume.

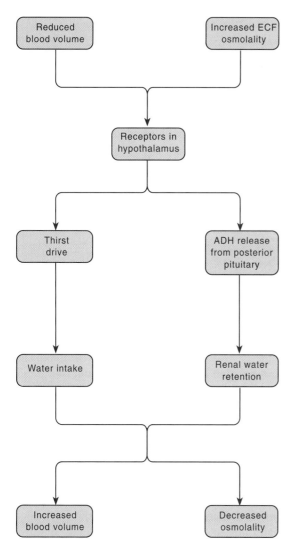

Figure 16.8 **Water Regulation.** ADH-mediated compensation can reduce losses when the body fluid osmolality or volume is increased. The thirst drive provides new input to aid the corrective response.

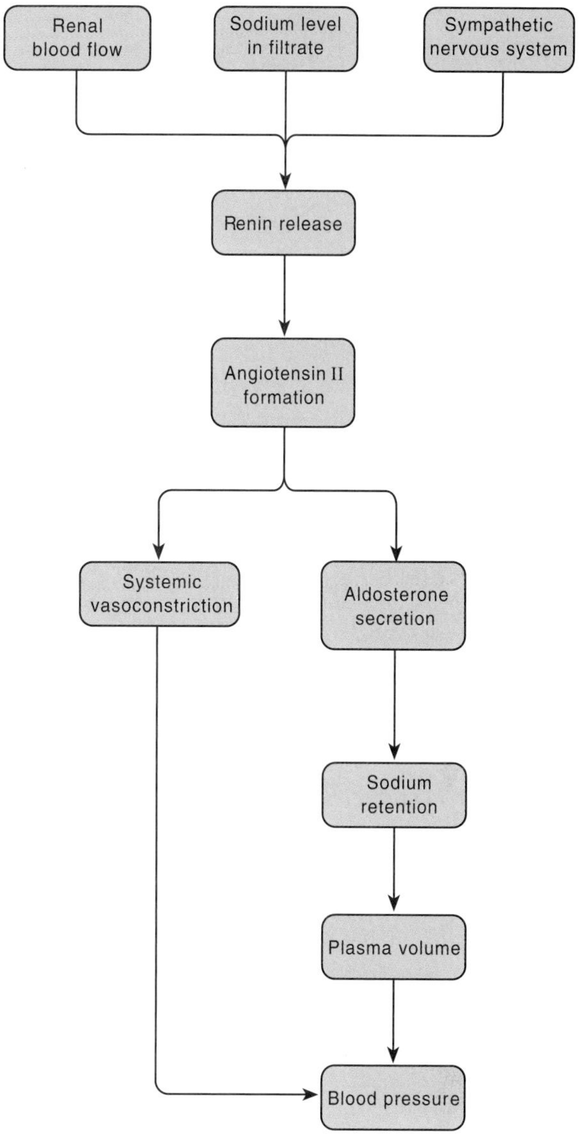

Figure 16.9 **Blood Pressure Regulation.** Reflexes that control blood pressure are mediated, in part, by the renin-angiotensin system.

Urinary water loss is regulated by **antidiuretic hormone** (ADH), also known as **arginine vasopressin,** which is released from the posterior pituitary gland. ADH increases the water permeability of collecting duct cells and, to a lesser extent, those of the distal convoluted tubule. Because the collecting duct is relatively impermeable to ions, water is drawn by osmosis into the hypertonic interstitial fluid of the renal medulla. ADH is therefore an important component of the system regulating the osmotic pressure of the extracellular fluid (fig. 16.8). ADH is released into the blood in response to input from pressure receptors, principally those in the heart, and osmoreceptors in the brain. Decreased BHP, cardiac pressure, and increased osmolality stimulate ADH secretion. Water reten-

tion tends to expand plasma volume and reduce osmolality. In water deficiency states, input to the thirst center in the hypothalamus activates the thirst drive, causing additional water intake.

Aldosterone secretion depends on the concentration of K^+ in plasma and on the renin-angiotensin system, which is sensitive to the Na^+ level in filtrate, to renal blood flow, and to sympathetic input from the CNS (fig. 16.9). Changes in BHP are related to plasma volume, which in turn is dependent on the overall volume of ECF. Should normal ECF volume or osmolality change, appropriate alterations in aldosterone and ADH secretion produce corrective responses in the nephron that restore fluid volume and osmolality.

Checkpoint 16.2

You might be wondering how ADH works, since there aren't any membrane transport systems that can directly move water molecules. A good analogy is that ADH operates something like a faucet. With a steady water pressure, opening or closing the tap allows more or less water to flow. In the case of the nephron tubules, there is a lot of water in filtrate and a steady osmotic pressure drawing it out of the tubule. Acting like a faucet, ADH adjusts membrane permeability by causing the tubule cells to move more pores to their membrane surfaces, allowing water to more easily flow through the membrane down its osmotic gradient. In this way, more water is retained. When low ADH levels cause cells to reduce the number of membrane pores, less water can flow through the membranes even though the osmotic pressure remains high. In this case, less water can be retained, and so it is lost in the urine.

BODY FLUID IMBALANCE

The preceding discussion of water and Na^+ regulation illustrates two essential factors that have a bearing on fluid imbalances. The first is the close linking of Na^+ and water. Since Na^+ is the dominant electrolyte in the ECF—indeed, contributing about half its osmolality—a change in Na^+ level has significant effects on water balance. Similarly, any gain or loss of pure water will soon have an effect on Na^+ concentration. The second factor worth noting is that fluid imbalance problems may arise from defects in the mechanisms that maintain body fluid concentration and volume homeostasis.

In the following sections, and in clinical situations, it is important to use appropriate terminology to describe fluid imbalance. The term **volume** implies that both water and Na^+ are involved. For example, you may encounter a patient who is threatened with hypovolemic shock due to **volume depletion.** On the other hand, if water loss or gain dominates the clinical picture, and Na^+ gain or loss is minimal, then **dehydration** and **water intoxication** are the correct descriptive terms. Let us consider these two conditions before we deal with volume derangements that involve both water and Na^+.

Dehydration

Dehydration is the condition in which there is decreased total body water, while total body Na^+ is near normal. It may come about as the result of reduced water intake or excessive losses. Lack of access to water is unusual, but may arise in those dependent on others to supply it. Children, the elderly, the bedridden or crippled, or those with some

compromised mental capacity, are particularly at risk. If there is no water replacement, skin, respiratory, and GI losses continue and dehydration results. Abnormally high water losses may be present in certain disease conditions. In diabetes insipidus, a condition described in chapter 17, ADH secretion is suppressed and the resulting inhibition of renal water reabsorption promotes heavy water loss. In untreated diabetes mellitus, high blood glucose increases the osmotic pressure of nephron filtrate, and thereby also inhibits water reabsorption.

Under the threat of developing dehydration, both increased ECF osmolality and BHP decreases can activate the thirst drive. This drive is usually able to restore normal ECF concentration even when losses are quite high, as in cases of heavy perspiration and diabetes. However, in members of the dependent groups indicated earlier, or in those with a defective thirst mechanism, correction of water depletion may not occur, and if losses are heavy, severe dehydration may develop quite rapidly.

In dehydration, Na^+ levels are near normal, but since there is a decreased water volume, the body fluids are hypertonic. Considered in terms of Na^+, the dominant ECF ion, the situation is one of **hypernatremia** (*natrium* is the Latin word for sodium). This condition is sometimes described as **relative hypernatremia** to imply that water loss, rather than Na^+ gain, is at the heart of the matter.

Water Intoxication

An increase in total body water, with no changes in the body's total Na^+ level, dilutes the ECF and produces the condition of water intoxication. Increased water intake is normally not able to dilute the body fluids significantly because the renal diuresis responses are so efficient. With normally functioning kidneys, an intake exceeding 10 liters per day can be cleared by a correspondingly large urinary output. Even if there is an extreme **polydipsia** (excessive water drinking), as might be found in some mental aberrations, water intoxication will rarely develop. Much more frequently, it arises from an impaired water excretion capacity based on excessive ADH secretion. When it occurs, nephron tubule water permeability is increased to produce excessive water retention at normal renal osmolality gradients.

Excessive ADH secretion produces the **syndrome of inappropriate antidiuretic hormone** secretion (SIADH). It arises because of excessive ADH release by the posterior pituitary when there is no physiological requirement for it. Various CNS disturbances, such as infection, trauma (including surgery), cerebral hemorrhage, pain, or anesthesia may be involved, as may various psychogenic disorders. The underlying mechanism seems to involve disturbances in the control system that regulates ADH secretion. These disturbances produce a lower set point for body fluid osmolality, and the posterior pituitary responds with increased ADH output.

Although ADH is normally secreted by the posterior pituitary, some nonendocrine tumors can also secrete ADH

Table 16.3   Changes Associated with Volume Depletion and Expansion

Precipitating Condition	Term Applied to Plasma After Loss or Gain	Volume Change		Sodium Change
		ECF	ICF	
Chronic diarrhea	Isotonic depletion	D	—	—
Intense perspiration	Hypertonic depletion	D	D	I*
Renal Na⁺ loss	Hypotonic depletion	D	I	D
Normal saline infusion	Isotonic expansion	I	—	—
Hypertonic saline infusion	Hypertonic expansion	I	D	I
Water intoxication	Hypotonic expansion	I	I	D*

D = decrease, I = increase, — = unchanged. Note that changes in intracellular fluid (ICF) volume are the result of osmotic flow between the ICF and ECF; water moves from the more dilute to the more concentrated compartment. *Indicates a 'relative' change.

or functionally similar substances. The tumors involved include oat cell carcinoma of the lung and certain tumors of the pancreas, intestine, or brain. Lung secretion of ADH is associated with some nontumor conditions, especially infections, COPD, tuberculosis, and asthma, but the mechanisms are unclear. Certain drugs can produce SIADH, either by directly stimulating ADH secretion or by increasing renal tubule sensitivity to it. Chlorpropamide (used by diabetics), carbamazepine (an antiepileptic), cyclophosphamide (a cancer chemotherapy agent), and various antidepressants are examples.

Like dehydration, water intoxication may be considered in terms of Na⁺. In that context, we refer to the situation as one of **relative hyponatremia:** the normal quantity of sodium is diluted by the abnormally high volume of water. In many clinical settings, the terms *dehydration* and *water intoxication* are not even used. Instead, attention is centered on Na⁺, and only the relevant "natremia" terms are employed.

Gains or Losses of Water and Sodium

Pure water loss or gain is much less common than conditions in which both water and Na⁺ are involved. Usually the fluid volume change is due to an initial Na⁺ change, with water effects following. Note that Na⁺ and water levels may not always be altered to the same degree. In some cases, Na⁺ loss may exceed water loss, producing a hypotonic ECF. In other cases, where water loss exceeds Na⁺ loss, the ECF becomes hypertonic. Of course, if water and Na⁺ changes are matched, then the ECF remains isotonic even though the volume may be increased (expanded) or decreased (depleted). Table 16.3 presents some common water and volume changes using this terminology.

Volume Depletion

When water and electrolytes are lost from the ECF, volume depletion is the result. Losses may arise through heavy perspiration, vomiting or diarrhea, or intestinal resection or GI

fistulas that reduce absorption. Renal losses may also be involved when kidney disease impairs Na⁺ reabsorption or in cases of adrenal cortex insufficiency, which reduces aldosterone output. Of course, diuretic therapy can also produce exaggerated volume losses via the kidney, if dosage is imprecise or if the drug is misused by the patient. Skin burns can also result in volume depletion as the skin's barrier function is lost and evaporative losses are exaggerated. A water-dominated organism in a dry environment relies heavily on the skin to prevent fluid loss, and burns are a serious threat if they are extensive. Whereas GI, kidney, and skin losses are true losses from the body fluids, various **sequestration states** (situations in which fluid is lost from vessels but remains in the body) can produce volume depletion effects. Acute peritonitis, pancreatitis, and internal bleeding are examples. Note that in edema and ascites, which are slow to develop, volume compensation reflexes are usually able to prevent volume depletion. Clinically, the sequestration of body fluids is called **third-spacing** (fig. 16.10).

Volume Excess

This condition is largely the result of renal Na⁺ and water retention, which may be due to kidney disease or to cardiac or liver conditions that promote water and sodium retention. In renal failure, the kidneys lose the ability to excrete Na⁺, usually as a result of declining filtration. Water retention follows, and ECF volume increases. In congestive heart failure, as well as in liver cirrhosis, edema and ascites are often present. In third-spacing, loss of fluid from the plasma activates reflexes that restore volume by retaining Na⁺. As they expand plasma volume, additional fluid is lost from the plasma and the cycle repeats. This can lead to serious consequences, as described in the earlier chapters dealing with congestive heart failure and liver cirrhosis. Urinary protein losses associated with the nephrotic syndrome can also produce edema as a result of the attendant decrease in plasma osmotic pressure. Cycling of volume expansion reflexes follows as in CHF and cirrhosis.

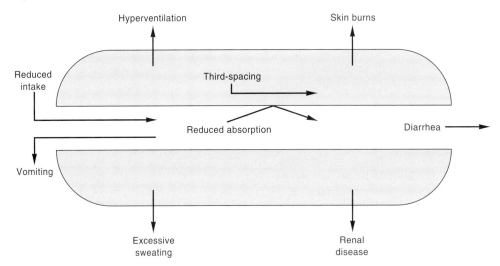

Figure 16.10   **Volume Depletion.** Principal factors contributing to the loss of fluid volume.

 Checkpoint 16.3

After studying the Volume Depletion and Volume Excess sections, take a minute to go back to table 16.3. If you can see how its indicated ECF and ICF changes are linked to the precipitating conditions and then see the logic of the relevant terminology, you can be confident that you have a pretty good grasp of the situation.

Fluid retention can also arise in cases of aldosterone hypersecretion. The cause may be adrenal cortex hyperplasia or a benign tumor. In other cases, excessive renin secretion may be responsible, often as a response to renal ischemia. Overall, these conditions contribute to fluid volume excess much less than do CHF, cirrhosis, and renal failure.

Consequences of Fluid Imbalance

The primary consequences of volume expansion or depletion are related to plasma volume changes and osmotic effects. Plasma volume changes are reflected in the blood pressure. At modest volume changes, pressure-regulating reflexes may be able to maintain normal blood pressure. If larger volume decreases develop, some pressure drop may result, or if increased plasma volume raises pressure beyond correctable levels, systemic edema will follow. Of course, if fluid losses are large and rapid, for example in badly burned skin or from hemorrhage due to massive trauma, then hypovolemic shock may arise.

In volume depletion states where the plasma remains isotonic, water retention reflexes will produce thirsty patients with dry oral mucous membranes, reduced perspiration, and lower urinary output. As well, there is usually a reduction in skin **turgor**—the firmness and fullness of the skin that results from a normal interstitial fluid pressure. If plasma volume is depleted, interstitial fluid moves from the tissue spaces to compensate, and turgor is reduced. Note that in the elderly, skin aging changes may make the assessment of turgor difficult. Reduced plasma volume is also reflected in an increased hematocrit.

In many fluid imbalance patients for whom plasma osmolality is not corrected, neurological signs and symptoms may be present. These are related to shrinking or swelling of brain cells and the resulting disruption of intracellular fluid concentration. When dehydration produces a hypertonic plasma (relative hypernatremia), the higher plasma osmolality draws water from the intracellular compartment (fig. 16.11). If volume depletion is due to Na^+ loss exceeding water loss, the plasma becomes hypotonic and water enters the cells, causing them to swell.

In volume excess states, similar osmotic swelling or shrinkage occurs. In water intoxication, the plasma becomes hypotonic, favoring osmotic flow into the cellular compartment (fig. 16.11). When Na^+ retention arises as a result of renal malfunction or aldosterone hypersecretion, water retention tends to exceed Na^+ retention, so the plasma is also hypotonic in such cases.

When CNS cells undergo mild osmotic shrinkage, the patient exhibits weakness, lassitude, and irritability. With progression to more profound levels of derangement, seizures, coma, and death may occur. If brain shrinkage develops rapidly, hemorrhage from torn cerebral veins may result to compound the problem.

In fluid excess states, the ECF volume is increased and is usually hypotonic. (Recall that when both are retained, water retention exceeds Na^+ retention to produce a relative hyponatremia.) The result is an osmotic shift to the cellular compartment and the swelling of the CNS. This condition is sometimes referred to as **cerebral edema.** Swelling in the brain produces headache, nausea, and vomiting. The relative intracellular hyponatremia also produces malaise

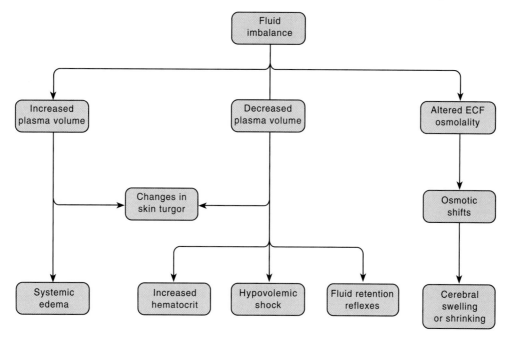

Figure 16.11   **Effects of Fluid Imbalance.**

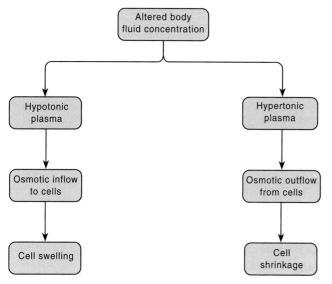

Figure 16.12   **Osmotic Effects of Body Fluid Concentration Abnormalities.** Cellular consequences of undesirable osmotic shifts when body fluid concentration is disrupted.

and lethargy at low levels, with seizures and coma more prevalent if swelling is increased (fig. 16.12).

Therapy in Fluid Imbalance

Volume depletion due to hemorrhage can be restored with carefully matched whole blood or an appropriate blood fraction. **Normal saline** (isotonic) solutions can readily restore volume and plasma concentration. If the kidneys are functioning, they will soon correct Na$^+$ and water imbalance as long as they have an adequate volume of infused saline on which to work. If fluid is present to excess, diuretic therapy

Focus on Iatrogenic Fluid Imbalance

If therapy is imprecise or overzealous, fluid imbalance may be worsened. An example of such an iatrogenic complication is fluid excess caused by excessive saline infusion during volume depletion therapy. Another example is the overly vigorous use of diuretics, intended to promote diuresis but unintentionally producing a depletion state. Unfortunately, these are significant factors in the fluid imbalances seen in clinical settings.

can restore volume if the kidneys are unable to compensate after the underlying problem has been addressed.

ELECTROLYTE IMBALANCE

For the sake of clarity, the major electrolytes are considered separately in the following sections. However, in clinical situations, excess or deficiency of one ion often produces imbalance in other ions. These effects, and those of the water imbalance that often accompanies them, combine to produce the pattern of signs and symptoms seen in a given patient.

Sodium Imbalance

The intimate relation between Na$^+$ imbalance and body water alterations has already been described in the context of fluid imbalance. The key points of Na$^+$ level alterations are considered in the following sections.

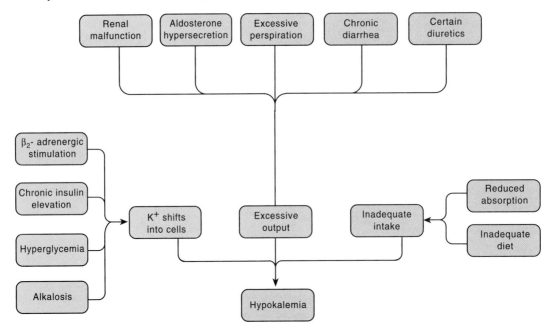

Figure 16.13   **Hypokalemia.** Principal factors in the pathogenesis of hypokalemia.

Hyponatremia

Na$^+$ deficiencies are almost always the result of body fluid loss rather than inadequate Na$^+$ intake. Na$^+$ is plentiful in even minimal diets, so meeting normal requirements is rarely a problem. Note also that much hyponatremia is relative—that is, the result of excessive body water rather than a true Na$^+$ depletion. Where renal defects prevent adequate Na$^+$ retention, or when aldosterone levels are depressed, Na$^+$ losses occur, but they are soon matched by compensating water losses that return the ECF to an isotonic state. Thus, even though Na$^+$ has been lost, and fluid volume reduced, ECF concentration is normal.

Hypernatremia

The Na$^+$ excess state most often arises when water losses exceed Na$^+$ losses, producing a relative hypernatremia. True hypernatremia is rare, but may arise where therapeutic administration of NaCl infusions is excessive (see focus box). If Na$^+$ is excessively retained, corresponding water retention produces systemic edema. The patient experiencing hypernatremia is thirsty, lethargic when undisturbed, irritable when aroused, and may exhibit various neurological signs ranging from mild disorientation to coma.

Potassium Imbalance

Potassium (K$^+$) is the dominant cation of the intracellular fluid compartment, which contains about 98% of total body K$^+$. Its concentration in the ICF is about 40 times that of the ECF, and thus it represents the principal osmotic determinant of cellular volume. K$^+$ also plays an important role in neuromuscular activity through its contribu-

tion to the membrane potentials on which neuron and muscle function depend.

Perspiration and fecal losses of K$^+$ are normally low. Most dietary K$^+$ is excreted in the urine by two mechanisms. In one, tubule cells directly respond to K$^+$ concentration in the renal interstitium, appropriately increasing or decreasing tubular secretion to match homeostatic requirements. The second mechanism depends on circulating aldosterone to regulate K$^+$ reabsorption via tubule transport systems. Increased aldosterone levels are followed by reduced reabsorption and increased renal K$^+$ excretion.

Hypokalemia

Hypokalemia is the condition of lowered K$^+$ concentration (*kalium* is Latin for potassium). It may be due to a total body K$^+$ deficit or to shifts of K$^+$ from the ECF into the cellular compartment. Such shifts may arise as cellular K$^+$ uptake is stimulated—for example, by insulin, glucose, or drugs that mimic certain sympathetic nervous (β_2-adrenergic) system effects. K$^+$ also shifts into cells in the imbalance condition called alkalosis, described in a later section.

K$^+$ deficiency may result from inadequate dietary K$^+$ intake. This is unlikely, but there is increased risk when appetite is depressed, as it commonly is in the elderly, those with CNS or GI disturbances that cause chronic nausea, and those with a psychogenic aversion to eating. Hypokalemia is more likely to be caused by excessive loss of K$^+$ in ways similar to those in which Na$^+$ is lost: in vomiting, heavy perspiration, and, particularly in cases of chronic diarrhea, as a component of the liquid stool. Laxative abusers are also therefore at risk of K$^+$ depletion (see focus box, p. 349). Absorption difficulties can lower K$^+$ intake in cases of intesti-

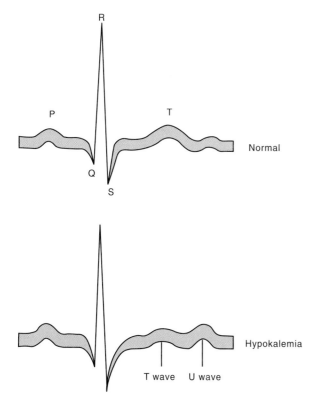

Figure 16.14   The ECG in Hypokalemia. The T wave is depressed and the U wave is elevated.

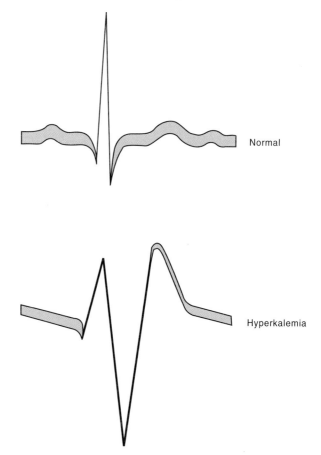

Figure 16.15   The ECG in Hyperkalemia. All elements are abnormal.

nal resection where absorptive surface is lost, or when a GI tract fistula allows absorptive surface to be by-passed.

Kidney tubule reabsorption defects or aldosterone hypersecretion states may also increase K^+ losses. Drugs can play a role as well, particularly diuretics such as furosemide, ethacrynic acid, acetazolamide, and thiazides. As in the case of most electrolytes, there is the potential for an imbalance following inappropriate administration of intravenous fluid, in this case a solution deficient in K^+ (fig. 16.13).

In hypokalemia, the dominant signs and symptoms are a reflection of disordered neuromuscular function. Weakness, muscle twitching, and depressed neuromuscular reflexes are typical. Skeletal muscles may lose their normal firmness—that is, they demonstrate a loss of neuromuscular tone. A characteristic electrocardiographic change is seen in hypokalemia. It involves depression of the S-T segment, flattening of the T wave, and a prominent U wave (fig. 16.14). The U wave is a minor deflection of the ECG that follows the T wave. Intestinal smooth muscle may be affected, causing paralytic ileus (deficient peristalsis) and vomiting.

Hypokalemia also has an impact on the kidney. Low K^+ levels seem to promote prostaglandin synthesis. They reduce the tubule's sensitivity to ADH, and diuresis and polyuria result.

Hyperkalemia

Hyperkalemia, the state of K^+ excess, is potentially life-threatening and may arise in aldosterone deficiency states

in which depression of renal excretion causes K^+ retention. Of course, renal failure or excessive intravenous fluid administration can also cause hyperkalemia. In cases of extensive trauma, especially crushing injuries, massive release of K^+ from damaged cells may produce a K^+ load that exceeds the kidneys' excretion capacity. In conditions involving extensive hemolysis, large amounts of K^+ may be released from damaged red cells.

K^+ shifts from the cellular compartment can increase K^+ level in the extracellular fluid. This occurs most often in acid-base imbalances, as described later in this chapter in the Acid-Base Imbalance section. Just as insulin and certain drugs promote K^+ uptake and hypokalemia, beta-blockers and insulin deficiency have the opposite effect, limiting K^+ uptake from the ECF.

Prolonged and severe hyperkalemia is potentially grave. Its major effect is on the myocardium, causing dysrhythmias. Characteristic ECG changes are present in hyperkalemia. Initially, the S-T segment is depressed, whereas T waves are increased. With progression of K^+ build-up, the P wave is lost, the QRS complex broadens, and the T waves become especially prominent (fig. 16.15).

Chloride Imbalance

Chloride (Cl⁻) is another of the principal anions in the ECF. It passively follows Na⁺, both when it is absorbed from the GI lumen and when it is reabsorbed in the nephron. For this reason, **hypochloremia,** the condition of Cl⁻ deficiency, is typically associated with Na⁺ deficiency. Thus, increased loss of GI fluids, perspiration, or renal failure can produce hypochloremia. In hypokalemia, compensating K⁺ retention mechanisms may produce a corresponding loss of Na⁺. When loss of Cl⁻ follows that of Na⁺, hypochloremia may result. In **hyperchloremia,** excessive Cl⁻ is usually present from increased intake. This might be the result of dietary excess, or, more commonly, excessive intravenous infusion of NaCl in Na⁺ depletion therapy. The influx of Na⁺ adequate to correct hyponatremia can easily produce hyperchloremia, because the Na⁺ and Cl⁻ in the intravenous infusion are present in equal concentrations. The exceptions to the similarity in conditions that give rise to Na⁺ and Cl⁻ imbalances are acid-base changes, which can affect Cl⁻ but not Na⁺. These are described in the Acid-Base Imbalance section later in the chapter.

Signs and symptoms of Cl⁻ imbalance are similar to those seen in Na⁺ imbalance—that is, they reflect fluid imbalance: edema and acute weight gain in hyperchloremia and dehydration effects in hypochloremia.

Calcium Imbalance

Most calcium ion (Ca⁺⁺) is present in the ECF with very little present in the ICF. Plasma Ca⁺⁺ is present in two forms, which exist in equilibrium. About half is present as a free ion in the plasma. The other half is bound to citrate ion or albumin. The unbound, ionized calcium of the plasma is its physiologically active component. When more of the ionized form is present, the equilibrium shifts to restore balance by binding more of the ionized form to protein or citrate. A deficiency of ionized calcium causes an opposite shift of the equilibrium as calcium is split from its binding molecule.

Ca⁺⁺ homeostasis is principally mediated by **parathyroid hormone** (PTH). Parathyroid cells modify their secretion of this hormone when ECF Ca⁺⁺ deviates from its normal range. PTH increases GI absorption and renal retention of Ca⁺⁺, and mobilizes Ca⁺⁺ from bone. The thyroid hormone **calcitonin** also affects ECF Ca⁺⁺ by promoting excretion when Ca⁺⁺ is present to excess.

The state of Ca⁺⁺ excess is called **hypercalcemia.** It may result from hyperparathyroidism or hypothyroid states, both of which favor Ca⁺⁺ retention. Since the kidney is our major means of calcium excretion, renal disease tends to cause calcium retention and hypercalcemia. Because vitamin D is required for Ca⁺⁺ absorption, hypercalcemia may be caused by excessive therapeutic intake of the vitamin. Increased ECF Ca⁺⁺ is also associated with the presence of various malignant tumors. This condition is **hypercalcemia of malignancy** and is caused by tumor

products that promote bone matrix degradation and by primary or secondary tumor growth in bone that causes it to release calcium. Because plasma calcium and phosphate levels are inversely related, hypercalcemia is often accompanied by phosphate deficiency, or **hypophosphatemia.**

Hypercalcemia typically causes nephrolithiasis (kidney stone formation), muscle cramps, and pain. Some GI hyperactivity is also common, producing nausea, abdominal cramps, and diarrhea. The widespread tissue deposition of calcium seen in chronic hypercalcemia is termed **metastatic calcification** and should not be confused with dystrophic calcification, the Ca⁺⁺ deposition at sites of necrosis, described in chapter 1.

Although abdominal cramps are also seen in **hypocalcemia,** hyperactive neuromuscular reflexes and **tetany** differentiate it from Ca⁺⁺ excess states. Tetany is a pattern of excessive muscle irritability involving intense muscle spasms in the extremities. A deficiency of Ca⁺⁺ may result from a dietary lack of vitamin D, suppression of parathyroid function, or hypersecretion of calcitonin. Sprue or other malabsorption states can also produce hypocalcemia. Because the absorption of Ca⁺⁺ depends on normal intestinal acidity, antacid therapy for peptic ulcers or gastric resection may so reduce intestinal acidity that absorption of Ca⁺⁺ is depressed. Widespread infection and pancreatic or peritoneal inflammation may also produce hypocalcemia because they promote the binding of Ca⁺⁺ so that its ionized form is less available to the ECF (fig. 16.16). Ca⁺⁺ also has effects on acid-base balance.

THERAPY IN FLUID AND ELECTROLYTE IMBALANCE

As in any therapy, in cases of fluid and electrolyte imbalance, an attempt is made to correct the initial cause of the imbalance. Then interventions promoting loss in excess states, or increased input in deficiency states, can proceed. In deficiency states, intravenous administration of the appropriate fluid and electrolytes can restore balance. Water movement from the plasma to the tissue spaces or to the ICF and vice versa can be accomplished by intravenous infusion to produce an appropriate change in plasma osmolality.

When total body fluid is excessive, diuretics are used to stimulate renal water loss. Most depress nephron Na⁺ reabsorption, so that water is lost and fluid volume is reduced. Note, here, the potential for excessive diuretic therapy that could produce hyponatremia and hyperkalemia. Other diuretics function by interfering with passive reabsorption of Cl⁻ in the nephron. This reduces the osmotic gradient between the nephron and the peritubular tissues and therefore limits reabsorption of water. Another approach involves diuretics that reduce the response of the nephron tubule to ADH. The resulting reduction of water permeability produces the desired water loss while at the same time retaining electrolytes.

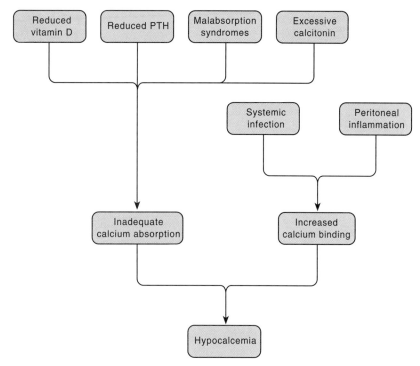

Figure 16.16   **Major Factors That May Contribute to Hypocalcemia.**

ACID-BASE IMBALANCE

The acidity of the body fluids is a critical variable in normal metabolism. Even small changes in acidity can produce major disturbances of function because many physiological chemical reactions are strongly influenced by pH. In particular, most cellular enzymes function only within a narrow range of pH change, beyond which reaction rates fall sharply. Changes in acid-base balance also affect several electrolytes—Na^+, K^+ and Cl^-, in particular—which can further disrupt homeostasis. The normal range of pH is between 7.35 and 7.45, with an average value of 7.40. When pH falls below 7.35, a condition of **acidosis** is said to exist; whereas above 7.45, the term **alkalosis** is used. The critical nature of pH is indicated by the fact that it need vary only slightly to produce disease. Symptoms develop when pH falls below 6.85 or rises above 7.65. Below pH 6.8 and above pH 8.0, death occurs.

The hydrogen ion (H^+) of the body fluids is produced directly or indirectly as a result of cellular metabolism. Protein and fat metabolism produces organic or inorganic acids, but these amounts are small. Aerobic energy metabolism contributes over 100 times more by constantly producing carbon dioxide, which affects pH via the carbonic acid equilibrium:

$$CO_2 + H_2O \rightleftharpoons H_2CO_3 \rightleftharpoons H^+ + HCO_3^- \quad \text{(Eq. 1)}$$

The essential requirement in maintaining correct pH is that H^+ be excreted at a rate that matches its production. The lungs are crucial to this process, in that by exhaling

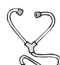

Focus on the Lab Report

The laboratory report plays a critical role in dealing with fluid and electrolyte imbalance. It must be carefully assessed before any intravenous fluid is administered. The essential principle is that one must have some insight into the patient's current fluid and electrolyte status before beginning an IV infusion. This avoids exaggerating any existing imbalance and also provides the data to guide selection of an appropriate IV solution. Even if you don't make the selection, your understanding can catch an error before some harm is done. Remember, inappropriate IV administration is a significant cause of water and sodium imbalance in hospitalized patients.

CO_2, the equilibrium (shown in Equation 1) shifts to the left. This favors the combining of hydrogen ion with bicarbonate ion (HCO_3^-) and the formation of carbonic acid (H_2CO_3). The result is a lowering of hydrogen ion concentration in the ECF. Because CO_2 gas is related to hydrogen ion through carbonic acid, it is referred to as **volatile acid.** Acids produced in protein and lipid metabolism are excreted in the kidney. These are known as **fixed acids.**

Although fixed and volatile acids can be efficiently excreted, a potential problem arises in the cells where H^+ is initially produced. Because only slight increases in [H^+]

can disrupt cellular function, it is necessary to cope with this newly produced acid until it can be excreted. This task is accomplished by a **buffer system,** which functions to resist changes in pH by taking up or releasing H^+ when its concentration changes. Only free, unassociated H^+ contributes to acidity. When taken up by another molecule, the hydrogen is no longer free and no longer acts as an acid. This is the essence of a buffer's function. In the following equilibrium, the buffer is represented by the anion B^-, which exists in equilibrium with its combined form HB. Changes in the H^+ level cause the equilibrium to shift in a direction that minimizes pH change. In (Eq. 2), acid levels are high and the indicated shift lowers the $[H^+]$.

$$H^+ + B^- \rightleftharpoons HB \quad (Eq. 2)$$

In the situation indicated in (Eq. 3), hydrogen ion level is low and the equilibrium shift raises the acid level.

$$H^+ + B^- \rightleftharpoons HB \quad (Eq. 3)$$

After formation of hydrogen ions in cells, intracellular buffers take up the hydrogen ions and transfer them to the major plasma buffer: the bicarbonate buffer system. In cells and in both ECF compartments, proteins, including plasma proteins and the hemoglobin in red cells, also function as buffers in that they can take up H^+ when it is in high concentration and release it should pH rise (fig. 16.17). It is the buffers of the ICF and ECF that take up and hold H^+ until it can be excreted.

Hydrogen Ion Excretion

Most H^+ excretion occurs indirectly when volatile acid (CO_2) is exhaled by the lungs. A system of systemic chemoreceptors sensitive to acid have input to the brain stem, where respiratory control centers are housed. When ECF H^+ level is increased, an increased ventilation response drives off CO_2 to lower the H^+ concentration. This system can effectively cope with the CO_2 generated by aerobic energy metabolism, but additional regulation capacity is needed for three reasons. One is to provide a backup system for acid excretion in situations in which respiratory insufficiency compromises CO_2 clearance. The second is the need to excrete the fixed acid produced by protein and lipid metabolism, which the lungs can't excrete. The third reason is the need to ensure the reabsorption of filtered bicarbonate and to generate additional HCO_3^- to replace the amount expended in buffering activities. Renal processes provide these needed regulatory capabilities.

In renal acid excretion, fixed acids derived from protein and lipid metabolism are passed to nephron tubule cells by the plasma buffers. The cells then secrete this H^+ into the lumen. In the process, sodium ion is exchanged for the H^+ to balance positive charge (see fig. 16.18a). Once in the lumen, H^+ combines with bicarbonate ion that has been filtered from the plasma. The carbonic acid formed in this way is promptly split into CO_2 and water by the enzyme carbonic anhydrase, which is present at the luminal surface

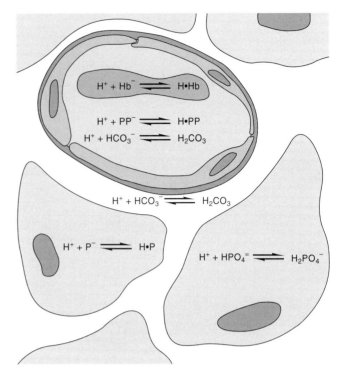

Figure 16.17 **Buffer Systems.** The principal buffer systems that take up H^+ in cells are cell proteins (P^-) and a phosphate system. Bicarbonate buffering occurs in the interstitium and plasma. Plasma proteins (PP) and hemoglobin (Hb) are other important buffers.

of the tubule (represented by asterisk in fig. 16.18). The carbon dioxide readily enters the tubule cell where carbonic anhydrase is also available to catalyze the formation of new carbonic acid inside the cell. Once formed, it dissociates to form additional H^+ that diffuses back into the lumen. In this way, there is a steady recycling of hydrogen ion between the cell and the lumen, which has two key effects. One is the production of HCO_3^- that is picked up by the blood to regenerate plasma buffering capacity. The other effect is on H^+ excretion, in that when secretion of H^+ exceeds the amount of filtered bicarbonate, the excess H^+ remains in the tubule lumen and is lost in the urine. In other words, when the plasma contains more than the optimum level of H^+, more will be filtered, but all won't find a bicarbonate ion with which to join. These are lost, and the H^+ returns toward the optimum homeostatic level.

Figure 16.18b illustrates the situation in which acid production is reduced so that the ECF is too alkaline. In such cases the secreted hydrogen ions are insufficient to combine with all the filtered bicarbonate. The result is an increased loss of the alkaline bicarbonate and restoration of optimal pH. So, whether acid production is increased or decreased, nephron mechanisms are able to make homeostatic adjustments.

Buffers, in cells and the ECF, can respond in a matter of seconds to shifts in pH, while respiratory responses take a bit longer: a few minutes. By contrast, renal excretion

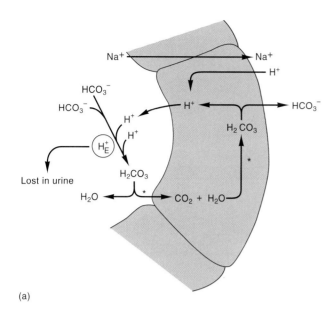

(a)

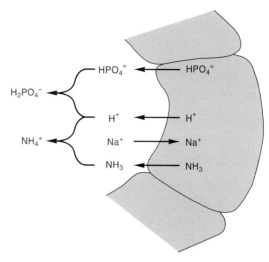

Figure 16.19   Acid in the Tubule. H^+ tends to diffuse out of the tubule unless combined to form the low-permeability ammonium and dihydrogen phosphate ions. The exchange of sodium for H^+ is also indicated.

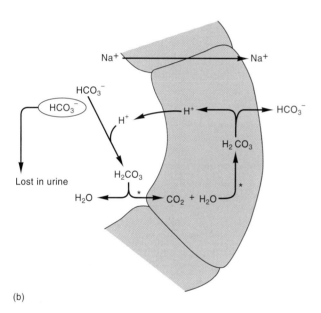

(b)

Figure 16.18   Excretion of H^+ in the Nephron Tubule.
The asterisk (*) represents the enzyme carbonic anhydrase, which catalyzes the reversible carbonic acid equilibrium. (*a*) Filtered bicarbonate combines with H^+ formed in tubule cells. H_E^+ is excess for which no HCO_3^- is available, so it is lost in urine. (*b*) In this case, since body fluids are too alkaline, less H^+ is available to combine with HCO_3^-, which is lost to make the body fluids more acidic.

may take hours to respond, but it can continue compensation for an extended period, with the added benefit that its action restores buffering capacity. This renal response, once fully activated, can excrete up to 500 mM of excess H^+ or HCO_3^- daily. This is roughly ten times normal daily production. If acid or base is produced above this level, excretion capacity is exceeded and a net accumulation results in a pronounced acidosis or alkalosis.

Following its excretion into the tubule lumen, the excess H^+ has a tendency to diffuse back into the peritubular

tissues. This is prevented by the tubule cells' secretion of ammonia (NH_3) into the lumen. There, the NH_3 and H^+ combine to form the ammonium ion (NH_4^+). Ammonium has a low permeability and can't readily diffuse back into the peritubular spaces. This renal process effectively confines excreted H^+, in the form of NH_4^+, to the lumen and ultimately the urine. The formation of dihydrogen phosphate ($H_2PO_4^-$) in the lumen has a similar effect (fig. 16.19). Note that in cases of renal disease, acidosis typically arises as a result of the kidney's reduced ability to excrete H^+. But if the dysfunctional kidney is also unable to secrete ammonia and dihydrogen phosphate, the acidosis will be aggravated because some of the H^+ the kidney has managed to excrete will be able to diffuse back out of the tubule to reenter the blood.

Related Ion Effects

Potassium   Altered pH in the ECF can produce secondary changes in the level of other ions. When acidosis is present, high ECF concentrations of H^+ cause it to diffuse into cells where H^+ concentration is lower. As a result of the accumulating positive charge inside the cell, positive ions move out of the cell, and since K^+ is the dominant intracellular cation, its passage to the ECF will be most significant. Hyperkalemia is the result. Similarly, in alkalosis, ECF H^+ concentration is reduced, favoring its diffusion from cells to the ECF. K^+ diffuses in to compensate for lost intracellular cations, the ECF K^+ level falls, and hypokalemia results (fig. 16.20).

In the preceding examples, the acid-base shift arises initially, with K^+ effects then developing in response. When K^+ imbalances are first present, secondary acid-base derangements may arise. Consider the situation in the nephron tubule cells generally. In hypokalemia, a reduced K^+ level

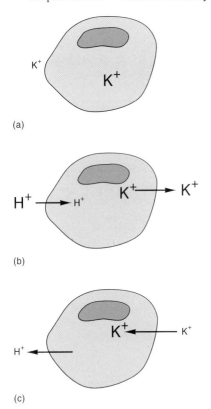

Figure 16.20   **Acid Effects on K⁺.** (*a*) Normal K⁺ gradient across the cell membrane. (*b*) Acidosis produces a secondary hyperkalemia. (*c*) Alkalosis favors outward diffusion of H⁺, which is replaced by K⁺ to cause a secondary hypokalemia in the ECF.

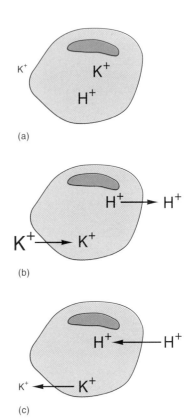

Figure 16.21   **K⁺ Effects on Acid.** (*a*) Normal concentration gradient of K⁺ across cell membrane. H⁺ is present as a product of metabolism. (*b*) Hyperkalemia favors K⁺ diffusion into the cell and H⁺ diffuses out to compensate for positive charge build-up. A secondary acidosis results. (*c*) Hypokalemia favors loss of K⁺ from the cell, and compensating H⁺ diffusion produces a secondary alkalosis in the ECF.

in the ECF causes K⁺ to diffuse out of the cell. The cation loss is answered by the diffusion of H⁺ into the cell. The resulting increase in intracellular acid triggers its excretion, and as the process continues, the ECF acid-base status shifts toward alkalosis. The opposite effect is seen in hyperkalemia, where the tendency is to acidosis (fig. 16.21).

Sodium   The relation between H⁺ and ECF volume regulation is based largely on renal reabsorption of Na⁺ ion. As Na⁺ is exchanged for H⁺ in the nephron, pH shifts may occur. If ECF volume is excessive, Na⁺ reabsorption falls and reduced H⁺ exchange occurs, meaning that H⁺ retention is increased and a shift toward acidosis develops. Similarly, when ECF volume is low, increased Na⁺ reabsorption occurs while H⁺ is passed to the lumen, and a tendency to alkalosis emerges (fig. 16.22).

Calcium   You may recall, from the earlier discussion of calcium imbalance, that Ca⁺⁺ is present in the body fluids as a free ion or bound to protein or citrate. This binding is acid-dependent, so that in acidosis more Ca⁺⁺ is taken up by protein and citrate, and hypocalcemia may develop. In alkalosis, hypercalcemia is also often present, as a result of the opposite effect of increased pH (fig. 16.22).

Other ion effects are mediated by aldosterone. Increased aldosterone secretion may occur in response to diuretic therapy. As diuresis proceeds, fluid loss activates the renin-angiotensin system, which increases aldosterone secretion, Na⁺ retention, and H⁺ loss to produce alkalosis. When aldosterone secretion is below normal levels, its stimulus to K⁺ and H⁺ excretion is reduced. The result is retention of both ions and concurrent acidosis and hyperkalemia.

Patterns of Acid-Base Imbalance

Intracellular buffers are responsible for most buffering, but the carbonic acid system is especially significant in determining the acid-base status of the plasma. Because the plasma is easily analyzed, the state of its bicarbonate buffer system is often used as an indicator of pH in the ECF generally, as well as in the intracellular compartment. In assessing pH in the extracellular fluid, a useful approach is based on the **Henderson-Hasselbalch equation.** It expresses pH in terms of the components of the bicarbonate buffer system:

$$pH = K + \log \frac{[HCO_3^-]}{[H_2CO_3]} \qquad \text{(Eq. 4)}$$

The value of the constant K is 6.1, and under normal circumstances the ratio of $[HCO_3^-]$ to $[H_2CO_3]$ is 20:1. The

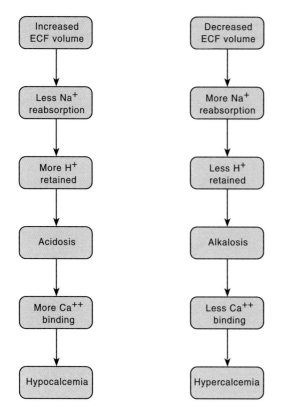

Figure 16.22 **Na⁺ and Ca⁺⁺ Links to Acid Imbalance.** Altered ECF volume can affect ECF acidity through sodium's exchange for acid in the kidney. Acid-base imbalance can produce ECF calcium derangements.

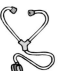

Focus on Diuretic Use and Acid-Base Imbalance

H⁺ shifts may be caused by diuretic therapy wherein the diuretic acts by suppressing Na⁺ or HCO₃⁻ absorption to promote water loss. The ion involved and the segment of the tubule where the diuretic acts determine the direction of the pH shift.

The popular **loop diuretics,** such as furosemide or ethacrynic acid, exert their effect by blocking Na⁺ absorption from Henle's loop. This leaves unusually large volumes of sodium-rich filtrate, which pass to the distal tubule. There, Na⁺ absorption proceeds at a high rate, linked to H⁺ loss. The potential side effect is a shift toward alkalosis. By contrast, the **thiazide diuretics** work by blocking Na⁺ absorption in the distal tubule segments. This means less H⁺ secretion and a lowered risk of alkalosis. The hypokalemia caused by thiazide diuretics may cause a secondary alkalosis (see fig. 16.21*c*).

The class of diuretics called **carbonic anhydrase inhibitors** functions by interfering with carbonic anhydrase activity at the nephron tubule's luminal surface. This reduces the formation of H_2CO_3 in the lumen, leaving HCO_3^- to exert an osmotic diuresis effect. With increased bicarbonate losses, acidosis may develop.

log of 20 is 1.3. Substituting these values, into equation (4) yields the normal extracellular fluid pH value:

$$pH = 6.1 + 1.3 = 7.4$$

Because the value of K does not change, any difference in pH is the result of a change in the ratio of the concentrations of HCO_3^- and H_2CO_3. Furthermore, because $[H_2CO_3]$ is related to the partial pressure of CO_2, equation (4) can take the form:

$$pH = K' + \log \frac{[HCO_3^-]}{PCO_2} \quad \text{(Eq. 5)}$$

The new constant, K', adjusts for the relationship between PCO_2 and H_2CO_3. Equation (5) is significant because it expresses pH in terms of PCO_2, which is altered by changes in ventilation, and in terms of plasma $[HCO_3^-]$, which changes in response to renal hydrogen ion excretion.

Acid-base imbalances are classified on the basis of equation (5). Those pH imbalances caused by changes in the elimination of CO_2 by the lungs are classified as respiratory imbalances. For example, as PCO_2 increases because of inadequate ventilation, the denominator of equation (5) increases. This produces a smaller value for the ratio $[HCO_3^-]$: PCO_2, and therefore a lower pH. This condition is termed **respiratory acidosis.** On the other hand, if PCO_2 is diminished, the ratio increases and so does the value of pH, to produce **respiratory alkalosis.** Alternatively, when pH imbalance is caused by changes in acid production, renal excretion, or gastrointestinal losses, the imbalance is said to be of metabolic origin. In such cases, the ratio $[HCO_3^-]$: PCO_2 will shift because of changes in $[HCO_3^-]$ indirectly linked to changes in H⁺ ion production or loss. So, in **metabolic acidosis,** increased H⁺ ion shifts the carbonic acid equilibrium to the left. This decreases the $[HCO_3^-]$, the ratio decreases, and therefore the pH decreases as well. In **metabolic alkalosis,** reduced [H⁺] forces a shift to the right in the carbonic acid equilibrium. The result is an increase in the $[HCO_3^-]$, an increased ratio of $[HCO_3^-]$ to PCO_2, and therefore a larger, more alkaline pH (fig. 16.23).

Respiratory Acidosis

In respiratory acidosis, faulty pulmonary function causes a build-up of CO_2 in plasma that lowers pH. The problem may be acute, as in the adult respiratory distress syndrome (ARDS), status asthmaticus, or pneumothorax, or chronic as in chronic airway obstruction (CAO). Respiratory acidosis may also follow traumatic or other damage to the brain stem where the respiratory control centers are located. Similar effects are also produced by inappropriate drug doses that depress CNS function. Because renal compensation is slow to develop, it may be several days before the kidneys are able to restore a normal pH.

A generalized weakness is characteristic of acidosis, with deranged CNS function the greatest threat. In severe cases, confusion and disorientation may be followed by coma and finally death.

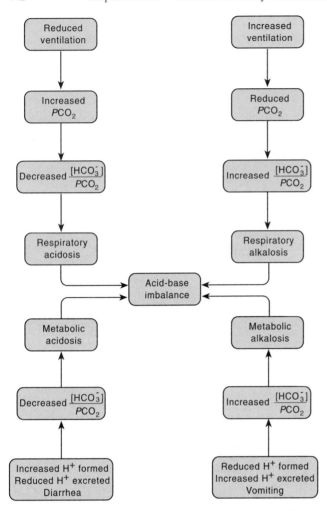

Figure 16.23   **Acid-Base Imbalance.** The development of the major patterns of acid-base imbalance starts at the top or bottom of each column.

Respiratory Alkalosis

Respiratory alkalosis is the result of excessive pulmonary CO_2 clearance. It is much less common than respiratory acidosis. It may arise as the result of hyperventilation that attempts to compensate for hypoxemia, or may be psychogenic, as for example, in anxiety states. High fever, brain stem damage, or pulmonary embolism are other conditions in which hyperventilation occurs. Patients may complain of numbness, a generally increased sensitivity (paresthesia), lightheadedness, and even tetany in extreme cases. They may also experience convulsions or lose consciousness.

Metabolic Acidosis

In this condition, declining pH is the result of a fall in $[HCO_3^-]$ or a rise in $[H^+]$. Most often this is the result of increased production of acid metabolic products, as in prolonged hypoxia, where the shift to glycolysis produces lactic acid. **Lactic acidosis** is also associated with certain tumors, drug or toxin ingestion, and respiratory failure. In those suffering from diabetes mellitus, altered metabolism produces keto acids (see chapter 17). Alcoholics may also produce

excess ketoacids. In renal failure, a decline in H^+ excretion capability often follows the loss of nephrons in glomerulonephritis, or the reduced H^+ secretion typical of pyelonephritis. In either case, normal H^+ production exceeds available excretory capability, and pH falls. Direct loss of HCO_3^- can also produce acidosis, usually in chronic diarrhea, since there is significant secretion of bicarbonate into the lumen of the distal small intestine. Intestinal fistulae may also cause acidosis due to the lack of intestinal surface on which bicarbonate (and all other) absorption depends.

In metabolic acidosis, respiratory compensation produces a rapid and deep pattern of breathing known as **Kussmaul's respirations.** As in respiratory acidosis, the symptoms include generalized weakness, fatigue, nausea, vomiting, and CNS depression.

Metabolic Alkalosis

In this condition, acid may be lost from the GI tract by vomiting or through nasogastric suction. Renal causes are most often related to the use of potassium-losing diuretics that induce hypokalemia (see fig. 16.21c). In response to the initial H^+ loss, HCO_3^- losses can rapidly provide compensation. For this reason, metabolic alkalosis is unlikely to develop without some factor that compromises renal HCO_3^- compensation. Volume depletion states, for example, involve pronounced Na^+ reabsorption, and HCO_3^- is retained to balance charge. In adrenal cortex tumors that hypersecrete aldosterone, H^+ is excessively secreted. In either case, alkalosis is sustained. Often, too-vigorous antacid therapy for gastric hypersecretion will produce a metabolic alkalosis.

Signs and symptoms in metabolic acidosis are nonspecific and are more the result of the secondary hypercalcemia—for example, muscle cramping and G-I hyperactivity. Hypoventilation may also be present as a compensation that tends to increase pH.

Compensation in Acid-Base Imbalance

The two mechanisms that have an impact on ECF pH—ventilation and renal H^+ and HCO_3^- excretion—are available to compensate for acid-base imbalances. If, for example, $[HCO_3^-]$ is decreased as a result of excessive acid production, compensation can be achieved by suitably reducing PCO_2. This can be accomplished by hyperventilation until the desired ratio, and therefore pH, is achieved. Alternatively, if lung disease causes a decrease in the $[HCO_3^-]$: PCO_2 ratio because of the accumulation of CO_2, then renal excretion of H^+ ion can be increased to elevate the $[HCO_3^-]$ until the $[HCO_3^-]$: PCO_2 ratio approaches the desired value. If the respiratory system causes pH to change, then renal hydrogen ion excretion and its indirect $[HCO_3^-]$ effects will compensate. When acid production changes, compensation is achieved by ventilation changes that alter PCO_2. This means that following compensation, both $[HCO_3^-]$ and PCO_2 will have higher or lower values, but they will still be within normal limits (fig. 16.24).

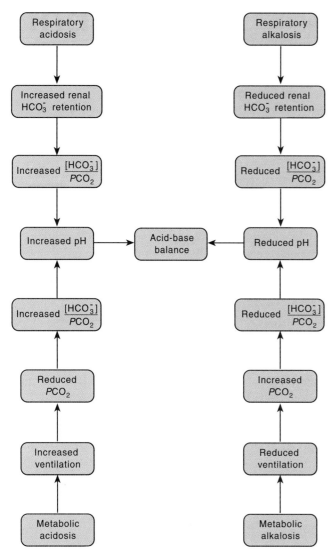

Figure 16.24 **Compensation in Acid-Base Imbalance.** Start at the top or bottom of each column.

Although compensatory acid-base shifts are important in minimizing the adverse effects of an elevated or depressed pH, they can complicate diagnosis if a compensation effect is confused with the original cause. For example, an acute metabolic acidosis that develops because of renal failure activates a hyperventilation response. This may reduce the acidosis, but since shifting the bicarbonate equilibrium has reduced [HCO$_3^-$], this effect may be taken as the original cause of the problem. Generally, the term **uncompensated** is applied to acidosis or alkalosis in which no compensation response is activated. In **partially compensated** imbalances, pH is abnormal, but it is closer to normal than if compensation had not occurred. **Fully compensated** (or chronic) acidosis or alkalosis involves restoration of a normal pH although other ion imbalances may be present. Generally, respiratory compensation in metabolic acidosis or alkalosis is less capable of restoring a normal pH than is the kidney in correcting for respiratory acidosis or alkalosis. Table 16.4 illustrates an approach to assessing acid-base imbalance that is based on an initial consideration of the PCO_2 and then pH. After you digest the previous sections, the table should pull things together for you.

Therapy in Acid-Base Imbalance

Therapy attempts to correct the cause of the initial imbalance, but often this is not possible. Efforts are therefore made to adjust the pH of the ECF via oral or intravenous administration of appropriate agents. These may have a direct effect, as in the oral administration of sodium bicarbonate (NaHCO$_3$) to correct acidosis. Alternatively, a substance may be used that is in itself not directly corrective, but that is metabolized to form products that produce the desired pH shift. In acidosis, for example, solutions containing sodium gluconate or sodium lactate ions are used, because their metabolism produces Na$^+$ to hold HCO$_3^-$ in the ECF. In alkalosis, ammonium chloride (NH$_4$Cl) is used because the metabolism of the ammonium ion produces acid products that offset the excessive alkalinity.

Table 16.4		Initial Assessment of Acid-Base Imbalance
PCO$_2$	**pH**	**Comment**
Normal	Abnormal	Normal CO$_2$ indicates adequate respiratory function, so pH disruption must have a metabolic cause. Later commpensation by the lungs will produce altered PCO_2 values.
Low	High	The low PCO_2 indicates hyperventilation that has raised pH via the bicarbonate equilibrium: **respiratory alkalosis.**
Low	Low	The ECF is acidic but the low PCO_2 indicates an active ventilation response, so this problem has a metabolic source: **metabolic acidosis.**
High	Low	A high PCO_2 indicates some inability to clear CO$_2$. The drop in pH results as more carbonic acid is formed via the bicarbonate equilibrium: **respiratory acidosis.**
High	High	Since elevated PCO_2 would tend to produce acidosis, the existing alkalosis must mean H$^+$ has been lost. The lungs are hypoventilating to retain CO$_2$ as a compensation: **metabolic alkalosis.**

Case Study

A 1-year-old child worried his parents when he ran a fever and refused any food or drink for 24 hours. The following day the child developed diarrhea and vomited periodically. The parents phoned their general practitioner, who advised them to give the child clear fluids only for a day and then to gradually reintroduce solid foods.

The child took the clear fluids offered, but vomited them soon after they were given. He also continued with intermittent diarrhea for the remainder of the day. On the next day the parents' concerns were worsened when the pattern continued and the child became listless and refused even liquids. With no improvement by evening, and six consecutive hours of dry diapers, the parents took the child to the hospital emergency room.

The attending ER physician's examination determined the child to be generally normal and well developed. The exceptions were dryness of the mouth, sunken eyes, a rapid pulse, and a generally diminished skin turgor. On the basis of these findings, a diagnosis of gastroenteritis with dehydration due to diarrhea and vomiting emerged. A viral etiology was suspected.

The child was admitted to hospital, and IV fluids were administered to rehydrate him. Nothing was given by mouth until the vomiting subsided, about 14 hours later. A series of blood analyses proved normal, and the child was released to his parents with instructions to continue with fluids and then slowly add increasingly solid food as improvement continued. They were also advised to monitor closely for any interruption of the recovery. The child's progress was rapid and no further complications developed.

Commentary

The night admission via the ER is not uncommon since, to concerned parents, all signs and symptoms in their children seem worse at night. In this case, all indications were consistent with a dehydration state. The suspicion of a viral etiology, without direct evidence, was based on the high incidence of transient and benign viral gastroenteritis among children. It was further supported by the lack of any travel or day care contacts where exposure to other infection sources was possible.

The blood studies were done primarily to assess whether metabolic acidosis or hypokalemia had resulted from the bouts of diarrhea and vomiting. Since most such viral gastroenteritis is self-limiting, more extensive stool studies for parasites or other agents would have been undertaken only if the signs and symptoms had persisted. Admission to hospital was prudent because if intervention is delayed, severe complications can develop rapidly, especially in children.

Key Concepts

1. If the quantity and composition of the body fluids is not maintained within homeostatic limits, serious functional disturbances and even death may result (p. 423).

2. Water and sodium are closely interrelated, and any deficiency or excess in one may well produce an effect in the other (p. 430).

3. Dehydration typically results from excessive water loss and rarely from inadequate intake (p. 430).

4. Water intoxication is typically produced by a defective water excretion mechanism and only rarely as a result of excessive intake (p. 430).

5. Most water intoxication is due to an excessive secretion of ADH, arising from faulty neurologic control, from the effect of certain therapeutic drugs, or by tumors (pp. 430–431).

6. Volume depletion may result from body fluid losses via the GI tract, kidneys, skin, or may develop in various sequestration states in which fluid is lost from vessels but retained within the body (p. 431).

7. Fluid volume excess is usually mediated via the kidneys when they are diseased, or through inappropriate fluid retention reflexes related to heart failure or liver cirrhosis (pp. 431–432).

8. Fluid volume expansion or depletion can affect plasma volume, and therefore arterial BHP, or induce osmotic effects to which cells of the CNS are particularly vulnerable (p. 432).

9. Therapy in fluid imbalance typically involves the intravenous infusion of fluids whose composition restores normal volume and osmolarity (p. 433).

10. A given patient's pattern of fluid and electrolyte balance is the result of complex interrelations among the various electrolytes dissolved in the body water, with deficiency or excess in one often producing imbalances among the others (p. 433).

11. Excesses or deficiencies of sodium are usually relative changes produced by excessive loss or retention of body water (pp. 433–434).

12. Most hypokalemia is due to excessive loss of potassium via the GI tract, skin, or kidneys, while the potassium excess state may arise from aldosterone hyposecretion, renal failure, or widespread cell damage associated with extensive trauma (p. 434).

13. Since chloride ion passively follows sodium ion, most chloride imbalance is a secondary effect linked to sodium deficiency or excess (p. 436).

14. Hypercalcemia, caused by excessive retention or impaired excretion, may produce nephrolithiasis, muscle cramps, and pain, while hypocalcemia, caused by a dietary deficiency, inadequate absorption, or excessive renal excretion, is typically accompanied by muscle hyperactivity and tetany (p. 436).

15. Therapy in electrolyte imbalance is directed at correcting the initial cause and at restoring balance by the intravenous administration of an appropriately balanced solution (p. 436).

16. Acidosis and alkalosis may produce secondary imbalances in both potassium and calcium (pp. 439–440).

17. Reduced pulmonary excretion of carbon dioxide produces respiratory acidosis, while excessive carbon dioxide excretion via the lungs causes respiratory alkalosis (pp. 441–442).

18. Increased metabolic acid production, or loss of bicarbonate, produces the condition of metabolic acidosis, while in metabolic alkalosis, acid is lost via the GI tract or the kidneys (p. 442).

19. Reference to a given patient's degree of pulmonary or renal compensation for an acid-base imbalance is indicated by the terms *uncompensated,* in which pH imbalance is not reduced, *partially compensated,* where the degree of imbalance is reduced, and *fully compensated,* in which pH is restored to normal (pp. 442–443).

REVIEW ACTIVITIES

1. From left to right across the bottom of a piece of paper, write the following five items: systemic edema, increased hematocrit, shock, fluid retention reflexes, and cerebral swelling or shrinking. Above the first four, add the plasma volume changes that would cause them. Above cerebral swelling or shrinking, add their cause. Does your page look like the bottom part of figure 16.11?

2. Look at the lower two cells shown in figure 16.6. If these were cells in the brain, what kind of problems might develop in each case?

3. Complete the following quick reference table, which will give you a quick check on some important links between the major electrolytes. All you need to do is to replace the question mark with an appropriate arrow in the right column. Pages 430–440 have all the information you'll need.

If	Then
↑H_2O	? Na^+
↓H_2O	? Na^+
↑Na^+	? Cl^-
↓Na^+	? Cl^-
↑K^+	? H^+
↓K^+	? H^+
↑H^+	? K^+
↓H^+	? K^+
↑Ca^{++}	? $PO_4^{\equiv}$
↓Ca^{++}	? $PO_4^{\equiv}$
↑H^+	Ca^{++}
↓H^+	Ca^{++}

4. Complete the following table by indicating the electrolyte change that each therapeutic agent might produce. The agents indicated by an asterisk often have effects on two ions. You needn't start looking in the text before page 430.

Therapeutic Agent	Possible Electrolyte Effect
Thiazides*	
Sodium bicarbonate	
Ammonium chloride	
Ethacrynic acid*	
Furosemide*	
Vitamin D supplementation	
Carbonic anhydrase inhibitors	
Sodium gluconate	
Antacids	
Acetazolamide	

5. Think back to the case study. If lab tests on the plasma had indicated that acidosis was present, would it have been respiratory or metabolic acidosis, and how would the ratio of bicarbonate to the partial pressure of carbon dioxide have changed to produce it?

Chapter

17

Endocrine Pathophysiology

Tie off pancreas ducts of dogs. Wait six or eight weeks. Remove and extract.

SIR FREDERICK BANTING, CO-DISCOVERER OF INSULIN,
FROM HIS EXPERIMENTAL NOTEBOOK

rubor
et tumor
cū calore
et dolore

The excessive or inadequate secretion of the body's many hormones produces a broad array of endocrine disorders. As background for a description of the major endocrine diseases, this chapter starts with a review of the endocrine system and the general principles that govern its function.

ESSENTIALS OF ENDOCRINOLOGY

The endocrine system consists of ductless glands whose secretions are delivered by the blood to the tissues they regulate. This is in contrast to the exocrine system, whose secretions are delivered to their sites of action by ducts (fig. 17.1). The endocrine system employs its secretions, called **hormones** (from the Greek word meaning "to set in motion" or "to excite"), to provide controlling input to cells. Hormonal control of cellular activities serves the overall somatic requirement for homeostasis and is the principal function of the endocrine system.

There are some variations on this essential endocrine mechanism. For example, **paracrine** cells secrete hormones that diffuse to adjacent cells and regulate their actions, and **autocrine** cells secrete substances that control their own function. Note that in these cases, the hormones never reach the general circulation in appreciable quantities.

The presence of many small deposits of endocrine tissue, in widespread parts of the body, supports the concept of a dispersed regulatory system. In this broad sense, a dispersed regulatory system would include the nervous system because of its release of chemical substances (at synapses and junctions) that elicit responses from adjacent cells (paracrine function). The nervous system also exerts broad regulatory and control functions: some directly, and others indirectly by its links to the endocrine system. Such **neuroendocrine** activity can be seen in the release of the posterior pituitary gland's hormones in response to nervous stimulus from the hypothalamus. The anterior pituitary gland is also largely dependent on the hypothalamus for its control, but in this case, control is mediated by **releasing hormones** rather than by action potentials. The hypothalamus secretes the releasing hormones, which travel directly to the adjacent pituitary to govern release of its hormones. When an endocrine gland's hormone controls the secretion of a second endocrine gland, the hormone is said to be a **tropic hormone.** In these ways the endocrine and nervous systems are closely linked in providing the body's requirements for precise regulation of its many functions (fig. 17.2).

Consider the example of sex cell production in either gender. It depends on the sex hormones secreted by the ovary or testis (endocrine glands in their own right, in addition to producing sex cells). Sex hormone production is dependent on anterior pituitary tropic hormones, which in turn rely on hypothalamic releasing hormones for their secretion. Here is a case of the nervous system influencing the release of three levels of control chemicals, which ultimately determine a single response: spermatozoan and oocyte production. In cases of infertility, the underlying de-

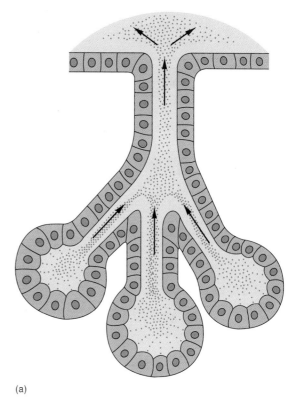

(a)

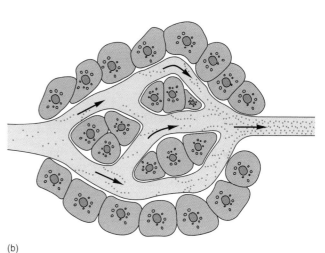

(b)

Figure 17.1 **Delivery of Secretions.** (*a*) In exocrine secretion, ducts deliver the gland's product to its site of action. (*b*) Endocrine glands secrete directly into the blood, which widely disperses their hormones.

fect might lie in the sex gland itself, its endocrine cells, the anterior pituitary, the hypothalamus, or other brain areas.

Despite the existence of paracrine and autocrine functions, most hormones depend on the blood for delivery. Many hormones are water-soluble and travel freely dispersed in the plasma, but the steroid and thyroid hormones have low water solubility and are carried in plasma complexed with albumin or specific carrier proteins. Protein-bound hormones exist in equilibrium with small amounts of unbound hormone. The protein-bound hormone seems to provide a reservoir of hormone that is available should secretion be

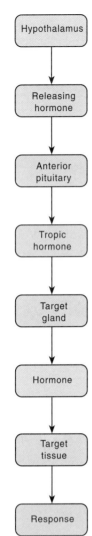

Figure 17.2   Neuroendocrine Control. Nervous and endocrine roles often combine to determine the regulatory input to a given target tissue. Note that the tissue's response is determined by three levels of endocrine control.

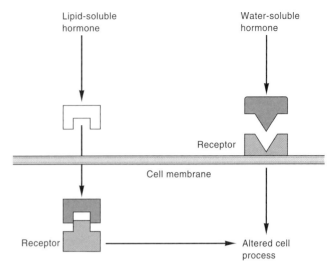

Figure 17.3   Hormone-Receptor Binding. Lipid-soluble hormones interact with intracellular receptors, since they can readily pass into the cell. Protein hormones are unable to enter the cell easily. Instead, they bind to surface receptors. In either case, hormone binding triggers the cell's responses.

reduced. In normal circumstances, it is the tiny amount of free hormone that is responsible for eliciting tissue effects.

Endocrine Specificity

Since hormones are carried throughout the body by the blood, they reach all tissues. However, not all tissues respond to them. Only certain tissues, and in some cases only one tissue, alter their activity in response to a particular hormone. These responding tissues are the hormone's **target tissues.** A given hormone's target, then, responds to that hormone, whereas all other tissues do not. This is an example of endocrine system specificity. It is based on the binding of hormones at specific cellular receptors. The receptor has a particular shape that is matched by only one of the many circulating hormones, and this match allows the two to fit closely enough for binding to occur.

There are two broad classes of target tissue receptor that are related to the two chemical categories of hormones. The **intracellular receptors** are present in the cytoplasm,

some at the surface of the nuclear membrane. These can bind steroid and thyroid hormones because they are lipid-soluble and can readily pass through the cell membrane to reach receptors in the cell's interior. For protein, peptide, and single amino acid hormones, the situation is different. Having low lipid solubility, they can't easily enter the cell. Instead, they are bound by **membrane receptors** at the cell's surface. The binding of hormone by either receptor type produces the same effect: an alteration of the target cell's level of activity (fig. 17.3).

The key to endocrine specificity lies in the differing patterns of receptor distribution among the many body tissues. A given cell has a particular array of receptors specific for many hormones. Other cells may have some receptors in common with it, but will also have some receptors that the given cell lacks. The differences explain the differing tissue responses to the particular hormones in the blood at a given time (fig. 17.4).

Mechanisms of Target Tissue Response

The frequency at which target tissue receptors bind hormone determines the tissue's activity: Increased binding rates induce an increased response. The response is, in some cases, greater cellular activity and, in other cases, inhibition of cellular processes; but basically, more hormone binding means more target tissue response, and vice versa. How, then, does hormone binding alter cellular functioning?

Two fundamental processes are involved. In the case of the steroid and thyroid hormones, their binding to intracellular receptors forms complexes that enter the nucleus. There they interact with regulatory elements of the chromosome's DNA. The result is an increase in the production of enzymes that will enhance a metabolic pathway's activity, thus producing an appropriate alteration of the target tissue's function (fig. 17.5a).

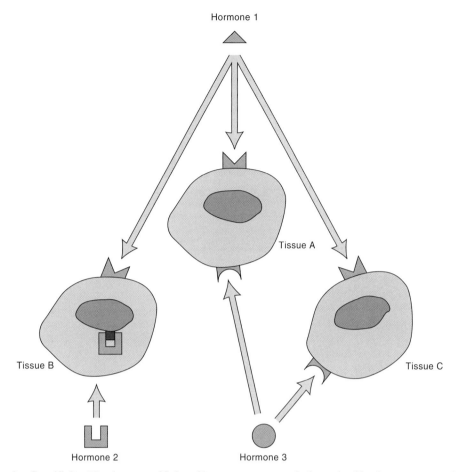

Figure 17.4   **Endocrine Specificity.** The tissue specificity of hormone responses is determined by the presence or absence of tissue receptors. Those with receptors (target tissues) are responsive to the hormone; those without receptors are not. Hormone 1 elicits responses from several tissues, while hormone 2 is highly specific, with one target tissue only. Hormone 3 controls the activity of two of the three tissues.

In the case of those target tissues that respond to binding of their surface receptors, membrane transport systems may be involved. These increase or decrease activity in response to receptor binding, altering cytoplasmic concentrations of various molecules or ions on which cell processes depend (fig. 17.5*b*). In most cases, membrane receptor binding is followed by the triggering of a sequence of activation steps that ultimately affect the cell's functions. Most hormones activate one of two receptor systems that are designated as **G proteins** or **protein kinases.** These systems in turn activate various intermediate processes catalyzed by specific enzymes (fig. 17.5*c*). Much research is devoted to clarifying these intermediate steps, in an effort to increase our ability to therapeutically manipulate cellular responses.

The Determinants of Plasma Hormone Level

From the preceding, you can see that the determining factor in an effector's response is the frequency of receptor binding. With greater binding frequency there is increased cellular response, and vice versa. The frequency of receptor binding is in turn dependent on the amount of hormone delivered by the blood. This amount is determined by the balance between the rate at which hormone enters the blood and the rate at which it is cleared from the blood by inactivation or excretion. Inactivation of hormones usually occurs at two sites. One is the target tissue, where enzymes degrade hormones and convert them to nonfunctional forms. The other inactivation site is the liver. Hormones reaching the liver are chemically converted to inactive forms by hepatic enzyme systems, a process related to the liver's detoxification functions. Hormones are also cleared from the body by the kidney. They are excreted in the urine, often entering the nephron tubule by tubular secretion mechanisms. The products of target tissue and hepatic hormone inactivation may also be excreted in the urine (fig. 17.6).

Hormone inactivation by liver and target tissues or hormone excretion normally occurs at steady rates. This means that the blood's level of a given hormone is primarily determined by changes in its rate of secretion. For increased target tissue response, more secretion increases the level of circulating hormone, whereas reduced secretion causes it to decline as inactivation and excretion continue.

Hormone secretion has two components. One is hormone synthesis from dietary or endogenous precursors. Controlling stimuli to the gland directly or indirectly affects synthesis of hormone, speeding or slowing the process. The

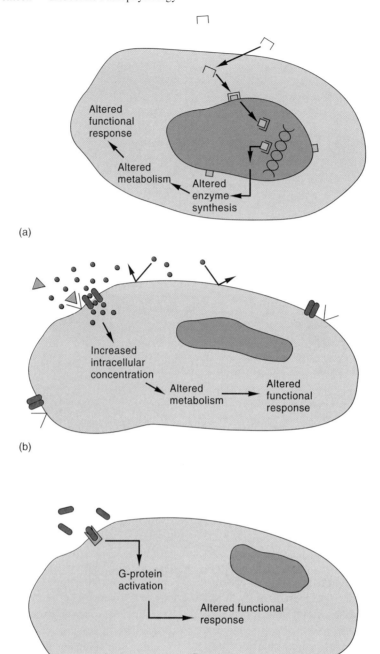

Figure 17.5 **Endocrine Response Mechanisms.** (*a*) Receptor binding linked to the synthesis of enzymes that regulate cell functions. (*b*) Surface receptors bind hormone and alter membrane transport of ions or molecules linked to key cellular responses. (*c*) Hormone bound at surface receptors triggers G-protein activation that alters cell activity.

second factor that determines secretion is the rate at which hormone is released from the endocrine cell. In some cases, hormone is stored within the gland, with release determined by nervous, hormonal, or other stimuli.

Secretion control is typically based on the principle of negative feedback. For example, the level of circulating hormone is inversely related to its own secretion rate. That is, when hormone level is excessive, secretion is inhibited; too low a hormone level acts as a stimulus to secretion. The thyroid and sex hormones are controlled in this way. Another regulatory input is the level of some homeostatic vari-

able that is controlled by a hormone. Calcium concentration in the plasma is an example. This variable is principally regulated by parathyroid hormone (PTH). As calcium levels change, parathyroid cells appropriately modify PTH secretion. Insulin is a similar example. Its secretion is regulated by the blood glucose level that it controls. The nervous system may also control hormone secretion directly, as in the interaction between the posterior pituitary and the adrenal medulla, or indirectly by way of anterior pituitary tropic hormones. Figure 17.7 summarizes these secretion control inputs.

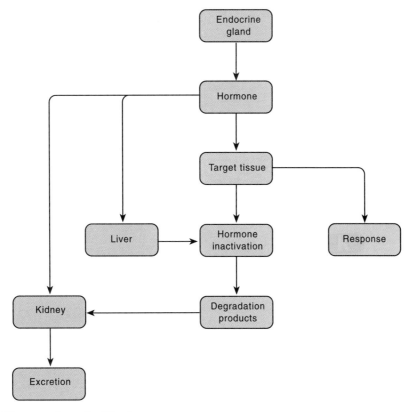

Figure 17.6 **Hormone Clearance from the Blood.**

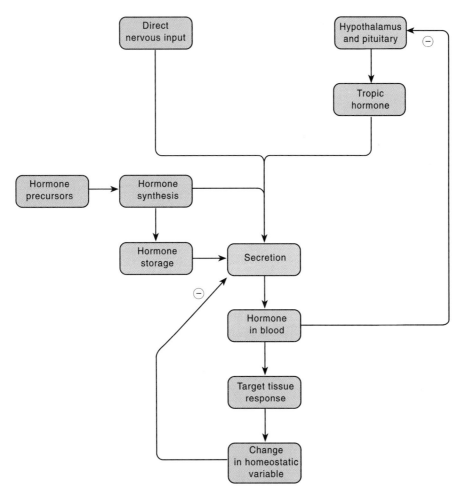

Figure 17.7 **Endocrine Secretion Control.** Once synthesized, hormone may be stored prior to secretion. The nervous system may control secretion directly or via the hypothalamus-pituitary link, which leads to tropic hormone secretion. The change in the variable may be monitored to control secretion, or the hormone level in the blood may be fed back to regulate tropic hormone secretion.

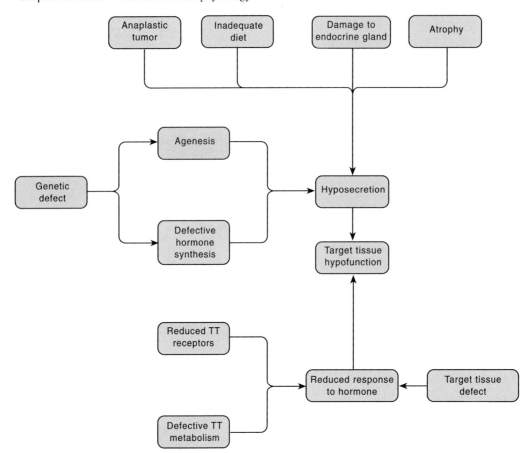

Figure 17.8   **Factors in Endocrine Hypofunction.** Inadequate secretion of hormone or a reduced target tissue (TT) response when hormone secretion is normal can both produce target tissue hypofunction.

ENDOCRINE DYSFUNCTION

Essentially, endocrine dysfunction produces only two types of defect: excessive or inadequate target tissue responses. In the case of exaggerated target tissue responses, hypersecretion of hormone is most often at fault. When target tissue responses are deficient, either endocrine hyposecretion is the cause or there is a defect in the tissues response to normal levels of hormone. Much endocrine pathophysiology rests on these basic concepts, and they should be the first factors to consider in clinical situations involving endocrine disorders. They are reflected in the descriptive terminology encountered clinically—for example, hyperpituitarism or the hypothyroid state.

The following section expands these principles of endocrine dysfunction, while the rest of the chapter is devoted to particular endocrine glands and their specific disorders.

Endocrine Hypofunction

In endocrine hypofunction states, target tissue responses are inadequate. The cause may be hyposecretion or it may be a loss of target tissue sensitivity to its controlling hormone.

Hyposecretion

In rare cases, inadequate secretion is due to **agenesis,** or lack of gland development. This is a clear-cut example of

hyposecretion, as no hormone source is present. In other cases, a genetic defect may produce a metabolic abnormality that prevents synthesis of normal hormone. Of course, hyposecretion may be due to a dietary deficiency that causes a lack of hormone precursors, but more commonly, it arises because a normally developed gland is damaged and is unable to maintain normal secretion. Infection, infarction, or autoimmune mechanisms are most often involved, with chronic inflammation less frequently responsible for the damage.

Another cause of hyposecretion is atrophy of an endocrine gland. This is most often due to a lack of tropic hormone input, which reduces demand for hormone secretion.

Tumor growth can be the cause of endocrine hyposecretion when tumor tissue replaces functional endocrine tissue. Secretion is reduced if the tumor cells are sufficiently anaplastic to produce no hormone, or if they secrete altered hormone forms that are nonfunctional or of reduced potency.

A special case of endocrine hypofunction is based on therapy for hypersecretion. Surgery to remove part of an excessively active gland may resect too much tissue, inadvertently producing a hyposecretion state. The essential factors in endocrine hypofunction are summarized in figure 17.8.

Hyposecretion states are often accompanied by elevated levels of control hormones. These result from the negative feedback stimulus presented by subnormal hormone levels (see fig. 17.7). Tropic hormones of the anterior pituitary or hypothalamic releasing hormones are typically involved. Following recovery or therapeutic restoration of normal hormone levels, secretion of control hormones is suppressed and their normal values are restored.

Hormone Resistance

Resistance is the term often used to describe insensitivity of a target tissue to its hormone. This phenomenon, which is increasingly recognized, often involves a hereditary defect that compromises the target tissue's ability to synthesize hormone receptors. Other genetic defects may be present in the intracellular systems activated by normal hormone binding. The consequence is a depressed target tissue response even though hormone levels are normal, or even elevated. Higher than normal hormone levels may be a reflection of the negative feedback response to reduced target tissue activity (fig. 17.8).

The immune system is often a factor in hormone resistance. In such cases, an autoimmune mechanism produces an antibody against hormone receptors that is similar to the normal hormone. Its shape allows the antibody to fit the receptor, but not closely enough to elicit the usual cell response. The result is reduced target tissue activity. Furthermore, since the antibody cannot be rapidly degraded by the target tissue's inactivation systems, it remains bound to the receptor for a longer period, blocking normal hormone access to the receptor and further reducing secretion.

Another resistance mechanism is based on what might be considered a fatigue factor. If faced with chronically high hormone levels, target tissues may respond by reducing their receptor numbers. The result is a lowered level of tissue activity.

Endocrine Hyperfunction

In hyperfunction states, exaggerated target tissue responses are present. The usual cause is hormone hypersecretion.

Hypersecretion

The second major pattern of endocrine dysfunction is hypersecretion, in which circulating hormone is present at levels that are inappropriately high. Excessive hormone secretion may arise when an endocrine gland is exposed to unusually high levels of its tropic hormone. Its response is an increased synthesis and release of hormone. In such cases, the gland may increase in size by hypertrophy or hyperplasia. Defective feedback control may be a factor in endocrine hypersecretion, but details of such mechanisms are scarce because of the difficulties of studying the disease in nonhuman systems.

Tumors of endocrine glands may produce hyperfunction states if the neoplastic tissue retains the ability to secrete functional hormone. Even if the tumor's hormone is only partially functional, its excessive secretion can produce exaggerated target tissue responses. The production of hormones or hormonelike substances by nonendocrine tu-

✓ *Checkpoint 17.1*

Although there is enormous complexity in the subtleties of endocrine dysfunction, don't overlook the basics. In dealing with excessive or inadequate target tissue responses, look to the source of the hormone that controls the tissue. The gland is either turning out too much hormone or is unable to secrete enough. If the gland is OK, the problem may lie in another gland that controls it. In hypofunction cases, if the gland and its controlling inputs are OK, target tissue resistance may be the problem.

mors was described in chapter 6. Such cases can confuse diagnosis. For example, when a small and difficult-to-locate tumor secretes excessive functional hormone, diagnosis may focus on the endocrine system while the unrecognized tumor continues to grow.

Because most hormones produce effects by speeding or retarding widespread metabolic reactions, it is not surprising that the signs and symptoms of endocrine disease often present a puzzling picture of altered function simultaneously involving many of the body's organ systems. The remainder of this chapter deals with the major endocrine glands and their most common disorders. The testis and ovary will be considered in chapter 20, in the context of reproductive disorders.

THE THYROID GLAND

The thyroid is involved in some of the most commonly encountered endocrine diseases. The associated functional disruptions may be quite extensive because of the widespread effects of the thyroid hormones. Before considering thyroid abnormalities, let us review the gland's normal structure and function.

Normal Anatomy and Physiology

The thyroid gland is positioned in the region of the throat. It consists of two lateral masses on either side of the trachea, joined by a connecting **isthmus** that crosses the midline, just inferior to the larynx (fig. 17.9).

The endocrine cells of the thyroid gland are cuboidal cells arranged in a single layer to form the wall of a hollow sphere. These are the **thyroid follicles,** which make up thyroid tissue. Secretion of thyroid hormones involves synthesis by the follicle cells, storage within the follicle, and then release into the blood (fig. 17.9b).

The two thyroid hormones are unique among the body's chemical regulators in that they contain iodine. Derived from dietary sources, especially seafoods, the iodide ion is taken up from the blood by the thyroid's follicle cells after its absorption from the intestine. This is an active

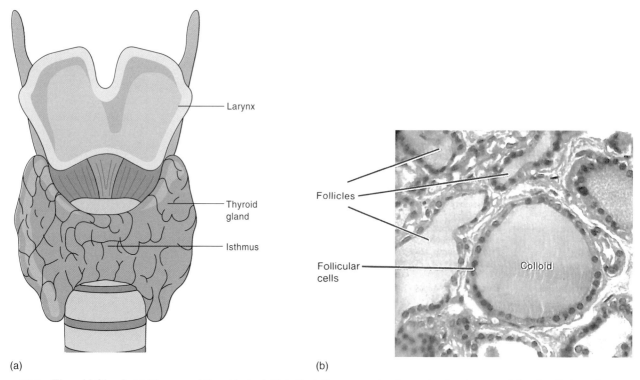

(a)   (b)

Figure 17.9   **Thyroid Gland.** (*a*) The normal thyroid gland. Note the isthmus crossing the center line to connect the gland's lateral masses. (*b*) Thyroid histology, showing characteristic follicles and hormone-containing colloid.

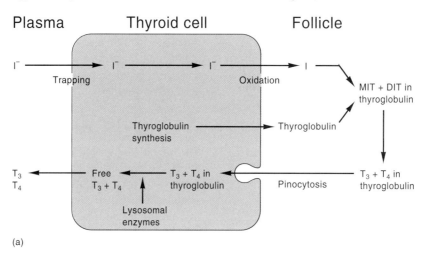

(a)

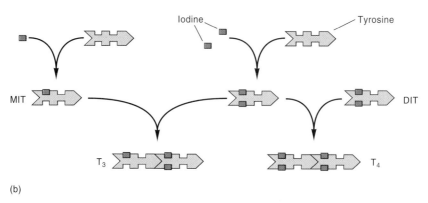

(b)

Figure 17.10   **Thyroid Hormone Synthesis and Secretion.** (*a*) Iodide trapping, thyroglobulin formation, and T_3T_4 secretion by the thyroid gland. (*b*) In the colloid within the follicle, iodine combines with the tyrosine of thyroglobulin to form MIT and DIT. These then combine to form T_3 and T_4.

transport process that concentrates iodide within the follicular cells. The process is called **iodide trapping.** Normally, the thyroid achieves an iodide concentration up to 50 times greater than that of plasma. In hyperactive states, the cellular concentration of iodide produced by iodide trapping may exceed 300 times the plasma levels. Because of iodide trapping, over half the total body's iodide is found in the thyroid (fig. 17.10*a*).

Once inside the cell, iodide is oxidized to iodine and released into the fluid of the follicle, which is called **colloid.** A major constituent of colloid is the protein **thyroglobulin.** It contains the amino acid tyrosine, with which iodide combines to form both monoiodotyrosine (MIT) and diiodotyrosine (DIT). These are then converted to the two active thyroid hormones, **triiodothyronine** (T_3) and **thyroxine** (T_4) (fig. 17.10*b*). The hormones remain a part of the thyroglobulin structure and are stored in the follicle in this form until needed for secretion. There is sufficient T_3 and T_4 stored in the thyroid's follicles to provide normal secretion for about three months, should all synthesis stop.

Prior to secretion, small quantities of colloid are taken back into the follicle cells by pinocytosis. There, the pinocytotic vesicles merge with lysosomes whose enzymes split T_3 and T_4 from thyroglobulin. Once freed, the hormones diffuse into the plasma for distribution throughout the body. In the blood, most T_3 and T_4 is transported bound to alpha globulins and albumin. The principal protein involved is known as **thyroxine-binding globulin** (TBG). This binding means that the thyroid hormones responsible for stimulating target tissues are the very small, unbound quantities that circulate in the plasma.

Control of Thyroid Secretion The control of thyroid secretion depends on the anterior pituitary and hypothalamus. **Thyroid-stimulating hormone** (TSH), also known as **thyrotropin,** is the immediate stimulus to thyroid secretion. It is secreted by the anterior pituitary gland and binds to follicle cells, triggering their release of stored hormones. It also increases both iodine uptake and hormone synthesis. TSH secretion is in turn dependent on **thyrotropin-releasing hormone** (TRH), which is produced in the hypothalamus. TRH reaches the pituitary directly via the portal circulation, which joins it to the hypothalamus. High levels of the thyroid hormones cause an inhibition of TRH and thyrotropin and therefore of T_3 and T_4 secretion. They also antagonize TRH by in some way decreasing TRH receptor numbers on TSH-secreting cells in the anterior pituitary. Very high plasma iodide concentrations (on the order of about 100 times normal) also suppress thyroid function.

Prolonged exposure to cold increases thyroid secretion, which in turn stimulates metabolism and generates body heat. Emotional states can affect thyroid secretion as well, with varying conditions stimulating or suppressing the gland's activity. These thyroid-controlling inputs are summarized in figure 17.11.

Thyroid Hormone Effects In systemic tissues, especially the liver and kidney, target cells convert most T_4 to T_3. T_3 binds much more readily than T_4 to nuclear hormone re-

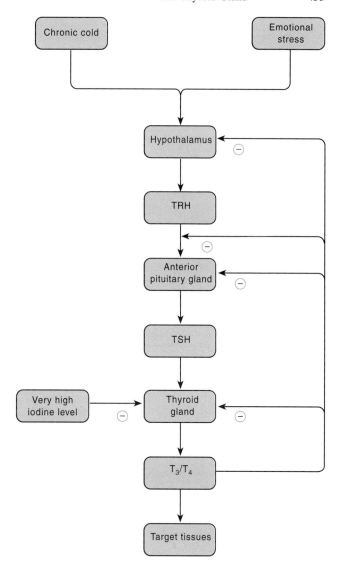

Figure 17.11   **Thyroid Secretion Control.** Normal controlling inputs and other factors that regulate thyroid secretion. T_3 and T_4 levels in the blood inhibit thyroid secretion and TRH and TSH release, as well as antagonizing the effects of TRH on the pituitary.

ceptors in target cells. About 90% of thyroid hormone effects are the result of T_3 binding, with the remaining 10% due to T_4. After binding, target tissue enzymes degrade T_3/T_4, removing its iodine, which is then recirculated. Most is taken up by the thyroid gland for reuse, and a small amount is excreted in the urine. Other degradation products are cleared in the urine and bile.

Thyroid hormones have a very wide range of target tissues—virtually all cells of the body. Their major effect is metabolic, generally promoting protein, carbohydrate, and lipid utilization. Aerobic energy metabolism is also affected, with changes in T_3/T_4 levels reducing it by half or increasing it to as much as twice the normal rate. Normal growth and development are also regulated by T_3/T_4. The nervous system is particularly dependent, so that infants exposed to deficiencies of the hormones in the first six months of life suffer irreversible mental retardation. Because of their widespread metabolic effects, thyroid

Table 17.1	Principal Effects of the Thyroid Hormones

Primary Effects

    Aerobic energy metabolism
    Glucose metabolism
    Protein metabolism
    Lipid metabolism
    Ion transport

Secondary Effects

    Growth/development
    Cardiac output
    Ventilation
    CNS activity
    Thermoregulation
    Muscle function
    GI activity
    Reproductive functions

hormones are important to many organ system functions. The most significant are listed in table 17.1.

Thyroid Pathophysiology

Broadly speaking, thyroid disorders produce excessive levels of T_3/T_4 and exaggerated target tissue effects, or depressed levels and reduced activity. The gland itself may be the source of the malfunction, or some defects in the hypothalamus-anterior pituitary control system may be at fault. Whatever the underlying etiology, the thyroid gland is a good example of endocrine dysfunction because the signs and symptoms of altered secretion are closely related to the effects of T_3/T_4 on target tissues.

Thyroid Hypofunction

The hypothyroid state is one in which thyroid hormone secretion is inadequate to maintain normal levels of target tissue stimulation. The result is a generalized fall in the metabolic rate. Less metabolic heat is generated, body temperature drops, and the skin cools as body heat retention reflexes are activated. The decline in metabolism also produces weaker, more sluggish muscular contractions throughout the body. In the gastrointestinal tract, the result is a slowing of motility, which can produce constipation, while in the myocardium, contractility is reduced and, hence, cardiac output may decline. In the hypothyroid state, an increase of body weight is typical because dietary habits continue to supply the usual number of calories to a metabolism that consumes fewer of them. The excess input is stored as fat. The lack of T_3 and T_4 also causes a rise in the blood cholesterol level, which, if maintained for prolonged periods, may contribute to the development of atherosclero-

sis. Hypothyroidism may also produce a decreased sex drive in both sexes and cause irregularities in the pattern and intensity of the menstrual flow.

Lack of thyroid hormone stimulation to the CNS produces a depression of overall mental functioning. Instead of responses that are quick and alert, in the hypothyroid state mental processes are slower and dulled. An affected individual also requires a great deal of sleep. CNS suppression also contributes to a decline in the heart rate and, hence, the cardiac output, although some of this effect follows the lowering of tissue demands for oxygen and waste removal by a depressed metabolism. A moderate decline in T_3/T_4 secretion is linked to relatively mild signs and symptoms. More pronounced hormone deficiency produces myxedema.

Myxedema When, in the adult, secretion of thyroid hormones is chronically reduced, the resulting condition is called **myxedema.** It is so named because of a characteristic edematous swelling around the eyes and lips and at the fingers. A metabolic derangement, assumed to be the result of thyroid hormone lack, causes **glycoprotein** to be deposited in the dermis. (Glycoprotein is protein with some carbohydrate incorporated into its structure.) The term *myxedema* refers to the presence of this glycoprotein, which binds water to form a gel in the dermis and thus produces the facial puffiness associated with severe and prolonged hypothyroid states. Because the water is chemically bound, it cannot move freely through the tissues, so no pitting edema is usually seen, nor does the tissue fluid settle to dependent regions of the body as in congestive heart failure. Edema of the fingers causes them to thicken, while vocal cord edema causes a lowering of the voice.

In myxedema, the usual signs and symptoms of hypothyroidism are exaggerated, with a greater decline in overall metabolism producing increased physical weakness. At the same time, mental functions become increasingly slow and confused. Because heat retention compensations are needed at even normal temperatures, the ability to adjust to cold environmental temperature is compromised in myxedema. In severe, untreated myxedema, the sufferer may lapse into a coma characterized by low body temperature. The elderly are particularly at risk of **myxedema coma,** which can be fatal. Table 17.2 lists the predominant clinical effects of adult hypothyroidism.

Cretinism When thyroid hypofunction occurs in the newborn, normal growth and tissue differentiation are impaired. If the condition is untreated, physical and mental retardation result. The affected individual is called a **cretin,** and the condition characterized by the abnormality is known as **cretinism.** Physically, a cretin is short because of greatly reduced growth. Somatic proportions are altered because skeletal development is retarded more than that of soft tissues (fig. 17.12). A stocky, thick body with infantile proportions is the result.

Obesity is typical, but some of the appearance of obesity is due to the presence of near-normal abdominal vis-

Table 17.2	Clinical Effects of Adult Hypothyroidism

Decreased Energy Production

Weakness
Fatigue
Cold intolerance
Lassitude
Weight gain
Decreased ventilation (decreased oxygen requirement)
Constipation
Bradycardia (slow heart rate)
Hypotension

Decreased Protein Synthesis

Anemia
Dry sparse hair
Dry scaly skin

Decreased CNS Activity

Memory loss
Drowsiness
Apathy

Mucoprotein Synthesis

Water retention
Nonpitting edema (myxedema)
Edema of vocal cords—husky voice

Decreased Liver Function

Elevated plasma lipids ⎫
Elevated plasma cholesterol ⎬ Atherosclerosis
Decreased Vitamin A Synthesis ⎭

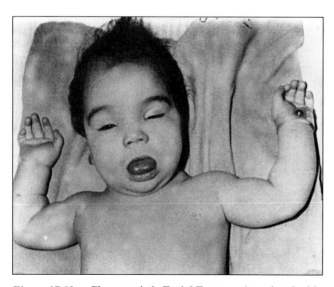

Figure 17.12 **Characteristic Facial Features Associated with Cretinism.**

Table 17.3	Clinical Effects of Juvenile Hypothyroidism

Myxedema
Mental retardation
Sexual immaturity
Delayed skeletal maturation
Short stature
Increased subcutaneous tissue
Protrusion of a thickened tongue
Dry, scaly skin
Slow growth and weight gain
Goiter

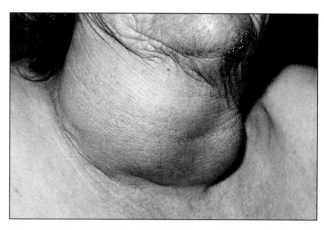

Figure 17.13 **The Goiter in This Woman's Throat Is Clearly Visible.**

cera in a smaller than normal body frame. Thickening of the tongue, which is also symptomatic of cretinism, may interfere with swallowing and presents the risk of choking, especially in infants. Tooth and hair development is faulty as well, and the cretin's skin has a characteristic coarseness and scaliness. A yellow tinge to the skin may be present from accumulating carotene pigments, which are normally metabolized under the influence of thyroid hormones. Sexual development is also retarded.

The CNS requirement for thyroid hormones is unsatisfied in cretinism. Brain development suffers and mental retardation is the result. Emotional derangements often accompany defective mental functions (table 17.3). In cretinism, maternal hormones can satisfy the newborn's earliest demands, but within a few weeks slowed mental response and lethargic behavior become noticeable.

Goiter Goiter is the condition of thyroid gland enlargement. Swelling may be minimal and difficult to recognize, or the gland may enlarge to over ten times its normal 30-g size (fig. 17.13). Goiter is typical of thyroid hyposecretion states since, as thyroid hormone levels fall, the inhibition of TSH is removed and its secretion is increased. In response to continued exposure to high TSH levels, follicular hyperplasia

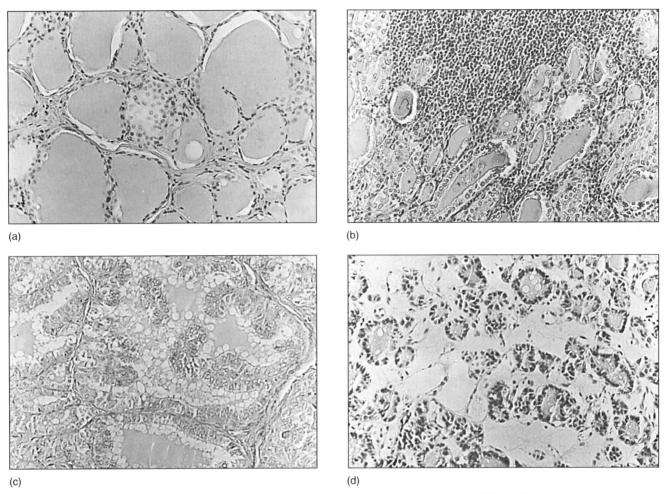

Figure 17.14   **Thyroid Follicles.** (*a*) Note the uniform colloid texture within each of these normal follicles. (*b*) In Hashimoto's thyroiditis, colloid deficiency and inflammatory cell infiltration are apparent. (*c*) Graves' disease. Note the hyperplasia of the follicle's epithelium, which produces the irregular folding. (*d*) Benign follicular adenoma.

develops, with follicle cells secreting abundant additional thyroglobulin. The result is a generalized enlargement of the thyroid called **diffuse colloid goiter.** The colloid reference is to the presence of the excess thyroglobulin.

Goiter may also be caused by a deficiency of dietary iodine. In such cases, although the gland is unable to maintain its normal output of hormone, thyroid secretion is usually sufficient to avoid or at least minimize symptoms. Iodine deficiency goiter has become uncommon since the practice of adding potassium iodide (KI) to table salt has been widely adopted.

Some goiter is characterized by the presence of irregular nodules within the thyroid tissue. This condition is called **multinodular goiter.** The nodules form when regions of follicular atrophy and fibrosis are present among normal or hyperplastic follicles. Nodular goiter has greater incidence in females past the age of 30. In some cases, a multinodular goiter will hypersecrete. This phenomenon complicates diagnosis because it suggests a thyroid tumor. In such cases, the condition is called **toxic goiter.** The threat imposed by the more common hyposecreting goiter, or **nontoxic goiter,** is secondary to its enlargement: compression of adjacent throat structures, with the esophagus, jugular veins, and larynx being at greatest risk.

Etiology of Thyroid Hypofunction   Much adult thyroid hyposecretion is the result of surgical resection or radiation therapy for thyroid hypersecretion states, usually Graves' disease (to be discussed later). Another hypothyroid state, cretinism, is rare in North America, with most cases due to a rare congenital defect that blocks thyroid hormone synthesis. Previously, higher incidence was linked to dietary iodine deficiency, but this has since been eliminated by supplementing the diet with sodium iodide. More cretinism is seen in areas of the world where there is no iodine supplementation to the diet. These are usually third-world countries at some distance from the ocean, the major natural source of iodine.

With these exceptions, hypothyroid states develop secondary to thyroid trauma and thyroiditis. This is most clearly seen in penetrating wounds of the neck that produce acute inflammation. However, bacterial or viral infections, especially in the mouth and throat regions, may produce subacute or chronic changes that are minor or even pass unnoticed. The most common thyroid hyposecretion state is a chronic granulomatous disease called **Hashimoto's thyroiditis** (fig. 17.14*b*). In this condition, fibrosis and infiltration of thyroid tissue by inflammatory cells occur at the expense of functional gland tissue. Hyposecretion is the

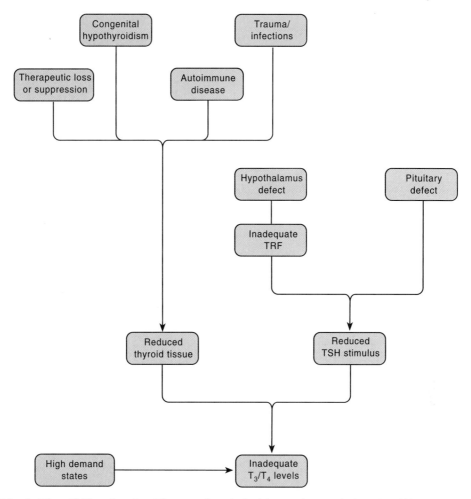

Figure 17.15   **Etiolgy in Thyroid Hypofunction.** These are the principal factors that may induce thyroid hyposecretion. Note that in high-demand states, the deficiency of hormone is relative and usually transient.

result, with glandular hyperplasia and goiter formation the result of falling thyroid hormone levels that stimulate TSH release. Even though hyperplasia occurs, tissue damage dominates to yield a net loss of functioning follicles.

Hashimoto's thyroiditis is an autoimmune disorder that has a an ill-defined genetic component indicated by its higher incidence in certain families. Abnormalities of T-cell activity are prominent in its pathogenesis, but antibody also contributes to the problem. The condition is usually mild, with symptoms of myxedema occurring if prolonged. In severe cases, pericardial and pleural effusion and myocardial dilatation may complicate the course of the disease.

In about 5% of hypothyroidism, disturbances of the hypothalamus or anterior pituitary produce insufficient stimulus to the thyroid, and hyposecretion follows. Some therapeutic drugs have thyroid-blocking side effects and may produce symptoms of hyposecretion. Examples are lithium preparations, phenylbutazone, and para-aminosalicylic acid.

Transient conditions of relative thyroid hyposecretion also occur. Periods such as pregnancy and puberty generate a high demand for thyroid hormones because of the rapid growth and development rates prevalent in those conditions. At such times, normal hormone levels are initially inadequate, and a condition of relative hyposecretion exists.

Mild, temporary thyroid hyperplasia usually provides the needed additional hormone to correct the deficiency. The etiological factors in hypothyroidism are summarized in figure 17.15.

Therapy in Thyroid Hypofunction Therapy for thyroid deficiency is straightforward. It is a matter of providing thyroid hormone, which is readily available in oral preparations. Once the appropriate dose level has been determined, a reversal of symptoms usually follows. Thyroid hormone preparations offer the further benefits of being inexpensive and having no significant toxic or other side effects. Many people have successfully maintained thyroid hormone therapy for decades without side effects. In the case of congenital thyroid hormone deficiencies arising at birth, therapy must be started promptly to avoid irreversible physical and mental retardation.

Thyroid Hyperfunction

When thyroid hormones are present to excess, exaggerated target tissue responses result. This condition is called **thyrotoxicosis,** or simply **hyperthyroidism.** With hypersecretion, several characteristic signs and symptoms develop. One is an increase in metabolic heat production. In

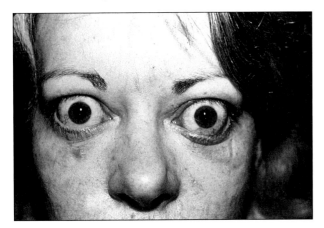

Figure 17.16   **Exophthalmos.** Protrusion of the eyes in hyperthyroidism.

Table 17.4	Clinical Effects Seen in Hyperthyroidism

Increased Metabolic Rate

Muscle wasting
Increased activity
Heat intolerance—sweating and skin flushing
Weight loss
Insomnia
Hyperventilation
Diarrhea, nausea, and vomiting
Tachycardia and congestive heart failure
Hypertension

Increased CNS Activity

Rapid speech
Emotional instability
Nervousness and irritability
Tremor of the limbs

Other Findings

Exophthalmos (protrusion of the eyeball)
Toxic goiter (enlargement of the thyroid gland)

response, heat loss reflexes produce a flushed skin and a high rate of perspiration. Many individuals suffering hyperthyroidism are almost constantly perspiring. Excessive production of metabolic heat also limits the ability to tolerate high environmental temperature, because heat loss compensations are already activated.

Another characteristic of the hyperthyroid state is nervous excitability. The affected person is highly active physically and mentally. In contrast to the victim of hyposecretion, who is lethargic, in hypersecretion states **insomnia** (the inability to sleep) is the problem. Such individuals may be highly irritable, emotionally unstable, and subject to attacks of anxiety and paranoia. Another characteristic neurological sign is a slow tremor of the hand.

Cardiovascular effects are also seen in thyrotoxicosis. The heart rate is increased, in response both to the increased metabolic demands for oxygen supply and waste removal and to the direct cardiac stimulation effects of thyroid hormones. Cardiac dysrhythmias may also be present, especially in the elderly. Blood hydrostatic pressure remains at near-normal values as increased cardiac output is countered by the systemic vasodilation needed to meet high tissue demands for blood flow.

Excessive energy demands produce metabolic shifts in hyperthyroid states. Plasma lipid levels fall as fat in the adipose tissue stores is consumed, and substantial weight loss often follows even though appetite and food intake increase. Thyroid hormone excess also stimulates breakdown of muscle protein for use as an energy source. This protein loss can affect muscle contractility in both skeletal muscle and the myocardium. The greatest threat in such cases is that of heart failure, because the myocardium is weakened at the same time that the demand for cardiac output is high. However, failure of the myocardium is a risk only when thyrotoxicosis is severe.

A distinctive sign in hyperthyroidism is **exophthalmos** (fig. 17.16). In this condition, the eyes protrude from their orbits. This seems largely due to cellular infiltration and edema of orbital tissues that thrust the eyes forward. If extreme, exophthalmos can prevent the eyelids from closing completely, increasing the risk of corneal damage.

Other typical signs and symptoms of thyrotoxicosis are hyperventilation, as a means of clearing the additional carbon dioxide produced by the elevated metabolic rate, and hyperactivity in the GI tract, producing attacks of diarrhea. The generally increased metabolic rate may produce vitamin deficiencies when demand outstrips dietary supplies. In males, impotence may develop, whereas in females, menstruation may decrease or stop entirely **(amenorrhea).** These effects are summarized in table 17.4.

Etiology of Thyroid Hypersecretion The most common thyroid hypersecretion syndrome, usually affecting young females, is called **Graves' disease.** In this condition, the thyroid gland exhibits a diffuse hyperplasia, with its size increasing to two to three times normal (see fig. 17.14*c*). The result is a toxic goiter condition in spite of normal or very low TSH levels. Onset of symptoms is slow and progression is gradual. Weight loss, hyperactivity, and the other components of the thyrotoxicosis syndrome are usually seen, with exophthalmos typically present to varying degrees.

An autoimmune etiology is involved in Graves' disease. One might reasonably expect autoimmune mechanisms to damage tissue and produce a hypothyroid state; yet, this condition involves thyroid hypersecretion. What is the explanation for this seeming contradiction? The answer is that the autoimmune response is not directed against the thyroid cells or thyroglobulin. Instead, antibodies against the TSH receptor are present. They are known as **thyroid-**

Focus on Terminology Variations in Graves' Disease

The reason why autoimmune response develops in Graves' disease is unknown. It has been suggested that a genetic defect is involved or possibly an unusual release of thyroid antigens that act as a stimulus to the system.

As with many diseases, as more information accumulates, new terminology emerges. In Graves' disease, use of the acronym TSAb is relatively new. Earlier, the term **long-acting thyroid stimulator** (LATS) was used, and it is still frequently encountered. In some cases, the acronym TSAb will be used, as it is in our description of the mechanism underlying Graves' disease. You may also find the acronym **TRAb** employed in this context. It refers to **TSH receptor antibody,** which appears to be an antibody subtype specific for the TSH receptor, which can be distinguished from another TSAb that promotes growth and secretion, but apparently not via the TSH receptor. Another variant that is also in use is **TSI,** referring to **thyroid-stimulating immunoglobulins.** More precision in terminology will emerge as our understanding is increased, but until then you can expect to find all of these terms used in clinical and laboratory settings.

---

stimulating antibodies (TSAb), and since they closely resemble TSH, they can bind to TSH receptors and stimulate thyroid secretion. They are also sufficiently different from TSH to resist enzymic degradation, and therefore remain active ten times as long as TSH. As well, the high plasma levels of thyroid hormones suppress TSH secretion (see fig. 17.11), reducing competition for TSH receptors and allowing TSAb to dominate.

A pattern of eye pathology specific to Graves' disease contributes to its characteristic exophthalmos. The eye is thrust forward because of an increase in the volume of the orbit's contents. Deposition of water-binding molecules, antibody, and infiltrating cells are all thought to play a part in enlarging the eye and its surrounding tissues.

Other, less commonly encountered hyperthyroid conditions are known that do not involve autoimmunity. One condition is toxic goiter, in which an initially undersecreting goiter develops regions of tissue that hypersecrete and do not respond to lowered TSH levels. For this reason, they are said to be secreting autonomously. The hypersecreting foci may enlarge to form one or more large nodules in the thyroid gland. Hemorrhage and fibrosis are also present and contribute to the nodularity. If hypersecreting, this condition is described as **toxic multinodular goiter.** Another, rare hyperthyroid condition is the result of idiopathic TSH hypersecretion, which leads to thyroid enlargement and toxic goiter. The excess TSH secretion may be due to an exaggerated anterior pituitary activity (of unknown origin) or because of hypersecretion of TRH by the hypothalamus.

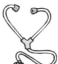

Focus on Lowering Surgical Risk in Thyrotoxicosis

Prior to thyroid surgery to deal with thyrotoxicosis, a regimen of iodide (I^-) therapy is instituted for a period of about ten days. The high concentration used has the effect of suppressing gland function (see fig. 17.11). The gland atrophies in response, forming a smaller mass with a reduced blood supply. A much lower surgical complication rate is the result.

Incorrect dosage of thyroid hormones in hypothyroid therapy can also produce the hyperthyroid state.

A major threat in thyrotoxicosis is **thyroid storm,** or **thyroid crisis,** in which high levels of thyroid hormones exacerbate the symptoms of a preexisting hyperthyroid state. Rather than a burst of secretion, a large release of hormone from TBG is thought to be responsible. The precise trigger for this release is unknown, but it is often associated with the postoperative state and systemic infections.

Thyroid crisis involves a dramatic further increase in metabolism, which abruptly drives up body temperature, producing **hyperpyrexia.** This can have adverse CNS effects, including delirium and convulsions. Loss of fluid from extreme perspiration and from the diarrhea and vomiting caused by pronounced GI hyperactivity can combine to produce electrolyte imbalance and hypovolemia. Of course, all of these critical events are superimposed on the problems associated with the original infection, trauma or postoperative condition. High thyroid hormone levels can also induce cardiac arrhythmias, which, with hypovolemia, can contribute to cardiovascular shock and death.

Therapy in Thyroid Hypersecretion Unfortunately, most therapy to counter hyperthyroidism cannot eliminate its primary cause. Instead, inactivation or removal of some thyroid tissue is sought. Although several drugs are known to suppress T_3 and T_4 synthesis, such as methimazole and propylthiouracil, the problems and cost of a lifetime of drug therapy side effects seem an unwarranted burden on the patient. Destruction of the thyroid's hypersecreting tissue is usually achieved by the use of ionizing radiation. Dose determination is difficult, however, and if excessive, can so depress secretion that myxedema results. Surgical removal of some hyperactive tissue is effective. Although it may also lead to a hyposecretion state as time passes, the problem is easily corrected because thyroid extract therapy is inexpensive and problem-free.

Tumors of the Thyroid Gland Most tumors of the thyroid are benign adenomas that derive from thyroid follicle cells (see fig. 17.14). The tumors are typically unable to secrete functional hormone, but since they grow only gradually and normal tissue is able to maintain adequate hormone output, hypothyroid states are usually avoided. Some thyroid tumors, however, have well-developed follicles. These retain the ability to secrete functional hormone and can produce thyrotoxicosis. Malignancies are rare and have the highest incidence in females past the age of 40. Invasion to adjacent throat structures and lymphatic metastases are typical. Although an unusual primary carcinoma site, the thyroid gland is often the site of secondary growth from breast and lung metastases.

As with most tumors, identifying a specific etiology is difficult. However, early exposure of the thyroid to irradiation, as in nonthyroid tumor therapy, and prolonged exposure to high levels of TSH are known to be associated with increased malignant tumor incidence.

PANCREATIC ISLET CELLS

Blood glucose is a variable that requires close regulation because it is the dominant fuel of cellular energy metabolism. The brain, with its numerous functions critical to survival, and a few other tissues, are absolutely dependent on glucose as an energy source. Most other tissues have alternative energy metabolism pathways that they can use when glucose is in short supply. However, in lacking this ability, the brain requires close regulation of the blood's glucose to prevent its fall below the critical value needed for brain function. Also, blood glucose regulation must prevent glucose excess, which increases extracellular fluid osmolality, causing water to be drawn from cells by osmosis. The resulting increase in ECF volume can lead to diuresis and dehydration.

Normal Histology and Physiology

The cells of the **islets of Langerhans** are the primary regulators of blood glucose. The islets are microscopic masses of endocrine tissue scattered among the exocrine cells of the pancreas. Each islet contains three principal cell types. One is the **alpha cell,** which secretes the hormone **glucagon.** These cells make up about 25% of the islet's total. The most common cell type is the **beta cell,** which is the source of the hormone **insulin.** This cell type makes up about 70% of islet cell numbers. The remaining 5% of islet cells are **delta cells,** which secrete the hormone **somatostatin** (fig. 17.17). This hormone suppresses secretion of insulin and glucagon. Together, glucagon, insulin, and somatostatin closely regulate blood glucose. A fourth hormone, **pancreatic polypeptide,** is also secreted by the islets. Although its regulatory functions are not well understood, its excessive secretion by islet cell tumors makes it a useful diagnostic indicator.

Functions of Insulin and Glucagon

Insulin is a polypeptide that is increasingly secreted into the blood when glucose is available for cell use. The beta cells are sensitive to glucose level and alter their secretion in direct response to its presence. They may also respond to hor-

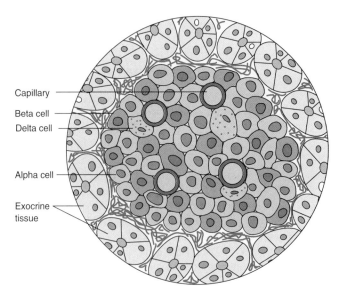

Figure 17.17 **Pancreas Histology.** Microscopic view of a typical islet of Langerhans and surrounding exocrine tissue.

mones that are secreted by the intestine when glucose is digested. This response allows some initial insulin secretion in anticipation of glucose absorption. Beta cells increase secretion of insulin in response to elevated blood glucose levels, and glucagon is secreted by alpha cells when blood glucose levels are depressed. The effects of glucagon are opposite to those of insulin. This functional antagonism allows for closer control of this important plasma variable. In the following discussion of insulin's functions, keep in mind that for each one, the effect of glucagon is usually its opposite.

Glucose is the primary energy source in cell metabolism. Following its absorption from the intestine, the blood's glucose level rises. The result is an increase in insulin secretion, which stimulates cell uptake, utilization, and storage of glucose. At the same time, insulin suppresses the use of fat as an energy source. When glucose levels fall, reduced insulin secretion favors the release of glucose from storage and the use of lipid-based energy sources.

One of the major effects of insulin is on cellular glucose uptake. Because it has low solubility in cell membrane lipid, glucose uptake depends on membrane glucose carriers. This system operates in the tissues that make up two-thirds of the body's weight: skeletal and cardiac muscle, adipose tissue, and connective tissue fibroblasts. The major exceptions are brain, liver, and red blood cells, whose glucose uptake is not insulin-dependent. The rate of carrier activity is insulin-dependent and normally accounts for 75% of a cell's glucose uptake.

In the liver, insulin has an important effect on **glycogenesis.** When ample glucose is available, higher insulin levels promote the formation of glycogen as a means of storing glucose for later use. In this process, numerous glucose units are polymerized to form the glycogen macromolecule.

Checkpoint 17.2

If you recall the mechanism underlying the effect of ADH on water movement through nephron tubule cells, it's interesting to note that insulin's effect on glucose uptake takes the same approach. That is, insulin affects the number of glucose carrier proteins in the cell membrane. There is a continuing cycle of glucose carrier movement from the cytoplasm to the cell surface and back to cytoplasm. Insulin modifies this cycle. More insulin increases this movement, with more carriers at the surface meaning more glucose uptake. When insulin levels fall, fewer carriers are present at the surface and glucose entry declines.

Table 17.5   The Antagonistic Metabolic Effects of Insulin and Glucagon

Cellular Activity	Insulin	Glucagon
Glycogenesis	↑	↓
Glycogenolysis	↓	↑
Gluconeogenesis	↓	↑
Ketogenesis	↓	↑
Lipolysis	↓	↑
Lipogenesis	↑	↓

At the same time, insulin activates the hepatic synthesis of free fatty acids (FFAs) from glucose. These are then combined with protein and enter the blood, which carries them to adipose tissue for storage. Insulin also inhibits the release of FFAs from adipose tissue. These are normally metabolized in the liver, but because the liver has sufficient glucose to make its own FFAs, those in adipose tissue are not required.

When glucose levels fall, insulin secretion declines, causing a reversal of the effects just described. That is, cell uptake and utilization of glucose in muscle and adipose tissue are reduced. The result is a tendency to maintain the plasma glucose level, making more available to the brain and other tissues that depend on it. In the liver, glycogen synthesis is suppressed, and the low level of insulin activates two other metabolic pathways. One is **glycogenolysis,** in which glucose is produced from the breakdown of glycogen. The other is **gluconeogenesis,** in which new glucose is synthesized. Both of these reaction pathways provide glucose to maintain an adequate plasma level. Also in the liver, lowered insulin levels activate lipolytic metabolism. In **lipolysis,** FFAs are converted to keto acids. These reach the systemic tissues, where they may be utilized as an energy source.

Glucose scarcity, with the drop in insulin that follows, stimulates the secretion of glucagon and other hormones. Their combined metabolic effects generally compensate for the lack of glucose. The hormones involved are glucagon from the islet alpha cells, growth hormone from the anterior pituitary, epinephrine from the adrenal medulla, and glucocorticoids from the adrenal cortex. Together, these stimulate protein breakdown to provide molecules needed for gluconeogenesis. They also increase the amount of lipid available for energy metabolism, indirectly producing an elevated plasma lipid level. The focus here is on the islet hormones, whose antagonistic effects are summarized in table 17.5.

Diabetes Mellitus

Diabetes mellitus (DM) is a major endocrine disorder involving the islet cell hormones. It is, in fact, the single most common endocrine disorder. Estimates of the incidence of DM range from 1% to 2% of the North American population. Of this number, many cases are undiagnosed and receive no treatment until the disease is well advanced. Although DM is recognized to have a genetic component, its precise pattern of transmission is not known.

DM is a metabolic disorder with wide-ranging and serious effects, many of which are life-threatening. It may occur in either of two forms, which differ in pathogenesis but produce essentially similar metabolic derangements. The more severe of the two forms, which typically affects the young, is the less common. It develops following failure of the beta cells and requires insulin therapy. This type of DM has been variously described as **juvenile onset DM, type I DM,** or, because insulin therapy is always required, **insulin-dependent DM** (IDDM). The last term is probably the best, because it makes reference to an unambiguous characteristic of the disease. The term *type I DM* is arbitrary and lacks descriptive value. The term *juvenile onset DM* is somewhat misleading, because some IDDM occurs as late as age 25. Of the two types of diabetes mellitus, IDDM makes up about 10% of the total.

The second type of DM has a slow, gradual development of symptoms, so that often years pass without the victim being aware of any change. Insulin therapy is required much less often in this type, so the term **non-insulin-dependent DM** (NIDDM) is descriptive. It is also called **type II DM,** or **maturity onset DM,** because most cases are diagnosed past the age of 40. In NIDDM, beta cells slowly lose their capacity to produce insulin, but target tissues also show reduced sensitivity to it.

Etiology of IDDM

The essential component of IDDM's etiology is autoimmune destruction of beta cells in the islets of Langerhans. As is so often the case in autoimmune disease, the precise reason why normal self-antigens in a particular tissue become altered and vulnerable to immune attack is unclear.

Familial patterns of IDDM incidence suggest a genetic predisposition to an immune recognition defect, but some environmental agent is thought to be required to take advantage of it. Several lines of evidence indicate that a beta cell viral infection is a factor. There is also some evidence that certain environmental chemicals or therapeutic drugs may contribute to the alteration of beta cell antigens. However the genetic and environmental factors interact, the result is that altered beta cell antigens are recognized by the immune system as nonself. A cell-mediated immune attack follows, with signs and symptoms emerging when most beta cells are destroyed and insulin levels fall (fig. 17.18). This may occur over a period of years without symptoms because of the beta cells' reserve secretion capacity.

Pathogenesis of IDDM

The chief signs and symptoms in IDDM can be directly traced to lack of insulin secretion. The immediate result is an increase in blood glucose **(hyperglycemia),** because without insulin, cellular uptake and utilization of glucose is limited. In the fasting state, blood glucose varies in the range of 70–100 mg/dl. In IDDM, this value is increased to exceed 180 mg/dl, and at extremes may reach 1,200 mg/dl. One effect of hyperglycemia is the urinary loss of glucose **(glucosuria).** When glucose levels are elevated, filtration at the glomerulus produces a filtrate with an abnormally high glucose content. Such high levels exceed the capacity of the tubule cells to reabsorb glucose, so that any glucose in filtrate that exceeds the maximum reabsorption limit is lost in the urine. Normally, only minute amounts of glucose reach the urine. Glucosuria, therefore, is a principal diagnostic indicator of IDDM.

The loss of glucose in the urine has further consequences. High levels of glucose in nephron filtrate increase the nephron tubules' osmotic hold on water, preventing its normal reabsorption and causing an **osmotic diuresis.** Polyuria and a compensating increase in thirst and water intake (polydipsia) are typical of untreated IDDM.

In IDDM, low insulin secretion stimulates hepatic glycogenolysis and gluconeogenesis, both of which produce glucose, which is released into the blood. Of course, most of this newly released glucose cannot be taken up by cells because of the lack of insulin. This means that the existing hyperglycemia is increased, as is the amount of glucose lost in the urine. Another complication follows chronically increased gluconeogenesis. This is the depletion of body proteins that are broken down to supply the subunits from which glucose is synthesized in gluconeogenesis. Essentially, this means that protein (from muscle, for example) is converted to glucose and then lost in the urine. The result is weakness, fatigue, and weight loss.

Lipid metabolism is also stimulated by low insulin levels, causing hyperlipidemia and the excessive production of **ketone bodies.** These products of lipid metabolism are **acetone** and the keto acids **aceto-acetic acid** and **hydroxybutyric acid.** As they accumulate, they produce a meta-

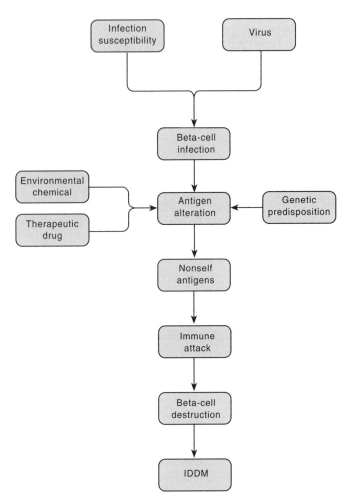

Figure 17.18   **Etiology of IDDM.**

bolic acidosis called **ketoacidosis,** which is often seen in the diabetic. They can produce nausea and vomiting and are toxic to brain tissue. Ketone bodies are volatile and have a characteristic odor that is often detected on the breath of the diabetic. In IDDM, there is a constant risk of **acidotic coma,** a result of the combined effects of ketoacidosis, dehydration, and the toxic effects of ketone bodies on the brain. The major signs in IDDM are presented in table 17.6. Figure 17.19 summarizes the pathogenesis.

Hypoglycemic coma is the result of brain glucose deprivation. It may be caused by inadequate dietary intake, high glucose utilization, as in exercise, or from an accidentally excessive insulin dose. In the last case, high insulin levels promote widespread glucose uptake, which can reduce the amount available to the brain. Deprived of its major energy source, it can't maintain normal levels of activity, and loss of consciousness results.

Etiology of NIDDM

There is a strong genetic component that operates in NIDDM, more so than in IDDM, with multiple genes thought to be involved. Evidence supports a genetic mechanism underlying an essential defect in beta cell function.

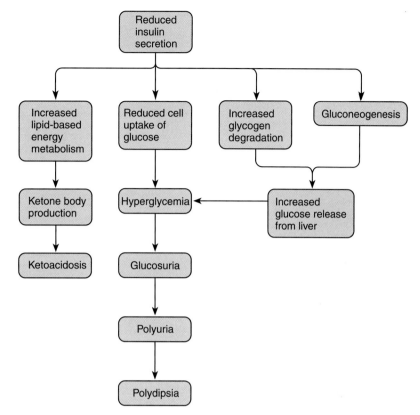

Figure 17.19   **Pathogenesis of IDDM.**

Table 17.6	Major Signs and Symptoms of IDDM

Signs and Symptoms	Comments
Hyperglycemia	High blood glucose from reduced cell uptake and increased release from liver
Glucosuria	From high blood levels of glucose
Polyuria	Hyperglycemia reduces renal water reabsorption
Weakness/fatigue/ weight loss	Caused by disordered protein and carbohydrate metabolism
Ketoacidosis	The result of excessive lipid energy metabolism and other metabolic derangements

Although able to secrete insulin, the beta cell response to glucose is muted and sluggish, so that fine control of blood glucose is disrupted. Another key element in NIDDM is **insulin resistance.** In essence, insulin resistance involves the inability of cells, in particular those of muscle and the liver, to normally take up and metabolize glucose. An aspect of insulin resistance is based on slower cycling of glucose carriers to cell surfaces. The result is reduced glucose uptake and hyperglycemia, even though insulin is being secreted. Insulin resistance also involves defective utilization of the glucose that does manage to enter the cells. (Note

that a genetic defect may be a factor in insulin resistance, but this is uncertain.) A key, nongenetic factor in NIDDM is obesity—over 75% of NIDDM sufferers are significantly overweight. The link seems based on insulin resistance in that those who are obese have fewer insulin receptors i.e., even obese people who are nondiabetic show this effect. When obesity and the genetic beta cell defect interact over years, NIDDM emerges. A lack of exercise is also a characteristic shared by many who develop NIDDM. A sedentary life probably contributes by reducing the need for glucose so that uptake is subnormal. Inadequate exercise may also be a factor in obesity and its associated insulin resistance. There are several other nongenetic variables that may contribute to the etiology of NIDDM and research into their precise role continues.

Pathogenesis of NIDDM

The essential, probably genetic, beta cell defect in NIDDM appears to be operating before any signs of the disease emerge. When tested, those without overt NIDDM, but with a family history of the disease, overreact to dietary glucose with an exaggerated insulin output. Then, in the early stages of the disease itself, the defective beta cells respond to glucose with insulin secretion that is sluggish and imprecise. This faulty insulin secretion combines with insulin resistance to contribute to the hyperglycemia that characterizes the condition. During the years over which the disease progresses, the hyperglycemia acts as a strong

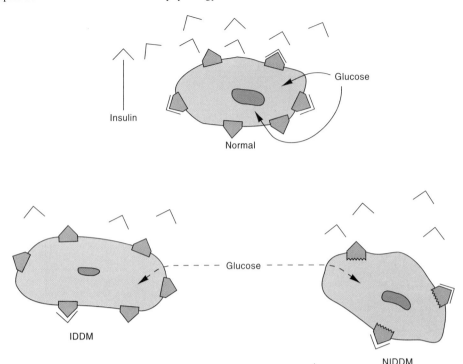

Figure 17.20   **Mechanisms in DM.** Glucose uptake in a normal cell depends on insulin binding cell surface receptors. In IDDM, insulin is deficient, and glucose uptake and metabolism are compromised. NIDDM arises when abnormal insulin secretion and insulin resistance (represented by fewer receptors) effect combine.

insulin-secretion stimulus to which the cells are increasingly unable to respond. It is as if the beta cells become fatigued by the constant demand for insulin.

Ultimately, the beta cells undergo apoptosis and are replaced by fibrous tissue. Note that this later loss of beta cells is fundamentally different from the earlier autoimmune destruction of beta cells in IDDM. (Figure 17.20 illustrates the essential distinction between the underlying mechanisms of IDDM and NIDDM.) In many cases of NIDDM, especially in those past the age of 60, there is prominent hyalinization of the islets, with a protein called **amylin** accumulating in islet tissue spaces. Amylin is secreted with insulin and is thought to be a hormone with an insulin-antagonist function, but its precise contribution to glucose homeostasis is unclear. It may be that its overproduction is an aspect of a genetic derangement of beta cell function. There is also uncertainty about the build-up of amylin between beta cells: Does it interfere with their function or is it excessively produced by cells that are already failing? To further demonstrate how the pieces of this puzzle don't all fall neatly into place, note that amylin also accumulates in the nondiabetic elderly, indicating, perhaps, that it is a normal aspect of aging. Figure 17.21 presents the essentials of NIDDM pathogenesis.

When first diagnosed, much NIDDM can be controlled with diet and exercise because both contribute to weight loss. As weight is reduced, insulin receptor numbers increase and insulin resistance is diminished. Of course, exercise also contributes to weight loss, but in generating an increased demand for glucose in skeletal muscle, the exer-

cise promotes an increase in insulin receptors. In spite of these beneficial effects, as the disease progresses, some insulin therapy may be required to offset the inevitable loss of beta cells. Table 17.7 compares the features of IDDM and NIDDM.

Another form of diabetic coma called **hyperglycemic, hyperosmolar, nonketotic coma** (HHNK), although uncommon, can arise in long-established NIDDM, particularly in response to some stress such as an infection or trauma. The stress creates an acute demand for insulin that overwhelms the already overtaxed beta cells, and insulin output drops to very low levels. This causes a dramatic rise in blood glucose and the blood becomes much more concentrated: It becomes hyperosmolar. Prior to the initiating stress, there is enough glucose metabolism to limit ketoacid production. Once underway, however, the situation progresses so rapidly that even though insulin levels are very low, there isn't time for ketoacidosis to develop before the onset of coma; hence, this is a nonketotic coma in contrast to the situation in IDDM. Glucose levels in HHNK can be as high as 2,000 mg/dl, producing a heavy diuresis that drops plasma volume significantly. Low plasma volume and the blood's hyperosmolarity combine to draw fluid into the blood. In the brain, the loss of fluid causes cerebral dehydration, which is responsible for the coma in HHNK.

Chronic Effects in Diabetes Mellitus

Both IDDM and NIDDM exhibit a pattern of long-term vascular and neurological change linked to the fundamen-

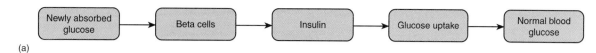

(a)

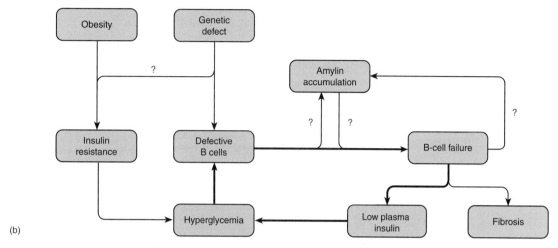

(b)

Figure 17.21 **Pathogenesis of NIDDM.** (*a*) Normal insulin response. (*b*) Genetic factors and insulin resistance combine effects in NIDDM. Heavy arrows represent the cycle of progressive hyperglycemia that causes fatigue and ultimate failure of beta cells. Question marks indicate uncertain relationships.

Table 17.7	A Comparison of Some Selected Features of IDDM and NIDDM	
	IDDM	**NIDDM**
Frequency among diabetics	10%	90%
Family history of DM	Less than 1/5	Over 1/2
Age of onset	Under 40, most under 20	Most over 40
Clinical course	Acute onset, rapid progress	Delayed recognition, gradual progress
Physique	Normal or lean	Usually obese
Plasma insulin	Low or absent	Normal early; later reduced
Sulfonyl urea stimulus	No insulin response	Insulin response
Acute threat	Ketoacidosis	HHNC
Therapy	Insulin, diet	Diet, exercise, some drug/insulin

tal metabolic derangements of diabetes. An important mechanism involves **glycated proteins.** These are plasma and tissue proteins that combine with glucose in conditions of hyperglycemia. After glycation, these proteins function abnormally to produce the various complications that threaten the later years of the person with diabetes. Hemoglobin, albumin, lipoprotein, eye lens protein, collagen, and cell membrane proteins are known to be involved in glycation.

Emergence of complications is variable, depending on the severity of the diabetes and the length of time its metabolic derangements have been present. In some cases systemic problems arise early; in others, not at all, but an average period of onset is 15 years or so after hyperglycemia develops.

Microangiopathy This is a characteristic pattern of small vessel change that accompanies diabetes. Most arterioles and capillaries are affected, with those of the skin, kidney, myocardium, and retina producing the most serious consequences. Thickening of arteriolar walls produces a type of arteriolosclerosis. Glycated proteins that escape from the lumen contribute to the thickening, as does excessive deposition of basement membrane. Systemic hypertension contributes to the problem, which affects half of adult diabetics. The arteriolosclerosis that accompanies high blood pressure adds to the diabetes-related wall changes to produce significantly compromised blood flow to systemic tissues. Particularly in the lower limbs, reduced blood flow interferes with healing. Minor wounds that would ordinarily heal quickly demonstrate a delayed and ineffective healing

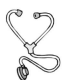

Focus on Diabetes Diagnosis in Ancient Greece

Both diabetes mellitus and diabetes insipidus are characterized by diuresis. In DM, the cause is the osmotic effect of high glucose levels in nephron tubule filtrate, whereas in diabetes insipidus, it is the lack of ADH. Even in ancient times, a patient complaining of large urinary water losses might be asked to produce a urine specimen. Lacking modern laboratory analytical machinery, and indeed, anything to plug it into, the canny physician would taste the specimen. The Greek word for honey is *meli;* so sweet-tasting urine would yield the diagnosis diabetes mellitus (the passing of sweet urine). On the other hand, insipid or flat-tasting urine would indicate a different condition and, hence, the distinguishing term diabetes insipidus would be applied.

Note that it was not necessary to ingest large quantities of urine to arrive at the diagnosis; a small taste was enough. Of course, urine is normally sterile, so no infection was likely to follow from such tasting. Although their knowledge was primitive in many ways, early physicians weren't fools, and we can be sure they would avoid tasting any urine that was cloudy, blood-tinged, or otherwise abnormal.

---

response. Because the compromised blood flow produces generalized hypoxia, anaerobic organisms can produce gangrene severe enough to warrant limb amputation. In the myocardium, microangiopathy adds to ischemia that is linked to the coronary atherosclerosis that occurs early and severely in DM.

The term **diabetic nephropathy** is applied to the characteristic microangiopathy of the kidney. Most arterioles and capillaries are affected, with progressive deterioration in renal function producing the nephrotic syndrome (see chapter 15) and, often, complete renal failure. In particular, pronounced renal ischemia can cause acute necrosis of the renal papillae, causing them to be shed. This **necrotizing papillitis** presents a serious threat. Older diabetics, in whom microangiopathy has been progressing for years, comprise the largest group of renal transplant recipients.

Fine retinal blood vessels are also affected in DM. Their walls and basement membranes are altered in ways that favor the formation of small aneurysms. These can rupture to damage the retina, producing progressive loss of vision. In some cases, the vessels proliferate, with tufts of tiny vessels encroaching into the eye's interior. **Cataracts** (clouding of the lens caused by alterations in its protein) and **glaucoma** (increased pressure within the eye) also have increased incidence in the diabetic. Some degree of blindness is 25 times more likely to occur in those with diabetes as compared to those without diabetes.

Atherosclerosis The major cause of death in diabetes is myocardial infarction due to atherosclerosis. The chronic glucose deprivation that cells face in DM generates an increased demand for lipid fuels that are drawn from fat stores and delivered by the blood. The resulting hyperlipidemia combines with the systemic hypertension that is common to diabetics to produce early and severe atherosclerosis (see chapter 9). As well, atherosclerosis in the large cerebral supply vessels adds to the brain ischemia that may be present as a result of the small vessel damage associated with DM. The result is an increased likelihood of CVA. Many of the heart attacks and strokes attributed to vascular disease in mortality statistics are, in fact, complications of DM.

The glycation of proteins may also contribute to the more extensive and rapid atherosclerotic involvement of the large vessels seen in diabetes. There is evidence that glycosylated collagen preferentially binds low-density lipoproteins (LDLs) at high rates. This might give rise to the increased deposition of LDLs in the intima to escalate the rate of atherogenesis. Glycated collagen may also enhance platelet binding and aggregation to promote thrombosis and infarction.

Peripheral Neuropathy Widespread effects in the peripheral nerves often accompany DM. They may affect neuron processes directly, or their supporting myelin sheaths, or both. Whatever the mechanism, the result is a variety of neurological disturbances, which may not be life-threatening but are a great source of distress to those who suffer from diabetes.

Sensory loss is often present, with skeletal motor dysfunction found less frequently. In either case, abnormal reflexes are common. Numbness, tingling sensations, or heightened sensitivity may be experienced, or sensory defects may produce deep and intense pain. When autonomic pathways are affected, a broad range of malfunctions may arise, including disturbances of GI motility, bladder dysfunction, impotence in males, and fainting from neurogenic vascular shock.

DM is known to affect the brain, but disturbances there are thought to derive primarily from small vessel changes that compromise circulation. For this reason, *peripheral neuropathy* is the term most commonly used in relation to the nervous system abnormalities associated with DM (table 17.8).

Diagnosis of Diabetes Mellitus

Diagnosis in DM is based on the presence of hyperglycemia, glucosuria, and polyuria resulting from lack of insulin secretion. This is a relatively straightforward matter in IDDM. In NIDDM, the situation is less clear, and in these cases the glucose tolerance test (GTT) is used. This test assesses the ability of an individual's cells to take up and metabolize glucose. After an oral dose of glucose is given, its level in the blood and urine is monitored. If blood glucose goes up and remains elevated, it is a sign that insulin secretion is inadequate to cope with the absorbed glucose (fig. 17.22).

In some individuals, GTT results are abnormal but below the level of clear-cut DM. Such individuals are said

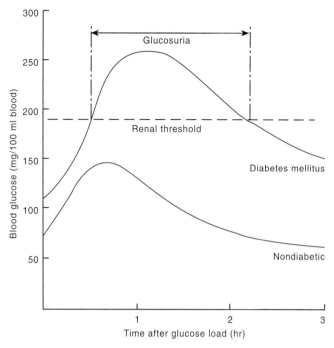

Figure 17.22 **The Glucose Tolerance Test.** The two curves indicate blood glucose level in the diabetic and the nondiabetic following oral administration of 100 g of glucose (glucose load). Note that when blood glucose level exceeds 190 mg/100 ml, renal reabsorption capacity is exceeded and glucose appears in the urine.

Table 17.8	Vascular and Neurologic Conditions Associated with Long-Term Diabetes Mellitus

Small Vessel Damage

Depressed peripheral healing response; gangrene risk
Impaired vision from retinal damage, cataracts, glaucoma
Depressed renal function; long-term renal failure
Impaired myocardial perfusion with increased MI risk

Large Vessel Damage

Early and severe atherosclerosis; higher incidence
   of MI and CVA

Peripheral Neurologic Abnormalities

Pain; bladder and bowel dysfunction

Focus on DM in Pregnancy

In **gestational diabetes,** impaired glucose tolerance emerges in 1–2% of pregnant women with no previous indication of the disease. The condition gives rise to delivery complications that are due to the large size of the infants born to mothers with diabetes. Associated derangements of maternal metabolism also produce congenital malformations in as many as 10% of newborns. Cardiovascular and neurological defects are most often involved. These may cause spontaneous abortion or death in the early postpartum period. As in other people with impaired glucose tolerance, mothers are more likely to develop NIDDM after about ten years.

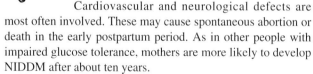

to have **impaired glucose tolerance.** About one-third of those with impaired glucose tolerance develop NIDDM after about ten years. The remaining two-thirds do not, but have a greater risk of atherosclerosis and its complications. High stress states, which place an increased demand on blood glucose control systems, may also produce transient glucose intolerance. Conditions such as trauma or infections are examples. Previously these cases were described by the terms **chemical, latent,** or **subclinical DM,** but the implication that DM was present, yet undiscovered, has led to the decline in the use of these terms.

Treatment of Diabetes Mellitus

Treatment of IDDM is predominantly by subcutaneous insulin injection. The aim is restoration of glucose metabolism, so that its dietary intake must be closely regulated and matched to insulin dose. This usually means that meals must be taken at regularly timed intervals, with frequent snacks between meals. Caloric levels are closely monitored for all food intake. Foods rich in sugars are strictly limited because they release glucose from the GI lumen into the blood more rapidly than insulin can cope with it.

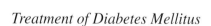

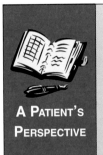

A Patient's Perspective

Compliance??: Living with Diabetes

—An account by Helene Jospe

Whoever came up with the concept of "compliance" was obviously not someone living with a chronic illness. For the notions of "disease" and "living with that disease" are very different.

My diabetes is only a part of me. This means that I must incorporate it into my life with all the other things that make up who I am. So, at any given moment, my mood, energy, motivation, stress, recent trauma or joys, physical status, personal relationship, financial status, job, etc., all influence everything I do. On top of these universal factors, my diabetes can add frustration (when my blood sugars are all over the place despite rigid adherence to diet and glucose testing), and feelings of deprivation when I get fed up with my controlled eating. So the idea of labeling my behavior according to a list found in an endocrinology textbook is ridiculous. The list is simple. I, as a human being, am very complex.

What makes me furious about the concept of compliance is the judgment that goes along with it. Adhering to the "rules" wins one the approval of his/her health care professionals. But with the label of "noncompliant" can come frustration, threats, punishment, disapproval, and even anger and ridicule on the part of these professionals.

Like every other human being, I make health-related choices many times a day. The dietary restrictions can be so limiting they can feel claustrophobic. I would sometimes choose to forfeit my dinner, and sit down with two cans of Diet Coke instead. Although I was well aware that this was not the best choice for me nutritionally, I did it because it kept me from wallowing in self-pity. At that moment, it was the best choice for my life. But ultimately, these are my choices. As long as I know the consequences to my actions, I am responsible for my behavior. This is the same issue for all the people who go on a diet. So, why is it that we accept dieter's situation as part of being "human," but not the person's with a chronic illness? In fact, why is it that in the latter case, it is labeled as noncompliant and often seen as a personal insult to health care professionals?

What I want from my health care professionals, aside from the information that I need to best manage my health in a way that suits my life, is empathy. There is a wonderful nurse on the diabetic day care unit. One day, as I was weighing in, I made a very disgusted face/gesture at the amount of weight I had gained. She said, "Don't be so hard on yourself. It must be so difficult to live with those diet restrictions. Give yourself a break." She did wonders for me with those words. She gave me the permission to not be perfect. She let me know the expectations around dietary restrictions were very difficult to follow. She allowed me to ease up on my judgment of my behavior. And knowing that another person was aware of how difficult this was for me on a daily basis gave me support and strength to watch my intake more carefully the next day. This was far better (and way more effective) than wagging a finger in my face and telling me I ate too much.

Recently, battery-powered insulin infusion pumps have been increasingly used. These provide a continuous insulin supply through a subcutaneous needle or intravenously. They have their own set of complications (e.g., battery failure or hypoglycemia from overdose) and are not indicated for all IDDM patients. Transplantation of the pancreas is also being explored, but the procedure is unlikely to become widespread because of immune rejection complications.

In NIDDM, insulin is required much less often. In many cases, the loss of excess weight provides a substantial correction of the problem. Moderate exercise also promotes carbohydrate metabolism and can contribute to normalization without drug therapy. If needed, one of several **sulfonyl urea** preparations may be used to stimulate insulin release from beta cells. Other drugs, which mimic the action of insulin, are finding increasing use in NIDDM therapy.

Secondary DM

When insulin hyposecretion is due to other than beta cell destruction or hormone resistance, the condition is de-

 ### Checkpoint 17.3

Reflect back on the large number of people affected by diabetes and the severe consequences that are associated with years of disease progression. Then note that therapy can only seek to normalize insulin and blood glucose levels, which of course is not a cure, but only a means of coping that attempts to slow the course of the disease. Now consider the North American trend to obesity that is linked to high-calorie, high-fat, high-sugar diets avidly eaten by people who spend increasing time in front of television and computer screens. Now speculate on the future of NIDDM incidence and rates of renal failure, blindness, and MI. It's not a happy prospect.

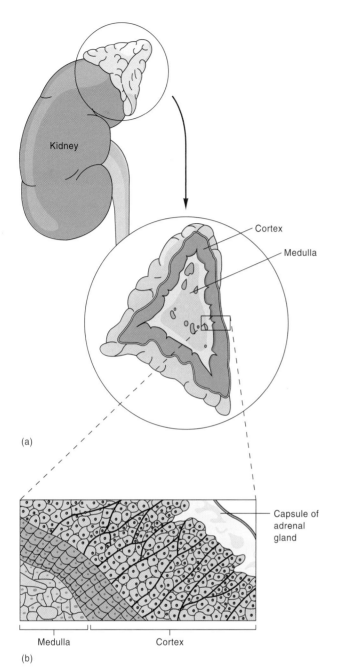

(a)

(b)

Figure 17.23 **The Adrenal Gland.** Its cortex and medulla can easily be distinguished in these (*a*) gross and (*b*) microscopic sections.

Table 17.9	Principal Adrenal Cortex Hormones

Mineralocorticoids

Aldosterone
Deoxycorticosterone

Glucocorticoids

Cortisol
Corticosterone

Gonadocorticoids

Dehydroepiandrosterone (metabolized to sex hormones in tissues)

Note that mineralocorticoids have some glucocorticoid effects and that glucocorticoids have some mineralocorticoid effects.

THE ADRENAL GLANDS

Broadly speaking, the adrenal glands produce hormones that enable us to better cope with a changing environment. Important homeostatic adaptations mediated by the adrenal hormones include the maintenance of body fluid balance and blood glucose level, as well as various cardiovascular responses.

Normal Anatomy and Physiology

The adrenal, or **suprarenal glands** are a pair of small (about 4 g each), approximately pyramidal masses that rest on the superior pole of each kidney (fig. 17.23*a*). Each gland is, in fact, two separate glands of quite different embryologic origins. The larger (85%) adrenal cortex is true glandular tissue, while the internal medulla develops from embryonic nervous tissue (fig. 17.23*b*). The glands' blood supply derives from the adrenal arteries and other branches of the abdominal aorta. A single vein drains each gland—the right adrenal vein joining the inferior vena cava and the left emptying into the left renal vein.

The hormones of the adrenal cortex are a closely related group of steroid hormones, known collectively as **corticosteroids.** Some of these, because they affect sodium and potassium levels, are called **mineralocorticoids,** while others, which regulate carbohydrate metabolism, are classed as **glucocorticoids** (table 17.9). Of the mineralocorticoids, the most important is aldosterone. It has high potency and is responsible for over 90% of mineralocorticoid stimulus to target tissues. The dominant glucocorticoid is **cortisol,** providing over 95% of glucocorticoid response. Note that cortisol also has some slight mineralocorticoid effect. The adrenal cortex also secretes small quantities of the male and female sex hormone precursor (**androstenedione**) that is converted to testosterone or estrogen in systemic tissues. Normally, only insignificant amounts are secreted, but they may be important in disease states.

scribed as **secondary DM.** In these conditions, a variety of conditions may contribute to the loss of pancreatic tissue and produce diabetes as a result of insulin hyposecretion.

Factors that are known to produce secondary DM are pancreatic inflammations or trauma, pancreatic surgery, or drug or chemical suppression of the insulin secretion. Various endocrinopathies may also affect insulin secretion, directly or indirectly. Examples are Cushing's syndrome, pheochromocytoma, and acromegaly, three conditions that will be described later in this chapter in the Adrenal Pathophysiology and Adenohypophyseal sections. Adrenocorticosteroid therapy may also induce secondary DM.

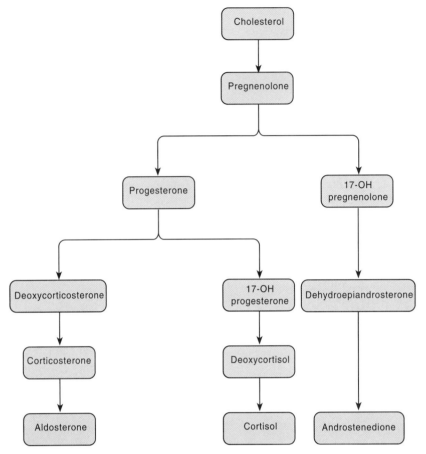

Figure 17.24   **Adrenal Hormones.** Synthetic pathways of the adrenal corticosteroids. Final estrogen and testosterone formation occurs from androstenedione in peripheral tissues.

Adrenal synthesis of the corticosteroids starts with the uptake of LDL by membrane LDL receptors. The cholesterol carried in the LDL is used to synthesize the three major steroid hormone types (fig. 17.24).

Control of adrenal secretion is achieved by two major controlling inputs. **ACTH (adrenocorticotropic hormone)** from the anterior pituitary gland regulates glucocorticoid and gonadocorticoid synthesis, while angiotensin II regulates the mineralocorticoid pathway. (The factors determining the feedback control of aldosterone were described in chapter 16.) ACTH is under the control of **corticotropin-releasing hormone** (CRH), produced in the hypothalamus and delivered to the pituitary by its portal circulation. Cortisol is the key to regulation. Its blood level exerts a negative feedback effect at the pituitary and hypothalamus to control both glucocorticoid and gonadocorticoid levels (fig. 17.25).

Once in the blood, cortisol travels bound to a specific transport protein called **cortisol-binding globulin** (CBG) and, to a lesser degree, to albumin. Only small amounts of unbound hormone are present in the plasma. Those corticosteroids not inactivated by target tissues are excreted in bile and urine.

In the small, internal core of the adrenal glands, the catecholamines norepinephrine and epinephrine are produced. The amino acid phenylalanine is the initial point in

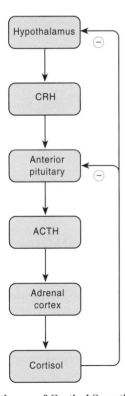

Figure 17.25   **Pathways of Cortisol Secretion Control.**

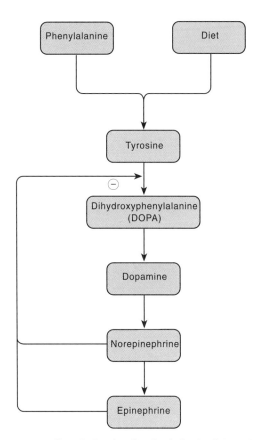

Figure 17.26 **Catecholamine Synthesis in the Adrenal Medulla.**

the synthetic pathway (fig. 17.26). The levels of norepinephrine and epinephrine exert feedback control at a key point in the metabolic sequence. Norepinephrine and epinephrine are stored in cytoplasmic granules, from which they are released in response to input from the sympathetic nervous system. Of the adrenal medulla's secretion, 80% is epinephrine, and the remaining 20% is norepinephrine.

General Adaptation Syndrome The adrenal cortex and the adrenal medulla have complementary roles in promoting a widespread adaptation to stress. Broadly, stress consists of either a significant deviation from some variable's homeostatic optimum or a more acute and immediate threat to physical or emotional well-being. Whenever stress occurs, a coordinated adaptive response follows, mediated by the adrenal cortex's increased secretion of cortisol and the adrenal medulla's enhanced release of catecholamines. This combined response has been termed the **general adaptation syndrome** (GAS). The surge in cortisol is so characteristic that those who study the response define a **stressor** as anything that triggers increased cortisol secretion.

Stressors vary greatly (table 17.10), but the GAS that follows provides a widespread and integrated response regardless of the stressor. On activation, the hypothalamus, the CRF-ACTH-cortisol pathway, and the sympathetic adrenal medulla responses combine to provide an integrated and widespread ability to meet the stressor's challenge (fig. 17.27).

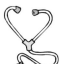

Focus on Side Effects of Corticosteroid Therapy

The therapeutic use of synthetic cortisol preparations to suppress inflammation is widespread. These anti-inflammatory effects emerge only at pharmacologic doses that are much higher than the physiological levels measured during the GAS. At physiological concentrations, cortisol may exert some role in inflammation regulation, but the degree to which this occurs is unclear.

Also, note that the prolonged therapeutic use of corticosteroids can promote the suppression or loss of normal cortical function. The high therapeutic doses have a suppressive effect on the hypothalamus and pituitary (see fig. 17.25). The resulting long-term decrease in ACTH stimulus can cause the cortex to lose sensitivity to ACTH. After a prolonged regimen of corticosteroid therapy, the cortex may require weeks or even months to recover from its highly suppressed state. Patients may be more vulnerable to stressors during this period.

Table 17.10	Stressors Capable of Inducing the GAS
Trauma (including surgery)	Pain
Intense/prolonged exercise	Emotional distress
Severe disease/infection	(anxiety/depression)
Systemic hypoxia	Severe hemorrhage
Temperature extremes	

The effect of these responses is to supply cells with increased cellular fuels (glucose, lipid), increased protein synthesis components (amino acids), and increased oxygen as a result of higher respiration rates, and to increase blood flow to deliver all of them more efficiently. The benefits of the GAS in coping with physiological disruption seem clear enough, but its adaptive aid in psychological or emotional stress is less clear. Indeed, as noted in earlier chapters, such long-term stress may contribute to atherosclerosis and systemic hypertension.

The GAS has been described as having three stages. The **alarm phase** is the initial response, involving the rapid release of catecholamines. This is followed by the **resistance phase,** in which corticosteroids provide a longer-term response that stabilizes to produce steady-state compensation for the high demands generated by the initial emergency. In the **exhaustion phase,** adaptive capacity has been overwhelmed, and unless the stressor is removed or therapy can intervene, the result may be rapid decline and death. This phase is characterized by loss of potassium as a result of its exchange for sodium in the nephron tubule, in

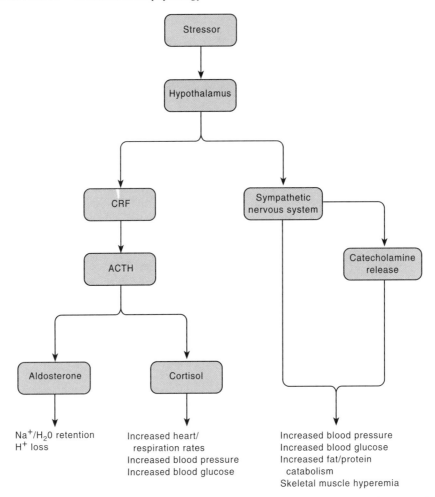

Figure 17.27   **General Adaptation Syndrome.** The GAS responses as mediated by the adrenals and the sympathetic nervous system.

 Checkpoint 17.4

You might try to evaluate in which GAS phase various of your patients find themselves. And consider that the diagnosis and treatment to which you contribute may be instrumental in prolonging your patients' resistant phase or in preventing them from moving into the exhaustion phase.

attempts to sustain blood volume and blood pressure. Those who ultimately succumb to long-term illness have enlarged adrenal glands caused by hyperplasia in response to the prolonged stress of the disease.

Adrenal Pathophysiology

Most adrenal disorders involve the cortex. Only two, relatively uncommon tumors produce hyperfunction of the adrenal medulla. We will consider these briefly after describing the more common cortical disorders.

Adrenocortical Hypersecretion

Since there are three classes of hormone produced by the adrenal cortex, there are three principal disorders related to their excessive secretion (**hyperadrenalism**).

Cushing's Syndrome The term applied to the glucocorticoid hypersecretion state is **Cushing's syndrome.** The signs and symptoms are predictable on the basis of the glucocorticoid effects already described. Victims of Cushing's syndrome are often obese, with a typical pattern of fat deposition in the face, at the base of the neck, and in the abdomen. A rounded "moon face" is characteristic of the Cushing's syndrome sufferer (fig. 17.28). Lipids made available by the action of cortisol are preferentially deposited in these areas, if they are not metabolized. Chronic protein catabolism produces muscle weakness, bone loss, as its protein matrix components are degraded, and bruising and striae (stretch marks) in the skin. High levels of cortisol also have mineralocorticoid effects, so sodium and water retention typically give rise to systemic hypertension and to hypokalemia. Prolonged hyperglycemia, induced by high levels of cortisol, can also produce insulin insensitivity and impair glucose tolerance. Increased androgenic secretion may also be present in Cushing's syndrome, with women

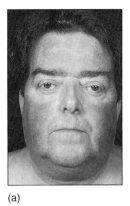
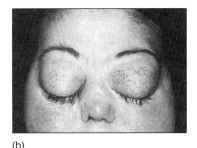

(a)   (b)

Figure 17.28   **Cushing's Disease.** (*a*) Characteristic facial roundness and florid (red) skin. (*b*) Deposition of lipid is responsible for the puffiness in the eyelids.

Table 17.11	Principal Signs and Symptoms in Cushing's Syndrome

Obesity	Altered GTT
Characteristic face appearance	Menstrual disorders
Weakness	Psychological disturbances
Systemic hypertension	Tendency to bruising
Hypokalemia	Striae

experiencing menstrual dysfunctions and some male-pattern hair growth and acne as a result. Mild to severe emotional or psychological disturbances may also be present (table 17.11).

The high levels of glucocorticoids in Cushing's syndrome arise most often as a side effect of prolonged ACTH or glucocorticoid therapy for other conditions. Other causes of hypersecretion are adrenal tumors. Benign adenomas and malignant carcinomas may produce a similar Cushing's pattern of signs and symptoms, but the carcinoma metastasizes extensively and so has a very poor prognosis. Note, however, that about half of cortical carcinomas are so anaplastic that no functional hormones are produced. In these cases, no Cushing's syndrome signs or symptoms are present, and the effects of local invasion and metastasis dominate the clinical picture. In secreting cortical tumors and therapeutically induced Cushing's syndrome, high glucocorticoid levels suppress ACTH production. In such cases, its low level can be useful in drawing diagnostic conclusions as to etiology.

By contrast, the two remaining causes of Cushing's syndrome are characterized by elevated plasma ACTH values. These may arise as a result of the ectopic secretion of ACTH by a nonendocrine tumor, usually bronchogenic carcinoma. Another, less common source might be the excessive ACTH output of a pituitary adenoma or a hypothalamic tumor that releases excessive CRF to stimulate ACTH secretion. In either case, the pronounced ACTH

stimulus to the adrenal cortex induces high cortical output, and Cushing's syndrome results.

Hyperaldosteronism In hyperaldosteronism, the problem is hypersecretion by the aldosterone-secreting cells of the adrenal cortex. This condition usually affects those 30–50 years of age, with men affected twice as often as women. It usually arises as the result of a cortical adenoma, sometimes referred to as **Conn's syndrome,** and rarely from a carcinoma's hypersecretion. In other cases, a nonneoplastic and idiopathic cortical hyperplasia is the cause. Excessive renal secretion of renin may also cause excessive aldosterone output. In such cases, a renal tumor or chronic volume depletion is the underlying problem.

The major effect of hyperaldosteronism is systemic hypertension due to sodium and water retention by the kidney. Hypokalemia and alkalosis secondary to sodium retention may also be present. About one in a hundred cases of systemic hypertension result from this condition.

Adrenal Virilism The result of androgen hypersecretion in females is **adrenal virilism.** In females, the excessive androgen induces various masculine traits such as beard growth, acne, voice deepening, and hair loss. Taken together, these changes are known as **virilization.** Menstrual abnormalities are also common. If androgen hypersecretion occurs in a young male, it leads to **sexual precocity.** In this condition, sexual development is rapid and premature. In such cases, the male sex organs and sexual drive of an adult may be present in a quite young individual. Etiology of the hypersecretion state is based either on hyperplasia or neoplasia of the androgen-secreting region of the cortex or a congenital enzyme derangement that promotes excessive androgen synthesis.

Adrenocortical Hyposecretion

Failure to secrete adequate amounts of corticosteroids gives rise to **hypoadrenalism** or **Addison's disease.** In this uncommon condition, corticosteroid deficiency may be due to destruction of the adrenal cortex or to suppression of ACTH by high therapeutic doses of glucocorticoids. In rare instances, a congenital enzyme deficiency is the cause. In most cases, destruction of the gland occurs by a poorly understood autoimmune mechanism, but infection, tumor invasion, or infarction may be also involved. Signs and symptoms emerge after loss of cortical tissue exceeds 80%.

The clinical pattern in Addison's disease is one of slowly developing weakness and fatigue, appetite and weight loss, and a characteristic pigmentation excess. The pigmentation increase is sometimes blotchy and is due to the pigment-stimulating effects of high ACTH levels caused by the feedback effects of low cortisol secretion (see fig. 17.25). Because Addison's patients have little ability to secrete cortisol and mount an adequate GAS, they are highly vulnerable to stress. If they are challenged by some stressor, an acute condition called an **addisonian crisis** may emerge. It typically involves fever, nausea, vomiting,

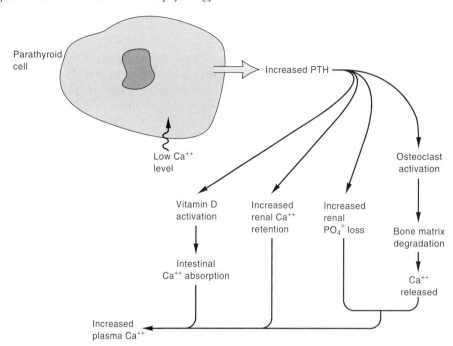

Figure 17.29   **Calcium Homeostasis.** In response to low Ca⁺⁺ levels, PTH elicits responses that increase plasma Ca⁺⁺ homeostasis.

hyponatremia, and hyperkalemia, as well as hypotension and dehydration, which pose the threat of circulatory shock.

Adrenal Medulla Pathophysiology

The derangements that arise in the adrenal medulla are rare tumors. One, **pheochromocytoma,** is usually benign, and the other, **neuroblastoma,** is malignant.

Pheochromocytoma This tumor arises in the catecholamine-secreting **chromaffin cells** of the medulla. Although most pheochromocytomas are benign, 10% are malignant. Sufferers typically develop systemic hypertension, with superimposed bouts of headache, heavy perspiration, tachycardia, and anxiety due to unregulated surges in catecholamine output from the tumor. Surgical resection has a high probability of success.

Neuroblastoma This highly malignant tumor occurs most frequently in children under the age of 15. It arises from undifferentiated cells present in nervous tissue. This tumor may develop at various sites in the peripheral nervous system, but over 80% occur in the adrenal medulla (recall the adrenal medulla's embryonic derivation from nervous tissue). In such cases, its effects are similar to those of pheochromocytoma in being caused by excessive catecholamine secretion, but its rapid and extensive metastasis is a more serious threat. If it is identified and surgically removed prior to an infant's first year, prognosis is quite good. After the first year, widespread metastasis makes the prognosis grim.

THE PARATHYROID GLANDS

The parathyroid glands are important regulators of calcium and other electrolytes and as a result, have significant impact on bone and indirectly on muscle function.

Normal Anatomy and Physiology

The parathyroid glands are small nodules of endocrine tissue held to the posterior surface of the thyroid gland by its capsule. Their number varies from two to eight, but four to six is typical. Their hormone is **parathyroid hormone** (PTH), also known as **parathormone.**

PTH is a peptide hormone synthesized in the **chief cells** of the parathyroids. Little is stored in the gland, and secretion is closely linked to synthesis. In the plasma, PTH travels as a free molecule, rather than bound to a carrier protein. Secretion of PTH is controlled by Ca⁺⁺ concentration in the extracellular fluid compartment (ECF). When Ca⁺⁺ concentration is low, PTH secretion is increased, and when high, it is suppressed (fig. 17.29). Magnesium ion (Mg⁺⁺) concentrations also affect PTH secretion similarly, but their input to the regulatory system seems less important than that of calcium. PTH acts directly or indirectly on various effector tissues to regulate plasma Ca⁺⁺ levels. It also affects Mg⁺⁺, PO₄≡, and HCO₃⁻. Its regulatory role is based on its effects on bone, nephron tubules, and vitamin D.

In response to a prolonged lowering of plasma Ca⁺⁺ levels, increased PTH secretion promotes Ca⁺⁺ and Mg⁺⁺ reabsorption by the nephron. This directly cuts Ca⁺⁺ losses to support the level of plasma Ca⁺⁺. PTH also activates osteoclasts in bone, stimulating their breakdown of bone matrix to make more Ca⁺⁺ available. This effect is enhanced by another PTH-mediated action, renal PO₄≡ excretion. This is effective because when calcium and phosphate are both elevated, they promote their incorporation into bone. Calcium alone does not have this effect so by excreting phosphate, bone deposition is not favored and the calcium released from bone remains in the ECF. A further PTH effect is the activation of vitamin D, which stimulates additional Ca⁺⁺ absorption from the small intestine. These last

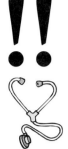

Focus on Anatomical Variability in the Hypoparathyroid State

Not only the number of parathyroid glands is subject to variation; their location also differs from one individual to the next. Some of these small nodules may not be associated with the thyroid gland at all. Instead they may be dispersed to various locations in the region of the neck in the superior mediastinum. Surgery or trauma involving these regions may produce an unanticipated hypoparathyroid state.

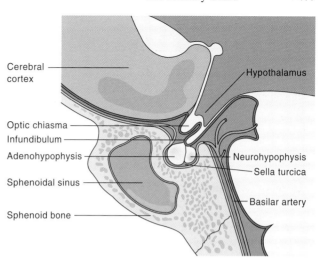

Figure 17.30 **Pituitary Gland.** Sagittal section through region of the pituitary gland. The adenohypophysis is distinct from the neurologically derived neurohypophysis.

two mechanisms are a new input of Ca^{++} into the plasma from body stores and the diet (fig. 17.29).

Hyperparathyroidism

Hyperparathyroidism is usually the result of a benign or malignant tumor or of parathyroid hyperplasia. These conditions arise more often in females than males and primarily produce loss of bone tissue from excessive osteoclast stimulus. The resulting bone weakness predisposes to bone pain, deformity, and fracture.

The result of chronic PTH hypersecretion is hypercalcemia, which may reach twice the normal Ca^{++} concentration of 8.5–10.5 mg/dl. It produces a range of muscular and neurologic defects (see the discussion on hypercalcemia in the Calcium Imbalance section in chapter 16) as well as predisposing to kidney stone formation. In extreme cases, widespread deposition of insoluble calcium phosphate in soft tissues may occur. This is known as **metastatic calcification.**

In renal disease, if $PO_4^{\equiv}$ is retained, then Ca^{++} is excreted. The resulting low Ca^{++} level activates PTH secretion, and bone degradation follows. When excessive secretion of PTH is caused by such a derangement, the condition is known as **secondary hyperparathyroidism.** If it is prolonged, parathyroid hyperplasia results. GI malabsorption or vitamin D deficiencies may also play a role in the etiology of secondary hyperparathyroidism, where inadequate Ca^{++} levels act as stimuli that induce PTH hypersecretion.

Hypoparathyroidism

Hypoparathyroidism is less frequently encountered than the hypersecretion state. Previously, the most common cause of hypoparathyroidism was the inadvertent removal of parathyroid glands during thyroid or other neck surgery.

More recently, awareness of the need to maintain parathyroid tissue, and the increasing application of nonsurgical therapies for hyperthyroidism, has reduced the incidence of hypoparathyroidism. Autoimmune destruction may also be involved in a lack of PTH output. A genetic condition in which the kidney is insensitive to PTH produces low calcium levels and is known as **pseudohypoparathyroidism** (PHP).

The principal result of diminished PTH secretion, or target tissue insensitivity to it, is hypocalcemia due to inadequate renal Ca^{++} retention or $PO_4^{\equiv}$ excretion. Impaired GI absorption and reduced Ca^{++} release from bone are also involved. Weakness, altered mental processes, and faulty muscular functions are the result (see the discussion on hypocalcemia in the Calcium Imbalance section in chapter 16).

THE PITUITARY GLAND

The pituitary derives its name from the Latin word for phlegm, since it was originally thought to be the source of the mucus that coats the nasal mucous membranes. This important regulatory gland has intimate structural and functional links to the hypothalamus, and we will therefore consider both in this section.

Normal Anatomy and Physiology

The position of the pituitary gland, suspended from the base of the brain, gives rise to its alternative name, **hypophysis,** which means "growing under" (fig. 17.30). The pituitary stalk (infundibulum) emerges from the hypothalamus to support the small (1-cm diameter) glandular mass, which projects into and is surrounded by a depression in the skull's sphenoid bone called the **sella turcica.** This elaborate protection gives testimony to the functional importance of the pituitary.

The gland consists of two regions: the **adenohypophysis** (anterior pituitary), composed of true glandular tissue, and the **neurohypophysis** (posterior pituitary), which derives from embryonic nervous tissue and is continuous with the hypothalamus. The posterior pituitary, rather than synthesizing and secreting hormone, acts as a storage site for hormones produced in the hypothalamus. These hormones

Table 17.12   The Principal Anterior Pituitary Hormones and Their Major Functions

Hormone/Abbreviation	Major Function
Human growth hormone (GH)	Stimulation of overall body growth and development
Thyroid-stimulating hormone (TSH)	Regulation of thyroid secretion
Follicle-stimulating hormone (FSH)	Stimulation of male and female gamete production
Luteinizing hormone (LH)	Stimulation of testosterone secretion; triggers ovulation and corpus luteum secretion
Prolactin (PRL)	Stimulation of mammary gland milk production
Adrenocorticotropic hormone (ACTH)	Regulation of adrenal cortical secretion
Melanocyte-stimulating hormone (MSH)	Stimulation of pigment production in skin melanocytes

migrate to the neurohypophysis along neurons that reach it via the pituitary stalk. From these, the hormones are released in response to action potentials from the hypothalamus. The two neurohypophyseal hormones are **vasopressin,** also called **antidiuretic hormone** (ADH), and **oxytocin.**

The adenohypophysis synthesizes and secretes seven major hormones from cells specialized for each hormone type. All but two of the anterior pituitary hormones are tropic hormones—that is, they control another endocrine gland's secretion. The exceptions are **prolactin** and **somatotropin,** or **growth hormone** (GH). Growth hormone acts on major metabolic pathways to generally promote growth in most body tissues.

Table 17.12 lists the pituitary's hormones and their principal functions.

Adenohypophyseal Hypersecretion

Hypersecretion of the anterior pituitary may be caused by a tropic-hormone-secreting adenoma. Malignancies or hypothalamic disorders are much less frequently involved. The adenomas are often tiny and cause no local invasive or compressive effects. However, because of the bony surrounding walls of the sella turcica, any adenomas that do enlarge significantly can compress the adjacent **optic chiasma.** This structure is formed by the merging of the two optic nerves prior to their entering the brain. The visual defects that accompany pituitary tumors are usually due to its compression or invasion.

The signs and symptoms in a given condition usually reflect hyperactivity in the pituitary's target gland. Cushing's syndrome is most often caused by ACTH hypersecretion and a thyroid hyperfunction state that resembles Graves' disease, but without its autoimmune component.

Hypersecretion of the two nontropic anterior pituitary hormones may also occur. When prolactin is present at high plasma levels, males experience impotence as a sole disturbance. In females, irregularities of menstruation are typical, often accompanied by varying degrees of breast milk production without pregnancy **(galactorrhea).**

Growth Hormone Hypersecretion

The effects of this condition depend on the age at which the hypersecretion state arises. If it is during childhood, prior to closure of the epiphyseal plates, rapid overall body growth is promoted by somatotropin's exaggerated stimulus to growth. The afflicted individual may reach a height of 8–9 feet with a proportionately large body. This is the condition known as **giantism,** or **gigantism.** If the pituitary tumor that causes this condition is not surgically removed or otherwise suppressed, it may completely destroy the pituitary by compressing it against the walls of the sella turcica. Death at an early adult age is the usual result if there is no intervention.

When somatotropic hormone hypersecretion occurs after adolescence, **acromegaly** develops. In this condition, although long bone length is fixed, bones enlarge by thickening. This change is accompanied by excessive growth of soft tissue, which produces a characteristic enlarging and coarsening of the features (fig. 17.31). Internal organs, such as the liver and kidney, are also affected. These changes occur quite gradually and may go unnoticed for some time.

Adenohypophyseal Hyposecretion

Hyposecretion may be the result of infection, primary or metastatic tumor damage, infarction, or various other injuries. The result is the suppression of all or most hormone secretion—the condition of **panhypopituitarism.** The resulting signs and symptoms are highly variable and generally reflect hypoactivity in multiple target tissues. In the case of tumors, various consequences of brain compression or invasion of the brain may be superimposed on endocrine hypofunction—for example, headache or visual disturbances.

Congenital or hereditary defects may produce hyposecretion of only a single anterior pituitary hormone. As you would expect, deficiency of a tropic hormone reveals itself as hypoactivity in its endocrine target gland. Hyposecretion of growth hormone is rare, but a prolactin hyposecretion

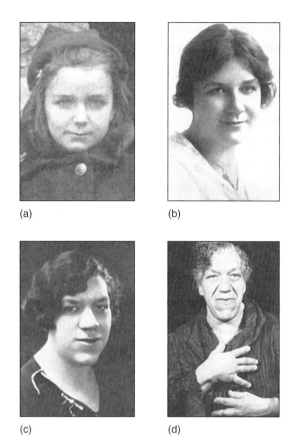

Figure 17.31 **Acromegaly.** The progressive coarsening of facial features in acromegaly is seen in this sequence of photographs taken at age 9 (*a*), 16 (*b*), 33 (*c*), and 52 (*d*).

state may arise as a result of hypotension related to perinatal hemorrhage. Because the adenohypophysis enlarges during pregnancy, it may compress the vessels that supply its blood. These vessels are arranged in a pattern that supplies the prolactin-secreting cells last, so they are at greatest risk of becoming ischemic as pregnancy proceeds. If at the time of delivery there is excessive blood loss, the fall in BHP can cause infarction of the prolactin-secreting cells. Of course, failure to lactate is the result, and at the very time when lactation is most needed. Abnormal menstruation is another consequence of inadequate prolactin secretion. This condition of perinatal pituitary infarction is known as **Sheehan's syndrome.**

Neurohypophyseal Dysfunction

Neurohypophyseal dysfunction, which is relatively rare, affects the secretion of ADH. Abnormalities of oxytocin secretion are unknown.

Diabetes Insipidus

This is a vasopressin hyposecretion state that may be caused by tumors, infection, trauma, or inadvertent damage from radiation therapy. The result is a significant diuresis due to a reduction of the nephron tubule's water permeability, which is controlled by ADH. Thirst and polydipsia are the expected responses, which can at least partially compensate for the sometimes enormous water losses (as much as 20 liters daily) that characterize this condition.

Syndrome of Inappropriate Antidiuretic Hormone Secretion

This condition was discussed in chapter 16 in the context of the excessive extracellular fluid that it produces. Most SIADH is due to production of ADH-like substances by nonendocrine tumors, usually of the lung, lymphoid tissue, or thymus. Other conditions that less frequently cause SIADH are disturbances of the hypothalamus, meningitis, infections, cerebral trauma, and infarction of the neurohypophysis.

Case Study

A 23-year-old female university student saw her general practitioner and complained of severe constipation, headaches, fatigue, and menstrual periods characterized by prolonged and excessive flow (**menorrhagia**). She had been experiencing fatigue and some degree of bowel irregularity for the past two years. These initially mild symptoms, combined with a slight swelling in her throat, had prompted a previous physician to measure her thyroxine levels, which were found to be normal. The diffuse nature of her complaints, combined with the emotional upset, at the time, of poor grades and a broken wedding engagement, prompted her previous doctor to suspect that her problems were stress-related.

She now reported that in addition to the general worsening of her symptoms, her throat was much more swollen and she was experiencing difficulty in coping with cold temperatures, saying she "had a hard time keeping warm." In view of these more recent developments, a blood test was done. It revealed that her thyroxine levels were abnormally low, and she was referred to an endocrinologist.

On physical examination the patient appeared generally well, with a normal body weight that had not recently changed. Her thyroid gland was diffusely enlarged, to approximately twice normal size, with no nodularity detectable on palpation. Her reflexes were normal, except for some delay in the relaxation phase of her biceps muscle. Other physical findings were normal. A blood test confirmed the depressed thyroxine levels: 2.3 μg% (normal: 4–10 μg%). A technetium radioisotope scan showed normal uptake in both thyroid lobes, with no obvious abnormal areas.

On the basis of these findings, a diagnosis of idiopathic primary hypothyroidism was made. Thyroxine replacement therapy was prescribed on a continuing, lifelong basis. The patient's signs and symptoms subsided and she suffers no side effects.

Commentary

The slow onset and progression of the initial thyroid changes produced no drop in plasma thyroxine levels, and the diffuse nature of the early complaints allowed them to be easily confused with psychological illness or stress-related disorders. Weight loss (in hyperthyroid states) or gain (in hypothyroid conditions) is common, but not always present, and any coincidental change in activity levels and appetite can affect body weight, to further confuse the picture.

Menstrual irregularities are also typical findings in thyroid disorders: amenorrhea with thyroid excess and menorrhagia in deficiency states. But since such irregularities also accompany a wide variety of other conditions, they may not provide much diagnostic help. In this patient, once the thyroid's hyperplasia response proved inadequate to maintain sufficient thyroxine in the blood, the emerging cold intolerance, constipation, and slowed muscle reflexes soon clarified the diagnostic picture.

Key Concepts

1. Endocrine disease is most often the result of excessive or inadequate hormone secretion, due to an imbalance in the gland's controlling inputs or to damage to the gland itself (p. 452).

2. Endocrine hyposecretion may be the result of a metabolic defect, gland agenesis, atrophy of a developed gland, or damage to an otherwise normal gland by infection, infarction, autoimmune mechanisms, or tumor growth (p. 452).

3. In response to endocrine hyposecretion, negative feedback reflexes produce increased levels of tropic hormones or hypothalamic releasing hormones, whose suppression may be monitored to confirm restoration of normal function (pp. 452–453).

4. Hormone resistance involves a reduction of hormone receptors, which produces target tissue insensitivity and hyposecretion effects (p. 453).

5. Endocrine hypersecretion is the result of excessive secretion of tropic hormones, defective feedback control mechanisms, or endocrine gland tumors (p. 453).

6. Thyroid hypofunction produces a systemic decline in the metabolic rate, causing cold intolerance, weight gain, and sluggish muscular and neurologic activity (pp. 456–457).

7. Chronically low plasma levels of thyroxine promote increased secretion of TSH, which induces the condition of thyroid hyperplasia known as goiter (pp. 458–459).

8. Thyroid hyperfunction produces a systemic elevation of the metabolic rate, causing heat intolerance, neurologic excitability, insomnia, weight loss, cardiac effects, and exophthalmos (pp. 459–462).

9. Diabetes mellitus exists in two forms: IDDM, the true islet hypofunction disease, and NIDDM, which involves defective secretion and insulin resistance (pp. 463–466).

10. A variety of chronic effects in DM involve small and large blood vessels and the nervous system, producing numerous and serious long-term consequences for the person with diabetes (pp. 466–468).

11. A range of adaptive responses to stress are mediated by the adrenal cortex and medulla, grouped under the title general adaptation syndrome (GAS) (p. 473).

12. Adrenocorticotropic hypersecretion may involve glucocorticoids, producing Cushing's syndrome, aldosterone, to yield hyperaldosteronism, or androgens in women, causing adrenal virilism (pp. 474–475).

13. The principal adrenocortical hyposecretion state involves a deficit of the corticosteroids, producing Addison's disease, which may compromise the GAS response (p. 475).

14. Hyperparathyroidism, which is usually caused by a parathyroid tumor, produces high levels of bone resorption, to the degree of compromising skeletal integrity (p. 477).

15. The numerous hormones of the adenohypophysis may be individually hypersecreted by an adenoma of a specific pituitary cell type, limiting effects to the target tissue regulated by each hormone (p. 477).

16. Hypersecretion of growth hormone prior to closure of the epiphyseal plates can so stimulate growth that body height might attain 8 or 9 feet, while hypersecretion after closure results in the enlargement and thickening of various tissues without any increase in height (p. 478).

17. Hyposecretion of adenohypophyseal hormones is usually due to tissue damage that affects all cell types to produce more widespread and variable systemic hypofunction effects (pp. 478–479).

18. In the neurohypophysis, disturbances of oxytocin secretion are unknown, but ADH secretion may be excessive, causing SIADH, or inadequate, causing diabetes insipidus (p. 479).

REVIEW ACTIVITIES

1. For each of the following situations, use upward or downward pointing arrows to show how each situation would cause plasma hormone levels to change.

   Tropic hormone hypersecretion

   Liver failure

   Target tissue hormone receptor damage

   Reduced target tissue hormone inactivation

   Kidney failure

   Anaplastic endocrine tumor

2. See figure 17.11. Why are the feedback effects of T_3/T_4 represented by minus signs? What would happen if they were plus signs?

3. The patient in this chapter's case study asks you to explain why she can't seem to keep warm. For help in answering her, see page 456.

4. Use page 464 to assist in laying out a flow chart illustrating the pathogenesis of IDDM. Start with "Reduced insulin secretion" at the top, and end with "Polydipsia" on the bottom. Refer to figure 17.19 when you're finished.

5. In figure 17.8, identify the section showing the steps that are thought to produce NIDDM. What is the name of this hypofunction mechanism? Page 465 may provide a clue. Which part of figure 17.20 would be useful to help make the point?

6. Write out a list of known or at least plausible links between each GAS response component in figure 17.27 and a physiological benefit that might contribute to coping with a stressor.

7. Prepare a giant quick reference list. For each major endocrine gland, indicate its principal hypo/hypersecretion states and the general pattern of target tissue problems that result.

Chapter

18

Skeletal and Muscular Pathophysiology

He knew the anguish of the marrow,
The ague of the skeleton;
No contact possible to flesh
Allayed the fever of the bone

*EXCERPT FROM "WHISPERS OF IMMORTALITY"
IN COLLECTED POEMS 1909–1962 BY T. S. ELIOT,
COPYRIGHT 1936 BY HARCOURT BRACE & COMPANY,
COPYRIGHT © 1964, 1963 BY T. S. ELIOT*
REPRINTED BY PERMISSION OF THE PUBLISHER.

rubor
& tumor
cū calore
& dolore

The osseous tissue that forms the skeleton and the muscle tissue of skeletal muscles are substantially different, but the organs they form have a close functional relationship. For this reason it is useful to consider their pathophysiology in a single chapter. This chapter also includes treatment of joint diseases, since most skeletal muscle action produces bone motion at joints. Since the emphasis here is on metabolic skeletal disease, bone fractures are described more appropriately in chapter 24, which deals with traumatic injury.

NORMAL BONE PHYSIOLOGY

Bone formation, or **ossification,** involves the deposition of inorganic ions, in the collagen-rich **osteoid** that forms a primitive bone model called a **template.** Calcium, phosphate, and hydroxide ions form plates of a water-insoluble salt called **hydroxyapatite.** The embedding of compression-resistant hydroxyapatite plates in osteoid, with its high-tensile-strength collagen, yields great strength. The principle is the same as the one applied in so much industrial technology: Materials with differing properties can be combined to form a new material with enhanced performance. Examples are fiberglass, which combines glass fibers in a resin matrix, and reinforced concrete, in which steel rods are embedded in a concrete matrix. Binding between the dissimilar components is based on interactions at the molecular level that yield pronounced increases in the material's strength, resilience, or other properties.

The process of bone formation starts prior to birth and continues throughout the period of growth and development. Elongation of the body's long bones occurs at a thin layer of cartilage called the **epiphyseal plate** or **growth plate** (fig. 18.1*a*). As full skeletal growth is achieved, ossification replaces the epiphyseal plate with bone. At this point, the length of the bone is permanently fixed (fig. 18.1*b*).

The skeletal structures formed during early development are crude approximations of their final, mature form. Following the initial formation of a bone, its structure is continually modified to better respond to functional demands. These are the result of altered patterns of weight-bearing, muscle tension, and other stresses that continually change during normal development. For example, the transition from a young child's crawling, through brief periods of standing upright, to unassisted toddling, and then to running over a playing field, places increased demand on the skeleton to increase its strength and weight-bearing capacity. As well, the tension generated by increasingly strong muscles requires modifications of the bone to form stronger muscle attachment points.

To accommodate these demands, a process of **bone remodeling** continues throughout life. In response to demand, bone remodeling involves a constant shifting of the balance between bone deposition by **osteoblasts** and its breakdown (resorption) by **osteoclasts.** The result is a continually active bone, which, once formed and remodeled to its mature configuration, remains sensitive to any changes in

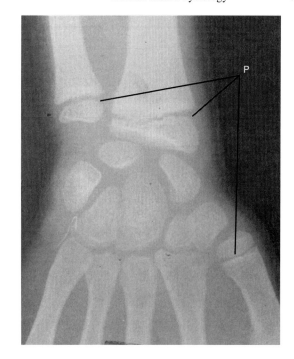

(a)

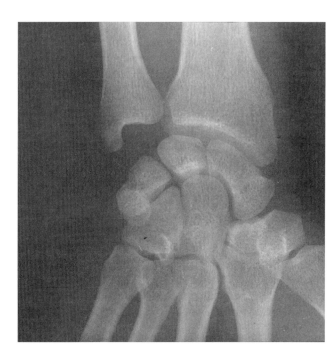

(b)

Figure 18.1   **Ossification.** (*a*) The epiphyseal plates (P) that can be seen in this radiograph indicate that ossification has not yet been completed. (*b*) This radiograph shows an adult's hand, with no epiphyseal plate visible.

demand that may arise. Vigorous body activity is matched by a stronger skeleton, while the skeleton that experiences lower activity levels, or is bedridden for a prolonged period, loses bone tissue and weakens in response. Even in an adult with an unchanging level of activity, remodeling continues

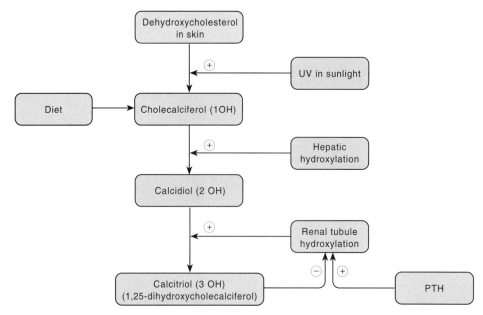

Figure 18.2 **Vitamin D Production and Regulation.** Hypoparathyroidism and renal or liver failure may produce calcitriol deficiencies, necessitating therapeutic supplementation to counter calcium imbalances.

in a steady state in which deposition is exactly matched by resorption. It is thought that this process continually renews bone structure to offset the aging of osteocytes, the cells resident in mature bone, and to replace or restore damaged **trabeculae.** These critical stress-bearing plates in the interior of bone may suffer microfractures in the course of normal loading that are repaired by bone remodeling.

Bone Metabolism and Its Regulation

Beyond its direct structural role in the skeleton, bone acts as a reservoir that can take up or supply calcium when its plasma level alters from the optimum. Accordingly, about 1% of bone's calcium is available to meet an immediate calcium demand. This **exchangeable calcium** is only loosely bound in the form of calcium phosphate and can be quickly released in response to short-term increases in parathyroid hormone (PTH) levels. When plasma PTH remains elevated over a longer period, it activates osteoclasts, and their resorption of bone makes further calcium available to the extracellular fluid. PTH also promotes the renal retention of calcium in support of falling plasma calcium levels and promotes intestinal calcium absorption through its indirect effects on vitamin D.

Vitamin D, **cholecalciferol,** was originally studied in the context of its natural occurrence in butter, eggs, and fish and was initially thought to be a vitamin—that is, an essential nutrient obtainable only in the diet. Now, it is known to be produced endogenously, so it can more accurately be regarded as a hormone. However, its status as a vitamin is so well established that the name persists. Of circulating cholecalciferol, about 20% originates in the diet while 80% is endogenous hormone.

The action of the sun's ultraviolet light on a cholesterol derivative in the skin produces cholecalciferol, with its single

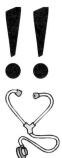

Focus on Dietary Supplementation of Vitamin D

During the winter in northern latitudes, the sun's angle may reduce skin activation of vitamin D to negligible levels for months. During this time dietary sources can meet most needs, provided that intake is adequate and well balanced. Across North America, cholecalciferol is widely added to milk, cereals, and various processed foods to ensure adequate dietary intake, particularly in children, whose growing skeletons have a high calcium demand. This practice has been effective in preventing deficiencies in children of low-income parents, especially those living in northern urban centers.

hyhdroxyl (OH) group. It, and any dietary cholecalciferol, is carried by the blood to the liver where it is modified by the addition of an OH group and in this form is given the name **calcidiol.** The kidney's nephron tubules complete formation of the fully active hormone with addition of another OH group to yield **calcitriol,** or 1,25-dihydroxycholecalciferol, the term that may appear on laboratory blood chemistry reports (fig. 18.2).

Calcitriol is 100 times more potent than calcidiol and 1,000 times more potent than cholecalciferol. The last activation step is controlled by PTH, so that increases in plasma calcitriol follow increases in PTH secretion. Once activated, calcitriol is principally taken up by the intestinal epithelium, where it indirectly promotes the active absorption of calcium from the lumen. Note also the feedback

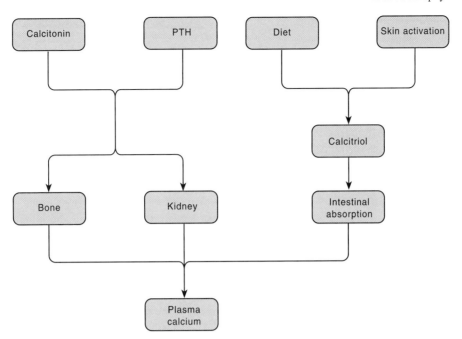

Figure 18.3   **Calcium Homeostasis.** Factors determining plasma calcium levels. Note that calcitriol has some additional systemic effects and that the role of calcitonin is minor.

regulation that calcitriol exerts: a direct effect on the kidney and an indirect input to the kidney via the calcium elevation that causes suppression of PTH secretion (fig. 18.2). Beyond its role in calcium absorption, calcitriol contributes to bone formation by influencing the deposition of some of the noncollagen proteins of osteoid. Various other nonskeletal functions of calcitriol are suspected, but they remain uncertain.

Calcitonin, from the thyroid gland, also has an effect on plasma calcium levels, opposite to that of PTH. Increased calcitonin triggers renal calcium excretion and suppresses osteoclast activity to lower calcium in the extracellular fluid. Beyond this, calcitonin's links to the other calcium-regulating mechanisms are unknown. Its role may be only a subsidiary one, in that no calcium derangements are caused by its excessive or inadequate secretion. Calcium homeostasis is summarized in figure 18.3.

Because it suppresses osteoclast activity, calcitonin has increasingly been used as a therapeutic agent to counter bone loss in osteoporosis and Paget's disease, both of which are described in the following section.

BONE PATHOPHYSIOLOGY

Bone disorders are essentially derived from infection, tumor growth, abnormal ossification, or an imbalance in bone remodeling. In metabolic bone disease, a net loss of bone **(osteopenia)** is the usual result, but conditions involving excessive **(hyperostosis),** irregular, or otherwise inappropriate bone formation also occur. Deficiency of an essential ossification factor or some derangement of its regulation may be involved, but some bone diseases remain

in the idiopathic category. Bone disorders are described here on the basis of whether they are inherited or acquired.

Genetic Bone Disorders

These rare conditions are transmitted by various patterns of inheritance. They usually involve a single factor essential to normal bone metabolism. Abnormal bone formation and skeletal defects are the result.

Osteopetrosis

This condition is also known as **Albers-Schönberg disease** or **marble bone disease.** Its most serious form is transmitted by a recessive pattern of inheritance and can therefore arise in the child of parents who have no skeletal disorder. The essential defect in osteopetrosis involves the osteoclasts. They are functionally deficient because of some abnormality of differentiation in the cell line from which they arise. In either case, the result is defective ossification, which produces excessive deposition of a bone tissue that is flawed in being brittle and easily fractured.

In mild cases, typical signs are short stature and weakened bones that fracture easily. Such cases may go unnoticed until adulthood, when an incidental radiograph reveals an unusually dense bone structure. Severe cases arise early and the victims have little chance of survival. In these conditions, excessive bone formation typically encroaches on bone marrow cavities to produce a progressively debilitating anemia and severe infections. Bone deformities in the floor of the brain case can cause increased intracranial pressure and can compress and damage cranial nerves, causing blindness, deafness, paralysis of the facial muscles, and various other cranial nerve disorders.

One therapeutic approach that has been tried is the use of marrow transplants to provide a source of normal osteoclast precursors. Although this has met with some success, the problems of suitable donor availability and the procedure's risks to anemic and otherwise weakened children are often difficult to overcome. Another approach takes advantage of the bone degradation effects of high levels of calcitriol. Administration of this substance has been beneficial in some cases.

Osteogenesis Imperfecta

The term **osteogenesis imperfecta** (OI) includes a number of related conditions that have in common an inherited defect in collagen synthesis. Specifically involved is the collagen that dominates the osteoid in which mineral deposition occurs. The result is faulty ossification, which produces osteopenia and brittle bones. In fact, you may encounter reference to these conditions as **brittle bone disease.** Defective tooth formation, a blue discoloration of the sclerae, and faulty hearing are also often present in OI.

Inheritance is by both recessive and dominant mechanisms, but scattered mutations also arise so that either, both, or neither of a victim's parents may exhibit signs of the disease. Several degrees of severity are recognized, from quite mild to an extremely severe form that is fatal prior to, or shortly following, the infant's birth (see Focus box: Worst Case OI). In mild cases, skeletal abnormalities may be noticed only as minor defects in radiographs. In those with a severe form who survive the perinatal period, pronounced stunting of growth, incomplete ossification, and various other skeletal defects may be present—for example, long bone shafts of variable thickness or length and **scoliosis** (lateral deformation of the vertebral column that can cause hypoventilation and a tendency to lung infections).

Achondroplasia

As its name indicates, this condition involves a defect in normal cartilage development. The problem is a lack of cartilage formation at the epiphyseal plates of long bones, which causes ossification to seal the plates early, preventing their further elongation. Normal ossification of other parts of the skeleton proceeds, but the abnormally short limbs and normal-sized spinal column and skull produce a characteristic skeletal disproportion. To exaggerate the effect, some bones may grow by thickening, even though they can't elongate.

The dominant inheritance of this condition means that an affected individual will probably have an affected parent. However, new mutations arise frequently, so an affected infant may have normal parents. Development of other organ systems proceeds normally, and a short but otherwise normal adult may achieve a full life span. In some cases, however, **lordosis** (anterior convexity) of the spinal column may

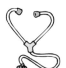

Focus on Worst Case OI

As noted, those with severe osteogenesis imperfecta who survive the early postnatal period face a difficult existence. Most will die young. Sadly, many severely affected individuals do not survive their period of intrauterine development. In these cases, spontaneous abortion often occurs, with the fetuses showing evidence of many bone fractures that occurred during early stages of development. Those who survive the gestation still must face the trauma of the birth process. Many do not survive the multiple rib and long bone fractures that result, or the brain damage that results from the lack of normal skull ossification.

---

arise, causing spinal cord and spinal nerve compression. In the very rare case in which each parent contributes a defective gene, the condition is quite severe and the affected newborn rarely survives much beyond birth.

Acquired Bone Disorders

We will consider bone infection and tumors of bone after describing the major metabolic bone disorders. In this group, osteopenia is typical, and only one disorder—Paget's disease—is characterized by significant bone deposition to compensate for increased bone resorption.

Paget's Disease (Osteitis Deformans)

In this condition, focal derangements of bone resorption and deposition occur over the course of the disease. In the initial stages during middle age, bone resorption dominates (the **osteolytic phase**). Later, in the **mixed phase,** bone deposition rates approximate resorption rates, but the newly formed bone is abnormal. It is coarsely structured and crudely organized, often forming dense, focal masses. This characteristic tissue is known as **pagetic bone** (fig. 18.4). In the late, or **osteosclerotic phase,** resorption declines and harder, more dense bone tissue is formed, again in a focal pattern.

Many individuals with Paget's disease are asymptomatic, but incidental radiographic studies may reveal the sites of pagetic bone deposition, as may elevations of serum alkaline phosphatase levels that result from the high bone turnover rates in Paget's disease. In later stages, patients may become aware of focal limb deformities or of skull thickening on the basis of a change in hat size.

Bones of the skull, vertebral column, and proximal portions of the major long bones are most typically involved (fig. 18.5). Skull weight can be significantly increased, so much so that patients carry the head in a characteristic bowed posture. In extreme cases, the heavy skull can cause compression fractures of the superior vertebrae.

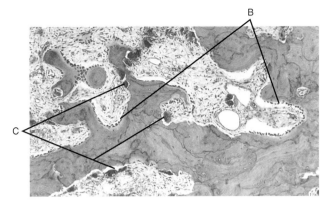

Figure 18.4 **Pagetic Bone.** Histologic examination of pagetic bone reveals a characteristic pattern of irregular and crudely structured bone. The dark spots aligned at the trabecular surfaces are the nuclei of osteoblasts (B), while the larger, multinucleated cells are osteoclasts (C).

Focus on Other "Paget's" Conditions

The term **Paget's disease** is also applied to a rare group of epithelial tumors that primarily affect the nipple, breast glands, vulva, penis, and scrotum. This section describes Paget's disease **of bone.** Once a bone context is clearly established, the term *Paget's disease* is descriptive and widely used. In other contexts, it is important to specify, say, Paget's disease **of the nipple** (a type of breast cancer) or **of the scrotum,** to avoid confusion with the bone disorder.

Hearing disorders are often present as well, and may derive from thickening of the ossicles or from compression of the eighth cranial nerve. Microfractures of pagetic bone and nerve compression are thought to be the principal causes of the pain experienced in Paget's disease. Bone fractures may occur at sites of bone resorption in the initial osteolytic phase. Because the bone is weakened, normally trivial stresses may cause the break. Although painful and delayed, healing does occur.

Note that because of the focal nature of these skeletal effects, even though various bones are affected, most bone is usually quite normal.

In rare cases, the abnormal blood vessel configuration of pagetic bone allows blood to by-pass normal capillary channels. The by-passed tissues become ischemic and, in response, local vasodilation triggers compensation reflexes that increase cardiac output. Where skeletal involvement is extensive, this extra cardiac demand can lead to high-output heart failure if the heart is already compromised by some other myocardial or valvular defect.

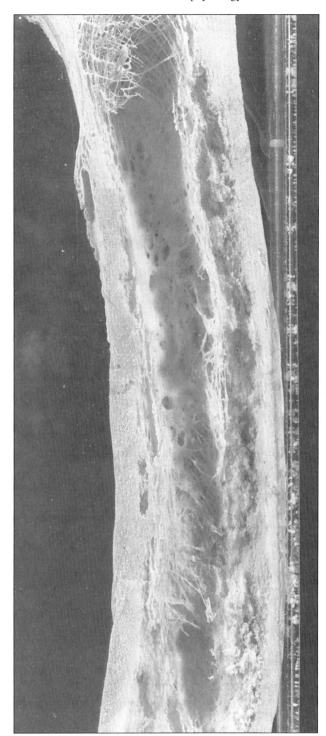

Figure 18.5 **Paget's Disease.** Note the excessive deposition of coarsely structured bone in this section of the tibia. The curvature is also abnormal.

This is the tibia of an 83-year-old man who died of respiratory complications of Paget's disease. Following diagnosis, the disease slowly progressed, causing various skull and long bone deformities, as well as a degree of vertebral collapse. In the sectioned and dried tibia shown here, elongation and anterior bowing can be seen, as well as significant thickening of cortical bone and coarsely structured cancellous bone.

Another serious threat confronts about 1 in 100 of those suffering from Paget's disease. In these, osteogenic or other sarcomas arise in affected bones, often at multiple sites. These tumors seem more resistant to therapy than the sarcomas that arise apart from Paget's disease. As a result, prognosis is poor.

Because it is often asymptomatic, much Paget's disease is undiagnosed. Estimates of incidence vary from 1% to 3% of adults, with significant worldwide variations. Most of those affected are over 60, and incidence increases with age, reaching as high as 10% of those age 80. Etiology is not clear, but a link to infection by a paramyxovirus has been established. Organisms in this group are responsible for measles, mumps, and various other infections. It may be that, following an initial viral infection, the virus becomes dormant. When activated in later life, it affects osteoclasts and disrupts the bone remodeling process.

Osteoporosis

Osteoporosis is the most common metabolic bone disease in North America. Its essential defect is gradual and progressive loss of bone mass. With steady loss of bone, a point is reached when weakened bones cannot resist the loads applied to them and they break. Bone fracture and its associated pain are the key features of osteoporosis. Most osteoporosis is idiopathic and is designated **primary osteoporosis,** while **secondary osteoporosis** involves bone loss due to some identifiable derangement.

Primary Osteoporosis After one's genetically determined peak bone mass is attained, it is maintained until the late 30s. After this, bone tissue is lost at the rate of about 0.5% per year. After many years, a critical point is reached at which bone is too weak to resist fracturing. Especially vulnerable are those with an initially lower skeletal mass, in that they will more quickly reach critical bone weakness. Groups with low skeletal mass are Caucasians and Asians; females lower than males. In males with large skeletal mass, fracturing is usually deferred until old age, or it may never occur. In women, generally, and Caucasian women in particular, an initially low skeletal mass mean aging effects start to produce fractures after about age 60. This age-related bone loss, designated **type II osteoporosis,** affects twice as many women as men. Bones most involved in this **senile osteoporosis** are the femoral neck, humerus, tibia, and hip. The essential, underlying defect is a slightly reduced degree of bone deposition during normal bone remodeling. Although small, over many years the net effect is loss of skeletal mass and weaker bones (fig. 18.6).

The key feature in **type I osteoporosis** is more rapid bone loss that causes fractures at an earlier age. The underlying problem lies in the osteoclasts that excessively resorb bone, causing a loss of bone mass. Postmenopausal women, espcially Caucasians with their lower skeletal mass, are at greatest risk, with fracture rates increasing about ten years following menopause. The link to menopause is the fall of estrogens, which triggers release

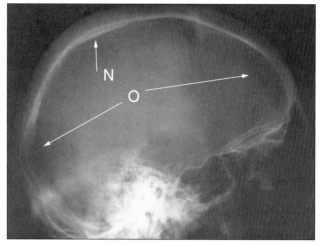

(a)

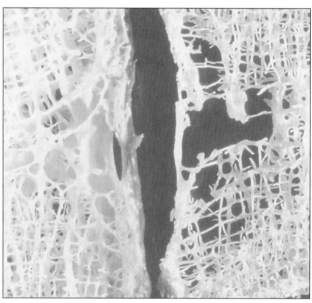

(b)

Figure 18.6   **Osteoporosis.** (*a*) This radiograph of the skull shows areas of osteoporotic bone loss (O), which can be compared with normal regions (N). (*b*) Normal trabecular bone at left for comparison with trabeculae in osteoporosis at right.

of various mediators (IL-6, TNF, PGE$_2$) that stimulate osteoclast activity. In such cases, bone loss rates can be maintained at ten times normal for years. The effect is most pronounced in cancellous bone, vertebral bodies, and the distal radii.

Etiology A variety of etiological factors combine in type I osteoporosis. Genetics seems to play a role—women from families with increased postmenopausal fracture incidence are themselves at greater risk. The exact genetic contribution is unknown; perhaps it is simply low bone mass, but more subtle effects may be involved, such as especially sensitive osteoclasts that become hyperactive once the inhibitory effects of estrogens are withdrawn following menopause. Of course, any factor that increases and maintains skeletal mass is beneficial in delaying bone loss to critical fracture levels, (e.g., physical activity and adequate intake of calcium and vitamin D). Note that obesity counters the development of osteoporosis by placing additional demand on the skeleton. Factors that promote osteoporosis are physical inactivity, calcium, phosphate, and vitamin D deficiencies; heavy caffeine and alcohol ingestion; and smoking.

Prevention and Therapy There is no known cure for osteoporosis. Current therapy aims at slowing the rate of bone loss and promoting new deposition in the hope of delaying the onset of fracturing. Various approaches are employed. Calcium and vitamin D supplements are used to support bone deposition during normal modeling. Calcitonin may be administered to support plasma calcium. Hormone replacement therapy (HRT) in postmenopausal women reduces bone resorption, as do the **biophosphonates,** a category of therapeutic agent that binds to bone to inhibit osteoclast action. The challenge of effective therapy is made more difficult because fractures usually occur before osteoporosis is diagnosed. This means that by the time the disease is recognized, loss of bone is already significant, and much more difficult to deal with. Diagnosis in osteoporosis has been aided by sophisticated techniques that assess bone density. In particular, **dual X-ray absorptiometry** (DXA) has been adopted as the diagnostic standard by the World Health Organization.

Indications are that, as with many conditions, prevention is the best means of coping with osteoporosis. The key, essentially, is developing the maximal skeletal mass, as determined by one's genetic makeup. This means ensuring that adequate dietary intake of calcium and vitamin D, as well as all the other nutrients, during the period of growth and development. Once the skeleton is fully developed, by about age 28 in most cases, its strength must be maintained through a lifelong pattern of physical activity that provides adequate skeletal loading, and by sufficient nutrient support for the remodeling process. It also makes sense to avoid cigarette smoking and heavy caffeine and alcohol use, which are associated with increased osteoporosis incidence. In an age in which modern therapeutics can offer rapid and effective responses to many medical problems, this recommendation may not seem like much, but an optimally developed skeleton is still recognized as the best defense against osteoporosis.

In the elderly, whose bone mass is already reduced, preventive measures that reduce the likelihood of a fall and fracture are important. Such measures must take into account the reduced vision, confusion, and altered balance and gait that are common among the elderly. Relevant side effects of medications must also not be overlooked.

Secondary Osteoporosis A loss of bone mass due to an excess of resorption over deposition may also arise as the result of some other derangement. This condition is known as secondary osteoporosis. The cause may be a nutritional deficiency, a genetic or endocrine abnormality, therapeutic drugs, certain tumors, or some other disease states. Various of these conditions are listed in table 18.1.

Focus on Rethinking HRT

For years, hormone replacement therapy (HRT) has been a mainstay of therapy for osteoporosis and much evidence clearly supported its ability to reduce bone loss and reduce fractures. As well, HRT has been routinely offered by well-meaning physicians to postmenopausal women because estrogens alleviated many of the side effects of menopause: hot flashes, memory problems, skin looseness and wrinkles, vaginal dryness, etc. Note that HRT was prescribed even for those women whose menopausal symptoms were mild and transitory on the assumption that estrogens also conferred a global protection against atherosclerosis and the MI and strokes associated with it.

A recent study has raised serious doubt about HRT and, as a result, its use is being reevaluated. The eight-year, U.S. government-sponsored study involved over 16,000 healthy women, half of whom took a commonly prescribed estrogen/progestin preparation while the other half received an inactive placebo. Since the benefits of HRT were well established in women with osteoporosis, independent monitors assessed the women during the study to be certain that those on the placebo weren't adversely affected by hormone deficiencies. Five years into the study, the monitors called a halt. While the women receiving the hormones had significantly lower rates of hip fracture, the alarm was sounded because they also suffered increased risks of myocardial infarction, CVA, thrombosis, and breast cancer.

Because this study was well designed and involved so many women, its results are having a significant impact. It would appear that HRT to reduce osteoporosis, atherosclerosis, and postmenopausal symptoms will be significantly modified. Lower-dose therapy for shorter periods will likely become more common to maximize benefits and minimize risks.

 Checkpoint 18.1

Because life expectancy is increasing, the coming years may well see epidemic levels of osteoporosis-related bone fracture. This may present a major public health problem. Currently, 50% of 80-year-olds suffer vertebral compression fractures, with 90% of hip fractures occurring in those past the age of 70.

Rickets and Osteomalacia

In these conditions, the defect in bone metabolism involves inadequate mineral deposition in an essentially normal organic matrix. The result is a softened bone that is subject to malformation or distortion, which causes pain. A broad

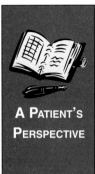

"The Long Road Back"—Osteoporosis

—Pamela Horner

It all started with three bone fractures occurring over a period of only a year and a half. A toe, a rib, and my wrist were all broken by relatively minor stresses that shouldn't have bothered normal bones. X-rays of my wrist showed some fuzziness, indicating possible loss of bone density. When the cast came off, my G.P. referred me to a specialist for possible diagnosis of osteoporosis. A month after this examination, since no more was said about it, I assumed there was no evidence of a problem.

Four months later, however, I began to have serious back problems. I wasn't alarmed on Friday, when I felt a twinge bending over the deep freeze. By the next Monday I was in such agony, I knew I needed help. I first saw a chiropractor and initially experienced some small improvement. But one morning, six weeks after that first twinge, I awoke barely able to struggle out of bed. I went to my G.P., who referred me to a physiotherapist, explaining that most back pain is muscular in origin and responds well to rest and physiotherapy. In my case these did no good at all. The mere getting to and from the office and climbing onto the table gave me excruciating pain. The therapist, obviously underestimating the degree of my disability, would blithely instruct me to "turn on your left side, now over to the right side," not knowing he was demanding the impossible. After two visits, I phoned my G.P., demanding some X-rays and some more definite diagnosis of my problem.

While awaiting the results of the X-rays and some other tests, I continued to suffer greatly. Getting in and out of bed was so agonizing that I spent most nights sitting in a chair with a heating pad at my back. I still dragged myself to my part-time receptionist job, but looking back it's hard to remember how I managed it.

When my diagnostic results were in, they spelled the end of my working days for a long time to come. They showed an alarming loss of bone mass and several compressed vertebrae. The doctor, extremely concerned, put me into the hospital for further tests. It was imperative to seek the cause of the extreme calcium depletion that was unusual for a woman only 54 years old.

I spent 12 days in the hospital, during which time I established a routine of sorts, although I was only truly comfortable flat on my back with pillows under my knees. Of course there were the added discomforts of daily blood withdrawal, 24-hour urine testing, and more X-rays. All of this confirmed the diagnosis of type I (postmenopausal) osteoporosis, and a regimen of calcium, fluoride, estrogen, and vitamin D therapy began.

On arriving at home, my back pain was still severe, so the first problem was where to sleep. The first couple of nights I opted for the living room sofa because I could curl my spine against its back for support. When the home therapist visited, she outlawed the couch because it was too soft. This sunny-dispositioned woman was the most helpful person the medical profession had yet offered in terms of helping me to deal with my pain. She showed me how to "log-roll" from side to side to avoid painful twisting and how to use my arms for support in getting in and out of bed.

While pain and general weakness forced me to bed for the greater part of the day, I interspersed these rests with "walk-abouts" through the house. Gradually, I worked my walking up a few steps down the walk to greet my husband on his return from work, then slowly increasing to three houses down the street. After a month of this I was getting all the way around the block.

The psychological stress associated with the acute phase of osteoporosis presented a major problem. It was difficult to be so utterly dependent on my family for the basic needs of life. For example, I couldn't shower or wash my hair without assistance, and being so helpless made me terrified of being alone. When I first ventured out on my own, I had an almost pathological fear of falling.

Over the next year I developed a more rigorous exercise program to which I credit my present near-normal mobility. I'm psychologically much more stable, partly because of the effects of becoming increasingly independent, but also due to the constant support of family and friends.

range of etiologies reflects the various nutritional requirements, regulatory functions, and tissues involved in calcium and bone metabolism.

Rickets

The condition of **rickets** is due to inadequate mineralization of the developing skeleton. It is primarily a condition of dietary vitamin D deficiency in infants and children and is rarely seen in the industrialized Western world, except in isolated pockets of poverty and among those ignorant of nutritional requirements. Softened bones in the developing skeleton are subject to deformity as soft tissue mass and skeletal loading progress. Shortened, deformed limbs are the result—bowed legs, for example (fig. 18.7). Characteristic deformities of the skull, chest, and teeth are typical, as is an increased tendency to bone fractures. Therapy to supply adequate vitamin D and calcium is usually successful in correcting the condition.

Osteomalacia   The term **osteomalacia** is applied to the condition of inadequate bone mineralization in the adult.

Table 18.1	Conditions Causing Secondary Osteoporosis

Endocrine Conditions	**Nutritional Deficiencies**	**Genetic Conditions**	**Miscellaneous**
Diabetes mellitus	Malabsorption syndromes	Osteogenesis imperfecta	Prolonged immobilization
Adrenocortical hypersecretion	Scurvy	Marfan's syndrome	Various metabolic bone diseases
Thyroid hypersecretion	Hypocalcemia		Rheumatoid arthritis*
Ovarian/testicular hyposecretion			Alcoholism*
Chronic steroid therapy			Chronic obstructive pulmonary disease*
			Epilepsy*

*Pathogenesis unclear

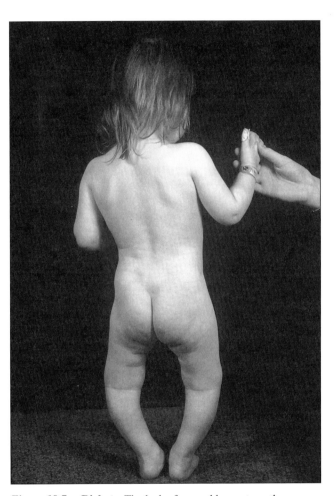

Figure 18.7 **Rickets.** The lack of normal bone strength causes the legs to bow under the weight of the upper body.

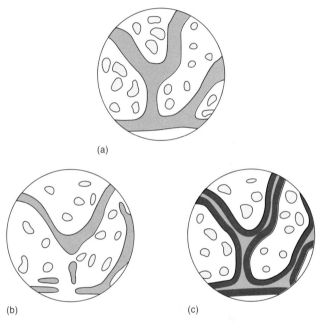

Figure 18.8 **Bone Loss.** (*a*) Normally ossified trabeculae are interconnected to isolate regions of yellow marrow, which contain deposits of adipose tissue. (*b*) Osteoporosis is characterized by loss of bone mass and thinning of trabeculae. (*c*) Osteomalacia. The darkened regions represent the surfaces at which abnormal remodeling has produced inadequately mineralized matrix.

Because initial skeletal development is normal, the later inability to maintain bone deposition during remodeling usually produces no bone deformities or other gross indications of the problem. A common symptom in later stages is bone pain, which may be accompanied by generalized muscle weakness and an increased predisposition to fractures.

In the general population, dietary vitamin D deficiencies are seldom the cause of osteomalacia, except for iso-lated cases in which the elderly or institutionalized receive improper care. More often, osteomalacia is due to a GI malabsorption problem, to a renal defect of phosphate retention that results in hypophosphatemia and defective bone mineralization, or to faulty activation of cholecalciferol in chronic liver or kidney diseases. The elderly are a population subgroup more often affected as a result of inadequate diet or, more commonly, a lack of outdoor activity, which reduces the sun's activation of vitamin D in the skin. Osteomalacia may accompany and complicate osteoporosis. Both conditions can be asymptomatic for years, but the bone aches and pains associated with osteomalacia may draw attention to the problem, which might otherwise be unnoticed until a fracture occurs. Figure 18.8 illustrates the essential changes from normal in osteomalacia and osteoporosis.

Osteomyelitis

This is the condition of bone inflammation, usually in response to its infection by a pyogenic (pus-producing) bacterium. Usually a staphylococcal or streptococcal organism is involved, but various other organisms are also known to infect bone. The source of such bacteria may be the blood, which delivers organisms from some distant infected site, but the widespread use of antibiotics to control infections has greatly reduced this cause. More often the organisms are introduced as a result of bone trauma involving a fracture, penetrating wound, or surgery. The long bones of children are most often involved, but in adults the spinal column may also be the focus of infection.

In acute osteomyelitis, proliferation of the bacteria is followed by the formation of a pus-filled abscess. Bone necrosis follows due to bacterial action, but also because of a reduction of blood supply at the scene. Supply vessels in marrow may be compressed as the abscess extends into adjacent marrow spaces. Blood vessels may also be blocked by bacteria and pus spreading through the bone's interconnecting blood channels. Also, as pus passes through damaged bone to its surface the periosteum can be forced up, tearing the blood vessels that pass through it to the bone's interior. Beyond the general effects of ischemia, the compromised blood flow not only reduces efficiency of the inflammatory response, it also restricts antibiotic access to the site where it is needed.

As infection progresses, subperiosteal osteocytes respond to the damage by forming new segments of **reactive bone** adjacent to the infection site. These can form a wall or sheath of new bone, isolating necrotic bone, pus, and bacteria from the phagocytes needed to clear the site. Surviving organisms can proliferate periodically to produce a pattern of chronic recurrence. In some cases, a permanent **sinus** may form. This is an epithelium-lined tract through which pus and necrotic bone fragments drain to the surface.

Clinically, osteomyelitis is characterized by pain and swelling at the infection site. Chills and fever are also typical, with lab reports confirming the presence of the infecting agent in only 50% of cases. Therapy often requires surgical clearing of necrotic bone and the draining of abscesses in addition to the administration of antibiotics. If therapy is unavailable or unduly delayed, complications can include rapid progression throughout the infected bone, joint damage, and pathological fracture (fig. 18.9). There is also a risk that organisms may be carried to other parts of the body to produce more extensive infection.

Bone Tumors

Bone provides a supportive environment for metastases and so is a very common site of secondary tumor growth. A carcinoma is the usual primary tumor, most often arising in the prostate, breast, thyroid, lung, or kidney. Access to bone is by way of the blood, rather than lymph, and the sites most often involved are the bones of the axial skeleton

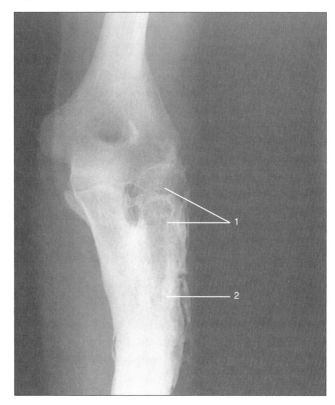

Figure 18.9   Osteomyelitis. Note the areas of necrosis (1) and reactive bone (2) in this radiograph.
A 12-year-old girl deeply lacerated her arm in the region of the elbow in a fall from a tree. The underlying bone subsequently became infected, producing the bone necrosis evident in this X-ray. Antibiotic therapy was able to arrest the process after surgery to clear necrotic bone and establish drainage of the infection site. Some permanent damage to the adjacent joint was unavoidable, however, and the patient was left with some restriction of movement.

(except the skull) and the proximal femur and humerus. Once established, a secondary tumor may grow and invade locally, disrupting the organization of the osseous tissue by inducing bone breakdown (**osteolysis**) or new bone formation. These effects are due to the release by the metastatic cells of substances that activate local osteoclasts, osteoblasts, or both. The result is a mix of growing tumor, resorbing bone, and new bone formation at the secondary site. Carcinomas, and some sarcomas, differ in their abilities to stimulate resident bone cells, so each produces its characteristic pattern of secondary growth, involving greater, lesser, or no effects on osteoclasts or osteoblasts.

Primary Bone Tumors These are much less common than secondary tumors, but can have devastating effects in that they arise most often in the young. Actively growing bone is much more likely to undergo a neoplastic transformation, and pain is an early indication of the tumor's expansion within the densely organized bone tissue. Like secondary tumors, primary bone tumors induce osteolysis, so that weakening of the bone, which produces a tendency to

Table 18.2   Selected Features of Principal Bone Tumors

Tumor	Status	Site	Affected Sex	Affected Age	Comment
Osteoid osteoma	B	Long bone diaphyses	Male	Under 25	Pain is significant
Osteochondroma	B	Metaphyses	=	Under 20	Common bone tumor
Chondroblastoma	B	Epiphyses	Male	Under 25	Rare, significant pain
Osteogenic sarcoma	M	Long bones, knee	Male	10–20	Most common bone tumor, lung metastases
Chondrosarcoma	M	Pelvis, ribs, proximal femur, and humerus	Male	Over 40	Second most common bone tumor
Ewing's tumor (sarcoma)	M	Distal femur and pelvis	Male	Under 20	Hemopoietic cell tumor, limited metastasis
Giant cell tumor	B/M	Epiphyses, knee	=	20–40	Benign form may damage locally

B: benign; M: malignant; =: equal incidence among males and females

pathological fracture, is a common feature. In addition, normal bone adjacent to the tumor may respond to tumor pressure by altering its pattern of remodeling. This response produces the altered and expanded contours of the bone's surface that are seen in the area of tumor growth. The danger in malignancies is, of course, metastasis, and in bone tumors, it typically involves the lung. In many tragic cases, amputation is necessary to cope with the primary tumor when other therapy is too little or too late. For unknown reasons, most bone tumors arise more frequently in males than females, with one exception—the giant cell tumor (table 18.2).

About one-third of primary bone tumors are benign. They arise from bone or cartilage cells and can be either of minimal significance or quite painful and predisposing to fracture. They can be surgically removed, and a bone graft used to restore the damaged site. Prosthetic devices are employed where a limb resection is unavoidable. Examples of benign bone tumors are the rare **osteoma,** which typically affects the skull, and the **osteoid osteoma,** usually seen in long bone diaphyses. Osteoid osteoma occurs more frequently in males and, although the tumor mass is small, it is usually quite painful. **Osteoblastoma** usually involves a larger tumor mass and primarily arises in vertebrae and long bones. A rare benign bone tumor arising from bone cartilage is the **chondroblastoma.** It usually develops in the epiphyses of the arm and leg bones.

Osteogenic sarcoma (osteosarcoma) is the most common malignant tumor of bone. It usually arises in those 10–20 years old and has a great predisposition to blood-borne metastasis to the lung. The region of the knee is most often involved, but the other long bones may be affected (fig. 18.10). The previously very poor prognosis for this tumor has improved with recent chemotherapy advances. By the time the diagnosis is made, metastasis has already occurred. However, chemotherapeutic agents are quite ef-

fective in destroying secondary growth, and up to 80% of patients remain disease-free after five years. Even when limb amputation is necessary, currently available artificial limbs offer far better possibilities for more normal mobility.

Chondrosarcoma, the second most common bone malignancy, is atypical in that it arises later than most bone tumors: after age 40. Many of these slow-growing malignancies are thought to arise in benign cartilage tumors in bone, some of whose cells become malignant. The tumor typically arises and grows in the interior of the pelvis, ribs, and proximal femur and humerus. It slowly expands, inducing osteolysis and sometimes breaking through the bone's surface. The cartilaginous tumor mass may contain variable regions of ossification. Although it is slow-growing, metastasis to the lung is not uncommon.

Ewing's tumor (Ewing's sarcoma) is a rare and highly malignant tumor of uncertain cellular origin. It arises principally in the limbs and pelvis of young males. Extensive and early metastasis, as well as rapid local bone invasion, contribute to the destructive effects of this condition. Although it is a threatening malignancy, refinements in therapy that combine surgery and radiation have significantly improved prognosis in Ewing's tumor.

Giant cell tumor is also known as **osteoclastoma.** The tumor's dominant cell type derives from precursors that resemble fibroblasts. Also present, and perhaps induced to form by the dominant tumor cells, are giant multinucleated cells that resemble osteoclasts. This tumor typically grows only locally, resorbing bone as it expands. It produces early local pain and swelling, often eliciting early surgical treatment that can completely remove the tumor. In such cases, prognosis is excellent, but if all tumor elements are not excised, recurrence at the original site is common. Some giant cell tumors metastasize early to cloud the prognosis.

Table 18.2 summarizes some of the features of the principal bone tumors.

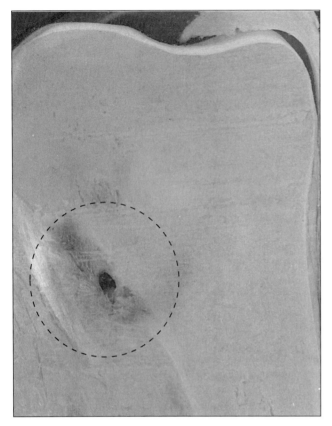

Figure 18.10   Osteogenic Sarcoma. The tumor and its necrotic core can be seen in the epiphysis of this long bone.

This osteogenic sarcoma of the tibia caused amputation of the leg of a 19-year-old woman. She had experienced some knee pain for two to three months before seeing her physician, who attributed the pain to a basketball injury. The pain persisted for six months, and when it increased to the point where she couldn't sleep, she saw another physician. She was five months pregnant by this time. No swelling or other surface abnormality could be identified, but X-ray studies and a biopsy confirmed the presence of the tumor. To spare her developing infant from exposure to chemotherapeutic agents, the woman opted for amputation of her leg above the knee. The infant was successfully brought to term, but the mother died of lung and liver metastases 18 months later. Figure 6.9 shows a microscope field from the biopsy specimen.

JOINT DISORDERS

Bones meet to form joints, or articulations. Most of these are freely movable joints known as **synovial** or **diarthrotic joints.** The less numerous **synarthrotic joints** are essentially incapable of movement, but provide strong binding of the bones. Pain and loss of mobility from joint disorders are very common around the world. The two most frequently encountered disorders are osteoarthritis and rheumatoid arthritis. This section will describe these and some less common conditions. First, however, a brief review of normal joint anatomy and physiology is in order.

Normal Diarthrotic Joints

The diarthrotic joint (fig. 18.11), which is most often involved in joint disease, is characterized by the presence of

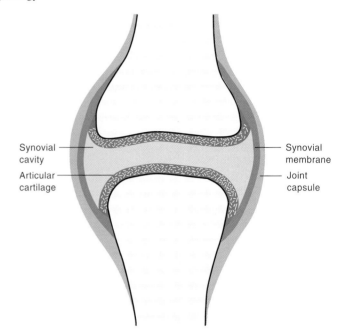

Figure 18.11   Joint Structure. The essential structure of a typical diarthrotic joint, seen in section. Synovial fluid is present in the synovial cavity.

a **synovial cavity** containing a lubricant, the **synovial fluid.** This fluid is also the nutrient medium that supplies the cells of the **articular cartilages,** which line the articular surfaces of the bones that form the joint. Synovial fluid is produced by the **synovial membrane** or **synovium,** which lines the **fibrous capsule,** the tough, protective sleeve of fibrous tissue that seals and protects diarthrotic joints. The synovial membrane or synovium lines all internal joint surfaces except those of the articular cartilages. Its villi and microvilli provide a very large surface area that favors the formation of synovial fluid. The free motion of diarthrotic joints is principally due to the smooth surface of the highly polished articular cartilages and the lubricating film of synovial fluid.

Providing for freedom of motion is one major joint function. The second is that of weight-bearing and weight transfer from one bone to another. The chief factors that make this possible are the related muscle masses that operate at the joint. These absorb much of the energy being transferred across the joint. Also a factor is the internal cancellous (spongy) bone architecture of the epiphysis, with its trabeculae arranged to efficiently distribute load. The resilience of cancellous bone combines with the effect of the joint's muscles to relieve most joint stress. This means that loading of the articular cartilages is normally kept to low levels, well tolerated by these thin (maximum 6 mm) layers of hyaline cartilage.

Osteoarthritis

Osteoarthritis (OA) is the most commonly encountered joint disease in North America. Despite its name, this disease has only a minimal inflammatory component, and so is often

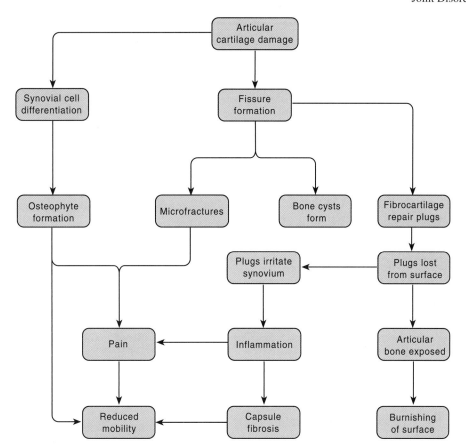

Figure 18.12   **Pathogenesis of Osteoarthritis.**

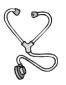

Focus on Terminology: A Clarification

Note that free, unrestricted joint motion is not the same as a joint's **mobility,** or **range of motion.** The shoulder joints and those between the articular processes of adjacent vertebrae are both diarthrotic joints. The range of motion is great in the shoulder and quite small between the vertebrae, but in both cases, what movement does occur is free and unimpeded.

---

called **degenerative joint disease** (DJD). It is osteoarthritis that is responsible for much of the pain and loss of mobility associated with the aging process. Its incidence is low in the young, but increasing age yields increasing evidence of joint damage. By age 65, over 85% of people have some degree of joint degeneration that is detectable in X-rays. Fortunately, only about 30% of these suffer pain or restricted joint function.

The underlying process begins in the articular cartilage, which becomes thin, irregular, and frayed. Cracks or fissures then develop in the articular cartilage, and with progression they fill with synovial fluid and penetrate to the underlying bone. Such fissures may extend through the thin surface of articular bone to form fluid-filled cysts, around

which reactive bone may form. Microfractures in the subchondral bone may also arise. The response to these changes is mitosis of chondrocytes and a new vascular supply to the damaged region, which leads to the formation of fibrocartilage repair plugs. As a result of the joint loading associated with normal activities, these plugs may be loosened and stripped away, exposing the bone's surface. Continued loading and friction over these surfaces causes them to become burnished; that is, they develop a smooth, hardened, ivorylike texture.

The synovial membrane is indirectly affected by these changes. Fragments of fibrocartilage, dislodged from their site of formation, can react at the synovial membrane's surface, inducing an inflammatory response. This may be a factor in the pain of osteoarthritis. Subsequent fibrous repair in the damaged, adjacent joint capsule may also restrict joint motion. To further complicate the problem, cells from the synovial membrane adjacent to the articular cartilage can develop into osteoblasts in response to the damage. The result is the formation of bony projections, called **osteophytes** or **bone spurs,** at the periphery of the joint. These are thought to be a significant factor in the pain and limitation of joint mobility that are characteristic of osteoarthritis (fig. 18.12).

The degenerative process primarily affects one or more of the larger weight-bearing joints, although finger joints are sometimes involved (fig. 18.13). Often, a link to long-term occupational or athletic joint stress is an underlying

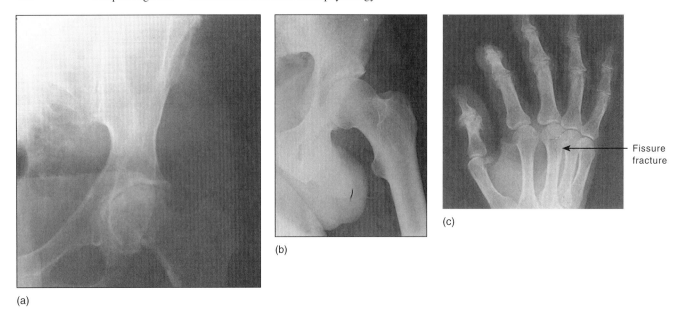

Figure 18.13   **Osteoarthritis.** Compare the articular surfaces of (*a*) a femur and hip damaged by DJD with (*b*) the normal hip joint. (*c*) Finger involvement; note the fissure fracture that extends from the distal articular surface of one of the right metacarpals.

factor. For this reason, osteoarthritis is considered to be related to wear and tear on the articular cartilages, although a biochemical defect in the joint cartilage may be an underlying aspect of the problem. In some cases, a malformed joint, obesity, or some postural defect may be the cause of excessive joint loading. There is also some evidence for a genetic component to this disease, but its exact nature is difficult to determine because patterns of activity in a family can influence joint use and wear. It may involve genetic factors that produce a weakened cartilage or destructive overreaction to joint loading.

When a contributing factor to joint stress can be identified, the term **secondary OA** is used. Such cases may involve young people who have suffered joint injury in athletics or automobile or other accidents, and who face the difficult prospect of many years of joint pain. Where no particular etiology is detectable, the condition is called **primary OA.**

Typically, joint aches and stiffness in osteoarthritis arise gradually in middle age, signaling that the process of degeneration has begun. These symptoms increase with activity and diminish with rest, and there is usually no pronounced inflammatory swelling or redness in the adjacent tissues. Osteoarthritis effects are confined to the joint and produce no systemic signs or symptoms. Increasing age finds the condition progressing, with pain and stiffness intensifying and becoming persistent. Most serious loss of mobility results from hip or knee involvement. When present in the distal interphalangeal joints, osteophytes are known as **Heberden's nodes.** At the proximal interphalangeals they are termed **Bouchard's nodes.**

Since there is no known way to prevent or arrest the degenerative process in OA, therapy is quite limited. For most sufferers, analgesics are helpful, as are activities that minimize joint strain. Of course, reducing any obvious ag-

Checkpoint 18.2

A Checkpoint in chapter 17 raised the issue of obesity as a cause of the rapidly rising incidence of NIDDM. Well, obesity is also a significant contributor to osteoarthritis in the knees. The extra weight excessively loads knee joints and the altered gait and posture needed to cope with the additional body weight often alters the angles at which forces are transmitted to joint surfaces. There is evidence that each 8 kg (17 lb) increase in weight adds significant risk of damage to the articular cartilage of the knee.

gravating factor, such as occupational joint stresses or obesity, will be beneficial. In severe cases, surgical removal of bone spurs or replacement of joints may be indicated.

Rheumatoid Arthritis

In contrast to osteoarthritis, **rheumatoid arthritis** (RA) is a systemic disease with prominent involvement of the joints. It initially affects the synovium, with later effects in articular cartilage and bone. It is an inflammatory condition that primarily affects the joints of the hands, wrists, ankles, and feet, with systemic effects involving the heart, lungs, skin, and other organs. It is variable in its severity—from so mild that it is almost unnoticed, to a severe condition that destroys and grossly distorts joints and reduces life expectancy. Also characteristic is its variable clinical pattern of remission and exacerbation. About 1% of the adult population is affected, with incidence among women about three times that among men. Age of onset is usually in the 20s or

30s, but RA has been known to arise as early as infancy or as late as the 90s.

Etiology

Rheumatoid arthritis is an essentially idiopathic disease that is characterized by immune-mediated destruction of joints. It appears that a genetic predisposition is in some way involved. In affected individuals, synovial macrophage receptors bind antigens, which in turn triggers the sequence of events that destroy the joint. The nature of the antigens that can induce this response in sensitive individuals is the subject of much research.

Some evidence suggests that the antigens are introduced by an infection, with suspicion falling on the Epstein-Barr virus, paroviruses, and mycobacteria. Other evidence suggests that RA may be an autoimmune disorder. In this proposed scheme, anticollagen antibodies are involved, but rather than causing the initial damage in RA, they may play more of a role in its progression. An autoimmune role is also indicated by the presence of **rheumatoid factor** (RF) in most cases of RA. RF is an antibody against immunoglobulin G (IgG), which plays a role in the pathogenesis of RA.

Pathogenesis of RA

Analysis of the joint changes associated with RA reveals a pattern of chronic inflammation that dominates in the synovium, with acute inflammation effects seen in the synovial fluid of the joint space. In the synovium, early changes involve cellular proliferation and damage to its microcirculation, perhaps due to an immune mechanism. Thrombosis and new vessel formation are also associated with the early joint changes in RA.

Synovial cells, T and B lymphocytes, and fibroblasts contribute to the increased cellularity in the synovium. The immune cells are activated, a fact suggesting that an immune stimulus is present, but its source is unclear. The thickening synovium becomes irregular, with its surface thrown into fingerlike projections that extend into the joint space. Its extension and covering of adjacent joint surfaces resembles a cloth, so the term **pannus,** from the Latin for cloth, is used to describe it. Swelling accompanies these changes, as does stiffness and pain.

The acute inflammatory component in these early stages of RA is seen in the excessive production of synovial fluid and the presence in it of large numbers of PMNs. Immune complexes, histamine, and other mediators are thought to induce the increased blood flow, neutrophil emigration, and fluid exudate formation. Pain, swelling, and joint stiffness are also produced by the acute inflammation effects.

If therapy is instituted at this early stage of the disease, inflammation can be limited and progression prevented, or at least delayed and reduced in severity. This stage is critical, in that beyond it, irreversible articular cartilage and

bone destruction occur. This is the result of an immune-mediated process involving T lymphocytes, macrophages, and neutrophils in the synovial fluid. These cells release cytokines that trigger the release of enzymes and destructive oxidants from cells of the pannus and the release of collagenase and other enzymes from articular cartilage cells. Their combined effect is the erosion of articular cartilage and destruction of the bone that lies deep to it. The various mediators also promote the breakdown of bone by osteoclasts to add to the destructive process.

B lymphocytes are also involved and form antibodies. Initially, RF is produced, but it is thought that the degradation of joint macromolecules may alter their antigenic configurations so that antibodies against them are also formed. In either case, phagocytosis of the immune complexes in joint cartilage and in synovial fluid triggers the further release of destructive enzymes and oxidants by the phagocytes and further joint erosion follows. Immune complex formation also activates the complement cascade, producing intermediates that are chemotactic for neutrophils. Their increased numbers at the scene continue the process as they engulf immune complexes and release the erosive contents of their cytoplasmic granules.

Cytokines in the pannus and joint space not only cause damage, but cause the release of cytokine inhibitors that antagonize their effects. This role may explain the different degrees of severity and rates of progression seen in RA. Mild or slowly progressive cases may be the result of higher levels of cytokine inhibitors than are present in the more severe and rapidly progressive conditions. Their periodically increased production could also explain the episodes of remission that characterize RA.

With continued hyperplasia and hypertrophy of the pannus, it encroaches further into the joint space. As it extends over joint surfaces, cartilage and bone erosion continue. Ultimately, the pannus may enlarge to fill the joint space completely. By this stage, the articular cartilages on both sides of the joint, and much of their underlying bone, will have been lost. In late stages, **ankylosis,** or fusing of the joint, may develop as fibrous tissue or bone replaces the pannus. Figure 18.14 summarizes the principal elements of the pathogenesis of RA.

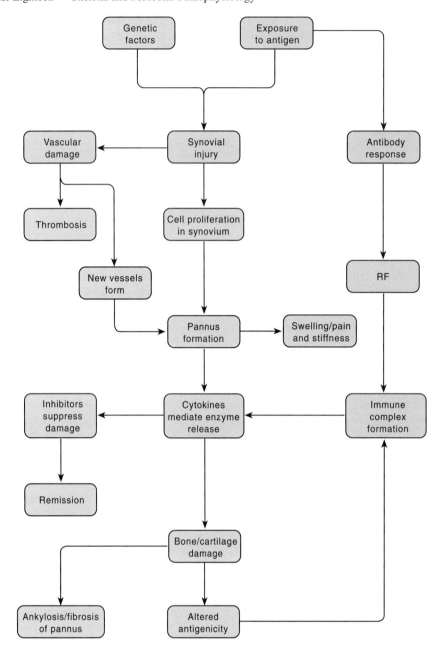

Figure 18.14   **Pathogenesis of Rheumatoid Arthritis.** RF is rheumatoid factor.

Joint distortion is a characteristic change in later stages of RA. It arises as ligaments and tendons adjacent to the affected joint are damaged. Joint pain often means reduced joint use, so muscle atrophy may also contribute to the loss of soft tissue support of the joint. With reduced support the bones are pulled from their normal positions, to severely distort the joint and restrict normal function (fig. 18.15).

Systemic Effects

A variety of systemic effects in RA are known, but their incidence is quite variable from one case to another. Most sufferers experience a generalized weakness and malaise, particularly in the early stages of the disease. Up to 35% develop characteristic granulomas called **rheumatoid**

nodules. These are regions of focal subcutaneous swelling found most often in the region of the elbow, heel, and the dorsal surface of the head. Other superficial sites are affected, especially those subjected to pressure, but internal nodules may also arise; for example, in the heart, pleural membranes, intestine, or meninges. Rheumatoid nodules consist of large concentrations of macrophages, lymphocytes, collagen, and granulation tissue that surround a central zone of necrosis and cellular debris. They may attain a diameter of 2 cm, but are typically painless and cause little functional disturbance. They are associated with high levels of circulating RF.

A systemic inflammation of the blood vessels, **rheumatoid vasculitis,** is also a common feature of RA, especially when RF levels are high. It may be related to

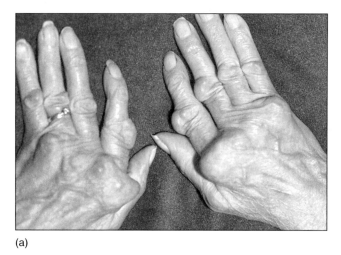 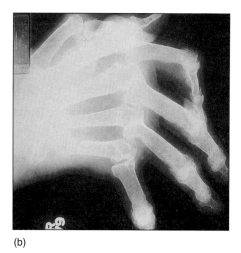

(a)   (b)

Figure 18.15 **Rheumatoid Arthritis.** The pronounced distortion of the finger joints is easily seen in both views.

nodule formation, but the precise link is unclear. Serous membranes may also be affected, producing effects in the heart (pericarditis) or lungs (pleural effusion). Eye involvement may occur but is rare. Most of these nonarticular conditions are thought to be related to immune complex deposition, but definitive evidence is lacking.

Therapy in RA

There is no cure for RA; the underlying cause can't be eliminated, and the destruction of joint structures can't be reversed. This means that therapy can only seek to relieve pain and reduce swelling, to allow the retention of as much joint function as possible. Generally, the treatment consists of anti-inflammation therapy, coupled with a regimen that reduces stress to affected joints. This may involve simply resting the joint, but in some cases binding or splinting to reduce movement may be indicated. Strengthening of associated muscles can be effective in maintaining joint mobility.

Drug therapy is based on agents whose analgesic and anti-inflammation effects can be quite beneficial. Table 18.3 lists the drugs that are commonly used in treating RA. Other agents seem able to alter the course of the disease, producing beneficial clinical results by other than an anti-inflammation effect. Recently, the use of **methotrexate** is showing much promise. The drug reduces symptoms and may also limit joint damage. The mechanisms underlying these effects are not understood. Methotrexate is known to block DNA synthesis and cell proliferation, and so may retard pannus formation. It may also work through some unrecognized immune suppression effects. Also used in support of NSAID therapy are antimalarials, hydroxychloroquinone, sulfasalazine and others (table 18.3). When NSAIDs and disease-altering agents are unable to produce relief, immunosuppression therapy may be successful, but as always, its application is associated with significant side effects. When joint damage is pronounced, surgery may be necessary to restore deformed joints and improve function. In severe cases, replacement with an artificial joint may be necessary.

Table 18.3	Drugs Employed in Therapy for RA
High Effectiveness	
Etanercept	Methotrexate
Infliximab	Prednisone
Moderate Effectiveness	
Cyclosporine	Leflunomide
Gold salts	Sulfasalazine
Hydroxychloroquine	
Low Effectiveness	
NSAIDs	

Other Joint Disorders

In osteoarthritis and rheumatoid arthritis, the principal focus of the disease is the synovial joint. In OA, the process starts in the joint cartilage and later affects the synovial membrane, while in RA, the initial damage arises in the synovium and only later affects the articular cartilage. By contrast with OA and RA, the less common conditions described next are those that have an initial derangement in some other part of the body, which produces secondary effects in the joints.

Gout

This disease is characterized by high levels of urate ions in the plasma. Uric acid is produced as a normal product of nucleic acid metabolism and is normally excreted in the urine and feces. If production is excessive, or excretion inadequate, urate ions accumulate in the plasma to produce a characteristic **hyperuricemia.**

Most hyperuricemia is related to defective renal handling of uric acid, usually for unknown reasons. Renal uric acid retention is also a side effect of various drugs, including

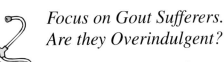

Focus on Gout Sufferers. Are they Overindulgent?

Because an initial episode of gout can be precipitated by episodes of excessive food or alcohol intake, the folk wisdom has it that gout is a disease of the overindulgent. In fact, various other factors not related to dietary or alcohol excess can trigger attacks. Examples are emotional stress, trauma (including surgery), drugs, various illnesses, or, surprisingly, periods of fasting.

---

aspirin, cyclosporine, and several diuretics. Hyperuricemia may also arise as an indirect side effect in various conditions (e.g., some malignancies, hemolytic anemia, and obesity). In some cases of gout, the underlying problem is excessive uric acid production. A long-recognized genetic component in gout may be linked to a defect in the system that regulates uric acid in the plasma.

The problems of gout arise from the deposition of monosodium urate (MSU) crystals in joint structures. These induce initial attacks of exquisitely painful arthritis in the foot, usually at a single metatarsophalangeal joint. In some cases, several joints may be involved. The initial episode is typically followed by an interval without symptoms, which may last from one to ten years. If no treatment intervenes to reduce uric acid levels, urate crystal deposition may become more extensive, affecting soft tissues, tendons, and synovial membranes. This deposition elicits a local inflammatory response that produces subcutaneous swellings in the forearm, elbow, ear, and other sites including internal organs. These resemble the rheumatoid nodules of RA and each is designated a **tophus** (pl. *tophi*). Therapy directed against hyperuricemia can usually prevent tophus formation. If therapy is delayed, a chronic arthritis from urate deposition can become more widespread and severe. Renal dysfunction is a common correlate of gout, often involving nephrolithiasis.

The incidence of gout is highest in adult males; only 5% of sufferers are female. Most initial attacks arise in the 40s. As indicated, timely therapeutic intervention can control progression and formation of tophi.

Pseudogout

In this condition, crystals of calcium pyrophosphate dihydrate (CPPD) are deposited in articular cartilage. The knee is most often affected, usually in the elderly with the wrist, shoulder, and ankle involved to a lesser degree. While crystal deposition is confined to the articular cartilage, the condition is asymptomatic. When crystals escape into the joint space, an acute inflammatory response produces painful episodes that resemble those of true gout. Pseudogout primarily affects the elderly and can be a cause of secondary osteoarthritis.

Ankylosing Spondylitis

In this condition, adolescent or young adult Caucasian males experience fusion of the vertebral column. The process usually starts at the sacroiliac joints and proceeds slowly up the spinal column, initially affecting the synovial joints between articular processes of adjacent vertebrae. As the disease progresses, joint structures are destroyed and replaced by fibrocartilage and bone. The process extends between adjacent vertebrae and fuses them together. As the dorsally fused articular processes are able to assume more weight-bearing, the vertebral bodies experience a corresponding reduction in weight-bearing demand (fig. 18.16). Bone resorption increases reducing their mass as they adjust to the situation. The result is an osteoporosis-like thinning, yielding a characteristic radiographic appearance that resembles a length of bamboo; hence, the term **bamboo spine.** Peripheral joints and some nonjoint structures may also be involved in ankylosing spondylitis, most often an eye inflammation.

Like rheumatoid arthritis, ankylosing spondylitis involves a genetic defect that predisposes to autoimmune attack on joint structures following infection. Because no rheumatoid factor can be detected in the serum of ankylosing spondylitis and some related joint diseases, they are described as being **sero-negative.** As with RA, therapy can only alleviate symptoms and seek to slow the progress of the disease. The early onset of the disease seems to provide more time for serious consequences to develop, and the prognosis is therefore less optimistic. A major problem in severe ankylosing spondylitis is spinal fracture, but most sufferers are able to maintain adequate mobility.

Systemic Lupus Erythematosus (SLE)

This is an autoimmune condition more fully described in chapter 5. It is characterized by the widespread deposition of immune complexes in various tissues, especially joints. Over 90% of cases involve joint pain and swelling related to the synovitis that develops in response to the immune complexes. The joints most often affected are those of the fingers, wrists, and knees. Deformation and destruction of joint structures is unusual.

As is typical of autoimmune diseases, females are predominantly affected, in particular those between puberty and age 40. A genetic predisposition is suspected to be a significant factor in this disorder.

DISORDERS OF SKELETAL MUSCLE

With its nerve and blood supply intact, skeletal muscle is remarkably resistant to disturbances that might compromise its function. Fluctuations in demand are met with hypertrophy or atrophy to provide a muscle mass adapted to changing circumstances.

In response to inadequate contraction stimulus, skeletal muscle atrophies and weakens. In most cases, the cause is a neurological defect involving CNS motor centers, PNS motor neurons (polio), or the neuromuscular junction (myasthenia gravis), all of which are treated in chapter 21.

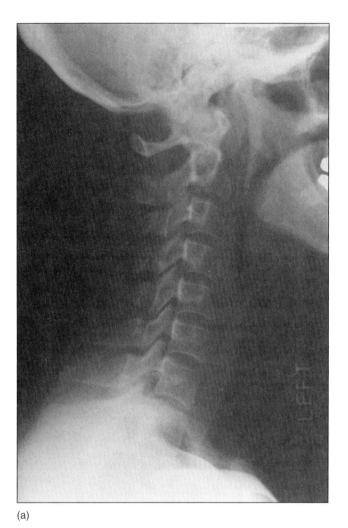

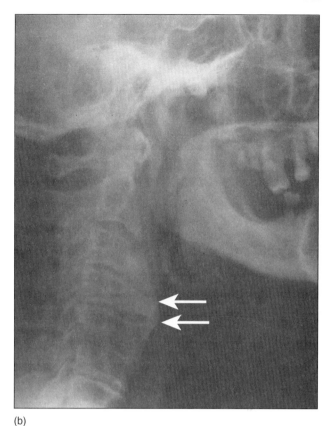

(b)

(a)

Figure 18.16 **Ankylosing Spondylitis.** Compare the clearly separate joint surfaces between adjacent vertebrae in the normal spinal column (*a*) with those in the ankylosing spondylosis patient (*b*). The arrows in (*b*) indicate points of vertebral ankylosis.

In **myositis,** inflammation may arise in response to systemic infections in which viruses, bacteria, fungi, or parasites gain access to skeletal muscle. Less commonly encountered inflammatory conditions involve a predominantly cellular infiltration in response to a suspected autoimmune defect. The term **polymyositis** describes the condition in which most signs and symptoms derive from muscle damage. In about 30% of cases, an accompanying skin rash is present, presumably due to dermal immune complex deposition. In these cases the disease is termed **dermatomyositis.** Because of their supposed, but not proven, autoimmune etiology, both of these disorders are considered in more detail in chapter 5.

Muscular Dystrophy

The term **muscular dystrophy** is used to denote a group of rare diseases characterized by a genetic etiology and the progressive degeneration of skeletal muscle. Differences in the degree of progression, pattern of inheritance, and age of onset are the basis for distinguishing among them.

Duchenne Muscular Dystrophy

This X-linked recessive defect is the most common of the muscular dystrophies. It arises in about 1 of every 3,000 live births (0.0003%) and, because of its pattern of inheritance, affects males almost without exception. Most cases arise in families with a history of the disorder, but there is no way to determine accurately whether a woman who is herself normal might be a carrier of the defective gene. To complicate matters, up to 30% of cases arise as the result of a new mutation, so there is no family history on the basis of which parents might anticipate the disease.

If suspected, the disease can be diagnosed immediately at birth on the basis of high serum levels of **creatine kinase** (CK). This enzyme is released from damaged muscle fibers at multiple sites. In affected children, it is possible by close observation to detect muscle weakness and delayed motor development quite early. Obvious loss of strength and motor skills emerges by age 5. From this point, the disease progresses to induce increasing muscle degeneration, in particular in the larger proximal muscle masses of the legs (fig. 18.17). By age 10, most victims require leg bracing to

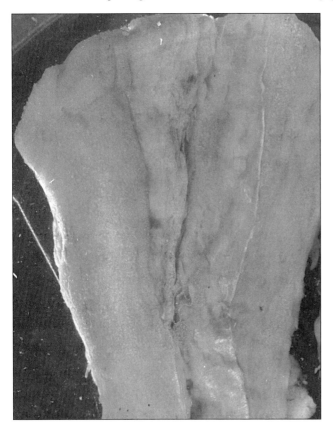

Figure 18.17 **Muscular Dystrophy.** The specimen shown here is pale because fat has replaced its muscle fibers.
Portion of the quadriceps muscle from a victim of muscular dystrophy who had been essentially bedridden since his early years. He died at age 19. The specimen contains only faintly visible streaks of muscle tissue, the atrophied fibers having been replaced by fat.

walk. Confinement to a wheelchair follows by age 12, and beyond age 15 most victims are completely bedridden.

Fibrosis, to repair degenerating or otherwise damaged muscle, is pronounced and is often followed by contracture, which produces distorting forces on the developing skeleton. Lordosis (anterior curvature) and scoliosis (lateral curvature) can result, leading to compromised respiration because the skeletal deformities prevent normal chest expansion. With muscle weakness also contributing, respiratory insufficiency is a major problem in the later stages of muscular dystrophy, with a superimposed respiratory infection often precipitating complete respiratory failure and early death. Survival to age 30 is unusual in those afflicted by this tragic disease. Cardiac muscle tissue is also involved in the degenerative process, with dysrhythmias and congestive heart failure developing in later stages of the disease. Mental sluggishness may accompany Duchenne muscular dystrophy, but its link to the mechanism responsible for the loss of muscle tissue is unknown.

The underlying defect in this condition is deficiency of a muscle protein called **dystrophin.** It seems to be involved in the system that links a muscle fiber's membrane with key elements in the extracellular matrix. This linking pro-

vides stability for the membrane during contraction. When dystrophin is lacking, this stabilizing effect is lost, causing damage and tearing of the muscle fibers, as they are unable to withstand normal contraction forces. The damaged portions of the fibers are cleared by macrophages, following which the remaining portions regenerate the lost regions. However, the essential membrane defect is still present in the newly regenerated regions, and so the stage is set for further damage. Ultimately, degeneration overwhelms the cell's regenerative capacity. Fibrous connective tissue and fatty deposits then replace functional muscle fibers. There is no known means of replacing the deficient dystrophin in this disease. Therapy can only intervene to sustain mobility and respiratory function for as long as possible.

A milder condition called **Becker's muscular dystrophy** is also due to abnormal dystrophin. It is essentially similar to Duchenne muscular dystrophy but has a later onset and is more slowly progressive, allowing survival to as late as age 40.

Myotonic Dystrophy

This is the second most common of these rare muscular dystrophies. Its transmission is by autosomal dominant inheritance, which means that it can more readily be traced through a family's history, since no carrier state is possible. In other words, if the defective gene is present, the disease is present, and affected individuals are easily identified. The genetic defect in myotonic dystrophy produces abnormal membrane ion channels that are linked to muscle atrophy, loss of strength, and a characteristic **myotonia** that distinguishes this condition from other muscular dystrophies. Myotonic muscle exhibits delayed relaxation after it contracts.

Myotonic dystrophy has a variable pattern of onset. Symptoms may arise in the teens and 20s, after which they follow a slowly progressive course. The muscles of the face, neck, and distal limbs are the focus of the degenerative process. In addition to its skeletal muscle effects, the disease may also produce myocardial degeneration, cataracts, atrophy of the testicles, and impaired mental functioning.

In the heart, defects in the conduction system pose the threat of serious dysrhythmias, while weakness in the respiratory muscles can compromise ventilation. In most sufferers, muscle defects are mild, producing only minimal interference with normal activity. In severe cases, severe disability may emerge as early as age 20–30.

Facioscapulohumeral Muscular Dystrophy

This genetic condition is transmitted by autosomal dominant inheritance, so males and females are affected equally. As its name indicates, the affected muscles are those of the face, shoulder, and upper arm, but the lower leg and foot muscles may also be involved. Their degeneration and weakness usually emerge between adolescence and age 40,

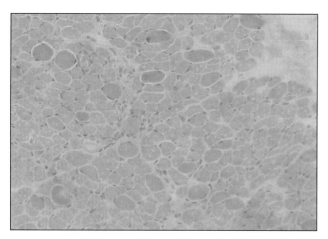

Figure 18.18   **Congenital Myopathy.** In this section through skeletal muscle, the individual muscle fibers are seen as rounded masses. The pale areas within each cell are characteristic of centronuclear myopathy.

with rates of progression slower than those seen in the Duchenne form.

No cardiac or other tissues are involved in facioscapulohumeral dystrophy, and mental development is normal. Although an early onset seems to allow time for more severe muscle involvement, the slow progression of the disease may make a near-normal life span possible.

 Checkpoint 18.3

Since the muscle disorders just described are relatively rare, you might think there's little point in knowing something about them. But note that rare conditions are rare only in the sense of having low frequency in the general population. Your career pursuit is likely to find you in the very sort of facility where these conditions are diagnosed and treated. So even though the average person-on-the-street may seldom encounter these conditions, you are much more likely to.

Congenital Myopathies

These are rare idiopathic conditions that are characterized by generalized muscle weakness that emerges soon after birth. Most diseases in this category progress slowly—many sufferers are able to cope relatively well with a life of muscle weakness. In severe cases, weakened respiration causes pulmonary disorders that are fatal within the infant's first year. One type of muscle damage seen in congenital myopathy, **centronuclear myopathy,** is shown in figure 18.18.

Case Study

Because of intermittent low back pain, a 22-year-old male student saw his physician. He explained that he had been troubled by low back stiffness when he got up in the morning, and that with his normal routine of activities the stiffness eased and he felt better. He had had no injuries, and he was rather sedentary, so it seemed unlikely that exercise strain could account for the problem. He described the pain as a "dull stiffness" with no radiation down the leg. When questioned, he recalled that his father, a construction worker, had suffered from back pain that was attributed to the rigors of his work, but he couldn't remember much since his father had died relatively young in a work-related accident.

On examination the patient was apparently healthy, with no grossly observable back defects, and had a full range of flexion, extension, and rotation at the waist. Palpation over the sacroiliac joints, however, revealed some tenderness.

X-rays of the chest and low back indicated no chest abnormalities, but did reveal some blurring of the sacroiliac joints and some degree of bilateral erosion of their bony margins. The erythrocyte sedimentation rate (ESR) was elevated. These findings were suggestive of ankylosing spondylitis. A blood test was returned as positive for

HLA-B27 antigen and negative for rheumatoid factor, verifying the diagnosis.

In addition to counseling as to the possibility of progression of the disease, the patient was given various exercises to build strength and support his posture. He was also advised to use a small pillow when sleeping and to follow a course of NSAID therapy. He was asked to return for annual assessment.

Commentary

The age and sex of this patient are typical. The common finding of a hereditary component is also suggested in the father's back problems, with his untimely death probably preventing development of spinal deformity at a time when the disease and its treatment were less well understood.

The chest X-ray was requested because, although the patient had not complained of chest pain, early changes at the manubriosternal joint are common in this condition. The elevated ESR is a nonspecific indication that an inflammatory process may be active. It involves increased time for RBCs to settle from plasma, presumably because in inflammatory conditions, the plasma's greater content of immune globulins and fibrinogen makes it more viscous. The HLA-B27 antigen is present in 90% of ankylosing spondylitis sufferers and confirmed the diagnosis in the context of the history and other findings.

The physician's pillow recommendation was aimed at reducing neck flexion to relieve strain on the lower back, while the exercise regimen was designed not only to build strength, but also to reduce the degree of deformation that might develop. NSAIDs have proven quite successful in limiting pain, but there is little more that can be done for ankylosing spondylitis patients. When the initial symptoms are as mild as these, they may well remain so for 10–20 years, offering only minor interference with work. With maintenance of an appropriate exercise program, much deformity can be avoided.

Key Concepts

1. Apart from infections and tumors, bone disease derives from abnormalities of bone formation or later imbalances in the bone remodeling process (p. 485).

2. Apart from infections and tumors, most of the more common bone disorders produce osteopenia, with the exception of Paget's disease, which involves both osteopenia and hyperostosis (p. 485).

3. Genetic bone diseases are rare and involve various patterns of inheritance of traits that produce defects in the cartilage template on which ossification depends or in the activities of osteoblasts or osteoclasts (pp. 485–486).

4. Pain, skeletal malformations, and pathological fractures are the principal derangements produced by acquired bone disorders (p. 486).

5. The most important factor in preventing the osteopenia that characterizes osteoporosis is the early development and maintenance of the maximum skeletal mass provided by one's genetic makeup, to counter the inevitable loss of bone in later life (p. 489).

6. Osteomyelitis is usually caused by a pyogenic exogenous bacterial infection that arises secondary to bone trauma, but organisms from previously established infection sites may reach bone via the blood (p. 492).

7. Most bone tumors are secondary carcinomas from various body sites; of primary bone tumors, two-thirds are malignant and one-third benign (pp. 492–493).

8. Osteoarthritis, the most common North American joint disease, involves the degradation of articular cartilage, often in response to long-term overloading of the larger weight-bearing joints (pp. 494–496).

9. Rheumatoid arthritis typically involves the joints of the wrists, hands, ankles, and feet and derives from inflammatory damage to the synovium, with later effects in articular cartilage and adjacent bone (p. 496).

10. RA is caused by the immune destruction of joint structures, and has a genetic component to its etiology (p. 497).

11. Superimposed on its alternating pattern of exacerbation and remission in affected joints, RA exhibits a range of variably occurring systemic effects (pp. 497–498).

12. Although essentially a systemic autoimmune disorder, 90% of SLE is accompanied by joint pain and swelling due to synovitis induced by immune complex deposition (p. 500).

13. With nerve and blood supply intact, skeletal muscle is remarkably resistant to disease, but with inadequate neurological stimulus, its cells atrophy and weaken (pp. 500–501).

14. Duchenne muscular dystrophy is the most common of a group of rare genetic diseases characterized by progressive degeneration of muscle tissue (pp. 501–502).

REVIEW ACTIVITIES

1. Write out the reasons that vitamin D can be considered a hormone as well as a vitamin. Refer to page 484 for help.

2. List all the factors that have a bearing on the etiology and pathogenesis of osteoporosis. There's no section labeled "Pathogenesis," so you'll have to dig around in the material on pages 488–489.

3. Complete the following table.

Essential Bone Derangement	Etiological Factor	Pathogenesis Factor	Disease
Focal loss and deposition	Possibly viral	Rare tumor incidence	
Osteopenia	Deficiency state	Adults affected	
Excessive deposition	Genetic	Little chance of survival if severe	
Shortness of stature	Genetic	Defective cartilage matrix	
Osteopenia	Vitamin D deficiency	Children affected	
Infection	Bacteria	Trauma	
Osteopenia	Low skeletal mass	Fractures in later years	

4. Since you're likely to encounter so much osteoarthritis, it's a good idea to be conversant with its pathogenesis. To see if you are, check figure 18.12 and verify that you know the following:

   (a) the link between fissure formation and bone cyst formation,

   (b) what osteophytes are and why they might affect joint mobility and cause pain,

   (c) what burnishing means,

   (d) the essential difference between osteoarthritis and RA (this emerges pretty clearly in figures 18.12 and 18.14 when the words "injury" or "damage" are used at the top of each).

   Pages 494–499 are the source for this material.

5. Given the information on pages 501–502, construct a flow chart that explains the current thinking on the pathogenesis of Duchenne muscular dystrophy. Lay it out top-to-bottom, starting with "Genetic Defect" at the top and "Muscular Weakness" at the bottom. Include the term "CK."

Chapter

19

Reproductive Pathophysiology

I would very much rather stand three times in the front of a battle than bear one child.

EURIPIDES
MEDEA

rubor

&'tumor

cū calore

&'dolore

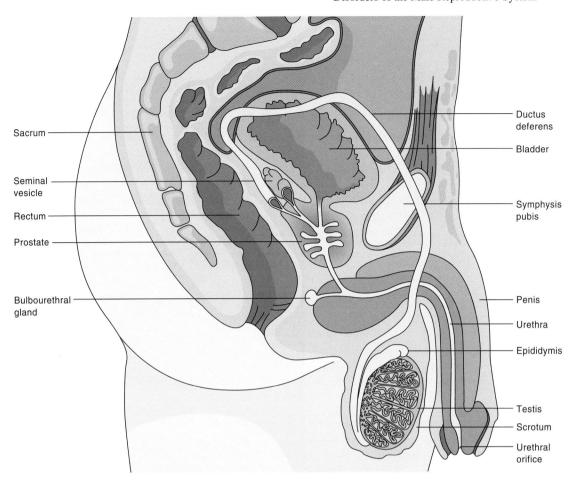

Figure 19.1   **Male Reproductive Structures.** Note the anatomic relation that facilitates palpation of the prostate gland via the rectum.

The reproductive system is distinctive in that its continued functioning is not as critical as that of other organ systems. In kidney, liver, or heart failure, for example, loss of essential functions is incompatible with life. Even when modern therapeutic resources sustain life, they bring their own burdens and demands to the survivor. In the reproductive system, by contrast, the failure of essential function usually produces only sterility or the inability to sustain normal prenatal development of offspring. However disappointing this may be, the physiological consequences are usually not serious. Furthermore, because a reproductive disorder may arise after one or more children are born, the inability to produce additional offspring has less impact. On the other hand, some disorders of the reproductive system do pose significant threats. For example, serious problems of bleeding and miscarriage can arise in pregnancy, and tumors of the reproductive organs, like most tumors, can have serious effects both locally and at sites of distant metastatic growth.

This chapter will consider only those reproductive disorders that arise in the testis, ovary, and uterus, and their associated ducts and glands. Disorders that arise in the hypothalamus and anterior pituitary, affecting neuroendocrine control of the reproductive system, were considered in chapter 17. Many psychological factors influence reproductive activities, but these are beyond the scope of this book, as are the rare genetic disorders that may produce sterility.

DISORDERS OF THE MALE REPRODUCTIVE SYSTEM

Of the male reproductive structures (fig. 19.1), disorders of the penis/urethra, bulbourethral glands, seminal vesicles, and vas deferens (ductus deferens) are rare. For example, the congenital abnormality called **hypospadias,** in which the urethral orifice opens at the upper surface of the penis, occurs only once in 50,000 live births. **Venereal infections,** those transmitted by sexual activity, may provide a threat to reproductive structures or distant organs (e.g., the brain in syphilis). These conditions, however, are usually readily controlled by antibiotics, which limit serious consequences. Most male reproductive disorders other than infection arise in the testis and prostate gland.

Testicular Disorders

The paired testes (singular, testis) are housed in the scrotum, outside the pelvic cavity. Although this location may expose the testes to a greater risk of damage from trauma, it appears to allow for closer temperature regulation of the

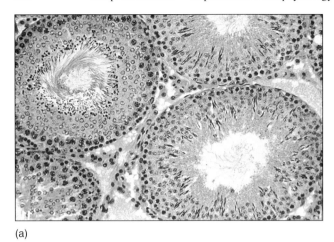

(a)

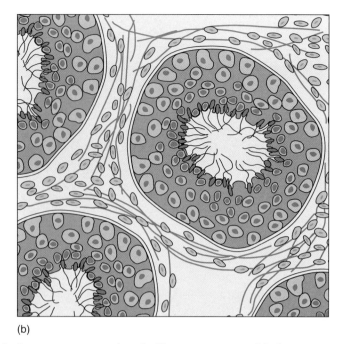

(b)

Figure 19.2   **Seminiferous Tubules.** (*a*) The numerous tails of developing spermatozoa produce the fibrous appearance of the lumen of the tubule at left. (*b*) The cells forming the tubule walls are involved in the cell divisions that produce fully formed spermatozoa. Note the cells in the space between the tubules. These are the interstitial cells that secrete testosterone.

process of **spermatogenesis**—the production of male sex cells, called **spermatozoa.** Scrotal temperature is about 2° C lower than that of the pelvic cavity, and this difference seems to be critical, for as testis temperature increases, spermatozoa production decreases. Spermatogenesis occurs within the testes, in the seminiferous tubules. These tiny, tightly coiled ducts have a total length of about 250 m and produce over 200 million spermatozoa daily (fig. 19.2).

Broadly, disorders of the testes are congenital or involve acquired abnormalities arising from infection, compromised circulation, or neoplasia.

Congenital Abnormalities of the Testes

Development of the testes normally proceeds within the pelvic cavity. Prior to birth, a passage, the **inguinal canal,** forms between the pelvic cavity and scrotum. The testes enter the canal and descend along it, through the abdominal wall, to take up their normal location in the scrotum (fig. 19.3). The **spermatic cord** remains as a link to the abdominal cavity and contains ductus deferens, that will ultimately conduct spermatozoa to the urethra, the testes' blood and nerve supply, and the **cremaster muscle.** This muscle alters its tension to draw the testes nearer to the warmth of the abdominal cavity in cold conditions, and to allow descent from it when temperatures are increased. In this way it helps to maintain optimal temperatures for spermatogenesis.

The most common congenital defect involving the testes is their failure to descend to the scrotum, a condition called **cryptorchidism.** In this term, Greek word elements refer to the testis (*orchido*) being hidden (*crypto*) within the

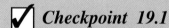

Checkpoint 19.1

The term *testis* is derived from the Latin word meaning "to swear"; that is, "to testify." In seeking to validate his testimony, a Roman male would place his hands over his testicles. He was swearing on something precious to him, much as the Bible or other sacred text is used in Western courts. Swearing in this way was a serious matter because if found to be lying, the offender was deprived of the glands on which he swore.

pelvic cavity. The condition usually involves only one testis, which remains inside the pelvic cavity or within the pelvic canal. The reasons why this might occur are difficult to establish, since the mechanisms underlying normal testicular descent are poorly understood.

An undescended testis seems able to maintain testosterone secretion, but spermatogenesis is suppressed by the warmer pelvic cavity temperatures to which it is exposed. As a result, the seminiferous tubules and the entire gland atrophy (fig. 19.4). Loss of fertility usually accompanies cryptorchidism. Without intervention to move an undescended testis to the scrotum (the procedure is called **orchiopexy**), a much greater danger emerges. Presumably because of the elevated temperatures to which it is subjected, an undescended testis is at an increased risk of developing tumors. After five years, the cancer risk in an undescended testis increases to 30 times normal.

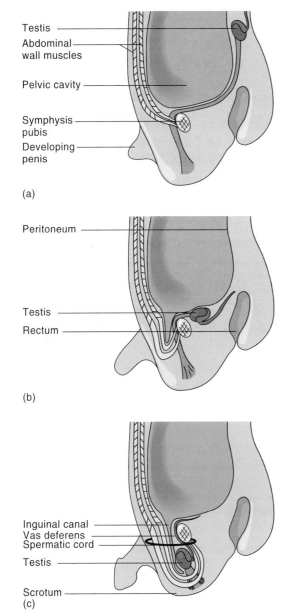

Figure 19.3 **Descent of the Testes.** The sequence of testicular descent from the abdomen to the scrotum: (*a*) Predescent position. (*b*) The descent under way. (*c*) Arrival at the developing scrotum. Note the components of the spermatic cord within black ring.

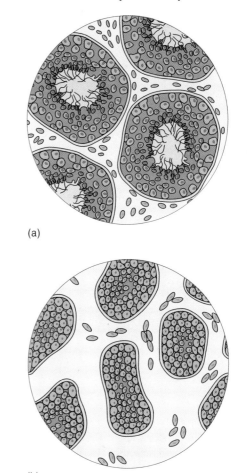

Figure 19.4 **Atrophy of Seminiferous Tubules.** Compare normal tubules (*a*) with atrophied tubules (*b*).

Table 19.1	Principal Types of Testicular Tumors

Germ Cell Tumors	**Stromal Tumors**
One cell type present:	Leydig (interstitial) cell
Seminoma	Sertoli cell
Embryonal carcinoma	Granulosa cell
Choriocarcinoma	Undifferentiated
Teratoma	

Testicular Tumors

Although the **interstitial cells (cells of Leydig),** which secrete testosterone, and the **Sertoli cells,** which support developing spermatozoa, are present in the seminiferous tubules, 95% of testicular tumors arise in the precursor cells that ultimately give rise to mature spermatozoa. For this reason they are known as **germ cell tumors.** The cells involved are largely undifferentiated, and when they become neoplastic, the tumor may develop along various paths of differentiation to produce differing cell types. In most cases, a single cell type is present, but in 40% of cases, two or more types can be identified. The major types are listed in table 19.1.

Germ cell tumors present the risk of local invasion to the epididymis and pelvic cavity. Metastasis via the lymph involves the chains of lymph nodes that lie alongside the aorta, while blood-borne metastases typically involve the lung, liver, brain, and bone. Initially, the only sign of a tumor may be testicular swelling caused by the increasing tumor mass. Pain incidence is variable, at least in the early stages, before swelling generates pressure against the testicles' essentially inelastic protective coat, **tunica albuginea** (fig. 19.5). Later invasion may produce urinary obstruction, and metastases often produce back and abdominal

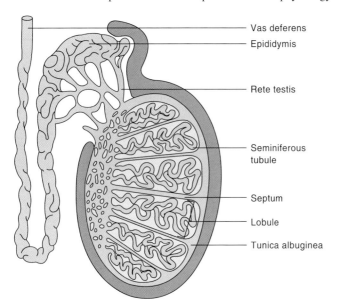

Figure 19.5   **The Testis.** Tightly coiled seminiferous tubules are isolated by septa of the tough tunica albuginea that protects the testis.

pain due to growth in secondary lymph nodes. Dyspnea from the effects of pulmonary metastases, weight loss, and gynecomastia (breast enlargement) may also be present to varying degrees.

The average incidence of germ cell tumors is 6 per 100,000 males, but peaks of higher incidence occur in the young, mostly related to cryptorchidism, and at age 15–35, perhaps because of the higher testosterone levels during these years. The most common germ cell tumor is the **seminoma.** Although malignant, this tumor is highly radiosensitive and cure rates are very high, even after metastasis has occurred. As with so many tumors, etiology in germ cell tumors is unclear. Different racial incidence, significantly higher in whites than blacks, suggests that a genetic factor is involved, and varying geographic distribution of the victims points to some role for environmental agents. It is interesting to note that in cases associated with cryptorchidism, the incidence of germ cell tumors is the same in descended and undescended testes. This finding seems to counter the idea that higher abdominal temperature plays an important role in the neoplastic conversion and suggests, instead, that a single underlying cause may be responsible for both the failure of descent and induction of the tumor.

Compromise of Testicular Circulation

Reduced blood flow to the testis is most often the result of twisting or **torsion** of the spermatic cord, which carries the testis' vascular supply. Often, particularly vigorous exercise or physical trauma produces the torsion, but if the scrotum is more loosely suspended, even moderately vigorous activity may allow the spermatic cord to twist.

If torsion only partially compresses the testicular veins, varying degrees of congestion and swelling occur as a result of restricted venous drainage. Pain arises and is due

Focus on hCG in Pregnancy Testing

! !

hCG (the "h" denotes "human" to distinguish it from therapeutic preparations derived from animal sources) is the normal product of trophoblasts present in a newly formed embryo. Its presence in a female's plasma or urine is therefore a sign of pregnancy. Since hCG is often produced by nonendocrine germ cell tumors, affected males could test positive for pregnancy.

both to the initial torsion and to the congestion and swelling that follow. If the torsion can't be resolved by manipulation or surgery, or if compression blocks all blood flow, necrosis, hemorrhage, and infarction follow.

Disorders of the Prostate Gland

The most common prostatic disorder is **prostatic hyperplasia.** It may be referred to as **benign prostatic hypertrophy** (BPH), but this term is inaccurate in that the essential problem is not enlargement of existing cells (hypertrophy), but the production of new tissue (hyperplasia). Since the same initials can also refer to **benign prostatic hyperplasia,** they are widely used.

Normally, at birth the prostate is a small mass weighing a few grams, which grows to a weight of approximately 20 g by age 20. This size is sustained until about the age of 45, when a second period of slow growth begins. By age 70, over 90% of males show some degree of prostatic hyperplasia. Symptoms indicating some degree of urinary obstruction by the prostate (fig. 19.6) emerge at an average age of 65. Such obstruction increases the risk of bladder infections and pyelonephritis, since longer urine retention favors bacterial growth.

If obstruction is pronounced, the excess prostatic tissue can be surgically removed to restore normal voiding. In the absence of surgical correction, the back pressure of urine can produce dilation of the ureters and can involve the kidney's calyces and pelvis. This is the condition of **hydronephrosis.** Not only does continued renal filtration add pressure to the system, which can distort the tissues involved, but the back pressures can compromise renal blood flow and precipitate renal failure.

Prostatic Carcinoma

In males, prostate cancer is the second most common malignancy (lung cancer is first) and the third highest cause of death from tumors (lung and colon tumors are first and second). Tumors of the prostate most often produce symptoms after the age of 50, with peak incidence emerging in the 70s. Although malignant, these tumors are usually smaller than the size reached in prostatic hyperplasia. Also, because many arise near the periphery of the gland, they cause little

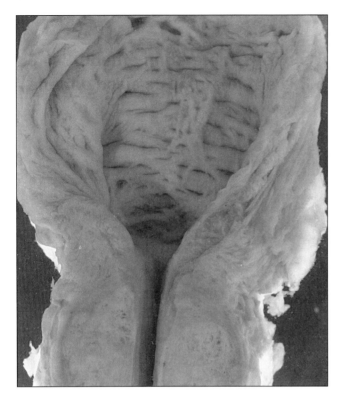

Figure 19.6 **Prostatic Hyperplasia.** The enlarged prostatic masses can easily be seen in this section. Cutting through the enlarged gland relieves its compression of the urethra, so its narrowing is not apparent in this photo.

Table 19.2		Staging of Prostatic Carcinoma
Stage	**Substage**	**Clinical Criteria**
A		No tumor symptoms reported Tumor discovered in biopsy of BPH
	A1	Focal growth of well-differentiated tumor cells
	A2	Diffuse distribution of poorly differentiated cells
B		Tumor palpable in prostate via rectal examination; mass confined within gland's capsule
	B1	Single mass palpable
	B2	More extensive gland involvement;
C		Invasion beyond capsule, based on evidence of local signs and symptoms and CT scan
	C1	No involvement of pelvic wall
	C2	Invasion of pelvic wall
D		Indications of metastasis
	D1	Secondary growth confined to pelvic lymph nodes
	D2	Distant metastases: lung, bone

urinary obstruction and may remain undiscovered until local invasion produces pain. Initially, metastasis involves the regional lymph nodes, then later, the lungs, bone, and other distant sites. A widely used staging system for prostatic carcinoma is based on the size and spread of the tumor. In stages A and B, growth is confined to the prostate, and in stages C and D, spread beyond the gland is involved (table 19.2). The TNM staging system (see chapter 6) may also be used in prostate cancer.

Like that of testicular germ cell tumors, the etiology of prostatic carcinoma seems to involve a genetic component, since incidence in blacks is greater than in whites. Environmental factors may also play a role, as indicated by a varying geographic distribution of age-adjusted death rates; Japan has a very low rate, Sweden's is very high, and the rate for North American males is between those extremes. There is no evidence that prostatic hyperplasia predisposes to prostate cancer.

Prostatic carcinoma growth is supported by testosterone. Therefore, after surgical resection of the tumor, treatment includes radiation and alteration of the tumor's endocrine support; both treatments are often effective in limiting further growth. One way to counter testosterone secretion is to administer estrogens, which antagonize testosterone's effects. In some cases, surgical removal of the testes—**orchiectomy**—is performed to abolish the source of the growth-supporting testosterone. Therapeutic agents that indirectly block testosterone secretion (leupro-

lide, goserel) or bind testosterone receptors to reduce its effects (flutamide, bicalutamide) show recent promise in limiting tumor growth.

The prognosis is better when therapy is instituted at stage A or B, with ten-year survival rates as high as 80% in some studies. Over half of prostate tumors are diagnosed at these earlier stages. If diagnosis and therapy are delayed until stage C or D, the prognosis is much poorer, with ten-year survival rates ranging from 10% to less than 50%. The secretion of **prostate-specific antigen** (PSA) by prostate tissue is useful in monitoring the effects of therapy. In prostate cancer, the increased volume of tumor tissue initially elevates PSA levels in the blood, but with effective therapy, and a declining tumor mass, PSA levels are gradually reduced. PSA assessment is also used for prostate cancer detection.

 Checkpoint 19.2

Disorders of the male reproductive system are relatively few, so the bulk of this chapter has to do with the larger number of problems associated with the female reproductive system. These consist of infections, menstrual cycle problems, tumors, and various disorders associated with pregnancy. Before continuing, you might do well to look back on the quotation by Euripides that introduces this chapter.

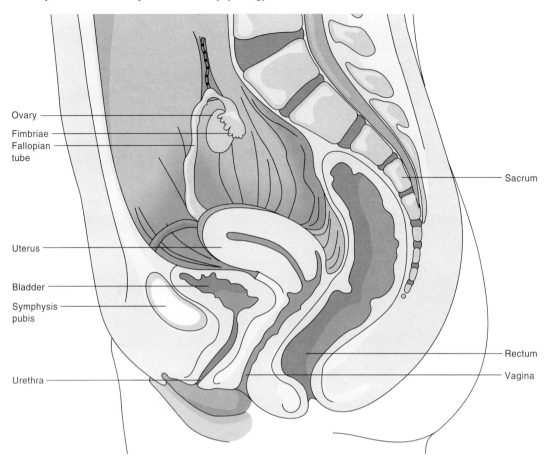

Figure 19.7   **Female Reproductive Structures.** Note the normal forward bending (anteflexion) of the uterus.

DISORDERS OF THE FEMALE REPRODUCTIVE SYSTEM

The emphasis in this discussion will be on the ovary and uterus (fig. 19.7), which account for the most serious reproductive system diseases suffered by women. Let us start, however, by describing the condition of ascending infection called pelvic inflammatory disease (PID). Since it can damage the reproductive structures, it often leads to sterility.

Pelvic Inflammatory Disease

Pelvic inflammatory disease (PID) is due to infection that usually originates in the vagina, ascends through the uterus and Fallopian tubes, and then spreads to the ovaries, broad ligaments, peritoneal surfaces, and various other abdominal organs, in some cases as far removed as the liver. The associated inflammatory response usually involves a purulent exudate, which may be discharged via the vagina or may be sequestered in tubal or ovarian abscesses. Postinflammatory scarring makes infertility a common sequela of pelvic inflammatory disease.

Most PID arises as a result of sexually transmitted organisms, usually *Neisseria gonorrhoeae* or *Chlamydia tra-*

Table 19.3	Organisms Typically Involved in PID
Neisseria gonorrhoeae	*Clostridium perfringens*
Chlamydia trachomatis	Coliform bacteria
Streptococci	*Actinomyces*
Staphylococci	*Mycoplasma*

chomatis. These organisms are quite virulent, and exposure to them is associated with a high rate of infection. Various other vaginal and cervical organisms may become involved when the initial venereal infection disrupts the balance of host factors that normally limit their growth (table 19.3). Less commonly, PID may originate with various medical procedures, such as insertion or manipulation of an IUD, (intrauterine device: a contraceptive uterine insert) **cesarean section** (surgical delivery of an infant through the uterine and abdominal walls when a normal delivery is not possible), or **dilation** and **curettage** (D and C: dilating the cervix to allow introduction of an instrument or suction device to strip away the endometrium, for the purpose of

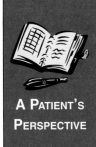

Coping with Chronic Pelvic Inflammatory Disease

—Anonymous

This account was recorded about ten years ago about a case of PID that was identified ten years before that. We can only hope that because PID is now part of the curriculum in med school and because aggressive antibiotic therapy is generally effective in its treatment, stories like this are a thing of the past.

M.   I've had chronic PID for just over ten years.

W.   Do you know how you got it?

M.   No.

W.   Did you ever use an IUD?

M.   Yes.

W.   Studies have shown that 3–8% of IUD users develop PID. Did your doctor warn you of this risk?

M.   No.

W.   Did you have any problems getting a diagnosis?

M.   Not for the first attack. However, the PID just kept recurring and finally became chronic. Then doctors thought I was just complaining, so a laparoscopy was done and they saw all the evidence of PID, all the scarring.

W.   In a 24-hour period, how much time do you have to spend lying down?

M.   About 22 hours. I can't stand for longer than ten minutes. So the time would be split into shorter periods of getting up and moving around. In an active day I might get up to go to the bathroom several times. I might heat some food. When I go to the physiotherapist, I walk to the car and lie down in the back seat. Then I get up and walk into the office. I count that being up.

W.   Do you have pain?

M.   PID pain is frightening. It's deep, sickening pain. Sometimes it feels like my reproductive system is being rubbed with ground glass. At other times it feels like I'm being punched in the abdomen again and again. It's hard to explain. It's much worse than labor pain or menstrual cramps. Sometimes I get sharp, stabbing pain that spreads slowly across my abdomen. It keeps me awake. I can't even sit in a chair or the knifelike pain becomes unbearable. I've awakened with pain. It's exhausting. Sometimes I'm in too much pain to be able to speak. The pain and isolation make life difficult to endure.

W.   The level of disability you have must put a strain on your relationship with your child.

M.   I worry about my daughter. She's 14 now. I've been sick since she was four. The few things we do at home consist mainly of watching television and playing board games. There have been times when my daughter's been really depressed and hasn't wanted to live with me. Getting regular in-home help from the government homemaker program took some of the burden off my daughter. I don't want her to feel she is responsible for me. I want to encourage her to live her own life and do the things she wants to do.

M.   PID is a hidden disability. I look "normal." And some people, including doctors, are suspicious of women who have chronic pain. The only people who really understand are women with chronic PID or people who have other disabling conditions. Able-bodied people have trouble understanding or being a friend partly because my situation makes them depressed. I find that I act a lot more cheerful than I really am so they are protected from the extent of my pain. They're afraid to try to meet my seemingly endless needs. They withdraw. Or they try to stay and we talk about their frustration.

W.   So you must feel sad and lonely.

M.   Yes. I'm only what you'd call happy once or twice a year. Having my house clean and tidy and being visited by friends help to keep up my spirits.

abortion or the removal of polyps or unexpelled placental remnants following an infant's delivery). From these facts, you can see that PID is a disease that is limited, almost without exception, to sexually active women. Younger women are more vulnerable than mature women, perhaps because of the thinner epithelium and less acidic epithelial secretions that are typical of younger women. Women who have never borne a child (nulliparous) are also at greater risk of developing PID. In rare instances, the precipitating infection may spread from an initially infected adjacent organ (e.g., the appendix or colon), or from a distant focus of infection via the blood.

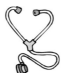

Focus on Vaginal Douching as a Risk Factor in PID

Many women routinely practice vaginal douching in regular hygiene or following menstruation or sexual intercourse. Unfortunately, this practice is associated with an increased risk of PID. Perhaps the process is irritating and provides sites of erosion where organisms can establish an infection. Alternatively, it may cause organisms from proximal sites to be flushed to deeper regions within the uterus.

The pathogenesis of PID is based on an inflammatory response elicited by the infecting organisms at the mucosal surfaces of the vagina and uterus, which produces an exudate that contains mucus and pus and thus is described as **mucopurulent.** The organisms' access and spread through the reproductive passages may be facilitated by their ability to attach to spermatozoa. Tissue culture studies suggest that, on reaching the Fallopian tube mucosa, gonococcal or chlamydial organisms are taken into its columnar cells where they produce damage, either by inducing the sloughing of ciliated cells or by eliciting an infiltration by PMNs, lymphocytes, and other host cells. Involvement beyond the tubes is common, with ovarian and peritoneal surfaces serving as sites from which the infection may spread to various adjacent and distant organs. Inflammations of the peritoneal surfaces of these various organs are denoted by specific terminology—for example, **periappendicitis, perigastritis,** and **perihepatitis.**

The inflammatory response in the Fallopian tubes **(salpingitis)** poses particular problems in that swelling can seal its ends, trapping the progressively increasing volumes of exudate. This causes the tubes to swell, distorting their shape and predisposing to abscess formation. The ovaries are also subject to abscess formation as a result of their close proximity to the Fallopian tubes. Such abscesses are known as **tubo-ovarian abscesses.** Abscesses may also arise at various other pelvic or abdominal sites, including the liver and inferior surface of the diaphragm. In such abscesses, various organisms, other than those of the initial infection, may proliferate and contribute to the destructive process.

Signs and symptoms in PID are related to the inflammatory process. Vaginal discharge of blood and mucopurulent exudate from vaginal and uterine surfaces is common. Pain associated with infection of the rectum and urethra may be present, and urethritis and bladder involvement may produce frequent urination and dysuria (painful urination). With extension to the Fallopian tubes and beyond, abdominal pain may arise—initially dull or aching, and later more severe and localized—depending on the infecting organisms and the organs involved.

The bleeding and abdominal pain of PID may cause the condition to be confused with various other disorders—for example, acute appendicitis, ectopic pregnancy, endometriosis, or an ovarian tumor (these last three are described in later sections). For this reason, it may be necessary to perform a **laparoscopy** (endoscopic viewing of the abdomen's contents) to arrive at a definitive diagnosis. Once the diagnosis of PID is established, treatment consists of various antibiotic regimens to suppress the infection. Usually, more than one antibiotic is required because multiple organisms may be involved. In some cases, the treatment may require surgical intervention to drain abscesses.

Long-term consequences of PID derive from postinflammatory scarring and the formation of adhesions between the tubes, ovaries, and adjacent organ surfaces. Stricture of the Fallopian tubes is also common. These changes can lead to infertility because they block the passage of

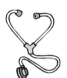

Focus on Dysfunctional Uterine Bleeding and Intense Athletic Training

Women engaged in vigorous and prolonged physical activity are subject to dysfunctional uterine bleeding and, in many cases, to cessation of all menstruation, **amenorrhea.** If a normal menarche is followed at some later time by cessation of menstruation cycling, the condition is called **secondary amenorrhea.** If the menarche does not occur, the condition is called **primary amenorrhea.** Intense physical training is associated with stress and with nutritional and metabolic alterations, which appear to contribute to the endocrine changes that interfere with ovulation. When exercise patterns are restored to more typical levels, apparently normal menstrual cycles return.

spermatozoa to the distal Fallopian tubes, the usual site of fertilization. When fertilization does occur, passage of the embryo to the uterus is also blocked, and implantation into the tube's mucosa (ectopic pregnancy) may occur. In the abdomen, adhesions can interfere with normal intestinal motility or cause pain when they restrain organs from shifting in response to body movements. In some cases, chronic abdominal pain and recurring bouts of salpingitis follow the initial acute attack and may continue for years.

Disorders of the Uterus

The normal uterus consists of the muscular myometrium and an internal lining, the endometrium (figs. 19.7 and 19.8). Broadly, the problems arising in these tissues relate to tumors of the myometrium and cervical epithelium and to various disorders of the endometrium, which are often characterized by uterine bleeding. Endometrial disorders are considered first.

Dysfunctional Uterine Bleeding

Uterine bleeding disorders are the most common problem affecting women of childbearing age. They may be related to various diseases, but when none can be identified, the condition is described as **dysfunctional uterine bleeding.** Abnormalities of bleeding that may occur during the menstrual period include prolonged, excessive, or meager flow. Another abnormality, bleeding between menstrual periods, is usually not associated with abdominal discomfort.

The cause of most dysfunctional uterine bleeding is failure to ovulate, as a result of some disturbance in the endocrine control of the ovarian cycle. Cycles that pass without ovulation are described as **anovulatory cycles.** They are thought to arise when the corpus luteum of one cycle continues to secrete beyond its normal ten-day life span

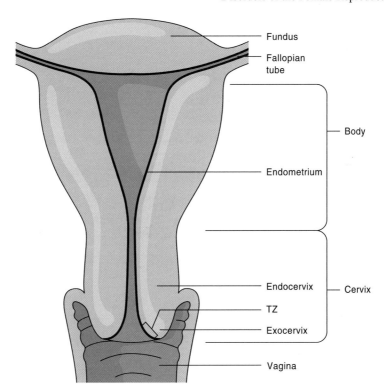

Figure 19.8   **Section through the Uterus and Proximal Vagina.** TZ: transformation zone.

into what would be the next cycle. High levels of hormones are thus prolonged enough to suppress normal follicle development in the ovary before the corpus luteum finally loses secretory ability. This means the next ovarian cycle is disrupted in that no graaffian follicle develops and no corpus luteum forms. The resulting lack of estrogen and progesterone provides an unusual hormone stimulus to the endometrium, which produces bleeding abnormalities.

Anovulatory cycles are more common around the time of the **menarche** (onset of menstruation) and the **menopause** (cessation of menstruation), probably because of delay in the acquisition of fine endocrine control as cycle patterns are established and because of its loss as cycles are ending. Between these times, anovulatory cycles may be caused by various metabolic disturbances, such as systemic disease, obesity, psychological stress, or some abnormality in the endocrine links between hypothalamus-anterior pituitary and ovary.

Endometriosis

In **endometriosis,** deposits of endometrial tissue are present at various sites external to the uterus. They are thought to arise from endometrial fragments that are expelled through the infundibulum of the fallopian tube into the pelvic cavity, where they become established. This seems to account for the high rate of ovarian involvement in endometriosis (80%), in that the ovaries are the first pelvic structures in the path of endometrial tissue as it is expelled from the fallopian tube. Alternatively, and less commonly, endometrial cells may gain access to lymphatics or veins

that carry them to regional lymph nodes or more distant sites (e.g., lung or bone).

Whatever their location, these extrauterine endometrial deposits are subject to changes induced by normal endocrine cycles. This means that they not only proliferate under the influence of rising estrogen and progesterone levels, but that they become necrotic and bleed when levels decline. This bleeding at pelvic sites typically causes peritoneal irritation and pain at the time of menstruation (dysmenorrhea). After bleeding, organization of the coagulated pelvic blood may produce adhesions between affected organ surfaces and pelvic walls. These can cause pain because they restrict normal visceral movements during exercise, defecation, urination, or sexual intercourse.

Infertility is a common consequence of endometriosis and results from disruption of the ovarian surface and blockage of the fallopian tubes. In some cases, cysts filled with coagulated blood **(chocolate cysts)** form within the ovaries. These can reach diameters of 10–15 cm.

Menstrual Pain and Premenstrual Dysphoric Disorder

The term **dysmenorrhea** describes the abdominal cramping that accompanies ovulation cycles in many women. In most cases, it is trivial or mildly uncomfortable, but in some individuals the pain is severe and interferes with, or prevents, normal activity. Dysmenorrhea is caused by exaggerated uterine contraction. The underlying mechanism appears to depend on the action of high levels of prostaglandins that are present during the second half of the cycle, when high

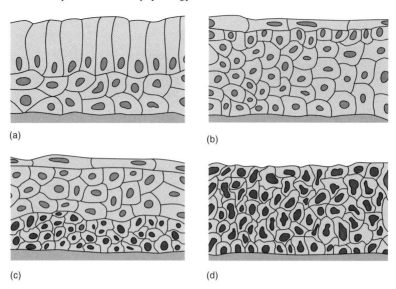

Figure 19.9   Cervical Epithelium. Representations of changes in the histology of the transformation zone. (*a*) Normal immature epithelium. (*b*) Squamous metaplasia adapts to the changed conditions of maturity. (*c*) Dysplasia, with deeper cells exhibiting pleomorphism. (*d*) Carcinoma in situ with all cells abnormal.

progesterone levels exaggerate their effect on the myometrium. Other smoooth muscle is also affected, producing headache, nausea, and vomiting. NSAID therapy is generally effective in the treatment of dysmenorrhea in that it blocks prostaglandin systhesis.

Premenstrual dysphoric disorder is the formal term for what is commonly known as **premenstrual syndrome** (PMS). Both terms refer to the array of signs and symptoms experienced by some women during the seven- to ten-day period that precedes the onset of menstrual bleeding. Those most commonly reported include edema, abdominal discomfort, breast fullness, and headache. A psychological component, involving varying degrees of irritability, anxiety or depression, aggressiveness, and alterations in libido, is often superimposed on the physical changes. The subsiding of PMS symptoms after the start of menstrual bleeding suggests an underlying hormonal mechanism that directly or indirectly produces them.

Hormonal effects on neurotransmitters, various metabolic pathways, salt and water retention, and other factors have been proposed as being involved in causing PMS, but there is no clear evidence for any of these. With no known etiology, therapy is usually directed at alleviating the particular combination of signs and symptoms present in each patient. Diuretics for systemic edema, NSAIDs for abdominal pain or headache, and various agents to reduce breast discomfort are typically employed. In severe cases, agents that act on the hypothalamus to block secretion of **gonadotropin-releasing hormone** (GnRH) are prescribed. These agents indirectly suppress the estrogen secretion that seems responsible for many of the signs and symptoms of PMS.

Endometrial Carcinoma

Endometrial carcinoma is a common malignancy of the uterus. It most often arises after menopause in conjunction with unexplained uterine bleeding. Exposure to high levels of estrogen seems to promote the development of this tumor. Conditions associated with such levels are diabetes mellitus, obesity, hypertension, and delayed menopause. In women who are born without ovaries, no endometrial carcinoma is observed until estrogen therapy is initiated.

If untreated, damaging effects in endometrial carcinoma are due to local invasion into the myometrium and at sites of metastatic growth, the lung in particular. Growth of the tumor may also extend along the Fallopian tubes to reach the ovaries. Therapy typically involves hysterectomy and removal of adjacent pelvic organs that have been invaded by the tumor. Radiation or hormone-suppression therapy is then directed against any smaller, secondary tumor growth. When endometrial carcinoma is detected early, therapy is usually highly successful.

Cervical Carcinoma

The cervix (neck) forms the lower third of the uterus. The portion of the cervix that projects into the proximal vagina is the **exocervix,** while the remainder, adjacent to the body of the uterus, is called the **endocervix** (fig. 19.8). The exocervix is protected by a stratified squamous epithelium, while the endocervix is lined by a simple columnar epithelium. In the young adult, the epithelium of the exocervix consists of a layer of columnar cells resting on a bed of reserve cells (fig. 19.9*a*), which are the source of new cells needed to replace those normally sloughed from the surface. With maturity, the exocervix is exposed to various vaginal irritants, as well as pH and estrogen changes, and to the trauma of coitus and childbirth. These induce an adaptive thickening and strengthening of the epithelium, termed **squamous metaplasia** (fig. 19.9*b*). Such adaptations produce the essentially normal adult epithelium of the exo-

Table 19.4	Grading of Cervical Intraepithelial Neoplasia (CIN)

Grade	Criteria
CIN I	Mild dysplasia
CIN II	Moderate dysplasia; less than two-thirds of epithelium's cells are dysplastic
CIN III	Carcinoma in situ; severe dysplasia in more than two-thirds of epithelium's cells

Table 19.5	Staging of Cervical Carcinoma*

Stage	Criteria
I	Tumor confined to region of cervix
II	Invasion to adjacent structures, but excluding lower one-third of vagina and wall of pelvis
III	Invasion to lower one-third of vagina or wall of pelvis
IV	Extension to bladder or rectum or structures beyond pelvis

* This is the essence of the system recommended by the International Federation of Gynecology and Obstetrics (FIGO).

cervix known as the **transformation zone**—the site where carcinoma usually arises.

The development of an invasive carcinoma from the metaplastic cells of the transformation zone occurs over a period of years and involves a predictable sequence of changes. (Before proceeding, you may find it useful to refer to chapter 6 for a brief review of terminology related to tissue growth abnormalities.) The early change from normal sees the epithelial cells exhibiting mild degrees of dysplasia. These initial changes are seen in the deepest layers, with the more superficial regions exhibiting pleomorphism in later stages (fig. 19.8c). Surface cells retain their normal appearance until the last, but ultimately dysplasia is in evidence in all epithelial layers. The next stage involves the critical transformation from dysplasia to neoplasia, with increasing anaplasia and more extreme pleomorphism characteristic of a full-blown carcinoma seen in all layers. Because the tumor is, at this point, confined to the epithelium, it is described as **carcinoma in situ** (CIS). Since the development of CIS is thought always to follow this sequence, all of these development stages are grouped under the title of **cervical intraepithelial neoplasia** (CIN), with an accompanying grading system that is widely used (table 19.4).

Unless there is intervention to interrupt the progression, tumor cells break through the basement membrane to invade locally. With more extensive invasion, adjacent organs are affected and access to lymphatics is achieved, followed by metastasis to regional lymph nodes, ultimately involving the lungs and liver. Blood-borne metastasis is a less common route for the spread of cervical carcinoma.

Previously more common, cervical carcinoma has been declining because of the ease with which a sample of cervical epithelium can be obtained via a Pap smear. Assessment of cervical cells can reveal the status of the epithelium in the context of the progressive changes that precede invasion. On findings of abnormal cytology, there is ample time to confirm the diagnosis and consider various interventions, given the long times involved in progression through the stages of CIN. Studies indicate that of all cases of mild dysplasia (CIN I), 40–50% will develop into CIS (CIN III) over a period of 5–20 years. Incidence of CIS has a peak at about age 30, while invasive carcinoma peaks in the early 40s. Most specialists recommend annual Pap smears starting at age 18 or at the onset of sexual activity.

Because CIN is confined to the cervical epithelium, it produces no symptoms. The tumor betrays its presence only when invasion has occurred, at which point there may be abnormal bleeding, vaginal discharge **(leukorrhea),** and pain from the irritation or compression of adjacent pelvic structures. Compression of the ureter, a common occurrence, may cause hydronephrosis, which can ultimately lead to renal failure and death. Invasion through the walls of the nearby rectum and bladder can lead to fistula formation between their lumina and the uterus. Although metastasis does occur, most of the serious consequences of cervical carcinoma derive from its invasion of pelvic structures.

Early detection is strongly related to therapeutic success in carcinoma of the cervix. When diagnosis is made while the tumor is confined to the epithelium, it is relatively simple to remove or destroy the lesion, and survival rates approach 100%. At later stages, the treatment may include **hysterectomy** (surgical removal of the uterus), excision of invading tumor, and radiation therapy. As expected, survival rates are higher in the earlier stages. The staging system for cervical carcinoma is indicated in table 19.5. Five years after diagnosis, survival rates are: Stage I—up to 95%, Stage II—up to 75%, Stage III—35%, and Stage IV—10%.

Studies of etiology in cervical carcinoma indicate that sexual transmission of a viral agent plays a key role. Incidence of the tumor is high when sexual activity starts early and involves multiple partners. A woman faces a particularly high risk when her partner has had previous sexual relations with a woman who had developed cervical carcinoma, the implication being that either he transmitted the oncogenic agent to the original partner or he picked it up from her and can now transmit it to others. The situation can be summed up in the stark contrast between the virtual nonexistence of cervical carcinoma in virgins and its very high incidence in prostitutes.

The principal viral agent implicated in cervical carcinoma is the human papilloma virus (HPV), although its exact role is unclear. Also suspected of contributing is a genetic predisposition to the action of the virus. Of course, an immune-suppressed status, for whatever reason, means reduced capacity to cope with the infecting HPV and a greater risk of neoplasia.

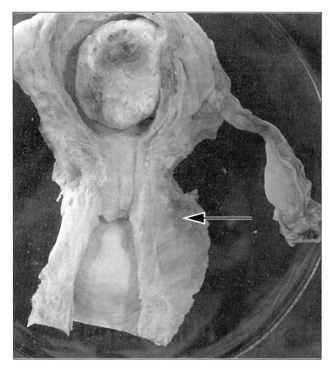

Figure 19.10   Leiomyoma. In this sectioned uterus a smaller, rounded leiomyoma is present at the arrow, causing a bulge in the uterine wall. The larger mass at the top is another leiomyoma projecting from the surface into the uterine cavity.

This uterus has been sectioned to reveal a leiomyoma, the size of a hen's egg, occupying the uterine cavity. Its presence was not betrayed by any signs or symptoms; at least none were reported. The mass was discovered incidentally, in examining a 50-year-old woman who had suffered a massive myocardial infarct from which she did not recover.

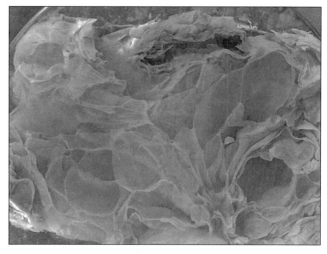

Figure 19.11   Ovarian Cysts. This section through an enlarged ovary reveals that its interior is dominated by numerous fluid-filled cysts.

A 15-year-old girl experienced three months of dysmenorrhea followed by a week of abdominal swelling. When fever developed, and persisted for 36 hours, she was examined and a large mass was found adjacent to her umbilicus. Exploratory surgery revealed a 6-kg (13-lb) growth, which had replaced her left ovary. It contained numerous cysts that were filled with a milky looking, mucinous fluid. The tumor was removed and postsurgical progress was satisfactory.

Disorders of the Ovary

Previous sections of this chapter have described secondary involvement of the ovary in PID and endometriosis. Apart from genetic defects in its ova, there are only two primary ovarian abnormalities of any significance: cysts and tumors.

Ovarian Cysts

The most common ovarian cysts are present in about 25% of women. They form from Graafian follicles that do not degenerate normally **(follicle cyst),** or that ovulate and then become sealed, forming an enlarged **luteal cyst.** These fluid-filled cysts are usually 1–2 cm in diameter, but at extremes may exceed 8 cm. Smaller cysts may present no signs or symptoms, but increasing size may be associated with abdominal discomfort. Since some cysts continue to secrete estrogens or both estrogens and progesterone, they are typically accompanied by anovulatory cycles and irregularities of menstrual bleeding. Although they may resolve spontaneously, they present the risk of rupture, at which point their released fluid contents and blood can cause acute irritation and abdominal pain.

A less common cystic condition of the ovaries is **polycystic ovarian** (PCO) syndrome, also known as the **Stein-Leventhal syndrome.** It is usually seen in young women and involves the presence of multiple cysts in both ovaries (fig. 19.11). Its essential characteristics are secondary amenorrhea, increased body and facial hair **(hirsutism),** infertility, and variable obesity.

Myometrial Tumors

Myometrial tumors are principally of two types: a rare malignant form, **leiomyosarcoma,** and a common benign form, **leiomyoma.** The benign form is also known as a **fibroid** and occurs in one in four women over age 30. The fact that many fibroids regress after menopause, whereas their growth is increased during pregnancy, suggests that estrogen is important to their development.

Leiomyomas vary greatly in size, from tiny growths to large, spherical, unencapsulated masses of over 25 cm diameter (fig. 19.10). In some cases, they take the form of a mass projecting into the uterine cavity. Depending on their size and location, they may be asymptomatic or produce varying patterns of excessive menstrual bleeding and discomfort or pain, which is due to their compression of other pelvic structures.

The leiomyosarcoma presents a much more serious prognosis, with survival rates of only 20–40% five years after diagnosis. Extensive metastasis contributes to the high lethality of these tumors. Incidence is highest at about the age of 50.

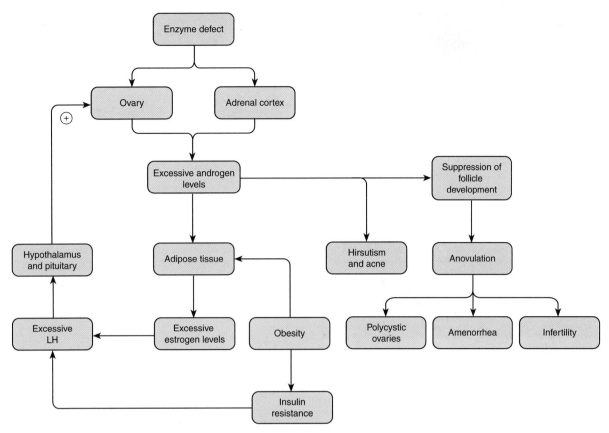

Figure 19.12   **PCO Syndrome Pathogenesis.** Once initiated by an intrinsic enzyme defect, positive feedback cycling (+) sustains the excessive output of androgens. Obesity and insulin resistance often contribute.

The root of the problem in PCO syndrome appears to be an enzyme defect that may initiate exaggerated secretion of androgens near the time of the menarche. Both ovary and adrenal cortex oversecrete androgens that are converted to estrogens in adipose tissue. The high estrogen levels that result have a stimulatory effect on the hypothalamus, which then begins steady secretion of an increased level of GnRH, which, in turn, stimulates secretion of **luteinizing hormone** (LH) by the anterior pituitary. The excessive LH induces an increased output of hormones from the ovaries, including androgen, which are, in turn, converted to more estrogen, establishing a positive feedback cycle that perpetuates the problem. The androgens are also responsible for inducing the growth of body hair.

Note that the normal interaction between elevated estrogen and the hypothalamus produces a short surge of LH output that triggers ovulation, which then subsides, but in PCO syndrome the high LH output is sustained. The exaggerated estrogen levels also exert the usual inhibitory effects on the anterior pituitary, suppressing its release of **follicle-stimulating hormone** (FSH). This means that no normal ovarian follicle development occurs, and amenorrhea, anovulatory cycles, and infertility result. The common association of obesity and PCO syndrome is thought to lie in the capacity of adipose tissue to convert androgen to estrogen. Obesity alone is not likely to produce high enough estrogen levels to initiate the cycling, but once ex-

cess androgen is present, obesity can add to the estrogen excess problem and exaggerate its effects. A complicating factor in PCO syndrome is insulin resistance in the obese (fig. 19.12). This condition produces an exaggerated secretion of insulin that directly or indirectly promotes androgen secretion. You may recall that insulin resistance often accompanies obesity. Although this is a second way that obesity can contribute, some women with PCO syndrome are not obese.

PCO syndrome is a common cause of infertility and is treated by reducing obesity and by various regimens of hormone therapy, which seek to restore a more normal balance and to interrupt the cycle of positive feedback that drives this derangement.

Ovarian Tumors

Ovarian tumors have a relatively low incidence (≈1/100 females), but they rank fourth in the list of tumor fatalities in females. The danger arises from the lack of signs and symptoms in the early growth stages of ovarian malignancies. By the time indications of abnormality emerge, the tumor's growth, invasion, and metastasis have developed to the point where aggressive combination therapy is required. In spite of improved therapy, prognosis in advanced cases remains poor, and as with so many tumors, the importance of early detection can hardly be overemphasized.

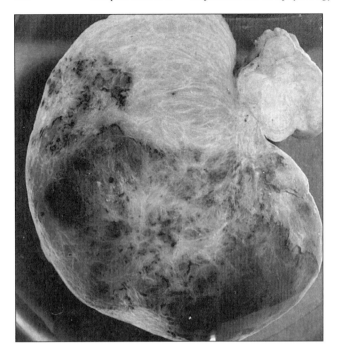

Figure 19.13 **An Ovarian Tumor.** This benign mass derives from the ovarian stroma (thecoma). It is about the size of a grapefruit. Compare with the ovary, which is about the size of an unshelled almond.
This thecoma was discovered arising from the ovary of a 57-year-old woman. She had complained of no symptoms that could be attributed to the tumor. After removal, the specimen could be seen to have a thin capsule enclosing its firm mass. Note the lighter-colored stromal bands interlacing the neoplastic tissue. Evidence of scarring at the sites of previous hemorrhage is also present.

Most ovarian tumors arise in those age 50–70, but no age is without risk. Various studies implicate genetics and various environmental factors in the etiology of these tumors, but specifics are few. Hormonal factors are also implicated in ovarian tumors. Studies indicate that bearing a child and oral contraceptive use reduce the risk of ovarian carcinoma.

Ovarian enlargement due to tumor growth may be substantial, involving one or both ovaries and producing significant and even enormous pelvic and abdominal bulk before signs and symptoms arise (fig. 19.13). The tumor's presence may first be detected in an incidental pelvic or abdominal examination, or it may reveal itself through various indications of abdominopelvic disturbance, such as pain or disruptions of normal intestinal or urinary function. In some cases, the bulk caused by a large tumor mass may be mistaken for simple obesity, while in other cases, preexisting obesity may mask the tumor's growth. A common feature of ovarian tumors is abdominopelvic distention, usually associated with the production of large volumes of fluid resembling serous fluid or mucous (see Focus box: "An Extreme Case of Ovarian Cyst"). These secretions are usually confined to large cysts within the bulky ovarian mass, but in some cases, a mucin-secreting tumor releases its gelatinous fluid into the peritoneal cavity. These prod-

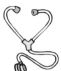

Focus on an Extreme Case of Ovarian Cyst

Recently, a woman diagnosed as having an ovarian cyst refused to allow its surgical removal because she was concerned she would die during the operation. It grew for ten years and reached a size that caused the woman to be bedridden for two years before finally agreeing to its removal.

After the resection, the cyst was found to have a diameter of 1 meter and to weigh over 300 pounds (137 kg). The mass consisted of 50 separate, benign ovarian cysts filled with mucous, serous, or fatty liquid contents. The 5-foot 10-inch woman weighed 200 pounds (90 kg) after the procedure and suffered no ill effects. You do the math to determine her pre-operation weight.

Table 19.6	Staging of Ovarian Cancers. Substages (not shown) carry A/B/C designation and indicate increasing tissue involvement and severity within a given stage.

Stage	Criteria
I	Tumor confined to ovaries
II	Extension of tumor growth to adjacent pelvic structures; one or both ovaries involved
III	Extension beyond pelvis to peritoneal surfaces, bowel, or liver
IV	Distant metastases

ucts may also accumulate at metastatic sites, extensively coating abdominal surfaces. Another factor producing abdominal distention is ascites, which develops as a result of the tumor's compression of lymphatic vessels. This blocks lymph drainage and leads to the accumulation of fluid in the peritoneal cavity.

The most optimistic situation arises when an ovarian tumor is sufficiently well-differentiated to retain estrogen and progesterone secretion. In such cases, the high hormone levels can produce early systemic effects that call attention to the tumor's presence before it can spread, thus allowing early therapeutic intervention.

Metastasis of ovarian tumors is by direct seeding onto adjacent pelvic surfaces and by way of the lymphatics. Lymphatic metastasis can give rise to widespread growth at secondary sites, some as far removed as the diaphragm. Metastasis by the blood to more distant sites, outside the abdominopelvic cavity, is less common. A widely used staging system for ovarian tumors is presented in table 19.6.

Table 19.7   Principal Types of Ovarian Tumors

Epithelial Tumors (70%)	Germ Cell Tumors (20%)	Stromal Tumors (10%)
Serous tumors	Teratoma	Granulosa cell tumor
Mucinous tumors	Dysgerminoma	Thecoma
Endometrioid tumors	Endodermal sinus tumor (Yolk sac tumor)	Fibroma
Clear cell tumor	Embryonal carcinoma	Sertoli-Leydig tumor
Brenner tumor		

There is great diversity in the various benign and malignant ovarian tumors (table 19.7). Each has its own specific diagnostic and therapeutic characteristics, but these are beyond the scope of this text. The following sections briefly describe the major features of the three principal categories of ovarian tumors.

Tumors of the Ovarian Epithelium Tumors originating in the ovarian epithelium constitute over 70% of ovarian tumors. For this reason, they are known as the ovary's **common epithelial tumors.** Differing lines of tumor cell development produce different types of epithelial cell tumors, which resemble various epithelia of the female urogenital passages. The **endometrioid adenocarcinoma,** for example, resembles endometrium, and the **Brenner tumor** resembles urinary tract epithelium. Among the epithelial tumors are the serous and mucin-producing tumors mentioned earlier. Epithelial cell tumors most often produce late signs and symptoms. Even when these emerge, they may be ignored or denied, allowing more extensive growth and spread and reducing the likelihood of successful therapy.

Ovarian Germ Cell Tumors These are mostly benign and typically arise in premenopausal women, but malignant forms can arise in children. Because they originate in the precursors of the female sex cells, they have the capacity for widely differing lines of differentiation. As a consequence, the tumors of this group are quite diverse, with varying sensitivity to radiation or chemotherapeutic agents. Some tumors of this group produce hCG and α-fetoprotein, but in amounts detectable only in the later stages of their development. This means these plasma tumor markers are of little help in making an early diagnosis; but once the diagnosis is established, their levels in plasma can be used to monitor the progress of therapy.

About one-quarter of all ovarian tumors are benign germ cell tumors, which have peak incidence in women aged 20–30. They are called **mature cystic teratomas** or **dermoid cysts,** and derive from a defect in meiosis that produces a diploid cell, which then proceeds to differentiate to form a cyst containing any number of mature tissue types. Most often the tissues are epithelial derivatives, with skin lining the cyst's interior. From this lining, hair and sebaceous glands may develop, and the cyst's interior may be filled with a sebumlike fluid or keratinlike material. Other tissues and organ elements may be found, including tooth,

bronchus, smooth muscle, nervous tissue, and various glands. Once discovered, these cysts can be surgically removed to effect a cure.

Tumors of the Ovarian Stroma These are the least common of the ovarian tumors. Microscopically, the stroma of the ovary has a fibrous appearance that is due to the presence of numerous spindle-shaped cells, resembling smooth muscle cells, and fibroblasts, which have some capacity for contraction and for collagen synthesis. Other cells of the stroma are more specialized in being able to secrete estrogen, progesterone, and in some cases, androgens. These, you will recall, can be critical as early indications of the tumor's presence. Stromal cell tumors constitute approximately 10% of all ovarian tumors and only 2% of the malignancies.

Pregnancy-Related Disorders

The following sections deal with the major abnormalities of pregnancy that threaten its successful outcome.

Ectopic Pregnancy

As the term **ectopic** implies, this is a pregnancy in which the fertilized ovum is implanted at a site other than the endometrium. Usually the cause is some defect or blockage along the uterine tube, leading to implantation in its wall. Most ectopic pregnancies, 90% or more, occur in this way and, in many cases, obstructions related to PID or endometriosis are responsible. However, in about half of ectopic pregnancies, the Fallopian tubes appear to be normal, so more subtle defects in the transport mechanism, or some exaggerated capacity for adherence on the part of the developing embryo, may be involved. In rare cases, instead of entering the infundibulum, a fertilized ovum may fall to a lower peritoneal surface, where it implants, or fertilization may occur at the ovarian surface, confining the embryo to the ovary.

Implantation in the oviduct raises the threat of rupture of its wall, followed by pelvic bleeding. This crisis usually induces pronounced abdominal pain and often leads to circulatory shock (fig. 19.14). Initially, there may be no sign of anything unusual because relatively normal development proceeds in the tubal mucosa. But the thin Fallopian tube wall can't sustain the embryo's presence, and rupture

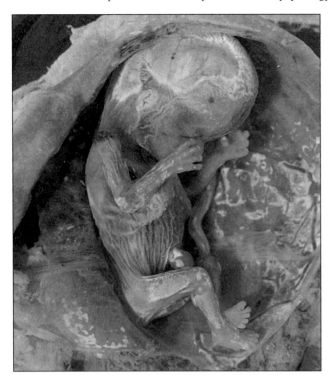

Figure 19.14   **Ectopic Pregnancy.** The fully formed fetus lies in the lumen of the uterine tube.

The fetus in this photograph developed for three months in the left Fallopian tube of a 23-year-old woman. At that time, the invading placenta broke through the tube's wall, causing intense lower-left quadrant abdominal pain. The hemorrhage that followed produced an acute drop in blood pressure, causing the woman to collapse. Pelvic examination revealed an orange-sized mass, lateral to the uterus, which was surgically removed. In the specimen, note the stretching of the tube in response to the expansion of the developing fetus, amniotic sac, and placenta. The woman's recovery from shock and surgery was uneventful.

usually occurs 2–12 weeks after fertilization. The variations of timing and degree of blood loss in ectopic pregnancies are due to differences in wall thickness and blood supply along its length.

In some cases, there is a seemingly spontaneous interruption of the ectopic development, followed by degeneration and absorption of the failed embryo. This occurrence may be related, not to the ectopic implantation, but to the fact that approximately 40% of all pregnancies abort spontaneously, presumably as a result of genetic defects or congenital factors such as infection or endocrine disorders.

Gestational Tumors

Three major tumors, which derive from the developing placenta and involve excessive chorionic gonadotropin secretion by its trophoblasts, are grouped under the term **gestational trophoblast disease** (GTD). One of these is a benign tumor composed of large masses of grapelike swellings of the placenta's chorionic villi. It is known as a **hydatidiform mole** (HM). (In this context, the term *mole*

refers to a formless mass and *hydatid* is a reference to water-filled cysts.) It forms as a result of faulty meiosis that produces ova with no chromosomes. The resulting embryonic cells carry only paternal chromosomes. Abnormal development and mole formation follow. With early detection by ultrasound imaging, the mole can be removed by suction curettage. Most are readily dealt with in this way.

A second type of GTD is the **invasive mole,** which does not metastasize but can invade from the endometrium into the myometrium. Extension of tumor to adjacent structures may also occur, but the greatest risk is perforation of the uterine wall and hemorrhage.

The third type of GTD is **choriocarcinoma,** a rare but highly malignant tumor that may develop in association with HM, spontaneous abortion, or even a normal pregnancy. The tumor mass is typically soft and bulky, with prominent areas of hemorrhage and necrosis. It metastasizes early and widely via the blood to the lung, vagina, brain, and liver. Both choriocarcinoma and invasive mole are quite susceptible to chemotherapy.

HM and choriocarcinoma are very rare in the Western world, but have higher incidence in Asia and Africa. Most cases occur in women younger than 15 years old and older than 40. Following curettage of a HM, 10% of GTD cases are found to be invasive moles, while 2–3% emerge as choriocarcinoma.

Abnormalities of Placental Attachment

Following fertilization, three or four days are required for transport of the developing embryo to the uterus. On arrival, it spends an additional three days or so at the endometrial surface, where it develops to the stage of a hollow cell mass called the **blastocyst.** It is this embryonic form that implants into the endometrium, which has undergone various changes to accommodate its further development of the embryo.

Implantation normally occurs in the upper portion of the uterus. While embryonic development proceeds, the endometrium underlying the blastocyst undergoes modification to become the **decidua basalis.** One aspect of this process involves formation of the early placental blood channels. The **placenta** provides for the passage of nutrients, blood gases, and fetal metabolic wastes between the maternal and fetal circulations. The exchange occurs via a particular arrangement of embryonic capillaries that occupy projections of the embryonic membranes called **chorionic villi** (fig. 19.15). These extend into pools of maternal blood present in the placenta. After the infant is delivered, the placenta separates from the supporting decidua basalis and is expelled by uterine contraction. (The lay term for the expelled placenta and its associated membranes is **afterbirth.**)

An abnormal implantation in the lower portion of the uterus positions the developing fetus, and sometimes the placenta, over the opening to the cervix. This condition, called **placenta previa,** presents the risk of serious hemor-

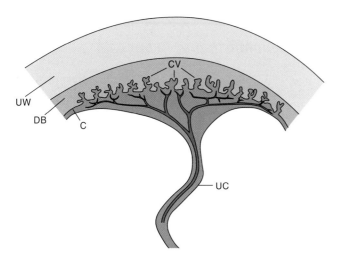

Figure 19.15   **The Placenta.** Projections of the embryonic chorion (C), the chorionic villi (CV), carry fetal capillaries that project into the region of the decidua basalis (DB), which contains pools of maternal blood. After exchange of nutrients and wastes between the two circulations, the umbilical cord (UC) returns blood to the fetus. UW: uterine wall.

Table 19.8	Grading in Placenta Previa

Grade	Determining Characteristics
I	Margin of placenta some distance from cervical canal
II	Margin of placenta at edge of cervical canal
III	Placenta partially blocks cervical canal
IV	Placenta completely blocks cervical canal

Grades II–IV involve bleeding prior to the child's delivery. Because the outlet from the uterus is obstructed, Grades III and IV are likely to require a cesarean section.

rhage because the elongation and thinning of the cervix that occurs in the later stages of pregnancy are exaggerated during the delivery. As the cervix elongates, the decidua moves from under the placenta, tearing the placental vessels and causing blood loss. The result is a reduction, or complete loss, of blood supply to the infant and the threat of hypovolemic shock to the mother. A cesarean section is often necessary in placenta previa. A system of grading in placenta previa is based on the site of implantation and the severity of complications (table 19.8).

When an endometrial abnormality at the site of implantation provides no decidua basalis to anchor the placenta, the embryo's chorionic villi invade the myometrium. This is the condition of **placenta accreta.** The lack of normal decidua formation may be due to endometrial abnormalities at sites of previous uterine disruption—for example, scarring caused by infection, previous curettage procedures, healing at the site of a previous cesarean section, or an underlying tumor. Placenta accreta may take the form **placenta increta,** where invasion is superficial and limited, or **placenta pancreta,** where there is penetration of the complete myometrial thickness. In the latter case, hemorrhage associated with rupture of the uterus is usually serious, occurring before or during the delivery. In all cases of placenta accreta, the delivery of the infant poses a serious risk of blood loss, since, in the absence of the decidua basalis, there is no provision for the orderly separation of placenta from uterus. When bleeding is severe, surgical removal of the uterus (hysterectomy) may be necessary.

The condition of **abruptio placentae** arises in the later stages of pregnancy, but prior to the actual delivery. In this disorder, a portion of the placenta may separate from its underlying decidua. The resulting disruption of the placental vessels causes blood loss that forms a hematoma within the placenta, compressing it and restricting fetal blood flow. As the blood coagulates, it rapidly consumes clotting factors, limiting the blood coagulation response at other sites where it may be needed. This interference with the coagulation response is especially threatening when delivery and the associated bleeding follow soon after abruptio placentae develops.

When blood is also lost to the pelvic cavity following a premature separation of the placenta, circulatory shock may present a serious threat to both mother and infant. Another danger, although rare, is pulmonary embolism by masses of fetal cells in the amniotic fluid that bathes the fetus. As these gain access to the disrupted maternal vessels, they can be carried to the right heart and then the lungs' vessels, where they become trapped. The amniotic cells also release thromboplastins, which can initiate disseminated intravascular coagulation (DIC) because the cells are widely distributed in the circulation.

Preeclampsia and Eclampsia

This is another condition whose descriptive terminology is in a state of transition. Previously known as **toxemia of pregnancy,** this term is falling into disuse since no toxins have been identified that might be involved in its etiology. Hypertension, albuminuria, and edema are often present, together forming the syndrome called **preeclampsia.** The term refers to the late occurrence of convulsions and coma, whose emergence in this context is described as **eclampsia.**

The hypertension, albuminuria, and edema of preeclampsia, usually arise 32 weeks into a first pregnancy, and are often accompanied by headache and disruptions of vision. Preeclampsia seems to originate from an implantation abnormality that affects placental blood vessels. The resulting placental ischemia may be severe enough to produce placental infarcts. More typically, ischemia triggers the release of vasoconstrictors and activates renal fluid retention responses that combine to produce a rise in blood pressure. Various mediators released from the ischemic placenta also disrupt endothelia, predisposing to disseminated intravascular coagulation (DIC; see chapter 7). It is this widespread blockage of blood flow in the systemic

Focus on Role of the Immune System in Preeclampsia and Eclampsia

Recent research has focused on the role of the immune system in preeclampsia. This research is based on the fact that although the placenta has different tissue antigens than the endometrium that supports it, a maternal response in some way masks the "foreign" placental antigens so that the placenta is not rejected. However, if the masking mechanism is disrupted, placental antigens are exposed to the maternal immune system's responses at the point where invading placental arterioles and anchoring cells are most intimately associated with the maternal tissues. The result is immune attack, with immune complex deposition, vasculitis, and necrosis of the vessels causing ischemic damage to the decidua. In response, tissue thromboplastins are released, followed by thrombosis and thromboembolism. Also released are prostaglandins and thromboxane A_2 (TxA_2), a vasoconstrictor that may trigger the characteristic systemic hypertension seen in this condition. One of the prostaglandins released may mediate ischemia by promoting platelet aggregation, while another may contribute to the uterine contractions also often seen in toxemia of pregnancy. Immune damage to the decidual anchoring cells would also explain the increased rate of abruptio placentae seen in preeclampsia.

Certain patterns of incidence of pregnancy-induced hypertension lend support to the idea of an immune system etiology. For example, a second pregnancy is less likely to involve a preeclampsia problem. Perhaps the masking factors that were induced by the first pregnancy, though inadequate at that time, proliferate to provide adequate masking in later pregnancies. The use of barrier methods of birth control appears to double the risk of pregnancy-induced hypertension. The explanation for this observation is that a component of semen provides an antigenic stimulus that functions to help activate the female's antigen-masking system. Apparently, blocking access of these seminal antigens (e.g., by condoms, diaphragms, or foams) means that there is less masking, and preeclampsia is more likely to occur. This is consistent with the observation that more toxemia of pregnancy occurs in the first pregnancies of women with minimal previous sexual intercourse. Presumably, although no barrier contraceptives are involved, minimal prepregnancy exposure to semen (or perhaps a particularly large and invasive placenta) results in a mismatch between the masking response and exposure to foreign antigens.

---

microcirculation that produces generalized tissue hypoxia. In the kidney, reduced blood flow through glomeruli causes damage that allows protein to escape to the urine. This loss of protein means a reduced blood osmotic pressure that combines with fluid retention to produce the characteristic systemic edema of preeclampsia. In severe cases, brain ischemia causes the later emergence of the convulsions and coma of eclampsia (fig. 19.16). Therapy to reduce hypertension and correct the edema often eases the situation. Signs and symptoms subside following delivery of the infant and the abnormal placenta, which may have to be induced to prevent progression to the more threatening eclampsia.

Breast Disorders

The significant breast lesions include lumps that may be either cysts or tumors, and that range from small, asymptomatic, and trivial, to life-threatening in their impact.

Fibrocystic Change

This very common breast condition is characterized by the presence of lumps in the breast. They consist, alone or in combination, of proliferated epithelium, fibrous stroma, or fluid-filled cysts. Cyst diameter may approach 5 cm with varying degrees of calcification developing over time. Many become tender during the time between ovulation and the beginning of menstrual flow.

Fibrocystic change is essentially idiopathic but estrogen-progesterone imbalance is known to be a contributing factor. Incidence is highest during a woman's reproductive years and is low before menarche and after menopause. Note also that oral contraceptives reduce the incidence of fibrocystic change, presumably because they improve the estrogen-progesterone ratio. Although they will occasionally be biopsied to remove any concern about potential malignancy, these fibrocystic lumps pose no threat.

Breast Proliferative Disease

This condition carries an increased risk of breast cancer. Breast stroma, glands, or duct epithelia not only are overproduced, but, as distinct from fibrocystic change, the tissues demonstrate greater dysplasia and anaplasia. In other words, they tend to resemble carcinoma. Most carcinoma risk is linked to epithelial tissue proliferation, but many lumps that show signs of breast proliferative disease remain benign.

Fibroadenoma

This benign tumor is the most commonly encountered form of breast neoplasia. The tumor mass is encapsulated and consists of varying combinations of fibrous tissue and glandular cells. Most fibroadenomas have diameters less than 4 cm, but some may achieve 10 cm. They typically arise in the reproductive years and, if not removed, they usually

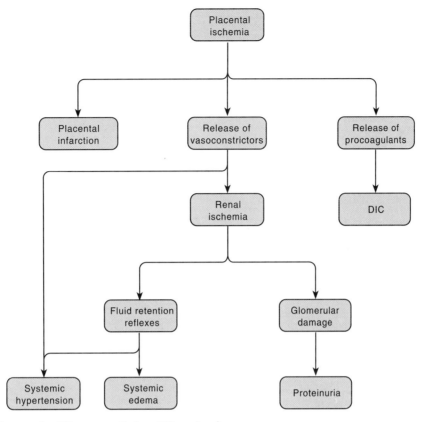

Figure 19.16   **The Pathogenesis of Pregnancy-Induced Hypertension.**

regress after menopause. This is due to the sensitivity of their glandular tissue to estrogen levels, which decline after the cessation of menstrual cycling.

Breast Cancer

Currently over 10% of North American women can be expected to develop some form of carcinoma of the breast. Most cases are diagnosed in menopausal and postmenopausal women, with much lower incidence prior to the mid-20s. Factors that predispose to greater risk are numerous. Genetic factors are involved in some breast cancer, with three specific defects in tumor-suppressor genes identified. These are involved in genetic transmission of a predisposition to cancer. Also important in some breast cancer is a dependence on estrogen as a growth stimulus. In such cases, over a woman's life, high exposure to the estrogen peaks that are associated with normal ovarian cycling seem to enhance breast cancer development. Since estrogen peaking is reduced during pregnancy, factors that prolong normal cycling, like an early menarche, a delayed first pregnancy, having no children at all (nulliparity), and an extended reproductive life span, are all associated with increased breast cancer incidence. Increasing age and exposure to radiation and the previously noted fibrocystic proliferative disease are additional risk factors. Ill-defined environmental factors are also likely at work. Their contribution is implied in the fact that when women from Asia, where breast cancer incidence is low, move to areas of high

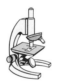

Focus on Breast Cancer Etiology

There is no evidence that breast cancer has a viral etiology in humans. Speculation about a viral role is based on the finding that in certain strains of mice, females develop breast carcinoma if exposed to a specific virus while they are nursing their young. However, no such link to a virus in humans has been found. Also, contrary to some suggestions, it seems unlikely that silicone breast implants play any causative role in breast cancer.

incidence such as North America or northern Europe, their breast cancer rates increase. Ultimately, breast carcinoma appears to result from a complex interplay between genetic predisposition and environmental agents interacting in a supportive hormonal milieu. Almost all cancers of the breast arise in its glands and are therefore adenocarcinomas.

Broadly, there are two classes of breast cancer: carcinoma in situ (CIS) is noninvasive, with its growth confined within the basement membrane of the duct or gland in which it arises. The other class is invasive carcinoma, where tumor cells infiltrate adjacent tissues, gain access to lymphatics, and metastasize (table 19.9). Most noninvasive

Table 19.9	Classification of Breast Cancer

Noninvasive	Invasive
Intraductal carcinoma	Invasive ductal carcinoma
Lobular CIS	Invasive lobular carcinoma
	Medullary carcinoma
	Tubular carcinoma
	Mucinous (colloid) carcinoma
	Adenoid cystic carcinoma
	Invasive papillary carcinoma

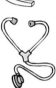

Focus on Breast-Feeding and Breast Cancer

It has been recognized that women who have more children have a reduced risk of developing breast cancer. Since there are many aspects of childbearing that might be responsible, a recent, large-scale study was undertaken to see if breast-feeding played any role in breast cancer incidence. Data from 47 studies in 30 countries, involving over 147,000 women, were subjected to complex statistical analyses that isolated breast-feeding from the other variables associated with childbearing. The results were clear: breast-feeding protects against breast cancer. Women whose children were breast-fed the longest had significantly lower risk of developing breast cancer. This result would seem to fit the long-recognized differences in breast cancer incidence between developed and developing countries. In developed countries where breast cancer incidence is high, women have fewer children and breast-feeding tends to be of short duration, if it occurs at all. Breast cancer incidence is lower in developing countries where women typically have more children and breast-feeding is common and of longer duration.

Of course, the nursing infant also benefits when supplied with the optimal nutrition offered by breast milk. Based on various studies, these benefits include reduced infections, less chronic disease (e.g., Crohn's disease), fewer allergies, less obesity, and higher IQ. Note also that cow's milk and "infant formula" are only rough approximations of human breast milk.

breast carcinoma arises in the ducts and grows without inducing changes that betray its presence; in particular, it induces no fibrous response in the stroma, since the tumor is isolated from the stroma by a basement membrane. Without fibrosis, the tumor is difficult to detect as a lump. In about one-third of cases, a noninvasive tumor acquires invasion capability and a stromal fibrous response follows, but by the time the resulting fibrous proliferation produces a palpable mass, some degree of metastasis may have already occurred.

Invasive tumors may produce various changes at the breast's surface due to contraction of the tumor's fibrous

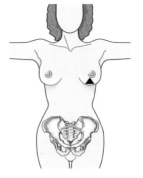

Tumor (T)
T_0–No evidence of tumor
T_1–Tumor diameter less than 2 cm
T_2–Tumor diameter 2–5 cm
T_3–Tumor diameter greater than 5 cm
T_4–Tumor of any size extending
    to chest wall or skin

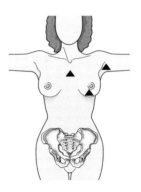

Nodes (N)
N_0–No lymph node involvement
N_1–Involvement of axillary lymph
    nodes that remain movable
N_2–Involvement of axillary lymph
    nodes that are fixed to each
    other or adjacent structures
N_3–Involvement of internal mammary
    nodes

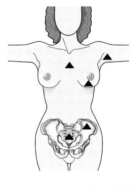

Metastasis (M)
M_0–No distant metastases
M_1–Distant metastases

Figure 19.17   **The TNM System in Breast Cancer Staging.**
▲: tumor growth.

stroma. Dimpling of the surface may result, or the nipple may be drawn inward. When the invading tumor cells reach the overlying dermis, they may infiltrate and obstruct its lymphatics. The result is a local reddening and hardening of the skin that is termed **peau d'orange,** since it has some resemblance to an orange peel.

Metastasis of most breast cancers is via lymphatic drainage to the regional nodes of the axilla, but blood-borne spread also occurs. The tumor emboli disseminate widely to grow at multiple sites, most often the lung, liver, adrenal glands, brain, and the skin, and bone (e.g., vertebral bodies).

The TNM system (see chapter 6) is commonly used in breast cancer staging (fig. 19.17). As you may recognize by now, intervention in early stages is related to better prognosis. In most centers, when a tumor's growth extends to the

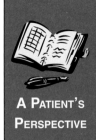

Breast Cancer

*". . . I said goodbye to my right breast
for the last time."*
—Ronda Moore

In the spring of 2000 while doing a breast self-exam, I felt a lump on my right breast. I knew it shouldn't be there and made an appointment to see my family doctor. She sent me off for a mammogram, an ultrasound exam, and a needle core biopsy. I was in shock because it never occurred to me that I might get breast cancer. I have relatively small breasts and back then, I was naive, thinking only big breasts were more susceptible. I was mistaken.

Shortly after, my family doctor called me with the bad news. She told me that I had breast cancer. I was in total shock, especially since I was home alone at the time. Ten days later I met with the oncologist who showed me the X-rays and my unwanted lump. He said it was a medium size, grade II invasive ductal carcinoma. He said I'd need a bone scan to be sure it hadn't spread. I was pretty scared about what the scan might show, but I had to know, so off I went.

At the hospital, the nuclear medicine technologist injected a small amount of isotope into my arm. It was mixed with another material that abnormal bone tissue likes. The exact recipe will not follow. A few days later, when the results came in, I met with the oncologist again. The news was good: no signs of metastasis . . . whew!

We talked about options and after he answered my many questions, I decided on a total mastectomy. This is when the breast and axillary lymph nodes are removed. After that I'd have a breast reconstruction procedure to restore the missing breast.

In early September I went in for my mastectomy. The first contact was with a preadmission nurse who took some information from me. She was all business and not very friendly. I felt like a hunk of meat ready to be processed. Next stop, blood work-up. I have not had blood taken that often and the nurse assured me that she was very experienced. I felt somewhat comforted until 15 minutes later she was still trying to find a vein.

My surgery was scheduled for 1:15 P.M. Now, I was really scared and sad at the same time. I said goodbye to my right breast for the last time. It has been my buddy for the last 43 years—I followed it everywhere; we were always together, day and night.

The surgery went well. The surgeon advised me that after the tumor was removed, my lymph nodes tested clear and my prognosis was excellent! This type of cancer is estrogen-sensitive and I would need to be on tamoxifen for five years as a preventive measure. I felt relieved that this unwanted cancer object was no longer part of me. I had said my goodbyes to my breast, so now I was facing the future a little lopsided.

In mid-October, I met with the oncologist who explained my follow-up chemotherapy. Of three options, two were certain to result in total hair loss. I have long hair that flows down to my waist and I also have many allergies, so I consulted with my family doctor and picked the third option, which would take longer but had less chance of hair loss.

Over the next six months, my eight chemo sessions started with a breakfast of some antinausea pills followed by a liquid lunch an hour or so later consisting of CMF fluid injections (cyclophosphamide, methotrexate, and fluorouracil). The stressful part was that before each session of CMF fluid, I had to have my blood tested for a certain level of neutrophils. When my counts were too low I had to wait until they came back up. That's why the eight sessions were spread over such a long time. And the good news was that I kept all my hair! The nurses at the treatment center were generally very attuned to the emotional needs of their patients. If it wasn't for their excellent bedside manner, it would have been very hard to get through the treatments. Although it took a long time, I got through it pretty well and was actually looking forward to the reconstructive surgery.

I had decided to have a TRAM procedure (transverse rectus abdominis myocutaneous). It uses a flap formed of a segment of abdominal muscle, and the skin over it to replace the lost breast without the need for an artificial implant. I was to be in the hospital for four to five days. The surgery was a success, but the next couple of days were *hell*. I couldn't drink fluids, nor could I keep down any food. My brain and I had a meeting of the topic "why was I vomiting so much?" We finally realized that the disinfectant used to clean the bedding was making me vomit. So, I convinced myself that I needed to leave the hospital while I still had the strength. If I didn't do something soon I'd die from dehydration. I talked to my surgeon and pleaded to go home. He and the nurses tried to convince me to stay but I said "no thanks." I got home and didn't vomit at all that day.

Before long it was clear that I wasn't healing normally. I had a rash and a boil that burst open and released yellow/green goop. I was put on various antibiotics that did not work, so I was sent to an infectious disease specialist. He said I had a new unwanted friend: the MRSA bacterium (methicillin-resistant *Staphylococcus aureus*). This is a strain that is resistant to the antibiotic that is supposed to kill it. I assume I picked it up in the hospital from someone who didn't follow the precautionary infection-control techniques plastered all over the hospital walls. I was put on special antibiotic pills that cost a small fortune. Two weeks later, I am told that I am MRSA free. Two weeks after that, I am still oozing goop and test results show that I am once again

(continued)

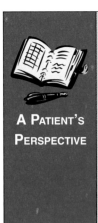

Breast Cancer—continued

MRSA positive. Subsequent tests showed the place that seemed to be harboring the MRSA villain. As I write this, I am scheduled to have an I & D abdomen (incision and drainage) operation. That story will have to wait until the next edition of this book.

One thing I can say about the whole experience is that lots of medical personnel overlook the power of humor. I would crack a joke about myself and was often met with a blank look. The nurses were generally better, but I think both docs and nurses should take the lead from the patient: If the patient can have a laugh during such a terrible ordeal, go along with it. We know it's a serious matter, but some of us try to take the edge off with humor. When I say "Everyone at the office thinks I should go for a 42 D," at least smile.

Looking back, it has been no picnic, but thanks to the support from my family and friends, I have survived and am looking forward to getting back to a normal life.

regional lymph nodes, therapy currently involves removal of the tumor mass or the entire breast (**mastectomy**). Affected lymph nodes are also removed, and postmastectomy radiation or chemotherapy is typical.

Treatment involves appropriate combinations of surgery, radiation, and chemical agents. Because many breast cancers retain their cell-surface estrogen receptors, a chemotherapeutic agent that binds to estrogen receptors, **tamoxifen,** is widely used. By acting as a blocking agent, it deprives the tumor of the estrogen stimulus that sustains it, and its growth is suppressed. As an added benefit, tamoxifen has few serious side effects and so is well tolerated by its users. There is also increasing evidence that it can prevent the initial development of breast cancer, and may therefore be suitable for prophylactic use in selected high-risk patients.

It is widely accepted that by the time of diagnosis, 50% of breast cancers have already metastasized. This means that once the primary tumor or mass has been removed, long-term survival is determined by growth at secondary sites. These secondary sites therefore are an important focus of therapy.

 Checkpoint 19.3

The importance of early diagnosis and treatment in breast cancer is well recognized, but there are many in our society who hold beliefs that can interfere with obtaining needed medical assistance. These beliefs are rooted in culture or are based on misinformation. In one study, women with late stage breast cancer reported holding beliefs such as *cancer is spread through the air; the devil is responsible for a person's cancer; breast surgery reduces attractiveness to men;* and *chiropractors are effective in treating breast cancer.* Holding such beliefs seemed to have caused those women to delay seeking medical assistance, allowing the disease to progress to the point where intervention was less likely to be successful.

Case Study

A 29-year-old woman reported to her general practitioner that for the past two months she had been experiencing lower abdominal pain, urinary frequency, and some nausea. She had stopped taking oral contraceptive pills four months ago, had a menstrual period immediately following, but had had no menstrual periods since. Her weight had been stable for the past two years.

On physical examination she looked generally healthy, but her abdomen was tender on the left side, exhibiting a slight fullness. She showed no obvious signs of vaginitis, and her cervix appeared normal. Blood tests proved normal, as did urinalysis, including a determination of chorionic gonadotropin (hCG).

The patient was referred to a radiologist for a pelvic ultrasound examination. It revealed the presence of a 5-cm ovarian mass. The radiologist recommended that she return in one month for reexamination. She returned as advised and reported that she had had an apparently normal menstrual period two weeks previously. The follow-up ultrasound scan showed that the mass had increased in size, and she was referred to a gynecologist.

On the gynecologist's recommendation, she was admitted to hospital, and during an exploratory laparoscopy procedure the cyst was located and removed. Postoperative examination of the excised ovarian mass revealed that it contained endometrial tissue into which bleeding had occurred, forming a chocolate cyst.

The patient was given the option of resuming oral contraceptive therapy to suppress the hormonal swings that could exacerbate the endometriosis. She had earlier stated her intention of becoming pregnant at some future time and was advised that endometrial deposits in the uterine tubes might affect the passage of ova or spermatozoa, reducing the chance of a successful pregnancy.

Commentary

In view of the patient's complaints, blood and urine tests were required to rule out urinary infections, while testing for hCG levels would reveal a normal or ectopic pregnancy.

Since oral contraceptives supply a small additional amount of hormones, sufficient to suppress follicle development and therefore endogenous estrogen secretion, this woman's use of the pill may have suppressed bleeding from the deposit of endometrial tissue that had reached her ovary.

The radiologist's recommendation to defer any action for a month was based on the fact that, given the patient's age, an ovarian tumor was unlikely to be present, and a delay might allow the resumption of normal hormonal and ovarian cycling. If the enlargement was a follicular cyst, it might well have regressed when estrogen and progesterone levels declined during a normal cycle. If that had occurred, the patient would probably have been spared surgery. Since after menstruation resumed the mass had not regressed, but had actually gotten bigger, surgery was necessary to ascertain its nature.

Key Concepts

1. Disorders of the penis/urethra, bulbourethral glands, seminal vesicles, and vas deferens are rare, with most male reproductive disease arising in the testis and prostate gland (p. 507).

2. The most common congenital defect of the male reproductive system is cryptorchidism, in which there is a failure of the testes to descend to the scrotum from the abdomen, where they initially form (p. 508).

3. The great majority of testicular tumors are malignant and are called germ cell tumors because they arise from spermatozoan precursors in the seminiferous tubules (pp. 509–510).

4. Torsion of the spermatic cord's vessels can compromise testicular venous drainage to produce congestion and swelling, or if extreme, infarction (p. 510).

5. Hyperplasia of the prostate, beyond the limited amount present in most males after age 45, can produce urinary obstruction and predispose to bladder infection, pyelonephritis, and hydronephrosis (pp. 510–511).

6. Carcinoma of the prostate is unrelated to benign prostatic hyperplasia and typically produces symptoms after age 50, with detection often delayed until local invasion causes pain (pp. 511–512).

7. Pelvic inflammatory disease usually involves an initial vaginal infection with subsequent ascent to involve the uterus, uterine tubes, ovaries, and other abdominal structures, often producing infertility due to postinflammatory scarring and adhesions (pp. 512–514).

8. Anovulatory cycles and their associated hormone imbalances are the principal cause of dysfunctional uterine bleeding (pp. 514–515).

9. The expulsion of endometrial tissue into the pelvic cavity can produce endometriosis, the condition in which the endometrial tissue becomes established and subject to proliferation and bleeding in synchrony with the uterine cycle, causing irritation, pain, adhesions, and the risk of infertility (p. 515).

10. High levels of prostaglandins seem to trigger myometrial ischemia, which causes the uterine cramping associated with menstruation (pp. 515–516).

11. An ill-defined hormonal imbalance is thought to underlie the array of signs and symptoms and psychological swings associated with premenstrual dysphoric disorder that accompanies the menstrual cycle in some women (p. 516).

12. Prolonged elevation of estrogen levels is associated with endometrial carcinoma, a relatively common malignancy that can spread to the ovaries (p. 516).

13. Cervical carcinoma usually originates in the endometrium's transitional zone after a slowly developing sequence of change: mild dysplasia through carcinoma in situ (pp. 516–517).

14. The ability to monitor changes in the cervical epithelium is largely responsible for the decline in the incidence of cervical carcinoma (p. 517).

15. Various nonbiological environmental agents and microorganisms are suspected of contributing to the etiology of cervical carcinoma, as indicated by incidence and transmission patterns (p. 517).

16. Graafian follicles are the most common source of ovarian cysts, which are associated with anovulatory cycles, irregular menstrual bleeding, and the risk of ovarian rupture (p. 518).

17. Polycystic ovarian syndrome, characterized by ovarian cysts, amenorrhea, hirsutism, enlarged ovaries, and obesity, derives from some imbalance in the complex interplay among estrogens, the hypothalamus, and the anterior pituitary, is triggered by an enzyme defect that causes excessive androgen secretion from the ovaries and the adrenals (pp. 518–519).

18. Ovarian tumors produce high mortality because of the lack of signs or symptoms prior to the point at which invasion and metastases have occurred (p. 519).

19. There are many types of benign and malignant ovarian tumors that exhibit a broad array of characteristics (pp. 519–521).

20. Ectopic pregnancy usually arises because of an obstruction that promotes implantation in the uterine tube, posing the threat of its rupture and the possibility of hypovolemic shock (pp. 521–522).

21. Hydatidiform mole, invasive mole, and choriocarcinoma are three tumors of the placenta that secrete high levels of hCG and that are grouped together as gestational trophoblastic disease (GTD) (p. 522).

22. Various abnormalities of placental attachment can cause bleeding sufficiently serious to produce hypovolemic shock in the mother and the fetus that depends on the placenta for blood supply (pp. 522–523).

23. Preeclampsia presents a picture of hypertension, proteinuria, and edema in response to placental ischemia (pp. 523–524).

24. A fundamental estrogen-mediated mechanism is thought to underlie the nonthreatening single or multiple masses formed of epithelium, fibrous connective tissue, or cysts that characterize breast fibrocystic change (p. 524).

25. Breast carcinoma appears to be the result of the interplay between a genetic predisposition and various suspected environmental agents in a supportive hormonal environment (p. 524).

26. Most breast cancer arises in the glands and ducts of the breast, rather than in its fibrous or adipose tissues, and is dangerous because metastases may occur prior to the development of the signs and symptoms that betray its presence (pp. 525–526).

REVIEW ACTIVITIES

1. Supply short, written answers to the following: In endometriosis, how is endometrial tissue thought to reach the pelvic cavity? How might it reach the lungs? What is the consequence of the presence of ectopic endometrial tissue? Check your answers against the information on page 515.

2. Carefully review the material on cervical cancer on pages 524–526. Make a ready reference list of relevant cervical carcinoma and Pap smear information. In chatting with anyone you know who isn't getting regular Pap smears, use the list to be informative and supportive, but in particular, persuasive (p. 517).

3. Write a list of the toxins known to be involved in toxemia of pregnancy. Now suggest a better name for this condition and identify why it is better. Reflect upon two ways that vasoconstrictors are implicated in the pathogenesis of preeclampsia.

4. List the essential differences among placenta previa, placenta accreta, placenta increta, and abruptio placentae. Check pages 522–523 if you have to.

5. Trace the outlines of one of the diagrams in figure 19.17. Add sites of tumor involvement for patients whose TNM staging is $T_2N_0M_1$ and $T_3N_2M_1$.

6. Complete the following table. If you use initials, be certain you know what they stand for.

Essential Problem	Name of Disease/Condition
Failure to ovulate	
Inadequate placental anchoring	
Myometrial ischemia	
Failure of testes' descent	
Grapelike placental tumor	
Pregnancy-related convulsions/coma	
Scarring and infertility	
Compromised testicular blood flow	
Embryonic implantation outside uterus	
Multiple, bilateral ovarian cysts	
Prostatic urinary obstruction	
Placenta obstructs cervix	
Albuminemia, edema, hypertension	
Nonneoplastic breast masses	
Ectopic menstrual responses	

Disorders of Central Nervous System Development, Vascular Support, and Protection

The brain is the highest of the organs, and it is protected by the vault of the head; it has no flesh, or blood or refuse. It is the citadel of sense-perception.

PLINY THE ELDER (AD 25–79)

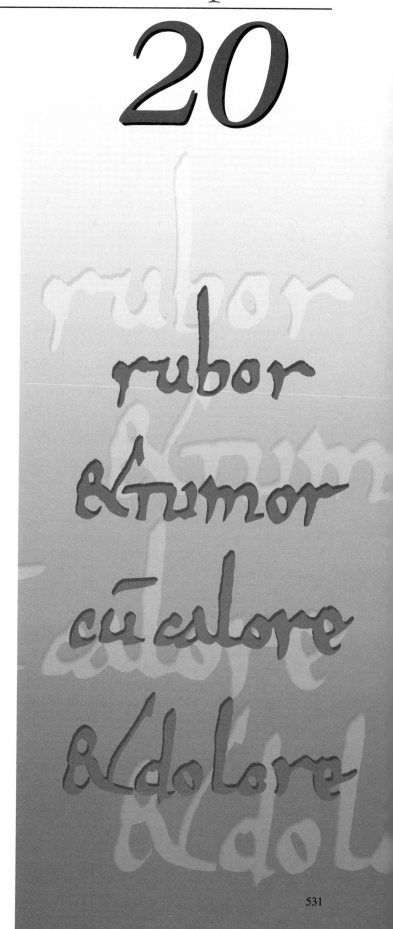

CENTRAL NERVOUS SYSTEM PROTECTION

Protection of the delicate tissues of the brain and spinal cord is normally ensured by the scalp, bony structures, and meningeal layers enclosing the cerebrospinal fluid. Trauma to or disease in these structures may compromise this protection.

Surface Landmarks

Surface structures are routinely used to localize brain and spinal cord features. The **nasion,** illustrated in figure 20.1, is the depression at the root of the nose where it joins the bones of the cranial vault. The **inion** is the point on the scalp that overlies the midpoint of the external occipital protuberance, which is a bony projection at the lower center of the skull, above the attachment of the posterior neck muscles. This point corresponds to the junction, on the inside of the skull, of the major venous sinuses draining blood from the brain. The inion also marks the most posterior extent of the loose connective tissue that allows the scalp to move freely and is part of the attachment of the

broad, thin sheet of muscle called the **occipitalis** portion of the **epicranius** muscle. Some people can voluntarily contract this muscle and shrug their scalp backward. The anterior portion of the epicranius, called the **frontalis,** is the muscle that enables a person to wrinkle the forehead or raise the eyebrows.

The **external auditory** (or acoustic) **meatus** (the ear canal) is easy to locate. Anterior and above it and just posterior to the area normally called the temple is the **pterion.** This is the area at the irregular, H-shaped meeting of the sutures of four bones: the frontal, sphenoid, parietal, and temporal (fig. 20.1). In this region (called the **temporal fossa**), the bones of the skull are at their thinnest and blows are likely to produce fractures, especially at the pterion. The anterior branch of the middle meningeal artery (one of the arteries that supply the skull bones with blood) underlies the skull at the pterion. Skull fractures in the region of the pterion may cause this artery and/or its accompanying veins to be torn, with resulting intracranial hemorrhage. Figure 20.2 illustrates the location of significant brain structures relative to the pterion.

The vertebral column, or spine, functions in three ways: it supports the head, trunk, and limbs; it allows movement of the head and trunk; and it protects the spinal cord. Certain landmarks are essential reference points (fig. 20.3). If you move your fingers down a person's neck with the neck flexed forward, you will feel a prominent bump in the spine at the base of the neck. This bump marks the **vertebra prominens,** which is formed by the spinous process of the seventh—the lowest—cervical vertebra (C-7). (The number of cervical vertebrae in humans is always seven.) A second prominent bump, which may be larger or smaller than the vertebra prominens, marks the first thoracic vertebra (T-1). Starting from this point and palpating firmly at the center of the spine, you can count the spinous processes of the thoracic (usually 12) and lumbar (usually 5) vertebrae. The lowest of the lumbar vertebrae (L-5) articulates with the top of the five fused vertebrae that form the sacrum. The delicate spinal cord extends down the meninges-lined vertebral canal from C-1 to about the disk between L-1 and L-2. It is protected dorsally by vertebral arches, ligamentous structures, and muscle.

During embryonic and first-year postnatal development, growth of the vertebral column outpaces the lengthening of the cord. Because of this disparity, the cord and its spinal nerve extensions appear to be "drawn up" the vertebral canal so that lower nerves must travel several segments before they pierce the dura (protective coverings of the cord) and exit through the lateral space between the vertebrae—the intervertebral foramen. Below L-2, therefore, there is a mass of spinal nerves, which arises at cord levels L-2 and lower and ends at coccygeal 1, that together is called the **cauda equina** (horse's tail). These nerves are contained in an extension of the dural sac that ends about

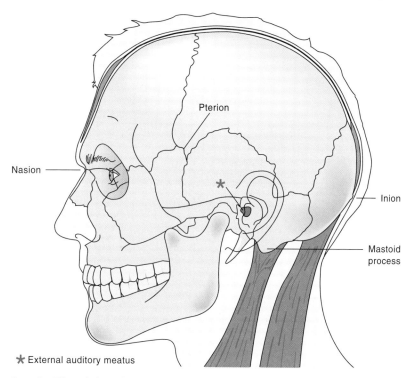

Figure 20.1   **Cranial Landmarks.** The relationship of key surface features on the head to underlying bony structures. The nasion, inion, pterion, external auditory meatus, and mastoid process are shown.

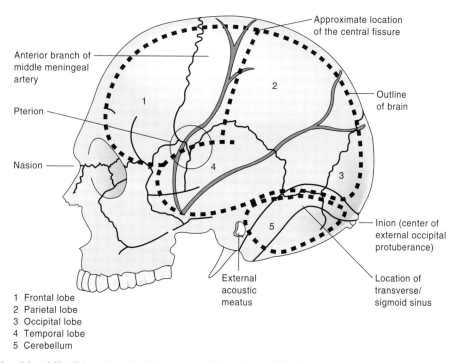

1 Frontal lobe
2 Parietal lobe
3 Occipital lobe
4 Temporal lobe
5 Cerebellum

Figure 20.2   **Relationship of Skull Landmarks to Important Vascular and Brain Structures.**

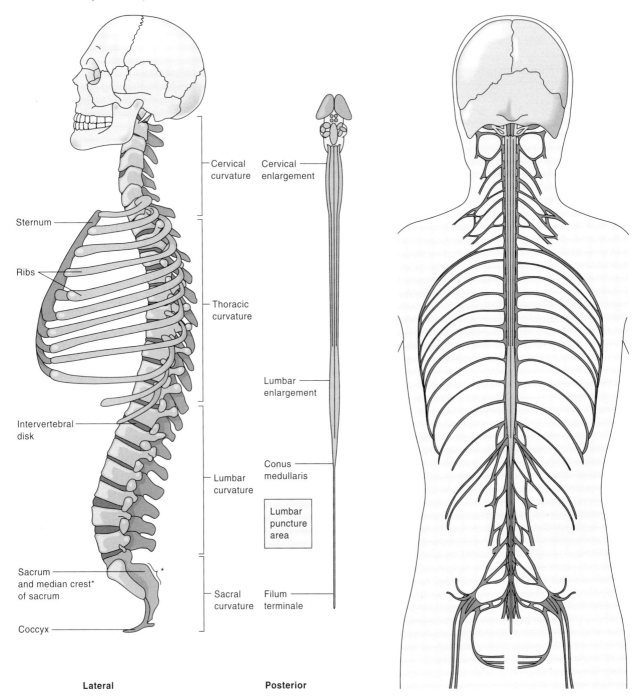

Figure 20.3   **Features of Vertebral Column in Lateral and Posterior Views.**

the middle of the sacrum. As illustrated in figure 20.4, a bevelled, large-bore needle can be pushed into this space, usually at the space between L-3 and L-4 or between L-4 and L-5, to sample an individual's cerebrospinal fluid (CSF) or introduce anesthetic drugs. (The procedure is called a **lumbar puncture** or **spinal tap.**) There is little danger of damaging these nerves. Contact with the needle creates distinct motor or sensory effects (e.g., muscle twitch or shooting pain), upon which the needle is withdrawn slightly, turned so the bevel is at a different angle, and reinserted.

Locating L-3 and L-4 by counting down from the vertebra prominens is a laborious process, and the result may be inaccurate because of variations in the number of thoracic and lumbar vertebrae. Two other approaches are commonly used. L-4 can be located directly because it lies at about the same level as the top of the iliac bones in a standing person. Alternatively, since the top of the median crest (formed by the fused spinous process of the sacrum) is S-2, L-4 can be located by counting up from S-2 (see fig. 20.3).

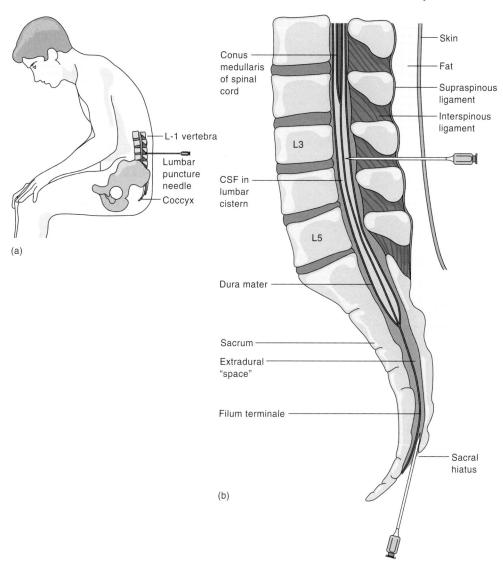

Figure 20.4   **The Technique of Lumbar Puncture (Spinal Tap).** (*a*) Note that the person's back is flexed; this is done to open the spaces between the spinous processes and laminae of the vertebrae. This procedure is usually done "side-lying." (*b*) Median section of the inferior end of the vertebral column, showing the spinal cord and its membranes. A lumbar puncture needle has been inserted at L3–4 for withdrawal of CSF. A needle is also shown in the sacral hiatus, the site sometimes used for extradural (epidural) anesthesia.

Protection of the Brain: The Scalp

The scalp has five layers (fig. 20.5), of which the first three (skin, connective tissue, galea aponeurotica) form the scalp proper. This part can be quite easily separated from the head in a car crash. The dermal layer (connective tissue) is richly vascularized and the arteries anastomose freely. Because this connective tissue is attached to the flat, fibrous sheet of connective tissue called the galea aponeurotica (*galea* is Greek for helmet, and an *aponeurosis* is a sheet of irregularly arranged, dense fibrous tissue), the arteries can't retract as they would in soft tissue. Thus, bleeding from superficial scalp wounds will tend to be profuse and prolonged. The galea is attached anteriorly at the frontalis muscle and posteriorly at the occipitalis. Deep wounds that split or cut the galea will gape widely because of the diver-

gent pull of the frontal and occipital parts of the epicranius muscle and, unlike superficial scalp wounds, will require deep sutures even though they may not bleed as profusely.

The **loose connective tissue** forms a subaponeurotic space or layer that is somewhat like a collapsed sponge. It allows free movement of the scalp proper. This layer can be easily torn in deep scalp lacerations and is capable of becoming distended with fluid if blood vessels are damaged or infection causes an accumulation of exudate. Figure 20.6 illustrates the attachments of the galea aponeurotica that limit fluid spread. Infection can be transmitted to veins and venous sinuses of the cranial cavity through emissary veins that pass from the scalp through the cranial bones or through veins draining the central face. Such an infection can set up an inflammatory process, with resultant thrombophlebitis and the possibility of infarction of portions of

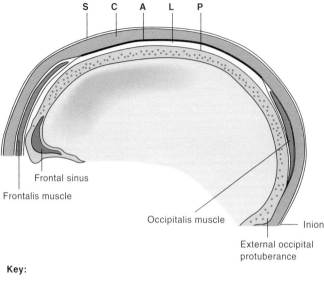

Key:

S— Skin (really, the epidermis)
C— Connective tissue (dense subcutaneous—the dermis)
A— Aponeurosis epicranalis (usually called the galea aponeurotica)
L— Loose (areolar) connective tissue
P— Pericranium (external periosteum)

Figure 20.5   **Scalp Structure.** Section through the scalp and calvaria, with a key to remembering the five layers of the scalp.

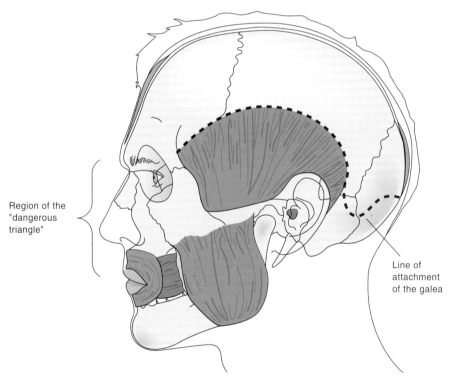

Figure 20.6   **Attachments of the Galea Aponeurotica.**

the cerebral cortex due to blocked venous drainage. Infection may also pass from the venous system to the cerebrospinal fluid or the neural tissue itself. All of the foregoing are potentially very serious conditions and have this given this layer the name **"dangerous space."** The triangle formed by the eyes and nose is an area of similar vulnerability (the **"dangerous triangle"**). Infected fluid from the

dangerous space or the face can pass into this area, which drains into the cranial vault. Here, infection and blood coagulation can occur with disastrous results (see the "Intracranial Thrombophlebitis" section later in this chapter).

The last layer of the scalp is the periosteum of the cranium—the **pericranium.** In contrast to the periosteum in other regions of the body, the pericranium has poor os-

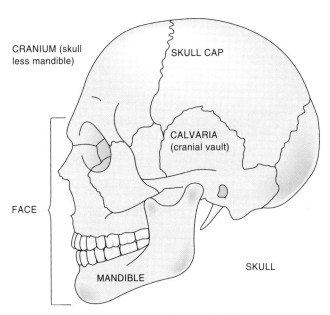

Figure 20.7   **Terminology Applied to Skull Structures.**

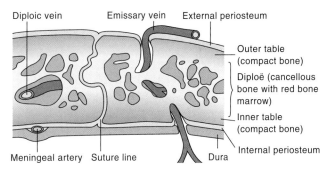

Figure 20.8   **Section Through Skull Bone.** A central spongy diploë is sandwiched between an inner layer (table) of compact bone and an outer layer. The diploë red bone marrow is a significant source of blood cells and platelets.

teogenic or bone repair properties. Hence, large traumatic insults to the cranial bones don't usually fill in and must be replaced with plastic (formerly metal) plates inserted to protect the brain. Burr holes drilled through the skull to monitor intracranial pressure or reduce a hematoma may be filled with cold-cure epoxy.

Nerves and vessels supplying the scalp enter from the neck, temporal area, and forehead (i.e., from below), and ascend through either of the two connective tissue layers. When a surgeon needs to expose the skull, surgical **pedicle flaps** are made—that is, a detached mass of tissue is cut away from underlying parts but is left attached at the lower edge. The numerous arterial anastomoses ensure that adequate blood supplies will continue to reach the detached scalp. The cranial bones are supplied from arteries within the cranium.

Protection of the Brain: The Skull

The **skull** is the most complex bony structure of the body and performs many functions. It encloses and protects the brain, which is the central concern here. But, as well, the organs of special sense (seeing, hearing, smelling, tasting, static and dynamic balance) are housed and strategically positioned within it. It also encloses the openings into the digestive and respiratory tracts.

The skull is composed of two parts. The first is the **calvaria** (not calvarium), which encloses the brain and is sometimes called the cranial vault or brain case. The second part is the **face,** which is attached to the anteroinferior part of the calvaria. While skull refers to the entire skeletal structure of the head, **cranium** implies the skeleton of the head excluding the lower jaw, or **mandible.** The roof of the calvaria is sometimes referred to as the **skull cap** (fig. 20.7) while the floor of the cranial vault is referred to as the **base** of the skull.

In cross section (fig. 20.8) the cranial bones have an outer and an inner table of compact bone, with an intervening layer of cancellous or spongy bone (the diploë). This structuring gives great strength to cranial bones while keeping weight to a minimum. It also raises the possibility, particularly with the younger patient, that the more elastic, outer table of the skull may remain intact, rebounding after a blow, even though the inner table and diploë have been broken into bits **(comminuted)** and forced into the meningeal and even brain tissues **(depressed).** So, manual inspection for suspected fractures is not sufficient and X-ray is routine.

Note the terms (fig. 20.9*b*) applied to the subdivisions of the floor of the cranial vault (anterior, middle, and posterior fossae). In Latin, **fossa** means "ditch" or "depression." The **crista galli** is in the middle of the anterior fossa. This is a spur of bone that extends from the relatively tiny ethmoid bone up about 1 cm into the brain case. It is the anterior point of attachment of a tough membrane **(falx cerebri)** that separates the two hemispheres of the brain. Rotational trauma may rip this membrane loose, and the spur of bone can do serious damage to the frontal lobes of the brain. The **cribriform plate** of the ethmoid bone is perforated. Filaments of the olfactory nerve pierce the protective membranes of the brain (the meninges) and pass through the cribriform plate into the upper portions of the nasal cavity, providing a sense of smell. A blunt blow to the skull, such as might happen when the head is driven into the windshield in a car accident, can cause the base of the skull to fracture (basal skull fracture). Such a linear fracture can cut through the cribriform meninges, allowing cerebrospinal fluid to leak into the nasal cavity, a condition called **rhinorrhea.** As will shortly be detailed, cerebrospinal fluid (CSF) contains glucose. Testing a posttraumatic nasal discharge with a ketostick (sometimes still used to detect sugar in a diabetic's urine) will allow one to discriminate between CSF, indicating a probable basal skull fracture with rupture of the meninges, and nasal mucous discharge, which contains no glucose. A basal skull fracture may also sever elements of the olfactory nerve, thereby leading to a loss of smell in one or both nasal cavities.

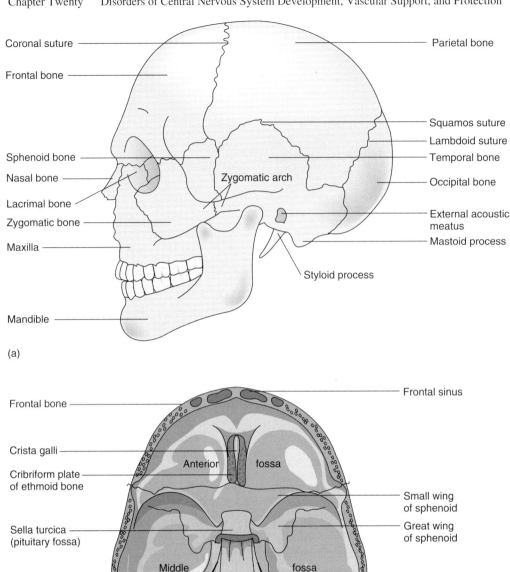

Figure 20.9   **Review of Skull Anatomy:** (*a*) Lateral view of the skull, showing principal bones and sutures. (*b*) View of the base of the skull from above, showing the internal surfaces and some of the cranial bones. Dashed line indicates course of the transverse and sigmoid sinus.

The bony recess of the **sella turcica** houses the pituitary gland, which is richly supplied with blood vessels to carry the trophic hormones released by this "master gland" to their target organs in all parts of the body. The sella is used as a reference point in viewing MRI or CT scans. Enlargement of the pituitary fossa and erosion of the sella turcica will accompany the expansion of a pituitary tumor and was diagnostic before assays of specific pituitary hormones

became common. It may still be the only way a pituitary tumor is diagnosed if it secretes hormonally inactive product.

The **sphenoid** (wedge-shaped) **bone,** which houses the sella turcica, is a major bone in the floor of the skull. The temporal lobes of the brain nestle into the middle fossa and are subject to trauma when accelerated against the ridge between the small and great wings of the sphenoid bone. The floor of the middle fossa is largely formed by the **temporal**

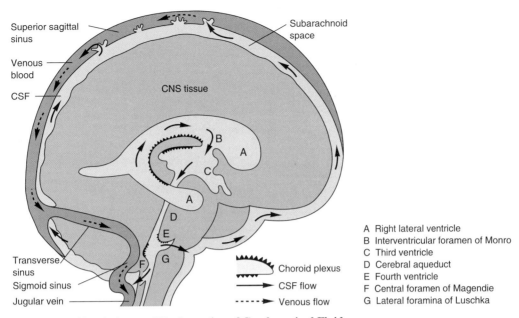

A Right lateral ventricle
B Interventricular foramen of Monro
C Third ventricle
D Cerebral aqueduct
E Fourth ventricle
F Central foramen of Magendie
G Lateral foramina of Luschka

Choroid plexus
CSF flow
Venous flow

Figure 20.10   **Production, Circulation, and Reabsorption of Cerebrospinal Fluid.**

bone, the petrous (rocklike) portion of which is often a site of linear fracture in basal skull fractures. It houses the elaborate structure of the semicircular canals and inner ear. Fracture through these structures can provide a potentially serious port of entry for infection of the central nervous system, as well as allowing CSF to leak into the middle ear or, with perforation of the eardrum, into the auditory canal. This condition is called **otorrhea.**

The spinal cord communicates with the brain stem through the foramen magnum (great opening), as do the arteries that travel up the spine and supply the posterior aspects of the brain. In figure 20.9b, the dotted line on the right side of the occipital bone indicates the groove that houses the major venous sinus (a specialized blood vessel) that drains the right side of the brain.

Meningeal Protection

If the brain were housed directly in the skull, brain on bone, any jolt or jar would be conducted immediately to the brain tissue. As well, the 1,500-g weight of the average brain would present a considerable mass, which, once moving, would tend to persist in its movement. This tendency could be disastrous if the skull suddenly stopped its linear or rotational movement, since it could lead to compressing or shearing of delicate nervous tissue. Further, the central nervous system has no lymphatic vessels. In the rest of the body, lymphatics carry any excess of extracellular fluid (that has passed out of the capillaries) back into the general circulation. What provisions exist in the central nervous system (CNS) to deal with these circumstances?

The brain floats in a thin pool of cerebrospinal fluid. This layer poses a significant cushion and, more importantly, reduces the effective weight of the brain to about 50 g. It has been estimated that CSF makes the brain about one-seventh as vulnerable to trauma as it would be in its absence. CSF

also distributes pressure evenly throughout the brain, which facilitates the perfusion of all brain tissues whether on the top, middle, or bottom of the brain. Much of the CSF is produced in specialized vascular tissue called **choroid plexus.** Concentrations of choroid plexus are found lining cavities deep within the brain. In its very early embryological development, the CNS is a hollow, tubelike structure. As the forebrain grows and elaborates, this central cavity, through which important blood vessels course, maintains its integrity and becomes quite complex in shape, forming four ventricles. The mature brain has two paired **lateral ventricles,** which are located in a continuous, C-shaped chamber from the frontal, through the parietal, occipital, and finally temporal lobes of the brain. They communicate with one another, and the **third ventricle,** at the approximate center of the brain (fig. 20.10), through the **interventricular foramen** of Monro. CSF is produced in the choroid plexus in both lateral ventricles and passes into the third (through the interventricular foramen), where additional CSF is added from further choroidal tissue. From the third ventricle, CSF passes down the narrow **cerebral aqueduct** (also called the aqueduct of Sylvius) into the **fourth ventricle.** More CSF is added and the entire production is pushed through three further foramina, out into the thin space that surrounds the entire brain and spinal cord. The traditional name of the **central foramen** was foramen of Magendie, while the **lateral foramina** were called foramina of Luschka. The circulation of CSF continues around the brain and cord structures to its eventual destination at the top of the cranial vault. Here, specialized structures called **arachnoid villi** pass the CSF into the venous blood. These are also called *arachnoid granulations,* as they have a granular appearance to the naked eye. The fluid is replaced three to five times per day.

Under normal conditions, CSF has stable characteristics that differentiate it from blood plasma or mucous secretions.

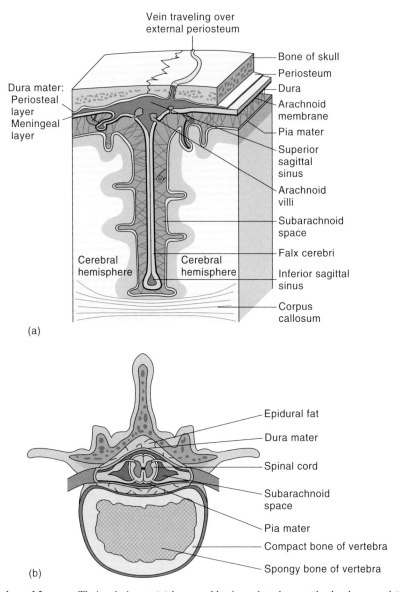

Figure 20.11   **Three Meningeal Layers.** Their relation to (*a*) bone and brain and to the vertebral column and (*b*) spinal cord.

It has approximately 60% of the glucose of plasma (mucous secretions have no glucose). It has almost no protein (20 mg/100 ml, versus 6,000 mg/100 ml for plasma) and about half as much potassium ion as plasma. The white blood cell count in CSF is below 5/mm³, and the fluid is clear and essentially colorless. In the context of diagnosis, note that bacterial infections of the protective membranes of the brain and spinal cord (meningitis) will deplete the glucose, increase the protein content, drive the white blood cell count up to perhaps 5,000/mm³, and cause the CSF to become cloudy. Recent hemorrhage will turn it bloody; older hemorrhage shows a shade of yellow (xanthochromia).

There are three distinct layers between the brain tissue and the bony calvaria (fig. 20.11). A delicate epithelium intimately covers the entire CNS, following all the convolutions of the brain and lining the passageways of the major vessels within the brain tissue. This is the **pia mater** (Latin for gentle or delicate mother). (The ventricles just described are lined with a different, single-cell-thick mem-

brane called the **ependyma.**) The cushioning, supportive pool of CSF is found in the narrow space between the pia and the tough outer membrane that actually makes contact with the bone—the **dura mater** (strong mother). This intervening membrane that actually allows for the circulation of CSF is called the **arachnoid mater,** or **arachnoid membrane.** If we strip off the outer dura, the arachnoid will appear as a delicate membrane, dark and irregular (*arachnoid* refers to its resemblance to tangled cobwebs). If we look at it in cross section, we will find that although it is a continuous membrane where it contacts the dura, most of its thickness is a tracery of short fibers that bridge the space between the outer membrane of the arachnoid and the pia mater. It is in this **subarachnoid space** that the CSF travels. As well, this space contains both veins and arteries that are supplying the brain and the meninges themselves. The pia and arachnoid together are referred to as the **leptomeninges** (light meninges) and are the site of meningeal infection (meningitis).

The dura mater makes direct contact with the inner periosteum of the calvaria. The two are histologically continuous. However, if a blood vessel traveling in the dura or passing through the skull were to rupture, particularly an artery, the pressure of the blood could tear the internal periosteum away from the skull and a bubble or pool of blood would form (a hematoma). Because of its location, this would be called an **extradural** or **epidural** hematoma. As a person ages, this connective tissue becomes less separable and the likelihood of this form of hematoma therefore decreases. Hemorrhage could also occur in the potential space between the dura and the arachnoid mater (**subdural hematoma**) or into the subarachnoid space itself (**subarachnoid hemorrhage**). The characteristics and effects of each will be discussed at a later point.

The CSF layer does a lot to protect the CNS. The structure of the meninges increases this protection by subdividing the cranial vault (and thereby the brain tissue) into smaller compartments. These partitions minimize the movement of neural tissue in response to lateral or rotational acceleration. One major reflection or fold of the dura (the **falx cerebri**) passes backward in the longitudinal fissure between the two hemispheres. The falx fuses with a second, transverse fold, called the **tentorium cerebelli,** that cradles the occipital lobes and forms a "tent" over the cerebellum. Both folds of dura carry large venous sinuses—vessels that are formed in the dura and are usually triangular in cross section. These large-diameter sinuses offer very little resistance to the passage of venous blood and thereby enhance cerebral circulation. A third, less significant reflection of the dura (**falx cerebelli**) separates the cerebellar hemispheres. These dural structures also can serve as referents; for example, a lesion is located **supratentorially** (above the tentorium) or **infratentorially** or **subtentorially** (below the tentorium).

A special feature of the tentorium should be noted (fig. 20.12). The **tentorial notch** provides an opening for the brain stem, as well as certain nerves and vessels. At the same time, it is tightly stretched in place. An expanding tumor, for example, could shift the brain stem to one side, pressing it against the side of the tentorial notch. Sensory and motor fibers generally cross over (**decussate**) below the level of the tentorium, so that left-brain lesions cause right-body symptoms. This normal expectation, that symptoms will appear contralateral to the lesion, reverses in the situation just described. That is, a mass on the right would push the left side of the midbrain against the tentorium, entrapping the fibers from the left hemisphere. Since the result would be right-sided symptoms, on the same side as the lesion, such findings are called **paradoxical.**

Like other connective tissue, the dura carries blood vessels and nerves. Many headaches are actually caused and felt in the dura. To illustrate, a spinal tap will temporarily reduce the volume of CSF. If a person stands up too soon after the spinal tap, the sagging that occurs as the brain is displaced slightly downward, in its only partially filled CSF pool, can put tension on the dura. This tension may be felt as a splitting headache. A fuller treatment of the role of the dura in headaches is given in chapter 23.

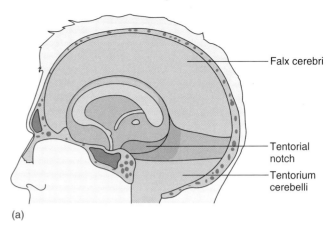

(a)

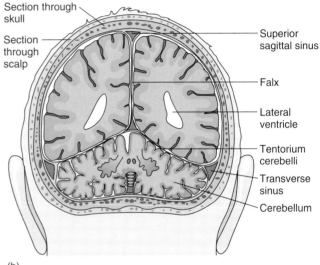

(b)

Figure 20.12   **Reflections of the Cranial Dura Mater. The** tentorium arches over the cerebellum and cradles the occipital and the posterior temporal lobes. The falx divides the cerebrum and extends between the inferior and superior sagittal sinuses. (*a*) Falx and tentorium with brain tissue removed, midsagital section. (*b*) Coronal view, brain and cerebellum in place.

Protection of the Spinal Cord: The Vertebral Column

The vertebral column protects the spinal cord. It has a host of other roles: articulation with the head, ribs, pectoral and pelvic girdles; a hemopoietic and immune system role, particularly in childhood; points of attachment for trunk and limb musculature; and an avenue for the vertebral arteries, which provide 30% of the brain's blood supply. Some of these tasks are made more precarious by the adaptation of the vertebral column to our upright posture. At the most obvious level, the lower vertebrae must bear more weight than those located higher in the vertebral column. This difference is dealt with by the increasing size of the vertebrae's bodies, but it still subjects lower intervertebral disks to large loads with attendant stresses. Second, the thoracic and abdominal cavities are obviously anterior to the vertebral column, so that the load on the spine is not distributed

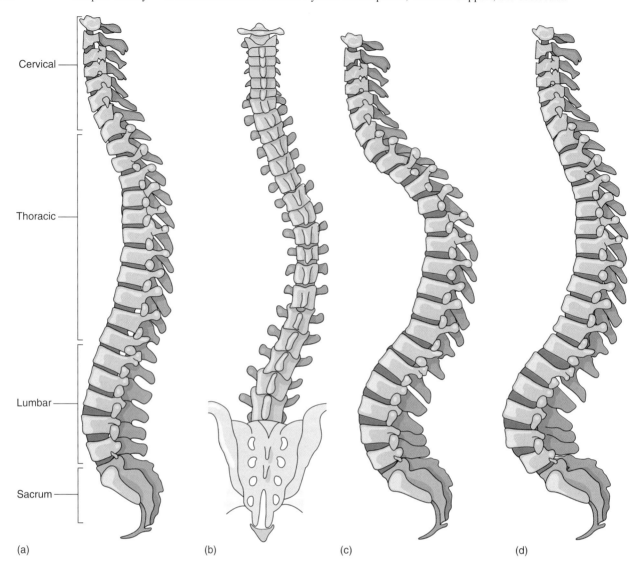

Cervical

Thoracic

Lumbar

Sacrum

(a)   (b)   (c)   (d)

Figure 20.13   **The Vertebral Column.** (*a*) The four natural curvatures of the vertebral column are achieved by the time the child has acquired mature walking and running gait (about age 3). (*b*) In scoliosis (Greek for crookedness), the curve is convex to the side (lateral curvature). There may be a single curve or complex curves, including kyphosis, as the vertebral column rotates to redistribute the altered load. This is a relatively common condition, particularly in adolescent girls, and often requires bracing or even surgical correction. (*c*) In kyphosis (Greek for humpbacked), there is abnormal dorsal curvature, usually in the thoracic region, which results in increased flexion in the upper back. This abnormality has been called "widow's hump" and is often associated with degeneration of vertebral bodies associated with osteoporosis. (*d*) In lordosis (Greek for backward bending), the curve is convex anteriorly, often in the lumbar region. The condition (called swayback) may be congenital or due to the weak abdominal musculature and excess abdominal fat.

symmetrically. Partial compensation for this load displacement is supplied by the abdominal musculature, which can make the trunk behave like a column that rests on the pelvic girdle rather than a mass suspended from the spine. The weakness in this design appears when the abdominal muscles themselves weaken. The back musculature must then take on an excessive load, which results in the **lordosis** identified in figure 20.13*d*.

The natural curvatures (fig. 20.13*a*), which develop to a certain extent to balance the loads on the spine, can become exaggerated as a result of excessive loads, muscular weakness, or degeneration of vertebral bodies. One of the effects of increased curvature is to place unusual loads and compression on the posterior side of the lumbar interverte-

bral disks, the consequences of which will be discussed shortly. Moreover, because the loads on the vertebrae are to some extent stacked, a load distribution problem in one part of the vertebral column may well be expressed throughout the spine. In **scoliosis,** a lateral displacement of the vertebral column in the thoracic area, which may have originated from unbalanced muscular strength, leads to extensive rotation of the thoracic and lumbar spine (fig. 20.13*b*). Major deviation from normal alignment can irritate and entrap spinal nerves and associated plexi and even impair the cord. Surgical correction of these orthopedic defects also carries a risk of cord or nerve dysfunction.

Figure 20.14 highlights relevant features of the vertebrae. The second cervical vertebra (the **axis**) possesses an

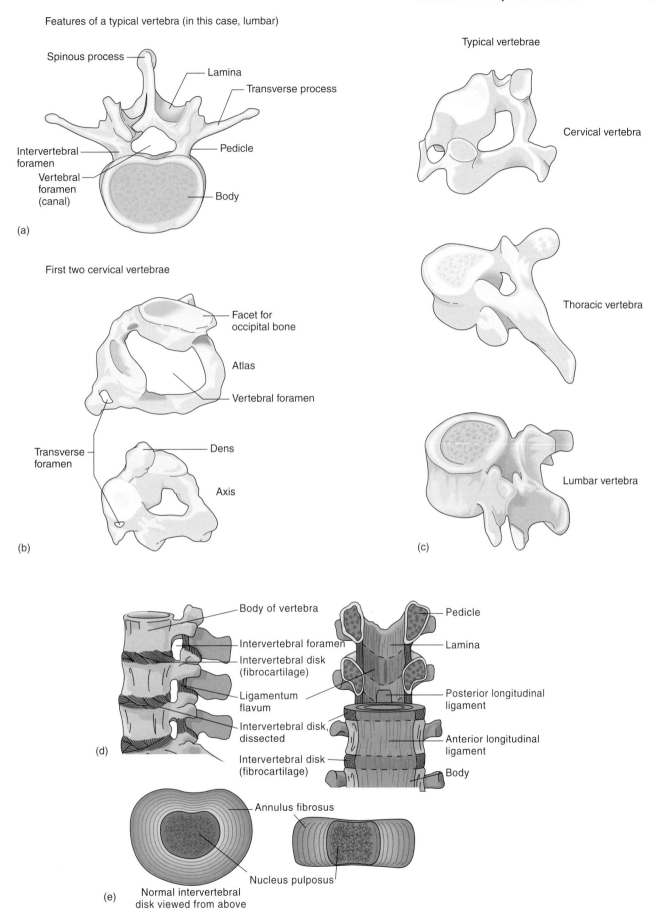

Features of a typical vertebra (in this case, lumbar)

Spinous process
Lamina
Transverse process
Intervertebral foramen
Pedicle
Vertebral foramen (canal)
Body

(a)

First two cervical vertebrae

Facet for occipital bone
Atlas
Vertebral foramen
Transverse foramen
Dens
Axis

(b)

Typical vertebrae

Cervical vertebra

Thoracic vertebra

Lumbar vertebra

(c)

Body of vertebra
Intervertebral foramen
Intervertebral disk (fibrocartilage)
Ligamentum flavum
Intervertebral disk, dissected
Intervertebral disk (fibrocartilage)
Pedicle
Lamina
Posterior longitudinal ligament
Anterior longitudinal ligament
Body

(d)

Annulus fibrosus
Nucleus pulposus
Normal intervertebral disk viewed from above

(e)

Figure 20.14   **Details of the Vertebral Column.** Vertebral (*a*–*c*) and ligamentous structures (*d*) and the intervertebral disk (*e*).

anterior vertical structure, the **dens** or **odontoid process,** around which the first cervical vertebra (the **atlas**) articulates. Severe hyperextension of the neck can fracture the dens and drive it into the cord. Such a lesion would prove fatal if immediate ventilation were not provided, because the phrenic nerve supplying the diaphragm originates below this (at levels C3 to C5) and would be isolated from its source of stimulation. The vertebral arch is formed by two pedicles, from which the transverse processes project, and two laminae, which produce the spinous process. A **laminectomy** involves the surgical resection of a part or all of the lamina and may include part of the pedicle. This is done to gain access to the vertebral canal or to relieve pressure on nerve roots or the cord itself. Spinal fusion involves removal of damaged intervertebral disks and fusion of adjacent vertebral bodies, with provision for enlargement of the consequently narrowed intervertebral foramina. Experimentation with the insertion of artificial disk material has not proven effective. Sometimes bone grafted from the person's pelvis has been used to replace the lost disk material.

The **intervertebral disks** are specialized points of articulation that allow limited flexibility between adjacent vertebrae while sustaining the weight of the body above them and incorporating substantial shock absorption and tensile strength. The intriguing design that meets these diverse challenges is also the origin of the most common pathologies affecting the vertebral column. The core of the disk (the **nucleus pulposus**) is relatively soft. It is cradled in a tough, fibrous capsule (the **annulus fibrosus**) that restricts the movement of the core. The collagen and elastin fibers that form the annulus extend out of the vertebrae themselves, thereby anchoring the disks and uniting adjacent vertebrae. During flexion the core acts like a pivot point in the center of the disk. This allows more movement, without unduly restricting the foramina between the vertebrae (through which the spinal nerves pass), than those possible if it were achieved by simply compressing the edge of the disk. Also, sudden compressive forces, such as those generated upon landing from a jump, can be absorbed. The core squashes by distending the annulus fibrosus, which then recoils, returning the core to its original shape.

As a person ages, the substance of the nucleus pulposus changes, reducing its capacity to bind water but increasing its strength. Between the ages of about 35 and 50, these trends (decreasing water and therefore size and resilience, but increasing strength) cause the intervertebral spaces to narrow, making nerve entrapment and resultant pain and hypofunction a possibility. Nerve root irritation can lead to inappropriate firing of motor neurons and muscle spasm. Altered relationships between articular surfaces (e.g., the inferior and superior articular facets) may be a source of pain. As well, one-time or cumulative injuries to the annulus fibrosus may cause it to rupture, allowing the still-soft nucleus to protrude or herniate. The layman's term for this condition, "slipped disk," is misleading, because the disk itself does not shift out of position. The anterior longitudinal ligament reinforces the anterior extent of the disk, while the narrower posterior longitudinal ligament limits disk protrusion directly onto the cord. These constraints favor herniation in a lateral/posterior direction. Limited herniation may press on the ventral (motor) roots of the cord, while more extensive herniation may affect dorsal (sensory) roots and the cord itself. These potential problems often lessen with advancing age, as the disk becomes thinner but tougher.

In another type of disk herniation, compressive trauma can cause the nucleus to herniate into the body of the adjacent vertebra. This is a relatively common condition with the uncommon name of **Schmorl's lesion.** It may go undetected unless the shift of nucleus pulposus and the resultant narrowing of intervertebral space causes nerve entrapment or pain. Pain may also arise from altered articulation of the facets on the transverse processes or the rib articulations on thoracic vertebrae. An X-ray would reveal an abnormal narrowing of the affected intervertebral space.

The normal treatment for disk herniation is bed rest with the knees over a support (most herniations occur in the lumbar region, and this position produces a sort of traction). Formerly, a proteolytic enzyme (e.g., chymopapain) was injected into the core of the ruptured nucleus pulposus to hasten retraction and reconstitution of disk structure. In difficult cases, surgical repair of the annulus and removal of herniated nucleus material may be done. Fusion of adjacent vertebral bodies may also be done. The current approach to back injury is highly pragmatic, with an emphasis on staying with or quickly returning to normal patterns of activity and exercise. If an activity—for example, running—can be performed without serious exacerbation of symptoms arising from disk herniation, it is likely to be recommended.

 Checkpoint 20.1

Make sure you have the essentials. Most CNS protections generally work very well, but create their own special vulnerabilities. Describe how this generalization holds for the scalp, the skull, the meningeal protection, and the vertebral column.

CENTRAL NERVOUS SYSTEM STRUCTURE AND FUNCTION

Metabolic Support: Cerebral Vasculature

Metabolism

The proper functioning of the central nervous system depends on appropriate blood supply and drainage. Three factors make the brain's continuous dependence on adequate blood supply more critical than that of any other organ. First, under normal dietary circumstances, the only fuel the brain is able to utilize for ATP production is glucose. (In a fast that lasts longer than three days, the brain will improve its ability to use fatty acids, products of fat breakdown, as an alternative fuel.) Second, there are only limited energy reserves in the brain analogous to the fat reserves in the body or the glycogen stores in the liver or skeletal muscle. This point leads directly to the third factor. The anaerobic capacity of neural tissue is very limited: the brain requires a constant supply of oxygenated blood. At the same time, the energy demands in the brain are high. It is a very metabolically active tissue.

What is this energy used for? Almost half goes to maintain the plasma membrane electrochemical gradients that are the basis of signal transfer. Another significant amount supports neurotransmitter manufacture and movement and the active transport of metabolites across the blood-brain barrier. These activities take place at comparable rates whether the brain is sleeping or alert and active. Because of these factors, the blood requirements of the brain are for a constant perfusion of 750–1,000 ml per minute (about 17% of the resting cardiac output) for a tissue mass (1,500 g) that is about 2% of the body's weight. As well, at rest almost 70% of the blood glucose and 25% of the oxygen carried are consumed by the brain. The only other organ that maintains such a steady metabolic rate is the heart, and, fortunately for the brain's glucose supply, the heart uses principally lipids during periods of low to moderate activity.

Cerebral Blood Flow

Cerebral blood flow (CBF), as we have noted, remains relatively constant. Factors both outside and inside the skull interact to maintain or challenge that constant blood flow. The overriding extracranial factor is the systemic blood pressure, monitored in the carotid baroreceptors at the vessels carrying the largest amount of blood to the brain. As well, there are vasomotor neurons in the medulla that fire in response to ischemia and massively increase sympathetic discharge, increasing heart rate and force of contraction and increasing systemic vasoconstriction. This is a backup system to ensure maintenance of cerebral blood flow. A second extracranial factor, cardiovascular function, is an issue when the cardiovascular system fails, as happens during ventricular fibrillation. The resultant brain ischemia can give rise to edema that can kill a person hours after heart function has been effectively restored.

Of intracranial factors affecting cerebral blood flow, the most important is **autoregulation.** This is an intrinsic capacity of healthy brain arterioles to regulate local blood flow, a capacity that they share, in degree, with arterioles in much of the rest of the body. There are two facets to autoregulation. First, cerebral blood vessels reflexively constrict when systemic blood pressure rises, thereby damping the potential increase in cerebral blood flow. Conversely, if blood pressure suddenly drops, as when a person quickly stands up, the vessels reflexively dilate, thereby compensating for the potential decrease in CBF. Second, when focused activity in one region of the brain increases its metabolic rate, and therefore its circulatory requirements, that region simultaneously increases its production of carbon dioxide, the single most potent dilator of cerebral blood vessels. The vessels in the area respond with vasodilation, increasing local perfusion and balancing glucose and oxygen requirements while clearing waste products. Decreasing pH and oxygen tension also cause vasodilation and local increases in CBF. NO (nitric oxide) plays an important role in the regulation of local blood flow in the brain. As well as the NO release from endothelia, specialized neural cells synthesize NO to appropriately enhance local perfusion. Autoregulation can maintain a constant cerebral blood flow even though diastolic systemic pressure may go as low as 60 mm Hg or as high as 140 mm Hg. This capacity for autoregulation is lost in severely hypoxic tissue and can worsen the degree and effects of ischemia.

The second major intracranial factor affecting cerebral blood flow is the intracranial pressure itself. This pressure might rise because of an expanding tumor, edema, or perhaps a hemorrhage. As the pressure within the cranial vault approaches the diastolic pressure of the arterial blood, CBF will be progressively compromised. The difference between the systemic arterial pressure (SAP) and the intracranial pressure is the **cerebral perfusion pressure** (CPP): CPP = Mean SAP – ICP, where Mean SAP = 1/3 (Systolic – Diastolic) + Diastolic. The normal range of CPP is approximately 80–100 mm Hg. If the CPP drops below 60 mm Hg, ischemia will develop. The effects of the resulting hypoxia are most severe in the boundary zones between the major arterial fields, areas known as the *watersheds.* There are also specific anatomical sites whose neurons are particularly sensitive to hypoxia—for example, the hippocampus (part of the limbic system and involved in memory and attention), the outer layers of the cortex, the sulci (grooves in the brain's surface), and certain critical cells in the cerebellum. A CPP of less than 30 mm Hg is incompatible with life.

Cerebral Vasculature

As shown in figure 20.15a, the brain is supplied by two pairs of arteries. The internal carotid arteries (which together carry over 70% of the cerebral blood) branch from the common carotids, which in turn arise from the aortic arch (left common carotid) or the brachiocephalic artery (right common carotid). As the internal carotid arteries enter through special foramina into the cranial vault, they take an S-shaped detour through a blood-filled venous sinus called the *cavernous sinus.* This site is significant because a variety of cranial nerves course through the sinus. They are vulnerable to pressure from an aneurysm in the carotid artery or infection of the cavernous sinus. As the internal carotids finally pierce the dura and enter the area at the base of the brain, each branches to form the middle cerebral

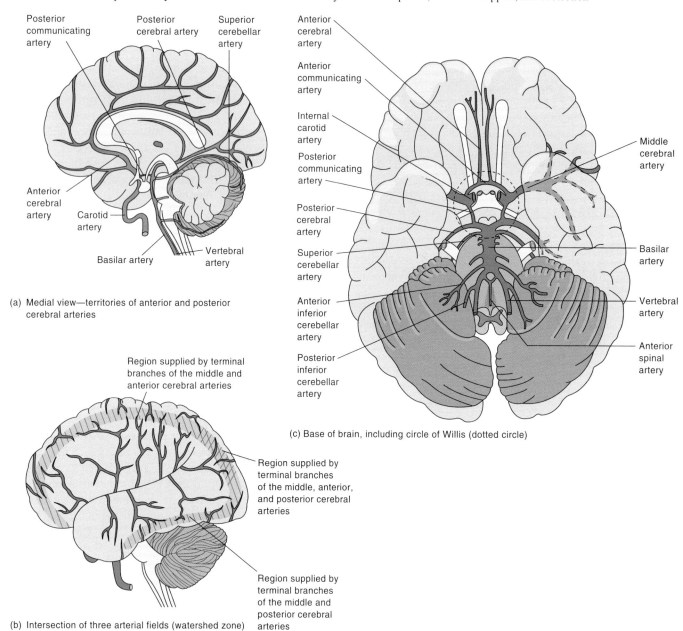

Figure 20.15   Cerebral Vasculature. (*a*) Arterial supply of the brain, medial view. The anterior cerebral artery supplies two-thirds of area of longitudinal fissure, while the posterior cerebral artery supplies approximately one-third, with a small area of overlap. (*b*) Arterial supply of the brain, lateral view. Most of the lateral hemisphere is supplied by the middle cerebral artery. Shaded area corresponds to the area of arterial overlap (anastomosis), the watershed zone. (*c*) Arterial supply, inferior view.

artery, the anterior cerebral artery, and the anastomotic posterior communicating artery.

The second pair of supply arteries are the vertebrals. These arise from the subclavian arteries, then pass up the transverse foramina in the cervical vertebrae and enter through the foramen magnum. They join to form the basilar artery, which throws off a variety of smaller arteries to supply the cerebellum and brain stem and finally branches into the two posterior cerebral arteries, which supply the posterior temporal lobe, the occipital cortex, and the pos-

terior longitudinal fissure. The branches of the internal carotids and two posterior cerebral arteries contribute to a unique vascular structure, the **cerebral arterial circle** of Willis **(circle of Willis).** This interconnecting system probably serves no anastomotic role in the normal functioning of the cerebral vasculature (i.e., it doesn't shift blood back and forth to meet demands). However, in the event of obstruction of a major cerebral artery, the alternative pathways it provides can make the difference between minimal functional loss and massive impairment.

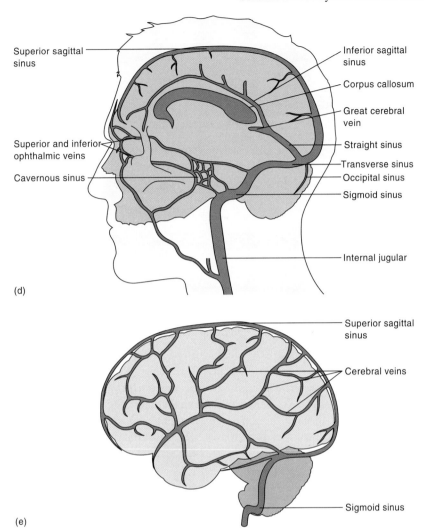

Figure 20.15, continued   Cerebral Vasculature. (*d*) Venous drainage of the brain, medial view. The medial hemisphere drains into the inferior sagittal sinus; deep structures drain into the great cerebral vein (of Galen). Together these form the straight sinus. (*e*) Venous drainage, lateral view. Most draining is into the superior sagittal sinus.

The details of the tissues supplied by specific arteries will be provided in the Cerebrovascular Accidents section later in this chapter.

The venous drainage of the brain is unique in that the veins have no valves and do not retrace the course of the corresponding arteries. Figure 20.15*d* shows the major venous sinuses that drain the bulk of the cerebral tissue. The **superior sagittal sinus** is the site of uptake of the CSF in the arachnoid villi. Many of the veins coming from deep in the tissue of the cerebral hemispheres course through the subarachnoid space to empty into this sinus. The blood passes posteriorly to the junction of the falx cerebri and the tentorium, where its flow is added to by blood passing from deep in the brain via the **straight sinus.** From this point of **confluence,** the sinus splits into a left and right **transverse sinus,** each of which takes an S-shaped course (now called the **sigmoid sinus**) until it passes out of the

floor of the cranial vault through the jugular foramen to become the **internal jugular vein.** Other veins drain the central structures of the cerebrum. Blood passes backward from the central core into the **great cerebral vein** of Galen to join blood coming from above the corpus callosum in the **inferior sagittal sinus.** Together, they form the straight sinus.

The Blood-Brain Barrier

The structure of capillaries in the CNS is quite distinct from that of capillaries in the rest of the body. The junctions between capillary endothelial cells in the brain are tight, unlike most systemic capillaries; brain capillaries are surrounded by and encased in the foot processes of glial cells called astrocytes; mitochondria are more numerous in the endothelial cells of brain capillaries. These mechanisms all

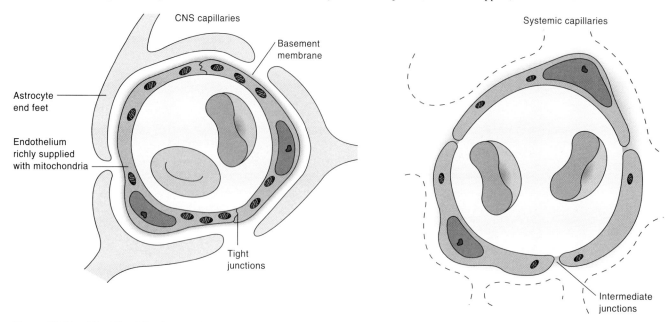

Figure 20.16   **The Blood-Brain Barrier Compared with Endothelial Junctions in Systemic Capillaries.**

contribute to an effective **blood-brain barrier.** The tight junctions limit movement of solute and water, as these must pass through the endothelial cells—not through the junctions, as can happen in other organs. The astrocytes form a transport system, picking up glucose, oxygen, and other metabolites and delivering waste products back to the capillary circulation. They also serve a structural support function (fig. 20.16). The endothelial mitochondria generate the ATP necessary to drive active transport. There is an analogous blood-CSF barrier that actively secretes the cerebrospinal fluid, which accounts for the fact that CSF normally has only 0.5% as much albumin as blood plasma. There is no corresponding CSF-parenchymal barrier, so if a substance or organism makes it into the CSF, it has unimpeded access to the brain tissue itself.

The blood-brain barrier functions to exclude substances that are of low solubility in lipid (e.g., organic acids), highly ionized polar compounds, large molecules, and substances that are not transported by specific carrier-mediated transport systems. These would include albumin and substances bound to albumin (e.g., bilirubin, many hormones, and drugs), many organic and inorganic toxins, and many drugs. Sugars, other metabolic substrates, and some amino acids have specific carriers within the endothelial cells. An example of a substrate normally excluded from the brain is penicillin. It is an organic acid that travels bound to albumin (a large molecule), and there is no transport carrier to move it into the brain. These factors limit its usefulness in treating CNS infection. Erythromycin, on the other hand, will pass easily through the capillaries. Dopamine, a neurotransmitter that is deficient in people with Parkinson's disease, will not pass, while L-DOPA, its

precursor, will. In summary, these barriers provide a system that preserves homeostasis in the nervous system by facilitating access of necessary metabolites while, at the same time, blocking entry or promoting the removal of unnecessary metabolites or toxic substances.

Typical Neuron

The cells of the nervous system that are specialized for response to stimuli, passage of signals, integration of information, and motor and neuroendocrine responses are called **neurons.** Neurons are not normally capable of dividing in the mature nervous system and are consequently not responsible for cancers in anyone but children. Although there are many different types of neurons, each with a characteristic structure and function, the motor neuron, the cell body of which is located in the anterior, central spinal cord, illustrates many common features (fig. 20.17a). Fine branches called **dendrites** carry signals toward the cell body, or **soma.** This contains the nucleus, numerous mitochondria, and noticeable granules of ribosomes on rough ER called **Nissl granules.** These are the site of manufacture of, amongst other things, **neurotransmitters,** the chemicals with which neurons communicate. These are pumped down the long process that allows the neuron to signal at a distance, the **axon.** Neurotransmitter is stored ready for release in vacuoles in the end processes of axons, called **end-foot processes** or **telodendria,** which contact the cells influenced by the neuron, whether muscle fibers, smooth muscle, glandular cells, or another neuron. The region where the soma fuses with the axon, called the **axon hillock,** is the site, at least in motor neurons, where the decision to

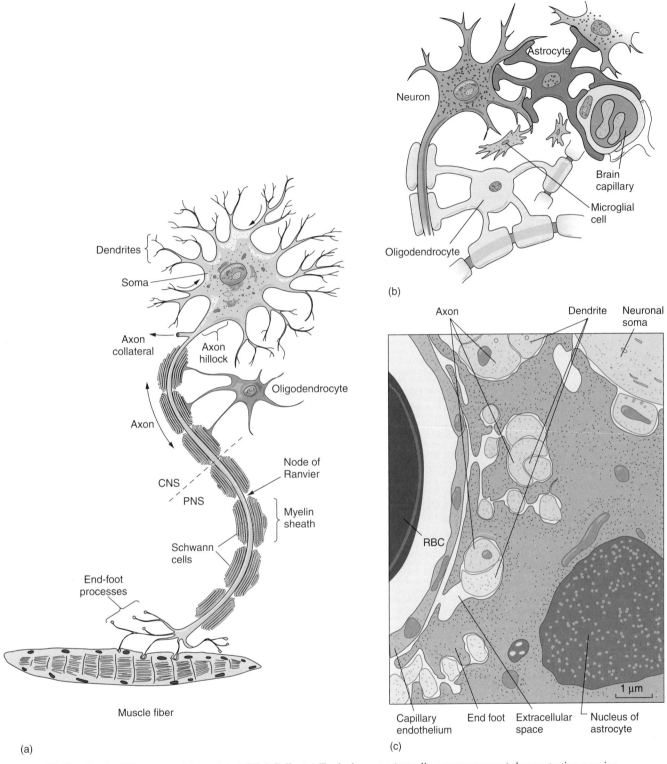

Figure 20.17 **Typical Neuron and Associated Glial Cells.** (*a*) Typical neuron (actually a motor neuron) demonstrating a major feature of specialization. (*b*) Simplified presentation of glial cells. (*c*) Relationship of brain capillary, astrocyte, neural processes, and neuronal soma.

produce a signal to pass down the axon is made. In this case, it is a simple summation of all the excitatory signals arriving at the soma, minus the inhibitory signals, most of which converge on the axon hillock.

The axon membrane, or **neurolemma,** is not exposed directly to the extracellular fluid, but is either embedded in a protective cell or wrapped in layers of cell membrane called **myelin sheath.** Within the CNS this myelin is produced by cells called **oligodendrocytes,** each of which may produce perhaps 20 individual segments of myelin wrapping several different axons. In the PNS, individual **Schwann cells** each wrap a segment of axon. Both oligos and Schwann cells are capable of multiplying in the adult and are therefore capable of producing cancers. Myelin serves to isolate most of the surface of the axon from the extracellular environment and insulate the electrochemical signal carried within it. Between the segments are zones called **nodes of Ranvier** at which there are dense concentrations of sodium channels. These act as booster stations for the signal traveling in the axon. A rapid diffusion of sodium within the axon raises the negative internal charge at the node to the point at which the sodium channels pop open. Sodium ions zip in, renewing the signal. Neurons that are only embedded in Schwann cells are called **unmyelinated,** while those that are wrapped in layers of Schwann or oligodendrocyte membrane are called **myelinated.** Signals travel much more slowly in unmyelinated axons because the sodium channels are distributed evenly along the axon: Channel opening is the most time-consuming event in signal conduction. Within myelinated neurons, there is a correspondence between size of axon and distance between nodes: The larger the axon, the greater the distance. Also, the larger the axon, the faster and more efficient the signal conduction. Because it jumps from node to node, signal conduction in myelinated axons is called **saltatory.** Neurons carrying pain and temperature information are either unmyelinated or lightly myelinated and therefore carry these signals slowly. Examples of large, well-myelinated axons, and therefore rapid, efficient signal conduction, are alpha motor neurons activating skeletal muscles and spindle fibers carrying information about tension in muscles and position in the joints and limbs.

Support or Glial Cells

The structure or function of neurons is supported by a variety of **glial** cells, including the oligodendrocytes and Schwann cells already described. **Astrocytes** (fig. 20.17*b*) are found everywhere in the CNS but are particularly prominent in the gray matter that composes the **cortex** and the central gray matter of the spinal cord called the **dorsal** and **ventral horns of gray matter.** Astrocytes enwrap the capillaries supplying the neurons and help ensure that only desired substances enter the extracellular spaces surrounding the neurons. In this way they contribute to a **blood-brain barrier** that protects the CNS. They also stabilize the environment around neurons by absorbing excess potassium and neurotransmitter released during neural stimulation, and can release glucose for the use of active neurons. Astrocytes can multiply in the adult and are therefore capable of producing cancers. **Microglia** are probably macrophages resident in the CNS. They are there to clear debris in case of any injury or infection. **Ependymal cells** line the tubular canal found in the center of the spinal cord and the C-shaped spaces in the center of each hemisphere (the two halves of the cerebrum) called ventricles. Ependymal cells wrap the capillaries of the **choroid plexus.** This tissue is found in each ventricle and the central spaces that unite them. It is responsible for production of the watery **cerebrospinal fluid** that acts to float and cushion the CNS. Ependymal cells can produce tumors called ependymomas.

Structure and Localized Function of the Brain

The Cerebrum: The Cerebral Cortex

The largest part of the brain is the **cerebrum.** It has two lateral halves: the **cerebral hemispheres.** The bulk of the mass of the cerebrum is formed of central white matter with nuclei of gray matter. Gray matter, whether of the superficial **cortex** or deep nuclei and central spinal cord, is the origin or destination and site of integration of all signals in the nervous system: It is the site of processing (fig. 20.17). Gray matter is colored by the dense presence of neural cell bodies and synapses. The **cerebral cortex,** which is the outer rim of gray matter, perhaps 3 mm thick, is thrown up in folds, or **convolutions.** These increase its total area and therefore the number of cells it can contain and the amount of processing it can do. The bumps are called **gyri** (singular, gyrus) and the grooves are called **sulci** (singular, sulcus). The nature of cortex in gyri and sulci is the same. Particularly deep sulci are called **fissures.** Four of these are important landmarks dividing the cerebral hemisphere. They are the **longitudinal fissure,** which divides the two cerebral hemispheres; the **central sulcus** (also known as the great central sulcus, the central fissure, or the fissure of Rolando); the **lateral,** or **Sylvian fissure;** and the **calcarine fissure** that divides the primary visual cortex in two. The central sulcus divides the **frontal lobe** from the **parietal lobe.** The lateral fissure demarcates the **temporal lobe,** while the **occipital lobe** lies between the parietal and temporal lobes.

The type of neuron in the cerebral cortex that responds to stimulation to produce perception, thought, decision making, movement, and so on is the **pyramidal cell,** so-called because its soma is somewhat pyramidlike in shape. These cells have elaborately specialized dendritic projections that support their function. Their single axon will project to a specific neuron in the brain stem, thalamus, basal ganglia, or spinal cord, through association pathways to a related area of cortex on the same hemisphere, or through commissural fibers to a related area on the other hemisphere. There is a direct relation between the precision of control or perception and the amount of cortex dedicated to a function or area of the body. As well, there is a general rule that function on one side of the body is processed on the cortex of the opposite hemisphere **(contralaterality).**

The following are the usual localizations of function on the cerebral cortex: the **primary motor cortex,** or area (also called the **motor strip**), is found on the **precentral gyrus;** the **primary somatosensory cortex** (where perception of skin sensation, limb position, and movement feedback occurs) is on the **postcentral gyrus** (fig. 20.19c gives more detailed information regarding localization of sensory and motor function); the **primary visual cortex** (which processes the raw visual information from the retina) is found on either side of the calcarine fissure deep in the posterior longitudinal fissure; the **primary auditory cortex** is found on the floor of the lateral fissure. Near the primary sensory areas are **sensory association areas** in which meaning is attached to the raw sensations. Likewise, anterior to the primary motor cortex, which can be seen as the keys of a piano involved in the direct production of sound (movement), lie other cortical areas essential for initiating and processing movement. These are the **premotor cortex** and the **supplementary motor area.** A lot of the cortex is taken up with processing the intercommunications between dedicated areas. For example, the **posterior parietal area** allows for the effective integration of motor, sensory and visual information to permit precise eye-hand coordination.

For the vast majority of people, language is specialized on the left hemisphere. **Wernicke's area,** on the cortex inferior and posterior to the lateral fissure, puts the sense into language, while **Broca's area** is where the movements required for speech are introduced before the message is imposed on the motor strip to produce audible or written language. A person with the rare, pure form of **Wernicke's aphasia** produces language that is unintelligible gibberish but that *sounds* like integrated language. Because Wernicke's area is damaged, victims are also unaware that they are producing nonsense. **Broca's aphasia** results in grossly impaired production of speech: The sense is there but the movements are impaired or absent; those affected just can't get the words out. (All of the foregoing are illustrated in fig. 20.19.)

The cerebral cortex can be considered in terms of the territory supplied by a given major artery. The **middle cerebral artery** supplies the lion's share of the lateral cortex (see fig. 20.15b). Functions that are mediated here include skin sensations; voluntary movement and awareness of movement, particularly above the waist; hearing and the interpretation of sound; awareness of taste; the production and reception of spoken speech (usually concentrated on the left hemisphere); the interpretation and labeling of visual perceptions; aspects of the control of eye movements; and some of our capacity for planning and foresight. Except for language, which is lo-

calized in the left hemisphere (and perhaps specialized capacities for music, mathematics, and creative thought, which are understood to be right hemispheric), these functional areas are on both lateral surfaces and act contralaterally (left hemisphere integrated with the right side of the body).

The territory of the **anterior cerebral artery** is largely the anterior two-thirds of the medial cortex. Functions here include voluntary movement, skin sensations and awareness of movement in the lower limbs, and an area that is involved in the initiation of movements called the supplementary motor area. This artery carries perhaps 10% of the blood feeding the hemisphere and is proportionately likely to be the site of pathology.

The **posterior cerebral artery** is part of an independent supply to the brain, the **vertebrobasilar system.** This feeds the primary visual cortex on the posterior medial surface and the posterior part of the corpus callosum (the splenium), which provides a pathway for the integration of images from both sides of the visual field (fig. 20.18). The vertebrobasilar system (see fig. 20.15c) also supplies the cerebellum, the inferior temporal lobes, and the brain stem, sustaining the crucial functions of attention, arousal, and consciousness, as well as swallowing, breathing, adaptation of heart function, and less conscious aspects of movement. Gagging, vomiting, eye movement defects, dizziness, and altered patterns of breathing may all indicate a lesion that affects the brain stem, as may altered consciousness (see chapter 22).

At the margins of these adjacent vascular fields there is a C-shaped area termed the **watershed zone** (see fig. 20.15b). Because this area is at the farthest extent of the vascular tree, it is more susceptible to factors that interfere with oxygenation, particularly impaired cardiac function, where both blood pressure and cardiac output are a concern. The classic problem here is the watershed zone infarct secondary to heart fibrillation, but infarcts may also be seen with carbon monoxide poisoning, near-suffocation, drowning, and severe anemia. Such infarcts may be quite limited and confined to the watershed zone and certain other susceptible brain structures. Figure 20.20 shows atrophy secondary to a bilateral watershed zone infarct. As you can see by inspection of figures 20.18 and 20.19, the damage would have little effect on critical motor or sensory function. Dysfunction would be more subtle in these cases. However, sometimes a fairly dramatic disorder called **unilateral neglect** arises. This results from a white matter lesion in the watershed zone that interrupts the integration of visual and physical-sensory information in one hemisphere (in the posterior parietal area). Affected individuals behave as though the opposite side of their body doesn't belong to them: the hair isn't combed and clothing is disheveled, even though motor control and sensation are intact. Other impairments of integrated function, such as in dressing or manipulating objects, can result from watershed zone and other scattered lesions. This is an example of a group of disorders often called **disconnection syndromes.**

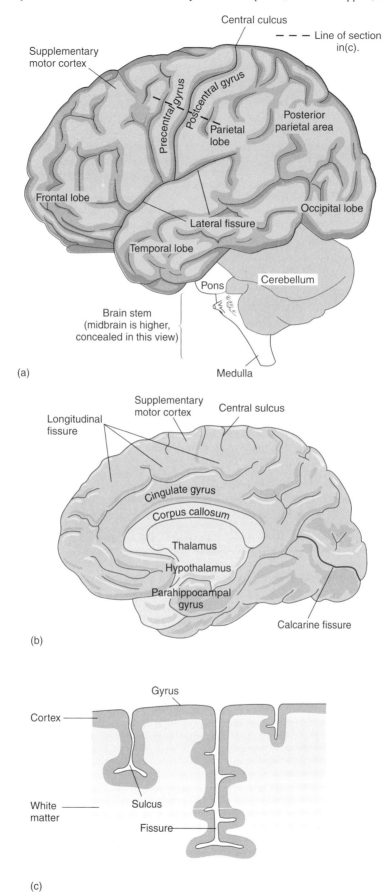

Figure 20.18 **Major Features of the Cerebrum (Shaded).** (*a*) Lateral view; (*b*) medial view—section along the longitudinal fissure through the corpus callosum; (*c*) section through the cerebrum to illustrate gyri, sulci, and a fissure.

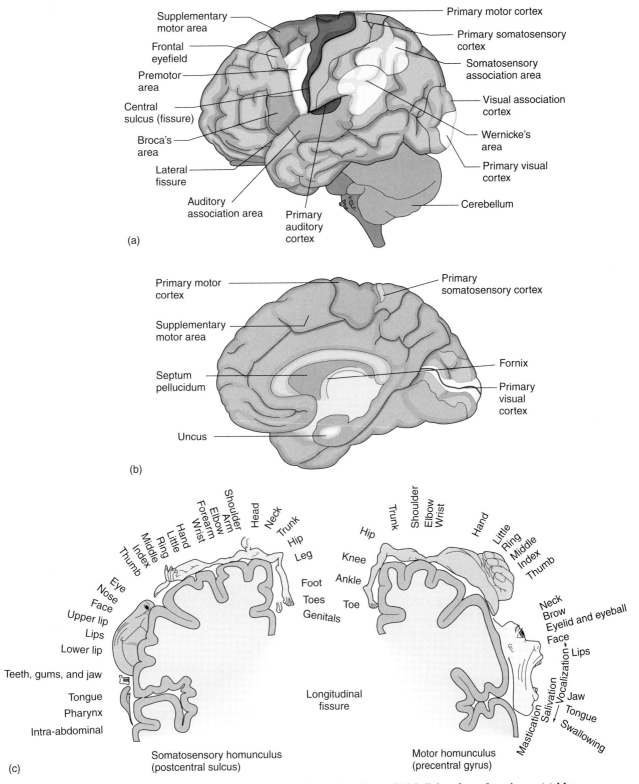

Figure 20.19 **Cortical Localization of Function.** (*a*) Lateral surface of cerebrum. (*b*) Medial surface of cerebrum. (*c*) Motor homunculus (little man) of the precentral gyrus and sensory homunculus of the post central gyrus (after W. Penfield and T. Rasmussen).

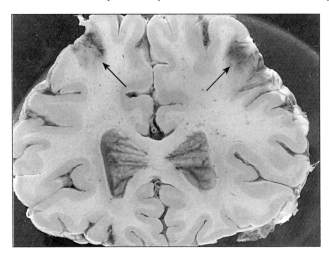

Figure 20.20   **Watershed Infarcts.** This coronal section of the brain shows atrophy secondary to resolution of old watershed infarcts (arrows).

The darkened and collapsed regions in this photo are watershed infarcts, which were caused by a rapidly progressive cardiovascular shock that could not be corrected before becoming irreversible. The hypotension-sustained blood deprivation also caused focal infarction in the kidneys. The shock was the result of an explosion in a small gas stove that a 60-year-old man was refilling with fuel. He was severely burned and survived only three weeks.

Deep Nuclei and White Matter: The Cerebrum in Coronal Section

Figure 20.21 shows some of the deep nuclei and white matter structures of the brain. The white matter is composed mostly of the myelin sheaths formed by oligos. Traveling in this protective environment are billions of axons interconnecting neural cells of specific areas of the overlying cortex (called **association fibers**), carrying signals from an area of cortex on one hemisphere to a corresponding area on the other hemisphere **(commissural fibers),** or carrying signals from the cortex to lower centers such as the brain stem or spinal cord or from lower centers to the cortex **(projection fibers).** It is this mass of white matter that allows for the immense variety of interconnections that occur in the CNS and makes possible the unique solutions that we call intelligence. One particularly prominent and important band of projection fibers, which passes between islands of gray matter deep within each hemisphere, is called the **internal capsule.** Much of the bulk of the white matter of the cerebrum can be referred to as the **corona radiata.** It is so-called because when one does blunt dissection of the cerebrum, the gray matter falls away, revealing a "radiating crown" of white matter tracts (bundles of myelinated axons). These may be any combination of association, commissural, and/or projection fibers.

Medial to the internal capsule and lateral to the central cerebrospinal fluid-containing space called the **third**

ventricle is a group of nuclei (functionally related island of gray matter) called the **thalamus.** (Actually there is a left and right set of thalamic nuclei.) The thalamus acts as an intelligent relay station, passing all sensory information (except smell) on to the appropriate area of the cerebral cortex. It is "intelligent" in the same sense that an old-fashioned switchboard operator was active in ensuring that calls with a higher priority (e.g., a call for the fire department), got passed on ahead of less critical information. Below the thalamic nuclei are two groups of nuclei called the **hypothalamus.** These monitor a wide range of homeostatic functions (water balance, temperature, levels of several hormones, etc.) and produce changes in endocrine and nervous system function that ensure survival. As well, they contribute to the expression of the **limbic system,** a brain system producing drives, stress responses, emotions, arousal, attention, and memory. The hypothalamus is often not visible in sections that show the thalamus well.

Another large set of nuclei within the cerebral hemisphere, in this case split by the internal capsule, are the **basal ganglia.** They are more widely distributed than the thalamic or hypothalamic nuclei. This is partly because the system is complex, involving many separate nuclei, and partly because these structures are separated or stretched in the developing brain. They are collectively responsible for co-processing the expression of voluntary movement, and are also involved in thought processing, imagination, the construction of spatial relations, and a variety of other important mental functions. If the basal ganglia are damaged, a person will have difficulty initiating movement, may tremble when inactive, and will experience rigidity. The major components of the basal ganglia (also called the **cerebral nuclei**) are the caudate nucleus, the putamen, the globus pallidus, and the substantia nigra. The **substantia nigra** is a major target of the pathological processes underlying Parkinson's disease.

An oblique section through the cerebrum may include portions of the brain stem. This view shows the substantia nigra, which is the anterior midbrain, the top of the brain stem. It also has the red nuclei, one of the sets of nuclei in the brain stem that are involved in movement. This section is located far enough forward to show the coiled **hippocampal formation** in the temporal lobes, one on each side. These are part of the limbic system and are essential in the formation of memory, which is processed here and then sent back to the area of cortex in which the original perception was formed. These hippocampal formations are affected early in the development of Alzheimer's disease.

The nuclei surrounding the third ventricle are vulnerable to hemorrhagic damage, particularly while the brain is developing (fig. 20.22). But while more prone to hemorrhage, the fetal brain is less susceptible to its consequences or can at least survive a hemorrhage that would prove fatal in an adult. This difference is due partly to the relatively low fetal blood pressure and the expandable nature of the

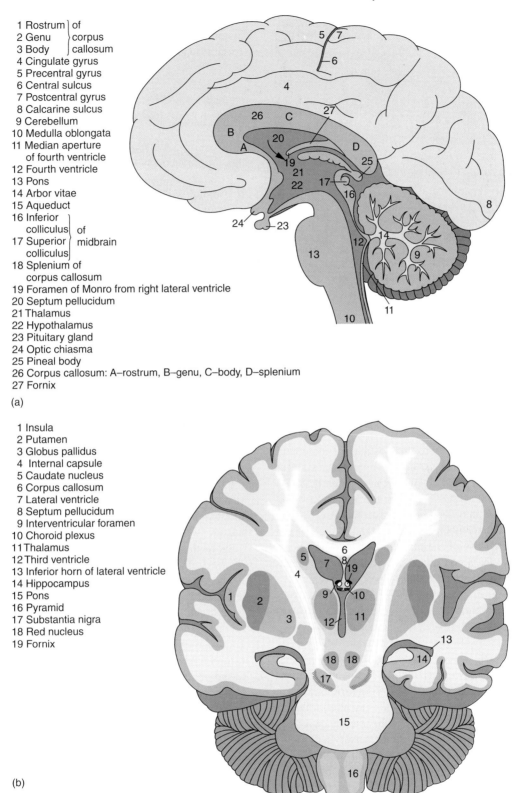

1 Rostrum ⎤ of
2 Genu ⎬ corpus
3 Body ⎦ callosum
4 Cingulate gyrus
5 Precentral gyrus
6 Central sulcus
7 Postcentral gyrus
8 Calcarine sulcus
9 Cerebellum
10 Medulla oblongata
11 Median aperture
   of fourth ventricle
12 Fourth ventricle
13 Pons
14 Arbor vitae
15 Aqueduct
16 Inferior
   colliculus ⎤ of
17 Superior ⎬ midbrain
   colliculus ⎦
18 Splenium of
   corpus callosum
19 Foramen of Monro from right lateral ventricle
20 Septum pellucidum
21 Thalamus
22 Hypothalamus
23 Pituitary gland
24 Optic chiasma
25 Pineal body
26 Corpus callosum: A–rostrum, B–genu, C–body, D–splenium
27 Fornix

(a)

1 Insula
2 Putamen
3 Globus pallidus
4 Internal capsule
5 Caudate nucleus
6 Corpus callosum
7 Lateral ventricle
8 Septum pellucidum
9 Interventricular foramen
10 Choroid plexus
11 Thalamus
12 Third ventricle
13 Inferior horn of lateral ventricle
14 Hippocampus
15 Pons
16 Pyramid
17 Substantia nigra
18 Red nucleus
19 Fornix

(b)

Figure 20.21 **Brain Anatomy.** (*a*) Sagittal and (*b*) coronal sections through the brain, showing relevant structures. The coronal section is through the interventricular foramen, midbrain, and pons.

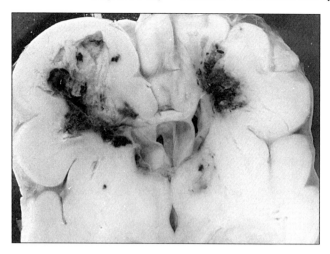

Figure 20.22 **Brain of Premature Infant Showing Hemorrhage in the Area of the Germinal Eminence.**
This brain came, not from a fetus, but from an infant born at 32 weeks. The difficulty in distinguishing between white and gray matter arises because the myelination is not yet complete at this early point of development. Also typical of premature infants are the periventricular hemorrhages that are clearly visible. These, and a variety of kidney and heart problems, combined to overwhelm the infant, who was able to survive only nine days.

fetal cranial vault, and partly to the plasticity of the developing nervous system. That is, if fetal brain tissues suffer hemorrhagic damage, their functions can apparently be assumed by healthy surviving tissue. In the adult, the blood from a hemorrhage into deep brain tissue can travel to the third ventricle, where it meets only the resistance of the CSF pressure. Because of the rapid movement of blood at arterial pressure, the blood dilates the ventricles and transfers pressure to the brain tissue itself, producing a massive back pressure against normal perfusion. This and the attendant movement of brain tissue are enough to cause rapid death in any significant intracerebral hemorrhage.

The internal capsule (see fig. 20.21*b*) provides a massive conduit for information flow in the brain. Descending signals that produce movement and modify incoming information and ascending signals that carry sensation, arousal, and information about the effects of movement all travel in the internal capsule. A hemorrhage in the internal capsule is prone to dissect along the lines of these sensory and motor fibers and extend to greater distances than might be expected. As well, a relatively small lesion that blocks the path of the internal capsule can have effects on movement and/or sensation out of all proportion to its size.

Some conditions—for example, hypertensive microaneurysms or leukemia, can cause widespread, tiny hemorrhages into white matter that isolate scattered areas of gray matter. The white matter that is infarcted undergoes liquefaction necrosis, leaving a cyst, or "lacune," hence the descriptive name **lacunar syndrome.** Its symptoms are highly varied and often very challenging to identify. MRI or CT

can be used to image the lacunae. These, coupled with a history of hypertension, make the diagnosis. Control of hypertension is the approach to avoiding further lacunae.

 Checkpoint 20.2

Most of this material should be a review of the basic anatomy and physiology you studied in previous courses. How well did you recall that material? Could you offer a pathological condition that arises in the vasculature, neural or glial cells and the cortex or deep cerebral nuclei? How does each of these disorders focus the need for this essential background material?

GENERAL CNS PATHOLOGY

Edema in the CNS

Edema is an increase in tissue mass that results from the excess movement of body fluid from the vascular compartment or its abnormal retention in the tissue. Although the basic mechanisms creating CNS edema are not unique to the CNS, certain conditions require that it be treated as a special case. For one, an increase in mass in the CNS, whatever its source, competes for the limited space within the meningeal and bony protection. The result may be destructive compression or movement of tissue or increased intracranial pressure (the next topic). For another, the CNS has no system for draining extracellular fluid that is analogous to the systemic lymphatics as already detailed. Most of the fluid that passes out of the capillaries to support neural function returns to the circulation via the capillaries and postcapillary venules. This dependence on adequate venous drainage is made more significant in the CNS by a relative absence of alternative anastomotic venous drainage. Blockage of veins or venous sinuses, such as may occur in thrombophlebitis, compression, or kinking due to shifts in tissue, may rapidly induce edema, which can interfere with function and further complicate the picture.

These differences give rise to distinctions in patterns of edema that aren't made outside the CNS. **Vasogenic edema** is closest to the pattern of edema typical of inflammation in the rest of the body. It is largely confined to the white matter of the brain and spinal cord. In this case, something perturbs the usually intact blood-brain barrier. The agent might be inflammation associated with infection, a toxic agent that damages capillary endothelial cells, or the abnormally permeable capillaries that are stimulated by and supply a malignant neoplasm. (The latter is the most common cause of vasogenic edema.) These situations favor the outflow of small plasma proteins that would normally be confined to the vascular compartment. With the resultant change in osmotic gradients, there is a net flow of fluid into the intercellular space, which causes swelling. As well, the plasma filtrate accumulates in the extracellular spaces, where the altered ionic balance impairs function.

Cytotoxic edema is, by contrast, an intracellular phenomenon. The typical agent is hypoxia. This may be secondary to ischemia that results from a cardiac arrest. Near-drowning and strangulation are other causes of generalized hypoxia. Focal edema will result from partial occlusion of an end artery; again, ischemia/hypoxia is the agent. Less common causes are toxic substances that directly impair the functioning of the sodium-potassium-ATPase pump or the metabolic processes that produce ATP. Since the neurons are the most active cells in the brain, cytotoxic edema tends to be focused here. The swelling therefore is largely cellular. It should be noted that some authors differentiate cytotoxic from hypoxic edema. Although the agent (toxin versus hypoxia) is different, the cellular mechanism is the same; so they are grouped together here.

In practice, edema is often a result of both vasogenic and cytotoxic processes. For instance, temporary ventricular fibrillation that results in grossly impaired cerebral perfusion will probably induce both neural swelling and a transitory breakdown in the blood-brain barrier. Where this distinction may be particularly important is in the treatment of cerebral edema. When the edema is principally cytotoxic (i.e., due to cellular swelling), passing a bolus of hypertonic solution (e.g., mannitol) through the cerebral vasculature will draw fluid out of the extracellular space. By reducing extracellular volume, this procedure will make more room for the swollen cells. As well, it will increase the osmotic concentration of the extracellular fluid, thereby arresting or reversing the movement of water into the cells. However, if the blood-brain barrier were defective, as for example in the swollen tissue of a neoplastic growth, this strategy could instead add to the problem. Mannitol would move into the extracellular space and, since it would act as an additional osmotic attractant, it would add to the swelling.

Increased Intracranial Pressure

The intact cranium and associated dural sheath are essentially inexpandable. The spinal dural sac in its protective vertebral cage is capable of a small amount of distention. These boundaries contain three incompressible elements: CNS tissue, cerebrospinal fluid, and blood. Expansion of any one of these elements must be balanced by proportional constriction of either or both of the other two, or there will be an increase in intracranial pressure. This relationship is known as the **Monro-Kellie hypothesis.**

The normal intracranial pressure is between 5 and 15 mm Hg. (For reference, this is slightly higher than venous pressure, but considerably lower than mean systemic arterial pressure of about 95 mm Hg.) Minor natural fluctuations occur that are linked to the respiratory cycle and the 24-hour cycle of rest and wakefulness. These largely reflect changes in intrathoracic venous pressure and resultant changes in CSF reabsorption. During exhalation there is a temporary increase in intrathoracic pressure. Reclining facilitates venous return from the extremities, which leads to a slight pooling of blood and an increased central venous pressure. Both of these impair cerebral venous drainage and thereby the reabsorption of CSF.

This will lead to an increase in CSF, which, according to the Monro-Kellie hypothesis, will lead to an increase in intracranial pressure (ICP) unless blood is expelled or brain tissue shrinks. Slightly increased ICP is what is observed. The same mechanism is responsible for the brief increase in ICP that is observed during the Valsalva maneuver (attempting to exhale against a closed glottis), coughing, sneezing, or straining at stool. Some of the potential increase is absorbed by the temporary distention of the spinal dural sac. These situations also generate brief increases in blood pressure and volume that are conducted to large and midsized cerebral arteries. For this reason they are to be avoided by people at risk of cerebral hemorrhage as well as those with increased ICP. (For example, stool softeners are prescribed for constipation.)

Chronically increased systemic arterial pressure has little impact on CSF volume and ICP because of the reflex constriction of precapillary arterioles that results in constant cerebral perfusion. However, supplying air enriched in carbon dioxide, such as used to be done for a patient with a recent cerebrovascular accident in an effort to improve perfusion of surviving tissue, can raise ICP. The carbon dioxide powerfully dilates arterioles, including those of the chorionic plexus, which increases CSF production *and* blood volume. This simply worsens the progression of the stroke, especially with hemorrhagic CVA by increasing cerebral perfusion, and does nothing for the damaged tissue as blood vessels there have lost their natural capacity for autoregulation. Blood flow increases to healthy tissue, perhaps at the cost of poorly perfused tissue at the margins of the stroke. By contrast, hyperventilation reduces PCO_2 and increases pH, which leads to arteriolar constriction and reduced CSF production. Decreasing blood and CSF volumes can bring down ICP, and mechanically assisted hyperventilation is commonly used in comatose or deliberately sedated patients to control increased ICP.

Increased ICP is a potential complication of a variety of pathological conditions. CNS edema and tumor masses are increases in CNS tissue volume that must be compensated for by expansion of the spinal dural sac and decreases in CSF and blood volume, or they will raise ICP. A slowly growing mass can also be accommodated by reabsorption of adjacent cranial bone. Such bone erosion is detectable in X-rays or CT scans and is suggestive of a tumor. In fact, erosion detected through these means was routinely used for diagnosis before CT and MRI became commonly available. Blocked venous return can increase ICP by impeding CSF reabsorption or generating edema, as can heart failure. Hemorrhage into tissue, or the subarachnoid space, or a subdural or extradural hematoma creates a trapped mass of blood that can increase pressure. If the source is arterial, this rise can be dramatic. Finally, increased CSF and hydrocephalus (see later discussion) can be responsible for raising ICP.

The mechanisms that can dangerously raise ICP—edema, tumor, hematoma, hydrocephalus, venous obstruction, and increased CSF volume—often produce their effects in a gradual, linearly increasing fashion. Rising ICP can be countered by specific compensations: expansion of the spinal dural sac, decreased CSF and blood volume, bone erosion, and atrophy of neural tissue. These compensations are capable of accommodating quite large increases in brain mass with little increase in ICP. This phase of the potential danger is sometimes referred to as stage 1.

As the mass continues to increase, a point is reached when compensatory capacity is exceeded. The result is a gradually rising ICP, characteristic of stage 2. As ICP rises, effective cerebral perfusion pressure drops. The resulting decrease in oxygenation stimulates the vasomotor centers in the medulla to induce peripheral vasoconstriction and to temporarily increase cardiac output through increased sympathetic discharge. The result is increased mean systemic arterial pressure and net cerebral perfusion pressure (treated in detail earlier in this chapter). If the source of pressure is a tumor, brain oxygenation will improve on a transitory basis. If it is a hemorrhage, however, the increased blood pressure will exaggerate the problem. It is likely that a patient will have lowered consciousness by stage 2.

Stage 3 establishes the conditions for a very rapid increase in ICP. This is sometimes called the point or stage of **decompensation.** Autoregulation is lost, so increased arterial pressure is expressed in an increased blood volume in the brain. Hypoxia, which becomes worse with the rise in ICP and the drop in cerebral perfusion pressure, leads to generalized cytotoxic edema and further increases in ICP. Coma deepens. Respiratory drive depends increasingly on arterial carbon dioxide levels, a system that normally acts as an "emergency backup." A pattern called **Cheyne-Stokes respiration** results: a period of apnea (15–60 seconds) is followed by deep, labored breathing that gradually becomes shallow and then apneic again. During the apnea, carbon dioxide accumulates until it triggers another breathing cycle, which clears the carbon dioxide and removes the drive to breathe. The raised arterial pressure that was caused by brain stem hypoxia and peripheral vasoconstriction stretches the pressure receptors in the carotid arteries. They signal the cardiac centers in the medulla, which in turn induces bradycardia.

Stage 4 is reached when the cerebral perfusion pressure falls below 30 mm Hg, and widespread necrosis begins. Compression of brain stem respiratory centers will then lead to respiratory arrest and death.

A quick assessment of ICP can be made by viewing the optic disk of the retina. In the past, ICP was directly assessed by performing a lumbar puncture. This procedure, however, creates the risk of making a zone of lower pressure below the foramen magnum, into which delicate brain and brain stem tissues may be driven by the higher pressure in the cranium. Now ICP is measured by drilling a small burr hole through the skull and introducing a pressure transducer, often into the space between the skull and the dura mater. Alternatively, it may be placed under the dura, or a large-bore needle may be introduced into a ventricle.

Where it is not possible to remove the cause of increased ICP, treatment consists of taking comfort measures while it runs its inevitable course. With treatable or reversible conditions, a variety of strategies are employed. It may be necessary to supply mechanical hyperventilation to a medicated and comatose patient. Blood pressure is reduced by the use of diuretics, to slow CSF production and reduce brain-blood volume. Drugs, usually barbiturates, are administered to slow brain metabolism so that hypoxia has a less destructive effect. An emergency craniotomy may be done to relieve pressure. The availability of ongoing monitoring and these other procedures may be critical to survival in cases where severely increased ICP may be a complication, as in near-drowning, carbon monoxide poisoning, prolonged cardiac arrest, and bacterial meningitis.

Herniation Syndromes

The correspondence between physical features of the brain and their adjacent bony and meningeal structures can produce a potential for lesion. Recall, for example, the situation of the brain stem in the tentorial notch. In general, any focal, expanding mass, whether edema, a tumor, or an area of hemorrhage, generates pressure on adjacent tissue. This sort of **compression syndrome** can result in localized impairment of function. It can also displace tissue, in which case it is referred to as a **herniation syndrome.**

If the increase in mass is in the frontal lobe, it can push the lower gyrus of the medial cortex, the cingulate gyrus, under the barrier of the falx cerebri (fig. 20.23). Such a **cingulate herniation** occurs deep in the longitudinal fissure and produces ambiguous symptoms until it is well advanced: clouded consciousness, perhaps partial complex seizures (see chapter 22). In another kind of herniation, a mass above the tentorium may push the medial temporal lobe down over the edge of the tentorium. A small hillock of tissue, the uncus, normally projects over the free edge of the tentorium. Since the uncus leads the advance of herniating tissue, this pattern is called **uncal herniation.** If swelling is either massive or generalized, the compression and herniation can be focused on the only sizable exit from the cranial vault, the foramen magnum. This condition may be referred to as **central herniation.** Because the midline cerebellar tissue, descriptively called the cerebellar tonsils, leads the advance and directly compresses the brain stem, it is also called **tonsillar herniation.**

In the context of central herniation, you may encounter the term **coning,** as in cerebellar coning. This outmoded usage implies that the concave cranial vault focuses the tissue displacement into a "pressure cone" that is some distance from the expanding lesion, much as rays of light are focused by a magnifying glass. In reality, pressure is conducted through the relatively soft brain tissue in the same way that it is conducted through fluid. As noted, the spinal dural sac is subject to slight expansion. What might be

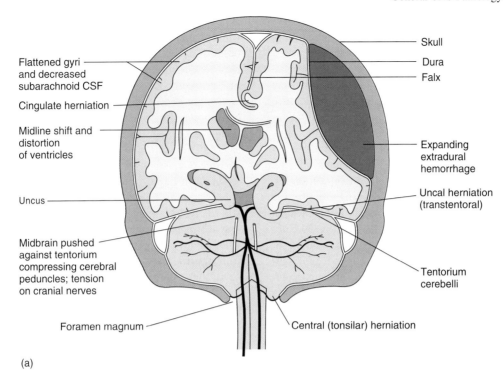

Skull
Dura
Falx

Flattened gyri
and decreased
subarachnoid CSF

Cingulate herniation

Midline shift and
distortion
of ventricles

Expanding
extradural
hemorrhage

Uncus

Uncal herniation
(transtentoral)

Midbrain pushed
against tentorium
compressing cerebral
peduncles; tension
on cranial nerves

Tentorium
cerebelli

Foramen magnum

Central (tonsilar) herniation

(a)

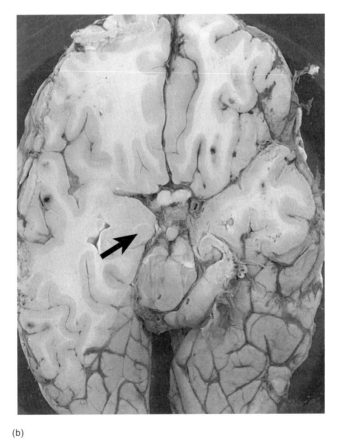

(b)

Figure 20.23 **Patterns of Herniation.** (*a*) The herniation pattern that might accompany the evolution of a massive extradural hematoma. A generalized swelling, on the other hand, may not produce a midline shift but would compress the ventricles and cause uncal and tonsillar herniation. Note, in this view the brain stem, which would lie behind the black "vessels," has been omitted to allow clear illustration of uncal herniation. (*b*) Photo of a low transverse section of a brain with fatally increased intracranial pressure. Uncal herniation is apparent at the arrow as is compression of the brain stem (level of the midbrain).

The enlarging mass of a glioblastoma, combined with cerebral edema that developed in response to it, led to the brain herniation pictured here. Midline distortions are the result of displacement by the enlarging tumor, which cannot be seen in this section. These distortions of the brain contributed to the death of a 76-year-old woman who developed left-sided paralysis and hemianesthesia prior to her death.

abnormally elevated but otherwise evenly distributed intracranial pressure is thereby focused at the foramen magnum as brain stem and cerebellar tissue move downward.

If the agent causing the increased pressure is generalized (e.g., edema due to hypoxia), brain displacement may be very even. Gyri may be flattened and sulci difficult to discriminate. The ventricles will be smaller as CSF is reduced to accommodate increased brain mass. If the pressure source is focal, chances are it will produce midline deviation. This may be detectable as off-center ventricles on a CT scan or a ventricle with an obvious protrusion into it. If the herniation causes kinking of the veins draining the central parts of the brain (where the great vein of Galen joins the straight sinus in the tentorium; see fig. 20.15*d*), edema can rapidly add to the expanding mass. Kinking or compression of the cerebral aqueduct will impede CSF outflow and lead to a rapid increase in ICP. Complete occlusion of the cerebral aqueduct will lead to fatal herniation in a few days.

Hydrocephalus

The term **hydrocephalus** indicates an increase in the volume of the cerebral ventricles. It is used whenever in the life span this condition might occur. A CT scan or MRI would reveal enlarged ventricles, their shape and evenness dependent on the cause of the hydrocephalus. There are three possible mechanisms: oversecretion of CSF, impaired absorption of CSF, and obstruction of CSF pathways.

Oversecretion, perhaps due to a tumor of the choroid plexus, is rarely encountered. Absorption of CSF can be impaired in many ways. Anything that raises venous pressure (e.g., venous or venous sinus thrombosis or severe congestive heart failure) will interfere with CSF reabsorption at the arachnoid granulations. These can be plugged or impeded by the protein and cellular and molecular debris that are produced in meningitis or subarachnoid hemorrhage, or by the high-protein CSF that may be produced from a spinal cord tumor or in Guillain-Barré syndrome. In obstruction, the pathways for the circulation of CSF can be blocked or narrowed sufficiently to produce back pressure in the CSF and distend the ventricles. The obstruction might result from a tumor or from fibrosis associated with inflammation and infection, or it might be the result of congenital malformation. If the ventricular enlargement is due to a loss of cerebral mass, such as might be the case in advanced Alzheimer's disease or adjacent to an old infarct, the condition is not accepted as hydrocephalus proper. Instead, it is sometimes called **hydrocephalus ex vacuo.**

Hydrocephalus can have the same clinical presentation while having varied causes. One example is a child who displays the **congenital** or **infantile** pattern of hydrocephalus. This child may be born with or develop an enlarged head (giving rise to the term *overt hydrocephalus*) with thinned skin over the cranium. The ventricles can be massively enlarged, with a corresponding thinning of the white matter. Since the fetal skull is normally deformable because of the fibrous fontanelles, distention of the ventricles can occur with little corresponding increase in intracranial pressure. Hence, there are few of the complications you might expect. As well, because of the plasticity in localization of function that appears to characterize the developing nervous system, normal function is possible as long as correction of the hydrocephalus is achieved before irreversible damage has occurred. Infantile hydrocephalus may result from impaired CSF reabsorption, which is perhaps due, in turn, to fetal or neonatal meningitis or hemorrhage. Alternatively, it may result from a congenital malformation that obstructs CSF circulation. An example is failure of development (atresia) of the foramina that allow CSF to exit from the fourth ventricle to the subarachnoid space. Two conditions to be discussed later—Dandy-Walker syndrome and Arnold-Chiari malformation (fig. 20.24)—may compress these foramina or the cerebral aqueduct, producing the same effect.

Children and adults are also subject to a number of nondevelopmental disorders that can produce hydrocephalus, by one or another of the three mechanisms that have been described. When the condition develops acutely, it is the resultant increase in ICP that creates a clinical emergency. Such a condition is referred to as **tension hydrocephalus.** Overproduction of CSF is very rarely the mechanism, while obstruction of CSF pathways is most common. The blockage is often at the cerebral aqueduct, and is often caused by a tumor mass or focal edema, but it may also be at the third ventricle, in the subarachnoid space, or in the arachnoid granulations. The inaccurate term "noncommunicating" hydrocephalus is sometimes applied to those cases in which the obstruction is more extensive. Complete obstruction (true "noncommunication") will cause fatally raised ICP in a matter of hours. Almost all hydrocephalus is in fact "communicating."

Some adults have enlarged ventricles without an increased ICP. They also may be confused or demented, walk with difficulty, and have lost bladder control. There is usually no headache associated with this condition. Such **normal-pressure** or **normotensive** hydrocephalus is now thought to result from a temporarily raised intraventricular pressure that stabilized and dropped. The cause for the increased pressure may have been head trauma, subarachnoid hemorrhage, meningitis, or a mass lesion like an abscess. The response to shunting is variable.

Shunting is the provision of an artificial passage for CSF flow to detour an obstruction. This is the treatment of choice for infantile hydrocephalus. As just noted, it is effective in reversing the symptoms of normal-pressure hydrocephalus. With cases of simple obstruction (e.g., aqueductal atresia), the shunt may consist of a short by-pass. With more complex obstruction or where CSF reabsorption is impaired, a sterile tube is laid from the lateral or third ventricle to the right atrium (ventriculoatrial shunt) or ab-

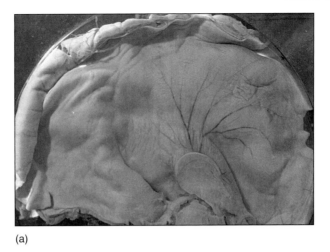

(a)

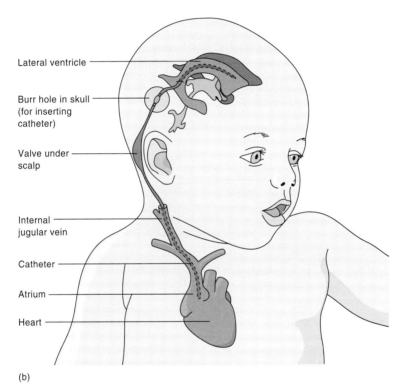

Lateral ventricle

Burr hole in skull
(for inserting
catheter)

Valve under
scalp

Internal
jugular vein

Catheter

Atrium

Heart

(b)

Figure 20.24 **Hydrocephalus.** (*a*) Enormous expansion of the lateral ventricle due to obstruction associated with Arnold-Chiari malformation. Vessels lie in the medial wall of the ventricle. The tiny corpus callosum is seen in the lower middle area of the photo with the brain stem and narrow cerebellum below. (*b*) Placement of a ventriculo-atrial shunt, which might have been used to arrest the progression of the hydrocephalus noted in (*a*). In this view the ventricles are pictured as they would be in a normal brain (i.e., not enlarged).

A child born with Arnold-Chiari syndrome had at birth an unusually large head, which continued to expand, reaching enormous size. He had only a small degree of motor activity, and even this declined. Only brain stem-level functions were sustained for six months until his death. The photo shows the left half of the brain, with cerebellum and pons visible in the lower section. Above is the enormously distended space formed by the lateral and third ventricles. The cerebral tissue is present only as a thin shell a few millimeters thick. The clearly defined blood vessels lie in the medial wall of the ventricle. Progression of hydrocephalus to this extreme extent is now uncommon, shunting being an effective treatment.

dominal cavity (ventriculoperitoneal shunt), where a one-way valve permits CSF outflow. An alternative is to place the shunt from the lumbar cistern, the same region from which a lumbar puncture is taken, to the abdominal cavity (lumboperitoneal shunt).

Coma

Normal and altered consciousness, and the description of the neurological structures that mediate consciousness, are covered in chapter 22. There the principal focus is the level of consciousness before, during, and after a seizure. But consciousness is affected by a wide variety of other medical conditions. The mechanisms responsible and the parts of the nervous system affected will vary with the disease. Remember that consciousness reflects the state of functioning of the nervous system, and that it can therefore be profoundly disrupted by a fully reversible and even very limited lesion.

It is not unusual for a patient to be delivered to the emergency department in a coma, the lowest level of consciousness, without benefit of a witness who knows the circumstances surrounding the coma. This situation presents a critical diagnostic puzzle. The possible causes range from alcohol or barbiturate overdose through craniocerebral trauma, stroke, epilepsy, or bacterial meningitis, to diabetes, kidney failure or heart disease. A sophisticated knowledge of the patterns of coma characteristic of each of these disorders guides the emergency room staff in arriving at an appropriate diagnosis and treatment plan. In general, the basic emergency interventions and the assessment of level of consciousness are similar from case to case. A patent airway is assured; cardiorespiratory status is assessed (Is the patient in shock? Is breathing adequate?); if bleeding has occurred, steps are taken to prevent further blood loss; and blood chemistry is assessed (e.g., blood glucose).

The description of level of consciousness requires some precision, as it indicates the status of the patient's medical condition and reflects the response to treatment (table 20.1). The most critical concern is with the patient who is in the deepest levels of stupor or coma itself. A widely used and effective scheme for standardizing the description of level of consciousness is the Glasgow coma scale, presented in table 20.2. It can be used with little instruction to give a regular (perhaps hourly) score that will reflect the progress of the condition or treatment.

The depth of coma is variable and is reflected in the level of integration of the response to stimulation. In the lightest levels of coma, the response may be integrated and purposive—for example, the examiner's hand may be pushed away. In somewhat deeper coma, withdrawal of a stimulated limb will be observed. The movement is largely reflex in nature. At deeper levels, only reflex behavior can be elicited, although a patient may still moan or stir in response to painful stimulation or a distended bladder. As coma becomes more profound, normal neuromuscular reflexes may be replaced by more primitive ones. For example, the response to firmly drawing a sharp object up the lateral surface of the sole of the foot changes from plantar flexion (normal plantar reflex) to a fleeting dorsiflexion

(extension) of the great toe with fanning of the other toes. This is called the **Babinski sign,** or a positive Babinski, and would be the normal reflex elicited in an infant less than 18 months old. In the deepest levels of coma, no reflex response is elicited even with intense painful stimulation, generated by pressing a pencil against the base of the fingernails (nailbed stimulation), pressing the thumbs into the orbits, or squeezing the testicles of a male.

For intense stimulation to elicit a reflex neuromuscular response, the reflex arc must be intact. That is, sense organs that pick up the stimulus must be functioning, and likewise the pathway that carries this signal, the center that mediates the reflex, the pathway that carries the signal out, and the structures that express the reflex. When using reflex responses, the examiner must be confident that the absence of a response is due to a lesion in the CNS where the reflex is mediated, rather than in reception or expression. Table 20.3 describes a variety of automatic or reflex behaviors that are commonly used to assess consciousness or localize the site or spread of a lesion in the CNS, particularly in the brain stem.

 Checkpoint 20.3

Study table 20.3 carefully. This is a very condensed synopsis. These diagnostic maneuvers and names have been in the neurologist's black bag for many decades and, in many cases, are less definitive than they appear to be. In this category are the breathing patterns. While the patterns are distinct and observable, their names derive from an outdated understanding of the neurological control of respiratory mechanics and their localization in the brain stem. Of the lot, only "Cheyne-Stokes" is consistent with current knowledge. The same comment can be made for the terms "decorticate" and "decerebrate" rigidity. "Decorticate posturing" during coma at least indicates a functional loss arising higher in the nervous system. As with the Babinski, eliciting these postures is at least partly "art": responses vary from moment to moment. You may see flexor (decorticate) posturing when stimulating the left side; with extensor (decerebrate) posturing on the right. Responses may also vary somewhat with the particular stimulus being used.

Table 20.1	Terminology Commonly Employed in Differentiating Levels of Consciousness

Term	**Comments**
Normal consciousness	Patient is fully responsive, with same awareness of self and surroundings as examiner.
Inattention	Patient has difficulty identifying and attending to relevant stimuli.
Confusion	Thinking is slower and less clear; patient is easily distracted.
Clouding of consciousness (obtundation)	Inattention and confusion are more profound; rousing patient is more difficult.
Stupor	Physical and mental activity is at a minimum; persistent and vigorous stimulation is needed for arousal; patient orients to examiner but responds minimally.
Coma	Patient can't be aroused, but may produce patterned behavior if the stimulus is intense.

Table 20.2	The Glasgow Coma Scale

The patient is rated on all three scales and scores are summed. The total (3 = deep coma, 15 = normal consciousness) is recorded.

Eyes Open

Never	1
To pain	2
To verbal stimuli	3
Spontaneously	4

Best Verbal Response

No response	1
Incomprehensible sounds	2
Inappropriate words	3
Disoriented and converses	4
Oriented and converses	5

Best Motor Response

No response	1
Extension (decerebrate rigidity)*	2
Flexion abnormal (decorticate rigidity)*	3
Flexion withdrawal*	4
Localizes pain	5
Obeys	6
Total	3–15

*These terms are explained in table 20.3.

Table 20.3	Functions or Reflexes Commonly Used to Assess Consciousness or Localize the Site or Spread of a Lesion to the CNS

Breathing Patterns

Normal breathing depends on a complex of stimuli in which both PCO_2 and PO_2 are important. Rhythms are generated in the respiratory center in the medulla, and respiratory rate and depth are modified by centers in the pons.

• Slow breathing	May indicate opiate or barbiturate intoxication.
• Rapid breathing	May be due to metabolic or respiratory acidosis or a lesion that affects brain stem regulation breathing.
• Cheyne-Stokes respirations (CSR)	Slow increase in rate and depth of respiration, which peaks and wanes, and is followed by 10–60 seconds of apnea. Due to bilateral cerebral lesion or metabolic disturbance. Respiration driven by PCO_2, which increases in apnea and begins respiratory drive. May be accompanied by snoring, so-called death rattle.
• Central neurogenic hyperventilation (CNH)	Also called Kussmaul respiration. Regular, increased rate and depth of respiration without pause. Due to lesion in lower midbrain or upper pons (respiratory center in medulla released from control of pontine centers).
• Biot breathing	Sometimes called ataxic breathing. Chaotic breathing rhythm; each breath varies in rate and depth. Lesion in the medulla. (Sometimes CSR changes to CNH and then to Biot as the lesion extends from upper to lower brain stem.)
• Apneustic breathing	Pause of 2–3 seconds after full inspiration. Lesion in lower pons (pontine centers do not function to limit inspiration).

(continued)

Table 20.3	Continued

Visual System—Eye Movements

- Corneal reflex

Stimulus: stroke conjunctiva with a wisp of cotton. Normal response: reflex eyeblink. Sensation travels via facial (fifth) cranial nerve, reflex is effected via oculomotor (third) cranial nerve. Lesion of either nerve or nucleus abolishes reflex.

- Pupillary response

Stimulus: shine bright light into one retina. Normal response: stimulated pupil constricts (direct reflex) and unexposed pupil constricts to same degree (consensual reflex).

- Doll's eyes

Stimulus: tilt the cradled head of patient. Normal response: compensatory eye movements (eyes will continue to look up despite position of head). Underlying mechanism maintains an image in the center of the retina (fovea) by moving eyes in the direction opposite and to the degree the head moves. Signal from semicircular canals is processed in the vestibular nuclei (dorsal-lateral junction of pons and medulla). Lesion abolishes doll's eyes.

- Caloric test

Stimulus: irrigate ear canal of reclining patient with cold water. Normal response: nystagmus—fast flicking (beating) of the eyes—away from the stimulated side. Warm water produces nystagmus toward stimulation. Same mechanism as doll's eyes. Temperature change in semicircular canal mimics fluid movement during head movement; lesion at pons-medulla junction abolishes response.

Neuromuscular Reflexes

- Babinski sign

Stimulation of lateral surface of sole of foot elicits plantar flexion in normal or light coma, fleeting extension of great toe and fanning of toes in deeper coma.

- Flexor withdrawal

Painful stimulation of limb evokes withdrawal in lighter coma.

- Decorticate rigidity

May occur spontaneously or in response to painful stimuli or passive movement; may be unilateral or bilateral. Posturing involves arm adduction, flexion at elbows, wrists, and hands; may include extension of lower limbs, plantar flexion of feet. Lesion has functionally isolated the cerebrum from the brain stem above the midbrain. Deepening coma progresses to decerebrate rigidity.

- Decerebrate rigidity

Stimuli same as decorticate rigidity. Posturing includes opisthotonus (rigidity and hyperextension of vertebral column), extension of arms with flexed, inturned wrists/hands, lower limbs extended, feet plantar flexed, toes inturned. Unilateral or bilateral. As in decorticate, may be sustained or fleeting response to stimulus or spontaneous. Isolation of higher function is between pons and midbrain.

- Primitive reflexes

These can emerge in lighter coma and in conditions with severe cortical impairment (e.g., late Alzheimer's disease). Characteristic of newborns, later normally inhibited. Rooting—turning mouth toward stimulated cheek; grasp (Darwinian) reflex—hand will close when palm stroked; sucking elicited by stroking cheek or object in mouth; Moro (startle) reflex—sudden change of posture, loud noise, or vibration elicits violent extension and then flexion of all limbs. Baby then cries. May be elicited in patient with cerebral palsy by a sudden drop or change in posture.

- Gegenhalten (paratonia)

An apparently "willful" resistance to passive movement of a limb. In contrast to Parkinsonian rigidity, this increases with the velocity of movement. In contrast with "clasp knife rigidity," this continues throughout the range of movement. It is due to diffuse cortical dysfunction (e.g., advanced Alzheimer's disease) and co-occurs with many of the primitive reflexes just noted (more detail in chapter 21).

DEVELOPMENTAL ANOMALIES: NEURAL TUBE DEFECTS

The central nervous system is one of the first structures observable in the developing embryo. By day 18 of gestation, the pancake of cells that will produce the body's organ systems, the embryonic disk, has begun developing a longitudinal **neural plate.** Ridges form along the margins of the length of this plate and thus produce a central **neural groove.** This deepens while the ridges grow to meet in the center, creating a **neural tube** that will subsequently elaborate to form the primary structures of the CNS. Associated islands of tissue running parallel and lateral to the neural tube contribute other central and peripheral nervous system structures, the muscles that some of them supply, and the vertebral column and bones of the skull.

The formation of the neural tube begins at the level of what will become the brain stem and then proceeds both rostrally and caudally. The rostral or cranial extent of the tube, which is completed and closes about day 26, produces the brain, while the central lumen and lining give rise to the system of ventricles. The caudal extension of the tube forms the spinal cord with its small central canal and is complete about day 30 (fig. 20.25).

The development of the neural tube can be interrupted at any point, producing a defect, whereafter the tube may form normally. Moreover, the disruption may range from very limited, perhaps a defect in skull closure or formation of a single vertebral arch, to extensive; for example, failure of brain development. Neural tube defects are responsible for the majority of fetal deaths and are an important source of congenital malformations and perinatal illness and death. They appear in a total of about 2 per 1,000 live births in the United States and Canada.

For the most part, conditions arising from neural tube defects are named descriptively, and the more limited the defect, the less serious and disabling the resultant condition. A general term referring to problems in the caudal neural tube is **spina bifida,** so named because the vertebral arch, which fails to close completely, may produce two palpable bases instead of the single, central spinous process. **Spina bifida occulta** is the least serious of these conditions. It is often asymptomatic, perhaps noted incidentally in an X-ray or at physical exam. In many cases, a mole with a tuft of coarse or silky hair or a small birth mark is evident over the vertebral column. Sometimes chronic back pain, enuresis (urinary incontinence), cold feet, or lateness in learning to walk is traced to this minor vertebral arch defect.

More extensive arch, meningeal, and cord malformations exist. One of these, **meningocele,** occurs with equal incidence at cervical, thoracic, or lumbar regions of the spine. A sac containing CSF, lined with meninges and usually covered with intact skin, protrudes from the vertebral column defect. There may be no neurological deficit, and surgical correction is often very successful. Such interven-

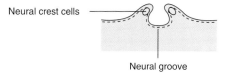

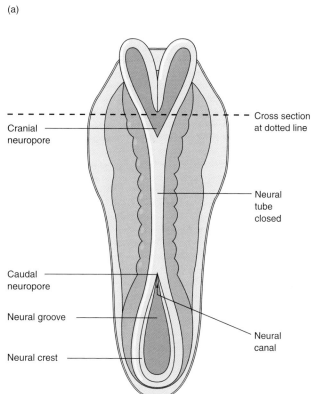

(a)

(b) 22-day-old embryo

Figure 20.25 **Structure of the Neural Tube.** (*a*) Cross section of the closing neural tube at the same level as (dotted line in *b*), showing neural groove and neural crest cells. (*b*) Embryo at 22 days. Much of the neural tube has closed. The cranial and caudal neuropore are in the process of closing.

tion is advisable because any breach in the skin may provide a portal for infection. The resulting spinal meningitis could readily spread to the cranial meninges, and secondary encephalomyelitis (infection of the brain and cord tissue) is a distinct risk. The protruding meningocele is also vulnerable to trauma, another argument for surgical correction. Figure 20.26 provides a diagrammatic overview of neural tube defects expressed in the spinal cord, and figure 20.27 shows an infant with meningocele.

In **meningomyelocele,** there is a similar protrusion, but it contains spinal nerves and part of the cord (or the cauda equina in the lumbar area) as well as the meninges and CSF. The condition may also be called myelomeningocele or spina bifida cystica. In this situation, fully normal neurological function is rare, and there is an increased tendency for loss of CSF and risk of infection. The majority of cases are in the lumbar and lumbosacral regions, and in about

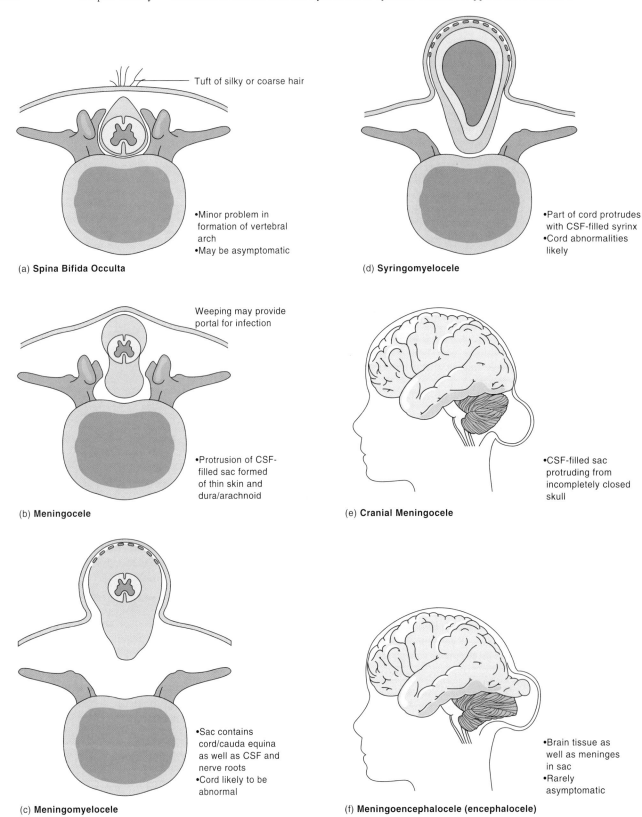

Figure 20.26 **Neural Tube Defects.** Spina bifida refers to problems in the formation and closure of the caudal neural tube and neuropore. Cranial meningocele and encephalocele result from problems in rostral neural tube/neural pore. Images (*a*) through (*d*) show spina bifida at the lumbar level of the cord.

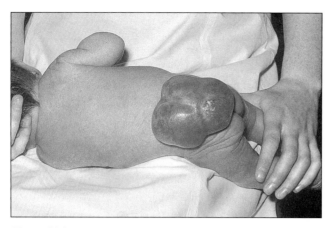

Figure 20.27   **Meningocele.**

half of these there is an associated brain stem defect called **Arnold-Chiari malformation.** Arnold-Chiari (II) is the specific form encountered. It is characterized by a lengthening and downward displacement of the vermis and tonsils of the cerebellum. These midline and medial structures are not accommodated in the abnormally small and shallow posterior fossa and pass through the enlarged foramen magnum to form a mass at the foramen magnum and over the upper cervical cord. An abnormal kink at the junction of the medulla and cord often combines with the foregoing herniation to produce hydrocephalus. As previously noted, hydrocephalus refers to any abnormal increase in the brain's cerebrospinal fluid volume. In this case, normal circulation is impeded by compression of the cerebral aqueduct. CSF then backs up and dilates the ventricles. Surgical introduction of a shunt may be required to manage the hydrocephalus. Besides Arnold-Chiari malformation, some meningomyelocele is complicated with encephalocele, yet to be described.

Neurological function below the meningomyelocele is usually altered. Partial or total paralysis (paraplegia) is common, as is partial or complete sensory loss. Voluntary control of bowel and bladder is often impaired. Sometimes there is an obliteration of bowel and bladder reflexes if the areas of the cord mediating these are involved. The impaired emptying that results may lead to bladder and bowel complications, for example, chronic bladder and kidney infections. The cord and nerve root lesions that are responsible may have been caused by a combination of impaired development, physical trauma due to displacement into the sac or consequent tension and abrasion, impaired perfusion, and/or fibrosis secondary to infection.

Another term you will sometimes see is **syringomyelocele.** In this condition, the central canal of the spinal cord is massively dilated, with parts of the dorsal cord protruding into the CSF-filled sac.

While meningomyelocele is found in a relatively high proportion of live births (about 0.3 per 1,000), **anencephaly** (at between 0.5 and 2 per 1,000) is the most common neural tube defect. It is also the most profound

compatible with survival to term. This is one of a group of neural tube defects that arise with a failure of the development of the cranial neural tube. In anencephaly, the roof of the cranium is missing, and there is only a small, undeveloped vascular mass lying in the base of the skull. Brain stem development may be normal and functional, so that while many victims are stillborn, some are capable of breathing and reflex swallowing. Although controversy exists around the care of these newborns, the common resolution is to maintain hydration and a humane level of physical care. Survival is usually only for a few hours or days. The rate of anencephaly varies rather dramatically, with Wales and Ireland showing peaks of up to 7 per 1,000 live births. This variation raises the possibility that the condition is a response to some factor in the environment. On the other hand, the three to seven to fold preponderance among female fetuses provides some balance of evidence for a genetically mediated basis. As with many developmental anomalies, solid explanations for an individual case are often elusive.

Cranial meningocele describes a meningocele in the cranial region. About 60% of those who are born with this condition and undergo surgical correction develop normal neurological and intellectual function. **Meningo-encephalocele,** less accurately but more commonly called **encephalocele,** is a rarer condition (1 in 6,500 live births). For the three-quarters of cases in which the defect is located in the occipital region, it is also more disabling, with only 10% developing normally after surgical correction. Those with the encephalocele into the nasal cavity or through the frontal or parietal bones have a somewhat better prognosis.

Dandy-Walker syndrome may be rarely found in association with any of the previously mentioned conditions or on its own. This is an impairment in the development of the midline cerebellar structures. Instead, there may be a cystlike structure in the center of the posterior cranial fossa. Hydrocephalus is found. Although impairment of function is variable, gait and eye movement disorders are common, as these are mediated by the midline cerebellum. Children born with this syndrome are also susceptible to seizure disorders.

Most neural tube defects can be detected prenatally by assaying maternal blood for α-fetoprotein. This substance is elevated in a normal pregnancy at weeks 16 to 18. It is produced by the fetus during neural tube and nervous system development and crosses the placental barrier into the mother's circulation. It is released in larger amounts when there are neural tube defects. Amniocentesis gives more accurate estimates of α-fetoprotein, and ultrasound can be used to detect major defects in the fetus.

The Arnold-Chiari and Dandy-Walker syndromes are often presented as posterior midline defects rather than neural tube defects proper. In specialized settings, it is common to encounter numerous other abnormalities of skull and brain development, but they are outside the scope of this text.

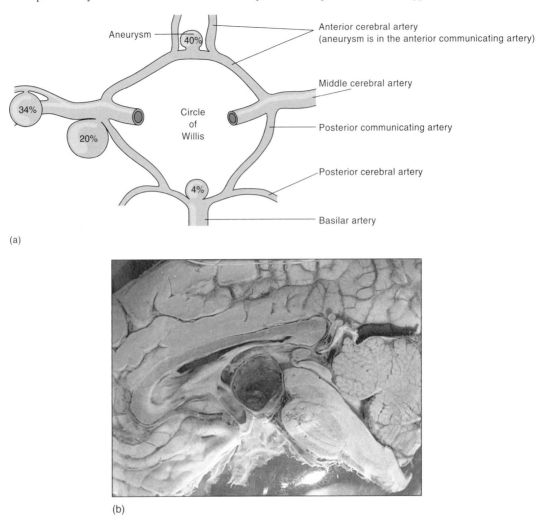

Figure 20.28   Common Sites for the Development of Berry Aneurysms. (See figure 20.15*a* for another view of the circle of Willis.) (*a*) Percentages of an aneurysm's relative frequency. (*b*) Berry aneurysm of the basilar artery, filled with coagulated blood.
This photo shows a ruptured berry aneurysm, filled with thrombus, which caused the death of a 53-year-old woman. It projected upward to block the outflow of CSF from the lateral ventricles, causing hydrocephalus to develop. Confusion and drowsiness prompted a scan of the ventricles. This revealed the hydrocephalus and a smooth, round mass thought to be an inoperable tumor. The obstructed CSF was bypassed to the subarachnoid space and she recovered. Soon after, however, symptoms recurred, the aneurysm ruptured, and she died. The error of diagnosing the aneurysm as a tumor might well have been avoided with more sophisticated imaging (MRI), but it was not available at the time.

CEREBROVASCULAR DISORDERS

This section will focus on a range of disorders that can bring people into cerebrovascular care or complicate their treatment for other conditions. You will be provided with a fairly brief treatment of topics including cerebral aneurysm, vasospasm, arteriovenous malformation, and thrombophlebitis. Then you will find a more extensive discussion of transient ischemic attacks and cerebrovascular accidents.

Cerebral Aneurysm

A **cerebral aneurysm** is a distention of a cerebral arterial wall that develops at a point of weakness. **Berry** (or saccular) **aneurysms,** which tend to develop at points of bifurcation, initially appear as small balloons (berries). **Fusiform**

aneurysms, as the name suggests, are elongated dilations developing along an artery and may be 3 cm or more in diameter. **Microaneurysms,** which are often associated with hypertension and will be discussed later, may be found diffusely in the brain parenchyma. The weakness that sets the stage for the development of berry aneurysms is usually thought to be a developmental defect in the muscle layer of the arterial wall, in which case the aneurysm may be present from a young age. Or the weakness may be due to wear and tear associated with hypertension (saccular and microaneurysms) or possibly head injury. Most berry aneurysms, about 90%, develop in or near the circle of Willis (fig. 20.28). Most other aneurysms (except microaneurysms) are located within the subarachnoid space. Berry aneurysms and microaneurysms are often completely asymptomatic, breaking their silence only if they happen to hemorrhage.

Large aneurysms behave like space-occupying lesions, which means that they can displace and compress nerves, nervous tissue, or other blood vessels. The signs and symptoms will depend on the size and location of the aneurysm: possibly cranial nerve dysfunction, headaches, lethargy, neck pain, perhaps a **bruit**—that is, a noise detectable over the site of the aneurysm, due to turbulence of the blood passing through. Although aneurysms may cause problems at any age, middle age is the most common time for aneurysms to enlarge or, more seriously, to rupture. Hemorrhage of preexisting aneurysms is the usual cause of bleeding into the subarachnoid space. Such bleeding is accompanied by violent (explosive) headaches, and by symptoms of nerve root irritation due to the blood in the CSF. These include stiff neck, Kernig's sign, and Brudzinski's sign, which will be described in the CNS Infection section. Mortality is in the range of 20–40%. If the hemorrhage occurs into the brain tissue, there is a rapid development of symptoms: explosive headaches again, and decreased level of consciousness as the intracerebral hematoma enlarges, leading to a mortality in the vicinity of 70%. This pattern is an example of a hemorrhagic cerebrovascular accident and will be discussed in more detail later.

Hemorrhage, as described, is a serious potential complication with cerebral aneurysms. Although a person may survive or recover from such a bleed, the risk of a serious, perhaps fatal, rebleed is high. Increased intracranial pressure, either with larger aneurysms or a hematoma, can be another serious complication. As well, cerebral aneurysms make an individual vulnerable to chronic or transitory cerebral hypertension. For this reason, control of essential hypertension is crucial. The person should also avoid any condition that raises intrathoracic pressure—for example, straining at stool (stool softeners are used) or exerting force with a closed glottis (Valsalva)—as well as circumstances that tend to temporarily raise systemic blood pressure—for example, stress, emotional shock, and so on.

Subarachnoid Vasospasm

Subarachnoid vasospasm is a transitory constriction or narrowing of an artery or branch of an artery. It may be localized or affect a large section of the artery. Of patients with subarachnoid hemorrhage, 30–50% will experience subsequent vasospasm, frequently in the vicinity of the ruptured aneurysm. It is a common potential complication (65%) of surgery done to evacuate a hematoma or correct an aneurysm. An initially localized constriction can spread to become a diffuse vasospasm that can lead to significant ischemia. The signs and symptoms will depend on the territory subjected to hypoxia and the duration of the vasospasm, with death being a possible outcome. A common occurrence with people surviving an intracerebral hemorrhage (with possible associated vasospasm) is that about ten days later there is a serious rebleed. At this point, vasospasm can again be a significant complication.

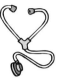

Focus on Lowering Temperature for Successful Reduction of Cerebral Aneurysm

In September 1997, neurosurgical history was made in Toronto, Canada. A man in his forties with a dangerously dilated cerebral aneurysm, while under sedation and general anesthetic, had his temperature greatly reduced to protect his brain and other vital organs. At this point, his heart was stopped to avoid potentially fatal hemorrhage from a very delicate and greatly distended cerebral aneurysm. The aneurysm was reduced, with excellent results. He was on the phone to his friends and relatives and visiting with family within ten hours of the surgery.

The pathogenesis has the following course. Although the initiation of subarachnoid vasospasm can apparently be spontaneous, most often it is in response to the irritation of blood breakdown products in the subarachnoid space. The vasospasm produces a decrease in cerebral blood flow that can complicate existing cytotoxic edema in damaged tissue. The subsequent swelling adds to the mass of the original bleed and further increases the intracranial pressure. In turn, a generalized drop in cerebral perfusion pressure will occur, with possible effects on cerebral blood flow. Vasospasm can put an additional stress on vasculature so that local autoregulation is lost as well. Through this chain of events it is possible that a relatively small, asymptomatic subarachnoid bleed could lead to subarachnoid vasospasm, thence to cerebral ischemia and a much broader pattern of symptoms.

Arteriovenous Malformations

An **arteriovenous malformation** (AVM) is a tangled mass of dilated blood vessels that pass from large or medium-sized arteries directly into a vein or venous sinus, bypassing the normal capillary bed (fig. 20.29). They range from small, local lesions to networks that may cover an entire hemisphere. They are varied in shape and location as well. They may be restricted to the subarachnoid space or dura, or they may form a cone-shaped tangle that extends from the surface of the cortex deep into the cerebrum. Dural AVM may have several arterial feeders. The veins or venous sinuses draining an AVM may be dilated or even form aneurysms because of the abnormally high pressure in the venous system.

Arteriovenous malformations are a congenital anomaly. As such, they grow in step with the developing nervous system, and even very large ones can be accommodated without disrupting normal neural function. The structure of

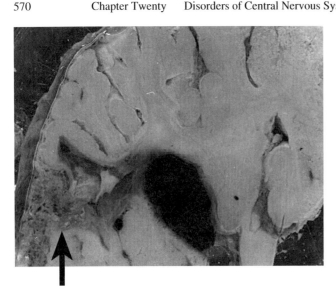

Figure 20.29   **Hemorrhage of an AVM.** Section of cerebrum with a moderate-sized arteriovenous malformation (arrow). Death was due to massive hemorrhage from this AVM.
Two seemingly unrelated cerebrovascular accidents, separated by 41 years, are involved in this case. At 25, this man suffered a cerebral hemorrhage from an arteriovenous malformation in his right parietal lobe. He recovered but suffered from residual partial paralysis and periodic seizures. At age 66, a second fatal hemorrhage occurred, causing the escape of blood into the ventricle pictured here. To the left is the cyst formed at the site of the earlier AVM bleed.

the vessel walls is also often abnormal, particularly with advancing age, being more permeable and more subject to hemorrhage.

AVM can cause problems in a number of ways. The blood shunted through the AVM is by-passing the tissue surrounding or underlying it. Especially if the AVM becomes progressively dilated, the result can be ischemia in that tissue. Second, the AVM itself and the dilated vein or venous sinus can compress adjacent tissue. Hemorrhage is the major potential complication. Depending on location and severity of the bleed, it could result in vasospasm (irritation), dissection and destruction of brain tissue, or the formation of an expanding hematoma. Particularly if an AVM aneurysm or expanding AVM mass deep in brain tissue is located above or surrounding the brain stem, compression of the cerebral aqueduct can lead to hydrocephalus and increased intracranial pressure.

Parallel to the varied routes of pathological impact, there can be widely varied signs and symptoms. Ischemia can lead to symptoms similar to those found in occlusive cerebrovascular accident (more later in this section). Local compression can give rise to a host of problems. Seizure activity due to local changes in brain tissue (e.g., gliosis, proliferation of glial cells) is one of the most common symptoms found with AVM. Headaches may be experienced. A bruit may be heard over the AVM. If there is a bleed from the AVM into the subarachnoid space, xanthochromia (yellow coloration of the CSF) will be detectable.

With regard to complications of AVM, there is a steadily increasing potential for (further) hemorrhage. As well, the continued expansion of the AVM, dural sinus, vein, or venous aneurysm has attendant effects on local compression of vessels, nerves, or brain tissue, and, as an expanding lesion, can increase intracranial pressure. Treatment of these congenital abnormalities may involve the introduction of small Silastic beads that occlude the AVM, use of proton beam radiation, or surgical excision.

Intracranial Thrombophlebitis

Intracranial thrombophlebitis is a condition marked by inflammation and clot formation in the dural venous sinuses, and perhaps invading the cerebral veins. It most often arises as a result of infections of the middle ear, the mastoid air cells within the temporal bone, the paranasal sinuses, the scalp, or the skin around the upper lip, nose, and eyes. Such an infection can enter the lymphatic vessels in the veins draining these structures and generate an inflammatory response in the walls of the veins, producing conditions that favor thrombosis. The thrombophlebitis may then extend along the emissary veins linking these areas with the dural sinuses. For example, an infection in the upper lip may cause thrombophlebitis in the facial vein, which then extends along the ophthalmic vein into the cavernous sinus (see fig. 20.15). Left and right cavernous sinuses communicate via the intercavernous sinuses, through which thrombophlebitis then commonly spreads. The infection that causes the thrombophlebitis may alternatively have been introduced during a basal skull fracture or a skull fracture, tearing the dural venous sinuses themselves. Streptococci and staphylococci are the bacteria most often responsible. Figure 20.15 shows the principal venous structures that may be implicated.

Signs and symptoms will depend to a certain extent on the site of the thrombophlebitis. A history of infected middle ear, mastoid bone, nose, face, or scalp is common, as is generalized headache. The patient may also have **papilledema**—a swelling of the region of the retina where the nerves and vessels enter the eye (due, in this case, to impaired venous drainage into a thrombosed cavernous sinus)—as well as eye movement abnormalities and pain (due to pressure on the third, fourth, sixth, and ophthalmic division of the fifth cranial nerves) and edema in the eyelids. If the thrombophlebitis is interfering with venous drainage of cortical tissue, the resulting back pressure will in turn impede arterial supply. Other effects may include focal abnormalities (due to local cortical hypoxia) and seizures.

In some cases, thrombophlebitis spreads to adjacent sinuses, thereby increasing obstruction to venous flow. Cortical infarction can result if drainage of cortical tissue is seriously compromised by the involvement of cerebral veins. The introduction of infectious agents frequently complicates these cases with other forms of intracranial infection (e.g., meningitis and brain abscess).

Cerebrovascular Accidents

Cerebrovascular accidents (CVAs) afflict approximately half a million North Americans a year. Although more a disease of aging people, no age group is spared. About one-third of those suffering a CVA (or "stroke") will die from it. Many of those who survive will be physically and socially disabled. On the positive side, there has been a significant decline in the incidence of CVA over the last 30 years, which is possibly due to more effective antihypertensive therapy. As well, with appropriate nursing and medical care, potential secondary complications of CVA can be limited and the post-CVA recovery enhanced.

What differentiates CVA from the other vascular disorders just reviewed is that the sudden onset of symptoms and neurological impairment associated with CVA are due directly or indirectly to a deficiency in blood supply. The "deficiency" can range from a transitory interruption that temporarily affects function to a permanent disruption that leads to necrosis of cerebral tissue and even death. Two mechanisms can alter blood flow: occlusion and hemorrhage.

Occlusive strokes can develop because an embolism lodges in a narrowing arterial vessel, obstructing downstream blood flow. More commonly, the obstruction has evolved at the site as a thrombus has formed about an atheromatous plaque. Hence, we have two forms of occlusive CVA: embolic and thrombotic. "Little" strokes that affect only function and last from a few minutes to less than a day are called transient ischemic attacks (TIAs). They are usually seen as symptoms associated with developing thrombosis and are therefore often classified as minor thrombotic CVA. Hemorrhagic CVAs can range from petechial to massive, with parallel damage to the CNS. They can result from hypertensive intracerebral hemorrhage (most commonly) or from a ruptured cerebral aneurysm or arteriovenous malformation.

Occlusive CVA: Transient Ischemic Attacks

Cerebral **transient ischemic attacks** (TIAs) are episodes of neurological dysfunction that develop suddenly, last from five minutes to usually less than one hour (never more than 24 hours), and clear completely. Certain risk factors for TIAs are common to *all* CVAs, presumably because they are related to the development of cerebral vascular disease: hypertension, heart disease, elevated plasma cholesterol, diabetes mellitus, atherosclerosis, increasing age, oral contraceptives, and smoking (particularly in combination with oral contraception use in women over age 35).

In 80% of people suffering a thrombotic CVA, there has been a history of one or more TIAs. This connection is rare (some say nonexistent) in other forms of CVA. The relationship of TIA to the developing thrombosis is, however, not entirely clear. It may be that bits of the thrombus (aggregated platelets, fibrin, and entrapped red blood cells) break off and are carried downstream to some point in the vascular bed (thromboemboli). These microemboli rapidly

fragment and are then transported through the capillary bed and into the venous circulation. The usually suspected site of the primary thrombus is at the bifurcation of the common carotid artery (just below the rear angle of the jaw). Other sources of emboli are the left atrium (emboli produced and thrown off during atrial fibrillation), thrombotic plaques formed on and then thrown off the mitral valves, and thrombi forming in the left ventricle as a result of endocarditis or myocardial infarction.

This account doesn't explain the common finding that successive TIAs often present with the same symptoms. How does a thromboembolism randomly end up plugging the same field in the arteriolar bed? An explanation consistent with this recurrence is that cerebral blood vessels are diseased and irritated beyond the site of the thrombosis. These areas induce an intermittent vasospasm, which, by reducing blood flow, leads to ischemia. Whether the immediate cause is embolism or vasospasm, the subsequent ischemia and hypoxia lead to the appearance of symptoms that are reversible when blood flow returns to normal.

Other causes of TIA include hypotension, "subclavian steal syndrome," which is due to the misdirection of blood down the left vertebral artery because of subclavian occlusion, and even anemia or polycythemia. Correction of these conditions resolves the TIAs.

The symptoms associated with TIA depend on the arteries involved. If the ophthalmic branch of the internal carotid artery is involved in embolism, the person might experience **amaurosis fugax** (literally, fleeting blindness). It will appear to the person as though a shade is being pulled down or up over one eye. When the microembolism clears the retinal capillary bed, vision will return to normal. Symptoms of cerebral ischemia in part of the field of the anterior or middle cerebral arteries may include contralateral monoparesis (weakness or paralysis of one limb) affecting a lower limb (with anterior cerebral artery occlusion) or hemiparesis affecting both limbs, but more dramatically the arm (with middle cerebral artery occlusion), localized tingling numbness, loss of vision in the left or right visual field, or aphasia (impaired language capacity). TIA of the vertebrobasilar arterial system may include drop attacks (the person suddenly loses postural tone in the legs), bilateral visual disturbance (dim, gray, or blurry vision or even total blindness), diplopia (double vision), vertigo, nausea, or dysarthria (difficulty forming or enunciating words).

By definition, there are no neurological impairments left when the TIA resolves. Nevertheless, a recent onset of TIAs is grounds for great concern. Since most TIAs are apparently related to evolving thrombotic lesions, there is always the danger of continued development of the thrombus, which may lead to permanent cerebral infarction. Note, however, that people do experience TIA without going on to develop full-blown thrombotic CVA. However, one-third of those with TIA will go on to *have* a full stroke within five years.

It has now become routine for people experiencing TIA to take an anticoagulant drug prophylactically, based

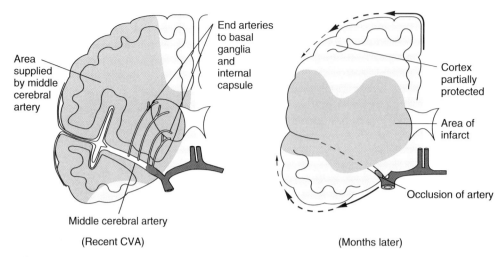

Figure 20.30   **Regions Vulnerable to CVA.** Internal structures supplied by end arterial branches tend to be more vulnerable to local arterial occlusion, while the cortex often has protective anastomoses. Arrows indicate this collateral perfusion. The occlusion pictured is of a major branch of a middle cerebral artery. Typically the area of impaired function is much larger immediately following the stroke and resolves to occupy the area actually infarcted or cortex that is isolated by the infarction of white matter.

Focus on TIA, PRIN, and CVA

The clear distinction between TIA and CVA (i.e., TIA resolves in less that 24 hours, leaving no residual neurological impairment) is more apparent than real. The closer we look for evidence, the more we find there is a "gray area" between no deficit and a clinically observable neurological deficit that would define "stroke." For example, a careful MRI study of TIA patients found small areas of acute ischemic injury (edema) in the white matter of two-thirds of the people who experienced symptoms for more than six hours. (Recall that this is far short of the 24 hours allowed for this condition to be called TIA. Also note that all of these people were free of clinical symptoms, another earmark of TIA.)

For the last decade, the term **prolonged reversible ischemic neurologic deficit** (PRIN) has been used to cover the gap between TIA and full-blown CVA. This term has been invoked to denote symptoms that persist beyond 24 hours and apparently or largely resolve within seven days. It is now clear that brain ischemia ranges in a continuum from very short-term hypoperfusion to complete failure of blood supply to an area with widespread infarction. Small areas of ischemic injury in the white matter, which by themselves are clinically silent, could coalesce with other small areas, at some point giving rise to symptoms that are detectable to an examining physician.

on the strong connection between TIA and thrombotic CVA (the next topic). Aspirin (one-half to one daily) acts to interfere with platelet aggregation and clot formation. It is sometimes combined with another antiplatelet drug, dipyridamole, which together work better than either in isolation. The use of clopidogrel (antiplatelet drug) avoids some of the gastric injury associated with aspirin. If the person has atrial fibrillation, a condition that predisposes to thrombus formation in the ineffectively perfused atrium, warfarin, which inactivates clotting factor proteins, is taken instead.

Occlusive CVA: Thrombotic CVA

A **thrombotic CVA** involves permanent damage to part of the brain, caused by ischemia that has resulted from the thrombotic occlusion of an artery. This is the most common form of CVA and is related to the risk factors cited earlier. The thrombosis is usually due to atherosclerosis, very often associated with hypertension, diabetes mellitus, and coronary or peripheral vascular disease. Alternatively, trauma to the head or neck may cause thrombosis of major arteries and subsequent CVA.

A thrombus (often at the bifurcation of the internal carotid or middle cerebral artery) usually takes a long time to develop, perhaps many years, and is usually asymptomatic until there is major stenosis of the arterial lumen. At this point, the symptoms of extreme ischemia will evolve over minutes or hours. Occasionally, the stroke progresses stepwise for a period of days or weeks (this condition is often called "stroke-in-evolution"). Anything that lowers systemic blood pressure will exacerbate the symptoms of ischemia (e.g., acute myocardial infarction, heart block, shock, surgical anesthesia, too vigorous treatment of chronic hypertension). The slight hypotension that prevails in sleep accounts for the fact that about 60% of thrombotic CVAs occur during sleep.

The area affected by the CVA will depend on the distribution of the artery occluded and the degree of anastomosis by other cerebral arteries. Internal structures supplied by end arterial branches are particularly vulnerable because there is little anastomotic supply from other arteries. Some of the cortex supplied by the occluded artery is protected from ischemic infarction by anastomoses of other cerebral arteries (fig. 20.30).

Focus on Brain Attacks

In the second edition, we reported on the pioneering use of backwards (venous) perfusion of an ischemic area of brain combined with the administration of tPA (conducted in 1997). Currently, this technique is only used in the circumstance of the treatment of a dissecting aortic aneurysm. In this surgery, the aorta has to be clipped temporarily as surgical correction is performed. Venous backperfusion of the brain avoids cerebral ischemia during aortic occlusion. The use of tPA, however, has become widespread. (Recall that tissue plasminogen activator, tPA, is a chemical that generates the enzyme plasmin, a powerful digester of thrombus fibrin. This plasmin is produced by the action of tPA upon the plasmin precursor plasminogen, which is already present within the thrombug.) This is part of an approach to the care for CVAs that has benefited from well-accepted advances in the emergency and long-term care of ischemic heart disease. Both stroke and ischemic heart disease are commonly the result of atherosclerotic arterial disease, and the need for and risks of immediate tissue reperfusion appear to be the same. This has made the half-hour after the first appearance of symptoms of a stroke a very critical window. Immediate administration of tPA significantly limits the tissue infarction secondary to thrombotic CVA and embolic CVA when the embolism is a fragment of a thrombus formed elsewhere. (Of course, tPA would worsen an evolving hemorrhagic stroke for obvious reasons.) Ischemia is injurious to tissue, whether heart, brain, or other. As noted in chapter 2, reperfusion creates a second source of injury through a variety of mechanisms. Extensive experimentation is being done with chemicals (e.g., allopurinol) that might help control this secondary injury; likewise for a variety of chemicals that are thought to be "neuroprotectants." This rapidly developing field shows great promise for limiting the damage done by stroke.

Again, taking its cue from strides made in the recovery from and avoidance of future heart attacks, CVA care includes addressing the primary risk factors in atherosclerotic disease. This includes controlling diabetes and high blood pressure, lowering total fat and cholesterol, improving diet, stopping smoking, increasing moderate exercise, nurturing supportive relationships, and controlling sources of stress. It is reasonable to expect that applying these practices throughout life will result in significant "stroke prevention."

The functional areas that immediately succumb to the CVA are typically much larger than the actual brain tissue that is infarcted. The edema responsible for much of this disruption results from two mechanisms. In the center, hypoxia compromises ATP production so that cytotoxic edema occurs (the neuronal and glial cells allow the influx of sodium and associated chloride and water, and thereby swell). This process is compounded by the loss of autoregulation. The same tissue vasculature loses its normal response to lowered oxygen, increased carbon dioxide, and increased lactic acid. So there is no compensatory dilation of arterioles and consequently no increase in blood flow. Formerly, carbon dioxide was administered to thrombotic CVA patients with the idea that this would increase focal vasodilation in the infarcted area. In fact, the reverse occurs: normal tissue is better perfused and the blood is diverted away from the infarcted area. At the margins of the infarcted zone, maximum vasodilation results from carbon dioxide accumulation in hypoxic tissue. This marginal region is then the site of vasogenic edema (arterioles dilate, tight junctions between capillary endothelial cells loosen). Besides broadening the area of functional impairment, this edema can contribute to increased intracranial pressure and consequent decreased cerebral perfusion pressure. This can, in turn, exaggerate the focal ischemia, or even precipitate further sites of thrombotic CVA.

Further serious complications may evolve in cases of extensive cerebral edema: displacement of brain tissue, herniation syndromes, possible brain stem herniation and death. Cerebral edema reaches its peak at 72 hours and resolves in approximately two weeks (fig. 20.31). Only then can the extent of infarction be known. Some people who experience profound temporary disablement (e.g., complete right hemiplegia and loss of speech), may recover with barely detectable sequelae. Once having had and survived a thrombotic CVA, however, a patient is at risk of suffering another.

The symptoms associated with thrombotic CVA will, to a large extent, depend on the specific area infarcted, although clinical syndromes will often overlap to some degree. Table 20.4 lists the symptoms that correlate with specific arterial occlusions. This information is of direct relevance to embolic and hemorrhagic CVA as well. Some of the terms will look unfamiliar, but do not be concerned at this point. The details of motor and sensory abnormalities are described in chapters 21 and 23, respectively.

Cerebral tissue that becomes infarcted undergoes a pattern of necrosis and resolution that is unique to the central nervous system: **liquefaction necrosis.** The support structure of organs outside the CNS is largely composed of a variety of connective tissue elements, both cells and extracellular matrix, and injury/necrosis results in an increase in these, through scarring. Except for the meninges and blood vessels, the CNS contains no connective tissue. The bulk of the brain and cord is made up of cells, particularly astrocytes and oligodendrocytes. Necrosis in the neurons and these glial support cells leads to their enzymatic and phagocytic destruction. Rather than being replaced by connective tissue as would happen elsewhere, they are replaced by a fluid-filled cyst. The area of necrosis may initially be pale to dark red (hemorrhagic infarct). The

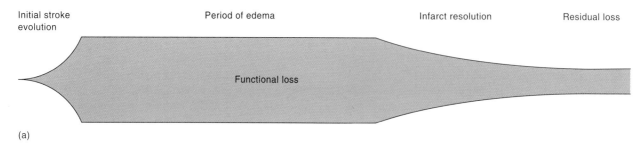

(a)

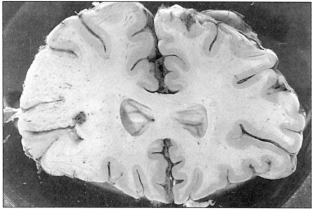

(b)

Figure 20.31   **Progression of a Thrombotic CVA in the Region Supplied by the Right Middle Cerebral Artery.**
(*a*) Edema and functional loss decline, but some loss remains after resolution. (*b*) Recent infarct in right cerebral hemisphere (left center). (*c*) Infarct after resolution (left center). Inset shows degeneration and atrophy in the corresponding cerebral peduncle.*

Thinning of the cortex and discoloration of the white matter deep to it can be seen in this eight-day-old infarct of the right cerebral hemisphere. The brain section is from a 71-year-old woman who was severely injured when she fell down stairs. She soon lost movement of her left arm, and after eight days, surgery was necessary to resect a segment of bowel infarcted by an embolus from her heart, which had formed as a consequence of cardiac trauma caused by the fall. She died in the hospital as a result of bronchopneumonia. The infarct was yet another sequela of the fall. (c). This section of a different brain shows approximately the area of infarct that would have remained if she had survived her first stroke and the pneumonia.

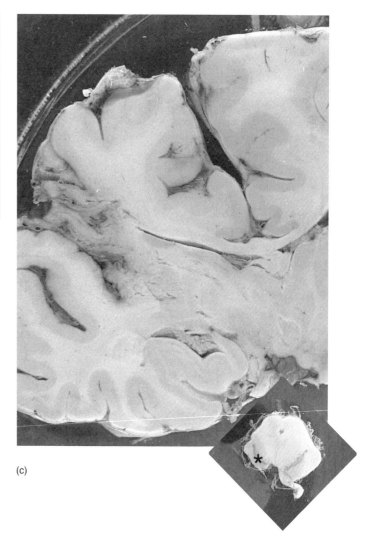

(c)

process of degradation takes some weeks, leaving a brownish soup that is eventually replaced by a clear, straw-colored fluid. In the surviving tissue adjacent to an area of injury or necrosis, there will be proliferation of astrocytes, a process called astrocytosis or gliosis. Gliotic cortical tissue can become epileptogenic, and seizures are a sequela for many with CVA.

Occlusive CVA: Embolic CVA

An **embolic stroke** results when an embolus, usually a fragment of a thrombus located in the heart, lodges in a brain artery and creates ischemia that leads to an infarct.

The second most common form of CVA, it is often associated with atrial fibrillation, a condition favorable to both the formation of thrombi in the atrium and their fragmentation. Another source of emboli is a mural thrombus associated with either myocardial infarction or endocarditis. Less commonly, bone fracture may allow marrow fat cells to enter the sinusoids in the medullary cavity and thereby the venous circulation. Fat emboli tend to lodge in the lung but are deformable and can pass through the lung vessels to reach the brain. Other emboli are tumor cells and septic emboli (particularly the vegetations associated with infectious endocarditis—composed of infectious bacteria, fibrin, platelets, and red blood cells). These infective emboli may

Table 20.4   Clinical Syndromes Produced by Occlusion of the Cerebral Arteries

Artery	Region Supplied	Symptoms Produced*
Internal carotid artery (supplies both the anterior and middle cerebral arteries)	Frontal, parietal, and temporal areas; basal ganglia; internal capsule; optic nerve and retina	**Acute:** coma, aphasia (if dominant hemisphere), contralateral hemiplegia, hemianesthesia, and homonymous hemianopsia, ipsilateral blindness due to occlusion of retinal artery on same side.
Anterior cerebral artery	Anterior part of internal capsule, tip of frontal lobe, anterior two-thirds of medial surface of cerebral hemisphere	**Chronic:** transient attacks of hemiparesis, hemianesthesia, etc., and monocular visual disturbances (amaurosis fugax) Dementia, confusion, or coma; contralateral hemiplegia and sensory loss affecting primarily the leg; urinary incontinence
Middle cerebral artery	Lateral cortex and much of white matter of frontal, parietal, occipital, and tip of temporal lobes. Perforating branches supply internal capsule, basal ganglia, and anterior thalamus.	Syndrome similar to internal carotid occlusion or stenosis except for absence of visual disturbances. **Total occlusion:** coma, contralateral facial weakness, hemiplegia, hemianesthesia, and homonymous hemianopsia with aphasia (if dominant hemisphere). **Occlusion of part of the territory:** partial contralateral involvement; sensory loss and weakness affecting arm more than leg
Posterior cerebral artery (supplied by the basilar artery, which is supplied by the vertebral arteries)	Midbrain, posterior part of thalamus, posterior part of internal capsule, base and posterior two-thirds of temporal lobe, medial surface of occipital lobe (visual cortex)	**Infarction of thalamus:** contralateral hemianopsia and hemianesthesia **Occlusion of branch to midbrain:** ipsilateral eye movement defects and contralateral hemiplegia with or without contralateral tremor
Basilar artery (vertebrobasilar system)	Structures of the posterior fossa (pons, medulla, cerebellum); inner ear	Clinical criteria of disease in basilar system: (1) signs of abnormality involving 3rd–12th cranial nerves in any combination, 3rd, 6th, 7th most commonly, (2) cerebellar dysfunction, and (3) various signs of upper motor neuron lesion. Some examples of symptoms associated with interruption of circulation: stupor or coma, eye movement defects, ipsilateral Horner's syndrome,† drop attacks, ataxia, complex sensory defects, dysphagia, dysarthria.

*Detailed explanations of symptoms are found in chapter 21 (motor) and chapter 23 (sensory).
†Horner's syndrome—eye affected has a narrowed pupil (miosis), the conjunctiva is reddened, the eyelid may droop (ptosis), the same side of the face is noticeably dry—is due to an interruption of sympathetic supply to that side of the face.

give rise to an abscess, as will be detailed shortly. Some emboli will arise intracerebrally from a developing thrombus or from a thrombus at the carotid bifurcation.

The mechanisms of pathological impact on brain structure and function are identical with those in thrombotic CVA once occlusion has been achieved: ischemia, broad functional loss, edema and infarction, resolution of edema, and then permanent functional loss. The feature that differentiates embolic CVA is the rapid development of symptoms (within seconds to one minute) and the absence of immediate warning signs (although embolic TIAs are sometimes seen, and one embolic CVA will often be followed by others). Emboli arising in the heart or passing the lung most often enter the brain via the internal carotid artery and tend to pass directly into the middle cerebral artery, as this is the most direct path of blood flow with the largest volume. Emboli entering through the vertebral arteries tend to lodge in the vascular bed of the posterior cerebral arteries for the same reasons. For symptoms, consult table 20.4.

Hemorrhagic CVA

Hemorrhagic CVA causes infarction by interrupting blood flow to a region of the brain downstream from the hemorrhage. Further damage is done if the hemorrhage creates an expanding hematoma, creating local shifts in tissue and perhaps elevating intracranial pressure. As well, the high-pressure pool of arterial blood can dissect delicate cerebral tissue, causing widespread damage (fig. 20.32). Intracerebral hemorrhages that result from cerebrovascular disease as opposed to trauma, can occur at some of the vascular defects described earlier in this section: berry and fusiform aneurysms and AVM. While hypertension may exaggerate the progression of these defects, it is not their cause. Hypertension can be directly responsible for hemorrhage within the brain tissue. This occurs when microaneurysms (named **Charcot-Bouchard** microaneurysms) develop in the small (< .3 mm) penetrating arteries of the brain. Hemorrhage is most common (50–60%) in the putamen (one of the nuclei in the basal ganglia) or the thalamus. In the posterior fossa, the pons and cerebellum are preferred sites. The onset of symptoms is rapid, but less abrupt than with embolic CVA, often evolving over an hour or two. Elevated blood pressure is evident in most cases (chronic hypertension), and BP may continue to rise as the stroke develops due to the increased intracranial pressure, resultant hypoxia, and reflex increase in sympathetic stimulation of the heart. About half of the individuals will report severe headache. The symptoms associated with hemorrhage into specific sites are presented in table 20.5 (again, explanations of some terms are postponed).

The intracerebral bleeding often enters the ventricles. There, as well as coloring the CSF (xanthochromia), it often causes rapid escalation of intracranial pressure. In about 70% of cases of intracerebral hemorrhage, the hematoma continues to expand and thus leads to destruction of vital brain centers and/or to large shifts of brain tissue, brain stem herniation, stupor, coma, decerebrate rigidity, and death.

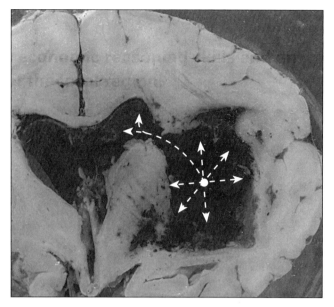

Figure 20.32 **Coronal Section through the Ventricles of a Brain after a Fatal Hemorrhage.** The approximate course of the expanding/dissecting intracerebral hemorrhage from the putamen through the internal capsule into the left ventricle is indicated by the dotted line.

This large hemorrhage in the left cerebral hemisphere has ruptured into the lateral ventricle. The victim was a 79-year-old male who was driving home from a wedding when his wife noticed him acting strangely. He was unable to find his way home without her direction. On finally arriving, he went to bed, but next morning was deeply comatose; his pupils were fixed and neither plantar nor brain stem reflexes could be elicited. His right side was found to be flaccid when he was admitted to the hospital, and he died a few hours later.

Table 20.5	Symptoms Associated with Hemorrhage into Specific Sites in the Brain and Brain Stem
Site	**Symptoms**
Putamen or internal capsule	Flaccid hemiplegia, hemianopsia, tonic deviation of eyes to injured side, speech is slurred, Babinski sign
Thalamus	Eyes may be deviated downward, hemorrhage may compress internal capsule causing hemiplegia and hemianesthesia.
Pons	Paralysis of conjugate gaze, pupillary miosis (constriction), flaccid quadriplegia, absence or weakness in response to caloric testing, absence of doll's eye responses, often coma
Cerebellum	Headache, vomiting, inability to walk or unsteadiness of gait, collapse

✓ *Checkpoint 20.4*

Let's do a brief summary. Intracranial hemorrhage can result from trauma, in which the hemorrhage may be into the tissue or the subarachnoid space, from a ruptured berry or saccular aneurysm, or from an AVM, which is usually into the subarachnoid space, or from a microaneurysm, which is usually into the brain parenchyma. CVA is the term applied to an interruption of CNS blood supply that develops within the arteries of the brain. This interruption can be achieved through hemorrhage, blockage by an embolism, or blockage by a locally evolving arterial thrombus. When the nature of the underlying pathology is known, appropriate therapy can be delivered (e.g., thrombolytic agents for thrombosis or thrombotic emboli, blood pressure control in hemorrhage). The principal cause of stroke is atherosclerotic disease and the principal manifestation of atherosclerosis is thrombosis downstream to an atheroma. The practices that are effective in reducing the incidence of heart disease will likely have the same general effect on CVA.

CNS INFECTION

Any interruption of the vascular, meningeal, and bony protection of the CNS can expose the brain and its meningeal tissues to infectious agents. Compared with the incidence of infection in the rest of the body, CNS infection is relatively rare. When it occurs, however, the effects can range from unpleasant but fully reversible, as is the case with some viral infections, to catastrophic. The protection that serves so well in isolating the CNS from infection has the downside of isolating an established infection from normal access and attack by the immune system. As well, it sometimes frustrates the pharmacological support that would effectively assist in the elimination of a systemic infection. Because there are growing numbers of people with chronically suppressed immune function (e.g., transplant recipients, people with AIDS), the management of nervous system infections is an expanding problem.

With any such infection, rapid identification of the infecting agent is a crucial first step. As described at the beginning of this chapter, usually a lumbar puncture is performed to determine the specific agent. The CSF findings associated with bacterial meningitis were noted earlier, in the discussion of meningeal protection. Viral meningitis produces a lymphocyte-rich exudate. Assuming that the agent is one for which effective therapy exists, treatment according to the sensitivities of the organism cultured must begin without delay.

Infections of the central nervous system may be limited to the subarachnoid space (**meningitis**), may affect the meninges and adjacent brain tissue (**meningoencephalitis**),

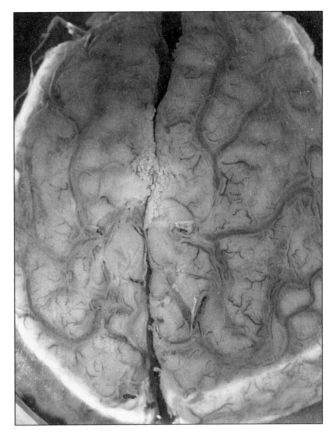

Figure 20.33   **Bacterial Meningitis.** The production of exudate has yielded the thickening and clouding of the meninges seen in this view of the superior surface of the brain.

may be focused in the brain tissue (**encephalitis**) or cord (**myelitis**), or may be focal (**abscesses**). The infective organisms, the mechanisms establishing infection and producing pathology, and the pathologic outcomes can be quite distinct.

Acute Bacterial Meningitis

Acute bacterial meningitis (also called **pyogenic meningitis**) presents a true medical emergency. If it is untreated, 50–60% of cases are fatal, and even with aggressive medical care, 5–6% succumb. The subarachnoid space, which is the focus of this infection, is continuous around the brain, spinal cord, and optic nerves. The CSF there contains very few lymphocytes and very little complement or antibody to attack microorganisms, but it does have glucose and electrolytes that can act as a medium. Any microorganism gaining entry can multiply and spread through the CNS with little host defense. Once established, an infection will induce an inflammatory response, producing the cellular and then fibrinous exudate that give the condition its name (pyogenic) (fig. 20.33). As well, veins and arteries traveling in the subarachnoid space become inflamed (vasculitis). The cellular debris and fibrin can block CSF outflow, which may rapidly raise intracranial pressure. Vasculitis may induce necrosis of vessel walls and thrombosis, which can lead to brain infarction.

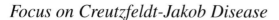

Focus on Creutzfeldt-Jakob Disease

While not a viral infection, Creutzfeldt-Jakob disease (CJD) merits mention here. This rare (1/1 million), progressive, and fatally destructive brain disease is caused by an abnormal form of a normal membrane glycoprotein called *prion protein.* The term derives from the initial belief that any *prion* was a *pro*teinaceous *in*fective particle. The agent is now called PrPC for "prion protein (Creutzfeldt-Jakob)." If these particles are introduced into the brain, two processes appear to occur. These PrPC cause a conformational change to take place in normal prion particles. There also appears to be a process whereby the PrPC induces the DNA to produce abnormal prions as well. Both lead to accumulations of PrPC sufficient to disrupt brain structure and function. Neurons die off and astrocytes multiply, probably producing some of the destruction of brain tissue that shows up as spaces in the brain tissue (giving rise to the older name "spongiform encephalopathy"). Remaining cells appear vacuolated, contributing to the spongiform appearance. After a very long incubation period in which no blatant symptoms are apparent, the person experiences a rapidly progressive (usually less than 12 months) dementia and motor impairment, leading to death. A characteristic EEG establishes the diagnosis (spike and wave complexes at 0.5–2.0 second intervals). Persons affected are usually between 40 and 60 years old. No treatment

is effective. Prions are remarkably resistant to conventional destructive techniques (autoclaving, formalin, caustic soda, chlorine bleach). A number of cases have been traced to infected depth electrodes used in EEG, pituitary extracts, surgery, or corneal transplant, and exposure to formalin-fixed, paraffin-embedded brain tissue (pathologists). Most cases are unexplained. Isolation of body fluids is the only precaution usually taken (as with hepatitis). Direct contact with brain tissue of any kind merits caution.

"New variant" CJD (vCJD) was first reported in ten cases in Great Britain in 1996, beginning the panic in Europe over "mad cow disease." There were several differences from the CJD that has just been described: Age of onset was younger, including teens; the EEG was not characteristic, some symptoms were different, and the course was longer, up to 22 months. The prion is also slightly different. Two other prion diseases (GSS and FFI) have also been identified, both with an autosomal dominant form of transmission (gene abnormality on chromosome 20), both ultimately fatal and untreatable at this point. Gerstmann-Sträussler-Scheinker disease (GSS) has a longer course (two to ten years). Fatal familial insomnia (FFI) has appeared at any age between 18 and 61 and many affected individuals have progressive insomnia. Again, the prions show slight differences.

The prognosis depends on whether rapid and effective antibiotic treatment can arrest the disease before any permanent damage has occurred. In such cases, full recovery is possible. Persistent meningitis can lead to cranial nerve damage, abscess, tissue infarction, or extension into the subdural space (empyema formation, explained later in the Subdural Empyema section). Acute death results from blockage of CSF outflow and edema, which cause increased intracranial pressure. Pneumonia or circulatory failure may be secondary causes of death.

The microorganisms responsible for bacterial meningitis vary with the age of the patient and the mechanism of infection. Epidemics among adults living in close quarters are often due to the meningococcal bacterium *Nisseria meningitides.* Pneumococcus (*Streptococcus pneumoniae*) and *Hemophilus influenzae* are common agents in both children and adults. They are frequently found among the normal bacterial flora of the nasopharynx. Immunization against *Hemophilus* is recommended for young children, especially those in close contact with many other children, as in day care. Newborns can develop a very resistant meningitis that is due to Gram-negative bacteria (especially *E. coli* and group B streptococci). Most cases of meningitis result from hematogenous spread from an upper respiratory tract infection, otitis media, or pneumonia. Direct spread

from an established infection or neurosurgical procedure is also possible.

Chronic Bacterial Meningoencephalitis

We will mention only three chronic bacterial infections of the meninges and adjacent brain parenchyma.

Syphilis enters the subarachnoid space usually only after a long presence in the body. The spirochetes (*Treponema pallidum*) of syphilis can plug and inflame the tiny vessels of the meninges, leading to inflammation of adjacent tissues of the brain and cord. They can enter the parenchyma to produce **paretic neurosyphilis,** which culminates in severe dementia, or they can selectively damage the sensory nerves in the dorsal roots, producing **tabes dorsalis** (see chapter 21). These disorders are only seen in about 10% of persons with untreated syphilis, but the emergence of AIDS has meant that conditions once rarely seen in our hospitals are now reappearing in their "classic" forms.

Lyme disease is caused by another spirochete carried by wood ticks. When affecting the nervous system, it can produce a variety of symptoms ranging from nonspecific meningeal signs, to specific (e.g., facial nerve) palsies, to mild encephalopathy. It has become a concern among hikers and people living in the mountainous countryside.

Tuberculosis can infect the meninges, producing a fibrinous exudate in the subarachnoid space. Arteries traveling in the subarachnoid space may become inflamed and obliterated. Sometimes large **tuberculomas** form in the parenchyma, producing a potentially significant mass effect.

Other Meningeal Inflammations

Viral (or lymphocytic) **meningitis,** while unpleasant (severe headaches, light sensitivity, malaise), is generally self-limiting. Treatment is symptomatic and almost all patients recover without problems. Individuals with a primary tuberculosis infection may develop tuberculous infection of the meninges and adjacent brain tissue (meningoencephalitis). Those with fungal and syphilitic infections may also develop meningoencephalitis.

Meningeal Signs

Some of the signs of meningeal inflammation are the light sensitivity, severe headache, and general malaise that were just mentioned. In acute meningitis, fever, vomiting, drowsiness, stiff neck, muscle aches, and backache are common. Rapid development of infection may lead to confusion, deepening obtundation, and coma. **Brudzinki's sign** is seen when abrupt flexion of the neck of a supine patient results in involuntary flexion of the knees. **Kernig's sign** is seen when an attempt to extend the knee while holding the thigh in a flexed position results in reflex resistance and pain in the hamstring group. Both of these responses probably result from irritation of motor and sensory nerve roots passing through the inflamed meninges. Brudzinki's sign is a hyperactive hip flexion reflex in response to neck flexion (this would be evident in a normal infant). Kernig's sign is simply a hyperactive deep tendon hamstring reflex. Both may be exaggerated by the position assumed, which may increase pressure within the spinal dural sac. In infants and old people, meningeal signs may not be distinct or clearly evident, and examination of CSF may be necessary to establish a diagnosis.

Viral Infections of the CNS

Viral infections of the CNS tend to be either acute, in which case the immune system usually mounts defense (poliomyelitis and smallpox are examples), or latent, chronic, and so-called slow virus infections. The latter can be very destructive. In this group, herpes simplex and varicella zoster can occur acutely, then appear to become latent. Recall that there is no CSF-brain barrier. This means that many of these viral disorders affect both the meninges and the brain parenchyma.

Herpes can recur as a potentially fatal encephalitis in infants. *Varicella zoster* produces chickenpox in its acute form and later can cause inflammation of cranial and spinal nerve roots and ganglia and the painful skin lesions charac-

Focus on CJD, Mad Cow Disease, Kuru Kuru, and Scrapie

The British slaughterhouse practice of feeding cattle with dead sheep, unknowingly infected with a sheep form of spongiform encephalopathy called scrapie, caused a major concern for the transmission of bovine spongiform encephalopathy in Europe in 1990. Reassurances were given as late as 1995 to the British public and the concerned European consumers of British beef that "some species barrier to the transmission of prion disease" exists. In 1996, the "mad cow disease" resurfaced with the horrifying possibility that infected cattle were infecting humans with a new strain of CJD. A number of cases seem to establish that, in fact, infective prions from other species can indeed cause the disease in humans. If particles succeed in passing the blood-brain barrier, they appear to induce the same conformational changes in normal prion proteins, which then continue the process at an increasingly rapid rate. At this point, there is good evidence of transfer of CJD from human patient to deliberately infected monkeys. Kuru kuru appears to be the same disease, only this time occurring in cannibals in New Guinea and transmitted by direct contact with the brains of infected individuals. Kuru kuru has almost disappeared since cannibalism was abandoned in the 1950s, only appearing sporadically in the older population. Scrapie is the form of the disease affecting sheep (they scrape themselves against fence posts, become demented, and die). The precise ordering of amino acids varies between species, and the pattern of pathology may vary in detail.

teristic of **shingles.** Rubella and cytomegalovirus can do extensive brain damage as congenital infections. Measles virus can also infect the nervous system. Because the nervous system produces only very small amounts of a protein (M protein) required by the virus for the formation of part of its viral coat, viral replication is exceedingly slow. However, eventually in two to three years this slow virus appears to produce a fatal chronic disease in infants and children called **subacute sclerosing panencephalitis** (SSPE). **Cytomegalovirus** (CMV) infects the nervous systems of fetuses and the immunosuppressed. The effects on the fetus can be catastrophic. CMV is the most common opportunistic viral infection found in people with AIDS. The nervous system is infected in perhaps 20% of cases.

Another relentlessly progressive (six months to one year) and fatal encephalitis, which is focused on the myelinating oligodendrocytes, is **progressive multifocal leukoencephalopathy** (PML). It is usually found only in debilitated patients with some form of immune suppression.

Reye's Syndrome

This potentially fatal postviral condition has recently received wide public attention because of the suspected role of aspirin in its pathogenesis. A minority of children in the age range 6 months to 15 years who have had a viral infection (usually influenza A or B or varicella), go on after four to seven days to develop **Reye's syndrome.** They have a (perhaps renewed) period of vomiting and lethargy. In about three-quarters of victims, the CNS effects might deepen to clouded consciousness or hyperexcitability, but then the condition resolves to full recovery, usually with in a week. One-quarter of the victims, unfortunately, experience degenerating consciousness due to progressive brain edema. This condition leads to deepening coma and death in 10% or more of Reye's syndrome cases. Aggressive intensive care, aimed at controlling the increased intracranial pressure secondary to edema, has resulted in this improved prognosis. Formerly, death rates were as high as 40%.

In a few cases, the cause of death is liver failure. This fact draws our attention to the underlying pathophysiology, which is still not understood. Early in its course, blood tests will show hypoglycemia, acidosis due to lactic acid accumulation, and increased free fatty acids. Within a week, signs of liver dysfunction appear: elevated ammonia, bilirubin, liver enzymes. Biopsy will show widespread (brain, liver, other tissues) mitochondrial injury and accumulation of fats in tiny intracellular vesicles, particularly in skeletal muscles, heart and kidneys. Although the cause is not clear, brain edema is the root of the CNS symptoms.

A variety of factors may contribute to the conversion of a viral infection to Reye's syndrome. Vomiting and resultant fasting lead to exhaustion of glycogen (glucose) stores and hence the mobilization of fatty acids. These may interfere with mitochondrial function and thereby cause hyperammonia. Genetic predisposition may play a role, as may endotoxins or lymphokines released in the immune response. Salicylates (e.g., aspirin) may simply tip the balance of an already disordered metabolism. With the exception of mitochondrial injury, the pattern in salicylate toxicity is similar to that in Reye's syndrome. However, children with Reye's, while often having been given aspirin to control fever and aches associated with flu, don't show toxic salicylate levels. Whatever the connection may be, the decline in use of aspirin to control fever in children has been accompanied by a lower incidence of Reye's syndrome, although this observation must be couched in the unexplained variability from decade to decade since it was identified in 1963.

Brain Abscesses

A **brain abscess** is a localized, fairly circumscribed area of necrosis and pyogenic (pus forming) bacterial infection principally found in the white matter (fig. 20.34). The presence of both necrosis and infection distinguishes this condi-

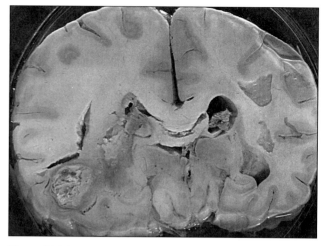

Figure 20.34   **Brain Abscess.** The circular mass at the left is a pus-filled abscess that has extended to the adjacent ventricle. *This is the brain of a middle-aged man who died of meningitis. He had suffered for several years from a chronic middle ear infection that had drained pus intermittently. Then he developed signs and symptoms of meningitis: headache, drowsiness, and vomiting. A lumbar puncture revealed that his CSF was clouded with pus, and it was cultured to determine the antibiotic sensitivity of the causative organism. Exploratory surgery to locate a suspected brain tumor was undertaken, but none was found. In spite of large doses of an appropriate antibiotic, death followed five weeks after the onset of meningitis. The specimen reveals the large cerebral abscess that had formed by extension from the infected middle ear. It was filled with a creamy pus, which had ruptured into the lateral ventricle. From the ventricle, the pus, containing infective bacteria, was carried to the subarachnoid space to produce the meningitis.*

tion from encephalitis and tells us something about how abscess formation takes place. The infection is introduced at the same time as an area of infarct is produced. This usually takes place in either of two ways.

In the first mechanism, a septic embolus may pass into the cerebral vasculature, perhaps by breaking off from an established set of valve vegetations that have developed in bacterial endocarditis. Infection in the lung is another common source. A distant infection (e.g., in burns, pelvic infection, or bones) is also possible. The embolus is composed of fibrin, trapped blood cells, and the sequestered infective organisms. It lodges in the narrowing artery or arteriole and produces a small ischemic infarct. In this region, the infective agent (*Staphylococcus aureus* is common, although a variety of bacteria, yeast, fungi, etc. may be involved) can get established in relative isolation from immune system interference. As the infection expands, the infected tissue will undergo liquefaction necrosis, and an extensive capsule of astrocytic gliosis may evolve. Inflammation and edema will surround this cystic space.

The other major mechanism for producing simultaneous infarction and infection is by spread from an established chronic infection. This will be in an area contiguous to the brain—for example, middle ear infection, mastoiditis, paranasal sinusitis, oral or dental infections, face or scalp infections. Spread is probably through thrombosed veins or their lymphatic drainage. The occlusion of veins impairs drainage and leads to infarction of cerebral tissue. Rarely, infection and infarction may be established by brain surgery or a penetrating head wound.

A person with an abscess may experience no distinct symptoms, in which case the condition may be identified as an incidental finding in a CT scan done for some other reason. Despite the primary infection and spread to the brain, about half of those affected experience no fevers. If the abscess expands or if there are multiple abscesses, as may be the case with hematogenous spread, symptoms related to the expansion of a mass lesion are likely to appear. Clouded consciousness, headaches, and more focal symptoms like seizures or neurological deficits may occur. There may be high fever and the possibility of very rapid progression, some people succumbing in 5–15 days. Symptoms may resemble those of CVA in nature and evolution. An abscess can break through to the surface of the cortex or the ventricular system and produce meningitis.

Treatment includes antibiotics, to eliminate both the primary and the abscess infection, and surgical excision or drainage. Seizures are a relatively common long-term result associated with the surrounding gliosis, and patients may require prolonged anticonvulsant therapy. Depending on the location and extent of the abscess, focal neurological deficits may remain after treatment.

Subdural Empyema

Subdural empyema is the collection of pus between the dura and the arachnoid membrane. The suppurative infection gets established here by spread from a contiguous infection as with abscess. It can expand, producing symptoms associated with a mass lesion, and can in turn induce thrombophlebitis in cerebral veins and infarction in their territory. As well, infection can spread to the brain or subarachnoid space (meningitis). Treatment consists of surgical drainage and antibiotic therapy. As with abscess, long-term disablement is variable. Many victims recover with only a thickened dural membrane.

CNS TUMORS

Tumors of the central nervous system constitute about 2% (20,000) of the over one million cases of cancer diagnosed in adults every year in North America. In children, cancer is much less common (perhaps 8,500 new cases per year), but by contrast, 20% of the cancers identified are in the eye, brain, or spinal cord (2,000 plus cases). A further distinction is that in adults, 70% of tumors are found above the tentorium (within the cerebral hemispheres, the thalamus etc.), while in children, 70% are subtentorial (brain stem, cerebellum, fourth ventricle).

Since tumors can arise only in tissues capable of mitosis, tumors in adults largely exclude those arising from neurons or primitive precursor cells. Mitotically active cells, therefore those capable of tumorigenesis, include **astrocytes,** which contribute to the blood-brain barrier and provide metabolic and structural support and stabilize the environment for neurons; **oligodendrocytes,** which provide the myelin sheaths in the CNS that ensure rapid, effective signal conduction; **ependymal cells,** which line the ventricles and central canal of the spinal cord; certain cells of the arachnoid membrane (giving rise to the meningioma); **Schwann cells,** which provide myelination in the peripheral nervous system; and connective tissue cells forming the endoneureal matrix surrounding peripheral nerve processes (giving rise to the neurofibroma). Cells producing blood vessels can also give rise to tumors (e.g., arteriovenous malformations). Infants and children are subject to neural and precursor cell tumors as well (e.g., neuroblastoma and medulloblastoma, respectively).

Outside the brain, the danger posed by a neoplastic growth is largely a function of its malignancy (see chapter 6). In the cranial vault, malignancy is only one factor that may affect morbidity and mortality. If it is located in or near strategic sites—for example, adjacent to the cerebral aqueduct or in the brain stem—even a small, slowly growing benign tumor can have devastating effects. Tumor excision is usually the treatment of choice in the CNS, as it is elsewhere in the body. However, CNS tumors may be physically inaccessible, may have infiltrated diffusely and require the resection of too much tissue, or may be small but located in vital brain centers. The blood-brain barrier makes chemotherapy ineffective for most tumors, and this fact, combined with the foregoing, often makes radiation the chief acceptable therapy. The limited capacity of the cranial vault is an additional variable that blurs the distinction between malignant and benign. Even though the malignant neoplasm will probably increase in mass faster, the ultimate impact of compression, herniation, and increased intracranial pressure from a benign but inoperable tumor will probably be the same.

Table 20.6 summarizes the relative incidence of CNS tumors. The bulk of tumors of the spinal cord arise from cells of the arachnoid membrane (meningioma) or the Schwann cells that myelinate spinal nerves (Schwannoma). They are slow-growing and create symptoms by compressing nerve roots or the cord. Surgical resection, with its attendant risks of cord and nerve damage, and radiation to kill actively dividing cells are alternative treatments. The spinal cord is also the destination of metastatic tumors, but to a lesser extent than the brain.

Most secondary brain tumors metastasize through the blood to the brain, where multiple, randomly distributed tumors may became established. The most common

Table 20.6	Approximate Relative Incidence of CNS Tumors

Adults

Spinal Cord—20%

- Majority are benign meningiomas and Schwannomas, with about 20% ependymomas and some gliomas

Brain—80%

Secondary (metastatic)—30%

- Malignant melanomas (from primary skin or other secondary), renal cell and intestinal carcinomas also a source

Primary (originating in brain)—70%

- Gliomas—48%
  (includes astrocytoma, glioblastoma, oligodendroglioma, and ependymoma)
- Meningioma—13%
- Neurilemmoma (Schwannoma) and neurofibroma—9% (mostly acoustic nerve tumors)

Children

Medulloblastoma—30%
Astrocytoma I and II—30%
Ependymoma—12%
Other—28%

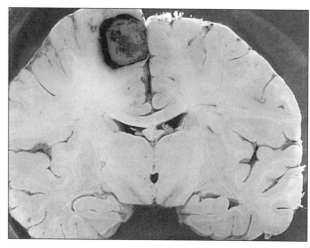

Figure 20.35 **Secondary Brain Tumor.** Malignant melanoma has metastasized from the skin to the brain.

In this photo, hemorrhage can be seen surrounding a tumor that had metastasized to the brain. It, and numerous other widely disseminated secondary tumors, caused the death of a 72-year-old woman who had initially noticed a lump on her back and then others on the abdomen and arm. Six months later, scans revealed the presence of a tumor in her lung and a biopsy of one of the skin nodules revealed it to be a malignant melanoma. This sort of progression of malignant melanoma is fortunately now relatively uncommon.

sources, in order of incidence, are carcinomas of the lung, breast, skin (malignant melanoma), kidney (renal cell carcinoma), and intestine. The incidence and distribution reflect both hemodynamics and tumor affinity for cerebral capillaries (see chapter 6). Usually the tumors are sharply demarcated from the surrounding brain tissue. Figure 20.35 shows a single malignant melanoma located near the falx. Occasionally, metastasis is to the subarachnoid space, where the tumor nodules can cover brain and cord surfaces **(carcinomatous meningitis).** Most metastasis is of highly malignant tumor types, so treatment is usually oriented to comfort and reduction of pain.

Of primary brain tumors, gliomas account for about 70%. Most of these arise from **astrocytomas.** Relatively benign astrocytomas (called I and II) are slow-growing and often broadly infiltrative. If solid and circumscribed, they may be surgically removed. While often resistant to radiotherapy, their growth may be slowed, giving five-year survival rates of about 50%. Astrocytomas III and IV are fast-growing and highly invasive. They are called **glioblastoma multiforme** because the appearance of the tumor is variable, with areas of necrosis, hemorrhage, and cyst formation dispersed through the white substance of the astrocytoma (fig. 20.36). These are usually inoperable because of

their size and infiltration. For glioblastomas, radiation therapy offers a distinct survival advantage, despite an ultimately poor prognosis. The tumor may spread across the corpus callosum into the other hemisphere. Survival beyond 12 months of the point when the tumor is recognized is unusual. Both astrocytomas I and II and glioblastoma multiforme are usually located in the cerebral hemisphere and may be diagnosed after they precipitate either a simple or complex partial seizure. While not appropriate to treat at length here, gliomas have been closely studied with respect to the factors involved in tumorigenesis and tumor progression (see chapter 6). The grading (astrocytoma I–IV) is paralleled by increasing genetic mutation, loss of chromosomal segments, and the overexpression of oncogenes, growth factors, and their receptors.

The **meningioma** is a usually benign, slow-growing tumor that arises from cells in the arachnoid membrane and accounts for about 20% of primary intracranial tumors. The tumor shown in figure 20.37 is flat and spreading, but focal, spherical growths are more common. They are highly vascular, so they show up well when CT scans are done with a contrast medium that passes the relatively permeable capillaries supplying the tumor and concentrates in the extracellular space. When focal, the pressure on adjacent bone can stimulate osteoclastic activity, and the resultant remodeling and thinning of bone may be evident on routine X-ray. Meningiomas tend to occur singly in the front half of the skull, in the superficial meninges or the falx or along the

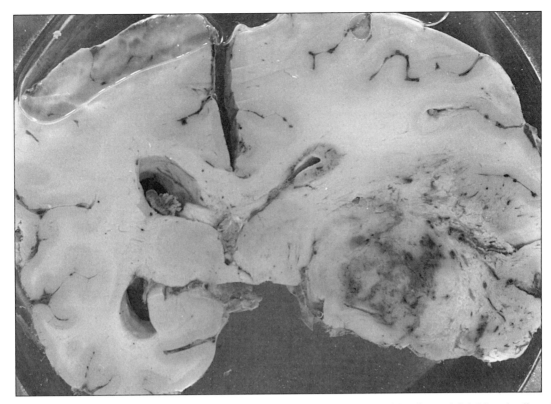

Figure 20.36   **Glioblastoma Multiforme.** The large tumor mass occupies the left temporal lobe (lower right). Note the distortion of the brain and ventricle and flattening of gyri that has resulted.
A 63-year-old cab driver was forced to give up his work because of progressive difficulty in speaking, reading, and making change.
A CT scan found the lesion pictured here in his left parietal and temporal lobes. A needle biopsy revealed the mass to be a glioblastoma.
No treatment was given and death followed four months after the diagnosis. This large, infiltrating tumor shows the scattered areas of
infarct and hemorrhage typical of glioblastoma multiforme.

ridge of the sphenoid bone or groove of the olfactory nerve. Association with the cavernous sinus makes effective resection problematic because of the complexity of cranial nerves and blood vessels traversing. Symptoms can occur over years and depend on the location of the tumor. They can include any of the following: paraparesis (weakness or paralysis of the legs), bitemporal hemianopsia if located near the optic chiasm (see chapter 21), or blindness in one eye. Surgical resection is usually effective, but its feasibility is, again, dependent on the location of the tumor. Meningiomas can be "graded" as to their malignancy. While most are benign with little chance (3%) of regrowth after resection, "atypical" tumors recur with an incidence closer to 80%. Viral antigens within those tumors suggest a role in oncogene activation or loss of tumor suppressor genes.

The **acoustic neuroma** (also called **acoustic Schwannoma** or **vestibular Schwannoma** because it is typically restricted to the vestibular component of the vestibulocochlear nerve) accounts for most of the peripheral nerve tumors that intrude into the cranial vault. It tends to develop in the foramen of the eighth cranial nerve, where pressure produces tinnitus (ringing) and progressive hearing loss. Protrusion into the cranial vault at the base of the brain, at the juncture of the medulla and pons, can stretch a variety of cranial nerves and press on motor tracts in the brain stem, producing unilateral sensory/motor deficits. Because it tends to grow off to the side of the vestibulocochlear nerve, resection with preservation of hearing and balance is possible. Bilateral tumor development is usually attributable to a **neurofibroma.** This mass grows more intimately into the nerve, so complete resection without nerve damage is unlikely.

Tumors of developmentally primitive cells or mitotically active neural cells produce about 40% of CNS neoplasia in children. The **medulloblastoma** is a highly malignant tumor arising in the cerebellum and spreading over its surface, often invading the fourth ventricle. Metastasis through the CSF is common. Symptoms result from destruction of functional cerebellum (see chapter 21) and restriction of CSF outflow (hydrocephalus). A combination of partial resection and radiotherapy currently yields a 50% ten-year survival rate.

Oligodendrogliomas form about 5% of all primary brain tumors. They are often (75%) identified as the cause of seizure activity as they develop in the cortex or subcortically. They tend to develop very slowly. Control of the seizures by the use of anticonvulsants may be all that is done. As they progress, chemotherapy, surgical resection, and radiation are

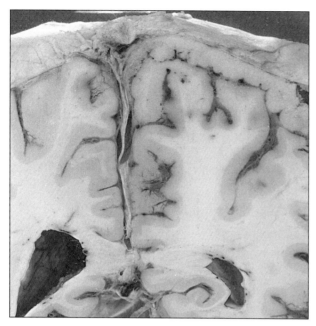

Figure 20.37   **Meningioma.** Although most are spherical, this meningioma is flattened and is spreading over the surface of the brain apparent at the right, superficial to the cerebrum.
The tumor shown here was an incidental autopsy finding.
A 73-year-old woman with a history of chronic alcohol abuse underwent rapid physical and mental deterioration. She developed pneumonia but was unresponsive to antibiotic therapy because of her state of debilitation. Death followed some weeks later. The flattened meningioma covers the vertex of the brain and extends into the longitudinal fissure. This difference from the usual spherical shape accounts for the lack of focal symptoms that a round and compressing mass would have produced. The widening of sulci and dilation of the ventricles result from generalized brain atrophy, probably due to aging and alcohol abuse. Thinning of the skull may be observed superficial to the tumor.

all used in their treatment. As the median age at diagnosis is 50 years, these are "life-shortening" tumors, requiring repeated treatment and monitoring.

Tumors of the **pituitary gland** merit a brief treatment here. While strictly endocrine, they are housed in the cranial vault, have close association with the hypothalamus, and can disrupt neural function through the compression or torsion of adjacent neural structures. The position of the pituitary within the meningeal-lined pituitary fossa, beneath the diaphragma sellae (a reflection of the dural membranes that covers the fossa and is pierced by the pituitary stalk, the infundibulum), and just posterior and inferior to the optic chiasma, sets the stage for some of the signs and symptoms of **pituitary adenoma.** This microadenoma (< 10 mm; 20% of tumors) or macroadenoma (> 10 mm; the other 80%) develops in the anterior pituitary, which normally composes the bulk (80%) of the pituitary mass. The less common "secreting type" releases one or more of the following hormones: prolactin (the most common, which produces symptoms in women but often goes unnoticed in men), growth hormone (which, in the adult, may produce acromegaly), ACTH (which is responsible for about 70% of Cushing's disease), and FSH or LH. Release of these hormones is the usual way that this endocrinely active tumor announces its presence. However, more tumors are "null cell," or nonsecreting, which means the tumor goes undetected until it creates mass effects. The classic in this context is the disturbance of peripheral visual field sensitivity that is described in chapter 22 as "tunnel vision," although a variety of other visual disturbances are observed. Cranial nerve compression affecting CN III, IV, and V can result as the tumor expands, eroding the sella turcica and entering the cavernous sinus space. Hypopituitarism may

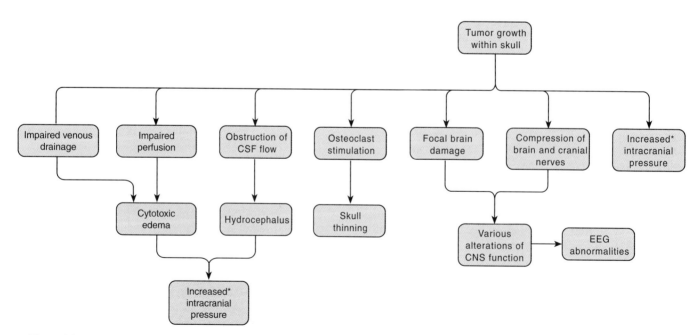

Figure 20.38   **Mechanisms of Symptom Production by Tumor Growth Within the Skull.** *A variety of mechanisms converge to increase intracranial mass and intracranial pressure, thereby exacerbating many of the conditions that led to the increased mass in the first place. At the point of decompensation, this positive feedback accelerates rapidly.

occur if the blood supply to the gland is crimped or compressed. Both types are typically slow-growing and don't get recognized until the third or fourth decade. The conventional treatment is surgical resection, particularly with macroadenomas. Radiation is also used. Tumors sometimes regrow when resected.

Many of the mechanisms whereby tumors produce symptoms have been covered earlier in this chapter. Figure 20.38 provides an overview. It should be noted that massive infiltration of functional brain tissue can occur (for example, by an astrocytoma) with few clinical signs. This means that tumor progression can take place without the patient's perception, a characteristic of tumors outside the CNS. Also, symptoms usually develop slowly, then dramatically accelerate to a crisis that may send the patient for diagnosis or be part of the final evolution of an untreatable condition.

Case Study

A frantic mother brought her 12-year-old daughter to a hospital's emergency room at 11 P.M. The child was rigid and in a stupor. Although the mother's English was quite poor and there was no one available to translate, it was determined that the attack was of sudden onset 30 minutes earlier. The child had experienced a mild, upper respiratory infection and an earache in the last 24 hours. When her temperature started to rise, her mother gave her an aspirin and put her to bed. On later checking on the child's condition, she noticed that the fever had risen significantly and she was unable to arouse the child.

In the ER, the patient's temperature was 39.5° C and she was unresponsive, showing increased muscle tone and unconscious irritability during her examination, which also uncovered evidence of otitis media. Her lungs were clear and her heart rate elevated. A well-healed scar over the upper left abdominal quadrant was present, and upon questioning the mother it was determined that the child had had her spleen removed following its rupture in a motor vehicle accident three years previously.

Blood and urine samples were obtained for testing and a chest X-ray was taken. A lumbar puncture was also done and indicated a cloudy CSF under increased pressure. An IV line was established, and a broad spectrum antibiotic was administered, pending results of blood and urine tests.

When test results were obtained, the urine and chest X-ray were normal, while white cell counts were elevated. In the CSF, the glucose level was depressed, protein and WBC counts were elevated, and there was Gram-positive diplococci present. The diplococci were identified and a diagnosis of pneumococcal meningitis was made. Tests showed the organisms to be penicillin-sensitive, and this antibiotic was substituted for the broad spectrum antibiotic.

Within 24 hours of the start of penicillin therapy, which was administered with another agent to increase the permeability of the blood-brain barrier to penicillin, the child's condition improved. After 48 hours had passed, she was sitting up in bed and communicating. In ten days she had fully recovered and was discharged from the hospital.

Commentary
Elevation of intracranial pressure is a hallmark of bacterial meningitis, which in this case can be assumed to have originated in the child's middle ear infection. The cloudiness of the CSF was due both to its elevated protein level and the presence of pus. The chest X-ray was important in establishing that there was no pneumonia or endocardial involvement, two common accompaniments of bacterial meningitis. Before the infecting organism is identified, ampicillin offers a broad effectiveness, but penicillin is more effective against most pneumococcal strains.

Although various bacterial species such as *Neisseria, Hemophilus,* or *Staphylococcus* may cause meningitis, in those who lack a spleen (and in those with sickle cell disease) it is particularly likely to be *Streptococcus pneumoniae.* The reasons for this are unclear, but the link is so well established that immediately following splenectomy, anti-pneumococcus vaccine is typically administered. The vaccine protects against the pneumococci responsible for about 90% of infections, but in the case of this child, the infecting strain was apparently one against which there was no protection. Her mother's quick response, in spite of a language deficit that might have deterred less assertive parents, was important, since pneumococcal meningeal infections are fatal in about 15% of cases.

Key Concepts

1. The scalp effectively protects the skull but can allow infection to enter the cranial vault through veins draining the face or loose connective tissue beneath the galea (pp. 535–537).

2. The skull may be subject to direct trauma, perhaps producing a hematoma or basal skull fracture that may expose the brain to infective agents (pp. 537–539).

3. Cerebrospinal fluid confers significant protection but is subject to infection, and the meningeal layers can be the site of hemorrhage and hematoma formation (pp. 539–541).

4. The vertebral column can be subject to dislocation, fracture, or disk protrusion, any of which can affect cord or nerve root function (pp. 541–544).

5. Infarcts may occur at the margins of adjacent vascular fields supplying the cortex (watershed zone) secondary to conditions that impair perfusion (e.g., fibrillation) or oxygenation (e.g., carbon monoxide poisoning, near-drowning) (p. 551).

6. Brain tissue can swell if capillaries become permeable and allow an extracellular accumulation of fluid in the white matter (vasogenic edema) or if cortical cells are injured and swell (cytotoxic edema) (pp. 556–557).

7. Any uncompensated expansion of brain, CSF, or blood within the relatively fixed cranial vault can lead to an increase in intracranial pressure, which can impair cerebral perfusion and compress, shift, or tear neural tissue (pp. 557–560).

8. Oversecretion, impaired absorption, or obstructed circulation of cerebrospinal fluid can lead to an expansion of the CSF compartment, particularly the cerebral ventricles, that is termed hydrocephalus (pp. 560–561).

9. Assessment and description of level of consciousness provides a significant approximate gauge of generalized neural function and the progression of pathology and treatment (pp. 561–562).

10. A variety of reflex and automatic functions can aid in the localization of CNS lesions and in monitoring their progression or resolution (pp. 562–564).

11. Problems in the closure and development of the neural tube can lead to defects in bony or meningeal protection or abnormal development of neural tissue. Defects of the caudal neural tube are termed spina bifida, while rostral defects range from minor to failure of brain development (anencephaly) (pp. 565–567).

12. An aneurysm is a dilation of a section of an artery that occurs at an injury or a site of congenital weakness of the arterial wall, in the case of berry or fusiform aneurysms, or secondary to hypertension in the case of microaneurysms (pp. 568–569).

13. Transitory constriction of subarachnoid arteries (subarachnoid vasospasm) can result spontaneously or secondary to subarachnoid hemorrhage, perhaps from an aneurysm, or surgery (p. 569).

14. Tangled masses of blood vessels that shunt blood directly from arteries to the venous drainage, called arteriovenous malformations, develop congenitally and are increasingly susceptible to hemorrhage (pp. 569–570).

15. Infection or inflammation in adjacent tissues can induce clot formation in cerebral veins or venous sinuses, thereby impairing venous drainage and cerebral perfusion and perhaps spreading infection (p. 570).

16. Cerebrovascular accident (CVA) is the term applied to a group of conditions in which localized cerebral blood flow is impaired by either occlusion or hemorrhage (p. 571).

17. In a transient ischemic attack, a brief vasospasm of diseased artery downstream from a developing plaque impairs perfusion of localized tissue, producing fully reversible hypofunction (pp. 571–572).

18. A thrombotic CVA evolves when the thrombus on a chronic plaque stenoses or occludes an arterial lumen, leading to downstream ischemia and necrosis (pp. 572–574).

19. Transitory edema usually produces broader impairment in a CVA than that eventually attributable to the necrosis of specific functional cortex or white matter tracts (pp. 573–574).

20. Occlusive CVAs are usually attributable to intra- or extracranial thrombotic emboli and produce symptoms similar to those of thrombotic CVA, but evolve more rapidly (pp. 574–576).

21. Hemorrhage interferes with downstream perfusion but also may produce a hematoma mass, dissect delicate neural tissues, or enter the ventricles or subarachnoid space (p. 576).

22. Bacterial infection of the subarachnoid space (pyogenic meningitis) is a medical emergency producing classic signs like stiff neck, fever, vomiting, and Brudzinski's and Kernig's signs (pp. 577–579).

23. Viral infections of the CNS vary from usually benign viral meningitis to fatal encephalitis (pp. 579–580).

24. The relative incidence, type, and location of CNS tumors vary between children and adults (pp. 581–582).

25. CNS tumors vary in cell type of origin, pattern and speed of development, and prognosis (pp. 581–585).

REVIEW ACTIVITIES

1. Without referencing the figures in your text, lay out a flow chart that terminates at a box labeled "Increased Intracranial Pressure" and that starts with boxes labeled "Abscess," "Intracranial Bleeding," "Tumor," "Blocked Arachnoid Villi," "Blocked Cerebral Aqueduct," "Trauma," and "Hypoxia." Be sure to include a box labeled "Cerebral Edema" somewhere in your chart. Then insert additional boxes so that the chart accurately reflects the pathogenesis of increased intracranial pressure.

2. Do another flow chart, this time starting with "Increased Intracranial Pressure" and ending with all of the logically expected outcomes.

3. Without referencing to the figures in your text, explain the processes of symptom production that are associated with the development of an intracranial tumor.

4. Construct a table that presents the progression of increased intracranial pressure to a fatal outcome.

5. Prepare a brief table summarizing the categories of neural tube defects.

6. Describe development of one of the CVA syndromes in such specific terms that it could be used in the exam question, "Identify the following clinically observed CVA and defend your answer."

21

Disorders of Movement, Sensation, and Mental Function

Man is the shuttle, to whose winding quest
And passage through these looms
God order'd motion, but ordain'd no rest.

HENRY VAUGHAN
(1622–1695)

rubor

&tumor

cū calore

&dolore

This chapter deals with disorders arising either centrally or peripherally that might disrupt normal movement or sensation, autonomic function, or higher mental processes. We begin with the background necessary to understand these.

CONTEXT FOR THE ASSESSMENT OF DYSFUNCTION

The Autonomic Nervous System

The **autonomic nervous system** is active in regulating a host of very important homeostatic, reactive, and sensory functions. Control of cardiac output, blood pressure, digestive processes and salivation, bladder contraction and micturition (urination), visual responses to changing light conditions or distance, temperature regulation: All are effected through the autonomic nervous system (ANS). So are the physical and physiological aspects of emotion, arousal, and stress response.

Somewhat arbitrarily, anatomists have defined the autonomic nervous system to be purely efferent; they include in this system only the nerves that travel out from the CNS to smooth muscle (in blood vessels, the lungs, digestive and urinary tract etc.), cardiac muscle, and glandular/secretory structures. In order to function normally, there has to be elaborate sensory input on this system. Information about blood pressure, filling of the stomach, intestine, or bladder, skin temperature, the availability of food, the presence of danger or sexual opportunity—all of this is constantly being relayed to the spinal cord and brain. There, central processing occurs, and at least some of the response to these challenges to homeostasis flows out through the nuclei and fibers that are properly termed the autonomic nervous system.

There are two clear divisions to the ANS, parasympathetic and sympathetic, which are distinguished by anatomical, functional, and neurotransmitter differences (fig. 21.1). The fibers of the **parasympathetic** branch begin in nuclei found in the brain stem and sacral portion of the spinal cord (craniosacral division). As is the case for all autonomic innervation except that to the adrenal medulla, there is a two-neuron chain between the nucleus and the effector organ. The first fiber, the **preganglionic fiber,** communicates with the second by means of the neurotransmitter acetylcholine. This is the case in both the sympathetic and parasympathetic branches. In the parasympathetic division, acetylcholine is also the neurotransmitter released from the second neuron (the **postganglionic fiber**) to affect the activity of the effector organ (smooth muscle, gland, etc.). Nuclei of the **sympathetic** division are found in the midlateral gray matter of the spinal cord between segments T-1 (first thoracic) and L-2 (second lumbar). In this case, most postganglionic fibers release norepinephrine (exceptions will be noted later).

Certain terms relating to these neurotransmitters require explanation. Fibers releasing acetylcholine from their end terminals are called **cholinergic.** Even though acetylcholine (ACh) is the same substance wherever it is released in the nervous system, the receptors for it (on muscle, postganglionic fibers, autonomic effectors, CNS neurons) can differ slightly. These differences make it possible to use a drug that is active in one set of receptors, but has virtually no activity at the rest. Atropine will be described as an example later.

Terminology associated with norepinephrine has its own peculiarities. Norepinephrine and epinephrine are closely related agents, examples of biological substances called **catecholamines.** Both are released from the adrenal medulla when it is subjected to sympathetic stimulation and are important agents in the very generalized "fight or flight" response to arousal. An older name for the substance now usually called epinephrine is **adrenalin;** hence, the term **adrenergic** when referring to its effects. For example, an **adrenergic agonist** is a substance, often a drug, that has the same effect on the body as do epinephrine and norepinephrine. Conversely, an **adrenergic antagonist** counteracts the activity of these two substances.

The autonomic nuclei just described, which are the avenues of activation of the ANS, must, of course, be acted upon themselves. Some impulses—for example, from the cardiovascular centers in the medulla—synapse directly with the appropriate sympathetic or parasympathetic nuclei. Most impulses originate in the hypothalamus. This complex structure integrates autonomic and endocrine control systems for maintaining homeostasis and responding to environmental demands.

Parasympathetic and sympathetic divisions of the ANS are often presented as having antagonistic functions—conserving versus activating responses, respectively. A more informative view is to recognize the range of autonomic innervation and function. Some structures have only parasympathetic innervation (e.g., bronchial glands) and some have only sympathetic innervation (e.g., the spleen, the adrenal medulla, sweat glands, and most blood vessels). Most structures are dually innervated. Some of these demonstrate complementary interaction of both divisions (e.g., parasympathetic stimulation is responsible for erection, while ejaculation depends on sympathetic activity). Other dually innervated organs do demonstrate antagonist action, but with many of these the interaction of opposite effects has a synergistic effect. For example, sympathetic stimulation increases heart rate and contractility, while parasympathetic stimulation decreases both; however, in a situation demanding increased cardiac output, not only does sympathetic outflow increase but vagal outflow is inhibited. (The vagus nerve carries parasympathetic impulses to the viscera.) This interaction greatly increases the effect of sympathetic stimulation beyond its isolated impact.

Autonomic responses are capable of being focused by the selective activation of fibers to one organ or system (e.g., sympathetic stimulation of the heart). But also, even the diffuse arousal implicit in the release into the general circulation of catecholamines (epinephrine and

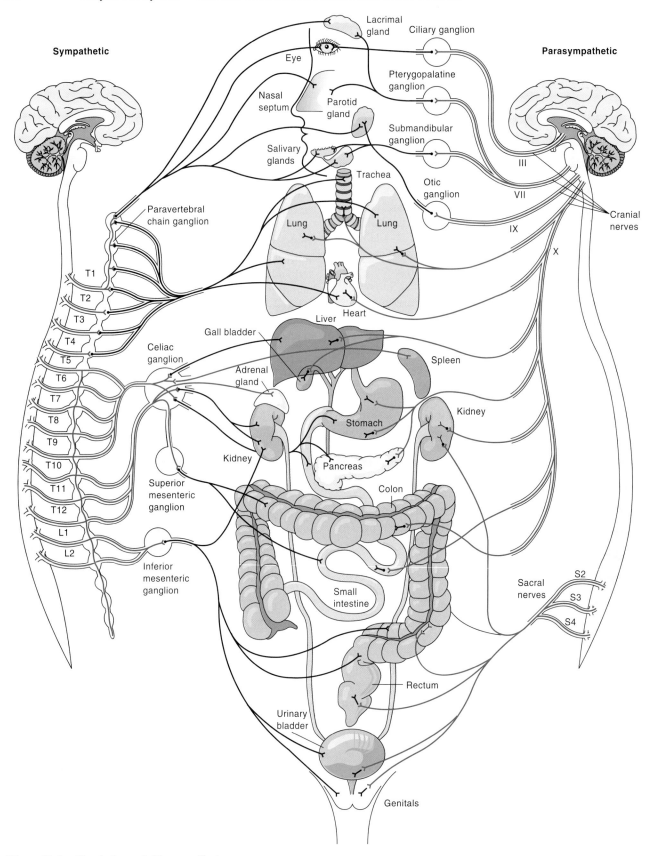

Figure 21.1   **The Autonomic Nervous System.**

Table 21.1   Major Responses of Selected Effector Organs to Autonomic Nerve Impulses

Effector Organs	Sympathetic Activation (Mostly Adrenergic Impulses)		Parasympathetic Activation (Cholinergic Impulses)
	Receptor Type	*Responses*	*Responses*
Eye			
Radial muscle, iris	α	Dilation (mydriasis)[+]	—
Sphincter muscle, iris	—	—	Constriction (miosis)[++]
Heart			
SA node	β_1	Increase in heart rate[+]	Decrease in heart rate; vagal arrest[+++]
AV node	β_1	Increase in automaticity and conduction velocity[+]	Decrease in conduction velocity; AV block [++]
Ventricles	β_1	Increase in contractility, conduction velocity, automaticity, and rate of idioventricular pacemaker[++]	—
Arterioles			
Skin and mucosa	α	Constriction[++]	—
Pulmonary	α, β_2	Dilation predominates[+]	—
Abdominal viscera, renal	α, β_2	Constriction predominates[+]	—
Skeletal muscle	α, β_2	Dilation predominates[+]	—
Lung			
Bronchial muscle	β_2	Relaxation[+]	Contraction[++]
Spleen capsule	α, β_2	Contraction[++]	—
Skin, sweat glands	ACh*	Generalized secretions[+]	—
Adrenal medulla	ACh[†]	Secretion of epinephrine and norepinephrine[++]	—

[+]Minor activation   [++]Moderate activation   [+++] Intensive activation

*Most sympathetic nerves ending on sweat glands release acetylcholine as a neurotransmitter.

[†]Sympathetic preganglionic fibers terminate directly on the adrenal medulla; all preganglionic neurons release acetylcholine.

norepinephrine) from the adrenal medulla has a different effect on different organs. This is because, like the cholinergic receptors, different receptors for the catecholamines have specific, different effects on their respective organs. Four different catecholamine receptors have been identified. Three of these have particular relevance. β_1 (beta one) receptors are found almost exclusively in the heart. When epinephrine or norepinephrine fills these receptors (having been released either from sympathetic fibers or from the adrenal medulla via the general circulation), the effect is excitatory. β_2 receptors, found on smooth muscle and gland cells, are inhibitory on the activity of these cells. α_1 (alpha one) receptors, found on smooth muscle and gland cells, have an excitatory effect. In this case, epinephrine would cause the smooth muscle cells to contract and, in arterioles, would thereby cause vasoconstriction. Table 21.1 presents a relevant selection of organs affected by autonomic activity.

Pharmacological Agents Acting through Autonomic Receptors

Agents Blocking the Effect of Parasympathetic Stimulation Atropine and atropinelike drugs have a strong affinity for the acetylcholine receptors on parasympathetic effectors, which they occupy without activating. They thereby block parasympathetic action. Atropine can be used to paralyze the sphincter muscle in the iris, thus allowing the unopposed action of the sympathetically innervated radial muscle of the iris to dilate the pupil (mydriasis) for fuller examination of the fundus (the area of the retina including the fovea, optic disk, and retinal blood vessels). It may be used preoperatively as a bronchodilator (blocks bronchial smooth muscle contraction) and to dry mucous membranes. It has a limited use in early myocardial infarction to relieve severe bradycardia (slow heart rate) or AV block.

Cholinergic blockers that have affinity for the whole range of acetylcholine receptors can be used to control the potentially fatal cholinergic crisis induced by certain insecticides that contain anticholinesterase agents. Without treatment, these substances allow acetylcholine to accumulate in autonomic pre- and postganglionic, neuromuscular, and central nervous system synaptic clefts, a condition that can lead to motor paralysis, lung congestion, convulsions, and death. Atropine, although not removing the anticholinesterase agent, blocks the action of the excess acetylcholine. Cholinesterase inhibitors are used to diagnose

(Tensilon) or treat (neostigmine) myasthenia gravis (see later section). Atropinelike agents must be available to reverse the cholinergic crisis that could result from the excess action of these drugs on the myasthenic patient.

Agents Acting Via Sympathetic Receptors to Increase Sympathetic Activity Epinephrine tends to act broadly on all sympathetic effector organs if used systemically, so it tends to be used locally—for example, to control superficial hemorrhage by constricting arterioles and precapillary sphincters. **Isoproterenol** attaches to all β receptors but has almost no affinity to α receptors, and therefore has a bronchodilator effect of value in respiratory disorders and a cardiac stimulant effect of value in heart block, cardiogenic shock, and after myocardial infarction. **Dopamine,** an agonist (stimulating agent) at mainly β1 receptors, produces increased contractility in the myocardium while maintaining blood flow through renal and intestinal vascular beds. These qualities make it useful in treating certain forms of shock. **Dobutamine,** a closely related β1 adrenergic agonist, increases contractility and cardiac output while producing little change in total peripheral resistance. This makes it a useful drug in treating congestive heart failure.

Agents Blocking the Effect of α-Receptor Sympathetic Stimulation One approach to reducing chronic essential hypertension is to inhibit sympathetic vasoconstrictor tone, thereby reducing peripheral resistance and, consequently, systemic blood pressure. **Prazosin** acts as an α1 blocking agent, selectively reducing vascular resistance without the inotropic (increased force of contraction) or chronotropic (increased heart rate) effects of a β agonist.

Agents Blocking the Effect of β-Receptor Sympathetic Stimulation A drug that blocks the cardiovascular effects of β sympathetic activity could reduce heart rate and contractility (β1), thus reducing the workload on the heart, and still compensate for reduced cardiac output by increasing resistance of vessels in lungs and skeletal muscles (β2), leaving sympathetic vasoconstriction of skin and mucosa (α) intact. **Propranolol** is such a nonselective β-blocking agent. These effects are desirable in treatment of hypertension, prevention of angina pectoris, and the control of cardiac arrhythmias. **Metoprolol,** a selective β1 blocker, is also effective in treating hypertension.

 Checkpoint 21.1

Medications that act on the usual targets of the autonomic nervous system are a mainstay in the medical management of a number of chronic conditions. Taking this perspective go back over this first section. Note a relevant medical condition, list the drugs that could be used to treat it, and explain how they work.

Brain Stem Structure and Function

The brain stem has three distinct anatomical regions (fig. 21.2). In order, descending from the cerebrum just posterior to the hypothalamus, they are the **midbrain,** the **pons,** and the **medulla oblongata.** These form a transition from the cerebrum to the spinal cord. Any information that enters the cerebrum (except vision or smell) and any efferent signals must pass through the brain stem. It has specific nuclei that mediate reflex and voluntary movements produced by the cranial nerves. Signals that arise in the hypothalamus and pass out along the nerves of the autonomic NS must travel through the brain stem. Centers that produce consciousness, arousal, and sleep are part of a network of neurons called the **reticular activating system** located in the core of the brain stem.

The *midbrain* is small—perhaps 2 cm long, 4 cm wide, and 3 cm deep—but absolutely essential for survival. The anterior portion **(cerebral peduncles)** is formed of descending motor fibers. Immediately posterior are two sheets of darkly pigmented **substantia nigra** (SN)2 which are a component of a larger, integrated system, the basal ganglia. Lesions to the SN produce the symptoms of Parkinsonism. Just behind the SN are the two spherical **red nuclei,** which are part of the brain stem motor nuclei system. Two sets of nuclei in the center of the midbrain (cranial nerves III and IV) control much of eye movements, while two other sets of nuclei in the posterior midbrain **tectum** are centers for integrating orienting responses to visual and auditory stimuli (the **superior** and **inferior colliculi,** respectively). The cerebral aqueduct passes through the posterior midbrain to conduct CSF from the third to the fourth ventricles. Below and continuous with the midbrain is the *pons.* Most of its bulk is formed of fibers crossing to or from the opposite hemisphere of the cerebellum, which sits on its posterior surface, but it also contains a center for regulating the breathing patterns that are generated in the medulla, and a nucleus to produce lateral eye movements. The **medulla** is inferior and continuous with the pons. Despite its slimmer size, it contains a number of essential nuclei (see table 21.2). The motor fibers that control distal musculature of the arms and legs to produce precisely controlled voluntary movements are called the **pyramidal tract,** or **lateral corticospinal tract,** in the spinal cord. The term *pyramidal* derives from the fact these fibers travel close to the surface in the medulla and form two pyramid-shaped bumps on the anterior, superior surface of the medulla. The widely branched neurous of the **reticular activating system** are scattered in the middle of the brain stem from midbrain to medulla. They participate in the regulation of cortical arousal, producing alert wakefulness and sleep. They also produce the motor paralysis that permits the uneventful experience of vivid dreams during REM (rapid eye movement) sleep.

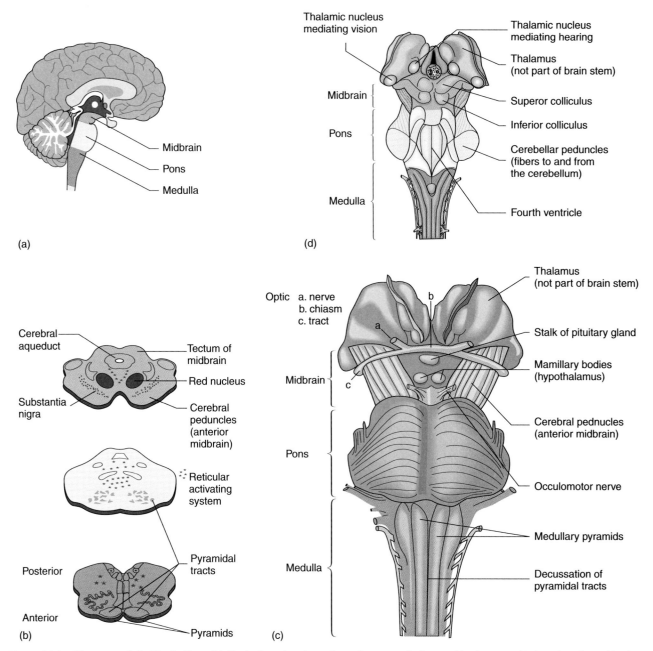

Figure 21.2   **Features of the Brain Stem** (*a*) Sagittal section through cerebrum, cerebellus, and brain stem. (*b*) Anterior view of brain stem. (*c*) Sections through midbrain, pons, and medulla. Note extent of the reticular activating system. (*d*) Posterior view of brain stem.

Cranial Nerve Function and Assessment

Cranial nerves (CN) are so named because they arise from the brain or brain stem. CN I (the olfactory nerve) and CN II (the optic nerve) are actually extensions of the brain, being myelinated by oligodendrocytes and possessing complex sensory end organs. In the case of the **optic nerve,** meningeal protection, typical of the brain, including dural sheath and CSF-filled subarachnoid space, extends to the eyeball.

The neurons that interact with the millions of photoreceptors in the retina are gathered together and leave the retina at the optic disk to pass along the optic nerve. Retinal blood vessels enter and leave at the **optic disk** and travel in the center of the optic nerve. The whole of the disk lacks photoreceptors, and their absence creates a blind spot in the lower temporal portion of each visual field that can become significantly enlarged in conditions like glaucoma (increased intraocular pressure). The normal disk is pinkish and round or oval, with sharply defined margins and a slightly cupped center. Increased intracranial pressure is conducted along the optic nerve in the CSF that surrounds it and can cause the disk to protrude. The margin of the disk will be swollen and less distinct, and the entire disk

Table 21.2   Functions Mediated at Different Levels of the Brain Stem

Found at all levels of the brain stem	Reticular activating system, (RAS) responsible for wakefulness arousal and sleep, activation of the motor system
	Ascending (sensory) and descending (motor) pathways

Midbrain

Superior colliculus	Posterior	Orienting responses to visual stimuli (turning the head, neck, and trunk)
Inferior colliculus	midbrain	Orienting responses to auditory stimuli
Red nucleus	(tectum)	Antigravity posture (arm flexion, toe extension)
Edinger-Westphal nucleus		Pupillary light reflexes
Oculomotor nucleus		Control of eye movements other than those of the trochlear and abducens
Trochlear nucleus		Movement of the eye down, inward, and outwards at lowest gaze
Cerebral peduncles		Descending motor pathways
Spinal lemniscus		Ascending sensory pathways (all superficial and deep sensation including pain and temperature)

Pons

Tegmentum (anterior pons)	Fibers bridging to or from one cerebellar hemisphere (somewhat analogous to the corpus callusum of the cerebrum)
Pneumotaxic and apneustic centers	Regulation of breathing patterns and lung inflation
Abducens nucleus	Lateral movement of the eye
Medial lemniscus	Superficial and deep sensation not including pain and temperature
Vestibular nuclei (junction of pons/medulla)	Integrate movements to maintain balance, produce arm and leg extension

Medulla

Cardiovascular center	Regulation of heart rate and force of contraction
Respiratory center	Generates a regular, rhythmic breathing pattern
Nucleus gracilis	Synapse of sensory information from lower trunk and lower limb
Nucleus cuneatus	Synapse of sensory information from arms, upper trunk, neck
Decussation below the pyramids	Decussation (cross-over) of the fibers of the pyramidal tract
Various centers	Gagging, vomiting, swallowing, coughing, sneezing, hiccuping

will have a reddish hue, presumably because the abnormal pressure interferes with venous drainage. It can also appear pale with microaneurysms at the periphery. This condition is called **papilledema** (choked disk). It is often referred to with the more straightforward name of **optic disc edema.** On the other hand, increased intraocular pressure may enlarge the depression in the center of the disk, a phenomenon called **cupping.**

Testing of cranial nerve function is a routine part of a neurological examination (the brief details are found in table 21.3). By combining the pattern and extent of deficits with a detailed knowledge of brain stem anatomy and the particular course of each cranial nerve (fig. 21.3), the clinician can localize a lesion and make educated guesses as to its nature.

Rinne's test can be used as an example. The subject has suffered hearing loss. The examiner strikes a special tuning fork and holds it next to the subject's ear. When the subject can no longer hear it, the stem of the fork is pressed against the mastoid process. If this allows the sound to be heard again, the deafness must be due to a problem in picking up vibrations at the eardrum or conducting them to the inner ear (conduction deafness). If there is no increased sensitivity, then deafness must be attributable to the inner ear (so-called "nerve deafness").

Visual Pathways

A variety of distinct problems can interfere with the processing of visual information: demyelination, tumors, emboli, edema, thrombosis, hemorrhage, contusion, for a not exhaustive list. Despite this variability in cause, the net effect will depend almost solely on the site at which the lesion interrupts the pathways of vision.

A quick review of visual processing from the retina to the visual association cortex is in order. First, what is

Table 21.3   Cranial Nerve Function and Assessment

Cranial Nerve	Function	Testing and Deficit
I. Olfactory	Sensory—sense of smell	Each nostril tested separately with aromatic substance; basal skull fracture a common trauma
II. Optic	Sensory—vision	Visual acuity tested with eye chart; to estimate extent of visual field, patient reports on object moved into field from periphery
III. Oculomotor	Motor—eye movements other than those attributed for CN IV and CN VI; raises eyelids, constricts pupil, focuses lens Sensory—state of contraction/tension in innervated external eye muscles	Ability to follow object, raise eyelids against pressure, constrict pupils to light
IV. Trochlear	Motor—superior oblique external eye muscle Sensory—state of contraction/tension	Difficulty shifting gaze in and down, a deficit noticeable when walking downstairs.
V. Trigeminal		
Ophthalmic branch	Sensory—surface of eyes, scalp, forehead, upper eyelid (motor to tear glands)	Whisp of cotton touched to surface of eyeball
Maxillary branch	Sensory—upper teeth, gum and lip, palate, face	Pinprick to face
Mandibular branch	Sensory—skin of jaw, lower teeth, gum and lip Motor—muscles for chewing and in floor of mouth	Pinprick to jaw, gum, lip; make chewing movements
VI. Abducens	Motor—lateral rectus external eye muscle Sensory—state of contraction/tension	Impaired lateral gaze in left eye when looking left, etc.
VII. Facial	Sensory—taste anterior tongue Motor—muscles of facial expression, tear gland, salivary glands	Taste tested (sweet, sour, salt); grimace, smile, purse lips; tearing in response to ammonia
VIII. Vestibulocochlear (auditory)	Sensory—hearing, balance, and movement	Rinne's test.
IX. Glossopharyngeal	Sensory—pharynx, tonsils, posterior tongue (taste), baroreceptors at bifurcation of carotids Motor—pharyngeal muscles used in swallowing, salivary glands	Gag reflex and swallowing tested; speech; taste for bitter
X. Vagus	Sensory—pharynx, larynx, esophagus, visceral organs of thorax and abdomen Motor—parasympathetic innervation of viscera including heart; swallowing and speech	Swallowing and speech.
XI. Accessory	Motor—muscles of soft palate, pharynx, larynx; muscles of neck and back	Speech, shrug shoulders, push forehead forward against resistance, turn head
XII. Hypoglossal	Motor and sensory for tongue movements	Tongue protruded and moved

the **visual field?** When our eyes are fixed on an object, everything to the left of the point of fixation is in the left visual field, and vice versa for everything to the right. **Macular** (or foveal) vision is very acute because the image is focused on the center of the retina (the **fovea**), where there is a particularly dense array of the photoreceptors responsible for the perception of color and detail. The image is inverted and turned left for right as it passes through the lens. Because of this, information in the upper portion of the right half of the visual field is cast upon the lower-left quadrant of each retina. That information is ultimately received and processed in the lower half of the left visual area in the occipital cortex. So, as a general rule, the neural pathways through which information from the visual fields is processed will be located top-for-bottom and left-for-right. Conversely, blindness in the left visual field will indicate disruption of the right visual pathways.

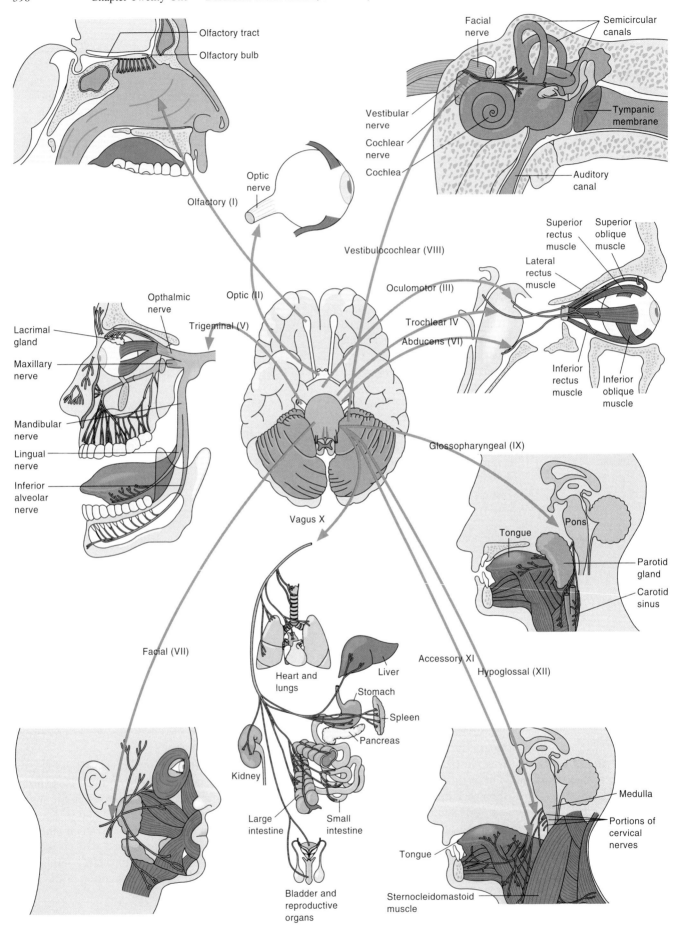

Figure 21.3   **Cranial Nerve Pathways and Innervation.**

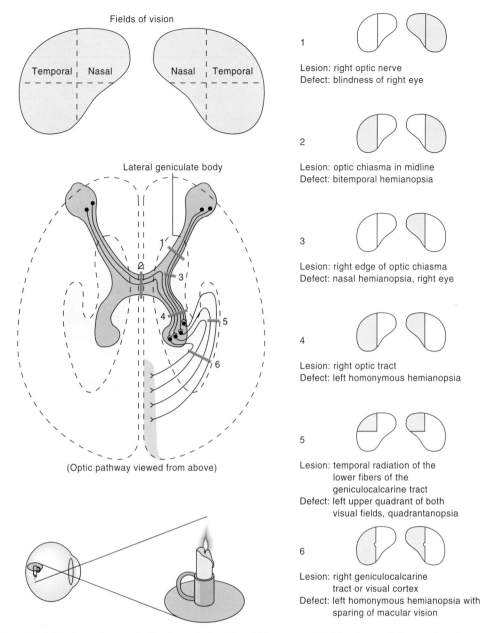

Fields of vision

Temporal | Nasal   Nasal | Temporal

Lateral geniculate body

(Optic pathway viewed from above)

1
Lesion: right optic nerve
Defect: blindness of right eye

2
Lesion: optic chiasma in midline
Defect: bitemporal hemianopsia

3
Lesion: right edge of optic chiasma
Defect: nasal hemianopsia, right eye

4
Lesion: right optic tract
Defect: left homonymous hemianopsia

5
Lesion: temporal radiation of the
lower fibers of the
geniculocalcarine tract
Defect: left upper quadrant of both
visual fields, quadrantanopsia

6
Lesion: right geniculocalcarine
tract or visual cortex
Defect: left homonymous hemianopsia with
sparing of macular vision

Figure 21.4 **Visual Field Defects Caused by Lesions of the Visual Pathways.** "Fields of vision" distorted ovals represent what is seen *not* the area of retina that is stimulated (which would be the exact opposite). The inserted figure of the candle illustrates the 180-degree rotation of the visual image that occurs through the lens.

Axons from the retina come together at the optic disk and pass into the optic nerve, which proceeds posteriorly through a fissure at the back of the orbit. At the base of the brain, just anterior to the stalk that connects the hypothalamus to the pituitary, the axons from the medial half of each retina cross over at the optic chiasm. For this reason, the information from the right half of each retina (i.e., the left visual field from both eyes), is now gathered together on the right side. This pathway is called the **right optic tract.** To restate this, axons from the left nasal retina are combined with axons from the right temporal retina to form the right optic tract (fig. 21.4). A lesion at the optic chiasm will most likely interrupt those crossing-over nasal retinal fibers. It

will therefore affect vision in the outside or temporal fields, leaving nasal fields intact and producing a sort of tunnel vision. The condition is called **bitemporal hemianopsia.**

Left and right optic tracts pass on to their respective thalamic nuclei (the left and right lateral geniculate bodies) for processing and routing to the primary visual cortex. (As well, they pass off collaterals that go to areas at the back of the midbrain called the superior colliculi, where this visual information makes possible certain visual reflexes and coordinated head and eye movements.) A lesion of the tract between the optic chiasm and the thalamus will wipe out sensitivity to an entire visual field for both eyes, a condition called **complete homonymous hemianopsia.** On their way from the lateral geniculate nucleus of the thalamus to the visual cortex, the fibers from the lower half of each right retina take an excursion around the lateral ventricle in the right temporal lobe (the temporal radiation of the optic tract). Here they may be subjected to lesions that would have no effect on the upper fibers that take a more direct route. This lesion would affect the upper *left* visual field (can you explain why?) and is called **upper left quadrantanopsia.** If the lesion occurs where the fibers have been reunited or at the visual cortex, we will have a condition called **incomplete homonymous hemianopsia.** In this case, there is apparent sparing of macular (central foveal) vision. This sparing is probably a result of incomplete clinical lesions rather than some bilateral representation of foveal information. For clinical purposes, the field defects that you should have at your fingertips are: single-eye blindness, bitemporal hemianopsia, and homonymous hemianopsia.

Checkpoint 21.2

Don't be disappointed if your comprehension of the details of the visual tracts and conditions that affect them takes you more time than some sections of comparable length. The concept here—that the "crossover" is of the light and that the nervous system operates to keep information cast on the right side *on* the right side—is intrinsically difficult. Try drawing your own wiring diagrams until you get it straight.

Peripheral Nerve Damage and Repair

A peripheral nerve is typically composed of the neuronal processes, or **axons,** from a variety of motor, sensory, and autonomic neurons. The larger, rapidly conducting axons are wrapped in multiple layers of myelin. This is produced by individual **Schwann cells,** which are interrupted at regular intervals by **nodes of Ranvier.** These exposed nodes are richly invested with sodium channels. It is this feature that produces the rapid, **saltatory** (jumping) signal transmission characteristic of myelinated axons. Motor neurons and the fibers carrying information about tendon and muscle tension, limb position, joint pressure, and the precisely discriminated skin sensations of light touch, vibration, and movement are examples of such well-myelinated axons. Unmyelinated or lightly myelinated fibers carry the sensations of slow and fast pain and temperature and autonomic signals to the sweat glands and blood vessels of the skin.

These axons are all imbedded in a fibrous connective tissue matrix that is named according to its location (epineurium, perineurium, endoneurium) (fig. 21.5). This connective tissue carries the blood vessels that maintain the axons and Schwann cells. The endoneurium conforms to the outer margin of the Schwann cell membrane and as such forms an **endoneurial tube,** which would remain patent if the axon and associated myelin sheath were removed.

Damage to a peripheral nerve can range from a temporary interruption of function, in which the axon and Schwann cell constituents are intact (neurapraxia), through interruption of the axon only, to severing of the entire peripheral nerve. To illustrate axon degeneration and repair, we will be using an example that is midway in this continuum—a crush injury that breaks the axons but leaves the endoneurial tubes intact. An even more desirable condition is set if the nerve is cleanly cut and then exactly repositioned, a distinct possibility with modern microsurgery.

Axon reaction is the term applied to changes that are seen in the neuron cell body (soma) within three days of the injury. The normal grainy appearance of the cytoplasm decreases (chromatolysis). This change is due to the dispersion and increased synthetic activity of protein-producing ribosomes preparatory to the repair process. As well, the nucleus swells and shifts out of its central position, and synaptic contacts from other neurons are withdrawn. The axon and its associated myelin sheath, for the whole length distal to the injury, begin simultaneous degeneration after about three days. This **wallerian degeneration** results in ellipsoids of myelin and axonal fragments that undergo rapid autolysis (self-digestion) and phagocytosis by macrophages normally resident in the endoneurium. At the same time, the myelin-free Schwann cells, which have contributed lysosomal enzymes to the breakdown process, multiply and fill the emptying endoneurial tube. After two weeks the process is complete and macrophages have withdrawn, leaving a Schwann-cell-filled endoneurial tube.

As soon as a day after severing, the end of the proximal section of axon, which has remained intact, begins sprouting. Effective regrowth occurs only in the environment of the Schwann cells, so the dominant sprout is drawn down the intact endoneurial tube to eventually reinnervate the appropriate end organ. Consult figure 21.6 for an overview of nerve degeneration and repair. The rate of regrowth varies with the nature of the injury and size of axon, but an average regeneration rate of about 1.5 mm per day is reasonable to expect.

In the adult central nervous system, the prospects of repair after a serious injury to neurons in the brain and spinal cord are very poor. Not only do the axons degenerate and not regrow distal to the point of injury, but most of their associated cell bodies will degenerate as well. Indeed, the preceding or subsequent neurons in a multineuron chain may also die back (processes called **retrograde** and **orthograde transneuronal degeneration,** respectively). Apparently neurons require functional interaction in the way of stimulation and the interchange of trophic (sustaining) factors to survive, in the same way that isolated muscle cells, having no workload, may atrophy and be replaced by fibrous connective tissue. The brain and spinal cord tracts (pathways) that are supplied by the degenerating neurons

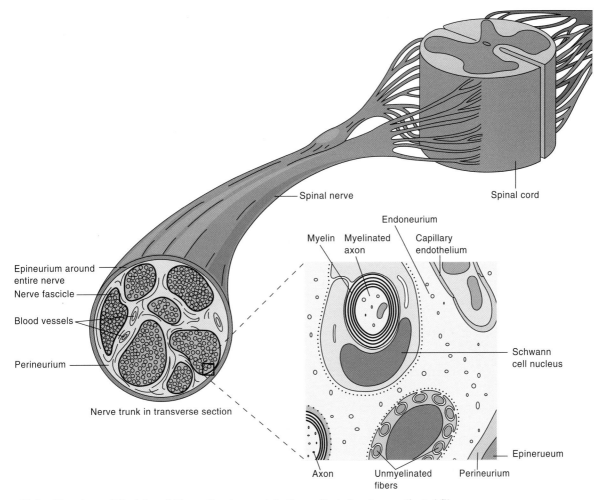

Figure 21.5   **Structure of Peripheral Nerve.** Inset presents both myelinated and unmyelinated fibers.

Focus on Neuron Regeneration within the CNS

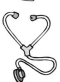

The arrangement of sense organs that are responsive to odors is intriguing in itself and of growing interest to researchers concerned with repair within the nervous system. The roof and adjacent walls of each nasal cavity bear a 2 cm² patch of olfactory epithelium that is populated by 5 million olfactory receptors. Each receptor has an elaborately ciliated end studded with specific odorant receptors that project into the nasal mucus. Odorant binding activates the associated axon that passes through the cribriform plate to synapse with the mitral cells of the olfactory bulb above, which, in turn, relays the signal directly to the olfactory centers of the brain. Unique among neurons, they are replaced every month or two by cells that arise from undifferentiated cells of the olfactory epithelium. Their axons make the relatively long (perhaps 1 cm) journey to the olfactory bulb,

which is within the central nervous system (as we have noted), and achieve appropriate synaptic association with unerring precision. This routine activity flies in the face of the unsuccessful struggle of severed nerve endings to make any progress in regrowth or reattachment in the CNS. These three qualities—replication, growth through the "hostile" environment of the CNS, and synaptic reconnection—are exciting the interest of researchers investigating CNS repair and regeneration. The cells that ensheath and guide the developing olfactory receptors, **olfactory ensheathing cells** (OECs), are the targets of interest. They have been transplanted into experimentally damaged rat spinal cord and have revived partial movement. They may also be helpful in repairing the persistently demyelinated plaques in multiple sclerosis (MS). OECs show more promise than peripheral Schwann cells, whose remyelinating and axonal regrowth contributions in the CNS have been disappointing.

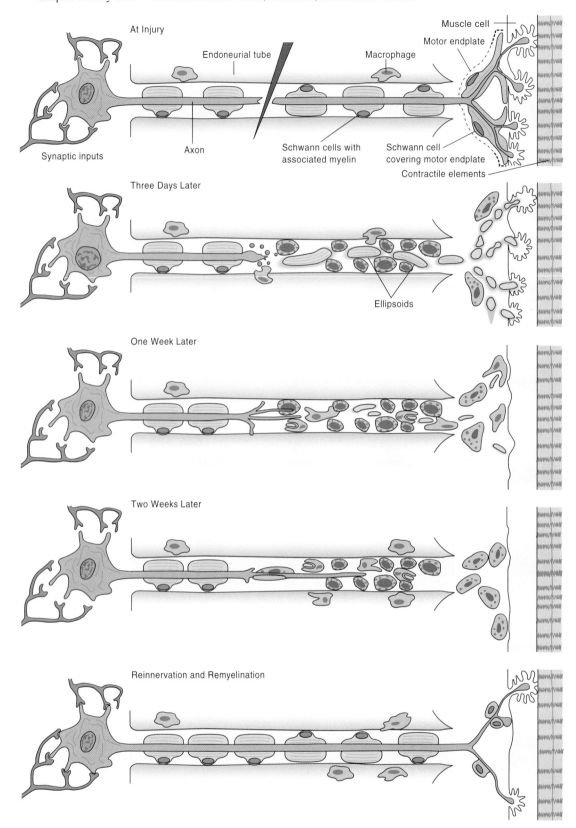

Figure 21.6 **Wallerian Degeneration and Peripheral Nerve Regeneration.** "Best-case scenario" is presented in which only severing of the axon has occurred. Resultant regrowth is perfect.

Focus on Crocodile Tears

Crush injuries result in slower sprouting but more effective reinnervation of end organs. If sensory axons sprout down a motor neuron tube, no reinnervation of the motor unit muscle fibers by the sensory axon will occur, although the abandoned fibers may be reinnervated by processes from an adjacent motor neuron. One patient, who in a fight had suffered traumatic separation of the facial nerve in its course through the cheek, developed a reversal of the expected pattern of innervation. When he was hungry and smelled food, his eyes teared up; when he was very sad, he salivated. This case of "crocodile tears" resulted from the growth of fibers normally associated with stimulation of the salivary glands into the lacrimal gland and vice versa.

Focus on Repair in the CNS

The failure of regrowth of axons in the CNS is a result of the unfavorable interaction between mature neurons and their microenvironment, formed principally by astrocytes and oligodendrocytes. Axonal growth proceeds as the molecules in the region of growth interact with molecules of the extracellular matrix in the presence of trophic factors such as neuron growth factor. Peripheral nerves that have been separated from their proximal axons create an environment favorable to axonal regrowth. This is partly due to the maintenance of a patent tube to guide the developing axon, but it appears to be mostly a result of trophic factors released by proliferating Schwann cells that fill the endoneurium. If a section of peripheral nerve is inserted into the spinal cord distal to severed motor neuron axons, axonal regrowth down this nerve will be rapid and effective. However, it will arrest as the normal cord environment is encountered. Active research proceeds into the trophic and extracellular matrix factors that might support CNS regrowth. For example, molecules given the eponym "NOGO" that are displayed on the outer surfaces of oligodendrocytes, including the myelin sheaths they produce, interact with receptors on the surface of severed axon's newly developing growth cone. Contact between the two immediately shuts down the extension of the growth cone, aborting axonal regeneration. Work is being done to interrupt the cellular signaling in the injured tissue, thereby allowing axons to bridge the gap and restore functional linkages.

The growth inhibition of the microenvironment appears to affect only mature neurons. Fetal neural tissue has been implanted into adult brains with apparently successful and appropriate axonal growth and synapse formation. Some patients with extreme parkinsonism (impoverished voluntary movement accompanied by resting tremor) have had extensive functional recovery after the midbrain implantation of fetal midbrain tissue. Scientific and ethical controversy surrounds these experiments. The use of autografts of tissue from the patient's own adrenal gland avoids these issues, as well as the prospect of tissue rejection (see focus box on OECs).

likewise atrophy, so the lesion may be apparent at some distance from its original source. A specimen of the spinal cord would have demonstrated atrophy in the opposite dorsolateral white matter, due to degeneration of the continuing fibers in the lateral corticospinal tract. (The term *lesion* is commonly used in neuropathology as a general term for some pathology that interferes with normal function. "Lesion" is also often used as a verb: for example, "The spinal cord was lesioned by the bone fragments.")

Recent discoveries have called these principles of retrograde and orthograde degeneration into question. Tetzlaff and co-workers at the University of British Columbia have demonstrated the long-term survival, in a dormant form, of cervical neurons whose processes were severed in the cord. Appropriate biochemical stimulation reactivated these neurons. Experimentation focusing on how to get them to grow functional connections with abandonded neurons proceeds at an intense rate.

Motor System Overview

The way a person moves voluntarily or in response to direct stimulation gives us a window into the integrity and state of functioning of that person's motor system and the sensory input necessary for its normal operation. When we tap the patellar tendon and elicit a knee jerk, we observe a fragment of an integrated motor system. The reaction we get (exaggerated, brisk, slow, reduced, absent), when put together with other relevant data, can tell us a lot about the general state of health, as well as the presence, location, and perhaps the nature of a lesion. By repeating our observations, we will have evidence as to whether the effects of the lesion are spreading. But, unlike the bits we regard as motor tests or signs, any adaptive movement involves the cooperative activation of diverse elements in the nervous system. Figure 21.7 presents a diagrammatic overview of

the elements involved in movement. These motor subsystems and a few of the important integrative pathways that connect them, including signs associated with their dysfunction, are the topic of this section.

A voluntary movement requires the cooperation of many interrelated centers and pathways. The intention is probably generated in widespread areas of the cortex that are not specifically dedicated to other functions. The intent is communicated to the caudate and putamen of the **basal ganglia,** which act like a sophisticated coach. The basal ganglia support behaviors that are likely to be on target— to produce rewards. These circuits run parallel to the cortical "intent" and facilitate or inhibit patterns of behavior by

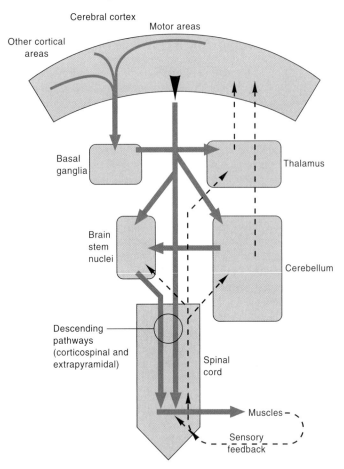

Figure 21.7 **Overview of Integrated Motor Function.** All elements are involved in any voluntary movement.

acting upon the thalamus. In this way, outflows from the basal ganglia are sent, via the thalamus, to an area called the **supplementary motor cortex** for review and editing. The cortex then imposes the motor program on the **primary motor cortex,** premotor cortex, and primary somatosensory cortex. These areas activate motor neurons in the **brain stem** and **spinal cord,** which in turn activate the muscles to produce the desired movement. The **cerebellum** acts to ensure that the desired movements occur smoothly in accordance with the motor programs. To do this, the cerebellum receives an ongoing copy of the motor program from the cortex. It runs a comparison between this and the actual movement as experienced in the muscles, tendons, and joints. This information is delivered to the cerebellum from these structures in an ongoing fashion so the comparison can take place and adjustments can be made in the expression of the motor program. The cerebellum alters the expression of the motor program by either reducing or increasing its inhibition of the brain stem motor nuclei, sort of like pushing or releasing the accelerator in a car. If the basal ganglia do not produce a functioning signal, as happens in Parkinson's disease, then thalamic facilitation of the cortex does not occur and movement is slowed or frozen.

Lower Motor Neurons

The cells that are attached to and activate skeletal muscles have their cell bodies in the anterior horn of gray matter in the spinal cord. They are variously called **anterior horn cells, motor neurons, alpha motor neurons,** and **lower motor neurons** to distinguish them from the fibers that connect them to the brain and brain stem. Their axons pass through the ventral root and out along the peripheral nerves, then branch and innervate the muscle cells with which they are associated. A motor neuron and the group of muscle cells it innervates are called a **motor unit.** It is these motor neuron cell bodies that are susceptible to attack by polio viruses.

The following clinical features are observed when lower motor neurons are injured. Muscle tone is reduced or absent and the muscle is paralyzed **(flaccid paralysis).** The absence or scarcity of motor neurons disrupts both voluntary movement and the expression of normal reflexes. For this reason, tendon jerks are weak or absent. Muscles supplied by the lesioned motor nerves atrophy rapidly **(neurogenic atrophy)** because they are deprived of stimulation and normal trophic factors. Tiny, spontaneous electrical discharges called **fibrillation potentials** will be noted within days of the denervation, using special electrodiagnostic techniques. Later, visible uncoordinated twitching and wriggling may be noticed in the denervated muscle. These are called **fasciculations.**

Healthy lower motor neurons in the vicinity of the denervated muscle cells may gradually reinnervate the denervated cells. These enlarged motor units are not capable of producing the finely graduated force generation characteristic of the original motor unit pool. As well, expansion of the motor unit taxes the motor neuron, making it susceptible to fatigue. In the case of polio, the phenomena of postpolio syndrome may be observed (see the focus box on polio).

Spinal Mechanisms

A great deal of important motor behavior is mediated in the spinal cord itself. Reflexive withdrawal from pain stimuli (heat, prick, etc.) can involve one or many integrated segments of the cord. The withdrawal is initiated before a person is consciously aware of the pain. **Tendon reflexes (myotatic stretch reflexes)** result when the action potentials generated in stretch sensors within the muscle pass into the cord, where they synapse with the large motor neurons in the anterior horn. These, in turn, will depolarize and pass an impulse to the stretched muscle, causing it to contract reflexively. The functional significance of these stretch reflexes is that they are in place to maintain adaptive muscle tone (tension). Upright posture is maintained, to an extent, by the unconscious action of these reflexes. They are also involved in complex ways with activities like walking, swimming, and so forth. Later we give some detail regarding the variety of motor reflexes that mature into function and then are "overridden" through the mastery of

Focus on Polio Victims Facing a Whole New Battle

Thousands of polio victims around the world who survived prevaccine epidemics of the crippling disease are battling a cruel second coming of problems.

Experts studying the syndrome agree it is not a recurrence of the actual polio virus. The syndrome is characterized by an onset of fatigue, pain, and muscle weakness caused by failing nerve cells that have been working overtime for 30 years or more to compensate for the damage done by the original disease.

In Canada and the United States, as many as a third of the polio victims who survived post-WWII epidemics of the disease are believed at risk for developing postpolio syndrome.

There are 55 clinics and 200 support groups in the United States devoted to the problem, in addition to another 50 support groups in Canada, Europe, Australia, New Zealand, and parts of Asia, says the International Polio Network in St. Louis.

"Fatigue seems to be one thing a lot of people are concerned about. People talk about the 'polio wall'—they hit it at maybe 3 in the afternoon and it's not just being tired. It's definite fatigue."

The syndrome is not life-threatening but it can be incapacitating.

---

voluntary movement (see table 21.10 for a reasonable catalogue). For now, it is enough to know that the adult cord and brain stem retain all the reflex structures that successively emerge as the newborn passes to young childhood. Walking provides a good synopsis. We consciously "intend" to walk at the broad cortical level. Signals are sent to a center in the dorsal midbrain (the **mesencephalic locomotor region**), which then generates a rhythmic gait (lower limb movements and arm swing) by "releasing" the integrated alternation of **central program pattern generators** associated with each of the limbs. These generators operate without sensory feedback from the limbs. The cortex monitors the success and appropriateness of the walking and intervenes when appropriate, perhaps a little faster and with more force when we are walking up a hill. The cortex is freed to do what it does best—that is, "think"—because of the smooth functioning of lower centers that, for the most part, operate without conscious awareness.

The functioning of the stretch reflexes can be isolated for diagnostic purposes. Tapping the tendon of a muscle rapidly stretches the muscle and initiates the events just described. The reflex reaction is reflected in joint movement or tensing of the muscle. **Hyporeflexia** indicates a weaker response than normal. This may be due to muscle weakness, damage to the stretch sensors, some impairment at the cord, or lesion of the motor neurons themselves. If the hy-

 Focus on the Dance with Madame Guillotine!

The following gruesome anecdote gives a dramatic illustration of the elicitation of spinal reflexes. The early days of the French Revolution were made monstrous, even by revolutionary standards, by the rush to execute the aristocracy by whatever means fell to hand. Improvised executions, very low-tech indeed, included smashing heads into walls, "defenestration" (people were flung out of windows), and smothering. Some "corpses" were found to still be alive, initiating another bout of savage execution. Out of his concern for the suffering of people he regarded as just as human as their executioners, Dr. J. I. Guillotin invented his famous instrument for humane execution. At first, the condemned were simply asked to place their necks beneath the suspended blade with no other preparation. The blade dropped. The headless body lurched upright, and sometimes staggered into the witnessing crowd, encountered a horrified peasant, and momentarily locked him in embrace: the legendary *Dance with Madame Guillotine!* An explanation for this complex series of behaviors lies in our understanding of action potential physiology and the presence in the cord of many centers for patterned reflex activity. Severing the spinal cord exposed the open ends of axons to the sodium-rich extracellular environment. Influx of sodium ions initiated action potentials that propagated down the cord, triggering a burst of activity in reflex centers and the central motor program generators associated with each limb—hence, the crude walking (leg straightening and stepping reflexes and patterned walking). Stimulation of the ventral surface elicited dormant but intact startle and grasping reflexes—hence, the embrace with the hapless spectator. Those of you who have some experience on a farm when its time to get the main ingredient for chicken pie may have seen similar behavior. The secret of the cord's subtle combination of persistent reflex structures and voluntary functional overrides is thus exposed for view. With experience, the executioners learned to tie the feet and hands of victims—at least easier on the crowd, if not the royalty.

---

poreflexia is exhibited bilaterally, we might suspect generalized depression of nerve function, perhaps due to electrolyte imbalance.

Hyperreflexia is an exaggeration of reflex response. This is seen transitorily in a very nervous individual as a normal facet of generalized nervous system activation. It emerges gradually as a pathological condition in individuals with significant damage to the motor neurons from the brain and brain stem to the anterior horn cells—for instance, in people with spinal cord injury. The intensification of reflex response can be extreme.

Areflexia is the absence of reflex action. This is seen in the posttrauma period for people with acute, complete spinal cord lesion. It appears to be due to the loss of the facilitating influence of upper motor neurons upon segmental reflex mechanisms. It is gradually replaced with normal reflexes if the lesion resolves or with hyperreflexia if it does not. It should be stressed that these spinal reflexes operate at the level of the cord under the facilitating or inhibiting influence of (particularly) descending motor impulses. Even if the cord above the specific segment has been completely destroyed, the basic neural machinery necessary to generate reflex actions can remain fully intact and functioning.

Cord Pathways (Upper Motor Neurons)

You may note, in figure 21.7, that there are two descending (upper motor neuron) pathways. The one that starts at the cerebral cortex (at the precentral gyrus) is called the **corticospinal tract** (origin—cortex, destination—anterior horn cells in the spinal cord). It is also called the **pyramidal tract** because most of its fibers cross over below two pyramid-shaped areas at the front of the medulla. Fibers course from the primary motor area, through the internal capsule (an extensive band of projection fibers communicating between the cerebral hemispheres and lower brain centers; see fig. 20.21b), through the midbrain and pons. Most decussate (cross over) below the medullary pyramids and then continue down the dorsolateral white matter in the cord (corticospinal tract) to finally enter the cord gray matter and synapse in the anterior horn. This tract is responsible for finely controlled movements, particularly of the hands and feet.

The other pathway (actually several distinct pathways) is called the **extrapyramidal,** or **multineuronal, tract.** These cord fibers originate in certain brain stem nuclei that are the target of motor impulses that arise in the cortex, particularly from the area anterior to the primary motor cortex. The cortical inputs activate or inhibit these brain stem nuclei, which in turn influence the alpha motor neurons. The extrapyramidal fibers are responsible for maintaining balance, adjusting to changes in position, and orienting to visual and auditory stimuli. As well, they mediate repetitive rhythmic movements (walking, bicycling, etc.) and maintain posture. They are particularly focused on proximal and axial musculature. In a sense they provide the background activity that makes possible the effective execution of the fine motor activities that are the domain of the corticospinal pathways. Figure 21.8 shows the origin, course, and destination of the pyramidal and extrapyramidal tracts.

Lesions of the upper motor neurons will give rise to the following clinical features. Voluntary movements of the affected muscles are absent or weak, while the tone of the muscles is increased. This is known as **spastic paralysis.** Normal stretch reflex arcs are intact and may become stronger, perhaps because of the formation of additional synapses. Tendon reflexes are increased (the **hyperreflexia** already noted). When the examiner attempts to passively extend a flexed joint, the limb at first resists extension and then suddenly relaxes **(clasp-knife rigidity).** Muscle atrophy is slow and not complete **(disuse atrophy)** as a result of the

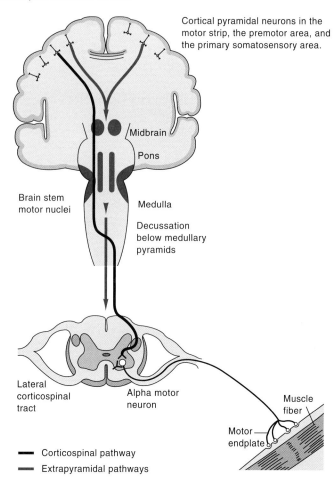

Cortical pyramidal neurons in the motor strip, the premotor area, and the primary somatosensory area.

Midbrain

Pons

Brain stem motor nuclei

Medulla

Decussation below medullary pyramids

Lateral corticospinal tract

Alpha motor neuron

Muscle fiber

Motor endplate

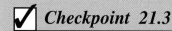 Corticospinal pathway
Extrapyramidal pathways

Figure 21.8 **Anatomical Pathways Involved in the Corticospinal (or Pyramidal) and Extrapyramidal Motor Systems.**

continued release of trophic factors and reflex stimulation of muscles. Abnormal plantar reflex **(Babinski sign)** is observed (see table 20.3). The Babinski sign in a person with cerebral trauma indicates that the upper motor neuron pathways are functionally (and perhaps structurally) disrupted.

✓ Checkpoint 21.3

To focus on the essential differences between the effects of damage to a lower motor neuron as opposed to those of an upper motor neuron, reduce the foregoing two sections to a simple table.

Brain Stem Motor Nuclei

Four distinct sets of nuclei in the brain stem mediate motor behavior via the extrapyramidal system (as just described). The precise location of a lesion within this relatively small area (about 1½ inches long) will have a profound effect on motor behavior. If it occurs very high, where the upper motor neurons traveling in the internal capsule enter the midbrain, the person, who is probably in a state of coma, will react to intense stimulation with decorticate rigidity, described in more detail in the section on coma (see chapter 20). A lesion ½ inch lower, which will isolate the top pair of nuclei plus the cortex, will produce decerebrate rigidity (see table 20.3). (See table 21.2 and figure 21.8 for the function and location of the following nuclei.)

The **red nuclei** (one on either side of the midbrain) are the origin of the **rubrospinal tracts.** These are apparently not of great functional significance in humans and appear to act in much the same way as the pyramidal tracts (activating distal, precisely controlled musculature). In animals, stimulation produces a powerful upper limb flexion and lower limb extension. This is suspiciously like what happens when someone with hemiplegia from a stroke attempts to walk: Their paralyzed arm flexes and their poorly controlled foot extends, making walking even more of a challenge. A stroke isolates or impairs the communication between the cortex and the red nuclei. Likewise, in the evolution of a generalized tonic clonic seizure, during the period of cortical disorganization, there is a brief "hands-up" arm flexion (similar to the decorticate rigidity just described)—more evidence for the involvement of the red nuclei.

This flexion phase of the seizure is followed by a powerful arm and leg extension (extensor phase), reminiscent of decerebrate rigidity, before the beginning of the clonic phase of the convulsion. This activity is similar to that produced by stimulating the **vestibular nuclei** that lie at the junction of the pons and medulla. These are the origin of a second set of extrapyramidal pathways, the **vestibulospinal tracts.** The normal function of this pathway is to produce relatively automatic adjustments of the whole body to changes in balance, posture, limb extension, and so forth. Movements, whether voluntary or externally generated, produce displacements in the semicircular canals and vestibular organs. These generate patterns of stimulation of the vestibular nuclei that reflexively produce compensatory movements to maintain balance and effective posture. Like all brain stem nuclei, these can be brought under voluntary control via the extrapyramidal pathways from the cortex. This occurs when we perform a task that requires these sorts of adjustments—dancing, for example.

The posterior midbrain, the **tectum,** houses two other sets of nuclei that are origins of another extrapyramidal pathway, the **tectospinal tracts.** The **superior colliculi** are the site of reflex orienting to visual stimuli. Stimuli in the periphery of the visual fields have a powerful capacity to "make" us look at them. Large-screen, Omnimax-type films with their intense clarity can produce enough reflex "pulling" of the eyes to make one nauseous. **Reflex orienting** involves turning the eyes, head, neck, and trunk toward the stimulus to better meet whatever challenge it might present. (Think of the last time you were aware that someone was looking at you even though the person was on the edge of your peripheral vision.) This area is also involved in fixating the gaze on a single target to produce a clear image on the retinae. The **inferior colliculi** manage the same responses to auditory stimuli. The adaptive advantage of quickly seeing what's making that sound is obvious.

The reticular activating system is an extensively branched meshwork ("reticulum") of neurons in the core of the entire brain stem. As well as mediating level of consciousness and cortical arousal, these neurons receive inputs from most of the axons that pass through the brain stem. This neural traffic has a role in consciousness and arousal (more in chapter 22), but is also has a motor function. An organism that is being bombarded by stimuli—for example, when it is under attack or in some intense social encounter—might usually benefit by being quicker in its reactions. This enhanced reactivity is accomplished by the **reticulospinal pathway.** A wide variety of information, from pain (see chapter 23) or intense visual or auditory stimuli to forceful muscular contractions, will "turn up" the activity in this system and thereby the reactivity of the motor neuron. Reticulospinal axons are one of the many inputs to the alpha motor neurons. Increased stimulation to the dendrites, while not sufficient by itself to cause the motor neuron to fire, will bring the entire field closer to depolarizing. In this context, an input that would have been insufficient on its own to cause a signal to the muscle, will achieve muscular contraction. Likewise, a signal that would have produced a weak contraction will elicit a powerful one. This can be demonstrated through the **Jendrassik's maneuver.** Test the knee-jerk reflex of a willing subject by tapping the patellar tendon and noting the rapidity and extent of foot swing. Next, get them to link their fingers in front of their chest and pull forcefully (Jendrassik's maneuver) while you repeat the same force to evoke a knee jerk. You should note a brisker and more exaggerated reflex. The enhancement of motor reactivity produced by chronic pain might be noted if we inadvertently bumped an old, apparently enfeebled, arthritic dog to find it flash around and nip us. The vestibulospinal, tectospinal, and reticulospinal pathways innervate principally proximal and truncal musculature, whereas the rubrospinal innervates mainly distal musculature. And a reminder: While these systems can be under significant unconscious or reflex control, they are all capable of being brought under voluntary control. In fact, it is hard to imagine a voluntary movement using the pyramidal tract—for example, writing—that doesn't involve the collaboration of most of these extrapyramidal pathways.

Cerebellum

The cerebellum mediates the coordinated contractions of agonist and antagonist muscles to produce a smooth, well-controlled movement **(synergy).** As well, it is significant in maintaining appropriate **muscle tone,** the slight constant tension of healthy muscles such that they offer modest resistance to movement when moved passively. In brief, the cerebellum performs these roles in the following way (fig. 21.9). When a motor activity is "decided upon" by the cortex, a copy of the motor plan is sent to the cerebellum, while the

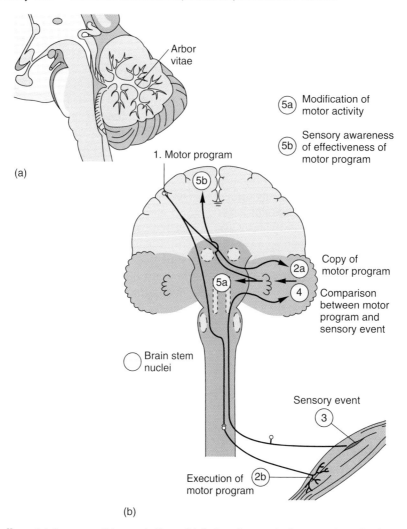

Figure 21.9   **The Cerebellum.** (*a*) Anatomy of the cerebellum. (*b*) Order of events in the execution of voluntary movement.

various brain stem nuclei and the alpha motor neurons receive the original. The motor units react by executing the directions from the corticospinal and extrapyramidal tracts. Information about how much movement of muscles and joints actually took place is fed back from the stretch, tendon, and joint capsule receptors to the sensory cortex (awareness of movement) and unconsciously to the cerebellum (via the ascending pathways shown in figure 21.7). The cerebellum is essentially a very elaborate on-line computer (it has as many nerve cells as the much larger cerebrum), and it does a comparison between what was expected and what was delivered. If there was either too much or too little movement, the cerebellum discharges to the appropriate cortical and brain stem areas to correct the error. This activity is very rapid and continually ongoing. Figure 21.9 summarizes cerebellar function and illustrates its anatomy.

The cerebellum mediates the smooth acceleration and then rapid deceleration characteristic of natural movements, whether of the limbs, voice, or eyes. Because it is particularly active in acceleration, deceleration, and arrest, func-

tional deficits show up most dramatically in these phases of movement. Lesions to the cerebellum may produce any of the clinical signs or symptoms indicated in table 21.4.

Basal Ganglia

The **basal ganglia** are nuclei of gray matter deep within the cerebrum. The term *basal ganglia* is actually a misnomer. A more accurate term might be *basal nuclei* or *cerebral nuclei*. Unfortunately, the older term still has predominance in medical circles.

The role of the basal ganglia has long been a neurological puzzle. Destruction of a tiny portion, such as the substantia nigra in Parkinson's disease, can be utterly disabling. But this disability can sometimes be ameliorated or reversed by further, deliberate lesions to other parts such as the subthalamic nucleus or related thalamic nuclei. The basal ganglia appear to work like a very effective coach. The athlete (the cortex in this case) is always responsible for the action. But the coach (the basal ganglia) focuses attention on the patterns of behavior that are most likely to

Table 21.4   Terminology Describing Signs and Symptoms Associated with Cerebellar Injury

Past-pointing: When rapidly reaching out to touch an object, the person overshoots the mark. The test for this may be to get the person to touch, in rapid alteration, her nose and your fingertip held 18 inches away.

Intention tremor: This tremor emerges during the execution of movement. As the limb reaches the end of its planned movement (say, to pick up a cup of tea), the tremor, which was present during movement, worsens, giving rise to the term **terminal tremor.**

Hypotonia: Muscle tone is abnormally weak.

Dysdiadochokinesia: Rapidly alternating movements (like patting the thighs with palms up and then palms down) are difficult or impossible.

Ataxia: Lack of coordination in movement, expressed in clumsiness, lack of precision.

Gait ataxia: Gait is characterized by a wide stance and unsteady walking ("drunken sailor" gait).

Dysarthria: Difficulty in speaking. With cerebellar lesions the result is sometimes called "scanning speech" because it resembles the struggles of someone who is having trouble reading out loud and develops a sing-song, emotionless sort of rhythm.

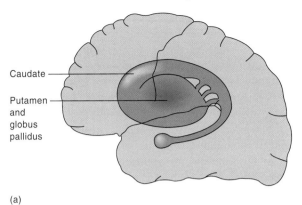

(a)

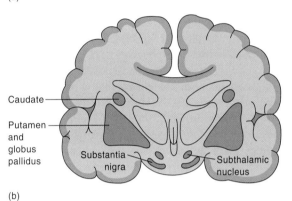

(b)

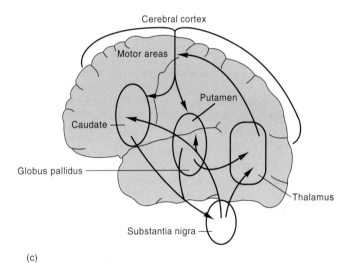

(c)

Figure 21.10   **Basal Ganglia Structures (*a* and *b*) and Functional Interrelationships (*c*).**

pay off or succeed, and helps trace a path through the infinite set of possibilities to the successful mastery of the overhand smash or the slide into third base. Although our attention will focus on the role of the basal ganglia in movement, there is a parallel processing of both cognitive and limbic system functions as well. This puts the basal ganglia in a linch-pin position in every significant operation of the brain, except perhaps lower-level homeostatic functions such as maintenance of temperature and blood osmolarity. And even these can be affected by stress and emotion, the domain of the limbic system, which, in turn, depends on the basal ganglia.

As far as is now known, the intention to move is formed diffusely at the cortex (particularly in the frontal lobes) and is communicated to the functionally integrated, yet physically divided, **caudate** and **putamen,** together called the **neostriatum** (fig. 21.10). The neostriatum, in turn, interacts with three other nuclei of the basal ganglia: the **globus pallidus** (called the **paleostriatum**); the **subthalamic nucleus;** and the dopamine-producing **substantia nigra** of the midbrain. Final output from the basal ganglia is directed through the substantia nigra and the globus pallidus to certain nuclei of the thalamus. These project *their* output to the **supplementary motor area,** back at the cortex. After processing here, these signals travel to the premotor, primary motor, and somatosensory areas, which are the origin of activity in the pyramidal and extrapyramidal

pathways, producers of the actual movements. The sequenced pattern of basal ganglia stimulation of the thalamus releases sequentially programmed patterns of movement from the motor areas of the cortex.

People who have lesions in the outflow nuclei of the basal ganglia (e.g., parkinsonism) have immense difficulty initiating movements. From this clinical finding, neurologists had formerly attributed initiation of movement to the basal ganglia. In fact, "facilitation," in the sense of coaching that has been described, is a more accurate description. Knocking out the substantia nigra removes the facilitating effect on the thalamus and leaves an indirect, inhibitory link involving the subthalamic nucleus intact. This locks in the motor programs of the cortex, preventing the normal cortical initiation of movement that always runs parallel to the activity of the basal ganglia. The behavior of "frozen addicts" illustrates the profound impact of lesions of the substantia nigra. These were a number of people discovered in San Francisco after taking illicit "designer" drugs inadvertently contaminated with the substantia nigra-specific toxin MPTP. Some were so disabled that they appeared to be comatose. In fact, they were fully alert with normal sensation—they were simply incapable of voluntary movement. Amazingly, if lifted to their feet and supported, they could walk, zombielike, between two attendants, stopping as soon as this outer impetus was removed.

Basal ganglia (fig. 21.10) lesions produce a very different pattern of clinical signs from those associated with cerebellar injury. A major disabling condition is **bradykinesia.** This is a general impoverishment of movement, in which the person finds it very difficult to initiate movement. **Tardive dyskinesia** (by definition, a slowly developing impairment of movement) is, however, the most prevalent disorder due to lesion of the basal ganglia. The lesions causing tardive dyskinesia usually arise from excess prolonged use of medications like tricyclic antidepressants. The person makes involuntary writhing movements of the face, tongue, head, and neck and may pull up the knees while sitting. It is often associated with dystonia, frozen movement.

Dystonia is second only to parkinsonism in the number of cases seen in movement disorder clinics. It apparently arises because of an imbalance in the subtle interplay of neurotransmitters (glutamate, dopamine, acetylcholine, norepinephrine, GABA) in the basal ganglia. It is more common in middle age, but may strike at any time. The earlier the age of onset, the more severe the progression and the more likely the spread to other parts of the body. An afflicted person experiences an involuntary drive in a muscle group that may be intermittent or continuous. This may result in a wry neck **(torticollis),** a twisted trunk, writer's cramp, and so on. The larynx may be involved, leading to whispering, breathy speech—the speaker often running out of air. Tremor, which can affect the limbs, may also be seen in the vocal cords, leading to a tremulous voice. The most severe form, Oppenhein dystonia, can progress to fixed torsion of the neck and trunk with limb flexion, which becomes reinforced over time by contractures. The genetic cause of this form has been established. Another form of childhood-onset autosomal dominant heritable dystonia, dopa-responsive dystonia (DRD), responds very well to medication. Although the cause of dystonia is not in the muscle or the neuromuscular junction, as is the case in most cramping, the preferred treatment focuses at this level. Tiny injections of botulinum toxin ("Botox" or "Myobloc") are made into the area of the motor endplate in the affected muscle. This toxin binds irreversibly to acetylcholine receptors and blocks muscle response to neural activation. Subsequent muscle atrophy weakens the force generated in the muscle sufficiently to relieve the dystonia. This is usually not effective in treating tremor of either the limbs or voice.

Resting tremor, a steady, slow (4 per second), involuntary tremor, is a common symptom. What differentiates this from the intention or terminal tremor of a cerebellar lesion is that it is repressed during voluntary movements. Many individuals develop strategies to make this resting tremor less noticeable. It is also absent in sleep.

Chorea (rapid, flicklike movements of the wrists and hands and face) and **athetosis** (slow, writhing movements of fingers and hands and sometimes the toes, feet, and proximal parts of the limbs, and even the face) are also found in people affected by diseases of the basal ganglia. As well, there may be a distinctive form of rigidity **(lead-pipe rigidity)** that presents a steady, exaggerated resistance to passive movement. Another possible effect is **cogwheel rigidity,** in which the flexed limb provides a rhythmically interrupted, ratchetlike resistance to extension.

A dramatic form of explosive involuntary movement may be observed in people who suffer a lesion, usually vascular, to the region of the small subthalamic nucleus. The limbs may be intermittently and violently flung outward without warning. These movements are called **ballisms,** and the most usual pattern is for one of the two nuclei to be affected, producing hemiballismus. The condition is usually transitory.

Before we leave this material, we should mention a form of tremor that may be mistaken for parkinsonian tremor, but derives from the "exposure" of the natural rhythmicity upon which much nervous system function appears to depend. We are speaking of **essential tremor** (or **familial tremor**). The former is probably the more accurate name, as many people experience this condition without any known family predisposition. We are talking about a fast (8 to 12 Hz) tremor of the arms and hands that is seen during movement and when a position is held, but is rarely seen at rest (in contrast to the tremor of Parkinson disease). This tremor sometimes makes bringing a drink to the lips a very unproductive activity. It can also involve the head and voice and, rarely, the legs. Most of us have experienced the situational emergence of this same tremor when we were nervous, underslept, or had overindulged in coffee or alcohol. In the present case, it is much more pronounced and far less "symptomatic." It is presently thought that essential tremor results from an exaggeration of an otherwise normal oscillation of signals between the cerebellum and a nucleus in the medulla called the **inferior olivary nucleus.** People with the condition may feel the need to reassure others that they are not nervous, etc. Most just live with it. Some want or badly require treatment, which is variably effective. It includes the use of beta-blockers and/or anticonvulsants, thalamic stimulation using implanted, deep thalamic electrodes, and limited thalamic lesions. Interestingly, drinking alcohol often temporarily abolishes the tremor.

Checkpoint 21.4

The symptoms of damage to the basal ganglia contrast nicely in many ways with those associated with the cerebellum. Describe how!

Thalamus

The thalamus is the part of the CNS through which all sensation except smell and all information about the form or results of movement are channeled. Small lesions here can produce many of the signs associated with cerebellar or basal ganglia dysfunction by interrupting the relay of signals from these systems. However, this sort of tiny focal lesion is very unusual. As just mentioned, the thalamus can be the target of treatments to address a variety of disorders.

Internal Capsule

As noted, the internal capsule is the major pathway for motor information flowing out from the cortex and for sensory and sensory-motor information flowing in. The effect of lesions here, which may be caused by trauma, vascular disorder, or toxin, depends on the position and extent of the lesion. **Locked-in syndrome** involves the functional or structural interruption of just the motor pathways and renders a person totally paralyzed except for the respiratory muscles, which are innervated spontaneously further down the brain stem. This person will have intact sensation and normal consciousness but complete paralysis of voluntary movement. The cause of locked-in syndrome might be the advanced progression of amyotrophic lateral sclerosis, a disease affecting both upper motor neurons traveling in the internal capsule, and lower motor neurons resident in the ventral gray matter of the cord.

Cerebral Cortex

The functions of the primary motor cortex and the premotor cortex have already been described. Lesions restricted to the motor cortex are rare. Usually a broader territory is involved, perhaps including some basal ganglia and part of the internal capsule or the underlying white matter. Given this background, we can describe some classic syndromes that include the motor cortex. **Hemiplegia** is paralysis restricted to the half of the body contralateral (on the opposite side) to the site of the lesion. The paralysis, since it is arising from an upper motor neuron lesion, will be spastic (rigid or hyperreflexive). As has been noted, because brain stem nuclei are isolated from cortical modulation, the person will assume a classic hemiplegic stance: The hand, wrist, and elbow are flexed and the toe is extended. This is reminiscent

of a unilateral decorticate rigidity (see chapter 20) and may be based on the same neural mechanisms. Hemiplegia would result if all the motor fibers in one internal capsule were disrupted. As well, a person would be functionally hemiplegic if the lateral precentral gyrus were lesioned, say by occlusion of the middle cerebral artery.

If the ischemia was on the language-dominant hemisphere (the left for most people), the person would most likely have a deficit in the ability to form and enunciate words—**productive aphasia,** specifically Broca's aphasia. There may also be a difficulty in finding the words to express the ideas in the first place—another form of productive and often receptive aphasia called **Wernicke's aphasia.** (**Receptive aphasia** implies a difficulty in comprehending written or spoken language.) Broca's area and Wernicke's area are identified in figure 20.19 in chapter 20.

Monoplegia (paralysis of only one extremity) could result from a very small lesion in the lateral precentral gyrus, in which case it could paralyze the arm and perhaps half the face (contralateral to the lesion). More probably the monoplegia is due to an interruption to the territory of the anterior cerebral artery deep in the longitudinal fissure, in which case the contralateral leg will be the area most affected by the paralysis. Bladder and bowel control would also be reduced.

Extensive diffuse injury of the cerebral cortex, as may occur in diffuse arteriosclerosis or Alzheimer's disease, can give rise to a strange form of rigidity called **gegenhalten** (German for "counter pull" or "hold against"). In this case, when a limb is passively moved, it gives an apparently willed resistance or opposition quite different from lead-pipe or clasp-knife rigidity. What appears to be happening is that the person, because of extensive cortical damage, can't cooperatively relax the limb.

Diagnosis in Movement Disorders

Something should be said about the diagnostic techniques commonly used to differentiate between the disorders that can affect movement. Degeneration of numbers of muscle fibers will release abnormal amounts of intracellular enzymes into the plasma, and these can be detected. For example, elevated creatine kinase is found in Duchenne-type muscular dystrophy. Electrical properties, assessed by inserting needle electrodes into muscle, give a variety of suggestive if nonspecific clues to the status of the muscle tissue and the health of its nervous supply. **Electromyography** (EMG) focuses on the muscle's response to needle insertion or movement (electrical activity should be crisp and brief), ongoing spontaneous activity (should be essentially electrically silent), the summed activity of a motor neuron and the hundreds of muscle fibers it supplies (the motor unit potential), and the massed activity that a person is able to induce voluntarily with varying effort (recruitment pattern). Muscle biopsies, which extract a tiny core of tissue,

Table 21.5   Assessment of Disorders of Movement

Note: In the assessment and diagnosis of movement disorders, few signs or symptoms are pathognomonic for a specific disease (i.e., symptoms associated with that, and only that, disease). One looks for patterns of signs and symptoms and other diagnostic findings to identify the disorder and determine what other signs and symptoms one might expect.

Visible or Palpable Signs

- Wasting (rapid versus slow; location) as opposed to hypertrophy or pseudohypertrophy
- Deformities of limbs, joints, trunk: e.g., **Charcot's joint** (neurogenic joint degeneration) due to failure to hold the joint in a physiologic position during movement because of muscle weakness and impaired sensation, latter also impairs protective feedback from the joint; e.g., **contractures** due to sustained limb position and formation of collagen cross-linkages that limits voluntary or passive movement (main or pied en griffe, talipes eqinovarus, etc.)
- Postural changes: stooped posture, sustained flexion or extension of limb, transitory twisting of trunk, neck, etc.
- Tremoring: resting, during movement
- Abnormal muscle tone: increased, decreased
- Apparent to patient: fatiguability, lack of energy, malaise, pain, parasthesias

Abnormalities of Force Generation or Relaxation

- Weakness: not necessarily universal, general versus diffuse, proximal versus distal
- Abnormalities of tone during passive movement: spasticity (resistance to movement related to rate of speed of movement; e.g., clasp-knife rigidity); rigidity (not related to joint angle or speed of movement, bidirectional; e.g., lead-pipe rigidity, cogwheel rigidity, gegenhalten); flaccidity (limb floppy)
- Fatiguability of muscle group: rapid in MG, increased force generation with repeated attempts in Lambert-Eaton, slow during the day in MG, very gradual in many disorders, exacerbating and remitting in inflammatory disorders and MS

Laboratory Findings

- Muscle enzymes in plasma in abnormal amounts related to muscle injury, inflammation, or degeneration. Isoform in myocardial infarction CK-MB (creatine kinase-heart form), in skeletal muscle injury, CK-MM (creatine kinase-muscle form). Presence depends upon a relatively intense process.
- Nerve conduction velocity studies indicate function in the peripheral nerve, mainly reflects function of large, well-myelinated axons (αmn, primary spindle afferents).
- Muscle biopsies: core of muscle is extracted in a large bore needle, examined using stains. Observation include variability in size of fibers, wasting, hypertrophy, patterns of type 1 versus type 2 distribution, abnormal constituents (fat cells; fibroblasts; hyalinized, amyloid-containing cells; inflammatory cells like lymphocytes or macrophages).
- Electromyography: expect insertional activity (injury potential, discharge when needle is inserted or moved) to be brief (1/10 sec) and "crisp"; expect spontaneous activity to be nonexistent (normal muscle is essentially electrically silent unless sampling near a neuromuscular junction); motor unit potential (electrical activity of the cells of one activated motor unit within the field of the needle; about 20 cells) of expected amplitude and duration, triphasic; interference pattern (summated activity in muscle under conditions of minimal to maximal voluntary recruitment) to be dense of appropriate amplitude.

are done to examine the tissue microscopically. Studies of nerve conduction velocities can localize slowing or loss of signal strength in a peripheral nerve. And sensory-evoked potentials can follow a peripherally generated signal to its destination in the primary somatosensory cortex of the contralateral hemisphere. Table 21.5 summarizes the assessment of disorders of movement.

IMPAIRED MOVEMENT THAT RESULTS FROM DISORDERS OF MUSCLE, NEUROMUSCULAR JUNCTION, NERVE, OR SPINAL CORD

The following disorders produce muscular weakness as their primary disability. If this occurs during musculoskeletal development, extreme joint deformities may develop along with the major disturbances of movement, including gait or grasp. In the adult frame, generalized or focal weakness can lead to less severe but recognizable limb or joint distortions. If a sensory deficit accompanies or causes the motor disability, neurogenic joint degeneration (called **Charcot's joint**) may occur. This is partly because the joint isn't held in the physiologic orientation for which it was designed. It is also probably due to increased wear and tear that ensues when normal sensation, including pain, is lost. The sensory phenomena that may accompany these disorders will be variable. In some cases, Duchenne-type muscular dystrophy—for example, ongoing pain—is not characteristic; on the other hand, in polymyositis about half of those afflicted experience significant pain. Motor deficits with a sensory component may produce a variety of sensory abnormalities, as detailed in table 23.4 in chapter 23.

Table 21.6	Disorders of Muscle Tissue (Primary Myopathies)

Dystrophies

DUCHENNE MUSCULAR DYSTROPHY—Transmission: X-linked recessive, almost all affected are males. Disease apparent by 2–5 years; begins with hip girdle weakness (waddling gait); weakness and wasting; rapidly progressive; death usual before 25 years. **Gower's sign** is a characteristic maneuver used to overcome weakness to get up from the ground: roll, over to kneel, push down on the ground with the forearms to straighten legs then "walk" up the legs to assume a standing posture. Cardiomyopathy often present. Elevated CK mm in patients; as many as 90% of adolescent female carriers have elevated CK mm. Also called pseudohypertrophic dystrophy because 80% show enlargement, particularly of calf, due to fibrosis and fat. Primary defect is in the failure to produce a cytoskeletal protein, **dystrophin,** normally associated with plasma membrane glycoproteins that secure it to the laminin protein on the outside surface of the muscle fiber. The membrane is therefore less stable and able to resist the forces generated in contraction, and the damage permits the entrance of excess calcium, which leads to excitotoxic injury to the muscle fiber. Eventually cell death ensues.

BECKER MUSCULAR DYSTROPHY—Same inheritance (X-linked) and mechanism as Duchenne-type, but rather reduced and abnormal laminin, less damaging to muscle fibers. Onset later (after age 12) and progression slower (still walking to age 20 or older).

FACIOSCAPULOHUMERAL DYSTROPHY—Transmission: autosomal dominant, both sexes equally affected. Onset in adolescence; mild and slowly progressive; course variable. Wasting of facial, pectoral, and shoulder girdle muscles. CK mm seldom elevated; heart uninvolved. Normal longevity possible.

LIMB-GIRDLE DYSTROPHY—Actually a group of disorders. Transmission: autosomal dominant or recessive; both sexes affected equally. Onset childhood, adolescence, or adulthood. Affects either shoulder or hip girdle; usually mild progression. Defect in membrane-associated glycoproteins.

Myotonias

MYOTONIA CONGENITA (THOMSEN DISEASE)—Transmission: usually autosomal dominant. Myotonia *without* weakness. No systemic disorder present (e.g., no cataracts or EKG abnormalities). Stimulated muscle maintains prolonged contraction. Early onset; compatible with normal longevity; affects all skeletal muscles. Muscle hypertrophy common. Exercise relieves symptoms. Decreased chloride channel density in muscle membranes slows repolarization.

MYOTONIC MUSCULAR DYSTROPHY (STEINERT DISEASE)—Transmission: autosomal dominant. Myotonia *with* weakness (major problem). Onset in adulthood. Variable expression and severity. Affects principally cranial and shoulder girdle muscles. Ptosis; sometimes eye movement disorder. Multisystem disease: baldness and testicular atrophy in males; cataracts in all patients.

Myositis

POLYMYOSITIS/DERMATOMYOSITIS—Multisystem immune-mediated diseases with muscle weakness major symptom. Half of patients experience rashes (dermatomyositis) on eyelids, extensor surfaces of joints. Begins with limb girdle weakness; can progress to neck weakness; impaired swallowing and breathing. Eyelid strength maintained (vs. myasthenia gravis). Elevated serum CK. Evidence for being distinct diseases: dermatomyositis seldom associated with another disease except carcinoma, rarely associated with collagen-vascular disease, occurs at all ages, myopathy more severe in contrast to polymyositis, which is associated with systemic disease in 50% of cases, often a manifestation of collagen-vascular disease (e.g., lupus), rare before puberty.

Primary Myopathies

Diseases intrinsic to the muscle fiber (**primary myopathies**) derive principally from either heritable or autoimmune disorders. The precise pathogenetic mechanisms and focus are subjects of active research and are largely beyond our scope. A traditional categorization produces dystrophies, myotonias, and polymyositis/dermatomyositis. Table 21.6 presents the relevant information.

Disorders of Neuromuscular Junction

Myasthenia gravis (severe weakness and malaise) is an autoimmune disorder in which antibodies are produced to acetylcholine receptors. These neurotransmitter receptors are produced on the folded surface of a skeletal muscle membrane where it is in intimate association with the end processes of a motor neuron axon (the motor endplate region). In normal function, the arrival at the end of processes of a nerve signal causes the release of perhaps 200,000 molecules of acetylcholine (ACh), which diffuse across the synaptic space or cleft, bind to ACh receptors, and open membrane channels. These allow the movement of sodium ions into the muscle cell and induce a second signal, this time in the muscle membrane, which triggers the contractile process in the muscle cell. After the signal is begun, the channels lose their affinity for ACh. It diffuses back into the synaptic cleft, is broken down by an enzyme called acetylcholinesterase that resides there, and the breakdown products are taken back up into the end processes for reuse. This chain of events allows for the rapid, controlled turning on of muscle tension and its equally important turning off. Binding of anti-ACh-receptor antibodies has no stimulatory effect, but neither is the antibody easily released. Two pathologic processes are instigated. Bound antibody stimulates neutrophil phagocytosis of the endplate muscle membrane. It also serves as a signal to the muscle cell and induces uptake and degradation of these receptor channels. The combined rate of degradation/phagocytosis exceeds the production capacity, and a net impoverishment of receptor channels occurs. Gradually, the muscle response to nerve stimulation is impaired and weakness increases.

Typical of many autoimmune disorders, the pattern is one of flare-up and remission. The classic form of MG (myasthenia gravis) affects the muscles of the face, neck, and limb girdles. It gets worse during the day and with fatigue. The eyelids droop (ptosis), the face becomes inexpressive, the head tips forward, the sternocleidomastoids become weak, the nasal voice becomes slurred, and it is difficult to raise the arms or climb stairs. As the usually chronic, progressive syndrome persists, it worsens and muscle wasting may occur. The course is highly variable. Some people develop only the eyelid and ocular muscle weakness (ocular myasthenia). Those with more generalized MG can respond well to therapy. Some have a very fulminant, progressive form with muscle wasting and poor response to therapy. These people can die within five years, usually of pneumonia secondary to immobility.

Chemicals that block the action of acetylcholinesterase allow ACh to accumulate in the cleft. This can compensate for the impoverishment of receptors and allow somewhat normal neuromuscular transmission. **Tensilon** (edrophonium) is a potent antiacetylcholinesterase drug. It is used only diagnostically. The patient suspected of having MG is given an injection of Tensilon. Within 10–30 seconds, life comes back to the face, the eyelids rise, and neck strength and shoulder girdle strength return, confirming a diagnosis of MG. Within ten minutes, the effects are reversed. Physostigmine and neostigmine are related drugs that can be used therapeutically. This chemical management has its downsides. ACh in relatively normal neuromuscular junctions is allowed to accumulate to excess amounts, producing muscle tetany. It can also produce abnormal patterns of autonomic discharge.

In this context, the emergency treatment of a person with a suspected **myasthenic crisis** is illustrative. This person would have an inability to swallow, clear secretions, or breathe adequately because of a sudden flare-up of myasthenic weakness. This condition must be discriminated from a similar-appearing **cholinergic crisis,** which is probably due to excessive plasma levels of antiacetylcholinesterase drug. These people would have excess bronchial secretions, excessive sweating, and impaired swallowing and breathing due to muscle paralysis. Life support must be available because the administration of Tensilon will deepen a cholinergic crisis, which can be reversed with the administration of an anticholinergic drug like atropine.

Other therapies focus on quenching the intensity of the immune response. Thymectomy was once performed fairly often and with varying results. (Thymic hyperplasia is a common finding.) More currently, management focuses on immunosuppressants and steroidal anti-inflammatories. Plasmapheresis, in which blood is circulated extracorporeally past a membrane that absorbs antibodies (gamma globulins) and then returned to the patient, is used to reverse a serious exacerbation. Because none of these techniques are selective for the anti-ACh antibodies, they render the person susceptible to infection, particularly bacterial.

Lambert-Eaton myasthenic syndrome (LEMS) produces many of the same symptoms as MG, particularly proximal muscle weakness, but also autonomic abnormalities (dry mouth, decreased sweating, perhaps impotence or constipation). It is usually a paraneoplastic phenomenon (associated with advanced progression of carcinoma, 60% of cases being associated with small-cell carcinoma of the lungs). The mechanism appears to be autoimmune mediated. Binding of antibodies directed against voltage-gated calcium channels in the terminal endings of peripheral nerves interferes with the calcium-influx mediated release of ACh. Recall that ACh is the neurotransmitter released at the neuromuscular junction and both the preganglionic terminals of all autonomic neurons, as well as all parasympathetic postganglionic neurons and sympathetic neurons associated with sweating. EMG distinguishes LEMS from MG: rather than the decrementing response seen to repeated stimulation in MG, LEMS shows an **incrementing response** to rapid, 10 Hz, stimulating ACh release.

 Checkpoint 21.5

It might be useful to draw yourself a simple diagram of a motor endplate (take part of figure 21.6 as a model and blow it up) and picture where MG is actually occuring. What *is* the process? How does it differ from Lambert-Eaton syndrome?

Peripheral Nerve Disorders

Diffuse Polyneuropathies

A variety of metabolic, toxic, and nutritional conditions can cause scattered peripheral nerve lesions, so-called **diffuse polyneuropathies.** These are usually chronic problems that may have a variety of mechanisms of injury. Vascular pathology in large and small arteries develops in diabetes, which may affect oxygenation of peripheral nerves. Substances accumulate in toxic levels in diabetes, in liver and kidney failure, in alcohol abuse, and in the chronic use of some drugs (e.g., isoniazid and hydralazine). Vitamin and substrate deficiencies can be associated with nutritional deficiencies or inflammatory conditions of the stomach or intestine.

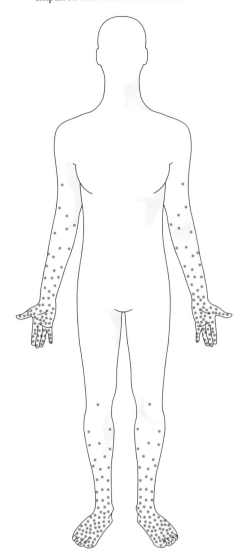

Figure 21.11   **Glove-and-Stocking Anesthesia Associated with Diffuse Peripheral Neuropathy.**

The pattern of motor and sensory loss is varied. **Glove-and-stocking anesthesia** can develop through the selective lesioning of pain receptors and lightly myelinated fibers in the distal extremities (fig. 21.11). Loss of larger fibers leads to impaired proprioception—that is, sensation of movement and limb position—and loss of function that depends on incoming, well-discriminated sensation. As a result, stretch reflexes will be diminished, vibratory sense in the periphery is decreased, and walking is impaired. The person may show foot drop due to impaired sensory input or muscle weakness that may develop peripherally. Paresthesias like numbness, tingling, or "pins and needles" (see chapter 23) are common.

Many of these conditions are irreversible at the late stage at which they are often detected, but progression may be halted if correction of the underlying pathology is possible. Electromyography and nerve conduction velocity tests are invaluable diagnostic aids.

Guillain-Barré Syndrome

This peripheral neuropathy results from an immune-mediated attack on the sheaths of well-myelinated fibers. Therefore, in Guillain-Barré syndrome (pronounced "gill-ann ba-ray"), both movement and well-discriminated sensation are affected. The typical course follows about a week after a flu or upper respiratory tract viral infection. In the United States, a rash of cases was noted after widespread vaccination in the swine-flu epidemic of the early 1980s. In its most extreme form, paresthesias—for example, tingling of the hands and feet—are followed by progressive weakness, areflexia, and distal sensory loss. Paralysis, including respiratory arrest, can occur, requiring mechanical ventilation. Survival of this crisis leads to a positive prognosis: 85% make a complete recovery in four to six months. Immunosuppressants and steroids or ACTH have varied efficacy.

The pathology results from infiltration of the endoneurial tube by lymphocytes and, later, macrophages. Demyelination is a direct result of the binding of antibodies to a variety of Schwann cell myelin proteins. The pattern of demyelination may be very focal. There may also be widespread axonal degeneration, which explains the slow recovery of function. Because the endoneureal tube remains intact for the most part, regrowth and reinnervation are usually effective. But the recovery of function may be incomplete, with enduring or permanent focal sensory or motor loss. Figure 21.12 provides a summary. Again, EMG and nerve conduction studies are a valuable diagnostic and prognostic aid.

Entrapment Syndromes

The general category **entrapment syndromes** groups together peripheral nerve lesions that are clearly due to local compression and trauma (e.g., Saturday night palsy or tardy ulnar palsy) with those that are related to overuse or repetitive motion injury (e.g., pronator teres syndrome) and with those that are probably a combination of overuse and genetic predisposition (e.g., carpal tunnel syndrome). The common problem in all these conditions is a focal slowing and loss of intensity of motor and sensory signals. Prolonged signal impairment will result in muscle wasting and eventually irreversible fibrosis; so prompt diagnosis and correction, if effective, are critical. More conservative approaches, including rest, physiotherapy, and learning ways of moving that don't irritate or compress the nerve, are usually considered before surgery. Surgery releases surrounding muscle tissue, removes connective tissue to facilitate vascular perfusion and reduce pressure, and repositions nerves that have been traumatized in their course. Particularly with carpal tunnel syndrome, the response to surgery is variable, independent of the chronicity of the condition.

Any peripheral nerve can be subject to compression or trauma. The common conditions of the upper limb are presented here. Table 21.7 summarizes these.

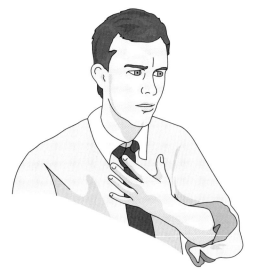

(a) Upper respiratory tract viral infection.

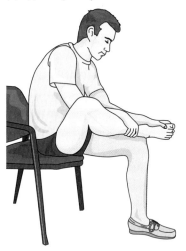

(b) Tingling and numbness in scattered areas, particularly the periphery.

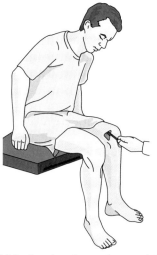

(c) Scattered weakness, decreased stretch reflexes (e.g.,↓ knee jerk).

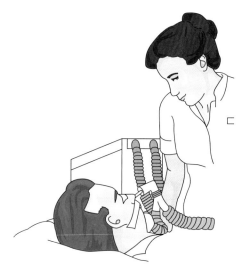

(d) On ventilator, complete paralysis.

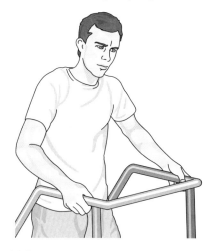

(e) Gradual recovery; walking with assistance (walker).

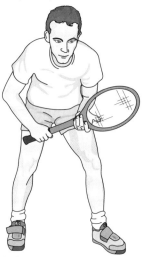

(f) Complete recovery.

Figure 21.12   **Stages in the Progression of Guillain-Barré Syndrome.**

Table 21.7	Summary of Major Peripheral Nerve Entrapment Syndromes Affecting the Upper Limbs, Presented in Order of the Site of Lesion (Distal to Proximal)

Radial Nerve

(Normally responsible for extension of elbow, wrist, and fingers, forearm supination, and sensation in the back of the hand, including proximal surface of thumb and first two fingers)

Posterior Interosseus Syndrome

Lesion in upper dorsal forearm (perhaps due to overuse of the supinator muscle in actions like that used in driving in a screw). Weakness in extension of wrist and fingers, supination strength intact, no noticeable sensory loss.

Saturday Night Palsy

Temporary (6–8 weeks) neuropathy due to compression in the posterior upper arm, named for common occurrence in people who have passed out and subjected nerve to prolonged compression. Triceps unaffected (normal extension at elbow) but extension of wrist and fingers impaired, as is forearm supination. Sensory loss restricted to back of hand, thumb, and first and second fingers.

Compression can also occur at the axilla, often from improperly used crutch; same symptoms as Saturday night palsy but includes impaired extension at elbow.

Median Nerve

(Normally responsible for forearm pronation; contributes to wrist flexion, finger flexion, and a complex variety of finger movements, sensation in palm and palmar surface of thumb, first two fingers and radial half of third)

Carpal Tunnel Syndrome

Lesion is in the ventral wrist where tendons, blood vessels, and median nerve enter the hand (carpal tunnel). Best-known and most common entrapment neuropathy. Incidence highest in fifth and sixth decades and in women. Frequently bilateral but dominant hand more affected; a majority of patients do considerable work with their hands. Painful paresthesias, which can awaken the patient, are often referred to elbow or shoulder; sensory loss in territory described above. Symptoms worsen after passive flexion or hyperextension of wrist of affected hand. Atrophy of thumb muscles causes flattening of palm called "ape hand."

Anterior Interosseus Syndrome

This nerve branches about halfway between elbow and wrist. Lesion causes pain in the forearm and elbow and impairs intrinsic hand muscles such that when patient is asked to form an "OK" sign, thumb and forefinger will make a "pinch sign" instead of an "O."

Ulnar Nerve

(Normally contributes to wrist flexion, innervation of a variety of muscles intrinsic to the hand, sensation of palm, little finger, and medial half of third finger)

Tardy Ulnar Palsy

Collective name for ulnar nerve lesions between shoulder and wrist. Two most common are cubital tunnel syndrome, where the nerve passes medially around the elbow (at the "funny bone") and lesion is due to repeated minor trauma (e.g., those who work long hours with elbows on a table) or immobilization following fracture, and a second in which the lesion is about 4 inches distal to the cubital tunnel where the ulnar nerve passes through the medial muscle contributing to wrist flexion (flexor carpi ulnaris), in which case overuse or congenital predisposition are explanations. Impaired sensation in territory described; weakness in a variety of abduction and adduction movements of fingers and thumb, and thumb flexion; wasting of hand intrinsics, when advanced called "claw hand."

General Comments on Treatment

If overuse is the cause, a change in activity or technique can reverse symptoms. Response to anti-inflammatory agents is variable. Response to surgical decompression and sometimes movement of nerve continues to improve with advances in surgical technique; in some conditions success is excellent, while in others it is variable.

Charcot-Marie-Tooth Disease

This heritable atrophy of peripheral motor and sensory neurons is usually passed by autosomal dominant transmission (see Huntington's disease later for an explanation). Degeneration of dorsal and ventral cord roots, the dorsal root ganglion, and alpha motor neurons is also observed. Both the axons and myelin sheaths are affected by this unexplained pathology. It begins with weakness and atrophy in the distal muscles of the lower limb, giving it the less complicated name **peroneal muscular atrophy.** Later the hands and arms are involved as the condition progresses proximally. Onset is usually in late childhood or adolescence but can be postponed until middle age in mild cases. The extent of progression is variable and usually arrests at the lower thigh and proximal forearm. A variety of limb deformities result from the muscle wasting. These require periodic orthotic correction.

Disorders of the Spinal Cord

Cord Structure and Function

The primary structural distinction in the cord (white matter pathways consisting of variably myelinated axons, surrounding gray matter consisting of cell bodies and their synaptic interconnections) is straightforward. The central butterfly of gray matter can be further subdivided into collections of motor neurons with related function in the anterior horns and sensory relay neurons in the posterior horns. The gray matter interconnections allow for the subtle modulation of both ascending sensory and descending motor information. Many distinct and consistent pathways have been identified in the white matter of the cord, each carrying its own information destined to initiate or modify nervous system outflow or inputs.

Outflow includes all movement excluding those of speech and facial expression, whose outflow signals leave the CNS along the cranial nerves before the cord starts. It also includes the modification of autonomic functions like digestion, cardiac function, vascular tone, sweating, and so on. Except for the small sacral parasympathetic portion, most cord autonomic discharge is sympathetic, a fact that can have profound consequences for a person with extensive spinal cord damage.

Input includes sensation arising in the skin below the head, as well as the joints, muscles, and tendons. All sensation from the organs of special sense (eyes, ears, nose, mouth) passes to the CNS along cranial nerves. Input also includes the sensory feedback upon which autonomic nervous system function relies. The presence in a cord isolated by spinal cord lesion of both feedback to the autonomic nervous system and unmediated sympathetic outflow sets the stage for a condition called **autonomic dysreflexia.** This is seen as a chronic problem in individuals with complete high cord lesions (quadriplegia). The smallest stimulus (cold, pressure from a blanket, bladder pressure) may elicit a **mass reflex.** There is massive sympathetic discharge, which

Focus on Brown-Séquard Syndrome

The different pathways of the spinal cord tracts are illustrated by observations of the 19th-century French physician Henri Brown-Séquard. He attended a young man who had been stabbed in the back in a barroom brawl. The lesion severed the right half of the cord in the midthoracic region (right hemisection of the cord). Most of the clinical findings were consistent with Brown-Séquard's common sense expectations: The man couldn't move his right foot; he had no awareness of light touch or whether the doctor had moved his right great toe up or down; stroking his right sole elicited a Babinski; and, in time, the right limb became hyperreflexive. The left leg, on the other hand, was normal. Well, not completely normal. He had lost his sensitivity to both pain and temperature in that leg. And even more curious, these sensations were intact in the right leg. What Brown-Séquard had stumbled on was the decussation of pain and temperature at the level of the cord at which it enters.

causes sweating, flushing, dangerously increased blood pressure, intense headache, and bradycardia. The latter requires explanation. The initial cardiovascular response to sympathetic discharge is vasoconstriction in arterioles (increased peripheral resistance and increased blood pressure) and increased rate and force of cardiac contraction. The increased blood pressure induces distention in the carotid baroreceptors, which are still normally functioning. Resultant increases in parasympathetic discharge from the cardiac center in the medulla are carried along the intact vagus nerve (CN X), which slows the heart rate. Uncontrolled sympathetic discharge is such that vasoconstriction maintains the elevated blood pressure. The violent headaches produced are an indicator of the extreme elevation of cerebral blood pressure. This condition must be medically controlled or the patient risks cerebral hemorrhage.

Table 21.8 and figure 21.13 present the clinically relevant cord tracts.

Spinal Cord Injury: Chronic Adaptation

The long-term response to cord injury will depend on both the level and the extent of the injury. Incomplete lesions will leave unaffected any sensation or movement for which open pathways remain. Conversely, if an area of gray matter is destroyed, so is any reflex activity it mediated. Individual assessment of all movement, sensation, and reflex activity is necessary to assess these issues. Complete lesions are simpler to assess in terms of the lowest level of intact sensation and motor control. But again, the possibility of cord damage below the point must be carefully assessed to predict the integrity of perhaps useful reflex function. An example is reflex emptying of bladder or bowel. If

Table 21.8   Summary of Ascending and Descending Cord Tracts

Ascending (Sensory) Pathways

Anterolateral Spinothalamic Tract

Carries information from pain, temperature, and crude touch* receptors to the thalamus (a relay station in the brain). It is then relayed to the cerebral cortex and conscious awareness. The first neuron passes from receptor to synapse in the dorsal horn (cell body in the dorsal root ganglion). The second neuron crosses the cord in the region ventral to the central canal and travels in this spinothalamic tract to the thalamus. The third neuron passes from the thalamus to the cerebral cortex. This is a crossed pathway, (i.e., damage to left pathway gives symptoms on the right side of the body; for example, a lesion to the left side of the cord in the spinothalamic tract will impair any temperature sensation from the *right* side of the body below the lesion).

Dorsal Columns—Medial Lemniscal Pathway

Carries information from receptors in the skin (light touch, vibration, capacity to discriminate between adjacent stimuli, pressure), particularly from the lower and upper limbs; also carries information from shoulder, arm, and finger on position and tension in muscles and tendons, movements, etc. The first neuron passes from receptor to the cord (cell body in the dorsal root ganglion) and then passes up the dorsal column of white matter (the fibers from the legs travel in the fasciculus gracilis and from the arms in the fasciculus cuneatus) to a nucleus in the medulla. The second neuron passes from this nucleus across the brain stem to the thalamus. The third neuron then passes from the thalamus to the cortex for conscious perception. This is an uncrossed pathway: damage to the left side of the cord results in sensory deficits in the left side of the body. This pathway also supplies the cerebellum with movement information from the upper limbs.

Descending (Motor) Pathways

Lateral Corticospinal Tract (Pyramidal Tract)

Carries movement signals from the cerebral cortex to the motor neurons in the spinal cord. A single neuron passes from the cerebral cortex, crosses over in the medulla, and travels down the cord in a lateral position. At the level of the motor neuron, the fiber passes into the gray matter of the cord to synapse with the motor neuron. This pathway is particularly significant in skilled hand and foot movements. Damage to the left side of the cord results in motor deficits on the left side. (Also called the "pyramidal tract.")

Extrapyramidal Pathways (Multineuronal Pathways)

These are pathways that provide for the support of movements of the lateral corticospinal tract. This includes movements of the trunk and proximal limb muscles, balance, posture, orienting to sight or sound and more. While working in coordination with the corticospinal tract, these tracts are distinct from it; hence, the name extrapyramidal. Because activation of these tracts requires the successive involvement of more than one neuron (versus the corticospinal), they are sometimes called the multineuronal pathways.

*This is mechanical stimulation that is intense enough to begin to cause tissue damage.

---

the centers mediating these are intact, then filling of the bladder beyond about 650 ml or distention of the rectum following an automatic mass peristaltic movement in the colon will elicit reflex relaxation of the internal sphincters and contraction of smooth muscle in the wall of the bladder or rectum, causing voiding. This tends to ensure, at least with the bladder, that emptying is more complete and the attendant risk of infection less. It also opens the possibility of "tricking" intact sensory and motor capacity to improve the quality of independent living. Manual pressure on the lower abdominopelvic area can stretch the bladder and bowel and induce reflex emptying. Intact reflex innervation of the bladder is not an unmixed blessing. Excessive blad-

der tone (neurogenic bladder) can restrict bladder filling and lead to constant overflow.

Complete lesion has a predictable pattern of functional loss depending on the level of damage. Table 21.9 provides an overview.

Sexual function and sensation are a major concern for the victim of a spinal cord lesion. Partial lesion may leave sensation intact, and as long as the level of the cord mediating sexual responses (parasympathetic—erection, at sacral 2–4; sympathetic—ejaculation, at thoracic 10–12) is unharmed, normal sexual function is a possibility even with motor impairment. Complete lesions prevent sensory awareness of genital stimulation, but intact reflex erection and ejaculation

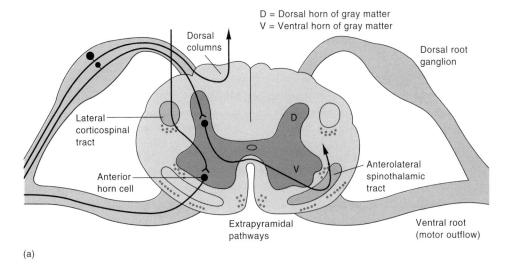

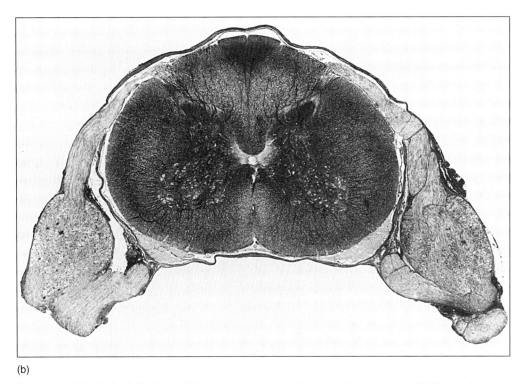

Figure 21.13   **Anatomy of the Spinal Cord.** (*a*) Principal cord tracts and regions of gray matter. (*b*) Photomicrograph of spinal cord.

may be a significant component of a paralyzed person's sexual repertoire.

Hyperreflexia, like the autonomic dysreflexia already described, may create a significant management problem, since it disrupts weak voluntary movement or interferes with the passive movement of limbs that is necessary when the person is dressed or positioned. It can be treated medically, or, if necessary, by surgical interruption of spinal nerve roots.

Syringomyelia

This condition, which produces a cavity (or "syrinx") in the central cord, is considered rare. Many cases are associated with the Arnold-Chiari malformation described in chapter 20. The usual location of the cavity is in the cervical gray matter of the cord just lateral to the central canal. When the cavity is simply a dilation of the central canal of the cord, the condition is sometimes called **hydromyelia.** As the **syrinx** expands, it first compresses the decussating fibers carrying pain and temperature information across the cord. This interrupts the function of these fibers and produces a classic pattern of pain and temperature insensitivity in the arms and upper trunk, called, because of its distribution, **shawl anesthesia** (fig. 21.14). Fibers that have decussated below the lesion continue uninterrupted in the anterolateral-spinothalamic tract, so pain and temperature sensation in the lower trunk and limbs are normal. If the cavity contin-

Table 21.9 Functional Capacity Associated with Complete Cord Transection at a Variety of Cervical and Lumbosacral Levels

Cervical Injuries

If these muscles are normal and	these muscles are weak and	these muscles are nonfunctioning, then	the level of the lesion is below
		Diaphragm	C1 or C2
	Diaphragm	Elbow flexors	C3 or C4
Diaphragm	Elbow flexors	Wrist extensors	C5
Elbow flexors	Wrist extensors	Elbow extensor	C6
Wrist extensors	Elbow extensor	Hand intrinsics	C7
Elbow extensor	Hand intrinsics		C8
Hand intrinsics			T1 or below

Dorsolumbar Injuries

If these muscles are normal and	these muscles are weak and	these muscles are nonfunctioning, then	the level of the lesion is below
		Hip adductors	L1 or above
	Hip adductors	Knee extensors	L2
Hip adductors	Knee extensors	Ankle dorsiflexors	L3
Knee extensors	Ankle dorsiflexors	Great toe extensor	L4
Ankle dorsiflexors	Great toe extensor	Ankle plantarflexors	L5
Great toe extensor	Ankle plantarflexors	Anal sphincter	S1
Ankle plantarflexors	Anal sphincter		S2

From Frank Netter, *Clinical Symposia,* vol. 30, no. 2. Reprinted by permission.

ues to expand, compression of motor and sensory neurons in the gray matter will depress motor behavior in the arms. Eventually obliteration of transmission in the outer white tracts will cause quadriplegia. Usually a person will go for care well before this point. Unexplained insensitivity to burns and cuts is the usual complaint. By-passing accumulated CSF (shunting) will usually arrest the progression of the dilation, although there is likelihood of permanent sensory deficits.

The other circumstance in which a syrinx forms is as a consequence of acute spinal cord trauma. An area of hematoma or necrosis is subjected to liquification necrosis, leaving a syrinx. This may expand to threaten residual cord function. The mechanism for the expansion of a cervical hydromyelia or syringomyelia is thought to be the abnormal directing of the pulsatile flow of CSF due to cerebellar and foramen magnum distortions associated with Arnold-Chiari. The fact that many syrinxes are not in communication with the fourth ventrical undermines this theory.

Subacute Combined Degeneration of the Cord

This generalized lesion of the posterior half of the spinal cord is often associated with a constellation of disorders that are related to its most common though not invariable cause: chronic alcohol abuse. The lesion gradually obliter-

ates the function of the lateral corticospinal tract, the dorsal columns, and the pathways carrying proprioceptive information from the legs. This results in impaired (particularly finely controlled distal) movement, ataxic (drunken sailor) gait, toe drop, impaired skin and proprioceptive sensation, and hyporeflexia. The pathogenetic mechanism is related to inflammation of the gastric mucosa, which impairs the secretion of the intrinsic factor that is essential for the absorption of vitamin B_{12}. This B_{12} deficiency gives rise to a severe form of anemia called **pernicious anemia,** which appears to be a mechanism of cord lesion. The pattern of cord lesion may result from an interaction between the anemia (hypoxia) and the vascular supply to the cord. The dorsal white matter is supplied by two small posterior spinal arteries, while the anterior cord and gray matter are supplied by the larger anterior spinal artery.

People who smoke and drink to excess are considerably more likely to develop this form of gastritis, although those who abstain can as well. The other disorders that are found in chronic alcoholics include cerebellar degeneration, lesions to the hypothalamus and hippocampal outflow paths that impair new memory formation, and a broad dementia called **Korsakoff's psychosis.** The latter may be more directly related to deficiencies in other vitamins, including thiamine, and to direct alcohol toxicity. Subacute combined degeneration is

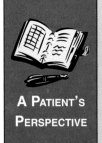

A Patient's Perspective

Experiences as a Quadriplegic

—John Callahan

There's absolutely nothing funny about a quadriplegic in a wheelchair—unless, of course, that person is John Callahan. For over 15 years, this irreverent cartoonist has been shocking us with his own special brand of wicked humor. In the world of Callahan, nothing is sacred, nothing is taboo, and nothing is funnier! He has graciously agreed to share a bit of his personal story with us in this Patient's Perspective.

THE LIGHTER SIDE OF BEING
PARALYZED FOR LIFE

CARTOONIST **JOHN CALLAHAN** HIGHLIGHTS SOME OF HIS EXPERIENCES AS A QUADRIPLEGIC

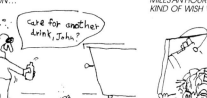

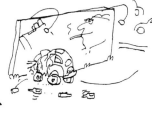

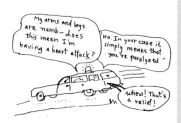

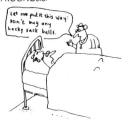

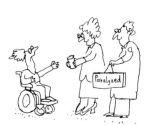

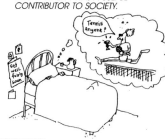

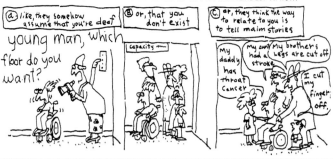

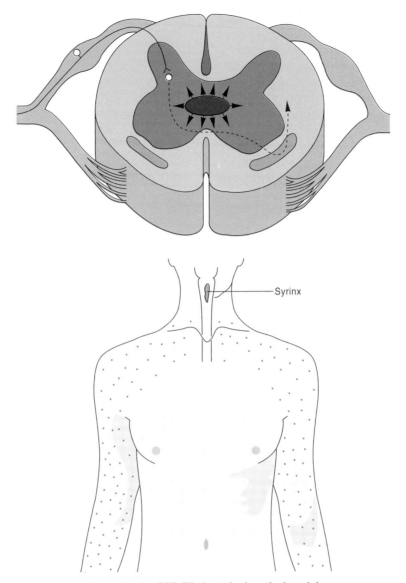

Figure 21.14   **Syringomyelia.** Syringomyelia produced a CSF-filled cyst in the spinal cord that compresses crossing spinothalamic axons. This gives rise to pain and temperature insensitivity in the area innervated, in this case a shawl anesthesia due to a cervical syrinx.

reversible in its very early stages by administration of B$_{12}$. This must be injected, as oral doses would not be absorbed.

In **tabes dorsalis** (dorsal wasting), a similar pattern is observed, with involvement of the dorsal root ganglia as well. Syphilis spirochetes are the agent in this case. As noted in chapter 20, they enter and damage the small dorsal arteries and produce deficits similar to those in subacute combined degeneration.

Amyotrophic Lateral Sclerosis

Variously called Lou Gehrig's disease and motor neuron disease, **amyotrophic lateral sclerosis** (ALS) is named because of the combination of loss of trophic factors to the muscles (lower motor neuron lesion) and the gross appearance of the cord at autopsy (lateral scarring because of lesions to the lateral corticospinal tract, upper motor neuron lesion). This ultimately fatal disorder is purely motor in nature. About 80% of

people with ALS die within three years of diagnosis. For the other 20%, the disease follows a slow course, taking ten or more years to progress. About 5% of cases are familial with an autosomal dominant pattern of inheritance. Rarely, people die within a year and some live more than 25. Stephen Hawking, the great physicist, is still a very active theoretician despite living with the disease for over 20 years.

The initial loss is particularly of corticospinal neurons, which produces clumsy and weakened hand movements and the signs one expects with a principally upper motor neuron lesion. Gradually more alpha motor neurons are involved, as are upper motor neurons innervating proximal and axial muscles. Muscle wasting, due to both disuse and denervation, becomes profound. EMG shows extensive pathology. Fasciculations may be observed. Breathing and swallowing are difficult. Death usually comes from intercurrent infection, choking, or aspiration in a severely debilitated person with fully normal cognitive capacities.

ALS is now seen as related to a variety of degenerative CNS conditions like Parkinson's disease. Mechanisms that are being explored as possible causes include environmental toxins, slow viruses, and excitotoxicity, the potentially destructive response of neurons to excessive and abnormal stimulation. No treatments are effective at present.

There are other patterns of motor neuron disease, the causes of which are equally mysterious. **Progressive muscular atrophy** affects lower motor neurons in an uneven pattern, with varied degrees of progression. **Bulbar palsy** affects mostly the motor neurons in the brain stem (ALS usually spares these until late in its course). It has a variable course but is, as well, ultimately fatal.

Spinal Muscular Atrophies of Infancy and Childhood

This group includes a variety of rare, heritable motor disorders that leave sensory capacities intact. They vary in age of onset, severity, and course and pattern of transmission. The pattern of lesion is similar to ALS. **Werdnig-Hoffmann disease** is the general name applied to those with onset in infancy. The most common form has early onset and sometimes rapid progression. The child is weak and limp from birth (called **floppy baby syndrome**). The classic presentation is an infant whose arms fall to the sides (jug handles) and whose legs relax in weak flexion (frog legs). Others show apparently normal development for several months, with subsequent motor degeneration. The baby has normal intelligence, and brain stem motor control is usually intact. The bright, responsive face is in contrast to the immobile body. All of these early onset forms are ultimately fatal. Transmission is by the autosomal recessive pattern.

Wohlfart-Kugelberg-Welander disease is a milder form of heritable motor neuron disease with two distinct patterns, onset before 2 years or in the range of 5–18 years. Males are more often affected, and the usual pattern of transmission is autosomal recessive. Proximal muscles are denervated, while bulbar and corticospinal tracts are spared. The earlier the onset, the more severe the progression, but the worst affected child is able to walk for at least ten years. Gradually, distal musculature is involved.

✓ *Checkpoint 21.6*

Current nomenclature sees the disorders discussed in the previous section as related disorders on a continuum. Using this framework, the classification is as follows: spinal muscular atrophy type 1 (**SMA type 1**) for Werdnig-Hoffmann appearing before 6 months, **SMA type 2** for the severe form arising 6 months to one year, and **SMA type 3** for the relatively mild form called W-K-W or K-W.

Friedreich's Ataxia

A fatal motor-sensory disorder with an average course of 15 to 20 years, **Friedreich's ataxia** is due to an autosomal recessive disorder affecting the production of a protein called *frataxin,* which normally associates with mitochondrial membranes. The deficiencies in frataxin that occur with these mutations may result in mitochondrial dysfunction and free-radical toxicity. The severity of Friedreich's ataxia appears to correlate with the degree of derangement of the gene. The cord is small. The posterior columns and corticospinal and spinocerebellar tracts are depleted of fibers. Bulbar motor neurons are largely spared. Cerebellar lesions are also noted. Gait ataxia is the initial symptom for most. There is difficulty standing steadily and running. A variety of joint deformities result from the sensory and motor impairments. Since the unconscious proprioceptive information doesn't ascend from the feet and legs, closing the eyes causes the person to sway and fall. Tremoring and choreiform movements are often seen. Intelligence is unimpaired. About half of those with this ataxia develop cardiomyopathies. Many die as a result of cardiac arrhythmias.

DISORDERS ARISING IN THE BASAL GANGLIA

Parkinson Disease

Over 180 years have elapsed since James Parkinson described the syndrome that now bears his name. The odd combination of slowed, reduced movement and restless tremoring suggested the name paralysis agitans. **Parkinson disease** (PD; also called parkinsonism) is a slowly degenerative CNS disorder affecting perhaps 80,000 middle-aged and older adults in North America. The disease has a course of 10–20 years, and twice as many men are affected as women.

The principal lesion in PD is in the substantia nigra, normally two darkly pigmented, dopamine-producing nuclei that are located in the midbrain. Their normal role is to provide an outflow pathway from the basal ganglia to the cortex via the thalamus and a feedback loop to the caudate and putamen. This loop appears to even out the discharge from these higher nuclei in the basal ganglia. Damage to the substantia nigra impairs the flow of motor programs from the basal ganglia, which is expressed as difficulty initiating movement and a general impoverishment and slowing of movement (bradykinesia). Loss of the feedback loop impairs the steady flow of programs and expresses itself as resting tremor.

In many cases, Parkinson disease is idiopathic; there is simply a gradual and unexplained loss of these dopamine-producing cells (fig. 21.15). In some cases, it can result from lesion by toxins like the MPTP that contaminated certain street drugs and produced the frozen addict syndrome described earlier. Although rare now, viral encephalopathy associated with the great influenza epidemic of 1914–18 produced hundreds of cases of postencephalitic parkinsonism. Lesions to other areas of the basal ganglia can also produce parkinsonism or a variety of other movement disorders.

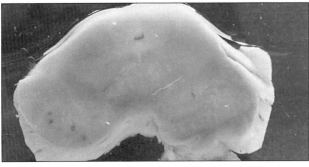

(a)

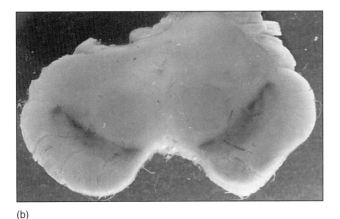

(b)

Figure 21.15   **Parkinson Disease.** Sections through the midbrain showing normal substantia nigra pigmentation (lower section) and the loss of pigmented neurons in Parkinsonism (upper section).

The top section through the pons is from a 50-year-old man who died in a nursing home. He had developed severe and progressive Parkinson disease in his thirties. Thalamic surgery to limit his dysfunction was unsuccessful, and he deteriorated until his death of a cerebral hemorrhage. The lower, normally pigmented specimen is provided for comparison with the victim's substantia nigra, whose neurons are almost completely lacking in pigment.

The most disabling symptoms in PD are muscle rigidity, which can be lead-pipe or oscillating cogwheel rigidity, and bradykinesia. The patient—typically an elderly male—experiences tiredness and weakness, but muscle strength is more or less normal. He has a slow (4–5 per second) resting tremor, sometimes with an alternating flexion-extension of the fingers called pill-rolling tremor. The tremor is typically suppressed during movement and exaggerated when the limb is held in extension. The person has poor balance and maintains a stooped posture with the neck flexed. He shuffles and may adopt a gait in which he chases his pitched-forward center of gravity (festinating gait). Arm swing is absent, and he turns the body as a unit (en bloc). Rolling over or getting up out of a crouching position or out of a chair is difficult. Fine movements like buttoning become laborious. Handwriting becomes small and speech quiet. The face becomes immobile and inexpressive ("masklike"), the skin becomes oily, and inflamed seborrhea is found at the hairline and crevices of the face. Autonomic function is al-

tered as well: patients experience orthostatic hypotension (blood pressure drops when they stand), excess sweating, constipation, and other autonomic disorders. Some patients suffer dementia similar to that found in Alzheimer disease (see Alzheimer Disease section). While not fatal, Parkinson disease shortens life expectancy significantly.

A variety of approaches are used to alleviate the symptoms as the disease progresses. Active exercise is encouraged, walking with swinging the arms, swimming, and so on. As well, the person is taught strategies to overcome the bradykinesia: "throwing" himself up to get out of a chair, lifting the toes when "glued to the floor," practicing rapid "explosive" activities. When symptoms have progressed to a point of severe disability, drug therapy with levodopa is begun. This is a dopamine precursor that will cross the blood-brain barrier, where it is converted to dopamine to augment the diminished production from the substantia nigra. It is administered with a substance (carbidopa) that blocks the enzymatic degradation of levodopa in peripheral tissue so lower, better controlled dosages can be given. Use of levodopa is postponed because of the risk of its common side and toxic effects: cardiac arrhythmias, gastrointestinal hemorrhage, the psychiatric problems experienced by about 30% of patients, and—the most serious and ironic problem—unpredictable involuntary movement disorders. Drugs affecting glutamate, acetylcholine, and norepinephrine pathways in the basal ganglia are used as adjuncts to levodopa therapy. Implantation of foreign or autograft tissue has been tested, but such procedures remain experimental. Lesions (either neurosurgical or functional lesions achieved by implanted electrodes) in the subthalamic nucleus, thalamus, or the internal segment of the globus pallidus have showed promising results.

Huntington Disease

Huntington disease (HD) affects about one person in 10,000 and produces characteristic rapid, writhing, flicklike contortions of the hands, arms, and face, truncal writhing, and a profound dementia. The dementia tends to consist of progressive loss of cognitive function. The movements, which have been characterized as dancelike, give this disorder its alternative name, **Huntington chorea,** which has gone out of usage because it doesn't describe the rigidity and tremor seen in younger patients or the bradykinesia that replaces choreiform movements with age.

The disease is due to a dominant genetic defect on chromosome 4 involving an abnormally large number of copies of a base sequence within the gene coding for the normal protein "huntington." Fathers who pass the disorder on to their offspring tend to pass genes with especially large numbers of repeats, therefore making it more likely that their affected offspring might have a juvenile onset form of HD. Heritable autosomal dominant conditions must be either relatively compatible with normal life if manifested early or delayed in expression if more severe; otherwise they would interfere with reproduction and

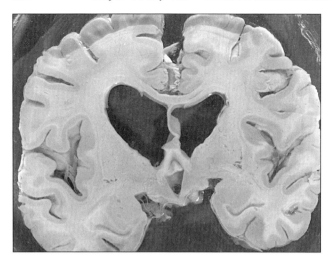

Figure 21.16 **Section through the Brain of a Person Who Died with Huntington Disease.** The basal ganglia, particularly the putamen, have atrophied and the cortex and underlying white matter have thinned. These conditions led to hydrocephalus ex vacuo.

Between ages 32 and 42, a woman progressed from neck pains, weakness, and tremor to confusion and significant intellectual deterioration. Although she was initially diagnosed as having MS, by age 42 choreiform movements indicated Huntington disease. She survived only a further ten years. No family history of the disease could be ascertained. This coronal section through the brain shows marked atrophy of the caudate nucleus, which allowed expansion of the ventricles.

consequently remove themselves from the gene pool. Huntington is an example of the latter case. Obvious clinical onset is usually at 35–45 years of age (range 20–50), and those who inherit it from their father show the disease earlier than those who inherit it from their mother (cytoplasmic constituents like maternal mitochondria appear to play a role). While the precise gene has not been localized, prenatal or postnatal predictive testing is accurate in almost 100% of cases. The uncertainty that used to hang over the heads of children of an affected adult can now be replaced with accurate information. In half of those tested, the news will be painful.

The pathology focuses on massive cellular loss from the caudate and putamen, with secondary loss of cells in particularly the frontal cortex. The ventricles are dilated (hydrocephalus ex vacuo), as indicated in figure 21.16. Current investigation of the pathophysiology concentrates on the role of excessive stimulation (excitotoxicity). Other medications are used to control chorea and tremoring, and antipsychotics are used to subdue the emotional outbursts that accompany the dementia. The average course of the disease to complete incapacitation and death is about 15 years.

COMPLEX DISORDERS

Cerebral Palsy

The term **cerebral palsy** (CP) is applied to a disparate collection of disabilities that derive from perinatal brain injury. Movement problems are prominent and readily ob-

servable, but sensory and cognitive deficits are also common. The mechanism, extent, and location of the injury will vary, but the child has survived and the injury is nonprogressive. The presence or severity of CP may not be evident in the young infant. But as deficits in voluntary movement and abnormally strong reflex patterns emerge, the original injury will become apparent. Also, in the absence of adequate supportive physiotherapy and training, the range of motor behavior may be restricted and musculoskeletal deformities may progress, but this does not indicate a worsening of brain function.

Because the term *cerebral palsy* has little descriptive or prognostic value and may carry a burden of erroneous meaning, many authorities would prefer more precise and specific terminology. Nevertheless, the term endures. Since its meaning can be so variable, however, neither the public nor the health care professional should be satisfied with less than a clear description of the extent of a given person's disability and a program of how best to work with it. Court cases over possible negligence or malpractice by those attending a birth have forced medical personnel to be much more precise in describing the timing and mechanism of the injuries that give rise to these disorders.

To understand the symptom complex possible in cerebral palsy, it is necessary to recognize that the injuries that cause it usually affect a relatively mature fetal or neonatal nervous system. The varied brain lesions generally act to separate well-developed and functioning components of the motor system (see the motor systems overview provided in figure 21.7). In this context, remember that the cord and brain stem, which are largely unaffected, house a host of motor reflexes that either are present at birth or emerge with the maturation of the infant and are overridden by voluntary motor behavior. Table 21.10 focuses on these normal reflex patterns that can become problematic in CP.

Infection, toxins, or anoxia can also damage highly cellular structures (areas of the cortex or hippocampus, the basal ganglia, the cerebellum, other smaller nuclei). This combination of disconnection and injury can result in impaired voluntary movement, exaggeration of reflex activity, and the development of abnormal movements. Interruption of pathways from the cortex to brain stem nuclei and the spinal cord similarly results in impaired voluntary movement. It also releases the reflex activity of the cord (hyperreflexia) and allows the unmediated activity of brain stem nuclei (e.g., increased flexor or extensor tone, reflex extension of the arms if the head is tipped back in dressing—symmetrical tonic neck reflex). The person's limited voluntary movement may itself excite these reflex behaviors. To these may be added impaired or abnormal movements symptomatic of either basal ganglia or cerebellar lesion (table 21.11).

These motor disabilities are the most obvious signs of cerebral palsy. However, the precipitating lesions are undiscriminating. It is reasonable to expect deficits in sensation from congenitally paralyzed or partially paralyzed limbs, although these will be difficult to assess and not, of course, apparent to the individual affected by CP, because he has only his own sensory experience to compare it to.

Table 21.10	Normal Reflexes in Infancy

Primitive Reflexes

These are present at birth or in the early months. Loss of certain of these (by CNS override or suppression) is necessary for development of other reflexes or conscious motor control.

    Stepping reflex: baby held under arms, held over a table with soles of feet pressed against it, produces stepping movement.

    Placing reflex: when dorsal aspect of foot is stimulated, leg is raised.

(These can be seen as preparatory to walking. They are replaced by "leg straightening" and "standing balance" reflexes as noted.)

    Moro response (startle response): arms and legs thrust out, then arms drawn in, crying. Stimulus is a sudden position change or thump on bed; fades by 5 months.

    Palmar grasp (Darwinian reflex): clasping response to insertion of object into palm. Fades at 3 months as grasp is more consciously controlled.

    Asymmetrical tonic neck reflex: baby supine; when head turned to one side, arm and leg on that side extend, opposite side flexes. May prevent rolling; fades by 6 months. Also called the "fencing reflex."

    Symmetrical tonic neck reflex: on all fours; extension of neck causes extension of arms and flexion of legs; flexion of neck elicits the reverse. Appears briefly at 6 months before infant learns to crawl; must be lost to crawl effectively.

    Landau maneuver: suspend infant horizontally in prone position; by 6 months most will extend neck and trunk. Flexion of neck will elicit flexion of hips, knees, and elbows.

    Crossed extension reflex: when the sole of the held foot of a supine baby is stroked, the opposite leg is flexed, abducted, and then extended.

Reflexes that Develop Postnatally and Persist

    Leg straightening: pressure to soles of feet elicits straightening of leg. Appears at 6–8 months.

    Balance reaction: sitting (appears at 6 months). } (These emerge when a seated or standing infant is thrown off balance;

    Balance reaction: standing (appears at 6 months). } the arms go out in the direction of the fall.)

    Parachute reaction: on sudden lowering of infant, arms extend over head and legs extend. Appears at 8 months.

(These reflexes are generally adaptive but must be suppressed in sports like tumbling and judo.)

Permanent Reflexes

    Babinski: before 2 years, extension of big toe and fanning of other toes. After 2 years, plantar flexion.

    Tendon jerks: can be elicited in any large muscle with narrow tendinous insertion; also called myotatic stretch reflexes or deep tendon reflexes.

Note: Abnormalities of reflex patterns (e.g., exaggerated, diminished, asymmetrical responses or delay in age of onset or disappearance) suggest cerebral damage or abnormalities of brain development.

Impairment of special sensation (vision, hearing, taste, and smell) will be variable, depending on the nature and location of the causative lesion. The mechanisms of injury are such that much cortical function can remain intact. Therefore, normal or superior intelligence is certainly possible, even in people with profound motor impairments. However, lesions sufficient to cause CP are also likely to impair general intelligence. With exceptions, there is a rough correlation between the degree of motor and mental impairment. Even those with normal intelligence may be hyperkinetic or distractable, have a short attention span, be subject to preseveration (getting stuck on one activity or stimulus), or have apraxias (inability to organize movements consistently in appropriate sequence).

It is common to classify CP on the basis of the area of the body most affected. Thus, you may encounter terms like quadriplegic CP (all four limbs affected more or less equally), diplegic CP (lower limbs more affected than upper), and monoplegic CP (only one limb affected). Alternatively, classification may focus on the predominant motor impairment—for example, spastic CP or athetoid CP.

The disconnections are largely due to a variety of vascular lesions in white matter. The relatively low blood pressure and expandable nature of the fetal skull allow fetuses and newborns to survive lesions that would threaten an adult. Perhaps 50% of preterm infants are subject to hemorrhage into the delicate germinal eminence (also called the subependymal plate), embryonic tissue that remains on the surface of the wall of the lateral ventricles until about 32–33 weeks into gestation. This hemorrhage may be confined to the immediate tissue and be asymptomatic. Rupture into the ventricles has more devastating and widespread consequences, compressing tissues including the internal capsule and basal ganglia. Cerebellar hemorrhage can occur in premature and full-term infants, causing damage to the cerebellar hemisphere. The white matter surrounding the ventricles is subject to both hemorrhage and ischemic infarct, which can damage the internal capsule or association fibers. Gray matter can suffer ischemic/hypoxic, toxic, or infective injury.

Although some CP can be attributed to birth trauma, these cases are in the minority. Many lesions arise well before or after delivery. The best preventive care is that

Table 21.11   Possible Symptom Complex in Cerebral Palsy Associated with Lesions to Motor Tracts, the Cerebellum, and the Basal Ganglia. For explanation, see section on motor system function.

Motor Tracts	Cerebellum	Basal Ganglia
Impaired voluntary movement (both fine and gross)	Hypotonia or atonia	Bradykinesia
Spasticity	Ataxia	Choreiform movements
Limb deformities due to unbalanced muscle tone (flexion at wrists, elbows, knees, hips, plantar-flexion of feet)	Intention/terminal tremor	Athetosis
Contractures	Nystagmus	Ballism
Hyperreflexia (stretch, crossed extension, symmetrical and asymmetrical neck, Moro)	Dysdiadochokinesia	Rigidity
	Dysarthria	Dystonia (athetoid movements frozen, usually, in extreme extension)

oriented to the prevention of prematurity or other complications of pregnancy, with emphasis on good maternal nutrition, postponing pregnancy until full adulthood, and healthy maternal life style.

Multiple Sclerosis

It is helpful to consider **multiple sclerosis** (MS) in the context of cerebral palsy. Unlike CP, MS arises through a single mechanism of lesion: focal, chronic, progressive, usually exacerbating and remitting demyelination of CNS tracts. As in CP, however, the lesions can occur in a wide variety of locations and, hence, give rise to complex symptom patterns. The areas of demyelination are called **plaques** and, while confined to white matter, can occur at any site where oligodendrocytes produce the myelin sheaths that facilitate the conduction of signals. This includes the cerebrum (where plaques tend to occur around the ventricles), the brain stem, the cerebellum, and the spinal cord. Involvement of the optic nerve produces monocular visual disturbance, which is the first reported symptom in about one-quarter of patients. While the plaques remain and mature, the specific symptoms usually worsen and then improve or resolve. The apparent movement of symptoms that is related to the development of new active plaques, and their emergence over time, gave rise to the older name for this disorder, disseminated sclerosis.

The clinical presentation depends on the location, extent, and pattern of development of the active plaques. This is a disease of young people (20–40 years old), rarely having onset before age 15 or after age 50. As noted, many people experience a transitory, usually unilateral visual impairment or blindness. About half of those who present with this **optic neuritis** go on to be diagnosed with MS. Double vision, caused by demyelination of the brain stem tract that coordinates the actions of the three nuclei responsible for eye movements **(internuclear ophthalmoplegia),** is common while not specific to MS. **Lhermitte's sign** (tingling in the back and anterior thigh upon neck flexion) is

frequently seen but again, not specific. A patient who becomes heated—either passively (from hot weather or from sitting in a hot tub) or actively (from exercise)—often experiences worsening of symptoms. This effect of heat is called **Uhthoff's phenomenon.**

Laboratory investigation of suspected MS often starts with a lumbar puncture. A slight increase in proteins may be noted, with a pattern of electrophoretic migration called **oligoclonal banding.** This finding, which is fairly specific to MS, is due to the presence of antibodies within the CSF, suggestive of an immune mediation of the disease. Changes in the conduction velocities along visual or auditory pathways in the CNS are detected by testing responses to visual and auditory stimuli. MRI is proving invaluable at imaging active and burned-out or silent plaques. Because the diagnosis of MS is problematic and has obvious import to the patient, the detection of a second plaque by means of electrodiagnostic tests, CT, or MRI is actively pursued.

The predominant pattern in MS is chronic exacerbation and remission (chronic MS). Symptoms become worse for two or three weeks, then partially resolve for perhaps one to five years, only to become worse again. The second occurrence can bring about a worsening of existing symptoms or the onset of entirely new ones. The third may be sooner and more extensive again. Various stresses can apparently trigger an exacerbation (infection, medication, stress, fatigue). The course of MS is unstable and unpredictable. About 10% of cases undergo a severe, rapid, progressive deterioration (acute progressive MS). Some individuals have died within seven months of first symptoms because of a combination of acute brain inflammation associated with the plaques and intercurrent infection. On the other hand, a significant number of people are never severely incapacitated, and some apparently experience a single episode that arrests and resolves (acute MS). Death, when it occurs, is usually attributable to the complications of MS (respiratory infection because of impaired ventilation, bladder and then kidney infection secondary to ineffective emptying, etc.).

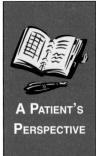

MS: Life on a Roller Coaster

*—Alicia Priest, The Vancouver Sun,
Monday, May 9, 1988.
Reprinted with permission.*

Seven years ago when Linda Young was 30, the world seemed to be singing her song.

Recently married to a New Zealander, Young was on the verge of emigrating to Kiwiland and, with her husband, sailing the South Seas on the 25-meter schooner he had built.

An avid dancer, sailor, bowler and occasional golfer, Young never imagined she'd be anything but socially and physically active.

Then everything changed. On a return visit to Vancouver, Young—who had experienced periodic episodes of numbness and blurred vision—was told she had multiple sclerosis.

A mysterious and incurable disease, MS is renowned for destroying people's dreams and plans for the future. It usually hits between the ages of 20 and 40.

A chronic, progressive ailment of the central nervous system, MS can cause blurred vision, loss of balance, slurred speech and paralysis. The course of the disease is unpredictable—sufferers often go through a cycle of remissions and relapses.

"The unpredictability of the disease makes coping very difficult," says April Lewis, a medical social worker and public awareness chairman for the B.C. division of the Multiple Sclerosis Society of Canada.

"I've had MS patients say to me 'it's like living on a roller coaster,'" Lewis says.

The disease has a reputation for tearing marriages and families apart.

"I was in shock . . . I thought What now?" Young says. "Travel was going to be the main focus of our lives but with a disease like this . . . every time I saw someone in a wheelchair I burst into tears and thought. "That's going to be me."

Young broke the news to her husband over the phone but because of her diagnosis, she was denied immigrant status in New Zealand. Her husband, who was physically fit but had two tumors removed from his leg, was denied immigrant status in Canada. The marriage dissolved.

"We were two medical misfits no one wanted," Young says. "Obviously, this marriage wasn't meant to be."

Now on a full disability pension, Young lives in a suburban co-op and is a single mother of a three-year old girl, Stacey.

"My lifestyle has taken a 180-degree switch," she says. "I used to thrive on stress—I loved the ups and downs. Now I can't handle crowds in a busy department store."

She says she went through the full range of emotions—from denial to anger to depression—before arriving at a point where she could cope with her illness.

Because she has a form of a disease called benign MS, Young's symptoms are largely invisible. While she uses a cane to maintain her balance—which her daughter calls "Mommy's walking stick"—she still gets dirty looks when she parks in a handicapped parking spot.

Her main complaint is excessive fatigue and weakness in her arms and legs. On a bad day, simple tasks like lifting a book are overwhelming.

Raising a child is exhausting at the best of times, but for someone with MS being a mother is especially taxing. Stacey is a typical, energetic toddler who sometimes leaves her mother far behind.

Resolute and determined to remain as self-reliant as possible, Young refuses to fit into the traditional MS mold.

"The general public has to realize that someone with MS is not someone old in a wheelchair," she says.

The symptom complex includes most of those on the list for cerebral palsy (table 21.11). Hyperreflexia is certainly detectable, but the exaggerated movements associated with basal ganglia involvement are not a problem (choreiform movements, athetosis, dystonia, ballism). The person may experience increased urinary frequency and urgency, and difficulty in urinating, as well as difficulty in swallowing, dysarthria, and extreme intolerance of heat. Large lesions in the frontal or temporal lobes may lead to emotional outbursts (swearing, weeping, laughing) that are unrelated to the situation or the person's apparent feeling state. Depression or euphoria can be a problem. This may have both a neurological and psychological basis. The unpredictable progression and attendant disability can overtax an individual's capacity to cope. Occasionally, an MS plaque

and associated edema can block transmission in the cord **(transverse myelitis),** causing paraplegia or quadriplegia.

Of the many drug therapies attempted, only corticosteroids and ACTH (adrenocorticotropic hormone) appear to have any effect. They can reduce the duration of an exacerbation but have no impact on the long-term outcome of the disease. Recent experimental work with interferon β (IFN$_\beta$) has shown some promising results in arresting the progression of MS. However, maintaining a healthy outlook and life style, while easy to prescribe and difficult to carry out, will benefit a patient more than any approaches at a cure that are currently available.

Study of the underlying pathophysiology is continuing. From such research it appears that the active plaque is a region of ongoing demyelination, in which myelin sheaths undergo breakdown and phagocytic destruction. The presence of antibodies against certain myelin proteins may play a role in this attack. The decreased signal conduction through a plaque is attributable to a combination of edema, disturbing the extracellular environment, and demyelination, exposing normally hidden potassium channels on the axons that short-circuit the signal. Resolution of edema and partial remyelination subsequently restore at least partial function. Eventually an active plaque is converted to a silent (burned-out) plaque in which widespread demyelination is again the rule, with extensive gliosis. Further exacerbation, however, produces new plaques. MRI has revealed that gradually plaques coalesce, expanding the area of impaired conduction and producing permanent dysfunction.

The epidemiology of MS hints at an interaction between a viral illness in the teen years and a genetic predisposition. People who grow up in northern temperate climates have increased risk, which they carry with them if they move after adolescence. Likewise, people from tropical regions are protected unless they move to a temperate clime as a child. Another finding in support of a genetic predisposition is the greater susceptibility of those not of Asian heritage, wherever they live.

Alzheimer Disease

Dementia, the loss of ordered neural function, is a major symptom in a number of unrelated disorders. Dementia is, in practice, a broad term that may denote disorder in many independent capacities: discrimination of and attending to stimuli, storing new memories and retrieving old ones, planning and the delay of gratification, abstraction and problem solving, judgment and reasoning, orientation in time and space, language processing, the appropriate use of objects, the planning and execution of voluntary movement. In **Alzheimer disease** (AD) there is a slow (usually five years or more) but inexorable progression of dementia in which mental function is surrendered more or less in the order just stated.

The memory loss initially affects only short-term storage and retrieval, but gradually extends to well-consolidated memories as well. Many people experience restlessness, sometimes almost a compulsion to move or walk. Combined with failing memory, this wandering can be a major problem for both the patient and those responsible for the patient. Many patients retain insight, at least in the early stages of the disease, which is another source of anxiety and depression. Ultimately the person is left mute and paralyzed. Death comes from infection of a weakened, dehydrated patient. In parallel, the personality—the combined qualities of cognition and temperament that are unique to a person—also suffers fragmentation. It is often this loss, perhaps years before the physical death of the person, that is most difficult for friends and family.

Senility—that is, age-related dementia—used to be evoked as a catch-all explanation for any disturbances of mental functioning that might appear in old age. The implication was that these were part and parcel of growing old, and could not be helped. But many such conditions are reversible, such as altered mental function due to depression, impaired heart function, or anemia. The bottom line is that no dementia should be seen as a normal concomitant of aging. The pathological basis should be vigorously explored and treated where possible. Of dementias that result from degenerative brain disorders (old term: **organic brain syndrome,** OBS), two have pathology concentrated in the cerebral cortex: Pick's disease and Alzheimer disease. **Pick's disease** is rarer and symptomatically indistinguishable from Alzheimer's. It tends to focus on the frontal and temporal lobes and leads to marked atrophy of the gyri, called walnut brain at autopsy. This difference from the more generalized pattern of atrophy in Alzheimer may be detectable in CT or MRI scans. The distinction may be academic, as the course is very similar.

Alzheimer disease may appear in patients as young as 50, in which case it used to be called presenile dementia. With advancing age the incidence of Alzheimer increases. About 6% of the population of older adults (post-65) are afflicted and almost half of those over 85 years of age are affected. Pathology is restricted to the cerebral cortex, the hippocampus, a nearby nucleus called the amygdala, and another called the basal nucleus of Meynert. Cells in the latter normally produce the neurotransmitter acetylcholine, which travels along widely branching axons to synapses in the cerebral cortex. Loss of cells in this nucleus results in widespread cortical depletion of acetylcholine and related chemicals, and presumably results in impaired neural function. A generalized loss of mainly pyramidal cells (see chapter 22) occurs in the areas named. As pyramidal cells die, so do their associated axons, which leads to loss of white matter. Gyri shrink and the ventricles expand (hypocephalus ex vacuo), reflecting the atrophy. The gyri thin while the sulci correspondingly widen, giving the brain a "walnut like" appearance at autopsy. The combination of clinical signs and MRI showing signs characteristics of these changes allows for accurate diagnosis in the majority (80–90%) of affected individuals. Early disease may be mistaken for a variety of conditions. Late disease is less ambiguous.

Three microscopic findings correlate with the severity and progression of the disease. **Neurofibrillary tangles** are cytoplasmic bundles of filaments that encircle or displace the nucleus of the pyramidal cells. They are apparent with silver staining methods. The major component is helically coiled phosphorylated **tau protein,** the same material that makes up the plaques about to be described. They can be seen as "ghost tangles" long after the neuron has died.

Neuritic (senile) plaques consist of a cluster of neural processes filled with filaments (such as are found in tangles) microglia and phagocytic astrocytes, surrounding a poorly staining core. This core is composed of a variant of proteins that, when deposited, are collectively called **amyloid** (starch-like) because they appear like clear starch. Neither the tangles nor the plaques are specific to Alzheimer's but are found in smaller numbers in normal aging brains and in other pathological conditions. Much research is now concentrating on the pathology that produces these plaques, with the intent of controlling or reversing it. **Amyloid precursor protein** (APP), although a normal constituent of cell membranes, is elevated in production in injured and Alzheimer brains. As well, it appears to undergo an abnormal breakdown in the Alzheimer brain. Instead of being processed into an integral protein that plays an unidentified role in the membranes of neurons, it is converted in lysosomes to an amyloid forming variant: **amyloid beta protein.** This substance is directly toxic to neural tissue and is involved in triggering or supporting a generalized inflammatory response. It can form small aggregations that produce an aberrant Ca^{2+} channel that may cause neurons to wear out. And it accretes as the major component of the amyloid that produces the senile plaques. **Amyloid angiopathy** is found only in cortical and small subarachnoid arteries. The amyloid is the same as that in the plaque cores and will be found as a clear zone in the muscle layer of these vessels.

About 10% of cases are familial, more commonly with early onset. The gene responsible is located on chromosome 21, as is the gene that produces the amyloid protein. Much research is investigating this and its connection to Down syndrome (trisomy 21). Interestingly, almost all people with Down syndrome who live beyond age 45 develop Alzheimer disease. Mutations identified in the APP gene in these people are correlated with both increased APP production and early onset of familial AD. The presence of mutations in two genes that code for intracellular proteins called "presenilins" (on chromosomes 1 and 14) has been related to the development of early-onset familial AD. More recently, research has advanced in identifying abnormalities in enzymes (secretases) that associate with presenilins and result in increased conversion of abnormal APP into amyloid beta protein. To date, no practical treatments have developed from this work.

This disease has thus far proved resistant to medical treatment. Potentially, knowledge of the formation, processing, and perhaps degradation of amyloid protein, may provide methods of treatment. In addition, the raised levels of aluminum found in the brains of Alzheimer's patients have been an active research focus. It is not clear whether aluminum levels are raised secondarily by release from dying neurons or play a direct or cofactor role, in combination with other toxins or a genetic predisposition. There is no evidence to support not using aluminum cookware or deodorants containing aluminum. Chelating agents that bind and remove aluminum have shown some promise, temporarily arresting or reversing some symptoms. THA (tetrahydroaminoacridine) has been used experimentally, particularly in the early stages, to enhance memory function. Despite major risks of liver toxicity, careful steps are being taken to make THA available on a limited basis because of its apparent effectiveness. And most recently, the observation that arthritics have a lower incidence of Alzheimer's has been translated into an apparently effective therapy at slowing progression. This is the use of as-

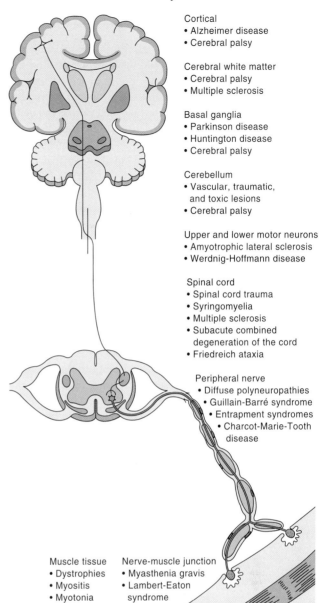

Cortical
• Alzheimer disease
• Cerebral palsy

Cerebral white matter
• Cerebral palsy
• Multiple sclerosis

Basal ganglia
• Parkinson disease
• Huntington disease
• Cerebral palsy

Cerebellum
• Vascular, traumatic,
  and toxic lesions
• Cerebral palsy

Upper and lower motor neurons
• Amyotrophic lateral sclerosis
• Werdnig-Hoffmann disease

Spinal cord
• Spinal cord trauma
• Syringomyelia
• Multiple sclerosis
• Subacute combined
  degeneration of the cord
• Friedreich ataxia

Peripheral nerve
• Diffuse polyneuropathies
• Guillain-Barré syndrome
• Entrapment syndromes
• Charcot-Marie-Tooth
  disease

Muscle tissue
• Dystrophies
• Myositis
• Myotonia

Nerve-muscle junction
• Myasthenia gravis
• Lambert-Eaton
  syndrome

Figure 21.17   **Overview of Pathologies That Affect Movement.**

pirin, which appears to arrest or slow the inflammatory component of this complex pathology.

In the meantime, the predominant therapy continues to center on minimizing the problems and frustration created by failing cognitive skills and on encouraging the exercise of remaining skills. A great deal can be done by simplifying the environment while maintaining elements that are familiar and personal. Remaining capacity can be exercised through intensely focused rehearsal and stimulation and the use of redundant cues (color coding plus labeling plus symbols, etc.). There is an emphasis on diet and exercise. Keeping the family involved by giving them the support and encouragement they require anchors this approach.

Figure 21.17 provides an overview of the various derangements that can affect motor functions.

Case Study

This case involves a 21-year-old cocktail server. She had been well previously and had no history of any serious illness. According to her statement, she "was into alternative, holistic lifestyle remedies" and had pursued various fad diets.

On her 21st birthday she celebrated by eating half of a box of chocolates, and a few hours later experienced a loss of vision in her left eye. She attributed this effect to the "heavy sugar rush" from the chocolates she had ingested, and so she initially sought no medical attention. She finally did see her doctor because, over the next four days, her eye became quite painful and her vision remained poor. She appeared generally healthy, and because no obvious abnormalities were detected by an eye examination, her general practitioner referred her to an ophthalmologist.

His diagnosis was optic neuritis, which, in the young and otherwise healthy, is strongly associated with multiple sclerosis. No treatment was given because the patient refused prednisone to alleviate her eye symptoms. She was referred to an MS clinic, where the diagnosis was verified on the basis of her history and the ophthalmologist's workup, but the patient refused any further tests. No treatment was prescribed, although annual follow-up examinations were recommended. She was then lost to the clinic and her GP's office follow-up procedures.

Six months later she was admitted to the psychiatric ward of a major hospital for aggression and psychosis. She was brought to the hospital by a neighbor, who reported that for the past three or four days she had been complaining of being unable to sleep and was combative, delusional, and paranoid, expressing bizarre and grandiose ideas. The neighbor didn't know the name of her GP (or even if she had one), so her medical records or history could not be obtained. She was diagnosed as manic-depressive, and lithium carbonate therapy was initiated.

Six months after this episode, she returned to her GP for treatment of a minor injury sustained in an aerobics workout. In the course of their discussions she reported her experience of being committed to a psychiatric ward and stated that she had discontinued her medication because "it wouldn't let me get tuned into my cocktail lounge customers and my tips were bottoming out." She refused her doctor's recommendation of further testing, left, and was again lost to further follow-up.

Eight months later she was again admitted to a psychiatric ward, and a diagnosis of manic/depressive illness was made. After reinstatement of lithium carbonate therapy, she improved and was released. She had no known medical contacts subsequently, and three months later committed suicide.

Commentary

The altered mental states experienced by this unfortunate woman are a common feature of MS—for example, emotional instability, depression, or euphoria. It was these that the lithium carbonate therapy sought to counter. Severe changes such as mania may also occur, but these are more often seen late in the course. The alternating pattern of remission and relapse seen in this patient is also typical.

Unfortunately, MS presents many diagnostic difficulties, and this patient was not unusual in rejecting further investigations for fear that a relatively minor problem might reveal some serious illness. In this case, the patient insisted that MS was an unlikely diagnosis on the basis of, in her words "the sorry evidence of a few little eye problems."

Key Concepts

1. Drugs that affect autonomic function can produce broad or focused effects by taking advantage of variability in naturally occurring receptors (pp. 591–592).

2. While peripheral injuries can undergo repair, this is generally not the case with central neuron lesions (pp. 598–601).

3. The symptoms associated with lesions of the peripheral nerves or alpha motor neurons in the cord (lower motor neurons) are decreased muscle tone, weakness or paralysis of voluntary movement, decreased or absent reflexes, rapid muscle atrophy, and electromuscular signs of denervation (p. 602).

4. The symptoms associated with lesion to the upper motor neuron (all motor pathways above the alpha motor neuron) are increased muscle tone, weakness or paralysis of voluntary movement, increased reflexes, slow (disuse) atrophy, and abnormal plantar reflex (p. 604).

5. Lesions affecting the cerebellum may produce any of a constellation of symptoms, including imprecision and tremor in directing movements and difficulty in walking, speaking, or performing rapidly alternating movements or eye movements (pp. 605–607).

6. Lesions affecting the basal ganglia may produce difficulty in initiating movement, as well as tremoring, writhing or flicking movements at rest, and rigidity (p. 608).

7. Diseases affecting muscle, which usually derive from genetic or autoimmune disorders and result from a variety of mechanisms, tend to produce muscle weakness (p. 611).

8. The principal disorder of the neuromuscular junction, myasthenia gravis, results from an autoimmune-mediated loss of neurotransmitter receptors (pp. 611–612).

9. A variety of agents can cause scattered lesions to the peripheral nerves, giving rise to a variety of symptoms of sensory and/or motor impairment (pp. 612–613).

10. Entrapment syndromes produce focal lesions in peripheral nerves, impairing signal transmission and leading to muscle weakness and wasting and impaired sensation, accompanied by characteristic paresthesias (pp. 613–616).

11. While injury to the spinal cord may interrupt sensory or motor pathways and destroy reflex or integration centers, the long-term adaptation involves increased reflex activity below the site of motor lesion and a variety of other problems (pp. 616–618).

12. The syndrome of symptoms accompanying a specific spinal lesion depends on the site and extent of the lesion (p. 619).

13. Parkinson disease results from lesion of cells in the substantia nigra and includes symptoms of muscle rigidity, bradykinesia, tremor, stooped posture, shuffling gait, and autonomic dysfunction (pp. 622–623).

14. Huntington disease results from an autosomal dominant inheritance of a defective gene which, at 35–45, produces symptoms of increasing motor dysorder and cognitive impairment and derangement leading to death in about 15 years (pp. 623–624).

15. Cerebral palsy results when an ante- or perinatal lesion to a normal nervous system impairs voluntary control while producing hyperreflexia and perhaps symptoms characteristic of lesions to either the basal ganglia or cerebellum (pp. 624–626).

16. Multiple sclerosis produces episodically progressive sensory, motor, and psychic abnormalities through an unexplained, immune-mediated attack on central myelin (pp. 626–628).

17. Alzheimer disease results in progressive loss of functional cortical neurons and is the dominant degenerative dementia, ultimately affecting all mental function (pp. 628–629).

REVIEW ACTIVITIES

1. Describe as completely as you can the difference between (a) the sympathetic and parasympathetic nervous systems, (b) acetylcholine and norepinephrine, (c) alpha and beta adrenergic receptors, (d) beta$_1$ and beta$_2$ blockers, (e) agonist and blocker.

2. Explain the difference between MS and Guillain-Barré syndrome.

3. Prepare a table that highlights the similarities and differences between (a) Huntington disease and Parkinson disease, (b) cerebral palsy and MS, (c) ALS and Werdnig-Hoffmann disease, (d) Alzheimer disease and Huntington's disease.

4. You are playing charades with your three best friends, who are all neurologists. You decide to act out a lower motor lesion. What would you actually *do?*

5. List the symptoms that lesions to either the cerebellum or basal ganglia have in common. Now list the symptoms that are different.

6. Differentiate between the weakness associated with polymyositis and that of myasthenia gravis.

Chapter

22

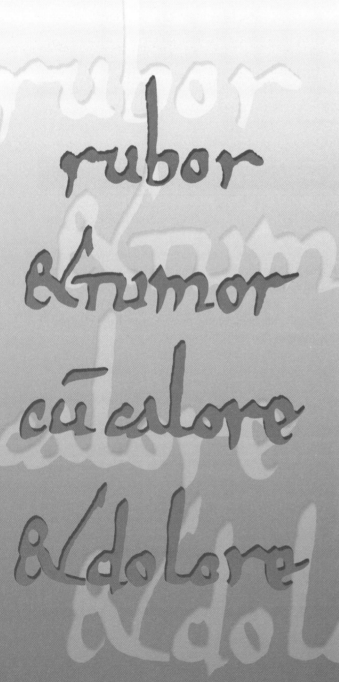

Seizures and Epilepsy

And when the fit was upon him, I did mark how he did shake . . .

WILLIAM SHAKESPEARE
JULIUS CAESAR

In North America, seizures are a relatively common occurrence, with approximately 2.5 million people subject to active epilepsy. That is, they have a continuing susceptibility to seizures that is not attributable to some other medical condition. Among acute neurological disorders, only stroke is more common. Epileptic seizures occur over a wide range of intensities from the trivial (e.g., a spontaneous perception of odor) to the life-threatening.

In addition to epilepsy, a large number of people experience convulsive states arising from another illness—for example, acute renal failure or cardiac arrest. This chapter is intended to provide information about both sorts of seizure activity and to establish the basis for understanding seizure development and progression.

SOME BACKGROUND CONCEPTS AND TERMINOLOGY

In discussing seizures and epilepsy, some familiarity with a core of basic terms and concepts is essential. The following sections deal with those most frequently encountered by health care professionals.

General Concepts

When dealing with seizures, a patient's level of consciousness can be of central importance, and any departure from full consciousness should be noted. Such **impaired consciousness** in a patient might be noted as "It was difficult to catch her attention" or "He appeared awake but didn't respond to questions."

A **convulsion** is an episode of widespread and intense motor activity. These may occur in isolation or in a series, and may often, but not always, be associated with a loss of consciousness. By contrast, a **seizure** is a rapidly evolving disturbance of brain function that may produce impaired consciousness, abnormalities of sensation or mental functioning, or convulsive movements. Because these may arise in combination, particular descriptive terms are used, such as **convulsive seizure** or **sensory seizure**, depending on which derangements are most prominent.

Epilepsy

Epilepsy is the condition characterized by a relatively long-term disturbance of brain structure and/or function that produces an increased susceptibility to seizures. The strict diagnosis of epilepsy requires a history of at least two seizures that can't reasonably be attributed to some other disease. In epilepsy, the underlying abnormality is centered within the brain itself. If seizure activity can be eliminated by correction of some metabolic disorder or by removal of a brain tumor, the diagnosis of epilepsy can't be made.

Seizure Terminology

The word element -*ictal* refers to activity during a seizure (*ictus* is Latin for a blow). **Interictal** is used in reference to the situation between periods of seizure activity. Another term encountered in the context of seizures is **photic stimulation.** It refers to the use of an intense flashing light to elicit an abnormal electroencephalogram (EEG) or an actual seizure, which is related to some underlying epilepsy-related abnormality. Photic stimulation, in combination with an EEG, can localize the focus of abnormal brain activity and may be encountered in the diagnosis of both epileptic and nonepileptic seizures.

A **partial seizure** is seizure activity that is caused by an abnormal discharge from a relatively restricted set of brain structures. For this reason it may also be known as a **focal** or **local** seizure. Partial seizures are characterized by only limited behavioral, mental, sensory, or motor expression. In contrast, a **generalized seizure** involves more widespread derangements arising from abnormal brain activity occurring over large areas of the cerebral cortex of both hemispheres at once. Such seizures may be varied, involving major convulsive activity or perhaps impaired consciousness accompanied by lip smacking or eye blinking. Generalized seizures affect both sides of the body, or at least produce bilateral abnormalities of brain wave activity.

A **tonic-clonic seizure** is a generalized convulsive seizure involving loss of consciousness. It starts with a stiffening of the muscles (tonic) and progresses to alternating spasms of contraction and relaxation (clonic). The term **myoclonic seizure** refers to muscle twitching and/or limb jerking movements due to abnormal cortical activity. Its actions are more localized than the coordinated whole body spasms seen in a clonic seizure. In the special case of the **myoclonic jerk,** the upper limbs or the entire body is thrown into one or two pronounced twitches. When serious progressive brain pathology induces myoclonic seizures, the condition is designated **myoclonus epilepsy.**

Hyperactivity of the stretch reflexes is known as **clonus.** An example would be brief, repetitive "pulsing" of the foot in reaction to sudden, passive dorsiflexion. It derives principally from defective functioning at the level of the spinal cord, although higher central nervous system pathology may also be the cause.

NONEPILEPTIC SEIZURES

Many seizures encountered in a health care setting will be **nonepileptic.** They will typically arise as a result of an extreme metabolic disruption associated with systemic disease, specific toxins, a deficiency state, or the local effects of a brain tumor. The following conditions produce most nonepileptic seizures.

Withdrawal from Sedative/Hypnotic Drugs

Generalized tonic-clonic seizures are a potential hazard complicating withdrawal from barbiturates and other sedative/hypnotic drugs, alcohol, and, interestingly, anticonvulsants (drugs used to suppress seizures or convulsions). The seizures may come in clusters, and victims are prone to convulsive **status epilepticus,** a life-threatening chaining

Focus on Alcohol Withdrawal and Seizures

Recent work has shown that chronic alcohol abuse induces the production and release of GABA, an inhibitory neurotransmitter. In time the brain adapts to this inhibition by increasing its level of excitation. Withdrawal from alcohol removes GABA's inhibitory effects, leaving the brain at a level of excitation that can produce seizures over the short-term. Drugs like phenobarbital and diazepam (Valium), which appear to have their anticonvulsant effect by raising GABA levels, are used temporarily to treat such seizures and then are slowly tapered off.

of seizure activity that will be discussed later. (About 3% of alcohol withdrawal patients who experience seizures go on to develop status epilepticus.) If acute withdrawal is the precipitating factor in the seizures, other symptoms should be evident, at least with alcohol and barbiturates: trembling, disturbed sleep, disorientation, illusions or hallucinations. (Also common is a high sensitivity to photic stimulation.) Gradual withdrawal, which is appropriate when removing a habituated patient from a prescribed barbiturate or other sedative drug, minimizes most of these symptoms and risks.

About 5% of those who have abstained from drinking alcohol after severe, chronic alcohol abuse will experience **delierium-tremens** (formerly called "the DTs"). This will occur following other phases of alcohol withdrawal (immediately after the phase in which the person is susceptible to the seizures just described) and occurs between three and ten days after the person has stopped drinking alcohol. The pathophysiological mechanisms is the same as that described for seizures (chronic loss of GABA inhibition). The person is agitated and confused, has vivid hallucinations, tremors, sweating, a racing heart, and elevated blood pressure. Treatment is largely symptomatic, but includes administration of diazepam (Valium) to increase seizure threshold and thiamine to offset the development of confusion and hallucinations. This is not a seizure disorder as such.

Bacterial Meningitis

Seizures often accompany bacterial meningitis, particularly with children. Meningeal signs (see chapter 20) and a lumbar puncture would have already established the diagnosis in most cases, but for some it is the myoclonic jerks or full tonic-clonic seizure that brings them to the emergency ward.

Renal Failure and Hepatic Failure

The crisis stage of renal failure follows about two or three days after the kidneys cease urine production (anuria). The resultant uremia and associated electrolyte changes can cause a dramatic convulsive display that includes twitching and trembling, myoclonic jerks, generalized convulsions, and possible tetany. This is the most dramatic seizure display to accompany an illness. These symptoms arise from complex metabolic derangements that include hyperkalemia, hypocalcemia, and elevated blood levels of urea and creatinine. Dialysis is used to control these conditions while the underlying renal failure either resolves (perhaps with transplant) or progresses to the end-stage, coma and death.

Hepatic failure, which is most usually associated with alcoholic cirrhosis but develops in any severe or advanced hepatitis, may produce **hepatic encephalopathy.** The symptoms may range from marked forgetfulness to impaired arousability to coma. The most characteristic motor symptom is a tremor ("liver flaps," "flapping tremor," "asterixis"). If an affected person stands with her arms extended and her hands outstretched the hands will collapse downward as there is a brief lapse in muscle tension, and then return to the extended position. This is not an seizure phenomenon (i.e., not generated by cortical discharge) and is found in association with severe hepatic, renal, and pulmonar disorders.

Hypoxic Encephalopathy

Individuals who have experienced cerebral hypoxia (resulting from cardiac arrest, carbon monoxide poisoning, near-drowning, suffocation, respiratory failure, etc.) often experience seizures when oxygen supply to the brain is restored. Myoclonic jerks affecting any part of the body or full-blown tonic-clonic seizures may result. Susceptibility usually lasts for a few days in association with stupor and confusion. A persistent **intention myoclonus**—which is not a seizure disorder—will develop in some people. In this condition, voluntary movements may elicit myoclonic jerks that can dramatically impair function. These people may also show sensory and motor deficits attributable to watershed infarcts (see chapter 20) and extensive memory and mental processing deficits.

Febrile Convulsions

The developing nervous system is somewhat more susceptible to seizures, including those induced by fever. Perhaps 5% of children three months to five years of age will experience seizures with fever (febrile convulsions or seizures), and in about one-third of that number, seizures will recur. Febrile seizures usually take the form of a brief, generalized motor convulsion, but focal seizures will be observed in 10% of patients. They occur in the absence of any brain infection or other CNS abnormality and are not usually classified as epileptic. Essentially three very different situations can give rise to seizures during fever: most commonly a normal brain may be destabilized by fever, or fever may trigger an epileptic brain's first seizure, or a brain with other serious progressive pathology can first generate a seizure during fever.

Historically, physicians have tended to suspect that febrile seizures, particularly recurrent ones, might lead to a permanent alteration of brain function and epilepsy and so have aggressively administered anticonvulsants (especially phenobarbital). However, only a small minority of children who experience febrile seizures subsequently develop epilepsy, and the connection between epilepsy and *recurrent* febrile seizures is only slightly stronger. Only 1–2% of children who have experienced a "simple febrile seizure" (i.e., brief seizure lacking focal manifestations) go on to develop prolonged convulsions or epilepsy. The risk escalates to about 10% for children who experience "complex febrile seizures" (focal signs, duration over 15 minutes, frequent recurrence within 24 hours), have a family history of seizures, or who had neurological abnormalities before their first febrile convulsion. Currently, therefore, the therapeutic approach is more conservative. Only those with abnormal neurological or other development, a family history of epilepsy, or unusually prolonged or focal febrile seizures are subjected to preventative anticonvulsant therapy. For the vast majority, standard care for the control of fevers appears to be appropriate.

Brain Tumor

A nonepileptic seizure may result from the effects of a brain tumor. Although the mechanism is not clear (compression and metabolic insufficiency or reactive gliosis), cortical tissue adjacent to a tumor may become a seizure focus. In fact, it is not unusual for a tumor's presence to be initially revealed by an abnormal EEG or a seizure. Where the tumor can be removed or otherwise suppressed, the seizure activity usually subsides. If these cortical changes persist after the tumor has been removed, then we can say the tumor has produced the epilepsy.

Cerebrovascular Accident

Seizures will infrequently accompany an embolic, thrombotic, or hemorrhagic CVA. A more common occurrence is for the cortical region adjacent to an area infarcted by a CVA to become a focus of seizure activity. As many as one-quarter of those who survive a CVA will have some continuing, usually focal, seizure activity. Note that in these cases the individuals have developed epilepsy. The risk of having or developing epilepsy secondary to injury, CVA, or other unknown cause, is about 3% by age 74, whereas the risk of experiencing a provoked or unprovoked seizure by that age is about 9%.

EPILEPTIC SEIZURES

While nonepileptic seizures present certain medical care challenges, they are usually not the primary concern. Treat the primary disease, and the seizure activity will cease (except perhaps as noted in the case of CVA). We now consider epilepsy, in which the seizure itself is the primary derangement.

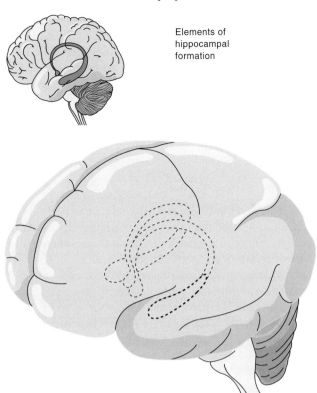

Elements of hippocampal formation

Figure 22.1   **Location of the Hippocampal Formation.** Dotted line indicates the hippocampal formation and its major extension into the hypothalamus. The hippocampus itself is outlined by the darker dotted line.

The term epilepsy is derived from the Greek, meaning "to seize upon" or "a taking hold of," an apt description of the seizures that occur with epilepsy. The storm of abnormal brain activity giving rise to a seizure may be experienced as a hallucination, an unprovoked set of sensations, limited involuntary movements, or twitching. In some seizures, the person may lose consciousness and have a major motor convulsion. Our understanding of epilepsy in some ways hasn't progressed significantly since John Hughlings Jackson proposed, a century ago, that seizures were caused by "occasional, sudden, excessive, rapid and local discharges of gray matter" and that a generalized convulsion resulted "when normal brain tissue was invaded by the seizure activity initiated in the abnormal focus."

Epilepsy: The Underlying Mechanism

Modern studies have confirmed Jackson's intuition that gray matter is the origin of seizure activity. More specifically, it is the cortical tissue that forms the outer layer of the entire cerebrum, forming its bumps (gyri) and its grooves (sulci and fissures) and also contributing a major part of the hippocampal formation. The hippocampal formation is crucial to memory processing and is one of the cortical regions that is inherently more prone to seizure generation. It is considered to be part of the limbic system and in common with certain other limbic components has a C-shape when viewed from the side (fig. 22.1). In contrast to the superficial cerebral cortex, the hippocampus (the principal cortical portion of the hippocampal formation) is located on the wall of the lateral ventricles, like the basal ganglia. The bottom of the C begins on the medial wall of the temporal horn of the lateral ventricle and extends around as far as the parietal lobe. Because of its deep location, seizures originating in the hippocampus are difficult to localize with the usual scalp electrodes used in a routine electroencephalogram (EEG).

The Epileptogenic Focus

Although some truly generalized seizures can begin with a sudden shift in the activity of millions of widely distributed cortical neurons, most seizures begin at an **epileptogenic focus.** This is a group of abnormal neurons that spontaneously depolarize, firing thousands of action potentials without an identifiable cause. In theory, any collection of neurons could become epileptogenic, but in practice, the focus usually develops in either the cerebral cortex or the hippocampus. If these cells are able to activate the relatively normal neurons with which they are associated, a seizure results. This recruitment of additional neurons can be quite limited, restricted perhaps to those cortical neurons immediately surrounding the focus, in which case the result is a partial seizure. If the recruitment is on a broader scale, causing a larger disruption of neural function, a more generalized seizure results. A seizure that begins focally, however, can spread in seconds or minutes to become **secondarily generalized.**

While the significance of the distinction between focal and generalized seizures should be clear, at least in terms of the impact on the person experiencing them, the therapeutic implications may not be so obvious. Most seizures fall between the two extremes: a strictly limited focal (partial) seizure with no secondary spread or generalization on one hand, and an apparently instantaneously generalized bilateral seizure on the other. Pure focal seizures have a discrete and limited focus. In theory, generalized seizures have no focus but develop from a more or less simultaneous disruption of normal cortical function. In practice, it appears that the vast majority of what seem from the outset to be true generalized seizures also originate from discrete foci, but in this case there may be multiple foci that show an extreme tendency to generalize secondarily. Many seizures that appear to be generalized, on the basis of behavioral and EEG criteria, are actually secondarily generalized from one or more foci.

An epileptogenic focus can be examined in detail by applying multiple, closely spaced electrodes on the surgically exposed surface of a section of cortex (electrocorticography). This technique reveals a relatively large area (16 cm^2 or more) in which innumerable random action potentials can be observed. On a routine EEG, such **spike foci** are too small to be individually recorded through the layers of meninges, bone, and scalp. Only when many small spike foci fire synchronously is their action observable at the scalp as a **spike-and-wave,** the electrical sign of an epilepto-

Focus on Considerations in Seizure Surgery

In a therapeutic context, the distinction between focal and generalized seizures is far from academic. The issue becomes more concrete when it is reduced to the questions, "Are all these seizures triggered from one focus?" and "If this focus were resected, is there a secondary focus capable of generating seizures?" Such questions are raised when considering surgery for disabling seizures that won't respond effectively to more conservative medical management (so-called "intractable epilepsy"). For surgery to be considered, the disruption of function that results from the removal of the affected cortex must not be worse than that created by the uncontrolled seizure activity.

genic focus (fig. 22.2). The absence of identifiable spike-and-wave phenomena in a routine EEG is therefore not evidence of the absence of an epileptogenic focus; that is, a negative EEG does not exclude epilepsy. The tendency for nerve cells in a focus to fire synchronously is related to their capacity to recruit other cortical tissue and produce a seizure. Individuals with frequent seizures are much more likely to have a focus that can be identified during a routine EEG. Beyond the spike-and-wave, there is an array of well-recognized abnormal EEG patterns that can be directly related to impaired consciousness and the behavior observed during a seizure. These details are beyond the scope of this text.

Epileptogenesis at the Cellular Level

The physical and physiological characteristics of the normal cortical **pyramidal cell** (the neuron in the cortex that produces its final excitatory outflow) give rise to the EEG and are the effectors for the disordered function that produces a seizure focus. Their name derives from the pyramid shape of the cell soma. Figure 22.3 presents the principal features of the pyramidal cell, a neuron that is densely distributed in the lower levels of the cortex. Axons from these cells project to the basal ganglia, cerebellum, brain stem, and spinal cord. Other, smaller pyramidal cells at different levels of the cortex relay activity to associated cortex in same and contralateral hemispheres and modify the activity of the thalamus.

Many neurons in the central nervous system respond to stimulation in an essentially additive way: If significantly more excitation than inhibition occurs, the cell produces a transmittable signal, an action potential. Signal generation in the pyramidal cell (PC) is a more complex and interesting phenomenon. Excitation typically occurs on the apical dendrite and its branches. Because of the presence of dendritic booster zones, relatively small input stimulus can produce an action potential in the apical dendrite that travels towards the soma (cell body). This activity, summated

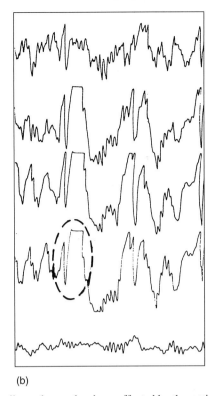

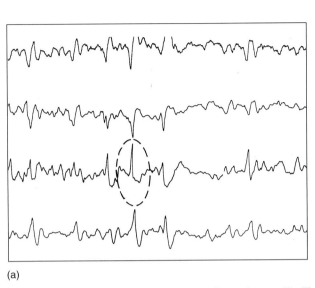

(a)   (b)

Figure 22.2   **Typical EEG Traces.** A spike (*a*) and a spike-and-wave (*b*). The spike-and-wave has been affected by the setting of the EEG in that the top of the wave is leveled off in several traces.

over millions of simultaneously depolarizing apical dendrites, is a major component of a normal EEG.

Most action potentials are arrested because of the high level of inhibition that is normally focused on the soma and basal dendrites. If excitation is intense enough, or if inhibition is removed, an action potential (AP) will be generated in the PC axon and a signal will leave the cortex. This interplay of excitation and inhibition allows for very subtle modulation of cortical activity; a very weak stimulatory signal can be "heard" while a very intense signal may be "ignored." In the context of epilepsy, a seizure might develop because of excess excitation or insufficient inhibition. The intense firing of an abnormally active pyramidal cell can readily recruit additional PCs. Conversely, if the normal inhibitory inputs to pyramidal cells are reduced in any way, these cells can become epileptogenic, that is, fire spontaneously.

Hippocampal PCs have an added characteristic that increases their epileptogenic potential. Rather than firing a single AP and then remaining in a resistant state as do most neurons, hippocampal PCs fire bursts of action potentials and then remain susceptible to subsequent activation for a brief period. Anything that destabilizes these cells or interferes with their physiological inhibition can, for this reason, be potentially epileptogenic.

Patterns of Seizure Activity

Because of the link between cortical activity and various observable seizure phenomena (behavioral, sensory, men-

> ### ✓ *Checkpoint 22.1*
>
> Activity in pyramidal cells underlies all cortical phenomena. In order for anything to be expressed or experienced, PCs have to fire and carry a signal out of the cortex, through the underlying white matter, to another destination. Despite this activity, the overwhelming balance of cortical stimulation is inhibitory.

tal, EEG patterns), it is important to make careful clinical observations of a given seizure's components. These can be useful both in diagnosis and in assessing a patient's response to therapy.

Typically, an epileptic individual's recurrent seizures have a relatively predictable pattern. He may experience a **prodrome**—that is, a set of symptoms that warns of a seizure's approach—minutes, hours, or even days before it occurs. As the seizure begins, an **aura** (from the Greek term meaning "breeze") may be experienced. Auras include mental, sensory, or motor phenomena that the person later remembers as signaling the onset of the seizure. Strictly speaking, these are part of the seizure, evidence that seizure onset did not disrupt either normal consciousness or memory. For the phenomenon to be an *aura*, the patient must recall this phase as distinctly different from what he regards as the *seizure*. The seizure will consist of a set of sensory,

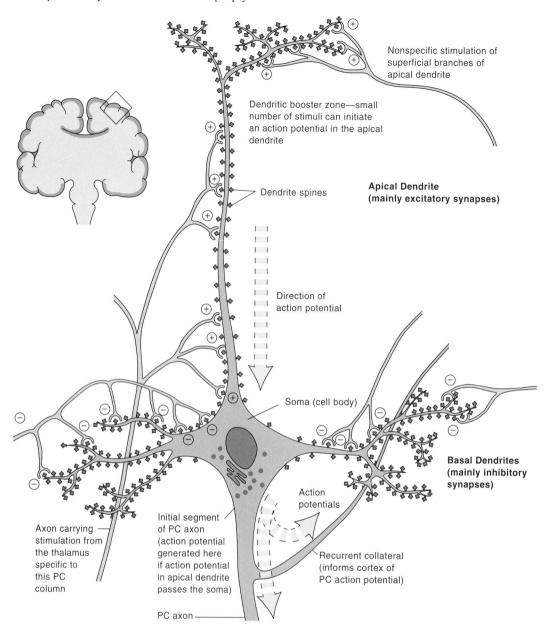

Nonspecific stimulation of
superficial branches of
apical dendrite

Dendritic booster zone—small
number of stimuli can initiate
an action potential in the apical
dendrite

Dendrite spines

**Apical Dendrite
(mainly excitatory synapses)**

Direction of
action potential

Soma (cell body)

Action
potentials

**Basal Dendrites
(mainly inhibitory
synapses)**

Axon carrying
stimulation from
the thalamus
specific to
this PC
column

Initial segment
of PC axon
(action potential
generated here
if action potential
in apical dendrite
passes the soma)

Recurrent collateral
(informs cortex of
PC action potential)

PC axon

Figure 22.3   **Principal Features of a Cortical Pyramidal Cell (PC).** The presence of "booster zones" that can readily initiate an action potential and the dependence on ongoing inhibition of the cell body and basal dendrites to limit discharge predispose the pyramidal cell to the "spontaneous" generation of action potentials that could cause a seizure.

mental, and/or motor activities that is fairly consistent for a given individual. These persist for a usually consistent period of time and then resolve. They are followed by a post-seizure state that differs for each person and seizure type. The aura that the patient notes and the characteristics first observable in the seizure are very useful in pinpointing the area(s) of the brain in which the seizure activity is initiated. Such localization is particularly important if the seizure is not medically correctable and surgery is contemplated.

Although the preceding generalization holds, variations in seizure patterns do occur. The most common variation, particularly if the person is on anticonvulsants, is a lesser version of the person's full-blown seizure pattern, often involving the aura or the aura and the first parts of the complete seizure pattern. As well, many people experience tonic-clonic seizures as

a complication of their fundamental seizure type. Less commonly, individuals may exhibit two or more distinctly different types of seizures, in succession or simultaneously.

 Checkpoint 22.2

Whatever your role in the health care team or whenever you encounter a person experiencing a seizure, watch closely what happens. Pay attention to the succession and, if possible, the timing of events. And note it down to support your memory. These observations may be the key to correct diagnosis and effective treatment!

Focus on Columns: The Functional Units of Cortical Organization

Each pyramidal cell is an element in the basic unit of cortical function, called a **column.** It consists of several hundred pyramidal and various associated cells organized around a single cortical input. This column has a unified function; for example, in the perception of a specific visual stimulus or tonal pattern, or perhaps the activation of a muscle group. Discharge of action potentials that affect the perception or movement is accompanied by a variety of other signals from the column that supply information to other areas of the cortex or promote coordination of contractions. Output from the column indirectly inhibits the surrounding cortical tissue. This limiting of cortical activity to the appropriate column is called **surround inhibition.** Box figure 22.1 presents the relationship between the principal cells contributing to the activity of a column.

If a number of cells in a column become abnormally excitable or are released from normal inhibition, they may serve as an epileptogenic focus, spontaneously and unpredictably emitting a burst of action potentials. This burst elicits and is immediately followed by surround inhibition. In theory, such a sequence accounts for the spike (action potentials) and wave (surround inhibition) characteristic of a focus. It may also provide the basis for the rhythmic alternation of massive excitation and subsequent inhibition that characterizes the convulsive tonic-clonic seizure. In this view, the synchronous firing of millions of pyramidal cells is followed by their reflex inhibition, which in turn passes, leaving them vulnerable to the next wave of excitation. These volleys may continue to the point of exhaustion of the majority of cortical pyramidal cells or of those pyramidal cells in the focus that are driving the seizure.

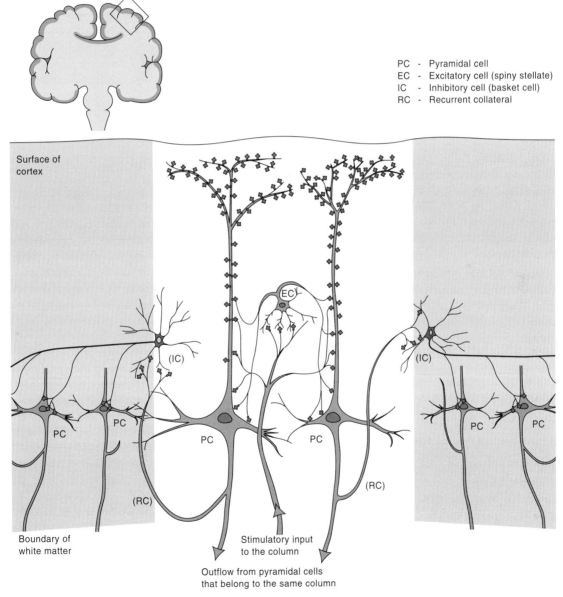

PC - Pyramidal cell
EC - Excitatory cell (spiny stellate)
IC - Inhibitory cell (basket cell)
RC - Recurrent collateral

Surface of cortex

(IC)

EC

(IC)

PC

PC

PC

PC

PC

PC

(RC)

(RC)

Boundary of white matter

Stimulatory input to the column

Outflow from pyramidal cells that belong to the same column

Box Figure 22.1 **The Relationship between the Principal Cells Involved in the Organization of Cortical Function.** Activation of a column of pyramidal cells (only two are indicated) through either stimulatory input (directly to PC apical dendrites or mediated by excitatory spiny stellate cells) or removal of inhibition (or both) induces action potentials in associated axons and inhibition of the cells surrounding the column (shaded area) through the activation by recurrent collaterals (RC) of inhibitory cells (IC).

Seizure Classification

The material in this section is organized around the classification of epileptic seizures proposed by the Commission on Classification and Terminology of the International League Against Epilepsy (1981), with certain clarifying modifications. Although there is considerable complexity in the various categories of seizure, only the essential types are considered here.

Partial Seizures

Partial seizures typically begin at a discrete and relatively limited focus. The specific seizure pattern depends on the function of the area of the brain that is stimulated by the focus. For example, **focal motor without march** denotes a seizure that arises in neurons in a specific part of the motor cortex and may involve twitching that is restricted to one hand or one side of the face, but does not spread. If there is limited spread (march), the seizure pattern will become more extensive, as in a **focal motor with march** seizure, in which case the twitching in the hand spreads to the forearm, then the upper arm, shoulder, and even one side of the face. This "Jacksonian motor seizure" beautifully illustrates the progressive involvement of contiguous areas of the motor cortex. It is, however, a very rarely observed phenomenon.

Simple Partial Seizures If the spread is very limited, the seizure will remain **simple,** with **elementary symptomatology.** These terms indicate that the seizure is relatively uncomplicated, affecting only limited aspects of neural function. Postural abnormalities or various sensory deficits are examples. In simple partial seizures, consciousness and memory are undisturbed.

Complex Partial Seizures In complex partial seizures (CPS), an alteration of consciousness follows the initial simple seizure. Although the victims may appear relatively alert and aware of their surroundings, their consciousness is definitely impaired. They typically appear confused or totally preoccupied and may exhibit various **automatisms.** These are purposeless and automatic behaviors are undertaken without intent or awareness. Typical automatisms include lip smacking, sucking, chewing or swallowing movements, fumbling with clothing perhaps undressing or incoherent talking, or the uninterrupted continuation of habitual acts like driving or turning the page of a book. It is estimated that 70% of complex partial seizures arise from a focus in the temporal lobe.

There are some other conditions that might readily be confused with a CPS. For example, a panic attack (phobic-anxiety syndrome) may produce psychic symptoms suggestive of the auras associated with CPS, such as a sense that everything has happened before (déjà vu), a sense of detachment (depersonalization), and various illusions or distortions of perception. When these are epileptic phenomena, they tend to be more stereotyped and vivid and of relatively rapid onset and brief duration (seconds to min-

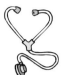

Focus on the Risk to Those Surrounding the Person Having a Seizure

Understandably, health care workers may be concerned for their safety when they see the restless, fearful behavior that a person in a complex partial seizure can display. By way of reassurance, you should be aware that unprovoked violence is very rare as an accompaniment of epileptic seizures. Of course, it is sensible to exercise caution when working closely with someone who could, in a confused state, lash out or defensively ward off a person who is trying to help. A directed attack, however, is so uncommon (19 cases out of 100,000 in one study of a group of the most difficult and potentially violent patients) that it is not a realistic concern.

utes). The evolution of a transient ischemic attack (TIA) may also produce symptoms that resemble a CPS or its aura, especially if the TIA alters the person's level of consciousness. Such a case may be a real diagnostic puzzle because the person may have developed an epileptogenic focus associated with an old embolic infarct and also be experiencing TIA. EEG recording during the experience usually settles the issue.

Simple partial and complex partial seizures may be observed in an acute care hospital setting, but rarely are they the reason for admission. Partial seizures that spread (secondarily generalize) into tonic-clonic convulsions are much more likely to be a reason for admission. Either the initial, less serious seizure pattern has begun to generalize or control of seizure spread may have broken down. For example, another illness or condition may make the person more susceptible to generalization, or the effectiveness of drug therapy may decline, either because the person has stopped taking the medication or because illness or another drug is interfering with its absorption. Many of the epileptic seizures encountered clinically arise for reasons such as these.

As was noted earlier, careful observation of the prodrome, aura, and details of the seizure is very helpful in establishing accurate diagnosis and effective treatment. Among seizures classified as generalized tonic-clonic, most are in fact secondarily generalized partial seizures. Often the generalization is so rapid that the true nature of the seizure can be confirmed only by very careful observations of behavior and correlation of these with EEG traces.

Partial Seizure Progression A simple partial seizure may exist on its own with no alteration of consciousness, and a complex partial seizure (consciousness altered from the onset) may be experienced without complication.

Apart from these cases, there are a limited number of ways in which seizure patterns can progress. A simple partial might progress to a complex partial seizure (at which point

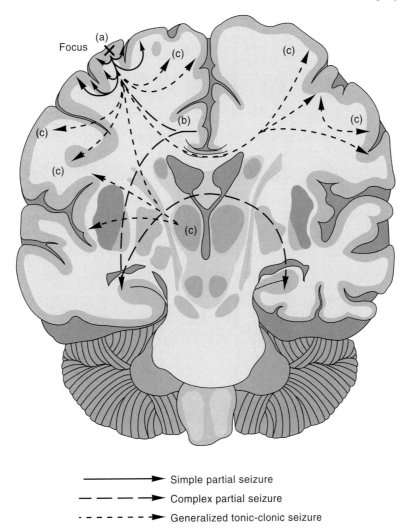

Figure 22.4   **Patterns of Seizure Progression.** Pathways whereby a simple partial seizure could theoretically spread to become complex and/or a secondarily generalized tonic-clonic seizure. (*a*) Epileptogenic focus recruits associated cortical tissue, producing a simple partial seizure. (*b*) Focal seizure projects to an association area connected to the hippocampal formation on the right side, which projects, in turn, to the left hippocampal formation. This results in a complex partial seizure. (*c*) Extensive spread leads to a secondarily generalized tonic-clonic seizure.

consciousness becomes altered) or to a generalized tonic-clonic seizure (fig. 22.4) with loss of consciousness. In similar fashion, a complex partial seizure might progress to a generalized tonic-clonic seizure. The most complex sequence would be found in an episode that begins with a simple partial seizure and progresses to a complex partial seizure (alteration of consciousness), which in turn progresses to a generalized tonic-clonic seizure (loss of consciousness).

Generalized Seizures

Generalized seizures are, by definition, incapable of being linked to a specific focus. That is, routine EEG tracings, observed behaviors, and patient recollections do not give any clues as to localization. The category commonly includes seizures that vary immensely in terms of their severity and the amount of brain tissue that is recruited into the abnormal paroxysmal discharge.

Absence Seizures Absence seizures ("absence" is usually pronounced as in French, so that "en" sounds like "on") may also be called **petit mal seizures** (again with a French pronunciation, similar to "petty mal"). They have a typical brain wave pattern and usually involve only minor impairments of neural function arising from changes in relatively small areas of the brain. A blank stare or other facial signs indicate the impaired consciousness (the person becomes "absent"). After two to ten seconds the patient suddenly resumes all preseizure activity, perhaps having lost only the thread of conversation. An abnormal EEG rhythm projected from the thalamus to the entire cortex stops the normal, integrated flow of cortical excitation. This disrupts intentional behavior, consciousness, and memory but usually leaves posture, muscle tone, ongoing automatic behavior like walking, and autonomic function unaffected. These typical absence seizures often include lip smacking, pouting, and eye blinking. They may also include clonic twitching of

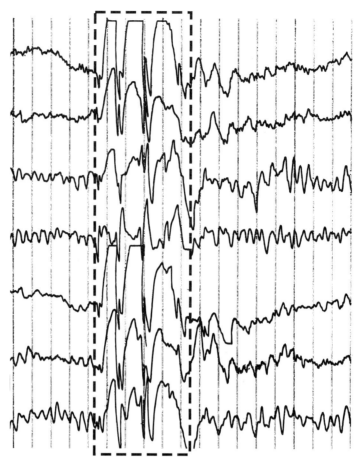

Figure 22.5 **Simple Absence.** Bilateral and synchronous 3-per-second spike-and-wave display associated with simple absence seizures. Note the sudden fully generalized onset and the similar, instantaneous resolution. This was a very brief seizure (approximately 1½ sec).

the fingers or both arms, postural tone may decrease or increase, and there may be autonomic components. The longer an absence seizure last, the more likely it will produce alterations in these latter activities. Because absence seizures may occur hundreds of times in a day, they can seriously interfere with learning or work performance.

Simple absence is typically an epilepsy of childhood or adolescence. Absence episodes begin in childhood (peaking at ages 6–7) or adolescence and produce a classic EEG display (fig. 22.5). The childhood form of the disease, which can produce frequent absence, often spontaneously remits as the nervous system matures. If it doesn't do so, generalized tonic-clonic seizures (GTCS) often develop in adolescence, but response to therapy is generally very good. The adolescent form (juvenile absence epilepsy) has a lower seizure frequency (less than daily), is also complicated with GTCS, and responds well to therapy. Above-average intelligence, normal background EEG, the absence of GTCS, and a negative family history of seizures are excellent positive prognostic factors.

Atypical absence or **absence variant,** although behaviorally indistinguishable from simple absence except perhaps for a slower resolution, has quite a different clinical course. It is associated with a clinical syndrome called Lennox-Gastaut that usually afflicts children of ages 1 year and older. These children exhibit a wide range of seizures (myoclonic, astatic, absence, tonic-clonic), are usually mentally retarded, and are typically difficult to treat effectively. The absence is accompanied by an EEG trace that is much more irregular and chaotic than that of simple absence. The course and outcome of this syndrome are variable, and some children perish from an underlying progressive encephalopathy.

Tonic-Clonic Seizures Tonic-clonic **(grand mal)** seizures are a fairly common type, representing a maximal seizure response of the brain in which all brain systems can be recruited into the paroxysmal discharge. The seizure is classified as "generalized" if it commences simultaneously in both hemispheres. This is the only feature that discriminates it from the secondarily generalized tonic-clonic seizure. Tonic-clonic seizures are the most serious seizures you will encounter in a health care setting.

The pattern of seizure is quite stereotyped (fig. 22.6), whether it is truly generalized from the start, secondarily generalized from another seizure form, or precipitated by alcohol or barbiturate withdrawal. Some patients have a

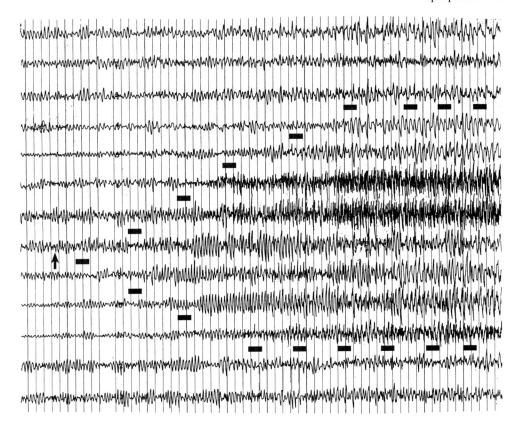

Figure 22.6   **Profile of a Grand Mal Seizure.** A generalized tonic-clonic (grand mal) seizure as it appears in a typical EEG. This trace shows generalization from a simple focus (→), as is typical of most tonic-clonic seizures. The generalization, however, is very rapid. Dark bars outline the abnormal EEG activity.

prodrome, which is some change that signals the subsequent GTCS. This may occur days in advance. The prodrome might include depression, irritability, apathy or malaise or, rarely, euphoria (the Russian novelist Dostoyevsky experienced such ecstasy that he considered his seizures a blessing!). The person may have one or more myoclonic jerks upon awakening the day of the seizure. About half of those whose principal seizure is the GTCS have a distinct aura a few seconds before the onslaught of the GTCS. This is evidence of the simple partial onset of their seizure and may be helpful in localization of the focus. Typically, the seizure itself goes through three phases: an initial **tonic phase** lasting 10–20 seconds, a 1/2–2-minute **clonic phase,** and then a **terminal phase** lasting about 5 minutes.

The tonic phase starts with a brief period of muscle flexing, which is accompanied by raising of the arms and opening of the eyes and mouth. Next there is a 10–15-second interval of pronounced extension, characterized by generally high muscle tension. During this period, the jaws close sharply and air is rapidly expelled to produce a characteristic **epileptic cry.** The arms and legs are extended, respiration stops with air fully expired, bladder tension may evacuate the bladder, and the pupils become unresponsive to

light. The end of the tonic phase is indicated by a short period of muscle tremor.

The onset of the clonic phase is indicated by an initial muscle relaxation, which is then followed by violent spasms of contraction and relaxation. In these, the strongest muscle groups dominate to produce a characteristic pattern of elbow flexion, leg extension, and torso hyperextension. These muscle spasms can be so intense that they result in torn muscles or bone fractures. During the clonic phase, respiration resumes but is ineffective, and cyanosis may develop. The autonomic system is also active, inducing pronounced perspiration, alternating constriction and dilation of the pupils, and heavy salivary secretion. The saliva may combine with blood from a tongue bitten during the tonic phase to produce a froth of blood in the mouth.

In the longer terminal phase that follows, the victim becomes limp and quiet, with normal breathing restored. This comalike state is characterized by a period of minutes during which the EEG is "flat." It may be followed by up to an hour of deep sleep, or the patient may become conscious with no recollection of the events of the seizure. Normal autonomic function is also restored during the terminal phase. Figure 22.7 presents an analysis of the various features of a typical GTCS.

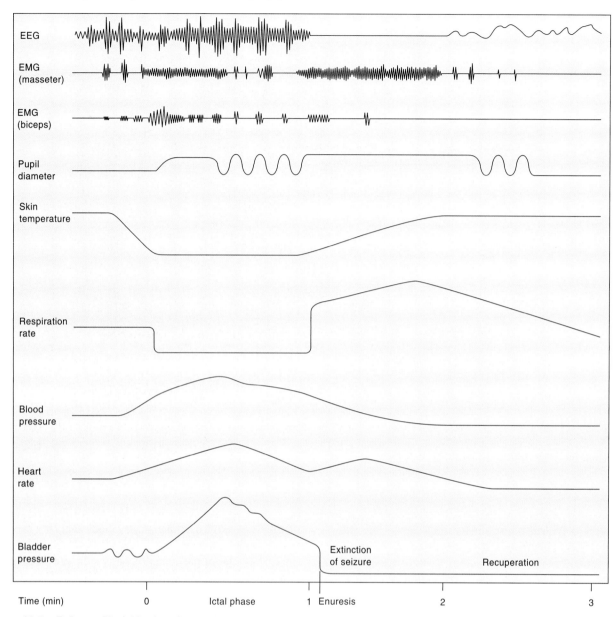

Figure 22.7   **Relevant Variables in a Generalized Tonic-Clonic Seizure (GTCS).**

Tonic-clonic seizures usually occur singly but may come in a cluster of two or three. A small proportion of patients (estimated at 5–8%) are at risk of lapsing into a series of GTCS without fully regaining consciousness. This condition, termed **status epilepticus,** is a severe medical emergency and is treated in a later section.

Other Generalized Seizures Two seizures can best be seen as subvariants of the complete tonic-clonic seizure. Both are more commonly found in children. The **clonic seizure** is like a tonic-clonic without the tonic phase. It is a generalized seizure characterized by rhythmic contractions of all muscles, loss of consciousness, and marked autonomic manifestations. **Tonic seizures** involve brief, generalized tonic extension of all four limbs and head extension with marked autonomic manifestations. These two are rare in adults. The sort of tonic-clonic variant likely to be en-

countered clinically involves a few massive myoclonic jerks that leave the person dazed or unconscious.

Atonic seizures are characterized by a sudden loss of muscle tone. The result will vary from head or body sagging, with full consciousness, to loss of consciousness, falling, and a complete loss of muscle tone. The term **akinetic** usually denotes a transient arrest of all motor activity, while the term **astatic** has been used to label drop attacks, sudden spells during which the person, usually a child, falls without warning. In current usage, the term *atonic* covers all of these variants.

Other patterns of seizure are usually seen only in infants or children and are often symptomatic of a broader clinical syndrome. The seizures expressed in very young babies may go unnoticed or at least unrecognized: horizontal eye movements, eyelid blinking or fluttering, sucking, smacking, swimming or pedaling movements, perhaps

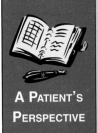
Just Get on With Life!

The Impact of Epilepsy
—M. Arthur

I had my first seizure when I was 22. It happened in the middle of the night before a final exam. I awoke in the morning on the bathroom floor. I knew something had happened, but I wasn't sure what. I had smashed my lip and cheek on a marble sink; there was blood all over and I looked and felt like hell. Since I had an exam that morning, I just got myself together as fast as possible and got to school. I was in a very intense and exciting theatre programme in Montreal and heavily involved in theatre outside school, in the evenings, and on the weekends. The exam was a disaster—I was so disoriented and what I call "hung over" from the seizure, that I couldn't finish writing the exam. My teacher said that I really should check in with medical services, but I didn't. I had stuff to do—work, school etc. This is typical of the way I have always handled things. I had two more seizures in quick succession at home in front of friends, and they didn't give me the option; they called the ambulance while I was unconscious.

I spent the next two weeks at Montreal General. They did every imaginable test on me. They (I found out later) were looking for a brain tumor. I was diagnosed with primary generalized tonic-clonic seizures without a warning aura. (No brain tumor!) I was put on Dilantin and phenobarbital. The phenobarbital made me feel just awful. I was tripping and falling, I couldn't walk upstairs, but I wasn't dizzy—I just didn't know where my feet were. And I started to tremor. This was associated with the Dilantin and has been with me ever since. Sometimes it's worse, sometimes better, but it is the only visual manifestation of the epilepsy. It's a sign to others: "She's got the DT's" or "She's really nervous." I'm not embarrassed about the epilepsy, but I am sure self-conscious of the shaking. They calm down sometimes when I'm doing fine handwork, or if I'm *really* relaxed, but otherwise they're usually there.

The only pattern that I've been able to notice in the 15 years I've had them is that my seizures sometimes come after periods of extreme tension, and often in the early morning, within an hour of waking. But not always. I get memory lapses—right after the seizures (for a day or two), they are profound—most of it comes back, but not all. I have lost big chunks of my life: I have no recollection of another guy living with my partner and I for the first two years of our marriage. My memory doesn't function in learning situations like it used to—but that could be other things. . . .

Two or three times seizures have happened in public. That's basically OK, I just have to handle the reactions of people who have witnessed it. It's often harder on them than me. The first time I saw someone having a seizure was strange, I was the first-aid person on the scene, and I helped the guy, but mostly I watched the reactions of others in the room.

I lost my driver's license 15 years ago. That's really frustrating. I used to go driving; it was a good release. I miss that a lot. I resent having to ask people for help, for a lift. and I get a little unreasonable when I have to deal with idiots (!) who think that I should limit my life because of the possibility of having a seizure. "You shouldn't climb ladders." Yah well, maybe I shouldn't get out of bed in the morning—it'd be safer! Basically, if I could seriously hurt myself or someone else, then I don't do it: for example, I don't use a table saw, or drive anymore (though I'd love to!). Having the epilepsy does make me think about things I wouldn't otherwise, but it does not rule my life. My Dad freaks out, "You're going to be living alone!" Both my parents still haven't come to terms with the epilepsy. My mum still has to be constantly reassured that it's not her fault in some way. She doesn't understand that it just isn't that big a deal to me. Honestly though, living on my own versus having a roommate has been a big issue for me too. I always have to bring up the epilepsy in every new living situation, every new job, just so people are prepared. It is only fair to them, but sometimes I don't feel that it is fair to me. But hey, what am I supposed to do, stop living my life?

---

spells of apnea. Slightly older children may show a variety of myoclonic jerks. These have been aptly called *lightning spasms*. The term **infantile spasms** refers to a varied expression of flexor, extensor, or lightning spasms or neck flexion (nods) that are associated with a condition called **West's syndrome** and affect infants over 8 months of age. While children who have no other evidence of neurological abnormality have been known to recover fully, many children with this syndrome suffer severe neurological impairment or progressive encephalopathy. Lennox-Gastaut, another childhood syndrome that affects slightly older infants (1 year plus), was described earlier.

An overview of the current system for classifying seizures is presented in table 22.1.

 Checkpoint 22.3

Even though the foregoing may seem like a complex descriptive categorization, the patterns of seizure are reasonably straightforward. The better you understand this scheme, the more effective and informative your observation of seizure activity will be. But be forewarned—you may find your first major seizure a disturbing event. One reaction will be that you lose track of time. What has taken seconds will "stretch": Keep one eye on the clock to get a realistic sense of how long the different phases last.

Table 22.1	Classification of Epileptic Seizures

I. *PARTIAL SEIZURES* (begin locally, also called focal or local)
  A. *Partial seizures with simple or elementary symptomatology* (consciousness is usually not impaired)
      1. With motor signs:
          a. Focal motor without march
          b. Focal motor with march (Jacksonian)
          c. Versive (also called adversive)
          d. Postural
          e. Phonatory (vocalization or arrest of speech)
      2. With *somatosensory* or *special sensory symptoms* (simple hallucinations [e.g., tingling, light flashes, buzzing])
          a. Somatosensory (superficial cutaneous, muscle, joint, and visceral)
          b. Visual
          c. Auditory
          d. Olfactory (smells)
          e. Gustatory (tastes)
          f. Vertiginous (sudden dizziness or vertigo)
      3. With *autonomic symptoms or signs* (including epigastric sensation, pallor, sweating, flushing, piloerection, and pupillary dilation)
      4. With *psychic symptoms* (disturbances of higher cerebral function—these *rarely* occur without impairment of consciousness and are therefore more commonly experienced as (part of) complex partial seizures. Examples are déjà vu, dreamy states, distortions of time sense, fear, anger, and more elaborate hallucinations.
  B. *Complex partial seizures* (with impairment of consciousness; may sometimes begin with simple symptomatology)
      1. *Simple partial onset, followed by impairment of consciousness*—may begin with simple partial features (A1–A4 above) followed by impaired consciousness or may include automatism (nonpurposive 'automatic' behaviors [e.g., fumbling]).
      2. With *impairment of consciousness at onset*—may only involve impairment of consciousness or may also include automatisms.
  C. *Partial seizures evolving to secondary generalized seizures* (tonic-clonic, tonic or clonic)
      1. Simple partial seizures evolving to generalized seizures
      2. Complex partial seizures evolving to generalized seizures
      3. Simple partial seizures evolving to complex partial seizures evolving to generalized seizures
II. *GENERALIZED SEIZURES* (seizure activity begins bilaterally, may be convulsive [e.g., B, C, D, and E or nonconvulsive; absence and atonic seizures])
  A. Absence seizures
  B. Myoclonic seizures (myoclonic jerks, single or multiple)
  C. Clonic seizures
  D. Tonic seizures
  E. Tonic-clonic seizures
  F. Atonic seizures (astatic, akinetic)
  (Combinations of B through F may occur [e.g., B & F, B & D])

Source: Abstracted from Gastaut (1970) with revisions proposed by the Commission on Classification and Terminology of the International League Against Epilepsy (1981). Only seizure patterns commonly found in adults have been included.

SEIZURES AND THE ALTERATION OF CONSCIOUSNESS

A major factor in monitoring a seizure in progress is the continual assessment of the patient's state of consciousness. This is an interactive process because, in this context, consciousness is equated with the capacity to respond. Appropriate responses depend, of course, on an intact capacity to orient, attend, receive, and process prior to producing a response. Additionally, normal consciousness implies mem-

ory, the ongoing running of a "backup tape" that may or may not be consolidated into lasting memory traces.

Components of Consciousness

A full discussion of consciousness is beyond our current focus. Suffice it to say that normal consciousness depends on the integrated function of at least these major components (fig. 22.8): appropriate sensory stimulation and their normal nervous system processing, appropriate output

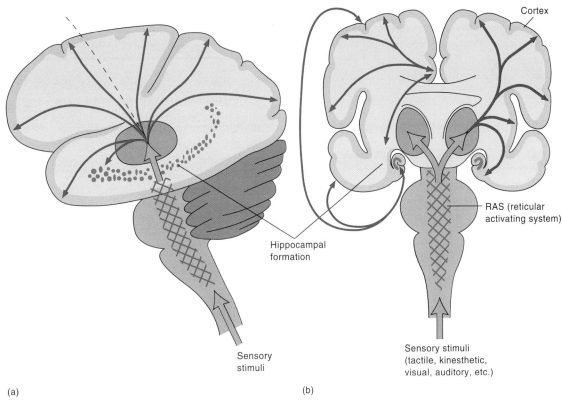

Figure 22.8   **Components of Consciousness.** (*a*) Lateral view illustrates four components described in text. Outflow from RAS passes to the thalamus and is then directed diffusely to the cortex to mediate level of consciousness. The relative location of the hippocampus is identified in heavy dots. (*b*) As well as tracing RAS outflow (right side of diagram), an attempt is made to suggest the inputs/outputs for the hippocampal formation (left side). Arrowheads at either end of lines suggest the reciprocal communications between cortical areas, where information arises and is eventually consolidated and stored, and the hippocampal formation. Pathways that unite the hippocampal formation with the autonomic nervous system and the pituitary have been omitted for simplicity. Dashed line in (*a*) indicates approximate section shown in (*b*).

from the reticular activating system (RAS), a functional cerebral cortex, and access to a functional hippocampal formation. To understand the ways in which consciousness can be altered in a seizure, a brief review of these is necessary.

Sensory Input and Processing

The effects of massive sensory deprivation have been investigated by suspending subjects in silent darkness in body-temperature tanks, with their limbs padded. These people have trouble concentrating within a few hours, and most experience the chaotic thought processes associated with outright psychosis within 12–18 hours. Such results illustrate our need for at least minimal sensory stimulation to maintain normal consciousness.

Reticular Activating System (RAS)

This is a network of brain stem neurons with extensive projections to almost every part of the central nervous system. In the RAS, sensory and cortical inputs are integrated with daily sleep and waking rhythms to produce patterns of out-

put that maintain our level of consciousness. Any altered RAS function produces changes in level of consciousness. These might range from hyperactivity to profound coma, including every intervening degree: aroused, normal, dull, stuporous, responsive only to painful stimuli, or unresponsive with exaggerated reflexes.

Physiological Cortical Functioning

The cerebral cortex is seen as the seat of consciousness, since this is where we presume it is experienced. Limited focal cortical damage appears to leave consciousness intact, although it may severely impair some other specific capacity. On the other hand, a massive diffuse derangement (as in Alzheimer's disease) or a severe systemic disorder (as in extreme liver failure) may completely abolish consciousness.

Hippocampal Formation

Each temporal lobe houses a hippocampal formation (see fig. 22.1). This elongated structure, which includes the hippocampus, is in communication with widely distributed brain structures, including large areas of the cerebral cortex. It is directly responsible for the ongoing consolidation of memory and for the attentional behavior that makes specific memories possible. If both hippocampal formations are disrupted simultaneously, attention and short-term memory are disrupted.

Seizure Type and Impaired Consciousness

The different patterns of seizure activity produce various impairments of consciousness. These result from the effects of abnormal electrical discharge on the CNS components that contribute to normal consciousness. The following sections explore some of the basics.

Impaired Consciousness in Partial Seizures

Simple partial seizures, because of their limited nature, do not impair consciousness directly, although they can produce mental states that so distract or disturb that much more effort is required to get and hold the patient's attention.

The impaired consciousness that characterizes the complex partial seizure derives from disruption of both hippocampal formations and perhaps other of the CNS centers noted earlier. Although varying depths of altered consciousness are recognized, *any* interference with a person's capacity to respond, if it can't be overcome voluntarily, leads to a diagnosis of complex partial seizure. For example, when asked a simple question, the patient may respond with a puzzled, uncomprehending, or blank stare. Depending on the extent of cortical spread in CPS, the alteration of consciousness may be profound, resembling the "away" of absence seizures, or it may be barely noticeable to a casual observer. In subtle cases, extensive questioning may be required to confirm the alteration of consciousness.

Impaired Consciousness in Generalized Seizures

By superimposing a widespread seizure-generated pattern of cortical excitation and inhibition, absence disrupts the normal rhythms that constitute normal consciousness. Because this disruption can be confined to the cortex, there may be no other evidence of neurological impairment. There is an "away" or "absence" (preseizure behavior ceases), but functions dependent on lower centers (maintenance of posture and muscle tone, autonomic function, routine behaviors like walking or cycling) can continue undisturbed. Because cortical memory functions are disrupted, no memory of the seizure is retained.

In tonic-clonic or grand mal seizures, the alteration of consciousness is by far the most profound. The massive volleys of seizure-generated excitation and inhibition dominate the entire central nervous system, seriously disrupting the normal function of all the centers to which we have attributed consciousness: the hippocampal formation, the cortex, and the reticular activating system. With these centers

Table 22.2	Factors That Can Precipitate Status Epilepticus

Infections, of the CNS or others (e.g., flu), that impair absorption of antiepileptic agents
Alcohol deprivation in chronic alcoholism
Withdrawal of antiepileptic therapy
Electroconvulsive shock therapy
Brain tumors
Acute withdrawal from sedative or depressant drugs
Various metabolic disorders (e.g., uremia, hypoglycemia, hyponatremia)

suppressed, attentional behavior, memory, thought, and consciousness itself are lost, with the victim temporarily lapsing into a coma.

Postseizure States of Consciousness

Particular attention must also be paid to the state of consciousness immediately after the seizure. After a grand mal seizure, the patient may not be rousable for five minutes and then awakens, looking confused and groggy. There is no memory of events during this immediate postseizure period, but with time, memory processes gradually resume normal function. In a CPS, the immediate postseizure state of consciousness allows an observer to differentiate between a CPS that arises in the temporal lobe (gradual return to normal consciousness) and one that arises in the frontal lobe (almost instantaneous restitution of waking consciousness). Similarly, restoration of normal consciousness can be helpful in discriminating simple absence (instantaneous) from absence variant (slower recovery).

GRAND MAL STATUS EPILEPTICUS

A relatively rare, but critical, occurrence in those with ongoing epilepsy, or those with seizures precipitated by drug or alcohol withdrawal or illness, is the prolonged continuation of their seizure state. A tonic-clonic seizure may recur with incomplete recovery between seizures, or the patient may experience continuous seizure activity. If the activity goes on for more than 30 minutes, major physiological changes occur. These are marked acidosis, significantly elevated PCO_2, hypoglycemia, and a fall in blood pressure that can further compromise glucose and oxygen supply to the brain tissue. If untreated, status epilepticus can lead to severe brain damage or death. The mortality in *treated* cases is 10–37%.

A variety of factors can precipitate a status attack (table 22.2). Once established, the massive, abnormal neural activity can itself cause brain damage by depleting oxygen and building up excess harmful metabolic by-products, as well as locally lowering the pH. As the systemic PO_2, PCO_2, and pH change beyond tolerable limits, the cardio-vascular centers in the medulla are compromised and the threat of progressive circulatory shock arises. In such cases, quick, aggressive therapeutic intervention is imperative.

Other types of seizure can also assume a status pattern. A person who is having 200–300 absence seizures in 24 hours is considered to be in **absence status epilepticus.** Although not life-threatening in the manner of status tonic-clonic, this is an entirely disabling condition and is aggressively treated in much the same way. When a focal (partial) seizure is maintained continuously (usually with no loss of consciousness), it is called **epilepsia partialis continua.** It also tends to be treated aggressively because of the risk of engendering further brain damage or generalizing into tonic-clonic seizures. **Electrical status** exists when, despite little or no clinical evidence of seizure activity, the EEG shows continuous, abnormal spike discharges. Electrical status is rarely encountered in a typical clinical setting, but it may be seen in the emergency room, where it may be confused with a street drug problem.

DIAGNOSTIC EVALUATION

The electroencephalograph was first used for diagnostic exploration of seizure disorders in the early 1940s, and it is still the chief evaluative tool. About 30–50% of patients with suspected epilepsy will have characteristic abnormalities on their first standard EEG, and follow-up studies increase that proportion to 60–90%. For the purposes of diagnosis, hyperventilation, which reduces cerebral perfusion, and photic stimulation are effective in inducing some seizures or interictal abnormalities. The more frequent the seizures, the more likely it is that the patient will show abnormalities on routine EEG. These are strong confirmations of epilepsy, since few normal individuals produce EEG patterns with epilepsy-related components.

Procedures that include placement of electrodes in the nasopharynx and sphenoid bone, as well as the use of depth electrodes that are surgically introduced into the cranial vault, increase the probability of detection and allow precise localization of seizure foci. Ideally, the EEG should be observed during the development and expression of a seizure. Most large, metropolitan centers have seizure monitoring units that make round-the-clock EEG and simultaneous videotaping possible. These are very helpful in the diagnosis of difficult cases and the precise localization required for surgical intervention. EEG monitoring of the target cortex during surgery (electrocorticography) is routine, since it allows resection of only that cortical tissue that is generating abnormal discharges.

A variety of other diagnostic techniques may also be employed. Although CT scans are often done, **magnetic resonance imaging** (MRI) has proven more effective at identifying structural abnormalities in the cortex (tumors, arteriovenous malformations, healed infarcts) or other lesions that may correlate with EEG abnormalities and an epileptogenic focus. Techniques that allow the imaging of neural function—for example, glucose metabolism—can be helpful in identifying areas of altered brain metabolism or perfusion during a seizure or during an interictal period. Such sites correlate well with areas that generate EEG abnormalities and with areas of structural change that are common at an epileptogenic focus. **Positron-emission tomography** (PET) and **single-photon-emission CT** (SPECT) are used in some centers for this purpose.

THE MEDICAL MANAGEMENT OF EPILEPSY

Accurate diagnosis of the seizure pattern or epileptic syndrome goes hand-in-hand with the effective management of epilepsy. For most individuals, management means the routine use of antiepileptic medication. The choice of drug depends on the individual's particular seizure type (table 22.3), because medications that are effective with one may be quite ineffective with another. The initial effort is to control the seizure with a single drug. This goal is achievable in more than 80% of the seizures that can be controlled with drugs. The major benefit of using a single drug is that there are fewer and less confusing side effects. Only after several single drugs have failed will combinations be tried, often in cases of epilepsy that involve several seizure types.

Currently, pharmaceutical agents provide excellent or at least quite acceptable levels of control in epilepsy. In the relatively small proportion of cases where they don't, surgical intervention may be indicated. In such procedures, the epileptogenic focus is first identified and then surgically removed. Of course, various factors can complicate the issue. For example, a focus may be identified but it may be in a location to which surgical access is limited. Another problem is posed by multiple or diffuse foci, whose removal would produce unacceptable functional losses.

As noted earlier, electrocorticography is used to monitor cortical activity during surgery to resect an epileptogenic focus. The goal is to limit the loss of cortical tissue to the volume responsible for the seizures, and no more. During the procedure, the patient remains conscious so that testing can monitor relevant neurological functioning. The aim, as always, is to balance any functional deficits against resolution of the seizure disorder.

Other, nonpharmacological approaches to seizure control are largely supportive. Patients need to learn to cope effectively with stress, eat well, and get sufficient rest. Avoidance of eliciting stimuli is effective in controlling some forms of what are called **reflex epilepsies.** Examples of these are the rare seizures brought on by gazing through the fingers while the hand is rapidly moved, hearing certain musical passages, reading, or tooth brushing.

Table 22.3   Drugs of Choice for the Pharmacological Control of Typical Seizure Patterns

Type of Seizure	Ease of Control	Antiepileptic Drug (in order of common usage)
Simple partial or secondary GTCS	Good	Carbamazepine or phenytoin; gabapentin over age 12; topiramate (lamotrigine as adjunct)
Partial complex	Moderate	Carbamazepine or phenytoin[#]; vigabatrin, gabapentin, clobazam, or lamotrigine; felbamate*
Simple absence	Good	Ethosuximide
Absence in conjunction with GTCS or myoclonic seizures	Moderate to difficult	Valproate[##] (perhaps lamotigine); clonazepam
Primary GTCS	Good	Valproate or ethosuximide (lamotrigine and valproate)
Lennox-Gastaut	Difficult	Valproate, felbamate*
Infantile spasms	Difficult	Ketogenic diet,** ACTH,*** vigabatrin
Myoclonic	Moderate	Valproate; clonazepam

[#]One may work, whereas the other worsens seizures or secondary generalization; "control" may mean control of generalization but continuation or worsening of complex partial phase.

[##]Valproic acid or valproate or sodium valproate

*High potential for liver toxicity and blood abnormalities

**High-fat diet induces moderate acidosis

***Stimulates the endogenous release of hydrocortisone (anti-inflammatory agent)

Case Study

The patient in this case was a 40-year-old male who had had seizures since he was 15, with their frequency recently increasing. Although his measured IQ was within normal range, he appeared slow, had poor general knowledge, and had short-term memory processing deficits. These, combined with seizures occurring up to six times daily, had made regular employment impossible, and he had been receiving a handicap pension for the past two years. He was referred for seizure investigation with the ultimate possibility of surgical intervention.

The patient was the fourth of ten children. There was no family history of seizure disorders except that his father had appeared to have a seizure secondary to a stroke that he suffered at 73. The only event in the patient's childhood that might be significant was a fall off a cliff, at age 8 or 9. He received a laceration but did not lose consciousness. A slight skull deformity in the left parietal region might be related to this accident. He had been quite slow in school even before his seizures began, at which point his performance worsened, and he left school after grade 10. He had attempted a variety of jobs since then, but frequent seizures interfered with success. He lived with a woman for seven or eight years in a common-law relationship and was married for two or three years, beginning at age 27 or 28, but eventually separated. He had one daughter who was medically

fine. Short-term memory had become worse lately, and social and sexual relationships were becoming more difficult. Medication (including phenytoin, methsuximide, and the antidepressant amytriptyline) was being taken regularly.

The seizure investigation covered almost five years, some of that time absorbed in waiting for specialist interviews and access to the seizure investigation unit. Observations by that unit showed that he appeared to experience two distinct patterns of seizure onset. With the first, he had a distinct aura that consisted of an undescribable cephalic sensation with a strong déjà-vu feeling. This was followed by visual searching, perhaps spontaneous vocalizations ("I, ah . . . ," "Oh," "Humh"), and fumbling with glasses or other objects. When questioned, he might be appropriately responsive, identifying objects and answering simple questions. He usually passed urine in the latter part of the seizure. He might change his underwear or bedding while still appearing to be in the state of altered consciousness. These seizures with a simple partial onset were usually mild, seldom generalized, and didn't leave him confused. He might remember some of the events of the seizure, but this was highly variable. His other seizures were without aura; they were clinically quite similar in their complex phase (i.e., during the fumbling, etc.) but left him feeling much more confused for longer periods of time (10–15 minutes). His responses to questioning were less integrated, and often he was nonresponsive. The seizures themselves were longer (2–3 minutes), and were much more likely to generalize. When this happened, the convulsion consisted of jerky movements of the head and eyes to one side, with raising and abduction of the ipsilateral arm.

His CT was normal, but MRI indicated an abnormality in the right medial inferior temporal lobe. Testing of speech lateralization and memory showed that his speech and language were localized to the right hemisphere (he was left-handed). Short-term memory was better in the right hemisphere than in the left. The findings from EEG monitoring during seizures were difficult to interpret, as there were widespread abnormalities in the traces. There was no clearly identifiable focus, although episodic sharp/slow wave activity in the anterior right temporal region was associated with drowsiness.

The patient was recommended for surgical investigation with the use of electrocorticography. This showed a fairly circumscribed focus, localized in the region identified by MRI (inferior, medial temporal lobe). While simultaneous memory and language testing and electrocorticography were done, tiny portions of abnormal cortex were removed. Most of the area identified on MRI was ablated, with no impact on language or language function. Drug therapy was continued after surgery, and a significant reduction in seizure frequency was noted (less than one per week). With this improvement, he was encouraged to attempt a preemployment program at a local college, and is currently enrolled in that program.

Commentary
This case is an example of a complex partial seizure with a poor response to usual medical management. For such patients, surgery is a possible and sometimes very effective alternative.

Key Concepts

1. Nonepileptic seizures are secondary to some other potentially reversible or transitory conditions such as alcohol withdrawal, bacterial meningitis, or liver or kidney failure (pp. 633–635).

2. Epileptic seizures result when a relatively permanent change in the environment, inputs, or nature of cortical pyramidal cells allows a portion of them (the focus) to discharge spontaneously and to recruit the involvement of larger portions of the cortex (pp. 635–636).

3. Physical and physiological characteristics of pyramidal cells predispose them to becoming seizure generators (pp. 636–639).

4. The majority of seizures begin focally, producing, at least temporarily, some evidence of limited recruitment—for example, an aura, localized EEG activity, focal abnormal movements or sensation, altered consciousness or psychic function (pp. 637–638).

5. A simple partial seizure may spread to become a complex or a generalized seizure (called a secondarily generalized tonic-clonic seizure) (pp. 640–641).

6. Generalized seizures (i.e., seizures that are generalized from the start, like absence, some tonic-clonic, and other rare seizures) arise more or less instantly with no evidence of focal origin (pp. 641–646).

7. Normal consciousness depends on appropriate sensory stimulation and processing and the integrated function of the reticular activating system, the cerebral cortex, and the hippocampal formation (pp. 646–648).

8. Consciousness is unimpaired in simple partial seizures and impaired in different and characteristic ways in partial complex seizures and specific generalized seizures (p. 648).

9. Grand mal status epilepticus (tonic-clonic status) is a medical emergency (pp. 648–649).

10. Evaluation of a tendency to have seizures involves minimally a routine EEG (a negative EEG does not rule out epilepsy) and perhaps further diagnostics including seizure monitoring, CT, or MRI (p. 649).

11. Drug therapy with a single anticonvulsant medication is the usual choice for medical management of epileptic conditions (pp. 649–650).

REVIEW ACTIVITIES

1. Explain what the following have in common and in what ways they are different:
   Simple absence seizures and atypical absence seizures
   Tonic-clonic seizures and simple absence seizures
   Simple partial seizures with psychic symptoms and complex partial seizures
   West's syndrome and Lennox-Gastaut syndrome
   Ethosuximide and carbamazepine

2. Describe what you would see if you observed the evolution of a seizure from a simple partial with motor signs to a complex partial to a full tonic-clonic seizure.

3. Imagine a worst-case scenario in which a person has the seizure pattern described in activity 2, and it is resistant to normal medical management. Describe the diagnostic procedures and choices that would probably be explored, from most conservative to most radical.

4. From memory, sketch a typical pyramidal cell and label the features that are relevant to its role as a seizure-generating cell. What are its normal inputs and where do its outputs flow?

Chapter

23

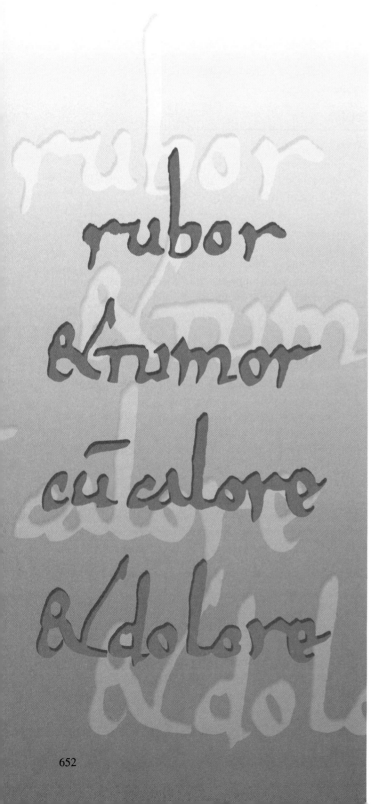

Pain and Pain Management

"We must all die. But that I can save (a person) from days of torture, that is what I feel as my great and ever new privilege. Pain is a more terrible lord of mankind than even death himself."

ALBERT SCHWEITZER

Pain is a significant, often central factor for many patients. In confronting pain, their experience will be highly variable. Procedures that induce agony in some will appear to be only mildly uncomfortable to others. Some will describe their pain in clear, precise terms, while others will have difficulty pinpointing the problem. Patients may regard their pain as a challenge, but too many are seriously debilitated, depressed, and almost broken by their experience.

Pain and pain management constitute a major focus for caregivers and diagnostic allied health professionals alike. In one study, 46% of patients with cancer reported poor or no pain control. In North America, almost 50 million people a year will require treatment for postoperative pain. Pain is a problem for people with sickle-cell anemia, AIDS, and MS. Perhaps 65% of nurses complain and may take time off of work because of chronic back pain.

PAIN: ACUTE AND CHRONIC

To begin our discussion, let us first note the distinction between acute pain and chronic pain. Although the term *acute* is often used in clinical settings to imply sudden and severe, in the context of pain, it refers instead to the transitory nature of the pain experience. Acute pain may range from mild to severe, but its overall duration is relatively short because the pain is usually related to the progression of disease and subsequent healing. An example is the pain associated with a fracture that heals satisfactorily or with a kidney stone successfully removed from its point of lodgement in a ureter. By contrast, chronic pain may also vary in severity but is of long duration (the usual rule of thumb is six months or more). It is often subclassified on the basis of its underlying cause. Where the pathogenesis of a well-characterized disease underlies the experience—for example, a poorly controlled cancer or a degenerative joint disease—the pain is termed **chronic malignant** or **symptomatic pain.** Where no such disease or degeneration can be identified, it is called **chronic benign** or **chronic nonmalignant pain.** Despite the use of the word *benign,* this type of pain can be a very disabling condition in its own right. Table 23.1 presents a pain classification scheme. Here, the focus shifts from the objective nature of the pain experience (acute versus chronic) to a combination of pain and supposed cause that occurs in individuals.

At least two important principles emerge from the acute/chronic categorization. The first is that in the neurophysiology of pain, significant differences exist in the neurological processing, perception, and impact of acute pain compared with that of chronic pain. The second principle is that different approaches to pain management are effective with different sorts of pain. This has a bearing on the selection of an appropriate therapeutic regimen to cope with it.

The Acute Pain Model and Pain Relief

In its most straightforward form, the experience of pain is based on the chain of events depicted in figure 23.1. Pain

Table 23.1	Classification of Patients According to Their Pain Experience and Underlying Pathology

Acute Pain

Underlying cause transitory
Treatment of pain symptomatic
Resolution based on resolution of underlying cause
Physiological: part of a natural or therapeutic process, vaccinations, injections, some activity related pain, childbirth
Posttraumatic or Postsurgery: examples: immediate response to whiplash, recovery from shoulder surgery
Secondary to Acute Illness: example: biliary colic associated with cholelithiasis

Chronic Pain

Underlying cause protracted or ongoing, perhaps untreatable or not identifiable
Long (six months?) duration
Pain is a (perhaps "the") major focus of care.

Chronic Malignant/Symptomatic Pain
(underlying pathology causes pain)

Recurrent Acute: unresolved cause, pain-free periods, only symptomatic care available (e.g., migraine headaches)
Ongoing, Acute: pain a significant component of chronic disease (e.g., joint pain in rheumatoid arthritis)
Ongoing, Time Limited: Example: cancer pain ends with death or control of disease.

Chronic Nonmalignant Pain
(pain itself and disablement that results are the major problem, response to drugs often poor)

May include conditions like chronic lower back pain that responds best to activity and exercise, and conditions like neuropathic pain and complex regional pain syndrome (see table 23.4)
Chronic Intractable Nonmalignant Pain Syndrome: same as above except patient is largely disabled by pain.

Source: Adapted from N. T. Meinhart and M. McCaffrey, *Pain: A Nursing Approach to Assessment and Analysis.* Copyright © 1983 Appleton & Lange.

stimuli may directly affect a tissue's nerve endings or indirectly cause tissue damage, releasing substances which then depolarize the nerve endings. These fine nerve endings are called **nociceptors** (*noci* is from the Latin for "to hurt"). The activation of the pain fibers associated with nociceptors is called **nociception.** Pain is the central sensory experience of nociceptive input. It has two quite separate components. Pain perception, like vision or audition, gives information about the nature, location, intensity, and duration of the nociception. Suffering, on the other hand,

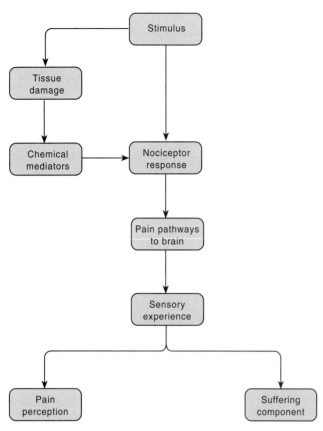

Figure 23.1   **The Essential Aspects of Acute Pain Processing and Experience.**

involves the reactions to pain, including varying combinations of autonomic, emotional, or behavioral responses.

Autonomic responses to intense pain typically consist of increased heart rate and blood pressure, increased secretion of epinephrine, raised blood glucose, decreased gastric secretions and motility, decreased blood flow to the viscera and skin, dilated pupils, and sweating. The emotional responses may involve fear, anger, anxiety, panic, depression, and even passive resignation. The simplest behavioral responses are spinal cord reflexes, but behaviors may range from lowered mobility to complex coping and avoidance behaviors. Behavioral responses may even include maladaptive patterns of adjustment that can complicate or even interfere with a person's recovery.

The model described in figure 23.1 best addresses the experience of acute pain that is based on trauma or disease, which is called **somatic** pain. In this case, pain is beneficial in that it informs us of danger and then mobilizes a drive state that attempts to remove the stimulus, correct the damage, or at least reduce the intensity of the pain or suffering. Treatment that is based on this model depends on a continued monitoring of signs and symptoms so that changes in a patient's status may be noted, providing the basis for a more refined or altered diagnosis. Any clinical consideration of pain and pain relief must assume that the underlying disease is accurately diagnosed and effectively treated.

This acute pain model is important to keep in mind because many current approaches to pain management may focus less on the causes of pain (since they may not be therapeutically accessible) and more on the patient's response to it. Reducing the patient's level of anxiety or tension and relieving depression or anger are a few examples. These are sometimes called **nonmedical, complementary,** or **alternative pain relief methods.** These methods are designed to alleviate pain, even if the underlying cause is not reversible. They exert their effects primarily by modifying reactions to the sensory experience (autonomic, emotional, or behavioral responses) or modulating the sensory experience itself in indirect ways.

THE PHYSIOLOGICAL BASIS OF PAIN PERCEPTION

With an understanding of the essentials of acute and chronic pain, and a basic model for acute pain, we can now turn to the structure and function of the specific neurological components of pain perception.

Nociception

Nociceptors, the finely branched nerve endings whose stimulation gives rise to pain, all appear the same when viewed with an electron microscope. In practice, however, some respond only to strong, mechanical stimulation, especially by sharp objects, or to temperatures above 45° C. These nerve endings converge on small, fine, myelinated fibers that conduct their action potentials relatively quickly (5 to 30 m/sec). Fibers of this type are called $A\delta$ **(A delta) fibers.** They are distributed only to the skin, mucous membranes, and selected serous membranes (e.g., the parietal peritoneum). They tend to fire immediately upon (intense) stimulation and cease firing when the stimulus is removed, producing the sensation of **sharp pain.** As well, they rapidly adapt to a stimulus—that is, you feel the needle pierce your skin but the sense of sharp pain soon goes away, even though the needle (stimulus) remains. You may experience some sharp pain again as the needle is withdrawn. Essentially, these fibers carry information about sharp, pricking, acute pain that is relatively well localized and discriminated (you know where it is and what's causing it!). Activation of a single $A\delta$ fiber is sufficient to cause pain perception.

A second population of pain fibers, smaller in diameter and unmyelinated, are called **C fibers.** They are distributed to the same areas as the $A\delta$ fibers, but with much greater density. In addition, they are very widely distributed in deep tissue: in muscle and tendon, visceral peritoneum, and the visceral organs themselves (e.g., the myocardium, the stomach, and intestines). Action potentials in these fibers tend to be generated by substances that are associated with tissue damage or insult. The entry, production, or release of bradykinin, serotonin, histamine, and potassium in injured tissue triggers pain receptors, while IL1, prostaglandin E_2, ception at the cord level triggers sympathetic discharge to the site of injury, enhancing the vascular and mediator response to injury, thereby enhancing pain stimulation.

Pain Fiber Connections in the Spinal Cord

Like those of other sensory fibers, the cell bodies of the Aδ and C fibers are found in the dorsal root ganglia. Their axons continue from the dorsal root ganglion into the spinal cord, where they synapse with the next neuron in the chain, called a **second-order neuron.** As Aδ and C fibers enter the cord, some send branches (collaterals) up or down the cord for short distances. They then travel deeper to their points of synapse (fig. 23.2a). This provides for the involvement of several cord segments in the mediation of complex pain reflexes (e.g., crossed extension; see table 21.9).

Most of the second-order neurons pass across the cord and then proceed toward the brain in the anterolateral-spinothalamic tract (fig. 23.2b). The term *spinothalamic tract* is somewhat misleading here, because the vast majority of second-order pain fibers traveling in the anterolateral-spinothalamic tract do not end up in the thalamus at all. Instead, they terminate in the reticular formation of the brain stem (fig. 23.2c). Here, through the reticular activating system, they mediate an increase in general consciousness, alertness, and attention. These are important orienting and defense reactions to pain. They occur whatever the specific nature of the pain stimulus and explain some of the jumpiness, irritability, and perhaps obsessiveness of pain sufferers.

A large number of the fibers in the anterolateral system enter an area of cells surrounding the cerebral aqueduct in the midbrain (called, therefore, the **mesencephalic peri-aqueductal gray matter**). From here, action potentials can be relayed to the hypothalamus and thence to the limbic system and cerebral cortex (fig. 23.2d). This is part of the neurological basis for the endocrine, autonomic, and emotional components of the reaction to pain. Extremely intense stimulation will activate neurons in this area. They, in turn, project to the dorsal horn of the spinal cord where they can inhibit the relay of subsequent pain signals. This may be the basis for the analgesia experienced by many who suffer extreme trauma.

The pain pathway, thought to be the evolutionarily most primitive, activates cells in the region of the dorsal midbrain (fig. 23.2e). (This area is called the **tectum** of the midbrain and is associated with orienting responses to visual and auditory stimuli.) In response, these cells appear to promote spinal cord motor mechanisms, thereby enhancing spinal reflexes and facilitating behavioral responses.

Neospinothalamic Pain Pathways

Many Aδ fibers synapse immediately upon entering lamina I and II (the area referred to as the **substantia gelitanosa**), the first two of five layers or laminae of the cord's dorsal horn. Axons from the cell bodies in this layer cross the cord and travel the anterolateral-spinothalamic system to

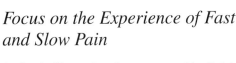

Focus on the Experience of Fast and Slow Pain

A simple illustration demonstrates this division of peripheral nociception into Aδ and C fibers. Using the nails of your thumb and index finger of one hand, pinch the web of skin between the base of two fingers on the other hand and note the sensations. First, and within a fraction of a second, you should have felt a sharp pain emanating precisely from the pinched area. Then, perhaps two seconds later, a duller, less clearly localized aching or burning sensation should have developed. It will probably slowly begin to throb. These sensations were mediated first by Aδ fibers and then by C fibers: hence, the commonly used terms **fast** and **slow pain.**

---

and leukotriene B$_4$ sensitize the same endings. Aδ fibers will respond to the same chemicals, but to a lesser extent. As noted, they tend to respond to specific mechanisms of injury like cutting, heat, intense pressure, etc. These impulses travel in a continuous fashion and are therefore much slower (0.5–2 m/sec) than those conducted over the Aδ fibers. As well, the initiation of firing is not as closely related to the onset or withdrawal of the stimulus. Firing is slow to develop, so pain may emerge some time after stimulus application, perhaps because of the slow release or formation of the triggering substances. Once initiated, action potential firing can persist long after the original stimulus has been removed. C fibers carry information related to long-lasting, burning, often called **dull pain,** which is poorly localized and more diffusely distressing.

A variety of events will potentiate pain transmission. Tissue injury (particularly burns in the skin) and subsequent inflammation can activate and sensitize "silent" nociceptors. This appears to happen in inflammatory bowel disease and will be familiar to some who have had unusual reactions to sunburn. Pain transmission itself facilitates the ease at which information immediately following pain is transmitted. This is called **primary hyperalgesia.** It is mediated through changes that occur in the dorsal horn of gray matter in the cord. Glutamate, the excitatory neurotransmitter that is released from the terminals of the C and Aδ fibers, binds to the NMDA class of glutamate receptors (the same receptors that facilitate short-term memory in the limbic system), and permits entry of Ca^{2+} into the second-order neuron. This in turn activates the formation of NO (which we have seen as a signal in inflammation and a vasodilator), which feeds back to the same terminals that released the glutamate in the first place. There can be a rapid expansion of the area that is sensitized to pain stimuli: **secondary hyperalgesia.** This "spreading pain" probably represents both central and peripheral adaptations. Another facilitation is accomplished by the autonomic nervous system. Pain re-

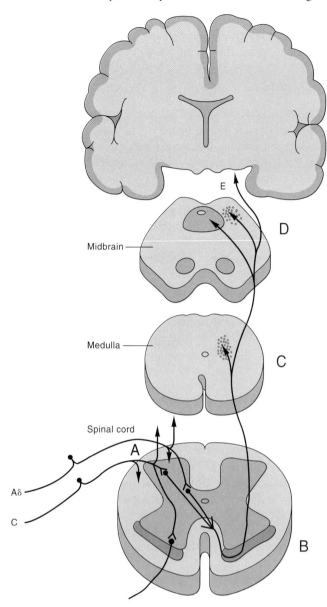

Figure 23.2 **An Overview of the Essential Neuronal Interrelations for Dull and Sharp Pain Perception.** Letters *A* through *E* are keyed to the text. The darker areas of the spinal cord represent the anterolateral-spinothalamic tracts.

Focus on Flexor-Withdrawal Reflex Physiology

The neural explanation of the flexor-withdrawal reflex involves action potentials generated in Aδ fibers by cutaneous receptors. The action potentials pass into the dorsal horn, where they synapse with excitatory second-order neurons, which in turn synapse with alpha motor neurons in the ipsilateral ventral horn. These motor neurons then stimulate the contraction of flexor muscles that draw the stimulated area away from the source of the painful stimulus. These same Aδ fibers simultaneously synapse with inhibitory interneurons (box fig. 23.1) that produce relaxation of the related extensor muscle group to facilitate the flexion of the limb.

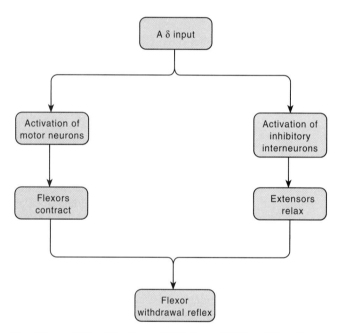

Box Figure 23.1 **The Flexor-Withdrawal Reflex.** This reflex depends on activation of flexors at the same time that extensors are inhibited.

their destinations (fig. 23.3). About one-third of Aδ fibers terminate in the **posterior nuclear group** in the thalamus. These fibers have been called the **neospinothalamic pain system** to denote that this is an evolutionarily advanced and sophisticated pain discrimination pathway. The effectiveness and specificity of neospinothalamic pain discrimination is due to the convergence on these same thalamic nuclei of the medial lemniscal fibers that carry highly differentiated sensory information for light-touch, two-point discrimination, stretch, and so on. Pain discrimination is enhanced through the addition of these sensations to the relatively well-discriminated Aδ impulses. Because the posterior nuclear group of thalamic nuclei provide direct access to the primary and secondary somatosensory cortex,

conscious appreciation of sharp, well-discriminated, and localized pain is realized.

Activity in Aδ fibers is the principal factor in eliciting pain-induced spinal reflexes. In the simplest of these, the **flexor-withdrawal** reflex, touching something sharp or hot causes rapid withdrawal of the stimulated limb. The withdrawal occurs so rapidly that it is accomplished even before we become conscious of the sensation of pain. This reflex minimizes exposure to the potentially harmful stimulus. In the **crossed-extension reflex,** reflex extension of the opposite limb is added to the flexor-withdrawal reflex. For example, if you step on a tack, you will simultaneously lift

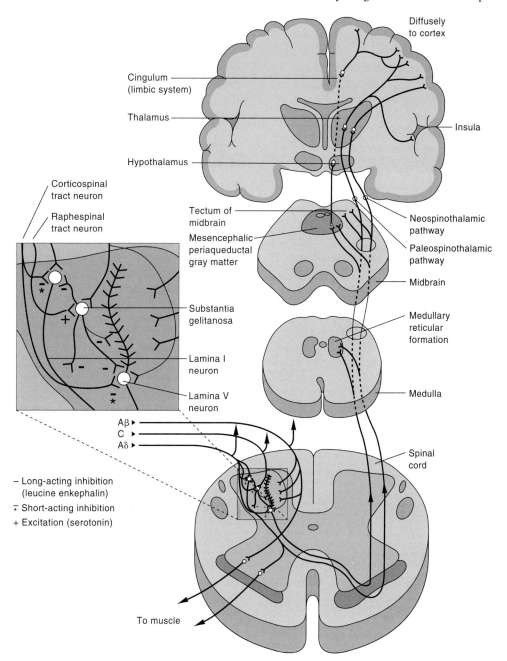

Figure 23.3 **Scheme of Aδ and C Nociceptor Synapses in the Dorsal Horn of the Spinal Cord.** Most output from lamina I and V passes to higher perception centers via contralateral spinothalamic tracts. Ipsilateral tracts are omitted for clarity.

the pricked foot and extend the other leg so that your weight is borne on the unstimulated foot.

Paleospinothalamic Pain Pathways

The C fibers have a slightly more complex fate in the cord: They synapse in either lamina I and II or V. But they form a major input to a much more complicated local processing system that feeds into a separate pain pathway that originates in lamina V. To make matters even more complex, lamina V appears to house two different families of neurons—those that respond to (and code for) the presence and inten-

sity of injurious stimuli and those that code for the nature of the injurious stimulus and, to some extent, its location. These lamina V neurons are critical in some pain syndromes as they can fire in bursts in the *absence* of stimulation in situations in which they do not receive "balanced" inputs.

Fibers from cell bodies in lamina V pass into the ascending reticular system, the mesencephalic periaqueductal gray matter, and the midbrain tectum, as do the fibers from lamina I and II. But, as well, some continue to the thalamus, particularly its **intralaminar nuclei,** from which they diffusely project to various parts of the cortex. The number of fibers arriving at the thalamus is small compared with the vast number of original C fibers, and there is also little overlap or convergence with fibers arising from Aδ. For these reasons, discrimination and localization of pain in this system are quite imprecise. The pathways involved are called the **paleospinothalamic pathways.**

The spinal cord processing of information that feeds into the paleospinothalamic pathway is shown in figure 23.3. It shows the array of interconnections in the laminae of the dorsal horn that make possible the varieties of pain fiber activity.

 Checkpoint 23.1

Let's pause here for a brief summary of the processing of pain as it enters and ascends the nervous system on its way to the cortex.

Much of the neural activity generated by pain stimuli feeds into the ascending reticular activating system to increase alertness, attentiveness, and the motor responsiveness of spinal cord mechanisms that enhanced reflex activity. Some excitation arrives at the tectum (posterior portion) of the midbrain and thereby increases the sensitivity of orienting responses to visual and auditory stimuli. The person can become highly distractible and jumpy (tectospinal component). These two (reticulospinal and tectospinal) account for some of the rawness and stimulus overload experienced by pain sufferers. A portion of the input ends up in the periaqueductal gray region of the midbrain, gaining access to the hypothalamus and therefore to both the limbic and endocrine systems. The strictly "spinothalamic" component is divided into two elements: a highly discriminated neospinothalamic pathway that provides direct access to the specialized sensory cortex, and a less well-discriminated paleospinothalamic pathway that appears to play an important role in the mediation of chronic pain. Check your understanding against the summary in Figure 23.4.

Figure 23.4 emphasizes the separation of information from C and Aδ fibers into paleospinothalamic and neospinothalamic pathways. This is a simplification of the actual cord processing *and* of the perception of pain itself. Many people with acute pain (postsurgical, for example) suffer from a great deal of dull throbbing and aching—phenomena we have associated with the paleo pathway. Likewise, chronic pain can include intense, stabbing, site-specific pain. A further complexity is that there are now known to be several distinct ascending pain pathways in the cord.

The thalamus has been described in its role of relaying pain information to the cortex—diffusely to the superficial layers of the cortex (general arousal and responsiveness) for the paleospinothalamic tract, and specifically to the cortex for the neospinothalamic tract. Thalamic injury can produce thalamic pain syndromes that are very challenging to treat. The final destination of pain information is, of course, the cortex. The centrally important areas for the arrival of pain at the cortical level are the primary somatosensory cortex, which principally serves a localization and discrimination role; the anterior cingulate cortex, which is implicated in thermal pain and in the emotional aspects of pain; and the anterior insular cortex, which may be involved in the perception of visceral pain. Of this list, the cingulate cortex has received the most attention. Psychosurgery, which has been performed for serious, intractable pain, focuses usually on the ablation of the cingulum bundle, which carries information to and from the cingulate cortex.

Endorphins and Descending Systems of Pain Inhibition

We have already noted the role of pain in alerting us to danger and activating some coping responses. Once this role has been served, however, it is desirable to limit the pain, and much therapeutic effort is devoted to this goal. One long-standing approach has been the use of narcotic agents (e.g., morphine) to dull the pain. Historically, narcotics are derived from plants and produce their effects by binding to specific receptors in the brain stem. Once the presence of such receptors was discovered, an intriguing speculation arose. Presumably, they would have developed in a system that used some internally produced substance that would bind to them; it was just a coincidence that plant-derived narcotics were sufficiently similar to bind to the same receptors (fig. 23.5). This speculation has proved to be correct, and the presence of *end*ogenous m*orphine*like substances is now well established. Certain of them, known as **endorphins,** are the subject of much study for their role as pain inhibitors.

The actual inhibitory effects of the endorphins are achieved indirectly. Endorphin receptors are richly distributed in the brain stem (in the periaqueductal gray and the nucleus raphe magnus). When activated by endorphins, they promote the flow of action potentials down the cord, to lamina I and II of the dorsal horn (the substantia gelitanosa). The arrival of these action potentials triggers the release of another member of the endorphin group called **leucine enkephalin.** This is a key step, in that leucine enkephalin exerts an inhibitory effect at the synapses between Aδ and C inputs to their second-order neurons. In this way, the descending pathways are able to limit pain inputs to the higher perception centers (figs. 23.6 and 23.7). The principal inhibitory effect of this descending system is on the paleospinothalamic pathways and their contribution to dull, aching pain. Since this is the case, we might predict

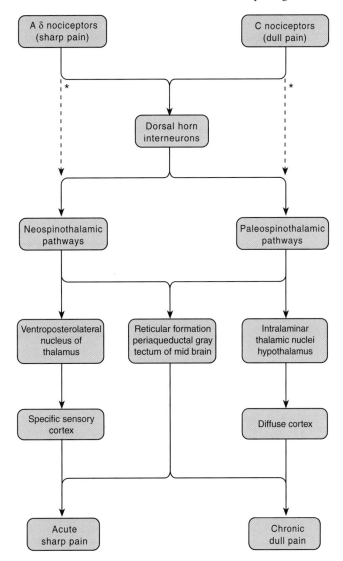

Figure 23.4   **The General Scheme for Underlying Perception of the Two Types of Pain.** *Dotted lines indicate a major contribution of Aδ fibers to the neospinothalamic pathway and C fibers to the paleospinothalamic pathway.

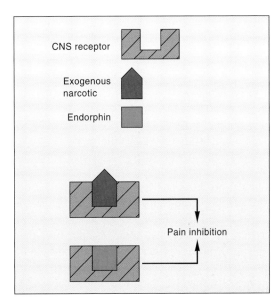

Figure 23.5   **Essential Mechanism Whereby Exogenous Narcotics Work Via the Endogenous Analgesia Receptors of the Central Nervous System.**

that exogenous substances that can bind to endorphin receptors would be most effective against this type of pain, and this is, indeed, the case.

Another technique, used when pain is severe and unresponsive to other analgesics, is **stimulus-produced analgesia.** It involves the placement of electrodes directly within the periaqueductal gray of the brain stem, from where their stimulus directly activates the descending pathways that induce pain inhibition, mimicking the effect of the binding of endorphins in the same area. This endorphin system is thought to be a major route for the pain-dampening effects of a variety of nonmedical pain interventions, including meditation, acupuncture, and distraction.

The endorphin system is only one of several descending systems that modulate pain transmission and perception. This may be the best place to discuss a poorly understood mechanism that is getting increasing attention. The autonomic system, specifically the sympathetic branch, has a role at two levels. We already noted the swelling and

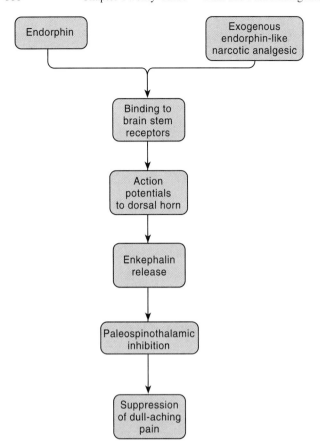

Figure 23.6   **Essential Elements of the Descending Analgesic System Used by Narcotics.**

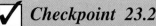

✔ *Checkpoint 23.2*

We will present a variety of medical and nonmedical pain management techniques later. Having read the preceding, can you think about the things you do to control pain of various types and place them into this framework? Predict the strategies, both pharmacological and nonmedical, that we will describe.

reddening that are not primarily inflammatory (injury instigated) in nature but may be induced by incidents of painful stimulation. The instant, cut-induced vasoconstriction discussed in chapter 1 is part of this sympathetic response. In more chronic situations; for example, some of the pain syndromes presented later in table 23.4, sympathetic reflex activation occurs as a feature, with swelling, increased blood flow and heat, and the excruciating presence of **causalgia** (burning sensation). We also mentioned the role of the hypothalamus in orchestrating emotional, endocrine, and autonomic responses to pain. Any approach that intercepts this autonomic reflex activity will enhance pain management.

Voluntary movement influences pain transmission by synapsing with interneurons in the dorsal horn of the cord and inducing short-acting inhibition (fig. 23.7). We have mentioned the damping impact that balanced stimulation of the so-called discriminative sensations (light touch, tickle, light pressure, limb position, vibration, etc.) has on pain transmission. Any voluntary movement induces this sort of peripheral sensory activity as well. These impulses arrive on Aα and Aβ fibers to the dorsal horn, where they tend to inhibit the relay of coexisting pain information. Cortical approaches probably express themselves through this pathway as well as the endorphin route already described.

Referred Pain

As a later section will show, adequate observation of a patient's pain experience requires a precise description of the pain and its localization. This can be quite straightforward—for example, a burning sensation at the incision site. But it can also be puzzling—for example, the radiating pains in the left axilla and arm that are associated with a heart attack. In such cases, it is important to recognize that all pain is really "felt" in the brain. The mind projects that perception of pain to an area of the body that is, in many cases, but not always, the same as the spot whose stimulation gave rise to the sensation in the first place. Sensations arising at the skin or in the mucous membranes and in some of the parietal serous membranes are quite accurately projected. When a mosquito bites you in the back of the leg you know exactly where to swat, without even looking. On the other hand, pain arising from internal organs, **visceral pain,** is not nearly this accurately projected. It may be perceived as arising on the skin surface or in muscles quite remote from the site of nociception. In this case the sensation is called **referred pain.**

The most widely accepted explanation for referred pain is based on the concept of **dermatomes.** Each of these is the area of skin supplied by a single spinal nerve. This means that cutaneous stimuli from a given dermatome produce action potentials that are always delivered to the corresponding spinal cord segment (figure 23.8). The relationship is very straightforward during early embryonic development (fig. 23.9a), when each of the dermatomes lies directly over its corresponding cord segment. However, as development proceeds and limb buds emerge and differentiate, the spatial relationship between dermatome and cord becomes distorted (fig. 23.9b). Even though some parts of the dermatomes are stretched some distance from their cord segment, the connecting nerves elongate to maintain the links previously established. As you might expect, the situation is actually somewhat more complex because there is some overlap in the actual distribution of dermatomes. The

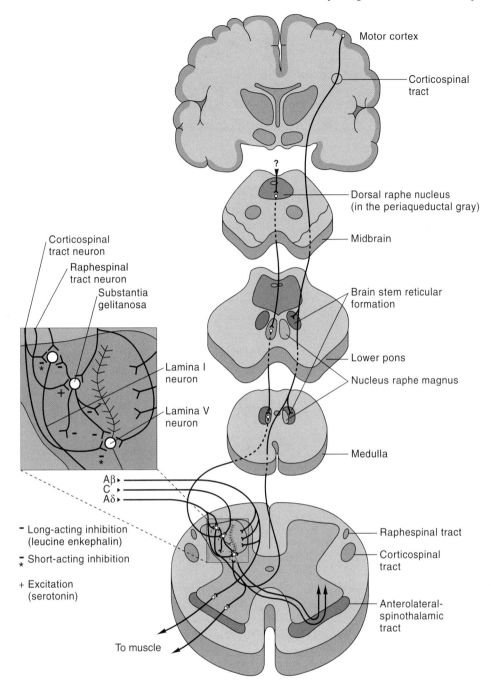

Figure 23.7   **Summary of Descending Pain Processing.**

treatment here is simplified only to make the point. Certain dermatomes serve as easy "neurological landmarks": C6—thumb, C8—little finger, T5—nipple, T10—navel, S2–5—perineum, S1—little toe.

The connection between this developmental pattern and referred pain is that the sensory nerves from various body organs enter the cord at points that coincide with those of a given dermatome. Early sensory input from a given dermatome seems to become a reference that higher

processing centers rely upon. Since most pain-related input is from the skin, interpretation centers seem to "assume" that all input is from the skin. When an organ is damaged, its pain afferents are interpreted as originating in the skin of the reference dermatome. For example, impulses entering the cord at levels T1–4 or T1–5 from pain receptors stimulated by myocardial ischemia are interpreted as impulses from dermatomes associated with T1–4. Hence, the referred pain that is characteristic of cardiac ischemia: chest

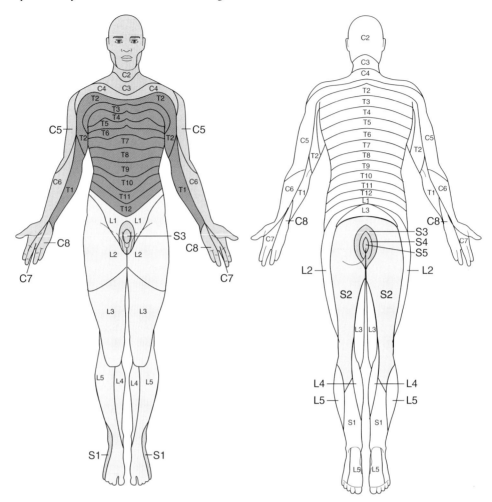

Figure 23.8   **Typical Distribution of the Dermatomes.**

pains on the left side (including the shoulder and axilla), which radiate down the left arm and perhaps from the base of the neck into the jaw. The general, but not invariable, left localization is presumably due to the entry of the majority of the fibers carrying pain information from the heart into the left side of the spinal cord. (Some people with myocardial ischemia will report bilateral pain, and—rarely—a person may report principally right-sided pain. Some typical patterns of pain referral are presented in table 23.2.)

Phantom Pain

In connection with the physiological basis of pain, we should touch on the puzzling pain experience called **phantom pain. Phantoms** are tactile and movement perceptions that remain after a part of the body has been amputated. There can be a very real sense that the leg, for example, is still there, has bulk and weight, can be moved at will, gets itchy, or, to the great distress of the amputee, is a

source of extreme pain. Phantoms can exist for any lost body part (e.g., breasts, hands, legs), but the greater the extent of cortical representation, the more likely it is that there will be a phantom.

Phantoms are more common in adults than children, and are thought to be quite unusual in young children. They may also occur when an area has been denervated—for example, in a spinal cord injury that severs all cord pathways at T–12. Some people with spinal cord lesions experience such realistic phantoms, capable of "movement" and apparent sensation, that the phenomena can be quite disturbing.

There is great variability in the persistence of phantoms. Some are only briefly apparent after an amputation, some fade or shrink gradually; some persist or recur for years. In emergency situations, a long-dormant but realistic phantom may arise with unfortunate consequences. For example, a person may reach out with a nonexistent arm to fend off a flying object.

Sensory reeducation can help a great deal in coping with phantoms connected to nerve damage. Where repeated

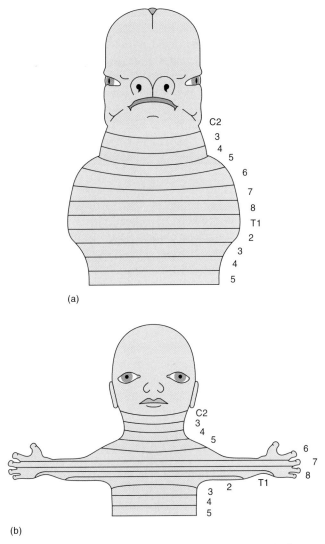

(a)

(b)

Figure 23.9 **Dermatome Migration During Embryologic Development.** (*a*) At about 4 weeks, the dermatomes are quite uniform and correspond closely to cord segments. Note early limb buds. (*b*) By week 16, dermatomes C6–T1 have migrated with the developing arms.

Table 23.2	Typical Surfaces to Which Selected Organs Refer Pain

Organ	Site of Referred Pain
Heart	Usually left shoulder and axilla, with radiation down inside of left arm; also radiation to neck and jaw (Note: reference to the right side is sometimes observed)
Esophagus	Pharynx, lower neck and arm, substernum near heart
Stomach	Epigastric region, usually between umbilicus and xiphoid process
Bile duct/ gall bladder	Midepigastric region, radiating to tip of right scapula
Pancreas	Midback, sometimes low epigastric region
Large bowel	Hypogastric region, lower abdomen, and periumbilical area
Kidney/ureter	Edge of rectus abdominis muscle below level of umbilicus, radiation to flank and groin
Bladder/testis	Suprapubic region
Uterus	Low abdomen or low back and side
Appendix	Initially near umbilicus, then shifting to lower right as parietal peritoneum becomes involved

opportunities for reeducation of the cortex exist—for example, in the paraplegic who repeatedly has his legs stimulated with clearly no corresponding sensation—the phantom tends to fade. Such reeducation may not be possible if the limb is missing, and the phantom may then persist; but the proximal portions (which are more poorly represented on the cortex than the distal portions) may fade, with a subsequent shrinking of the phantom.

Pain is not associated with all phantoms but when it does occur it can be a very troubling problem. Many amputees have transient phantom pain, and about 5–10% of this special population has serious, persistent phantom pain. The circumstances that bring on the phantom pain will vary. For some, it comes without warning, or it may be as-

sociated with fatigue, pressure sores, or a poorly fitting prosthesis. In other cases, stimulation or irritation of certain consistent trigger points will be the cause.

The approaches that have been used to treat phantom pain present a catalogue of modern pain treatment, ranging from physical and electrical stimulation (including acupuncture), through peripheral and spinal nerve sections and blocks, psychosurgery, psychotropic drugs, and megavitamin therapy, to a host of psychologically based approaches. The results vary from approach to approach, and even more from patient to patient. Individuals experiencing such pain will possibly require extensive and highly specialized referral, assessment, and care.

Cancer Pain

Part of the problem with cancer is that many forms can be well advanced before they produce definitive symptoms, including pain, and some people never experience pain generated by their cancer. The pain, when produced, can be extremely variable, depending on its specific source. Tumor masses impinging on neural structures can cause

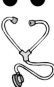

Focus on Impediments to Accurate and Complete Pain Reporting

Effective communication about pain requires a positive desire and capacity on the patient's part to send accurate information and an equivalent capacity and desire in the health care team to receive it. The following points are worth considering if pain assessment or management is not going well.

The first step is to look more closely at the person who is in pain. Some complaints about pain control derive from the erroneous expectation that the person will be entirely pain free, a challenge for patient education. Some individuals may be playing the good patient role, not wishing to trouble you; or, at a simpler level, they may simply be misinformed about the sort of pain to expect and what input from them is required. On the other hand, the patient who has learned to cope with the chronic pain associated with arthritis or chronic pelvic inflammatory disease may well have a fear of wearing out the listener. This person is probably at least as common as the person who likes to complain. And some unfortunate people will have lapsed into a learned helplessness, defeated by their pain and without the optimism that an attempt at communication requires.

Other patients may have specific reasons for concealing pain. Perhaps they are anxious to protect their family from the severity of their pain or the progression of disease they think it represents. Perhaps they fear that a report of intense pain will cause postponement of long-awaited surgery, in the same way a systemic infection might. Some people harbor common misconceptions about narcotic analgesics: that they will become addicted; that taking narcotics for pain when it is less severe will build up a tolerance so that the drug will not be effective later when they really need it; that the withdrawal from the narcotic will be worse than the pain. Or they may associate narcotics with addicts and degeneracy. Whatever the underlying concern, by sensitive and supportive questioning, you may be able to help the patient to identify it so that you can address it. Again, patient education may be the issue. Does the person understand the differences among tolerance (the requirement for increasing dose to achieve the same control), physical dependence (requiring gradual withdraw of medication), and addiction (psychological craving)?

A more subtle problem arises when dealing with people of different cultures and social backgrounds, whose behavior may be affected by deeply ingrained differences in the ways they understand, relate to, and express themselves about pain. If people produce pain behaviors that are recognizable and familiar to us, we are more likely to believe the expression as genuine and act to alleviate it. It is important, therefore, to make allowances for social and cultural differences when interpreting pain reports.

pain ranging from sharp and stabbing neuralgias (see table 23.4) to diffuse paresthesias. Invasion and displacement of functional tissue (bone, muscle, skin) can result in dull, aching pain that becomes more severe with tumor progression. Compression of or growth into a tubular structure can cause pain in a variety of ways. Backing up of glandular secretions can cause distention and pain before the organ slows or shuts down its secretion. If the tube is a ureter, pain may be the only sign before the kidney is irreparably damaged. Masses in or near the esophagus can render swallowing painful, and stenosis of the gut can lead to distention and diffuse pain. Arterial occlusion may result in ischemic pain, the nature of which will depend on the structure or organ occluded (if visceral, then referred pain, etc.). Venous or lymphatic blockage can lead to diffuse dull aching. A lung tumor growing into a bronchus can lead to infection in the unventilated region. This can produce dull chest pain or extend to the pleural membranes, producing the sharp pain of pleurisy. Advanced cancer, especially that accompanied by extensive necrosis as tumors outgrow their blood supplies, can produce excruciating pain. Potent central analgesics like morphine, given in appropriate doses and intervals, are necessary to help the patient cope. These efforts may be supplemented with therapeutic blocking of peripheral nerves where appropriate. In some cases, even these measures are inadequate.

DESCRIPTION OF PAIN PHENOMENA

Compared with sights or sounds, the perception, expression, and effect of pain sensations are subject to great variability both between individuals and within a given person. But this complexity shouldn't be allowed to interfere with effective clinical observation. Pain associated with disease processes or trauma can provide important clues to suggest or confirm diagnoses. And here, every detail can be meaningful: What is it like? Does it change or move? Is the pain clearly localized? To what events or circumstances is it related? What makes it better or worse? All of this data has to be evaluated in the context of the medical, personal, and social history within which it occurs. When evaluating what the patient says, it is helpful to bear in mind that "real pain" can't be distinguished from "imaginary pain," since the only true pain to the patient is what is felt.

The Patient's Description of Pain

The patient's verbal description of pain can present problems, either because the pain itself is difficult to describe (diffuse, wandering, etc.) or because of imprecision or variation in the patient's use of words. Some commonly used words that seem to denote clearly different subjective pain qualities are presented in table 23.3. The clusters of adjectives denote particular qualities of pain perception (e.g., in-

Table 23.3   Adjectives Used to Describe Pain. The clusters suggest differing intensities of a variety of independent qualities of pain.

Onset or Specific Nature of Pain?

1) numb	2a) penetrating	2b) tearing
dull	boring	rasping
tingling	piercing	gnawing
pricking	stabbing	lacerating
sharp	(referred to as	
cutting	"lancinating")	

Intensity?

"The pain is"	"The painful area is"
mild	tender
bothersome	sore
discomforting	hurting
moderate	smarting
intense	aching
horrible	splitting
excruciating	blinding
unbearable	

Time Component?

1) constant	3) steady
periodic	flickering
intermittent	pulsing
	throbbing
2) brief	pounding
enduring	

Spatial Quality?

1a) generalized	1b) deep	2) fixed
diffuse	superficial	spreading
focal		radiating
		jumping
		shooting

Tension or Pressure?

1) tugging	3) tight
pulling	pinching
taut	pressing
	heavy
2) cramping	squeezing
wrenching	crushing
	suffocating

Temperature?

1) hot	2) cool
burning	cold
scalding	freezing
searing	
(referred to as	
"causalgia")	

Emotional/Visceral Aspects?

1) haunting	3) sickening
fearful	nauseating
frightful	
terrifying	4) miserable
	punishing
2) distressing	wretched
agonizing	cruel
killing	vicious

Impact of Pain?

annoying
troublesome
nagging
tiring
grueling
exhausting
debilitating

Adapted and modified from R. Melzack, *The McGill Pain Questionnaire,* McGill University, Montreal, 1975.

tensity, timing, or location, etc.) and, where appropriate, the specific words have been scaled. With regard to one quality, changes in the intensity may be quite clear to the patient, especially when they are rapid, but this aspect of pain perception is greatly affected by fatigue, stress, lack of effective support, or inadequate management. The sensation of pain may be constant, while the perception of its intensity increases as the person becomes worn out.

In clinical settings where pain diagnosis and management is a central task, protocols incorporating such verbal and other pain assessment scales and questions are often used to standardize the documentation of the patient's pain experience. These ensure consistency and thoroughness and, with the inclusion of pain pictures like the one in figure 23.10a, give the patient an easier vehicle for self-expression than simple self-report. With children, the use of a pain intensity

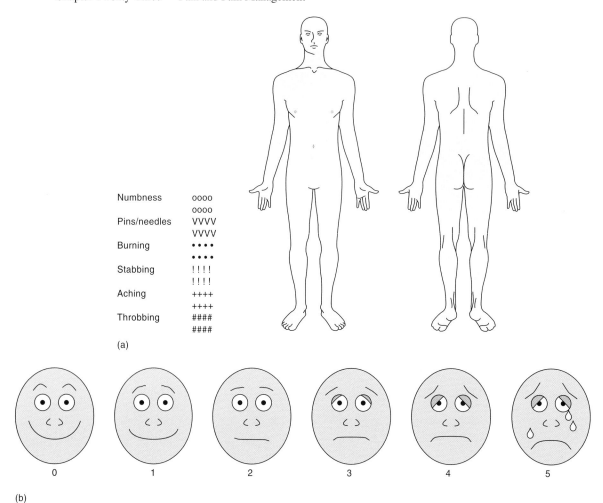

Numbness   oooo
           oooo
Pins/needles   VVVV
               VVVV
Burning   • • • •
          • • • •
Stabbing   ! ! ! !
           ! ! ! !
Aching   ++++
         ++++
Throbbing   ####
            ####

(a)

(b)

Figure 23.10   **Examples of Graphic Representations Useful in Helping Patients Describe Their Pain.** (*a*) A system for adults, which localizes and indicates intensity. (*b*) A method designed for children.

rating scale like the faces in figure 23.10*b* ensures a consistency and accuracy well beyond that from verbal reports.

Clinical Terminology

The need for precision in describing the varieties of pain experience has given rise to an elaborate terminology (table 23.4). For a phenomenon as complex as pain, a variety of medical terms have evolved. We can relate to many of these terms because we have experienced the acute pain with which they are associated.

The term **somatic pain** describes a potentially tissue-damaging stimulus that leads to the activation of nociceptors, the transmission of this information to the brain, and its interpretation there. This transmission and interpretation can be straightforward, as it is with stepping on a tack, or more complex, as with the referred pain of myocardial infarction.

In every such case, there is a significant stimulus (e.g., myocardial ischemia) and a fairly predictable response (e.g., perception of pain in the left axilla and superficial chest, etc.). In chronic pain, the satisfactory explanations for an individual's pain experience are most often made in terms of a complex interaction between altered neural input and/or processing and social/psychological and behavioral factors. The special case of pain that is due to altered neural input or processing, is sometimes called **neuropathic pain** (i.e., pain associated with neuropathy). Table 23.5 contrasts the characteristics of somatic and neuropathic pain.

Although acute pain and somatic pain are often associated (as are chronic pain and neuropathic pain), we must be clear that the terms are not synonyms. Acute and chronic strictly denote patterns of onset and duration, while somatic and neuropathic propose different physiological mechanisms for the production of pain.

| Table 23.4 | Definitions for Medical Terms Applying to Selected Peripheral and Central Neuropathics and Altered Perception of Sensation Sometimes Associated |

Symptoms	Definitions
Paresthesias	General term referring to any of a variety of spontaneous abnormal sensations and sensitivities including (but not restricted to) burning, numbness, pricking, tingling, increased sensitivity to somatic sensation.
Dysesthesia	Ongoing background aching or burning sensation in the absence of apparent stimulus.
Hyperpathia	General term applied to increased and sometimes abnormal sensitivity to stimuli (includes hyperesthesia, hyperalgesia, and allodynia).
Hyperesthesia	Extreme sensitivity to touch.
Hyperalgesia	Exaggerated sensitivity to painful stimuli.
Allodynia	Condition in which a variety of stimuli (e.g., light touch, breeze on the skin) are perceived as intensely painful.
Formication	A spontaneous sensation like insects (ants) crawling on the skin.
Causalgia	Continuous burning, searing sensation in which a variety of stimuli can cause pain (allodynia) often initially accompanied by flushing of the skin; most common following peripheral nerve injury. Chronic causalgia is associated with vasoconstriction.
Hemianesthesia	Loss of sensation from one side of the body, usually from a CVA.

Peripheral Nerve Syndromes

Focal peripheral neuropathy	Peripheral nerve damage due to trauma, vascular compromise, compression, etc; will affect sensory and motor function; not necessarily painful.
Neuralgia	Pain in the distribution of a single peripheral nerve; usually combines ongoing aching and burning with intermittent, sharp pain.
Trigeminal neuralgia (Tic douloureux)	A neuralgia in the distribution of the fifth (trigeminal) cranial nerve; principal symptom is intermittent intense, paroxysmal, lancinating pain; triggered by eating, cold air current, talking, or spontaneous.
Root avulsion	Severe trauma to spinal roots at the level of the cord caused by wrenching trauma to a limb; chronic pain common.
Generalized peripheral neuropathy	Damage to peripheral nerves, may be principally sensory or sensorimotor, symmetric or asymmetric, diffuse or focal; classically a diffuse peripheral neuropathy is symmetric and distal with a "glove-and-stocking" anesthesia (i.e., loss of sensitivity to pain first in the feet, then the hands) accompanied by a variety of paresthesias.
Postherpetic pain	Following or during active herpes zoster infection; sudden lancinating pain, perhaps background of causalgia; can be elicited by light touch, cold, sometimes spontaneous.
Myofascial pain	Following injury or disease in a joint and/or associated muscles, some patients develop "fibromyositis" with pain elicited by muscle contraction. This myofascial pain may be a factor in lower back and neck pain, and temporomandibular joint disorders.
Complex regional pain syndrome	Characterized by continuous pain with combination of throbbing, burning, allodynia, sensitivity to cold, increasing pain by repeated mild stimulation. May include "sympathetic signs" (edema, erythema, blotching, or blanching) and atrophy of muscle, soft tissue, bone.

Syndromes Attributable to Central Lesions

Multiple sclerosis	Often associated with a variety of paresthesias.
Tabetic pain	Associated with lesions to posterior roots and dorsal columns caused by syphilis (tabes dorsalis); skin and joint sensation impaired, paresthesias and dysesthesias.
Acute spinal cord trauma	A variety of paresthesias and dysesthesias as well as autonomic dysfunctions occur.
Thalamic pain syndrome	Damage to the thalamic nucleus involved in the referral of discriminative sensation (ventroposteriolateral nucleus) causes intense, paroxysmal pain, often causalgia, in the limbs opposite the lesion.

Table 23.5	Comparison of the Principal Differences between Somatic Pain (Arising from Tissue Damage) and Neuropathic Pain (Arising as a Result of Faulty Neural Input and/or Processing)

Somatic Pain

1. Pain stimulus usually identified easily.
2. Surface pain well localized; if visceral, felt in predictable referral areas.
3. Pain characteristics match previous pain experience.
4. Conventional analgesics usually effective.

Neuropathic Pain

1. Pain stimulus difficult to identify.
2. Pain often difficult to localize, felt in unusual referral sites.
3. Pain qualities unusual in patient's experience.
4. Poor response to NSAIDs and opioid analgesics.

PHARMACOLOGICAL MANAGEMENT OF PAIN

Pharmaceutical agents that limit pain, **analgesics,** are the mainstay of pain management in most medical and non-medical settings. Broadly speaking, analgesics act peripherally, attenuating or blocking the generation of pain signals in the tissues, or they act centrally, raising thresholds for pain transmission at a variety of sites in the central nervous system.

Peripheral versus Central Analgesics

Peripheral analgesics act by blocking the production of prostaglandins, particularly prostaglandin E_2 (PGE$_2$). PGE$_2$ appears to mediate nociception by sensitizing pain receptors to the stimulating effect of bradykinin. Blocking PGE$_2$ formation therefore leads to reduced peripheral pain stimulation for a given level of pain-producing bradykinin. You may recall from chapter 2 that both PGE$_2$ and bradykinin are produced in an inflammatory response. Along with other substances, they are responsible for the delayed but prolonged vasodilation and increased vascular permeability that promote the delivery of cells and plasma products to the site of injury. Bradykinin is generated from a plasma precursor. Prostaglandins, on the other hand, are generated from cell-membrane-derived arachidonic acid. Cyclooxygenase, the enzyme responsible for prostaglandin production from arachidonic acid, is inactivated by aspirin, acetaminophen, and nonsteroidal anti-inflammatory drugs. These drugs will produce analgesia (by raising the threshold for bradykinin

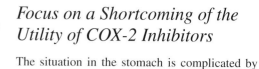

Focus on a Shortcoming of the Utility of COX-2 Inhibitors

The situation in the stomach is complicated by the important role of COX-2 in repair of a *damaged* mucosa. Mucosal injury induces COX-2 activity, which is an important source of the prostaglandins that mediate vasodilation to enhance repair. COX-2 inhibitors mute this response and thereby impair the healing of ulcers. So, healthy maintenance and repair of the gastric mucosa requires the unimpeded action of both COX-1 and COX-2 enzyme-mediated processes.

stimulation of nociceptors) at levels lower than those required to reduce the inflammation (fig. 23.11).

Cyclooxygenase comes in two isoforms that are differentially distributed in tissues. COX-1 is found in the gastric muscosa where it is responsible for healthy maintenance, including the secretion of protective mucus; in the kidneys where it regulates perfusion; and in platelets where it is involved in platelet aggregation, a key event in coagulation. COX-2 is richly available at sites of inflammation where it mediates, among other things, prostaglandin production. Aspirin, acetaminophen, and NSAIDs are nonselective blockers of COX activity; hence, their tendency to damage the gastric mucosa, in the case of acetaminophen to be toxic to the kidneys at doses over 4 g per day, and, in the case of aspirin, to irreversibly impair platelet function (the mechanism that allows aspirin to be used effectively to reduce the formation of platelet aggregates to impede atherosclerosis but predisposes the susceptible person to bleeding). COX-2 selective inhibitors (e.g., celecoxib and rofecoxib) leave COX-1 uninhibited and therefore don't have these specific downsides. Despite their immediate popularity, these COX-2 inhibitors do not have analgesic effects any better than those of NSAIDs and may not be entirely safe for the renal and cardiovascular systems. They are probably best used for pain control in patients who have a high risk of gastric bleeding.

Central analgesics, by contrast, are narcotic drugs. As noted earlier, narcotics bind to a variety of receptors in the cord, brain stem, and cerebrum that are the normal receptors for certain endogenously produced, morphinelike neurotransmitters, including the endorphins. These receptors are thought to be involved in mediating pain and some aspects of pleasure or reward. A variety of natural and synthetic narcotics are used, alone or in combination with substances intended to focus their action more effectively, to impede or block pain signals once they have entered the central nervous system.

Unfortunately (as has happened more often in this chapter than I'm sure you would like), the simple and useful classification of analgesics into central and peripheral has

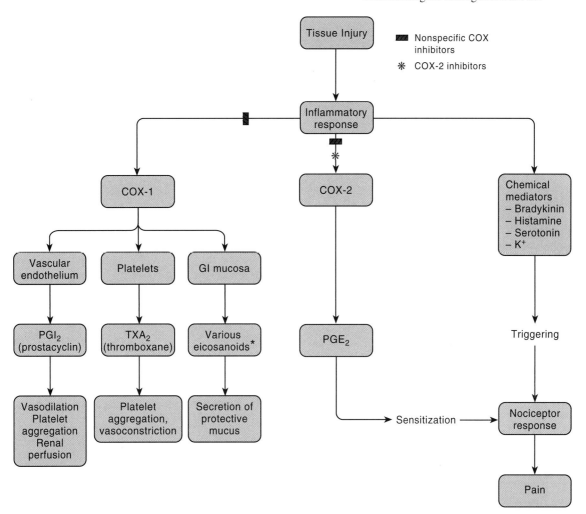

*Prostaglandins and thromboxanes are members of the eicosanoid family

Figure 23.11 **Mechanisms Underlying the Analgesic Effect of Cox-2 Specific and Nonspecific Cox Inhibitors.** Blocking Cox-2 inhibits PGE_2 production which reduces the sensitivity of nociceptors to stimulation by bradykinin and related chemicals present in inflamed tissue.

been shown to be inconsistent with reality. The local application of opioids to a site of injury provides potent analgesia, and cells that migrate to the site of injury also have opioid receptors. Whether these findings are normally relevant is still not clear (e.g., how would opioids get to the site of injury from the brain or spinal cord?). "Peripheral analgesics" also apparently act within the spinal cord and brain.

Nonnarcotic Analgesics

Although usage does vary, it is typical to refer to aspirin, acetaminophen, and nonsteroidal anti-inflammatory drugs (NSAIDs)—in other words, to the peripheral analgesics—as nonnarcotic analgesics. Aspirin (acetylsalicylic acid—ASA) is one of a group of salicylates that are potent peripheral analgesics. Unfortunately, it tends to irritate the gastric mucosa more than other salicylates (enteric-coated preparations avoid some of this); it can also depress platelet numbers and function, and is associated with Reye's syndrome

in children. Acetaminophen doesn't have these risks, but on the other hand, it is not a very effective anti-inflammatory agent.

Nonsteroidal anti-inflammatory drugs (NSAIDs) are generally equal or superior to ASA in analgesia. They act by interfering with prostaglandin production in the same way as ASA. Their antiplatelet effect is rapidly reversible, unlike that of ASA, and some are less irritating to the gastric mucosa. They are used with low back pain, migraine, postoperative pain, cancer pain, and dysmenorrhea.

Table 23.6 lists some common nonnarcotic analgesics. There is a limitation to the analgesia provided by these drugs, so they are best used to control mild to moderate pain. Also, unlike narcotics, many are effective antipyretics (i.e., they can control fever). They do not cause sedation, nor do they lead to tolerance or dependence. For these reasons, it is usually recommended that maximum use be made of nonnarcotic analgesics for any pain that has a peripheral component. Incidentally, as far as we know,

Table 23.6	Selected Analgesic Agents Commonly Encountered in Clinical Settings

Nonnarcotic Analgesics

Acetylsalicylic acid (ASA, aspirin)
Magnesium trisalicylate
Acetaminophen
Nonsteroidal anti-inflammatory drugs (NSAIDs):
    Ibuprofen
    Naproxen
    Indomethacin

Narcotic Analgesics

Mild to moderate pain:
    Codeine
    Oxycodone
    Propoxyphene
Moderate to severe pain:
    Meperidine
    Pentazocine
    Morphine
    Hydromorphone
    Methadone
    Levorphanol
    Nalbuphine

headaches are generated in tissue external to the brain's neural tissue (i.e., vessels, the dura, muscles, etc). In this sense, headache is "peripheral" and therefore often responds to nonnarcotic analgesics. (See the more detailed discussion in the Headache section of this chapter.)

Narcotic Analgesics

By binding to the central nervous system endorphin receptors, narcotics activate the descending analgesia pathways, which work at the level of nociceptor input to second-order neurons in the pain pathways. There are different endorphin receptors distributed throughout the CNS. Each narcotic (or "opioid") (see list in table 23.6) will have a different pattern of affinities with these receptors and thereby a different set of actions mediated by the receptors. Commonly encountered side effects include nausea, sedation, and constipation.

There is no significant foundation to the fear of developing addiction from the use of narcotic analgesics. Appropriate dose levels, to meet the need for analgesia, can be closely monitored and any dependence that does emerge can be readily dealt with by gradual withdrawal. Prolonged administration of narcotics does, however, lead to **tolerance,** the decreased effect of a given dose over time. When it occurs, as in cancer patients, it can be overcome by adjusting

dosage and frequency of administration while monitoring for any CNS effects, such as respiratory depression. In this regard, respiratory depression is an extremely rare complication of opioids. When it occurs, it is usually due to a too rapid dose escalation or perhaps to the removal of the powerful respiratory drive of pain itself.

Although opioids are usually restricted to the treatment of moderate to severe acute pain, they have recently been shown to be effective in the treatment of certain chronic conditions. Examples of conditions that have been successfully managed with opioids are neuropathic pain, osteoarthritis, and low back pain. It is useful to remember that, while used for pain control, many opioids have anti-inflammatory effects similar to those of NSAIDS.

Although widely used, the synthetic narcotic meperidine (Demerol) has significant hazards. Normeperidine is produced as a metabolite of the breakdown of meperidine. It is much more slowly cleared from the tissues than meperidine and therefore accumulates in the plasma. It can produce tremors, anxiety, myoclonus (exaggerated tendon reflexes), and generalized seizures, particularly in patients with compromised kidney function, who can't excrete it. Codeine and oxycodone are morphinelike substances suitable for treating moderate pain. They are often used effectively in combination with nonnarcotic analgesics.

Potentiators

Potentiators are medications administered with an analgesic to enhance the effect of a given dose. The theory is that, in this way, greater analgesia can be achieved without increasing side effects or risk of toxicity. In fact, these drugs may act in different ways. Some are actually additive drugs; that is, medications that have an analgesic effect on their own that is added to that of the primary analgesic. Hydroxyzine (Atarax, Vistaril), an antihistamine, is probably an example. Other drugs—for example, cimetidine (Tagamet)—appear to potentiate by interfering with the normal metabolic breakdown of analgesics in the liver. The result is slower clearance and higher plasma drug levels. The same effect can be achieved with more control by simply increasing the dose of analgesic or its frequency of administration, or both.

Other potentiators (e.g., phenothiazines) have varied effects on pain. The phenothiazine chlorpromazine (Thorazine), a drug whose primary use is as an antipsychotic, has some analgesic effect. However, the most popular phenothiazine (Phenergan), an antihistamine, is ineffective and may even be an antianalgesic. There probably are no dependable pure potentiators for narcotics, with the possible exception of aspirin and acetaminophen, which appear to potentiate codeine. On the other hand, adding 100–200 mg of caffeine (a strong cup of coffee contains about 150 mg) to either acetaminophen or ASA (650 mg) will significantly improve analgesia.

Anticonvulsants and Tricyclic Antidepressants

These drugs are sometimes called "adjuvants" because their utilization for pain control was discovered after their approval for other applications. Neuropathic pain presents real challenges to pharmacological management because it seldom responds to either narcotic or nonnarcotic analgesics. The sharp, stabbing pain of trigeminal neuralgia and some other focal neuralgias is often controlled by anticonvulsants (ganapentin, carbamazepine, or phenytoin), while tricyclic antidepressants (amytriptyline, imipramine) can be effective in controlling the pain arising in postherpetic neuralgia and peripheral nerve injury. Recall that one of the descending pain limitation systems causes the release of leucine enkephalin in the dorsal horn of the cord. Some tricyclic antidepressants enhance this effect. Whatever their route of action, these substances appear to be analgesic, whether or not the person is depressed.

NONMEDICAL/ALTERNATIVE APPROACHES TO PAIN MANAGEMENT

Intense, short-term pain—the prototype would be postsurgical pain—is best dealt with by the intelligent, short-term, and closely monitored use of analgesics as just described. Effective pharmacological pain control in the postsurgical or posttraumatic patient, or in the case of uncomplicated, intermittent back pain, allows the person to maintain fitness levels and engage in routines of work and socialization that are themselves therapeutic. But, however careful, the medical management of pain treats the person as a physiological organism and administers drugs or therapies to the person's body. It minimizes the role of the individual's expectations, personal involvement, choice, and voluntary action. Some estimates are that patient expectations alone are responsible for perhaps 50% of the effectiveness of doctor's office medical intervention. This is the so-called **placebo effect.** This term derives from clinical trials that routinely contrast the treatment effect of a trial drug against the effect of a **placebo** (a pill or treatment that has been demonstrated to have no effect; subjects can't discriminate the placebo from the pill or treatment that is being tested and believe the placebo has some desired treatment effect). Perhaps 30% of subjects are "placebo responders," yet pharmacological pain management leaves this out of the equation. (Incidentally, many psychoactive drugs on the market achieved FDA approval with an efficacy 10 or 15% above placebo.) **Alternative** or nonmedical approaches to pain management capitalize on the patient's expectations and utilize his choice, personal involvement, and voluntary action. They range from simple touch to hypnotic techniques. We present them here briefly because they operate mostly through neural pain processing structures already described but not utilized by the conventional NSAIDs and opiates. These are also the approaches available to the majority of our readers.

It is important to remember in the rush of "getting the meds out" or "taking blood" that there are effective and safe approaches that have a clearly delineated basis in our current understanding of the physiology of pain management.

General Principles

There are certain common principles underlying the effective application of alternative pain management strategies. In situations in which the helper and the pain sufferer do not have a prior relationship and there is little time for teaching, the approach must be simple—the helper must take charge in an unambivalent, confident, and practiced fashion. Likewise, the person in pain has to cooperate with the approach being tried and must be in moderate distress. These techniques are not going to work with the person who is either indifferent or numb with terror or convulsed with pain. Free choice is an essential ingredient, as is active participation. The focus is on things over which the person *can* have control when there is so much that is out of control or *feels* like it is out of control. All of these approaches engage in the practice of behaviors incompatible with pain. We tend to do only one thing at once: if we are acting in a relaxed, pain-free way, we are less likely to experience the anguish of pain. If we are acting brave and self-confident, we are less likely to feel afraid and to engage in the selective attention and thought processes that feed our anxiety. Conversely, if we are engaging in shallow breathing, are rigid and immobile, have drawn our attention narrowly inward, and are anxiously awaiting the next stab of pain, we intensify the pain experience. The focus should be on a noticeable difference rather than the complete elimination of pain. Attention should be drawn to how the technique *modifies* the feeling of pain, not on the expectations that pain will be magically removed. Practice and familiarity breed success. The more experience one has with a particular method, especially the more sophisticated psychological approaches, the more effective and dependable it is likely to be. And, finally, the availability of a coach or peer circle can make a tremendous difference. Everybody's experience is different. But having contact with someone who has a sense of the natural trajectory of this experience—how it is likely to unfold—and a confidence that transcendence is possible, lends people the courage to persist and survive. It must be emphasized that these alternative strategies are not a substitute for determining and treating the underlying cause of the pain. They are brought to bear when medical approaches are insufficiently effective, as in chronic pain, and when medical interventions are inappropriate because the pain is transitory or the risks of medical intervention outweigh their benefits (for example, with children undergoing repeated needle sticks for blood tests or chemotherapy).

We will not attempt to relate each of these approaches to a specific locale or mode of action. These approaches tend to use, in an overlapping fashion, many of the mechanisms we described in the section on the "Inhibition of Pain Perception": Cortical focusing, motor inhibition of ascending information, generation of complex, discriminative sensation from the periphery, interruption of autonomic pain facilitation, and endorphin release all play a role.

Comfort Measures

The caregiver can utilize a variety of actions and provisions that help to ease the patient's distress and assist in other management strategies. These measures communicate concern and caring and demonstrate that noticeable differences can be achieved through choice and activity. Such measures can include inquiring how the patient is doing, creating a soothing environment with pillows, comfortable seating, or a place to lie down, adjusting lighting and music, ensuring privacy). Caregivers can also provide patients with an opportunity to move about when procedures take longer than expected and distractions that the patient can control (magazines, card games, watching fish in an aquarium, etc.).

Counterstimulation

This includes a wide variety of approaches that introduce other stimuli to counteract pain. Gentle, firm, persistent touch (which, of course, must be acceptable to the individual) can have the effect of helping the patient compose himself. This approach communicates concern and caring, and helps patients engage in more adaptive behaviors. Icing involves the rubbing of ice (or, alternatively, placing an icepack) directly on the surface of the skin in the painful area, or in an area in which the helper is going to produce pain, for a maximum of ten minutes (more will induce inflammation and more pain). This approach has the added benefit of limiting the inflammation that may coexist with the pain. Simple vibration of the skin is effective in reducing the pain associated with injection (many dentists will pull repeatedly on the cheek during the injection of analgesic to great effect). Acupuncture requires the intervention of a licensed practitioner and can be very beneficial. Acupressure utilizes the same theoretical framework as acupuncture, but concentrates massage at the same meridian points. Trigger point massage focuses intense, and quite painful, massage on sensitive points in the musculature that can be palpated as "knots." Massage continues, relatively gently, until the pain subsides. This can produce long-lasting pain relief. In TENS (transcutaneous electrical nerve stimulation), electrodes are placed to the side of the vertebral column (or may be placed near or contralateral to where the pain is felt) and low-voltage, rhythmic pulses of electricity are introduced. Responses, as with all pain interventions, are variable.

Behavioral Approaches

These methods depend upon engaging in behaviors that are incompatible with pain behaviors. They expose the person to a variety of distracting stimuli. Activity itself can have both an antidepressant effect and can produce activity in the nervous system that has the effect of blocking the transmission of pain. They have all the added benefits of choice and control. Simply blowing gently during a painful or distressing event often helps patients cope and damps the intensity of the sensation. Small children can be involved in blowing bubbles when all else fails. The action of blowing is slow, deliberate, and sustained and produces some noticeable effects to which the child's attention can be directed (sound, muscular force, the feelings). Painful breathing is shallow, rapid, and guarded. Sustained patterned breathing is the exact opposite. Usually the breathing is slow, relatively deep, expansive, and deliberate. Simply counting breaths may be enough. LaMaze birthing techniques utilize intense "pant, pant, pant, puff" alternations to deal with intense pain without hyperventilating. Increased mobility resists the *natural* impulse to withdraw and be still, which certainly has a valid role, but can stabilize and prolong maladaptive responses. Patients should remain physically active and deliberately and progressively increase both physical and social activity. Keeping accurate records allows for reinforcing progress. Deep muscle relaxation involves the alternation of intense contraction and relaxation of major muscle groups, working systematically through the body from toes to head.

Psychological Approaches

In all of these approaches, attention is focused, narrowed, and absorbed. The strategies capitalize on enhanced choice, activity, control, and activity incompatible with pain behaviors. They vary from techniques that anyone can do instantly to those for which practice and personal compatibility are important. Distraction can be achieved through the use of pop-up books, storytelling, picture books, and fish tanks for kids, and magazines, card games, and information sheets for adults. Regular and extensive practice can make meditation an effective approach to pain management. Guided visualization, on the other hand, can be introduced to a novice who is talked through a comforting fantasy of his own making. Children can be helped to "anesthetize" their back for lumbar puncture by imagining a pain switch that they "turn down" or a magic glove that might be "pulled on" to damp the sensation of pin prick for a blood test.

 Checkpoint 23.3

You have engaged in nonmedical management of your own or someone else's pain, or perhaps someone has extended this assistance to you. Look back over the last section and identify the specific techniques used and note the "general principles" applied.

HEADACHE

Headache is a relatively common form of pain experience. Although headache may be temporarily completely disabling, the vast majority of headaches are benign, nonprogressive disorders. Headaches associated with excess alcohol use, smoking, stress, or fatigue are best treated by taking two aspirin and, rather than calling the physician in the morning, avoiding the cause in the future. Headache is the unfortunate accompaniment of a variety of medical disorders: fever of any cause, food poisoning, carbon monoxide poisoning, diseases producing hypercapnia (e.g., chronic lung disease), hypothyroidism, and others. In some syndromes, headache is the central complaint. These are various forms of migraine, cluster headaches, and tension headaches. Finally, in some cases headache is symptomatic of some serious underlying pathology.

Pain-Sensitive Structures

A knowledge of the structures of the head that are capable of generating pain is helpful in understanding the pathophysiology of headache. The bone of the skull and much of the dura, arachnoid, and pia are insensitive, as is all the brain itself. By contrast, the venous sinuses and tributary veins, the dura at the base of the brain, and the arteries within the meninges and the subarachnoid space are highly sensitive to any stimulation that can produce the sensation of pain. Similarly, certain nerves (e.g., trigeminal, vagus, upper cervical) generate pain when inflamed, compressed, or under tension. Superficial tissues are also capable of generating pain that is experienced as headache: skin, connective tissues, muscles, arteries, and periosteum of the skull. Other sensitive structures are the eye, the ear, and the nasal and sinus cavities.

Headaches can thus be produced by mechanical stimulation (traction, dilation, distention) of intracranial or extracranial arteries, large intracranial veins, venous sinuses or associated dura, the nasal cavity, and the paranasal sinuses. Inflammation or irritation of the meninges and raised intracranial pressure, as well as spasm, injury, or inflammation of extracranial muscles, can also result in headache. For an intracranial mass to generate pain, it usually has to stretch or displace vessels, nerves, or dura at the base of the brain. This can occur well in advance of any change in intracranial pressure (that is, while the tumor may still be quite small).

Symptomatic Headaches

Brain tumor produces headaches in about two-thirds of all patients. Most headache associated with brain tumor is not severe. Sometimes the pain is triggered by activity or postural changes (e.g., stooping), but there may be no provoking factor. Typically, headaches due to tumors are deep seated, variably throbbing, perhaps "aching" or "bursting," and occur with increasing frequency and severity. They may last minutes to an hour or more and occur once to many times per day, in some cases accompanied by forceful (projectile) vomiting. Rest will sometimes diminish the pain.

Headaches that are precipitated by cough or exertion are usually benign, although they raise the question of some intracranial mass (e.g., a tumor, an arteriovenous malformation—AVM) or developmental abnormality. The mechanism is presumably the increase in intrathoracic pressure during cough or exertion, which both raises the intrathoracic blood pressure and impedes venous drainage.

With arteriovenous malformation or aneurysm, there is little correlation between the size and the progression of the pathology and the nature of the symptomatic headache. Hemorrhage of an AVM or aneurysm, however, produces a highly symptomatic headache: rapidly developing, extremely severe, lasting many days, and localizing in the occiput and neck. Blood turbulence detected by auscultation and blood in the CSF are diagnostic. Those that survive the hemorrhage are candidates for surgical correction of the defective vasculature before a more serious rebleed occurs.

Headache that follows trauma (e.g., concussion or whiplash injury) is varied. It can be severe and chronic, with either continuous or intermittent pain. There is often also giddiness, vertigo, or tinnitus (ringing or whistling in the ears), and sometimes there is **posttraumatic nervous instability,** a condition of agitated restlessness and hypersensitivity not directly associated with headache. Headache immediately following trauma may signal the development of a subdural hematoma. In such cases, the headache is supplanted by drowsiness, confusion, stupor, and then coma.

Headache that is due to inflammation and blockage of the paranasal sinuses can result from the pressure of accumulated fluid; alternatively, as fluid is reabsorbed, the exit may remain blocked from tension on the mucous membranes, a condition leading to the so-called vacuum sinus headache. Headache of ocular origin (perhaps due to eyestrain) tends to be steady and aching and located in the orbit, forehead, and temple. It often occurs after sustained use of the eyes in close focusing and resolves with appropriate corrective lenses.

The headache of meningeal irritation, whether caused by inflammation from infection or by irritation from the breakdown of blood from a subarachnoid bleed or other cause, has an acute onset and becomes severe and generalized (or bioccipital or bifrontal). As with other meningeal signs, it worsens if the head is bent forward and is often accompanied by a stiff neck. Lumbar puncture produces an immediate headache upon arising from the procedure; in this case the pain is attributable to the loss of fluid and consequent tension placed on dural, venous, and arterial structures at the base of the brain as it sags within the cranial space.

Some general comments can be made about the discrimination between benign and symptomatic headaches. Remember that "benign" includes some pretty terrific headaches, including migraine, but they are not indicative of more serious, underlying pathology. Headaches are more likely to be benign if they are provoked by red wine, sustained exertion, strong odors, hunger, lack of sleep, a change in the weather, or the onset of a menstrual period. As well, diarrhea accompanying a headache is usually indicative of migraine, while a brief cessation of the headache upon waking or during pregnancies is also an indicator that the headache is benign.

Headache Syndromes and Their Treatment

There are several headache syndromes that, while nonprogressive and for the most part benign, can be cruelly disabling. They require diagnosis and appropriate symptomatic care.

Tension Headaches

This is one of the most common of headache syndromes. It is also one of the most poorly understood, and is often ineffectively treated. The sufferer experiences a bilateral, generalized sense of nonthrobbing pressure, fullness, or tightness that is characteristic. Onset is gradual and the headache can persist in continuous or variable intensity day and night for days, weeks, even years. At one time, the pain was thought to develop from muscle tension associated with stress, but careful studies using electromyography have failed to support that theory. In some cases, however, relaxation training using muscle tension biofeedback has apparently been effective in treating these hard-to-manage headaches. Since fatigue, nervous strain, and worry tend to provoke episodes of tension headache, strategies that reduce stress, improve coping, or restrain reactions, as with antidepressant or antianxiety drugs, will tend to reduce their incidence or severity. Nonnarcotic analgesics (e.g., aspirin or acetaminophen) may lessen the intensity of the pain but rarely get rid of it, and sufferers often take 6–8 pills a day with little effect.

Migraine Headaches

These headaches, with throbbing-to-dull pain often accompanied by nausea and vomiting, are frequently localized to one side of the head, perhaps behind one eye or ear—hence, the French term migraine, derived from the Latin hemicrania, meaning half the skull. Perhaps 20–30% of the population has some degree of migraine, with females being three times as susceptible. About 60% of migraine sufferers have a relative in the immediate family that has shared the complaint. Onset is often in childhood and adolescence or young adulthood, and most people experience extensive relief with middle age. Women are more likely to have the migraine begin during the premenstrual part of their cycle. During pregnancy the headaches typically lessen. Although the pathophysiology has yet to be fully defined, all the variants of migraine appear to result from arteriolar constriction and decreased cerebral blood flow. These variants include classic migraine, common migraine, and complicated migraine.

Classic migraine follows a typical course. The person may have premonitory symptoms hours before the attack: a sense of elation or energy or foreboding, cravings, drowsiness, or depression. Visual disturbances like scintillations, light sensitivity, bright zigzag lines or scotomas (blind spots) affecting one or both visual fields and even extending to blindness, or dizziness and tinnitus signal the start of the attack. These symptoms, sometimes called the prodrome, develop slowly, at least over minutes, and may spread or change. A duration of 20–30 minutes is very common. As with other symptoms of migraine, the gradual time course of development allows us to distinguish these symptoms of onset from epileptic phenomena. The pain and photophobia that follow the prodome are often so extreme that the person must withdraw to a darkened room to wait it out or sleep it off. The throbbing pain behind one eye or ear becomes a dull generalized ache, and the scalp may be sensitive. The duration is hours to one or two days, and bouts may recur at irregular intervals of weeks or months.

The **common migraine,** which now includes those headaches that used to be called tension headaches, follows the same course as classic migraine, but lacks the visual and other classic prodrome symptoms. It is often precipitated by tension. The most common form of benign, periodic headache—common migraine—is often accompanied by nausea, and occasionally by vomiting, giving it the name sick headache.

Complicated migraine, also sometimes called neurological migraine, is distinguished by the presence of neurological symptoms other than (and perhaps in addition to) the visual symptoms of classic migraine. These may include unilateral numbness and tingling of the lips, face, hand, or leg, which may deepen to weakness or paralysis imitating a stroke. The person also may have difficulty speaking or understanding speech. Such symptoms may occur before or during the aching phase of the headache and may spread slowly over a period of minutes; they usually resolve in minutes or hours.

The condition is termed "complicated" for another reason. Some people experience long-term, even permanent neurological deficits: hemianopsia, hemiplegia or hemianesthesia, or eye movement defects. Furthermore, some people experience the neurological symptoms without headache. Children may have nausea, abdominal pain, and vomiting without headache or may have intense spells of vertigo. Adults may have these symptoms or localized pain, bouts of fever, or mood disturbances. Migraine must be considered when other explanations for these symptoms have been ruled out. Diagnosis is made even more difficult because some older adults, with no earlier history of migraine, will develop migrainous neurological symptoms that resemble those of transient ischemic attacks.

The pathophysiological basis to migraine has not been established. The older theory was that the pain is caused by the vasodilation and vascular distention that follows a prodromal episode of vascular spasm and ischemia, but this theory has been shown to be incorrect. During the evolution of an attack, studies of cerebral blood flow show a slow drop in cerebral perfusion, usually beginning in the occipital region. Throughout the attack there are areas of modest (25–30%) hypoperfusion, and there is no evidence of localized or generalized dilation or hyperperfusion. The wave of only cortical hypoperfusion spreads anteriorly at a rate of 2 to 3 mm/min, following the convolutions of the brain's surface, independent of the distribution of the cerebral arteries. It remains unilateral, and spreads to the frontal cortex via the insula. This pattern of "spreading depression" must have its origin in neural (projections from the brain stem?) control and then expresses itself in vascular changes that ultimately trigger platelets to aggregate and release serotonin. Somewhere in this sequence, the trigeminal nerve releases vasoactive peptides on blood vessels both within and outside the cranial vault, producing the swelling and vessel sensitivity often experienced in migraine. It may be that a region in the periaqueductal gray, which we encountered in the discussion of the endorphin-mediated relief of pain, is central in the production of the pain of migraine. This area has the highest concentration of serotonin receptors in the brain. Antiserotonin drugs like methysergide are effective in arresting attacks, while drugs that trigger serotonin release, like reserpine, precipitate attacks. Many other neurotransmitters that affect vascular tone are being considered for their contribution to migraine.

Mild or slowly developing migraine may respond to aspirin, acetaminophon, or NSAIDs, with the addition of caffeine being effectve. Conventional medical control of severe migraines depends on treating the acute attack at its first sign, using ergot preparations (ergot is derived from a mold affecting rye grain). Once the pain becomes intense, codeine sulfate may control it, but aspirin and acetaminophen are ineffective.

The new antiserotonin drug sumatriptan, unlike other migraine medications available by prescription, can often arrest a migraine even after it has started to evolve. While expensive and not universally effective, for some it offers control that was formerly accessible only through the emergency ward. A variety of drugs can be used for prophylaxis when headaches are occuring frequently (two to three times per month or more). To be effective, these must be taken daily for at least a couple of weeks. Medications include propranolol, amitriptyline, valproate, and others. Feverfew, a herbal preparation, is used by some with satisfaction.

Cluster Headaches

These headaches are so named because they tend to occur nightly for weeks to a few months (in a cluster). Although the underlying mechanisms may be quite different from those causing migraine, cluster headaches are usually described as a migraine variant. Men are four times as likely as women to have them, in contrast to the pattern with migraines. Two or three hours after falling asleep the person awakens with steady, intense pain in one orbit and flowing tears. The nostril on the same side is plugged and later begins to run. The affected pupil may be constricted, the eyelid drooped, and the cheek flushed and edematous. The attack may last from ten minutes to two hours. The majority of people with cluster headaches show no history of migraine.

Cluster headaches are very difficult to treat effectively. If stress or fatigue is implicated, efforts are made to reduce it. Some people can interrupt an excruciating attack by administering oxygen or using an inhaled ergot preparation. Prophylactic administration of the tricyclic antidepressant amitriptyline is the method of choice, while methysergide, corticosteroids like prednisone, and the antidepressant lithium are used with very resistant cases.

Case Study

A 35-year-old male carpenter suffered an injury at work while lifting a heavy object. He stopped work and saw a physician, who identified muscle spasm and a reduced range of spinal mobility. Based on her diagnosis of low back strain, she prescribed a benzodiazepam drug as a muscle relaxant and a codeine/acetaminophen agent for pain, and recommended rest and a return for evaluation in two weeks. At that time, improvement was minimal and a regimen of physiotherapy was implemented, along with continuation of the drug regimen, which the patient requested for his pain. Improvement failed to materialize over the next several weeks, and an orthopedic specialist was called in for an assessment. X-rays and a CT scan indicated some evidence of low lumbar degeneration. The specialist recommended that the man not return to his occupation and that he approach the worker's compensation agency, which provides benefits in cases of work-related disability, for retraining in some less strenuous work.

The carpenter's approach to the compensation agency led to an assessment by an agency physician some 16 weeks after the initial injury. He found the patient to have been continuing with his medications and to have developed a marked degree of hostility and depression. He further found significant disagreement between the patient's complaints of pain and loss of movement and any objective findings. The patient was also quite deconditioned from the lack of normal activity during the past weeks. On some probing interrogation and reference to the agency's files, the physician discovered that the patient had a history of a broken home, work injury claims, and alcohol and drug abuse. Because he couldn't work, his wife had been forced to work in a disagreeable, low-paying job, and their family was rapidly becoming dysfunctional.

Rather than defer to the man's demands for further medical consultations and surgery to prevent his becoming a cripple, the doctor prescribed a low-dose antidepressant and withdrawal of the narcotic medication, suspecting it had been enhancing the patient's pain by endorphin depletion. He also arranged for a program of physiotherapy aimed at restoring conditioning and persuaded the man to accept some family counseling. As a result of this regimen, the patient reported loss of half his pain two weeks after withdrawal of the narcotics, and significant overall improvement after six weeks of gradually increased physical activity. Between family counseling and the employer's willingness to accommodate a gradual return to work, he achieved full resumption of work and a greatly improved home situation 25 weeks postinjury.

Commentary

Had this patient had a family physician aware of his history, recovery might have occurred much sooner. The pattern of an insecure upbringing, substance abuse, and depression are indicators of an increased likelihood of developing the pattern of chronic pain and disability behavior seen in this case. The depletion of endorphins and a resulting increase in passive pain should have been recognized earlier as being related to the extended use of narcotics and benzodiazepine agents. Endorphin replenishment following withdrawal of these agents was speeded by the antidepressant agent prescribed. It was also sound practice not to assume too quickly that the patient was motivated solely by a desire for a large insurance compensation award, and to attempt some degree of rehabilitation and renewal of self-esteem. Unfortunately, not all such cases resolve as successfully.

Key Concepts

1. Acute and chronic pain differ in their neurological processing, impact, and treatment (pp. 653–654).

2. Pain stimuli can produce physiological and psychic arousal, a variety of orienting responses, precise localization (via the neospinothalamic pathway), or chronic pain responses (via the paleospinothalamic pathway) (pp. 654–658).

3. Narcotics produce their analgesic effects by binding to endorphin receptors in the brain stem, and spinal cord, thereby stimulating fibers that release a neurotransmitter that inhibits pain signals as they enter the cord. TENS and stimulus-produced analgesia probably induce the same neurotransmitter release (pp. 654–660).

4. Referred pain is of great clinical diagnostic utility (pp. 660–662).

5. Phantom pain illustrates the role of central processing in pain perception and is a significant clinical problem (pp. 662–663).

6. The pain that may accompany cancer is highly variable in both nature and pathological basis (pp. 663–664).

7. The complexity and variability of the experience and causation of pain have given rise to a precise and detailed vocabulary (pp. 664–667).

8. Peripheral analgesics inhibit the production of prostaglandins, thereby raising the pain threshold (pp. 668–670).

9. Narcotics act centrally and, depending on their binding characteristics, can produce constipation, nausea, euphoria, and other effects (p. 670).

10. A variety of effective, nonmedical techniques can be used to ameliorate pain and support medical interventions (pp. 671–672).

11. A minority of headaches are symptomatic of serious underlying pathology, and in some conditions the pattern and localization of pain is quite characteristic (pp. 673–674).

12. A variety of headache syndromes, while nonprogressive and not life-threatening, can produce significant disability (pp. 674–675).

REVIEW ACTIVITIES

1. Recall your last significant experience with pain. Go through each cluster in table 23.3 and choose the appropriate terms to describe your experience.

2. Make a copy of table 23.4. Cut up the paper in such a way as to separate all the symptoms from their definitions, and keep them in one pile. Do the same with the peripheral and central syndromes, only mix them up. Now attempt to unite symptoms and definitions, separate peripheral from central syndromes, and unite each syndrome with its definition.

3. The point was made that acute pain is processed preponderantly by the neospinothalamic pathway, while chronic pain is processed via the paleospinothalamic pathway. In table form, list the features common to both pathways. Then list the ways in which they differ.

4. Find a few people who experience migraine or tension or cluster headaches (if you're unfortunate, one of them may be you!). Question them about their pain experience and try to classify their headaches.

Trauma

For he breaketh me with a tempest, and multiplieth my wounds without cause.

The Book of Job

rubor

& tumor

cū calore

& dolore

Chapter 1 defined trauma as physical injury and considered the mechanisms and tissue effects by which various physical agents (heat, radiation, mechanical force, etc.) produce injury. There, emphasis was on trauma causing cellular changes that could lead to disease. In this chapter, emphasis is on mechanical trauma and burn trauma, and the damage they produce at the organ and somatic levels of organization. These types of trauma are the most common types encountered in emergency services.

OVERVIEW OF TRAUMATIC INJURY

Automobile accidents, fires, falls, explosions, criminal assaults, and athletics are frequent sources of often severe physical injury. They typically involve an interruption of a tissue or an organ's surface to produce a **wound.** We begin the chapter by describing the essentials of wound production and the various wound types.

FACTORS AFFECTING WOUND PRODUCTION

Wound production is most often the result of the transfer of **kinetic energy**—energy of motion—from one object to another. Four factors contribute to wound production by mechanical trauma: the amount of energy involved, the duration of the impact that causes energy transfer to body tissues, the surface area over which the transfer occurs, and the physical characteristics of the tissue that receives the energy.

Amount of Energy

The kinetic energy of a moving object is expressed by the equation

$$E = \frac{MV^2}{2}$$

where E = kinetic energy, M = mass (or, for our purpose, weight), and V = velocity. For the case of simple forward motion, figure 24.1 illustrates the impact between the human body and an object. From the kinetic energy equation you can see that a heavier moving object possesses more kinetic energy; for example, doubling the weight produces twice the energy. Note, however, that because the velocity's value is squared, a doubling of velocity produces four times the energy. Applying this principle to baseball, you can appreciate that a batter develops more energy by increasing the bat's speed than he does by using a heavier bat.

Duration of Impact

This is the time over which energy is transferred to body structures to produce a wound. For a given amount of energy, if the duration of energy input is longer, there is more time for an organ to absorb it without damage. If the dura-

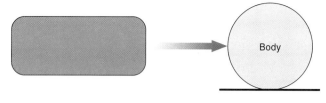

Kinetic energy = 1/2 mass × velocity²

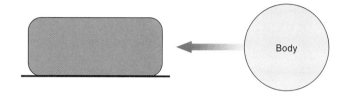

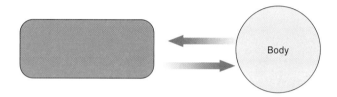

Figure 24.1   **Mechanical Injury.** Damage results when the body strikes or is struck by another mass. Either or both may be in motion prior to impact.

tion is short, there is more chance of overwhelming the organ's energy absorption capabilities. In other words, it is the rate of change rather than the amount of change that is significant in wound production. For example, if the total mechanical energy in the sound waves produced by a typical rock band in five minutes were delivered at the ear in half a second, the eardrum would rupture. Listening over the duration of five minutes, on the other hand, might produce only the awareness of uncomfortable loudness. (Note that chronic exposure to such sound intensity can cause permanent damage to internal ear structures.)

Surface Area

The third factor that has a bearing on wound production is the body surface area over which the force is applied. Generally, the greater the surface area, the less serious the mechanical injury. When a force is spread over a large surface area, any specific region receives a smaller portion of the total. If the same force is applied over a small surface area, each specific region is forced to absorb much more energy, with greater risk of its being overwhelmed. Generally, a blow of given force is more damaging when delivered with a pointed object than with a blunt object because of the much smaller surface area across which the energy is transferred. A protective helmet operates on this principle, reducing energy tranfer to the skull. It offers a large surface area over which impact is dissipated.

Note that what a helmet does for the skull is an extension of what the skull does for the brain. In providing a strong enclosure for the brain, the skull is able to dissipate energy and reduce risk to the brain's delicate tissue. By further extension, the cerebrospinal fluid, confined under pressure within the meninges, dissipates energy that exceeds the skull's coping capacity. Of course, all of these protections can be overwhelmed, as described in the later section, Craniocerebral Trauma.

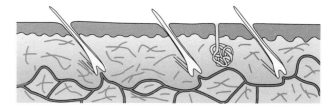
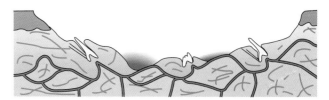

Figure 24.2 **Abrasion.** *Top:* Normal skin. *Bottom:* Abraded skin. The epidermis and superficial dermis are lost, but residual accessory structures provide islands of cells from which regeneration can proceed.

Tissue Characteristics

The resilience of an organ is its ability to absorb energy and recover with minimal effect. This property allows a tissue to resist mechanical trauma. When a force is applied, a less resilient organ is less able to dissipate it without damage. For example, when equal forces are applied to their surfaces, the less resilient liver is more likely to be damaged than the more flexible and elastic pancreas. Similarly, a tightly contracted muscle is less resilient than a relaxed one. This may explain why, in auto accidents and falls, those who are asleep, unconscious, or in an alcoholic stupor seem to receive less traumatic injury than those who are conscious and bracing to resist injury. Of course, if muscles were contracted to produce resistance to acceleration or deceleration in the precise direction required, injury would be reduced. Unfortunately, in situations involving mechanical injury, it is usually impossible to predict the timing or the exact angle at which impact forces will be applied, so that appropriate contractions are seldom brought into play.

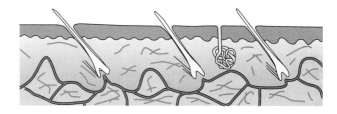
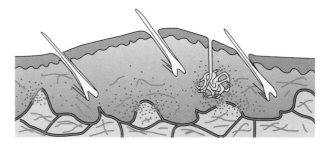

Figure 24.3 **Contusion.** *Top:* Skin is normal. *Bottom:* The epidermis is unbroken, but there is damage and hemorrhage beneath the surface.

WOUND CLASSIFICATION

The following sections describe the various wound types caused by mechanical forces.

Abrasion

One type of wound is produced by friction, usually applied at a low angle or parallel to the body's surface. As an object scrapes over the surface of the skin, the epidermis is forcibly removed. The resulting wound is called an **abrasion** (fig. 24.2). Deeper layers of the skin may also be involved.

Abrasions occur frequently and are usually minor. In fact, it would be unusual for a normally active schoolchild to go through a week's play without receiving several minor skin abrasions. More severe abrasion is typical in automobile accidents in which an occupant is thrown from the vehicle or when a pedestrian or a cyclist is struck by a car.

The result is rapid body motion along pavement, gravel, or similarly rough surfaces. Deep and extensive abrasion in such cases is common.

Contusion

A **contusion** is a bruise. It is a wound in which damage to small blood vessels allows blood loss into the tissue spaces. Usually, a contusion is the result of a blow delivered over a large surface area, at the skin or an organ's surface. Falls, other whole-body collisions, and blows with a blunt instrument usually produce much contusion, because forces are distributed over a wide surface. Although tissue and vessel damage occurs, the surface remains unbroken (fig. 24.3). Blood loss from the vascular system is usually minimal because blood hydrostatic pressure (BHP) in small vessels is low. As blood leaks into the tissue spaces, tissue hydrostatic pressure soon rises to exceed BHP and stop further escape of blood. Of course, once it leaves the vessels the blood coagulates because exposure to tissue thromboplastins activates the extrinsic coagulation pathways (see chapter 7). When vessel damage is more severe, focal pooling of blood within a tissue produces a **hematoma.**

The characteristic discoloration of a skin contusion is caused by various pigmented substances that are derived from hemoglobin. Just deep to the skin's surface, blood in the tissue spaces first appears as a dark red-blue. Later, purple, brown, and yellow-green colors emerge as phagocytes continue the sequence of hemoglobin breakdown. When contusions occur at greater subcutaneous depth, longer periods may pass before blood is visible at the skin's surface. In some cases, there is no surface discoloration, and only swelling and pain give evidence of injury.

Bruising of internal organs may occur secondary to body surface trauma. The heart, for example, may suffer bruising following thoracic wall trauma, because the ventricles are immediately deep to the sternum. Contusion is even more severe if the force is applied during systole, when the contracted tissue is in a less resilient state. The brain's surface may also suffer contusion. An abrupt blow to the skull can produce a force that is transmitted through the bone to reach the brain. If the skull remains intact, it dissipates the force over a greater surface, producing a contusion. This is referred to as a *coup injury* (pronounced *koo*), from the French word for blow. A single blow may produce contusion at the brain's surface below the point of impact, but since the brain can move slightly within the skull, the force of the blow may also cause the brain to be abruptly forced against the skull at an opposite point. The result is a second contusion at the brain's surface, called a **contrecoup** injury, from the French word meaning counterblow (fig. 24.4).

Laceration

The wound that results from a tearing or splitting of the skin or an organ's surface is called a **laceration.** It should be distinguished from a cut, or **incision,** in which a sharp edge slices through the surface. A laceration is a surface split that results from forces that stretch the skin or an organ's surface until it tears apart. Lacerations may have different configurations. They may be straight, curved, or star-shaped **(stellate),** depending on the organ's physical characteristics and the direction in which force is applied. A laceration's edge may be regular or ragged. If especially deep, or when a hollow organ's wall tears completely through, the laceration is called a **rupture.**

Surface lacerations can be produced in several ways. A strong blow with a blunt instrument can cause laceration of the skin. An irregular stellate tear, surrounded by an area of extensive contusion, is often produced by crushing injuries

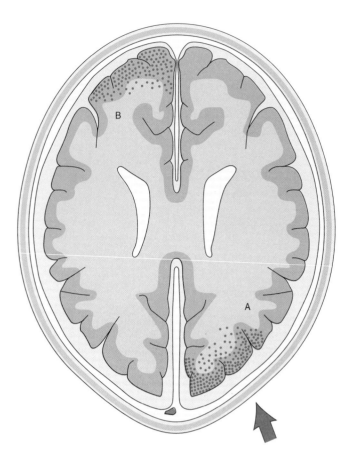

Figure 24.4 **Contrecoup Injury.** Because the brain can move relative to the skull, a blow at one point (A) may produce a contusion at an opposite point (B).

where high pressure is applied over a large body surface. The abrupt application of force involved in high-speed automobile collisions often produces lacerations of internal organs. At impact, the vehicle's speed is immediately reduced while the occupants continue to move until they strike some obstacle such as the dashboard, roof, or floor. The rapid deceleration subjects internal organs to forces that can cause their laceration and rupture. The lung and liver can be damaged in this way. In the case of hollow organs, rapidly building forces are more likely to produce rupture when the organ is filled. This effect is seen most frequently following large meals, when the stomach is quite full, and in accidents that involve forces applied to a full urinary bladder. An improperly worn lap seat belt, stretching across the abdomen instead of the bones of the hip, can produce a sharp pressure pulse in the abdominal cavity in head-on collisions. Laceration of the mesentery and intestinal rupture may be the result.

Explosions often produce extensive lacerations of internal organs. As a blast abruptly applies forces that are then just as abruptly released, it produces compression of organs, followed by their immediate decompression. The result is surface tearing and often rupture (fig. 24.5).

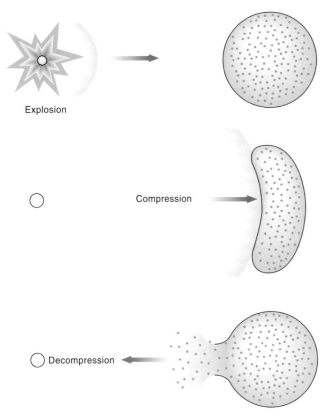

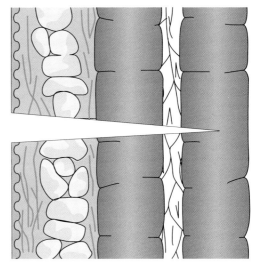

Figure 24.6   **Penetrating Wound.** A sharp object, such as a knife, produces damage that is limited to its path through a tissue.

Figure 24.5   **Organ Rupture.** Laceration and rupture may result when the pressure wave generated by an explosion produces an abrupt compression of a hollow organ followed by an equally abrupt decompression.

Penetrating Wounds

A **penetrating wound** does most of its damage below the surface. It is usually caused by a sharp, elongated object and is typically deep and narrow (fig. 24.6). Bleeding is often more serious in penetrating wounds, although damage to deep vessels may mean that the lost blood is not visible at the surface. Knife stab wounds are good examples in that at the skin's surface, they often appear less serious than they later prove to be. If sufficiently long, the penetrating object may reach various vital organs, causing severe hemorrhage when major vessels or the heart are entered, or extensive peritonitis should gastric or bowel contents escape via a penetrating wound of the abdomen.

A gunshot wound is a special case of a penetrating injury (fig. 24.7). Damage from a bullet is produced by the large forces that derive from its high velocity. (Recall the significance of the velocity in the kinetic energy equation.) For two penetrating wounds of equal depth, one produced by a knife and the other by a bullet, the bullet wound will produce more tissue destruction and more bleeding. In such cases, damage is produced not only by the bullet's tearing through organs, but also because it rapidly rotates around its long axis while in flight. This rotation releases energy into tissues at a right angle to its path, producing blood ves-

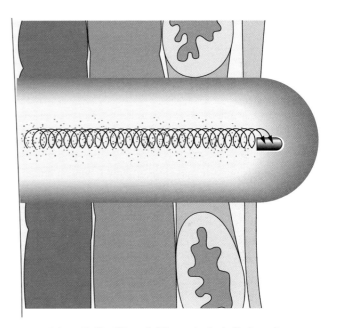

Figure 24.7   **Bullet Wound.** Tissues in the bullet's path are directly destroyed. Energy from the bullet's rotation is also released into adjacent tissues causing damage at some distance from the bullet's path.

sel rupture and other mechanical trauma, even though there is no direct contact with the bullet (fig. 24.8a).

A bullet's passage through the body can also produce secondary effects. For example, in striking bone, the bullet can produce sharp-edged fragments. These are capable of producing lacerations in structures at an appreciable distance from the bullet's track (fig. 24.8b). Bone fragments driven up near to the skin from deeper sites within can also produce contusions at a surface that shows no other sign of injury. Similarly, in striking the body, the bullet itself may fragment to disperse its destructive effects (fig. 24.8c).

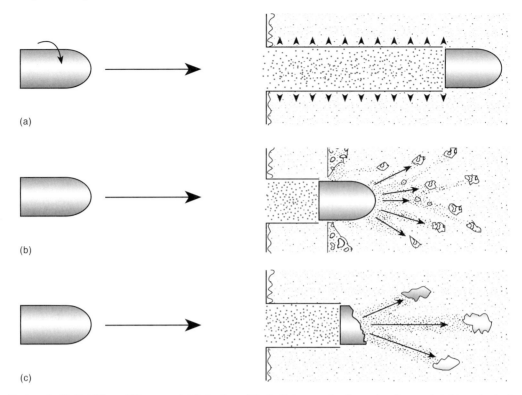

Figure 24.8   **Factors in Bullet Wound Damage.** (*a*) Spinning of the bullet generates damaging forces at right angles to the bullet path. (*b*) Bone fragments act as secondary projectiles when shattered by the bullet. (*c*) The bullet itself has fragmented. Such fragments may lacerate or compress tissues, vessels, or nerves. They may also enter vessels to be transported as emboli.

After striking some firm structure, usually a bone, a bullet or its larger fragments may start to tumble. This results in a enlarged and often distorted pain of destruction through body organs. There are so many factors that can affect a fragment's path through the body that emergency personnel never assume a straight track between entrance and exit points.

Bone Fracture

When forces that overwhelm its substantial strength are applied to a bone, it breaks. Bone fractures take different forms determined by forces that are differently applied to the bone (fig. 24.9). Some are **incomplete fractures,** in which the break does not produce complete separation of the two ends of the bone. For example, the break might appear only as a crack along a bone's surface (**fissure fracture),** or a bone might be punctured, by a bullet or other penetrating object, for example (*puncture fracture*). A third type of incomplete fracture is the **greenstick fracture,** which results from bending forces applied to a bone, with breakage occurring at the convex surface of the bend.

Simple fractures are breaks that form two quite separate bone fragments. If three or more pieces are produced, the fracture is described as **comminuted.** In extreme cases, such as a bullet striking a bone, comminuted fractures may involve large numbers of separate small bone fragments. When a fracture causes a bone edge to pierce the skin's sur-

face it is called a **compound fracture.** In a **depressed fracture** of the skull, a blunt instrument causes a portion of the skull to be driven down from the adjacent intact region (fig. 24.10). If a disease process, such as neoplasia, weakens a bone so that normal stresses cause breakage, the fracture is said to be a **pathological fracture.**

Fractures are common examples of trauma. They are frequently the result of falls, athletic injuries, and automobile accidents. Pedestrians struck by automobiles often first suffer lower leg fractures from the impact of the car's bumper. Other fractures may subsequently occur as they strike the pavement, often from some height. Skull fractures are common in such cases. Occupants of a vehicle involved in a head-on collision frequently experience knee, hip, and shoulder fractures. The knees are often driven forward to strike rigid dashboard structures. Joint fractures occur as the arms and legs are braced in anticipation of impact. When collision follows, large forces are transmitted by bones to cause fractures at the joint.

Following bone fracture, the potential for damage to adjacent soft tissues is high. Ragged bone edges and small fragments can move against nearby vessels or other organs to lacerate their surfaces. Rib, hip, and skull fractures are all associated with secondary damage to the more vulnerable soft tissues they protect.

Because cartilage also has a certain rigidity, it is also subject to fracture. The cartilage of the tip of the nose is

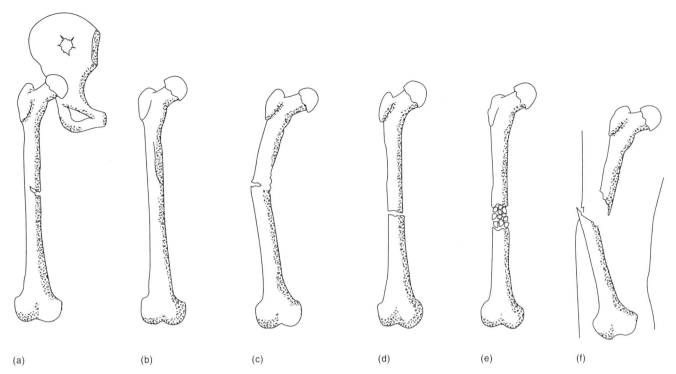

Figure 24.9 **Bone Fracture Types.** (*a*) Puncture fracture of pelvis and incomplete femoral fracture. (*b*) Fissure fracture. (*c*) Greenstick fracture. (*d*) Simple fracture. (*e*) Comminuted fracture. (*f*) Compound fracture; the sharp edge of an oblique fracture has penetrated the skin overlying the fracture site.

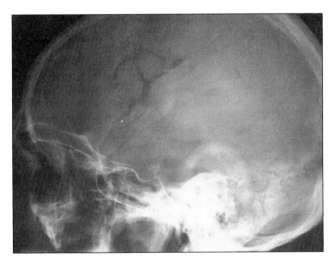

Figure 24.10 **Depressed Skull Fracture.** The fragments produced by a blow to the skull have been driven below the level of the cranial surface.

A 24-year-old male was drinking with friends in a hotel bar. He was pushed sideways in a scuffle, struck his temple on the corner of a metal chair, and briefly lost consciousness. Bleeding was minor but a lump rapidly developed at the site. En route to the hospital, his consciousness became clouded. This radiograph confirmed a depressed fracture of the skull. CT indicated an expanding extradural hematoma developing from laceration of the anterior meningeal artery. Immediate surgical evacuation of the hematoma and cauterization of the artery restored intracranial pressure and consciousness, with no neurological sequelae.

often broken. The cartilage segments of the larynx and trachea may also fracture in cases of neck or thoracic trauma. Such an injury is serious when collapsed airways block air flow to the lungs.

SYSTEMIC RESPONSES TO TRAUMA

Severe trauma of any kind produces not only local damage, but also an integrated series of systemic coping responses. These promote blood pressure maintenance and the metabolic responses that make adequate fuel and repair molecules available for distribution to traumatized tissues and the body generally.

The threat of circulatory shock is often present when trauma is severe. Its key elements, and the cardiovascular reflexes that counter it, were described in chapter 11. It is worth recalling that when the heart or the brain stem's cardiovascular regulatory centers are damaged, the threat of a progressive and irreversible decline in blood pressure is high. In cases in which trauma involves the kidney, its sodium and water retention capacity may be compromised. The resultant loss of ability to support plasma volume, and therefore blood pressure, may allow shock to develop more rapidly and severely.

An array of coping responses mediated by the endocrine system is a valuable resource in confronting severe trauma. The general adaptation syndrome (GAS) was described more fully in chapter 17. Essentially, it produces widespread metabolic responses that provide increased

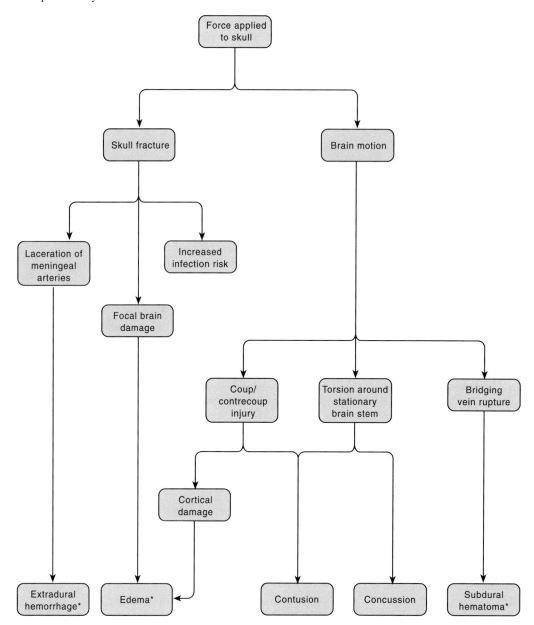

Figure 24.11   **Craniocerebral Trauma.** Asterisks indicate conditions involving intracranial pressure.

supplies of cellular energy sources and the amino acids needed for healing. As part of the GAS, the liver releases glucose to produce a characteristic posttrauma hyperglycemia. The GAS also produces a period of weight loss following trauma, as body proteins are expended to sustain the elevated rates of gluconeogenesis. Subcutaneous adipose tissue is also reduced as fat is metabolized in many tissues as an alternative to glucose. A characteristic hyperlipidemia results. Protein and fat lost in this way are replaced after recovery.

PATTERNS OF REGIONAL TRAUMA

With basic concepts and terminology established, we can now turn to the principal body regions and give a more de-

tailed treatment of their major patterns of trauma. In considering these, note that whereas the protection of the skeleton is an important factor in preventing injury, when mechanical forces are extreme, fragmented skeletal elements can themselves become injurious or even lethal.

Craniocerebral Trauma

Figure 24.11 illustrates the destructive mechanisms operating in head injury. A blow to the skull can fracture it. Immediate possible consequences are laceration of meningeal arteries, or brain contusion or laceration. The rapid linear or rotational acceleration of the skull can cause loss of consciousness and further vascular or neural damage. These effects are all considered **primary brain injury.** They can

Table 24.1   Evidence of CSF as a Sign in Skull Fracture

CSF Leaks

Fracture is near ear.
   CSF leaks into middle ear. If eardrum perforates, clear or bloody CSF is present in ear canal **(otorrhea).**
Fracture involves paranasal bones.
   CSF drains via nose or into nasopharynx **(rhinorrhea).**

Other Indications of CSF Loss

Halo sign on dressing or bed linen: blood circled with yellowish stain from CSF in blood.
Nasal secretions
   Watery versus normal viscosity may mean CSF is present.
   Glucose is detected (with KetoDiastix); glucose is normally in CSF but not in nasal secretions.

set the stage, singly or collectively, for a variety of delayed complications that can cause secondary brain injury. The one emphasized in figure 24.11 is the increase in brain mass that can develop from hemorrhage (hematoma) and cerebral edema, because these can produce a dangerous rise in intracranial pressure (see chapter 20). Other serious complications associated with craniocerebral trauma are CSF leakage (see table 24.1), locally introduced infection, and hypoxia due to vascular disruption. Together, they can cause **secondary brain injury** such as local infarction and loss of function, epilepsy, diffuse encephalopathy, posttraumatic hydrocephalus, and psychiatric disorders. Thus, a person may survive the primary injury only to succumb to the secondary complications.

In studying craniocerebral trauma, you should be aware that despite the alarming nature of the material presented here, only about 20% of cases of craniocerebral trauma require referral to a neurologist.

Concussion

Concussion is a period of lost or altered consciousness that follows a brain injury, In mild cases, rather than a loss of consciousness, one may experience a feeling of being stunned or losing mental focus. It is a common, though not inevitable, accompaniment of craniocerebral trauma. Concussion is characterized by the abrupt transfer of energy to the brain, producing an immediate, usually reversible, paralysis of nervous function. The effects of concussion can range in severity from a very brief disturbance of mental functioning to deep coma, but always involve a period of amnesia. Severe skull and brain trauma can occur without concussion if the force is delivered very rapidly and in such a focused way that the mass of brain tissue is not significantly moved. The classic demonstration of this possibility goes back to 1868 in the case of Phineas Gage. He was engaged in tamping explosives with an iron rod when an accidental detonation drove the rod through his cheek, frontal lobe, and skull. He covered the wounds with his

hands, got on a horse-drawn wagon, and was driven to the nearest doctor, being fully capable of conversation.

The mechanism of concussion is thought to involve rotational brain movement, focused at the juncture of the midbrain and subthalamic region, that disrupts the function of the reticular activating system of the brain stem (see chapter 22). The resulting amnesia is experienced as both retrograde (loss of memories extending back in time from the point of injury) and anterograde (impaired production of memories until some point after the injury). From the patient's perspective, loss of consciousness extends from the beginning of the retrograde memory loss to the end of the anterograde impairment. The length of this period of amnesia is the most reliable indicator of the extent of injury, with longer duration reflecting more severe injury.

In more severe concussive injury that results in coma, there is immediate loss of consciousness and depression of reflexes. The person falls to the ground and has a transitory (seconds) arrest of breathing and a fall in blood pressure. Immediate testing would produce a positive Babinski reflex. The return to normal consciousness is gradual. Reflexes return, as do responses to pain, simple commands and questions, and then conversation. Finally, normal memory returns and the person recalls conversation and events.

Coup and Contrecoup Injuries

Even minor concussion demonstrates the principle of coup/contrecoup injury. If the impact causing the concussion is to the *right* side of the head, the greater deficit in function (even if very short-lived) will arise because of functional changes on the *left* side of the brain. Typical signs to look for are weakness in right hand grip (contralateral), perhaps slurring of speech and difficulty finding words (left localized), and the sensation of "pins and needles" on the right of the body. More severe injury, where there is actual contusion (demonstrable bruising, particularly of cortical tissue), will follow this pattern. Some

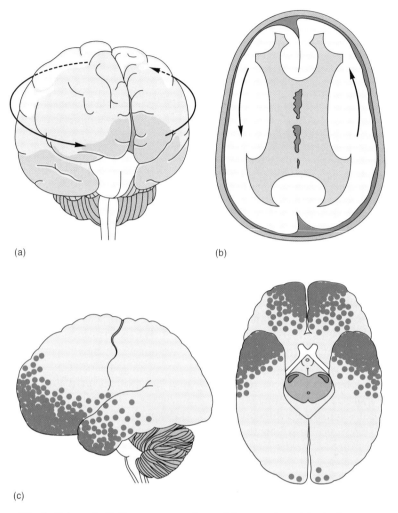

(a)

(b)

(c)

Figure 24.12   **Mechanisms of Brain Injury.** (*a,b*) Damage occurs from violent rotation of the brain, in which shearing forces cause injury to the centrally located corpus callosum. (*c*) Shading indicates the sites where contusions were found in a study of 40 brain trauma cases.

contusion will be at the point of impact (coup), but more will tend to concentrate opposite the blow (contrecoup). The explanation for this phenomenon is that much of the force of the blow is transferred to the scalp and skull, which then accelerate brain tissue in the protective pool of CSF. At the end of its arc of movement, the motion of the brain is arrested against the cranial vault. The brain tissue then absorbs this compressive force and violently rebounds off the skull, setting up distorting forces that produce further damage (see figure 24.4). These forces can produce edema, tiny petechial hemorrhages, laceration, and larger scale hemorrhage; if combined with rotational forces, they can also produce shearing of structures as large as the corpus callosum. In fact, in 20–30% of fatal head injuries, the skull remains completely intact.

In this context, figure 24.12c presents the accumulated evidence of the brain areas that suffered contusion in a series of brain trauma cases, mostly motor vehicle accidents. The superimposed dots show that the frontal and temporal lobes received extensive injury. The occipital lobe showed

less involvement, as blows to the dorsal skull produced more contrecoup than coup injury. The medial frontal damage may be attributable to collision with the falx or with the superiorly projecting crista galli of the ethmoid bone.

Basal Skull Fracture

Have you ever dropped a watermelon onto a table or floor? If this accident has happened, you have probably observed the mechanics behind basal skull fracture. At the point of collision, the skull experiences compressive forces that it is well designed to withstand. It is the opposite side of the skull (the equivalent of the split top of the watermelon) that is subjected to expansive forces, where the fracture occurs.

In this way, a blow to the forehead (like that produced by the head hitting the windshield) may cause a fracture of bones in the base of the skull, at some distance from the point of impact. The strong bones of the skull absorb the forces without fracturing and conduct the force to the face or the back of the skull. The consequences of comminuted and

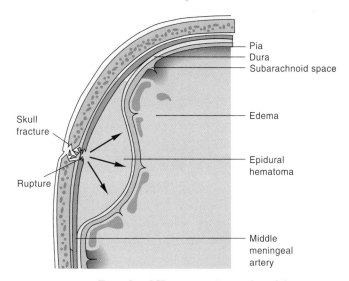

Figure 24.13   Extradural Hematoma. Laceration of the middle meningeal artery by skull fragments has allowed arterial blood to accumulate compressing the adjacent brain.

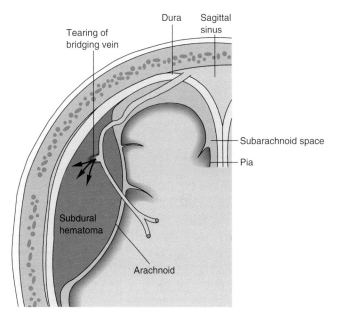

Figure 24.14   Subdural Hematoma. Abrupt rotational forces or a blow to the skull can produce tearing of the bridging veins that cross from the brain through the meninges. The resulting bleeding produces a subdural hematoma.

!! Focus on Babies, Boxers, and Brain Damage

Because of combined torsional forces, coup/contrecoup injury, and the limited development of the supporting falx and tentorium in young children, a baby or young child can receive sometimes fatal brain injuries when shaken violently. The effect is aggravated since the child's head tends to swing more extensively than would an adult's because the neck is relatively weak.

At the other extreme of physical development, strong, healthy boxers can experience a variety of brain and brain stem injuries in response to repeated high-energy blows. Sometimes boxers are referred to specialists by the licensing commission or their doctors because of questionable neurological or CT scan findings. In a group of boxers who were studied using both CT and MRI, MRI proved better at imaging abnormalities, at least after 24–48 hours posttrauma. Findings included frontal lobe atrophy, small cysts in the cerebrum and brain stem, subtle changes in periventricular white matter, subdural hematomas, and evidence, in a retired 66-year-old boxer, of several areas of contusion or hemorrhage. MRI also ruled out some suspicious findings from CT. So, babies, because of delicacy of structures, and boxers, because of the intensity and repetition of blows, are both at risk of brain damage.

depressed fractures and the need for routine X-rays were discussed in the section on bony protection in chapter 20.

In the content of general skull fracture, **closed head injuries** are fractures in which there is no breach of vascular or meningeal protection of the brain. The term **open head inury** implies only that the fracture has caused some break in this protection, not that there are gaping wounds. Prophylactic antibiotic treatment is routine when an open head injury is suspected.

Hematomas

One of the possible consequences of craniocerebral trauma is hemorrhage. As blood escapes a damaged vessel, it coagulates, forming a hematoma. The **extradural hematoma,** sometimes called **epidural hematoma,** is an extreme medical emergency because the usual source of blood is arterial (typically the middle meningeal) and therefore at great pressure (fig. 24.13). Treatment includes emergency evacuation of the hematoma and usually requires ligation of the torn artery. This can be done with no permanent disablement (see fig. 24.10). Sequelae may involve increased intracranial pressure and herniation.

Subdural hematomas can have a more varied presentation. The usual source is a ruptured **bridging vein.** These carry venous blood from the brain's surface through the subarachnoid space to reach the superior sagittal sinus within the dura (see fig. 20.15). Because of this "bridging,"

trauma that lacerates the veins allows blood to escape to the space between the dura and the arachnoid (fig. 24.14). The resulting **acute subdural hematoma** typically develops over 24–48 hours. Subdural hematomas often form bilaterally because of brain movement within the skull that tears veins in both hemispheres. This development time is slow compared to an extradural hemorrhage, which typically plunges the victim into a coma shortly after recovery from the original concussion. Routine instruction after any head injury thought to be serious enough to have possibly caused a hemorrhage, whether or not concussion occurred, is to

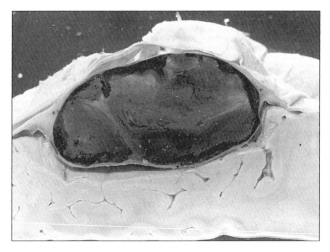

Figure 24.15   **Chronic Subdural Hematoma.** The mass of coagulated blood is trapped within the meninges.
This subdural hematoma was confined within the meninges of an older woman. The compression of the brain that resulted caused left-sided paralysis, which was misinterpreted as being due to a stroke. Because of her hemiplegia, she was confined for many years to a nursing home, where she died at age 86 of a severe attack of gastroenteritis, unrelated to her neurological dysfunction. At autopsy, no indications of infarction were found. Her last years might have been much different had the subdural bleeding not been allowed to become chronic. Regions of the hematoma appeared fresh, indicating that some further recent bleeding had occurred. It seems likely that some supposedly trivial trauma was initially responsible for the bleeding.

have a friend stand by for the first 24 hours and awaken the patient at least a few times during the night. This precaution is taken to monitor the possible evolution of an acute subdural bleed. The treatment is identical to that for extradural hematomas, as is the pathology of the expanding mass (see the sections on edema, increased intracranial pressure, and herniation syndromes in chapter 20). Even with appropriate care, both extradural and subdural hematomas are grave conditions.

Subacute subdural hematoma is the term applied when the hemorrhage develops slowly (more than 48 hours, less than two weeks). Typically the person has experienced concussion but recovered normally. Then symptoms associated with a growing mass lesion gradually appear. These often occur bilaterally, and their surgical evacuation, with ligation as necessary, can restore normal function.

The **chronic subdural hematoma** presents a diagnostic puzzle. This is usually found in older patients or debilitated people like chronic alcoholics. The initiating trauma may have been so minor that the patient won't remember the incident (fig. 24.15). The development of a chronic subdural hematoma is more complex than that of the other subdurals described. A slow leak from a bridging vein produces a small hematoma. Enzymatic activity within the clot breaks down larger molecules, thereby increasing the osmolarity of the solution and causing water to enter from the

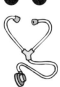

Focus on Blowout Fractures of the Orbit

Head trauma may be associated with injuries determined by the peculiarities of the orbit's structure. Although the orbit protects the eye on all but its anterior surface, its internal bony plates are quite thin. A direct blow to the eye, such as is increasingly common in squash and racketball, can generate very high orbital pressures. Such pressures can force the inferior orbital wall to fracture, driving orbital fat and parts of the inferior rectus and oblique muscles through it into the maxillary sinus below. In extreme cases, the entire eye has been forced into the maxilla. This injury is called a **blowout fracture of the orbit.** Even at such extremes, with prompt attention there is a high likelihood of completely restoring vision.

The prognosis is less favorable when a sharp object is driven superiorly through the orbit. Although thicker than the inferior wall, the superior wall is nevertheless quite thin and can be easily penetrated, allowing access to the brain.

 Checkpoint 24.2

If you have access to a demonstration skull that allows for removal of the cranium, inspect the floor of the brain case. Note the surprisingly jagged surfaces and consider the effect on a rather delicate brain that is forced to twist or slide over such a surface. Then recall the blood vessels situated at the base of the brain. It's not hard to see how strong blows to the head can produce tearing and intracranial hemorrhage.

surrounding tissues (CSF and blood being adjacent). The water expands the hematoma, causing more trauma to bridging veins, which tear to cause further bleeding and expansion of the hematoma. This stepwise process can continue for months. Chronic subdural hematoma is often called the *great imitator* because the symptoms produced mimic a variety of CNS disorders: epilepsy, stroke, demyelinating disease, and so on. CT scan is often essential for diagnosis. Treatment involves craniotomy and evacuation of the hematoma. Because of its long-term evolution, permanent neurological deficits are typical.

Acute Spinal Cord Trauma

Acute spinal cord trauma occurs in approximately 10,000 North Americans each year. These cases are the result of a

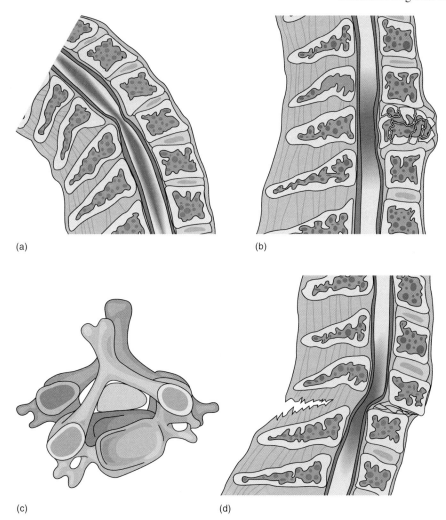

(a)

(b)

(c)

(d)

Figure 24.16 **Spinal Cord Trauma.** (*a*) Hyperextension of cervical spine causing central and intradural hemorrhage with edematous swelling of spinal cord above and below compression (see focus box: "Whiplash Injury"). (*b*) Crush fracture with fragmentation of vertebral body and projection of bone fragments into spinal canal. (*c*) Vertebral dislocation compromising the spinal cord. (*d*) Anterior dislocation of cervical vertebra with compression of spinal cord.

variety of injuries: motor vehicle accidents, industrial and sports injuries, domestic accidents, military actions, and criminal assault.

Characteristics of the vertebral column and the mechanism of injury combine to produce different patterns of injury. The vertebral column is most vulnerable at its points of greatest mobility: at C-1 and C-2 and C-4 to C-6 and at T-11 to L-2. The odontoid process (dens of C-2) is susceptible to fracture and displacement into the cord. Further, in the area of the spinal cord's cervical and lumbar enlargements, there is less room in the dural canal to accommodate splinters from fractured vertebrae, the movement of dislocation, or the swelling that often complicates injury. The velocity and force of the impact are also factors. A sudden blow to the head may shatter C-1 and the dens, whereas slower impact more often results in vertebral dislocation. Gunshots may drive bony fragments into the cord or, if near the cord itself, reduce it to a pulp. Extreme flexion/extension may cause diffuse contusion over a wide area, while a knife may sever cleanly. The nature of the injurious activity is a further factor. For example, diving accidents commonly injure the cervical region of the cord. Industrial accidents commonly damage dorsolumbar vertebrae. Figure 24.16 presents some of the common mechanisms of injury.

The care delivered immediately after injury and in the weeks that follow is crucial. Effective emergency and acute care can limit the secondary injury that might otherwise occur. It is important to stabilize the vertebral column with minimal movement in the process, to limit further extension of the cord injury from dislocated vertebrae or bone splinters. Surgical intervention to remove bone fragments, clear a hematoma, or relieve compression may be necessary. Because of the cord's extreme susceptibility to edema

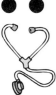

Focus on Whiplash Injury

A special case of a hyperextension injury is an acceleration stress to the neck, commonly called a **whiplash injury.** These typically arise when an automobile is struck from behind. The head is snapped posteriorly as the body is given an abrupt anterior acceleration. The head is then snapped forward in a recoil, which adds to the damage. Direct injury to the spinal cord is unusual in such accidents, although some brain injury may be involved. Most symptoms seem related to local spinal ligament damage, stretching of nerve roots, and stretching damage to anterior neck muscles and other throat structures. Headache, dizziness, and ear and eye disorders in whiplash injuries are thought to be caused by irritation of adjacent sympathetic ganglia or by altered cerebral blood flow through the affected neck.

---

and the secondary complications that edema can produce, aggressive control of inflammation, by means of corticosteroids, is routine.

Traction is commonly used to stabilize the vertebral column and avoid compression. With high cord damage, which may be ultimately more disabling, the patient's vertebral column can accept weight-bearing with the assistance of a halo brace much sooner than is the case with a trauma lower in the vertebral column. This is because the lower vertebrae must bear greater loads.

The characteristic response to cord trauma is a profound loss of cord function below the injury, called **spinal shock.** Not only are conscious movement and sensation lost, but reflex behaviors like deep tendon jerks and autonomic function (e.g., temperature regulation and vascular tone) are lost as well. Spinal shock is apparently the response to a sudden cessation of descending motor input to the cord from the cortex and brain stem motor nuclei. The loss of the excitatory component of these descending inputs leaves inhibitory influences in the cord unopposed. It is not due to edema or other responses to the injury itself, and its extent is not predictive of eventual cord function. If the disruption is purely functional, movement, sensation, and reflexes will return as spinal shock resolves, along with reversible conditions like inflammation and edema (within a few weeks for most people, much longer on occasion). Regular assessment of voluntary movement and the dermatomal distribution of sensation loss (see chapter 23) is an integral part of clinical care during this acute phase. The return of reflex behavior (i.e., resolution of spinal shock) *before* the return of sensation or voluntary movement is an indication of more extensive cord damage and less hopeful prognosis since information isn't reaching the brain and brain output isn't reaching cord gray matter.

The most common pattern of cord damage is diffuse injury, although very focal injury can occur. The nature of any permanent deficits depends on the extent and location of cord damage. Localization of cord function was considered in chapter 21, as were the long-term changes that follow cord trauma.

Thoracic Trauma

Because the vital functions of the lungs and heart may be compromised by thoracic trauma, it is a major cause of trauma-related death in North America. It is frequently accompanied by some degree of spinal cord injury. This section describes the principal patterns of traumatic injury to the thoracic cage, lungs, and heart.

Thoracic Cage Trauma

Most commonly, thoracic trauma produces rib fractures and raises the threat that jagged rib edges may tear through the soft underlying lungs and their abundant vasculature. Such injury is most likely to occur directly deep to the point of impact, as rib edges or fragments are forced into the pleura and lung. Less serious trauma may be resisted at the point of impact, with forces then transmitted to the weaker posterior ribs, where an outwardly directed break occurs. These are less likely to damage underlying structures.

Most often, the fifth through ninth ribs are fractured, probably because the more superior ribs are guarded by the shoulder girdle and the lower ribs are more heavily protected by muscle. For this reason, fractures of the upper ribs and the strong sternum are uncommon. When they do occur, they indicate greater impact forces and the potential for greater secondary damage to underlying tissues. Fractures of the first three ribs can cause lacerations of the great vessels of the heart or of the heart wall itself. Lower rib fractures tend to damage the diaphragm, the liver, or spleen.

The combination of jagged rib surfaces, lacerated lung veins, and respiratory movements set the stage for the development of an air embolism. As described in chapter 8, the chief threat in such cases is a fatal cardiac airlock.

When three or more adjacent ribs are fractured, so that a section of the thoracic cage can move independently, the result is the condition of **flail chest,** which was described in chapter 13. Hypoxemia and hypercapnia can then arise because of hypoventilation of the lung underlying the detached wall section, the **flail segment** (figure 24.17). The lung contusion beneath the flail segment is probably a bigger factor in disrupted respiratory function.

Lung Trauma

Pneumothorax, previously described in chapter 12, arises in thoracic trauma when the rough surfaces of fractured ribs cut through both pleura and lung, allowing air to enter the pleural space. The result is lung collapse. This condition is

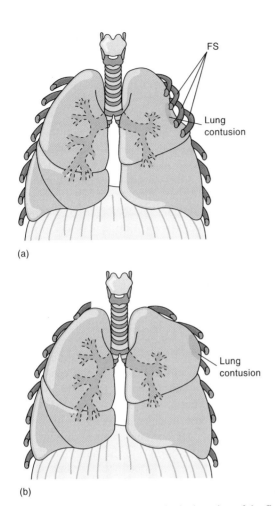

(a)

(b)

Figure 24.17   **Flail Chest.** The paradoxical motion of the flail segment (FS). (*a*) On inspiration, the rib cage should expand, but the lowered thoracic pressure draws the detached flail segment inward. (*b*) During expiration, the ribs are drawn in, but higher pressures move the flail segment outward.

called a **closed pneumothorax,** since the chest wall is not directly open to atmospheric air. Instead, the air enters the pleural space through the lung airways and the lung's severed surface (see fig. 12.32). Blunt trauma to the thoracic wall may also produce a closed pneumothorax when it induces abrupt pressure peaks that burst alveolar walls and the visceral pleura, allowing air to enter the pleural space.

An **open pneumothorax** exists when atmospheric air can directly enter the pleural space via an opening in the chest wall. If the wall defect allows air flow during both inhalation and exhalation, the sound produced gives rise to the descriptive term **sucking chest wound.** If the defect is forced closed during expiration, a valvelike action is produced. That is, air can be drawn in to the pleural space but can't be exhaled. The result is a continually increasing pressure in one pleural cavity, which relentlessly forces the collapsed lung, heart, and other mediastinal structures into the opposite pleural cavity. This is the condition of **tension pneumothorax** (fig. 24.18). It is potentially lethal, in that its high pressures can compress airways to restrict pulmonary

Focus on Neck-Cracker Neuropathy

Voluntary and habitual "cracking" of the cervical spine can be annoying to those within hearing distance. The motivation for this activity is unclear, but participants relate a vague sense of discomfort in the neck that is relieved by forceful lateral flexion. We recently evaluated a patient whose case illustrates that such neck cracking may be injurious.

A 20-year-old college student recalled making an unusually vigorous cracking maneuver of forcing his neck to the left. He immediately experienced right-neck pain, which subsided over a week. A month later he noted winging of his scapula and limited abduction of the arm. Neurologic examination revealed depression of the right shoulder. The upper and middle fibers of the trapezius were weak and atrophic. Spinal accessory-nerve conduction studies and electromyographic examination confirmed a spinal accessory neuropathy. It seemed likely that the right spinal accessory nerve had been stretched by extreme neck flexion to the left.

Habitual neck crackers should be advised of the possible consequences.

A cautionary letter to the *New England Journal of Medicine.* K. R. Nelson, MD and P. Tibbs, MD.

air flow and compress pulmonary vessels to impede blood flow. Not only does this produce inadequate oxygenation of the blood, but vascular compression can severely limit venous return to the heart, thereby compromising cardiac output and posing the threat of circulatory shock.

Penetrating or blunt trauma to the thorax may produce contusions that are often of little clinical significance. Lacerations of the lung, however, may affect both airways and blood vessels, raising the possibility that blood will enter an airway, flow to its distal extremities, and interfere with respiration. Alternatively, blood may form a hematoma at the site of the injury. If the laceration also involves the visceral pleura, blood may enter the pleural space to produce the condition of **hemothorax.**

Ruptures of the Diaphragm

Penetrating wounds or blunt trauma can rupture the diaphragm, disrupting its function of isolating the thoracic and abdominal cavities. If sufficiently large, the opening in the diaphragm can allow herniation of the spleen, stomach, or bowel into the thoracic cavity. The driving force for this displacement is the pressure gradient across the diaphragm between the higher-pressure abdomen and the lower-pressure thoracic cavity. Herniation usually involves the left portion of the diaphragm (**left hemidiaphragm**), since

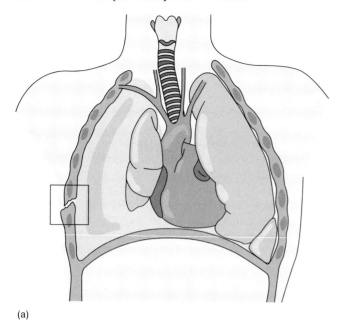

(a)

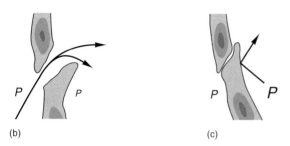

(b)   (c)

Figure 24.18   **Tension Pneumothorax.** (*a*) Injury to thoracic wall allows air to enter pleural space, and lung collapses. Trapped air causes displacement of thorax contents to the left. (*b*) On inhalation, pressure gradient draws air into thorax. (*c*) Valve action of wall defect on exhalation prevents relief of pressure.

the liver is too large to herniate and it presents an obstacle to smaller organs on the right side of the abdomen.

Cardiac and Great Vessel Trauma

Automobile steering wheels present a threat to the anterior thoracic wall and the heart, which lies just under it. Particularly in those without a restraining seat belt, the heart is often subjected to blunt trauma in head-on collisions. Contusions of the myocardium are a common result. They have the potential to cause cardiac dysrhythmias or reduced cardiac output due to a lowered stroke volume. As in myocardial infarction, a contused myocardium releases enzymes that can assist diagnosis. Contusions may be severe enough to produce a ventricular aneurysm or complete myocardial rupture, but these are rare events.

Penetrating cardiac wounds are much more serious because they may lead to more severe damage and a rapidly progressive cardiogenic shock. If the wound allows ventricular pressures to force blood through it, the condition may be promptly fatal. In some cases, the torn pericardial sac may not allow blood to escape as rapidly as it fills. Cardiac

tamponade (see chapter 10) follows, with trapped blood raising pericardial pressures and providing an external compression of the heart. This compression limits the heart's filling during diastole and can be fatal if it is not promptly treated.

In some cases, penetration of the heart may be achieved by a small bullet or bone fragment to cause only a minor myocardial wound. However, once within the heart, the object may lodge in a position that interferes with a valve's function, blocks a coronary vessel, or interferes with a component of the cardiac conduction system. In such cases, the immediate threat may be reduced, but only in exchange for the longer-term prospects of congestive heart failure.

Penetrating thoracic wounds that sever or lacerate the aorta or vena cavae are usually immediately fatal. Massive blood loss into the chest cavity is typical, or if the wound is at the base of the aorta, cardiac tamponade develops.

Nonpenetrating thoracic trauma commonly causes rupture of the aorta. Most often, high-speed automobile collisions are involved, but any source of high-impact forces to the thorax, such as falling from a height, can produce the same result. Most often the site of the aorta's rupture is in its arch, near the point where it is supported by the ligamentum arteriosum, the ligament derived from the ductus arteriosus (see fig. 10.39). The ligament provides a line of support between the aorta and the pulmonary trunk and seems to restrict the aorta's free motion. When an impact at the thoracic wall causes abrupt displacement of the aortic arch, the ligament acts to restrain its motion. When severe impact is involved, the aorta can tear near the point where the ligament is attached (fig. 24.19). Surviving such an event is unlikely, as loss of pressure is pronounced and immediate. In some patients, survival may be prolonged if the inner wall layers tear but the tougher tunica adventitia remains intact. In these cases, the vessel may withstand the high aortic blood pressure long enough to allow therapeutic intervention, but without such intervention, complete rupture is inevitable.

Abdominal Trauma

Nonpenetrating abdominal trauma can produce contusion, laceration, or rupture of the abdominal viscera. Factors affecting such injuries are the organ's resilience, whether it is hollow (and more likely to rupture) or solid, like the liver, and more likely to be lacerated. Also relevant is the organ's position in the abdominal cavity with respect to overlying bones, the ribs, pelvis, and spinal column. The vertebral column can contribute to injury. When traumatic force is applied to the abdomen, internal organs can be damaged as they are compressed against the strongly resistant spinal column. If vertebrae themselves are fractured, sharp bone edges can lacerate the aorta or venae cavae, causing serious hemorrhage. Also, because of their size, fractured pelvic bone edges can produce large-scale tearing of the pelvic viscera when trauma is severe.

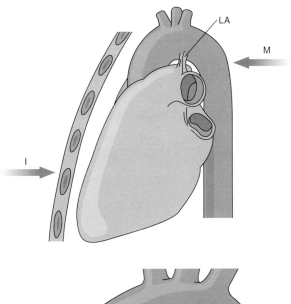

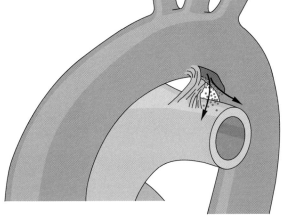

Figure 24.19   **Rupture of the Aorta.** This lateral view of the thorax shows the heart and great vessels. Also shown is the ligamentum arteriosum (LA) fixing the aorta to the pulmonary artery. Below it, the aorta has some degree of movement. Abrupt impact to the thorax (I) when the body is moving in the direction M can tear the vessel wall near the ligamentum arteriosum.

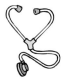

Focus on Seat Belt Trauma

Nonpenetrating trauma to the abdomen from improperly positioned automobile lap safety belts can cause contusions to the abdomen's wall and laceration and rupture of the intestine. Lap seat belts must be positioned so that restraining forces are spread over the iliac crests. When they are, the risk of abdominal trauma is very low.

Better protection against injury is provided by a three-point restraining system that supports with both lap and shoulder straps. Even when impact is high enough for the shoulder strap to cause rib fractures, such an outcome is far better than the results of ejection through the windshield onto pavement, and perhaps into the paths of other vehicles.

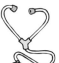

Focus on Overuse Syndromes

In athletics, it is helpful to distinguish acute traumatic injuries from the long-term, low-level injuries categorized as **overuse syndromes.** These typically produce inflammatory symptoms of pain and swelling, and most resolve with rest, which allows for healing to occur. In many cases, the risk of reinjury can be significantly reduced by adjusting training loads, improving technique, and supporting critical stress points. An example is **tennis elbow,** or **lateral epicondylitis,** which involves inflammation of the region where forearm muscles join to the distal humerus near the elbow. This injury responds well if the forearm is supported with tape or elastic sleeving, but if playing technique is faulty, the condition may continue to interfere with play.

The variety of overuse disorders is indicated by the layman's terminology that describes them: handlebar palsy, tennis leg, bowler's thumb, runner's knee, golfer's elbow.

The spleen is particularly vulnerable and is the most frequently damaged organ in cases of blunt trauma to the abdomen. The spleen's rich vascular supply makes intra-abdominal hemorrhage and hypovolemic shock the major risks in splenic rupture. The large blood flow through the kidney and liver make them similarly vulnerable. Note, in particular, the vulnerability of the alcohol abuser's liver. Its cells are typically engorged with fat (fatty change), making the organ's surface tense, less resilient, and more susceptible to laceration. Note, also, the same abuser's high likelihood of involvement in a motor vehicle accident that can deliver blunt trauma to the abdomen and its vulnerable liver.

In breaching the abdominal wall, penetrating wounds raise the threat of abdominal infection. In cases where a large wall defect allows abdominal organs to escape from the abdomen, an **evisceration,** the risk of infection is greatly increased.

The bowel, because of its length and its coiling within the cavity, can sustain injuries at multiple points from a single penetrating wound. When accompanied by damage to the high-volume abdominal blood vessels, such wounds present the risk of serious hemorrhage. As well, the spilling of bile, pancreatic or gastric juice, and intestinal contents onto peritoneal surfaces may cause widespread peritonitis and more extensive organ involvement.

Trauma in Athletics

Trauma in athletics can include any of the injuries described in the previous sections, such as when falls, racket injuries, ice skate blade severing injuries, and so on, produce blunt or penetrating trauma to the head, chest, and abdomen. Most athletic injuries, however, affect the bones, ligaments, muscles, and tendons of the peripheral limbs when acute stresses overwhelm these structures.

The incidence of traumatic injuries in athletics is increasing because of the large numbers of individuals engaged in fitness or recreational activities who may not be adequately trained or outfitted, or whose assessment of their abilities or capacities is unrealistic. Among those more skilled, advanced training and technical developments, together with the increasing height and weight of athletes, combine to produce greater risks of athletic trauma. For example, downhill skiing previously involved long, graceful, more horizontal arcs that took the skier to the bottom of a slope in a leisurely fashion. In recent years, much more aggressive skiing and snow-boarding has become popular as a result of improvements in equipment and technique, which allow more abrupt and frequent turns in steep high-speed descents. These place much more stress on the legs and greatly increase the risks of knee injuries and bone fractures in falls. To add to the risk, higher-speed falls onto ski or board edges or ski pole points are likely to be more damaging.

Another example related to improved equipment can also be taken from downhill skiing. Previously, ski boots were worn to ankle height, where normal joint flexion could absorb shock. More recently, ski boot design has featured rigid, much taller boots, which, while supporting the ankle well, transmit stresses to higher, less-yielding sites. As a result, there has been a significant increase in fractures of the tibia at the level to which the rigid boot extends, the so-called **boot top fracture.**

The principal athletic injuries encountered can most conveniently be described on the basis of the structures involved.

Bone Trauma

The various types of bone fracture were considered earlier in this chapter. In this section, we will note only that particular athletic activities often produce typical patterns of injury as a result of their characteristic limb and joint loading.

A special case of the overuse syndrome is the **stress fracture,** sometimes known as a **fatigue fracture.** It most commonly arises in the tibia, femur, distal fibula, or the foot's second and third metatarsals as a result of repeated long-term application of stress. In such cases, the level of loading is insufficient to produce an acute fracture, but just exceeds the level that the bone can absorb without damage.

With a stress fracture, pain may arise during exercise, but is relieved during rest between activity sessions. Initially, X-rays may show no signs of damage, but later, callus formed in healing bone may be detected to verify the presence of the stress fracture.

Ligament and Joint Trauma

Ligaments are bands or sheets of dense, fibrous connective tissue whose collagen provides the high tensile strength needed to stabilize and strengthen joints. When impact or excessive joint stresses stretch or twist ligaments beyond their limits, they will tear. A **partial tear** leaves a portion of the ligament intact, usually enough to provide some degree

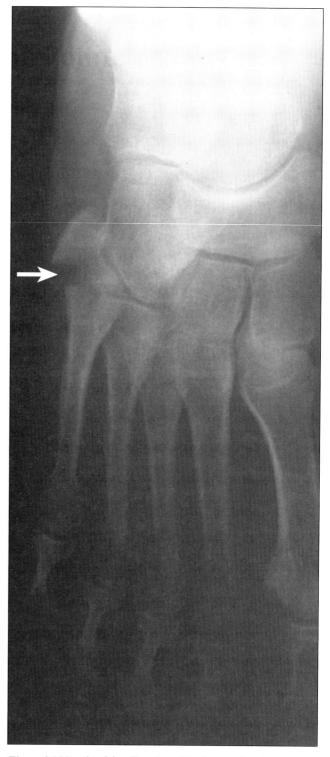

Figure 24.20   **Avulsion Fracture.** The bone defect (arrow) was caused by an abrupt and forceful tension exerted by the attached tendon.

of stability. In a **complete tear** or **rupture,** the ligament is completely separated and joint strength and stability are compromised. In cases in which a pulling force is applied to a tendon or ligament, it may remain intact but pull off a section of bone at its attachment site. This special case of a bone fracture is called an **avulsion fracture** (fig. 24.20).

Bleeding follows most ligament tears. When the damaged ligament lies within the joint capsule (e.g., the knee's cruciate ligaments), bleeding into the synovial fluid can delay healing. Restoration of a ruptured ligament may require surgery. More often, the tear is partial, and resting the joint can be expected to promote healing, although the process may take anywhere from six weeks to several months.

Forces applied to a joint may be sufficient to separate its bones, usually stretching or tearing joint ligaments in the process. If the ligaments return the bones to their original positions, the injury is described as a **sprain.** If the bones remain displaced, the joint is said to be **dislocated.** A dislocation may be total—a **luxation,** where articular surfaces are no longer apposed, or it may be a **partial dislocation** or **subluxation.** In this case, the articular cartilages may be in partial contact but are usually misaligned. Some degree of ligament and joint capsule tearing always accompanies a dislocation, but healing proceeds normally once the opposing bone ends have been **reduced**—that is, restored to their original positions.

Twisting at the knee joint may impart shear forces to the lateral and medial meniscus. These are incomplete rings of fibrocartilage that promote joint stability. Shear involves the application of two forces at 180° to each other in the same plane (fig. 24.21a). In the knee joint, the result is a tearing apart of the meniscus, sometimes producing fragments that move about in the joint space. Because the medial collateral ligament of the knee is attached to the medial meniscus, forces applied to the ligament often produce tears in the meniscus (fig. 24.21b). Surgical removal of torn cartilage segments may be necessary to restore function. If damage to the menisci is severe, their complete removal may be necessary. In such cases, knee loading may traumatize the articular cartilages and promote the development of osteoarthritis (see chapter 18).

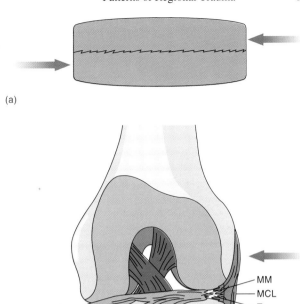

(a)

(b)

Figure 24.21   **Meniscus Tear.** (*a*) Shear forces applied to a structure, with the jagged line representing the plane in which tears are likely to develop. (*b*) Shear forces applied to the knee can produce tears (T) in the medial meniscus (MM) because the medial collateral ligament (MCL) is firmly joined to it.

Checkpoint 24.3

In this context of traumatic injury, don't overlook the important relationship between ligaments and bones. If a damaged ligament lets go, the bone it supported is at risk. For example, forces abruptly applied to the ankle joint can cause extreme eversion of the foot. This results in forces in the supporting ligament that are large enough to produce an avulsion fracture of the tibia's medial malleolus (remember, that's the prominent lump on your ankle's medial surface). Free of the ligament's restraint, the talus and tibia can be forced out of position to cause secondary fractures in the fibula and the tibia's lateral malleolus (the lump of the other side of the ankle). This is known as a Pott's fracture-dislocation of the ankle.

Tendon Trauma

The high tensile strength of tendon is adapted to its function of transmitting a muscle's contractile force to bone. Tendons are more susceptible to damage from shear forces and compression than to damage from tension, but abrupt or severe stretching can cause them to tear or completely rupture. Aging and disuse contribute to a tendon's loss of resiliency and strength, so those no longer young need to build tendon strength before applying the heavy loads of a new activity.

As with ligaments, a long healing time is required when tendon damage occurs, in particular because injuries often occur at poorly vascularized sites such as the insertion of the Achilles tendon on the calcaneus or the insertion of the supraspinatus muscle's tendon on the humerus.

Muscle Trauma

A muscle can suffer structural damage when it generates high intrinsic contractile loads or is excessively stretched. Such injuries are known as **distraction ruptures.** By contrast, **compression rupture** is trauma that results from

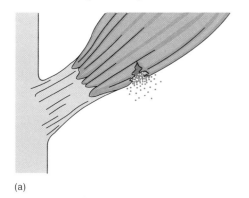

(a)

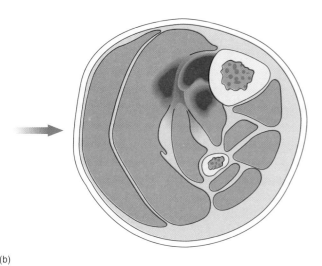

(b)

Figure 24.22 **Muscle Trauma.** (*a*) Distraction rupture near tendinous muscle attachment with bleeding from the torn muscle. (*b*) Transverse section through leg. Impact from left has driven muscle against bone to produce a deep compression rupture and hematoma.

a direct impact to the muscle, which often forces it against an underlying bone. In either type, the rupture may be partial or complete.

Distraction ruptures typically result from abrupt loading beyond the muscle's resistance capacity. Actions that involve quick acceleration or deceleration can provide such overloading. Tearing the muscle will usually involve tearing blood vessels as well, and bleeding into the area of damage is common (fig. 24.22*a*). In trauma to exercising muscle, bleeding is more severe because very high blood flow is required to meet the demands of vigorously active muscles. Bleeding is limited in trauma to resting muscle (e.g., in auto accidents) since blood flow rates are much lower. Scar tissue usually forms after phagocytes clear the coagulated blood because, when torn, the muscle's connective tissue architecture allows fiber ends to draw back from the wound site, making regeneration difficult.

In muscle compression ruptures, an underlying bone provides a rigid resistance that prevents dissipation of impact force. The impact can therefore cause deep contusions or hematomas in the muscle tissue adjacent to the bone

(fig. 24.22*b*). Because compressive trauma leaves more of the muscle's connective tissue framework intact, there is more likelihood of muscle fiber regeneration, if bleeding is not too severe. Excessive bleeding between fiber ends that need to grow together can delay or prevent regeneration and may necessitate repair by fibrosis. After the injury, an appropriate program of rehabilitation can induce hypertrophy in the remaining tissue so that the muscle's original strength is restored.

BURN TRAUMA

The wound produced by thermal injury to the skin is called a burn. It arises when thermal energy is applied to the skin at a rate greater than that at which the energy can be dissipated. Several factors affect the skin's ability to absorb and dissipate thermal energy: its thickness (thin on eyelids and ventral forearms, thicker on soles and palms), blood supply, water content, the degree of pigmentation, and the presence of hair or extraneous surface matter (e.g., cosmetics, dirt, etc.). Another factor is the time over which the energy is delivered. The same energy delivered to the skin over a longer period produces less damage than if all the energy must be dissipated in a brief interval. The combined effect of these variables determines the degree of skin damage.

Two systems of descriptive terminology are widely used in dealing with skin burns. In one system, a **first-degree burn** involves only mild injury to the epidermis without significant necrosis. Inflammatory vasodilation, swelling, and pain are present, but are usually limited. A typical sunburn is an example of first-degree burn. A **second-degree burn** involves destruction of the epidermis and part of the underlying dermis. Accumulating fluid between the epidermis and dermis may initially produce blisters, but subsequent loss of the necrotic epithelium exposes the deeper layers. In second-degree burns, intact sensory receptors can produce much pain as healing proceeds. However, residual hair follicles and other skin appendages provide sites from which newly formed epithelial cells can spread over the surface. **Third-degree burns** are most serious because they damage the epidermis, all of the dermis, and even some subcutaneous tissues. The lack of any functional remnants of the skin's follicles or glands as sources of epithelial regeneration usually means that skin grafting is needed to restore the surface.

The alternative system of burn classification ignores first-degree burns, since they heal readily without disruption of essential skin function. In this system, a skin burn that destroys the epidermis and some portion of the dermis is said to be a **partial-thickness burn** (essentially equivalent to a second-degree burn), while one that involves loss of all of the epidermis and dermis is said to be a **full-thickness burn** (essentially equivalent to a third-degree burn) (fig. 24.23).

In second- and third-degree burns, the surface regions are directly destroyed by heat effects that denature and coagulate protein, melt down lipids, and caramelize or "toast"

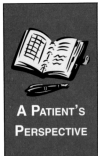

A PATIENT'S PERSPECTIVE

Severe Limb Trauma

" . . . it looked like it had been chewed by a shark."
—Kerry Calder

I started my job at the paper mill as a laborer. My work station was close to where one conveyor belt passed over another. One night, I was shoveling scraps of wood next to the conveyors. I lost my balance and, before I knew it, I fell onto the belt. It was carrying me to where it crossed under the other belt. It was all I could do to get one leg to the ground, but my other leg was drawn between the two wheels that drove the upper belt. As my foot was pulled in, I could feel my bones breaking. I was pulled in up to my hip but my crotch was forced against a metal support that prevented me from being pulled in completely. I was scared and in excruciating pain as the rotating wheels continued to grind my leg. My screaming was hard to hear over the high noise level in the mill, but help finally came after 15 or 20 minutes. A cutting torch was needed to free me before I could be rushed to the hospital.

My parents were called and, after being examined, I was told that my leg would have to be amputated at the hip. I still recall how violently I reacted to that suggestion and insisted that my dad promise he would try to persuade the doctors to try to save my leg.

When I awoke after surgery, I tried to sit up and couldn't. I couldn't even raise my head off the pillow. I tried to move my leg to see if it was still there and the pain was so intense I knew it was. Over the next ten days, the pain became more intense and I was heavily drugged. I became highly emotional and resisted the hospital staff's efforts to help, with the exception of one nurse whose name I can't even remember. She would come and whisper in my ear, telling me I would be alright. Over the next ten days, the pain continued and I developed several pockets of infection. A doctor came in and pulled off the blanket so I could see my leg for the first time. It was swollen to two or three times its normal size. It was brownish black above the knee and wrapped in bandages below. It smelled bad and I knew that wasn't good. They had given me some morphine, but when the doctor used a scalpel to open the infected spots, the pain was terrible. Every place the knife cut a yellow ooze came out. It was like watching a horror movie. I was terrified, but after everything was cleaned up I could finally sleep.

Two months later, four days after my 19th birthday, I saw my leg below the knee uncovered for the first time. I cringed at what I saw—there was little or no skin on my leg and it looked like it had been chewed by a shark. I remember feeling horrified and so depressed that all I could do was cry.

Over the next months, I had seven surgeries and although I felt stronger and the pain was becoming more tolerable, I was becoming more depressed—partly because my friends would visit and tell me of all the fun they were having. I resented this and felt it would be just fine if they didn't come to visit anymore.

The only real pleasure I had during this time was by way of the nurses. Since they were all older than me, they treated me like their baby and went out of their way to see I was well cared for. Some would sit with me on breaks and show me pictures of their families and vacations they'd just returned from. I regret never telling those women how much they meant to me and that if it weren't for them, I don't know how I would have gotten through the experience.

There was one incident in the hospital that changed how I viewed myself and my situation. I got a new roommate—an elderly man who was weeping all the time. He had diabetes and had only one arm left because his legs and an arm had been amputated. He had just learned that his last arm also needed to be amputated. This got me pretty depressed, but then I realized that I had far less to feel sorry about and that I was lucky to have my arms and legs. Over the following months of my rehabilitation, I realized that this event changed my life forever. As time passes, I realize I've become a better person for the insights I've gained into coping with a disability, pain and altered self-image.

---

carbohydrates. Adjacent regions may initially remain intact, but they absorb enough energy to damage heat-sensitive enzymes and they become necrotic after one or two days. Tissues beyond this region remain intact, and from them inflammatory and healing responses can develop.

There are three serious consequences of severe burns: shock, infection, and deformity. Hypovolemic shock can develop as a result of the formation of large volumes of inflammatory exudate. This is an important factor, but extensive necrosis also increases the osmotic pressure in the wound to draw water more rapidly from adjacent vessels. A third factor in loss of the skin's protective barrier is the increased rate of evaporation that contributes to fluid loss.

Infection is a second problem arising in burns, also following from loss of the skin's barrier function and its antibacterial secretions. Exogenous organisms and those that normally colonize the skin and its appendages can both become established in a burn wound. Their proliferation is particularly favored by the nutrient-rich exudate and tissue debris in the area of damage. Wound dressings also contribute by maintaining a warmer temperature within the exudate, which promotes bacterial growth. At the wound

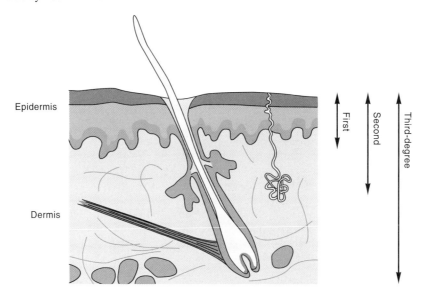

Epidermis

Dermis

First

Second

Third-degree

Figure 24.23   **Skin Burn Classification.** A partial-thickness burn is essentially the same as a second-degree burn, while a full-thickness burn is the same as a third-degree burn.

site, bacterial destruction of tissue can transform a partial-thickness burn to a full-thickness wound. A more serious consequence is **invasive burn wound sepsis,** in which bacteria enter the blood and are widely distributed. Secondary infection sites in the kidney, liver, and brain are responsible for the high mortality associated with invasive burn wound sepsis.

The third consequence often associated with burn trauma is the psychological and emotional impact of skin deformity and restricted mobility from extensive contracture in the healing skin. Even when surgical correction is possible, the prolonged period of healing that follows severe burns, and the often multiple grafting and other restorative procedures, can significantly delay ultimate resolution. Without continued psychological support, the loss of self-esteem in such cases can produce serious, long-term psychological effects.

Although burns to the skin are most common, burns of the respiratory passages can occur when intensely heated air and combustion fumes are inhaled. The generally thinner respiratory epithelium is vulnerable, and burns at airway surfaces are usually more serious than skin burns. In such cases, apart from direct airway surface trauma, lung damage may be followed by large-scale fluid loss from pulmonary capillaries, raising the threat of adult respiratory distress syndrome (ARDS) and its potentially grave consequences. Pulmonary damage allows lung infections to arise, with bronchopneumonia offering yet another challenge to the already heavily burdened victim.

Smoke Inhalation

Many cases of skin burns are complicated by the pulmonary and systemic effects of smoke inhalation. The drawing of hot, irritant gases into the lung airways causes more fire-related deaths than skin burns. The principal damaging effect is respiratory failure that produces sys-

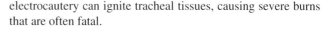

Focus on Tracheal Burn Risk

A bizarre combination of circumstances can produce iatrogenic burning of the tracheal surface. Following throat or chest trauma, patients often require sustained ventilation support with oxygen. Surgical procedures to repair tracheal trauma may rely on electrocautery to prevent bleeding. This technique uses electrically generated heat to sear vessels shut. In an oxygen-rich environment, the tiny sparks associated with electrocautery can ignite tracheal tissues, causing severe burns that are often fatal.

temic hypoxia and acidosis. Superimposed on these difficulties are the effects of the various toxic components of the smoke that enter the blood through damaged alveolar surfaces. Many home furnishings and commercial and industrial facilities contain plastics and other materials and produce highly toxic fumes on combustion.

Following smoke inhalation, obstruction of pulmonary airways is produced by the inflammatory response to mucosal injury. Pronounced exudate formation quickly produces significant swelling of the mucosa to reduce airway size and restrict air flow. With mucosal damage comes destruction of its cilia. This reduces particle clearance capability at a time when particle burden is high and predisposes to infections that can complicate recovery. In alveoli, accumulating fluid and smoke components inactivate surfactant. This increases alveolar surface tension to produce atelectasis, further compromising respiratory function. An additional threat in smoke inhalation is circulatory shock.

The smoke can affect alveolar capillaries so that their permeability is rapidly and profoundly increased, allowing large-scale fluid movement into the pulmonary interstitium to produce an abrupt drop in blood pressure. When the resulting shock is not fatal, the effects of the rapidly developing pulmonary edema and ARDS may well be.

Case Study

Following a head-on motor vehicle accident in a rural area, three people were admitted to a small local hospital. Two victims had immediately threatening injuries that demanded the attention of the limited staff. The other victim, a 45-year-old male, had walked into the ER. A quick assessment showed that he had been wearing his seat belt and so was spared any facial or other head injury, although he did complain of chest pain on his right side and of difficulty in breathing.

On physical examination, there was pronounced local tenderness in his right thoracic wall, suggesting a possible rib fracture. His blood pressure was low, 100/50, but this and the patient's pallor were attributed to his localized chest pain and the emotional impact of the accident. He was left to rest quietly while the other victims' pressing needs were attended to.

When staff and the X-ray facilities became available, the patient was prepared for a chest X-ray. During these preparations, about 30 minutes after his arrival in the ER, it became evident that his dyspnea had worsened and that his trachea was deviated from the midline toward the left. Suspecting a tension pneumothorax, the doctor passed a needle through the right thoracic wall, expecting to release air trapped within the thoracic cavity. Instead, he obtained blood.

At this point the patient rapidly lost consciousness and collapsed. Resuscitation procedures were started immediately, IV lines were placed, ECG monitoring was established, blood volume expanders were administered, and a blood sample was sent for typing in the event that blood transfusions were necessary. The patient became increasingly pale and his skin cool and clammy.

His blood pressure was declining rapidly when the ECG indicated ventricular fibrillation and BP became undetectable. Vigorous resuscitation measures, including electrical defibrillation, were unsuccessful.

At autopsy, a rib fracture and lacerated internal mammary artery were found, in addition to a penetrating wound to the thoracic wall.

Commentary

It can be very difficult to cope when high demand arises without warning and facilities and personnel are limited. In this case, the staff had so much to do in so little time that they could not immediately and thoroughly assess the status of this patient and detect his hypovolemic shock. Only after someone noticed the trachea's deviation, indicating the likelihood of a tension pneumothorax, did the hemothorax and massive blood loss become evident. Unfortunately, by then it was too late to intervene successfully.

This is an example of the rapidity with which cardiovascular shock can produce grave consequences; recall that the patient had actually walked into the ER. The case also illustrates that in some circumstances very little can be done to interrupt a deteriorating condition and prevent a patient's death.

Key Concepts

1. Severe traumatic injury usually results from burns or mechanical injury, which typically produce wounds by disrupting organ surfaces (p. 678).

2. Wound production is influenced by the interplay of four variables: the amount of energy applied, the duration of impact, the surface area over which force is applied, and various factors related to the physical properties of the tissues involved (pp. 678–679).

3. Wounds are classified according to the type of damage produced by forces applied to body or organ surfaces (pp. 679–682).

4. An extensive terminology is employed to describe the various patterns of bone fractures that can result from motor vehicle accidents, falls, and many other sources of bone trauma (pp. 682–683).

5. Various systemic responses combine to maintain blood flow and metabolic support in the face of traumatic injury (pp. 683–684).

6. Craniocerebral trauma is particularly serious because the brain is especially delicate and is encased in a skull whose internal irregularities can damage the brain's surface (p. 684).

7. Torsion of the cerebrum around the brain stem may produce concussion, a reversible interruption of cerebral functions that is always accompanied by some degree of amnesia (p. 685).

8. Hematoma formation has varying effects, which are determined by the vessels involved, their relation to the meninges, and the time over which the bleeding occurs (pp. 687–688).

9. Spinal cord trauma is closely linked to vertebral column trauma because the cord is readily compressed in the narrow vertebral canal and because the column is vulnerable at its most mobile sections (pp. 688–690).

10. Trauma to the thoracic cage can disrupt respiratory movements or produce sharp bony edges capable of lacerating the lungs and heart (pp. 690–692).

11. The heart and great vessels are subject to traumatic injury that can produce contusions, dysrhythmias, or serious bleeding (p. 692).

12. Nonpenetrating abdominal trauma may result in contusion, laceration, or rupture of the abdominal viscera, while penetrating wounds add the risk of hemorrhage and infection (pp. 692–693).

13. Trauma is strongly associated with athletics, where forces are often focused at the peripheral limbs (pp. 693–696).

14. Thermal injuries to the skin result from the delivery of energy at rates faster than the skin can dissipate it, and are classified on the basis of the depth of skin damage (p. 696).

15. The most threatening sequelae of burns are related to fluid loss from burned surfaces and to infection, both aspects of the loss of the skin's barrier function (pp. 697–699).

REVIEW ACTIVITIES

1. Jot down the effects on wound production when a given force is applied: (a) over a shorter time, (b) over a larger area, (c) to an organ of lower resilience, (d) over a longer time, (e) to a highly resilient organ, (f) over a smaller area.

2. Think back to your youth and list the various traumatic injuries that were a part of your growing up. Assess each as to its type: laceration, contusion, burn, fracture, and so on, and note any lingering effects.

3. Make two lists showing the consequences of different penetrating wounds to the same body region: one for effects caused by a sharp object, the other for effects caused by a bullet.

Photo Credits

Chapter 1

1.6*b:* © NIBSC/SPL/Photo Researchers, Inc.; **1.14***a-b:* Boyd Museum of the Department of Pathology, Faculty of Medicine, The University of British Columbia; **1.22***a-***1:** © Larry Mulvehill/Photo Researchers, Inc.; **1.22***a-***2:** © Mediscan/Visuals Unlimited; **1.22***b-***1:** © Larry Mulvehill/Photo Researchers, Inc.; **1.22***b-***2:** © Science Photo Library/Photo Researchers, Inc.

Chapter 2

2.12: © Dennis Kunkel/PhotoTake; **2.19***b:* Boyd Museum of the Department of Pathology, Faculty of Medicine, The University of British Columbia.

Chapter 4

4.5: British Columbia Institute of Technology, Medical Laboratory Technology; **4.10:** © Ken Kajiwara; **4.15:** © Division of Biomedical Communications/Southern Illinois University; **4.18:** Boyd Museum of the Department of Pathology, Faculty of Medicine, The University of British Columbia.

Chapter 5

5.6*b-***1:** © Dr. John Ortaldo/Peter Arnold, Inc.; **5.6***b-***2:** © Dr. John Ortaldo/Peter Arnold, Inc.

Chapter 6

6.6: Boyd Museum of the Department of Pathology, Faculty of Medicine, The University of British Columbia; **6.7, 6.9, 6.11***a:* British Columbia Institute of Technology, Medical Laboratory Technology; **6.11***b,* **6.12, 6.24***a-b,* **page 150:** Boyd Museum of the Department of Pathology, Faculty of Medicine, The University of British Columbia.

Chapter 7

7.3*b:* © Manfred Kage/Peter Arnold; **7.14:** Boyd Museum of the Department of Pathology, Faculty of Medicine, The University of British Columbia; **7.22***a:* © Ed Reschke/Peter Arnold; **7.22***b,* **7.23:** British Columbia Institute of Technology, Medical Laboratory Technology; **7.27***a:* © Ed Reschke/Peter Arnold; **7.27***b:* © SIU/Peter Arnold; **7.30:** British Columbia Institute of Technology, Medical Laboratory Technology.

Chapter 8

8.1, 8.2: Boyd Museum of the Department of Pathology, Faculty of Medicine, The University of British Columbia; **8.8:** © Richard Anderson.

Chapter 9

9.2: © Prof. P. Motta, Dept. of Anatomy, Unversity "La Sapienza", Rome, SPL, Photo Researchers, Inc.; **9.6, 9.9, 9.10***a-b,* **9.11, 9.13:** Boyd Museum of the Department of Pathology, Faculty of Medicine, The University of British Columbia; **9.23:** British Columbia Institute of Technology, Medical Radiography Technology; **9.24, 9.26:** Boyd Museum of the Department of Pathology, Faculty of Medicine, The University of British Columbia.

Chapter 10

10.8: © McGraw-Hill Higher Education/Karl Rubin, Photographer; **10.9, 10.11***b,* **10.15, 10.16, 10.17, 10.19:** Boyd Museum of the Department of Pathology, Faculty of Medicine, The University of British Columbia; **10.28***a-b:* British Columbia Institute of Technology, Medical Laboratory Technology; **10.40, 10.41***a,* **10.42:** Boyd Museum of the Department of Pathology, Faculty of Medicine, The University of British Columbia.

Chapter 12

12.16*a,* **12.16***b,* **12.17***a-b,* **12.21***a-b,* **12.28, 12.33:** Boyd Museum of the Department of Pathology, Faculty of Medicine, The University of British Columbia.

Chapter 13

13.9, 13.10*b,* **13.11, 13.12, 13.17, 13.18, 13.21:** Boyd Museum of the Department of Pathology, Faculty of Medicine, The University of British Columbia.

Chapter 14

14.11*a,* **14.11***b,* **14.12, 14.13, 14.16, 14.18, 14.19, 14.21, 14.23, 14.24:** Boyd Museum of the Department of Pathology, Faculty of Medicine, The University of British Columbia.

Chapter 15

15.7*a-d,* **15.14, 15.15, 15.18, 15.22:** Boyd Museum of the Department of Pathology, Faculty of Medicine, The University of British Columbia.

Chapter 17

17.9*b:* © Martin Rotker; **17.12:** © Project Masters, Inc./The Lester Bergman Collection; **17.13:** © Dr. P. Marazzi/SPL/Photo Researchers, Inc.; **17.14***a-d:* Boyd Museum of the Department of Pathology, Faculty of Medicine, The University of British Columbia; **17.16:** © Project Masters, Inc./The Lester Bergman Collection; **17.28***a-b:* © Biophoto Associates/SS/Photo Researchers, Inc.; **17.31***a-d:* Albert Mendeloff. "Acromegaly, diabetes, hypertension, proteinuria, and heart failure." © *American Journal of Medicine* 20:1 (January 1956) p. 135.

Chapter 18

18.1*a-b:* British Columbia Institute of Technology, Medical Radiography; **18.4:** © Richard Anderson; **18.5:** Boyd Museum of the Department of Pathology, Faculty of Medicine, The University of British Columbia; **18.6***a:* British Columbia Institute of Technology, Medical Radiography Technology; **18.6***b:* © Dr. Michael Klein/Peter Arnold, Inc.; **18.7:** © Biophoto Associates/Photo Researchers, Inc.; **18.9:** British Columbia Institute of Technology, Medical Radiography Technology; **18.10:** Boyd Museum of the Department of Pathology, Faculty of Medicine, The University of British Columbia; **18.13***a-c:* British Columbia Institute of Technology, Medical Radiography Technology; **18.15***a:* © Logical Images/Custom Medical Stock Photo; **18.15:** © Richard Anderson; **18.16***a-b:* British Columbia Institute of Technology, Medical Radiography Technology; **18.17:** Boyd Museum of the Department of Pathology, Faculty of Medicine, The University of British Columbia; **18.18:** © BioPhoto Associates/Photo Researchers, Inc.

Chapter 19

19.2*a:* © Biophoto Associates/Photo Researchers, Inc.; **19.6, 19.10, 19.11, 19.13, 19.14:** Boyd Museum of the Department of Pathology, Faculty of Medicine, The University of British Columbia.

Chapter 20

20.20, 20.22, 20.23*b,* **20.24***a:* Boyd Museum of the Department of Pathology, Faculty of Medicine, The University of British Columbia; **20.27:** © Biophoto Associates/Photo Researchers, Inc.; **20.28***b,* **20.29, 20.31***b-c, c***(inset), 20.32, 20.33, 20.34, 20.35, 20.36, 20.37:** Boyd Museum of the Department of Pathology, Faculty of Medicine, The University of British Columbia.

Chapter 21

21.13*b:* © Per H. Kjeldsen; **21.15***a-b,* **21.16:** Boyd Museum of the Department of Pathology, Faculty of Medicine, The University of British Columbia.

Chapter 24

24.10: British Columbia Institute of Technology, Medical Radiography Technology; **24.15:** Boyd Museum of the Department of Pathology, Faculty of Medicine, The University of British Columbia; **24.20:** British Columbia Institute of Technology, Medical Radiography Technology.

Index

702

ACRONYMS USED IN THE TEXT

μg	Microgram
ABO	A, B, O system of red cell antigens
ACh	Acetylcholine
ACTH	Adrenocorticotropic hormone
ADA	Adenosine deaminase
ADCC	Antibody-dependent cellular cytotoxicity
ADH	Antidiuretic hormone
ADP	Adenosine diphosphate
AER	Agranular endoplasmic reticulum
AFP	Alpha-fetoprotein
AIDS	Acquired immune deficiency syndrome
ALG	Antilymphocyte globulin
ALL	Acute lymphocytic leukemia
ALP	Alkaline phosphatase
α_1-AT	Alpha$_1$-antitrypsin
ALS	Amyotrophic lateral sclerosis
AML	Acute myeloblastic leukemia
ANA	Antinuclear antibodies
ANF	Atrial natriuretic factor
ANP	Atrial natriuretic protein
APC	Antigen-presenting cell
APP	Amyloid precursor protein
ARC	AIDS-related complex
ARDS	Adult respiratory distress syndrome
ARF	Acute renal failure
AS	Atherosclerosis
ASA	Acetylsalicylic acid
ASH	Asymptomatic septal hypertrophy
ASHD	Atherosclerotic heart disease
AST	Aspartate amino transferase
AT-III	Antithrombin III
ATG	Antithymocyte globulin
ATN	Acute tubular necrosis
ATP	Adenosine triphosphate
AV	Atrioventricular
AVM	Arteriovenous malformation
AZT	Azidothymidine
B$_{12}$	Vitamin B$_{12}$
BCG	Bacillus-Calmette-Guerin
BHP	Blood hydrostatic pressure
BM	Basement membrane
BOP	Blood osmotic pressure
BP	Blood pressure (same as blood hydrostatic pressure)

BPH	Benign prostatic hypertrophy
BSP	Bromsulphthalein
BUN	Blood urea nitrogen
C1, C2, etc.	First, second cervical vertebrae, etc.
C	Centigrade
C′	Complement
CAD	Coronary artery disease
CAH	Chronic active hepatitis
CAL	Chronic airway limitation
cAMP	Cyclic adenosine monophosphate
CAO	Chronic airway obstruction
CAPD	Continuous ambulatory peritoneal dialysis
CB	Conjugated bilirubin
CB	Chronic bronchitis
CBD	Common bile duct
CBF	Cerebral blood flow
CBG	Cortisol-binding globulin
CD	Cadaver donor
CDC	Centers for Disease Control
CEA	Carcinoembryonic antigen
CF	Cystic fibrosis
cGMP	Cyclic guanosine monophosphate
CHF	Congestive heart failure
CIN	Cervical intraepithelial neoplasia
CIRLD	Chronic intrinsic restrictive lung disease
CIS	Carcinoma-in-situ
CJD	Creutzfeldt-Jacob disease
CK	Creatine kinase (same as creatine phosphokinase)
CLL	Chronic lymphocytic leukemia
cm	Centimeter
CML	Chronic myeloblastic leukemia
CMN	Cystic medial necrosis
CMV	Cytomegalovirus
CN I,	Cranial nerve I, II, etc.
CN II, etc.	
CNH	Central neurogenic hyperventilation
CNS	Central nervous system
CO	Carbon monoxide
COLD	Chronic obstructive lung disease
COPD	Chronic obstructive pulmonary disease
COX-2	Cyclooxygenase-2
CP	Cerebral palsy

CPH	Chronic persistent hepatitis
CPK	Creatine phosphokinase (same as creatine kinase)
CPP	Cerebral perfusion pressure
CPR	Cardiopulmonary resuscitation
CPS	Complex partial seizure
CRH	Corticotropin-releasing hormone
CSA	Cyclosporin A
CSF	Cerebrospinal fluid
CSR	Cheyne-Stokes respiration
CT	Computerized tomography
CTZ	Chemotactic trigger zone
CVA	Cerebrovascular accident
D and C	Dilation and curettage
DIC	Disseminated intravascular coagulation (clotting)
DJD	Degenerative joint disease
dl	Deciliter
DM	Diabetes mellitus
DNA	Deoxyribonucleic acid
DVT	Deep vein thrombosis
DXA	Dual X-ray absorptiometry
EBV	Epstein-Barr virus
ECF	Extracellular fluid
ECG	Electrocardiogram
ECM	Extracellular matrix
EDTA	Ethylenedia-minetetraacetic acid
EDV	End-diastolic volume
EEG	Electroencephalogram
EF	Ejection fraction
EKG	Electrocardiogram
ELISA	Enzyme-linked immunosorption assay
EMG	Electromyogram
EP	Endogenous pyrogen
EPO	Erythropoietin
Eq	Equivalent
ER	Emergency room
ER	Endoplasmic reticulum
ESR	Erythrocyte sedimentation rate
ESV	End-systolic volume
F	Fahrenheit
Fab	Antigen-binding fragment (of an antibody)
Fc	Crystallizable fragment (of an antibody)
FCD	Fibrocystic disease
FEV$_1$	One-second forced expiratory volume
FFA	Free fatty acids

FPC	Familial polyposis coli
FSH	Follicle-stimulating hormone
FUO	Fever of undetermined origin
GABA	Gamma-amino butyric acid
GAS	General adaptation syndrome
GER	Granular endoplasmic reticulum
GF	Growth factor
GFR	Glomerular filtration rate
GGT	Gamma-glutamyl transferase
GH	Growth hormone
GI	Gastrointestinal
GN	Glomerulonephritis
GnRH	Gonadotropin-releasing hormone
GP	General practitioner
GSE	Gluten-sensitive enteropathy
GTCS	Generalized tonic-clonic seizure
GTD	Gestational trophoblastic disease
GTT	Glucose tolerance test
HAART	Highly active antiretroviral therapy
HAV	Hepatitis A virus
Hb	Hemoglobin
HbA	Hemoglobin A
HB$_c$Ag	Hepatitis B core antigen
HbS	Hemoglobin S
HB$_s$Ag	Hepatitis B surface antigen
HBV	Hepatitis B virus
hCG	Human chorionic gonadotropin
HCV	Hepatitis C virus
HD	Hodgkin's disease
HDV	Hepatitis D virus
HDL	High-density lipoprotein
HEV	Hepatitis E virus
HHNC	Hyperglycemic, hyperosmolar, nonketotic coma
HIV	Human immunodeficiency virus
HLA	Human leukocyte antigens
HM	Hydatidiform mole
HOCM	Hypertrophic obstructive cardiomyopathy
HPV	Human papilloma virus
HR	Heart rate
HRT	Hormone replacement therapy